Sleep and Movement Disorders

SLEEP AND MOVEMENT DISORDERS

SECOND EDITION

SUDHANSU CHOKROVERTY, MD, FRCP
PROFESSOR AND CO-CHAIR OF NEUROLOGY
PROGRAM DIRECTOR, CLINICAL NEUROPHYSIOLOGY AND SLEEP MEDICINE
NJ NEUROSCIENCE INSTITUTE AT JFK MEDICAL CENTER
EDISON, NJ

RICHARD P. ALLEN, PHD, FAASM
DEPARTMENT OF NEUROLOGY
THE JOHNS HOPKINS UNIVERSITY SCHOOL OF MEDICINE
BAYVIEW MEDICAL CENTER
BALTIMORE, MD

ARTHUR S. WALTERS, MD
DEPARTMENT OF NEUROLOGY
VANDERBILT UNIVERSITY MEDICAL CENTER
NASHVILLE, TN

*PASQUALE MONTAGNA, MD
DEPARTMENT OF NEUROLOGY
UNIVERSITY OF BOLOGNA SCHOOL OF MEDICINE
BOLOGNA, ITALY

*Deceased

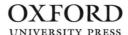

OXFORD
UNIVERSITY PRESS

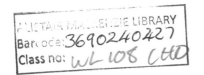
OXFORD
UNIVERSITY PRESS

Oxford University Press is a department of the University of Oxford.
It furthers the University's objective of excellence in research, scholarship,
and education by publishing worldwide.

Oxford   New York
Auckland   Cape Town   Dar es Salaam   Hong Kong   Karachi
Kuala Lumpur   Madrid   Melbourne   Mexico City   Nairobi
New Delhi   Shanghai   Taipei   Toronto

With offices in
Argentina   Austria   Brazil   Chile   Czech Republic   France   Greece
Guatemala   Hungary   Italy   Japan   Poland   Portugal   Singapore
South Korea   Switzerland   Thailand   Turkey   Ukraine   Vietnam

Oxford is a registered trademark of Oxford University Press
in the UK and certain other countries.

Published in the United States of America by
Oxford University Press
198 Madison Avenue, New York, NY 10016

Library of Congress Cataloging-in-Publication Data

Sleep and movement disorders / [edited by]
Sudhansu Chokroverty, Richard P. Allen, Arthur S. Walters.—2nd ed.
p. ; cm.
Includes bibliographical references and index.
ISBN 978–0–19–979516–1 (hardcover : alk. paper)
I. Chokroverty, Sudhansu.   II. Allen, Richard P.   III. Walters, Arthur S.
[DNLM: 1. Sleep Disorders—physiopathology.   2. Movement Disorders.
3. Sleep—physiology.   4. Sleep Disorders—psychology. WL 108]
LC Classification not assigned
616.8'498—dc23
2012040879

ISBN 978–0–19–979516–1

1 3 5 7 9 8 6 4 2
Printed in the United States of America
on acid-free paper

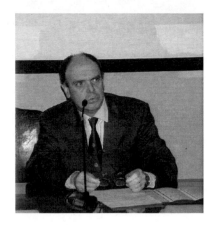

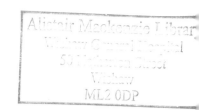

We dedicate the second edition of Sleep and Movement Disorders *to our esteemed colleague, an outstanding neuroscientist and a leader in the field of Sleep Medicine, Pasquale Montagna, MD, who died prematurely on December 2010 at the height of his career. A few months before death he signed the agreement to be one of the coeditors of this volume and made valuable suggestions for the contents, but fate took an ugly turn. Pasquale was born on September 11, 1950, in a picturesque small town in Muro Leccese in the southeastern part of Italy. After graduating first in his class in medicine from the University of Bologna in 1974, he received training in neurology at the same University. He traveled to Copenhagen, Denmark, to receive postgraduate training at the famous laboratory of Clinical Neurophysiology headed by Professor Fritz Buchthal. He returned to his alma mater in Bologna, first as a researcher and later rising to the rank of full professor in 2001 and succeeding Professor Elio Lugaresi as chairman of neurological sciences in 2007.*

Pasquale Montagna's contributions to understanding sleep-related motor events will remain his ever-lasting legacy. Pasquale was a prolific writer, contributing approximately 500 full scientific papers in peer-reviewed journals, over 227 presentations, and 59 book chapters in addition to two volumes of Sleep Disorders *(part of the* Handbook of Clinical Neurology *series) as senior editor and a book entitled* Fatal Familial Insomnia: Inherited Prion Diseases, Sleep and the Thalamus *as the sole editor. Pasquale Montagna's breadth of knowledge reached beyond neuroscience and sleep medicine as evidenced by his profound knowledge not only of Greek and other European cultures but also of the great Eastern civilizations. Despite his commitment to work, Pasquale remained devoted to his family and remained concerned about his wife and son until the very end of his life, as reflected in one of his last emotional e-mails: "It is indeed a troubled time for me and my family." We will remember you, Pasquale, forever, not only for your superb scientific contributions but also for being a great human being, a passionate and caring physician, and an inspiring teacher.*

Sudhansu Chokroverty
Richard P. Allen
Arthur S. Walters

Contents

Preface

MOTOR CONTROL in sleep is a complex phenomenon that is different from that in wakefulness. We are only beginning to understand the transformation of motor mechanism from an active state in wakefulness to a mixture of passive and intermittent activity in sleep. Many abnormal movements seen in daytime continue in sleep but to a lesser degree than in wakefulness. In addition, adventitious movements are triggered by sleep, causing the paradox of a sleeping brain with an active body. The purpose of the first edition was to address the difficulties in understanding and differentiating different types of abnormal movements during sleep. Since that volume published in 2003, there has been an explosion of knowledge stretching from molecular biology and genes to newer hitherto unknown nosological entities and phenomenology. Exploration of the human brain by sophisticated noninvasive neuroimaging techniques has shed light on the pathophysiology of much sleep-related movement disorders and in particular the dopamine abnormalities in the restless legs syndrome. Animal studies have been unraveling the mysteries of rapid eye movement (REM) sleep by precisely pinpointing the anatomical structures and neurotransmitters responsible for REM muscle atonia and electroencephalographic desynchronization. This paved the way to explore the pathophysiology of REM behavior disorder, a unique precursor to many neurodegenerative diseases. This also intensified the research to develop possible therapies to halt or prevent progression of such neurodegenerative diseases. Another important recent development is the publication of scoring guidelines in an attempt to standardize and quantitate various types of movements seen during sleep. All these advances in clinical and laboratory methods, molecular neurobiology, genetics, as well as therapy for movement disorders in sleep are brought together in this single unique volume.

The basic layout of the book remains same as in the first edition with slight modification. We have added several new chapters in this edition (e.g., Chapters 2, 11, 12, 13, 17, 20, 23, 29, 30,

31, 32, 36, 38, 46, 47, and 58) in light of new understanding of some entities. We commissioned new authors for Chapters 4, 18, 27, 33, 34, 43, 44, and 48. We discarded six chapters from the first edition (e.g., old chapters 2, 8, 25, 30, 36, 37, and 44).

As in the first edition, the book is directed at all sleep and movement disorder specialists. However, it should also serve neurologists, internists (particularly subspecialists in pulmonary, cardiovascular, or gastrointestinal medicine), psychiatrists, psychologists, otolaryngologists, pediatricians, neurosurgeons, and family physicians who deal with many patients suffering from undiagnosed or underdiagnosed sleep disorders. It may also be quite useful to those neuroscientists and other health care workers who have an interest in sleep and its disorders.

We end this preface with a sad note of announcing the untimely death of two of our outstanding contemporary neuroscientists and scholars, Wayne Hening and Pasquale Montagna. We will miss their robust scientific contributions, but they will remain forever in our memory not only for their scholarly contributions to the field but also for their humane qualities, gentleness, and passion for the welfare of fellow human beings. Our dear friend and colleague Wayne Hening was one of the coeditors for the first edition. Our esteemed friend and colleague Pasquale Montagna signed the agreement with Oxford University Press as one of the coeditors for the second edition, but shortly after that prematurely passed away. We dedicated the book dealing with *Restless Legs Syndrome* published by Elsevier in 2009 to Wayne Hening. We would like to dedicate this second edition of *Sleep and Movement Disorders* to Pasquale Montagna. We miss them both.

Acknowledgments

WE MUST thank all the contributors for their scholarly contributions that will make this volume an attractive and coveted exposition of a topic that we believe is a critical but often neglected area in the field of Sleep Medicine. The dedication and professionalism of the publishing staff at Oxford University Press (OUP) in New York and overseas made this production possible. Craig Panner, associate editorial director of medicine, neuroscience, neurology, and psychiatry at OUP, New York, steered us at every step of the production. We must also express our appreciation to Kathryn Winder, assistant editor at OUP, New York, for her dedication and care in the making of the book. It is a pleasure also to acknowledge the help of John Shinholser, Rachel Slaiman, and Samantha Staab who took over as editorial assistant to the journal *Sleep Medicine* as well as Jenny Rodriguez, secretary to the division of sleep medicine at our institute. Last but not the least, the senior editor (SC) must express his gratitude and love to his wife, Manisha Chokroverty, MD, for her unfailing support and encouragement, and for sacrificing all the precious weekends during the production of this volume. The coeditor (RA) also desires to express thanks to his colleagues, especially Dr. Christopher Earley, for their support and forbearance for the time he spent on this project but even more deeply appreciates the loving and understanding support from his best writing coach: his wife, Roberta Allen.

Contributors

Md. Noor Alam
Departments of Medicine
David Geffen School of Medicine
University of California
Los Angeles, CA
and
Research Service
V.A. Greater Los Angeles Healthcare Systems

Richard P. Allen
Department of Neurology
School of Medicine
Johns Hopkins University
Baltimore, MD

Radhika Basheer
Laboratory of Neuroscience
VA Boston Healthcare System and Harvard
    Medical School
940 Belmont Street, Research 151-C
Brockton, MA

Susan Benloucif
Technology Evaluation Center
Blue Cross and Blue Shield Association
Chicago, IL

Klaus Berger
Institute of Epidemiology and Social Medicine
University of Muenster
Muenster, Germany

Pierre J. Blanchet
Associate professor
Department of Stomatology
Faculty of Dentistry
Université de Montréal
Neurologist, Université de Montréal
    Hospital Centre
Consultant, Louis-H. Lafontaine Hospital
Montréal, Canada

Lindsay Boothby
Sleep Research Institute
Madrid, Spain

Lana Jeradeh Boursoulian
Department of Neurology
Vanderbilt University
Nashville, TN
Cumberland Medical Center
Crossville, TN

Oliviero Bruni
Department of Social and Developmental
    Psychology
Pediatric Sleep Center
Faculty of Medicine and Psychology
Sapienza University
Rome, Italy

Giovanna Calandra-Buonaura
IRCCS-Institute of Neurological Sciences of
    Bologna and
Department of Biomedical and NeuroMotor
    Sciences (DIBINEM) – University of Bologna
Bellaria Hospital
Bologna, Italy

Charles R. Cantor
Medical Director
Penn Sleep Centers
Associate Professor of Clinical Neurology
Perelman School of Medicine of the
    University of Pennsylvania

Michael H. Chase
WebScience International
Los Angeles, CA

Ronald D. Chervin
Professor of Neurology
Michael S. Aldrich Collegiate Professor
    of Sleep Medicine
and
Director, University of Michigan Sleep
    Disorders Center
University of Michigan
Ann Arbor, Michigan

Sudhansu Chokroverty
Professor and Co-chair of Neurology
Program Director, Clinical Neurophysiology
    and Sleep Medicine
Nj Neuroscience Institute at JFK
    Medical Center-Seton Hall University
Edison, NJ

Cynthia L. Comella
Department of Neurological Sciences
Rush University
Chicago, IL

Pietro Cortelli
IRCCS-Institute of Neurological Sciences of
    Bologna and
Department of Biomedical and NeuroMotor
    Sciences (DIBINEM) – University of Bologna
Bellaria Hospital
Bologna, Italy

Antonio Culebras
SUNY Upstate Medical University and the
    Sleep Center at Upstate University Hospital
    at Community General
Syracuse, New York

Alex Desautels
Center for Advanced Research in Sleep
    Medicine and Neurology Service
Hôpital du Sacré-Coeur de Montréal
Faculty of Medicine
Université de Montréal
Montréal, Québec, Canada

Martin Desseilles
Cyclotron Research Centre
Université de Liège
Belgium

Thien Thanh Dang-Vu
Assistant Professor of Clinical Imaging
Center for Studies in Behavioral Neurobiology
Department of Exercise Science
Concordia University
Montreal, Canada

Nico J. Diederich
Department of Neurological Sciences
Rush University
Chicago
Department of Neuroscience
Centre Hospitalier de Luxembourg
Luxembourg
and
Centre for Systems Biomedicine
University of Luxembourg
Luxembourg

Claudia Diederichs
Institute of Epidemiology and Social Medicine
University of Muenster
Muenster, Germany

Mark Eric Dyken
Professor of Neurology
University of Iowa
Roy J and Lucille A Carver College of
    Medicine
Director of the University of Iowa Hospital and
    Clinics (UIHC)
Department of Neurology Sleep Disorders
    Center
Director, UIHC Sleep Medicine Fellowship
    Program
Director, UIHC Clinical Neurophysiology
    Fellowship Program

Stanley Fahn
Department of Neurology
Columbia University Medical Center
New York, NY

Raffaele Ferri
Sleep Research Centre
Department of Neurology I.C.
Oasi Institute (IRCCS)
Troina, Italy

Nancy Foldvary-Schaefer
Associate Professor of Medicine
Professor of Medicine
Cleveland Clinic Lerner College of Medicine
    of Case
Western Reserve University
Director, Cleveland Clinic Sleep Disorders Center
Staff, Cleveland Clinic Epilepsy Center
Cleveland Clinic Neurological Institute
Cleveland, Ohio

Joanna Fong
Cleveland Clinic Sleep Disorders Center
Cleveland Clinic Epilepsy Center
Cleveland Clinic Regional Neurosciences
Cleveland, OH

Birgit Frauscher
Department of Neurology
Innsbruck Medical University
Innsbruck, Austria

Simon J. Fung
WebScience International
Los Angeles,CA

Christian Guilleminault
Stanford University Medical School
Stanford Sleep Medicine Center
Stanford,CA

Nancy Gadallah
New Jersey Neuroscience Institute
JFK Medical Center
Edison, NJ

Jean-Francois Gagnon
Centre d'Études Avancées en Médecine du
    Sommeil
Hopital du Sacre-Coeur, Montreal
Canada
and
Department of Psychology
Université du Québec à Montréal
Québec, Canada

Diego Garcia-Borreguero
Sleep Research Institute
Madrid, Spain

Mark Hallett
National Institutes of Health
Bethesda, MD

Philip A. Hanna
New Jersey Neuroscience Institute
JFK Medical Center
Edison, NJ

Timothy F. Hoban
The Michael S. Aldrich Sleep Disorders Center
University of Michigan
Ann Arbor, MI

Birgit Högl
Department of Neurology
Innsbruck Medical University
Innsbruck, Austria

Nelly T. Huynh
Assistant research professor
Faculty of Dentistry
Université de Montréal
Montréal, Canada

Alex Iranzo
Neurology Service, Hospital Clínic and Institut
    d'Investigació Biomèdiques August Pi i
    Sunyer (IDIBAPS), Centro de Investigación
    Biomédica en Red sobre Enfermedades
    Neurodegenerativas (CIBERNED)
Barcelona, SPAIN

Joseph Jankovic
Professor of Neurology
Baylor College of Medicine
Houston,TX

Takafumi Kato
Associate professor
Department of Oral Anatomy and
    Neurobiology, Osaka
University Graduate School of Dentistry
Osaka, Japan

Paola A. Lanfranchi
Department of Medicine
Division of Cardiology
Hôpital du Sacré-Coeur de Montréal and
    Université de Montréal
Québec, Canada
Center for Advanced Studies in Sleep Medicine
    Hôpital du Sacré-Coeur de Montréal
Montréal, Québec, Canada

Gilles J. Lavigne
Dean
Faculty of Dentistry
Université de Montréal
Center for Advanced Studies in Sleep
    Medicine
Hôpital du Sacré-Coeur de Montréal
Montréal, Québec, Canada

Jun Lu
Department of Neurology and Department of
    Sleep Medicine
Beth Israel Deaconess Medical Center and
    Harvard Medical School
Boston, MA

Elio Lugaresi
IRCCS-Institute of Neurological Sciences of
    Bologna and
Department of Biomedical and NeuroMotor
    Sciences (DIBINEM) – University of
    Bologna
Bellaria Hospital
Bologna, Italy

Beth A. Malow
Professor of Neurology and
    Pediatrics
Burry Chair in Cognitive Childhood
    Development
Director Sleep Disorders Division
Vanderbilt University
Nashville, Tennessee

Pierre Maquet
Cyclotron Research Centre
Université de Liège, Belgium

Robert W. McCarley
Laboratory of Neuroscience
VA Boston Healthcare System and Harvard
    Medical School
Brockton, MA

Damian McGovern
Department of Neurology
Vanderbilt University
Nashville, TN

Deborah McIntyre
Department of Neurology
Rush University Medical Center
Chicago,IL

Martin Michaud
Center for Advanced Research in Sleep
    Medicine
Hôpital du Sacré-Coeur de Montréal
Université de Montréal
Montréal, Québec, Canada

Pasquale Montagna*
Department of Neurology
University of Bologna School of Medicine
Bologna, Italy
*Deceased

Jacques Y. Montplaisir
Professor of Psychiatry and Neuroscience
Center for Advanced Studies in Sleep Medecine
Hôpital du Sacré-Coeur de Montréal,
Montréal, Canada
Director, Canadian research chair in Sleep
    Medicine and Professor of Psychiatry and
    Neuroscience
Faculty of Medicine
Université de Montréal
Montréal, Québec, Canada

Seiji Nishino
Professor
Stanford University School of Medicine
Department of Psychiatry & Behavioral
    Sciences Sleep and Circadian Neurobiology
    Laboratory Center for Narcolepsy
Palo Alto, CA

Maurice M. Ohayon
Professor of Psychiatry & Behavioral Sciences
Director
Stanford Sleep Epidemiology Research Centre
    (SSERC)

Masashi Okuro
Assistant Professor
Department of Geriatric Medicine
Kanazawa Medical University
Ishikawa, Japan

Marie-Helene Pennestri
Center for Advanced Research in Sleep
    Medicine
Hôpital du Sacré-Coeur de Montréal
Université de Montréal
Montréal, Québec, Canada

Liborio Parrino
Department of Neurosciences
Sleep Disorders Center
University of Parma
Italy

Tasneem Peeraully
New Jersey Neuroscience Institute
JFK Medical Center
Edison, NJ

Philippe Peigneux
Neuropsychology and Functional
    Neuroimaging Research Unit
Université Libre de Bruxelles
Belgium

Giuseppe Plazzi
Department of Neurology
University of Bologna
Bologna, Italy

Ronald B. Postuma
Department of Neurology
McGill University
Montreal General Hospital
Montreal, Québec, Canada.
Centre d'Études Avancées en Médecine du
    Sommeil
Hopital du Sacre-Coeur
Montreal, Canada

Mark R. Pressman
Director
Sleep Medicine Services
Lankenau Medical Center
Clinical Professor
Lankenau Institute for Medical Research
Clinical Professor
Department of Medicine, Jefferson Medical College
Adjunct Professor
Villanova School of Law

Federica Provini
IRCCS-Institute of Neurological Sciences of
    Bologna and
Department of Biomedical and NeuroMotor
    Sciences (DIBINEM) – University of
    Bologna
Bellaria Hospital
Bologna, Italy

Rodney A. Radtke
Professor of Neurology
Duke University School of Medicine
Medical Director
Duke University Hospital Sleep Center
Duke University Medical Center
Durham, NC

Pietro-Luca Ratti
Department of Neurology
Centre Hospitalier Universitaire de Toulouse
    and INSERM U825
Toulouse, France

Robert L. Rodnitzky
Department of Neurology
University of Iowa hospitals and Medical Center
Iowa City, IA

Richard J. Ross
Professor of Psychiatry at the Philadelphia VA
    Medical Center
Perelman School of Medicine of the University
    of Pennsylvania

Jacob I. Sage
Professor of Neurology
Robert Wood Johnson Medical Center
New Brunswick, NJ

Barbara Schormair
Institute of Human Genetics
Helmholtz Zentrum München -German
    Research Center for Environmental Health
Neuherberg, Germany

Denise Sharon
Department of Medicine
Tulane University School of Medicine
New Orleans, LA

Anita Valanju Shelgikar
Assistant Professor of Neurology
Sleep Medicine Fellowship Program Director
University of Michigan
Ann Arbor, Michigan

Michael H. Silber
Professor of Neurology
Center for Sleep Medicine and Department
    of Neurology
Mayo Clinic College of medicine
Rochester, MN

Rosalia C. Silvestri
UOC Neurologia e Malattie
Neuromuscolari Policlinico G. Martino
Messina, Italy

Narong Simakajornboon
Professor, Division of Pulmonary and Sleep
    Medicine
Director, Sleep Disorders Center
Cincinnati Children's Hospital
    Medical Center
Cincinnati, OH

Rajdeep Singh
Department of Neurology
Duke University Medical Center
Durham, NC

Shannon Sullivan
Stanford University Medical School
Stanford Sleep Medicine Center
Stanford,CA

Ronald Szymusiak
Departments of Medicine and Neurobiology
David Geffen School of Medicine
University of California
Los Angeles
Research Service
V.A. Greater Los Angeles Healthcare Systems

Desislava Tzonova
Sleep Research Institute
Madrid, Spain

Lunliya Thampratankul
Division of Neurology
Department of Pediatrics
Ramathibodi Hospital
Mahidol University
Bangkok, Thailand

Mario G. Terzano
Department of Developmental Neurology and
    Psychiatry
Center for Pediatric Sleep Disorders
Sapienza University
Rome, Italy

Michael J. Thorpy
Director Sleep-Wake Disorders Center
Montefiore Medical Center
Professor of Clinical Neurology
Albert Einstein College of Medicine
Bronx, NY

Josep Valls-Solé
EMG Unit. Neurology Department
Hospital Clínic
Institut d'Investigacio Biomedica August Pi i
    Sunyer (IDIBAPS)
Facultad de Medicina
Universitat de Barcelona

Jana Vâvrovâ
1st Faculty of Medicine
Department of Neurology
Charles University
Prague, Czech Republic

Aleksandar Videnovic
Circadian Rhythms and Sleep Research
    Laboratory
Parkinson's disease and Movement Disorder
    Center
Department of Neurology
Northwestern University
Chicago, IL

Arthur S. Walters
Department of Neurology
Vanderbilt University School of Medicine
Nashville TN

Anne-Marie Williams
Anne-Marie Williams
Sleep Research Institute
Alberto Alcocer 19
Madrid, Spain

Juliane Winkelmann
Institute of Human Genetics
Helmholtz Zentrum München-German
    Research Center for Environmental Health
Neuherberg, Germany
Institute of Human Genetics
Klinikum Rechts der Isar – Technische
    Universität München (TUM)
Munich, Germany
Department of Neurology
Klinikum Rechts der Isar – Technische
    Universität München (TUM)
Munich, Germany

Ming-Chu Xi
Research Physiologist
Department of Physiology
UCLA School of Medicine
Los Angeles,CA

Jack Yamuy
Research Physiologist
Department of Physiology
UCLA School of Medicine
Los Angeles,CA

Phyllis C. Zee
Professor of Neurology
Director Sleep Disorders Center
Northwestern University
Chicago, IL

Marco Zucconi
Sleep Disorders Centre
Department of Clinical Neurosciences
San Raffaele Scientific Institute
Milan, Italy

PART ONE

Introduction

1

Introduction

SUDHANSU CHOKROVERTY, RICHARD P. ALLEN,
ARTHUR S. WALTERS, AND PASQUALE MONTAGNA*

IN THIS volume, we examine an aspect of human motor control that has been largely neglected, mostly because it lies at the intersection of two medical and scientific disciplines—the studies of movement and its disorders, on the one hand, and the study of sleep and its disorders, on the other. For both fields, issues of how the nervous system controls movement are a primary and paramount focus. Motor control in humans is a complex act resulting from an intricate and finely balanced mechanism involving cerebral cortex, basal ganglia, brainstem motor center, cerebellum, spinal cord, and peripheral neuromuscular system.[1,2] Disorders of movements may result if there is a breakdown in this delicately balanced mechanism involving either the afferent, interneuronal, or efferent structures. Such disintegration may cause disorders of normal voluntary movements or the appearance of abnormal movements causing both negative and positive symptoms.

Akinesia (absence of movement), bradykinesia (slowness of movement), and paralysis are some of the important negative symptoms, whereas hyperkinesia (excessive movement) and dyskinesia (disordered movements), in addition to rigidity and spasticity, are considered positive symptoms. Motor mechanisms during wakefulness include several circuits: cortico-basal ganglionic-thalamo-cortical circuit, cortico-ponto-cerebello-thalamo-cortical circuit, descending brainstem motor pathways, and brainstem and spinal segmental circuits. All these circuits are influenced by peripheral afferent inputs. To summarize, the cerebellum participates in the initiation, timing, and coordination of the movements; the basal ganglia help in influencing the direction, force, and amplitude of the movements, as well as the internal generation and assembly of movements; and the cerebral cortex selects, plans, programs, and commands the movement.

---

* Deceased.

The corticospinal system then distributes the commands, and the segmental spinal motor apparatus drives the muscles to execute the movements. There is considerable modulation of the motor mechanism during sleep. Sleep in general is dominated by central inhibitory drive, but the excitatory mechanism intermittently breaks through the inhibitory phase in normal individuals, giving rise to physiologic motor activities during sleep (e.g., body movements, hypnic jerks). The dominant inhibitory mechanism of sleep is manifested by a progressive decrease of motor activity, including muscle tone during non–rapid eye movement (non-REM) sleep stages N1 to N3 and by marked decrease or absence of motor activity in rapid eye movement (REM) sleep. When this delicate balance between inhibitory and excitatory mechanisms breaks down, pathologic or abnormal motor activities emerge during sleep.

Movement disorder specialists generally are familiar with the involuntary or abnormal motor activities during the day, which may be associated with a variety of sleep abnormalities. In contrast, abnormal motor activities during sleep at night are encountered generally by the sleep specialists, and these abnormal movements may disturb sleep causing impaired daytime function. Because of their nocturnal occurrence, they may cause added diagnostic dilemmas. The question often arises whether these abnormal movements are diurnal movements persisting during sleep or parasomnias (abnormal movements intruding into sleep) or epileptic events at night. We briefly mention in this section two entities—REM behavior disorder and nocturnal seizure—to highlight such a dilemma. For a long time the movement disorder and sleep specialists viewed the events at night from different perspectives, but there is a growing realization that there are considerable overlaps and similarities between nocturnal and diurnal motor events, and sleep may be adversely affected by both diurnal and nocturnal involuntary movement disorders. Many neurologic disorders present with abnormal movements, both during daytime and nighttime, suggesting that both diurnal and nocturnal abnormal movements may result from a common neurobiologic alteration in the molecular mechanisms of sleep-wakefulness and motor control. It is now a challenge for both the movement disorder and sleep specialists to unravel the mysteries of such nocturnal movements so that we will have a better understanding of jerks and shakes during wakefulness and sleep. The ultimate beneficiaries of this insight will be our patients.

REM BEHAVIOR DISORDER—AN EXPERIMENT IN NATURE

An important entity that is often encountered by both the movement disorder and sleep specialists is REM behavior disorder (RBD). In 1965, Jouvet and Delorme[3] experimentally produced pontine lesions in the perilocus coeruleus alpha regions bilaterally in cats to produce abnormal motor activities during sleep and oneiric behavior in these cats, which in retrospect can be viewed as the animal counterpart of human RBD. In 1975, Tachibana, Tanaka, Hishikaway, and Kaneko[4] described abnormal REM sleep without muscle atonia (called stage I REM sleep) and motor dysfunctions in patients with acute alcohol withdrawal syndrome. However, in 1986, Schenck, Bundlie, Ettinger, and Mahowald[5] first described the human counterpart of the Jouvet and Delorme's experiment in cats as a new parasomnia syndrome, and this has later come to be known as REM behavior disorder. Subsequently, numerous cases appeared in the literature (see Chapters 29–31). Initially, it was thought that RBD was mostly idiopathic, but as more cases were described, it was realized that most cases are secondary and associated with neurodegenerative diseases. RBD occurs with great frequency in a number of neurodegenerative diseases, for example, Parkinson's disease (PD), multiple system atrophy (MSA), diffuse Lewy body disease (DLBD), olivopontocerebellar atrophy, progressive supranuclear palsy, and corticobasal ganglionic degeneration. In a number of these neurodegenerative diseases the alpha-synuclein inclusions have been noted (e.g., PD, MSA, DLBD), and some authors have proposed that RBD may be an alpha-synucleinopathy disorder.[6] In addition, RBD has been described in many cases of narcolepsy. Finally, RBD has been linked to dopamine cell dysfunction as clearly shown by the neuroimaging findings of reduced striatal presynaptic dopamine transporter in the iodopropane tropane single photon emission computed tomography (SPECT) scan with no reduction of postsynaptic dopamine D_2 receptors in the iodobenzamide (IBZM)-SPECT study.[7] RBD may precede many of these neurodegenerative diseases (e.g., PD, MSA, DLBD) or coexist with these diseases.[8–14] There are several reports trying to identify preclinical markers during the so-called cryptogenic or idiopathic stage of RBD.

NOCTURNAL SEIZURES OR ABNORMAL MOVEMENTS DURING SLEEP?

Abnormal motor activities may be the manifestations of some types of seizures or movement disorders, and if seen predominantly during sleep these may cause diagnostic problems. Movement disorder specialists, therefore, must be aware of such presentation. A case in point is nocturnal paroxysmal dystonia (NPD), an entity in search of an identity for a long time. The name derived from the abrupt, "paroxysmal" onset of episodes featuring dystonic (twisting, distorting) movements during sleep. This condition was probably described first by Horner and Jackson in 1969[15] when they described two families with several members presenting with hypnogenic nocturnal dyskinesia. Lugaresi[16–18] and his group, however, brought the entity of NPD to the forefront of the medical community. Later Meierkord, Fish, and Smith, et al.,[19] based on a comparative study between groups of NPD patients and those with undisputed frontal lobe seizures, supported the contention that NPD patients may have frontal lobe seizures.

Two other entities—paroxysmal arousals and awakenings and episodic nocturnal wanderings—share common features with NPD of abnormal paroxysmal motor activities during sleep and favorable response to anticonvulsants.[20] All these entities most likely represent partial seizures arising from discharging foci in the deeper regions of the brain, particularly frontal cortex. Because these events are distant from the scalp where electroencephalogram (EEG) is recorded, there is no associated scalp EEG evidence of epileptiform activities. Later an autosomal dominant nocturnal frontal lobe epilepsy (ADNFLE) was described by Scheffer, Bhatia, Lopes-Cendes, et al.[21] in five families. Attacks are characterized by brief motor seizures in clusters during sleep similar to those noted in NPD. Molecular neurobiologic studies suggested that the genes for ADNFLE are localized to chromosomes 20q13 and 15q24 with mutations in the neuronal nicotinic acetylcholine receptor (nACHR) alpha-4 subunit (CHRNA4),[22] beta-2 subunit (CHRNB2),[23] and alpha-2 subunit (CHRNA2). Since the original report, several other families have been described with autosomal dominant nocturnal frontal lobe epilepsy (see Chapters 26 and 35). This entity has been mistaken for sleep apnea and other involuntary movements or parasomnias.

MECHANISM OF ABNORMAL MOTOR ACTIVITIES DURING SLEEP

The mechanism of emergence of abnormal motor activities such as jerks, shakes, and screams during sleep differs in different conditions and is often not well worked out. Non-REM parasomnias or sleep-wake transition motor disorders may result from a combination of dysfunction of the arousal mechanism (which includes cholinergic ascending arousal system) associated with arousal fluctuations mediated via central motor pattern generators in the brainstem, an excessive activity of higher cortical center, and a failure of descending inhibitory system. In addition, disordered modulation by cholinergic, noradrenergic, serotonergic, or other neurochemically driven projections (e.g., glycinergic, glutamatergic, GABA-ergic) from the brainstem centers plays a role in all these abnormal motor disorders during sleep.

Suggested mechanisms for REM sleep muscle atonia[24] in normal individuals include activation of nucleus reticularis pontis oralis located ventral to locus coeruleus in the pons causing excitation of nucleus magnocellularis and paramedianus nuclei in the medial medulla via the lateral tegmentoreticular tract. Impulses from these inhibitory medullary regions are transmitted via the reticulospinal tract and inhibitory interneurons to motor neurons of the spinal cord. There is marked motor neuron hyperpolarization causing REM sleep muscle atonia. Intermittently, excitatory drive from the brainstem to the spinal motor neurons breaks through hyperpolarization causing intermittent myoclonic bursts (small, jerk-like movements) during REM sleep. Lesions in the peri-locus coeruleus alpha and the medial medullary regions involving the paramedianus nuclei cause REM sleep without muscle atonia. Other suggested mechanisms for REM motor disorders include a deficiency in the brainstem inhibitory system and a shift in the critical balance between excitation and inhibition.

Dissociation of all three states of human existence (wakefulness, REM, and non-REM sleep) with intrusion of one state into another or rapid oscillations of all three states may produce bizarre dissociated states characterized by abrupt motor activities and behavior during sleep at night.[25]

Mechanisms of seizures include cerebral cortical hyperexcitability, a failure of inhibitory mechanism, and excessive neuronal synchronization.[26,27] During non-REM sleep there is an excessive diffuse cortical synchronization mediated by the thalamocortical input, whereas during REM sleep there is inhibition of the thalamocortical synchronizing influence in addition to a tonic reduction in the interhemispheric impulse traffic through the corpus callosum. Factors that enhance synchronization are conducive to provocation of seizures in a susceptible individual. Non-REM sleep thus acts as a convulsant by causing excessive synchronization that predisposes to activation of seizures in an already hyperexcitable cortex. In contrast, during REM sleep there is an attenuation of epileptiform discharges and limitation of the propagation of generalized epileptiform discharges to a focal area.

PROMISING START AND RECENT CONTRIBUTION

There has been a promising start in the understanding of the neuroanatomic substrates of abnormal movements and motor control during sleep-wakefulness, as well as neurophysiologic mechanism of motor disorder. There have also been some recent advances in the understanding of molecular mechanisms of sleep and sleep disorders such as narcolepsy, fatal familial insomnia, and restless legs syndrome, but there still is a long way to go to answer the fundamental questions of why humans sleep and determining the function of sleep. One function of the motor system in sleep is to reduce movement so that sleep is undisturbed. Many neurotransmitters and neuromodulators control motor system and sleep-wake regulation, and there is considerable overlap in this control. Therefore, it is not surprising that a breakdown in this control encourages abnormal movements to emerge in sleep-wake states. Sleep-wake states also cause distinct modulation of abnormal movements.

In recent years there have been a number of exciting discoveries that have opened further pathways to the understanding of sleep and the motor system. One such recent contribution is the new understanding of the role of the pedunculopontine tegmental (PPT) and laterodorsal tegmental (LDT) nuclei.[28] Recent evidence suggests that PPT and LDT with their ascending projections to the thalamus; basal forebrain, including limbic cortex; substantia nigra; and descending projections to locus coeruleus, dorsal raphe nuclei, and other parts of the brainstem reticular formation; and spinal motor neurons appear to be placed in a crucial role to control motor activities during sleep-wakefulness. This knowledge has an implication in the understanding of sleep disturbances in PD and other neurodegenerative diseases.

Another exciting recent discovery concerns the role of the hypocretin (orexin) peptidergic neurons in the lateral hypothalamus and perifornical regions in regulating sleep-wakefulness and modulating motor control. Based on the widespread projections to the brainstem and forebrain arousal and sleep promoting neurons, it is most likely that the hypocretin system plays a crucial role in control of sleep-wakefulness. At least in one sleep disorder, narcolepsy-cataplexy syndrome, there is an intriguing suggestion that hypocretin cells participate in the mechanisms of abnormal intrusion of muscle atonia during wakefulness, causing cataplexy or absence of muscle atonia during REM sleep in many patients with narcolepsy and giving rise to manifestations of RBD.

Finally, the recent concept of "agrypnia excitata" offered important insights into the pathophysiology of prion disease and rekindled the role of the limbic thalamus in sleep-wake regulation.[29] This entity defines striking and distinctive behavioral and polysomnographic features combining the characteristics of fatal familial insomnia, morvan's fibrillary chorea, and delirium tremens.

Progress in Laboratory Techniques and Therapy

Simultaneous with the understanding of the basic science of sleep-wakefulness and motor mechanism, there has been concomitant progress in the laboratory techniques to evaluate motor disorders during sleep. In addition to the time-honored techniques of polysomnographic recordings and multiple sleep latency tests (MSLTs), video polysorrmography (PSG), computerized PSG, actigraphy, and newer neuroimaging studies (e.g., positron emission tomography, SPECT, functional magnetic resonance [MR] imaging, MR diffusion tensor imaging, and voxel-based MRI morphometry) are increasingly playing a significant role in evaluating motor disorders during sleep by uncovering their neural substrates. Actigraphy, in particular, is a promising new technique to measure body movements throughout the day and night for days or weeks at a time. Actigraphy is thus poised to play an important role in evaluating abnormal movements during sleep (see Chapter 15).

Increasing understanding of the nature of the abnormal movements during sleep has helped us, the sleep and movement disorder specialists, treat our patients more efficiently than before. There has been an explosive development in psychopharmacology, in our understanding of benzodiazepine and nonbenzodiazepine hypnotic drugs, and in pharmacotherapy of diurnal movement disorders and seizure disorders. Many of these drugs have been useful in treating some of the nocturnal movement disorders.

Organization of the Monograph

All of the recent advances in the field of sleep and movement disorders have been highlighted throughout this monograph. The book is divided into three major sections: basic science, laboratory evaluation, and clinical science. In addition to an overview of normal sleep, the basic science section addresses the role of orexin (hypocretin) in sleep and movement disorder, neurobiology of sleep, motor control during sleep and wakefulness, circadian neurobiology, and neuropharmacologic control of motor activity during sleep and genetics of sleep and its disorders. The section dealing with laboratory evaluation highlights the role of PSG, including video-PSG, MSLT, actigraphy, EEG monitoring, scoring of sleep staging, breathing and sleep-related movements, measurement and clinical significance of cycling alternating pattern in the EEG, autonomic evaluation, neuroimaging techniques, and other neurophysiologic methods to evaluate abnormal movements. The clinical section begins with an introduction, an approach and classification of movement disorders during sleep, differential diagnosis of abnormal movements during sleep, and epidemiology of sleep-related movement disorders. This section is further divided into two subsections—sleep-related movements (normal and abnormal) and movement disorders and sleep—to describe a variety of clinical disorders to highlight the emergence or triggering of abnormal motor activities during sleep and the impact of movement disorders on sleep. This section concludes by reminding readers not to neglect psychiatric aspects of movement disorders and sleep, as well as pediatric sleep-related movement disorders.

REFERENCES

1. Brookhart JM, Mountcastle VB, Brooks VB, et al. *Handbook of Physiology. Section 1. The Nervous System, Vol 2. Motor Control. Part 2.* Bethesda, MD: American Physiological Society; 1981.
2. Chokroverty S. An approach to a patient with disorders of voluntary movements. In: Chokroverty S, ed. *Movement Disorders.* PMA Publishing Corp; 1990:1.
3. Jouvet M, Delorme JF. Locus coeruleus et sommeil paradoxal. *J Soc Biol* 1965;159:895.
4. Tachibana M, Tanaka K, Hishikaway, Kaneko Z. A sleep study of acute psychotic states due to alcohol and meprobamate addiction. *Adv Sleep Res* 1975;2:177.
5. Schenck CH, Bundlie SR, Ettinger MC, Mahowald MW. Chronic behavioral disorders of human REM sleep: a new category of parasomnia. *Sleep* 1986;9:293.
6. Boeve BF, Silber MH, Ferman TJ, et al. Association of REM sleep behavior disorder and neurodegenerative disease may reflect an underlying synucleinopathy. *Mov Disord* 2001;16:622.
7. Eisensehr I, Linke R, Noachtar S, et al. Reduced striatal dopamine transporters in idiopathic rapid eye movement sleep behavior disorder compared with Parkinson's disease and controls. *Brain* 2000;123:1155.
8. Plazzi G, Corsini R, Provini F, et al. REM sleep behavior disorders in multiple system atrophy. *Neurology* 1997;48:1094.
9. Schenck CH, Bundlie SR, Mahowald MW. Delayed emergence of a Parkinsonium disorder in 38% of 29 older men initially diagnosed with idiopathic rapid eye movement sleep behavior disorder. *Neurology* 1996;46:388.
10. Uchiyama M, Isse K, Tanaka K, et al. Incidental Lewy body disease in a patient with REM sleep behavior disorder. *Neurology* 1995;45:709.
11. Turner RS, D'Amato CJ, Chervin RD, Blaivas M. The pathology of REM sleep behavior disorder with comorbid Lewy body dementia. *Neurology* 2000;55:1730.
12. Boeve BF, Silber MH, Ferman TJ, et al. REM sleep behavior disorder and degenerative

dementia: an association likely reflecting Lewy body disease. *Neurology* 1998;51:363.

13. McKeith IG, Ballard CG, Perry RH, et al. Prospective validation of consensus criteria for the diagnosis of dementia with Lewy bodies. *Neurology* 2000;54:1050.

14. Olson EJ, Bradley FB, Silber MH. Rapid eye movement sleep behavior disorder: Demographic, clinical and laboratory findings in 93 cases. *Brain* 2000;123:331.

15. Horner FH, Jackson LC. Familial paroxysmal choreoathetosis. In : Barbeau A, Brunette JR, eds. *Progress in Neuro-genetics*. Amsterdam, The Netherlands : Excerpta Medica Foundation; 1969:745.

16. Lugaresi E, Cirignotta F. Hypnogenic paroxysmal dystonia: epileptic seizure or a new syndrome? *Sleep* 1981;4:129.

17. Lugaresi E, Cirignotta F, Montagna P. Nocturnal paroxysmal dystonia. *J Neurol Neurosurg Psychiatry* 1986;49:375.

18. Tinuper P, Cerullo A, Cirignotta F, et al. Nocturnal paroxysmal dystonia with short-lasting attacks: three cases with evidence for an epileptic frontal lobe origin of seizures. *Epilepsia* 1990;31:549.

19. Meierkord H, Fish DR, Smith SJM, et al. Is nocturnal paroxysmal dystonia a form of frontal lobe epilepsy? *Mov Disord* 1992;7:38.

20. Montagna P. Nocturnal paroxysmal dystonia and nocturnal wandering. *Neurology* 1992;42(suppl 6):61.

21. Scheffer IE, Bhatia KP, Lopes-Cendes I, et al. Autosomal dominant nocturnal frontal lobe epilepsy. A distinctive clinical disorder. *Brain* 1995;118:61.

22. Barrantes FJ, Aztiria E, Rauschemberger MB, Vasconsuelo A. The neuronal nicotinic acetylcholine receptor in some hereditary epilepsies. *Neurochem Res* 2000;25:583.

23. Phillips HA, Favre I, Kirk Patrick M, et al. CHRNB2 is the second acetylcholine receptor subunit associated with autosomal dominant nocturnal frontal lobe epilepsy. *Am J Hum Genet* 2001;68:225.

24. Sakai K, Sastre JP, Salvert D, et al. Tegmentoreticular projections with special reference to the muscular atonia during paradoxical sleep in the cat. An I-1RP study. *Brain Res* 1979;176:233.

25. Mahowald MW, Schenc CH. State boundary dyscontrol and complex (including violent) sleep behaviors. In: Chokroverty S, Hening WA, Walters AS, eds. *Sleep and Movement Disorders*. Philadelphia, PA: Butterworth-Heinemann; 2003:417–29.

26. Chokroverty S, Montagna P. Sleep and epilepsy. In: Chokroverty S, ed. *Sleep Disorder Medicine. Basic Science, Technical Considerations and Clinical Aspects*. 3rd ed. Philadelphia, PA: Saunders/Elsevier; 2009:499.

27. Engel J, Jr., Pedley TA. *Epilepsy: A Comprehensive Textbook*. 2nd ed. Philadelphia, PA: Lippincott, Williams & Wilkins; 2008.

28. Rye D. Contributions of the pedunculopontine region to normal and altered REM sleep. *Sleep* 1997;20:757.

29. Montagna P, Lugaresi E. Agrypnia excitata: a generalized overactivity syndrome and a useful concept in the neurophysiopathology of sleep. *Clin Neurophysiol* 2002;113:552.

PART TWO

Basic Science

2

Non-REM Sleep

For Charging Our Batteries

ROBERT W. McCARLEY AND RADHIKA BASHEER

SEVERAL SLEEP-RELATED movement disorders (SRMDs) with stereotypical movements of the limbs (e.g., restless leg syndrome [RLS], periodic limb movement disorder [PLMD], rhythmic movement disorder [RMD], sleep-related leg cramps) and jaw movements (bruxism) result in impaired sleep quality and fatigue.[1,2] Repeated stereotypical movement-related arousals prevent restful sleep depriving the brain of the beneficial restorative effects of sleep. As Lavoie et al.[3] have shown, PLMD may hinder the production of deep slow-wave sleep (delta sleep), which this chapter shows is key for "recharging our batteries" and for the restorative aspects of sleep. This chapter may thus form a link between the fatigue and sleepiness experienced by PLMD and other movement disorders patients and the disturbed functions of non–rapid eye movement (non-REM) sleep. This chapter targets the role of increasing brain energy levels as an important function of non-REM sleep. If one equates the brain currency of energy, adenosine triphosphate (ATP), with the "batteries

of the brain," the data we present here will offer experimental evidence that the anecdotal expression is true on a deeper level.

INTRODUCTION AND HYPOTHESIS

The subjective experience of sleep as restorative of energy is a commonsense observation, but one not directly studied physiologically with modern technology. The importance of sleep and suggestions about its physiological role have been better documented as a negative, by what happens without sleep, since prolonged sleep deprivation (SD) or sleep restriction adversely influences metabolic processes,[4] general emotional and physical health,[5] and neurocognitive behavior.[6] An often postulated, although not directly measured, the function of sleep is to restore brain energy expended during active waking.[7,8] Although constituting only 2% of body mass, brain oxygen and glucose utilization account for approximately

20% of those of the whole organism.[9] Compared with wakefulness, indirect evidence that sleep reduces brain energy demands is a 44% reduction in the cerebral metabolic rate (CMR) of glucose[10] and a 25% reduction in the CMR of O_2.[11] Our previous report [12] also indirectly supports a link between wake-related neural activation and energy expenditure, since felines showed an increase in extracellular levels of a metabolic by-product of energy, adenosine, in a wake-active brain region, the basal forebrain,[12] and a decline during spontaneous sleep, a pattern also observed in rodent basal forebrain.[13] Moreover, adenosine levels increase markedly if sleep is prevented (i.e., SD).[14,15]

These adenosine studies prompted us to examine the actual "currency of brain cellular energy, ATP, since adenosine may be an indicator of neuronal activity-dependent energy use, by reflecting ATP breakdown. Steady-state ATP levels were once considered to be stable. However, recent brain studies indicate that electrical stimulation, glucose deprivation, or manipulations of $Na^+/K^+ATPase$ activity induce detectable changes in ATP levels.[16–18] ATP concentration might not only reflect the energy state but may also play an additional role in neurotransmission. For example, ATP concentration-dependent signaling mechanisms have been shown to regulate excitatory (glutamatergic) and inhibitory (GABA-ergic) neuronal activity through low- and high-affinity ATP-sensitive K+ channels.[19] Moreover, extracellular breakdown of released ATP could also contribute to increased adenosine levels.

DATA SUPPORTING THIS HYPOTHESIS

To summarize, our data indicated that there is a surge in directly measured ATP concentration during the initial hours of natural sleep, coinciding with an increase in non-REM delta activity, and supporting the hypothesis that a function of sleep is to provide the brain with an increase in energy availability for sleep-dependent processes.

Our study examined ATP levels in the brains of rats maintained under 12 hours light/12 hours dark periods. Every 3 hours for 24 hours, starting from 7 am (lights on, onset of normal sleep period), ATP levels were determined using a validated luciferin-luciferase ATP detection assay. We examined ATP changes in four brain regions important in sleep-wake physiology: basal forebrain (BF), frontal cortex (FC), cingulate cortex (CCX), and hippocampus (HIPP) (Fig. 2.1A). Within each of the four brain regions, the steady-state ATP level was stable during the wake period (7 pm–7 am, lights off), but ATP levels dramatically altered values in all four regions during the sleep period (7 am–7 pm, lights on). The average ATP values for a 24-hour period, calculated as μmol per gram tissue wet weight (molality), varied between regions. During the dark period the values were lower but constant within each region. On the other hand, during the light period, when rats were asleep most of the time (66.7 ± 6.3%), ATP levels in each brain region were elevated and, most important, were not constant but showed significant alterations in values within each brain region as compared with waking (Kruskal-Wallis ANOVAs, N = 6 in each region: average values in μmol/g wet tissue (p's < .006 for each region).

The increase in ATP during sleep followed a distinct pattern. The lowest levels were seen at 7 am. In the initial sleep period in all four brain regions, ATP levels surged significantly, showing highest values at 10 am (N = 6; $p < .01$), which declined slightly by 1 pm (N = 6; $p < .01$) (Fig. 2.1A). Using the diurnal average as baseline for diurnal comparisons, the percentage increase at 10 am was comparable in FC (219%) and BF (172%), which were greater than the increases noted in HIPP (154%) and CCX (151%) (Fig. 2.1A). The levels declined to baseline values by 4 pm. This initial surge coincides with the pattern of slow wave activity (SWA, delta activity, 1–4.5 Hz) that, like ATP, showed significant variability during sleep (Fig. 2.1B). A similar profile of slow-wave activity during the sleep period was also described by Dash et al.[20]

To further distinguish whether the surge in ATP was associated with the time of day (diurnal) variation or with sleep behavior, we subjected rats to 3 hours of SD by gentle handling starting at 7 am and examined the ATP levels at 10 am, the time when ATP levels were highest in diurnal control animals. This SD blocked the ATP surge seen in controls (Fig. 2.2A). When the rats were allowed 3 hours of recovery sleep (RS) after the 3 hours of SD, only in BF did the ATP levels surge to match the levels of the diurnal controls (1 pm). In other brain regions, 6 hours of RS was needed to induce the surge in ATP levels as shown for frontal cortex in Figure 2.2. Thus, SD postponed the ATP surge, although with variable time lags.

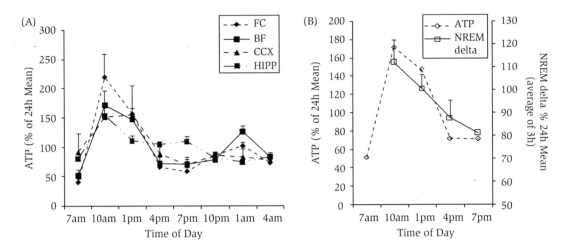

FIGURE 2.1 Diurnal variations in the ATP levels. (*A*) During the first 6 hours of spontaneous sleep the steady-state ATP levels surged, showing a maximal value at 10 am in all four brain regions with highest increase in frontal cortex > basal forebrain > hippocampus> cingulate cortex. (*B*) The changes in ATP levels closely correspond with the changes in the non-REM delta during the light period. (Adapted from Dworak et al.[24])

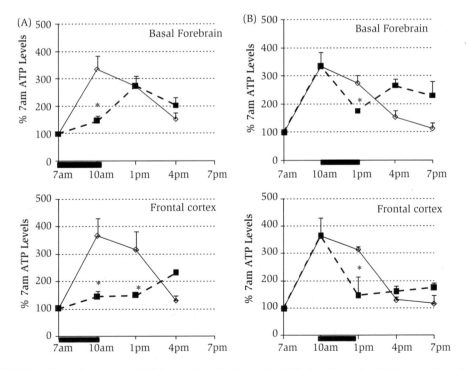

FIGURE 2.2 Sleep deprivation (SD) prevents the surge in ATP significantly. (*A*) Preventing sleep for 3 hours starting at light onset (7 am) also prevents the ATP surge at 10 am. (*B*) Three hours of SD following 3 hours of sleep decreases the ATP, suggesting the effect of SD on ATP is independent of time of day. SD performed after 3 hours of sleep also results in ATP decrease, indicating the effect of SD on ATP is independent of the time of day. (Adapted from Dworak et al.[24])

Next we addressed whether an interruption of the sleep period after onset would also influence the pattern of ATP change observed in normally sleeping animals. Rats were allowed to sleep during the first 3 hours of the light period (7–10 am), allowing the initial ATP surge to occur, and then underwent 3 hours of SD. In normally sleeping control animals, the ATP levels during 10 am to 1 pm begin to exhibit a slow decline, although still considerably higher than the diurnal average. SD from 10 am to 1 pm in the sleep period increased the rate of decline in ATP, so that ATP levels reached a low level at 1 pm, while transition to this low level was reached much later, at 7 pm in the normally sleeping animals. ATP levels after the 10 am to 1 pm SD were significantly lower in all four regions (p's < .022; Fig. 2.2B). When this 3 hours SD was followed by 3 hours of recovery sleep (RS) (1 pm–4 pm), ATP levels in all brain regions increased during the RS to levels higher than those in their diurnal controls at 4 pm, again demonstrating the sleep dependence of the ATP increase. Taken together, these results indicate that during waking (either spontaneous or due to 3 hours of SD) ATP levels remain close to the 7 am baseline values, while sleep onset results in a rapid and significant surge in ATP levels. Thus, these effects of sleep and wake behavior on brain ATP levels are independent of the time of day.

To determine whether the increase in ATP was related to regional neuronal activity patterns associated with sleep and wake, in a separate experiment ($n = 5$ rats/group) we compared the 7 am to 10 am SD-induced changes in the levels of ATP in two functionally diverse regions of hypothalamus, namely the lateral hypothalamus (LH) known to predominantly contain wake- and REM-active neurons,[21,22] and the ventrolateral preoptic nucleus (VLPO) that predominantly contains sleep-active neurons.[23] In the same rats we also re-examined FC. After the 3 hours of SD, ATP concentrations were significantly reduced in FC ($-53.36 \pm 8.01\%$, $p = .007$) when compared to sleeping controls, as was observed in the previous group of rats. ATP also showed a significant decrease in LH ($-40.17 \pm 19.8\%$, $p = .048$). Importantly, no significant change was observed in the sleep-active VLPO ($+10.69 \pm 20.36\%$, $p = .719$) (Fig. 2.3).

To furnish an experimental manipulation of SWA that would further test our hypothesis of non-REM delta-ATP association and to rule out potentially confounding diurnal effects, such as light, we use microdialysis to perfuse adenosine (300 µM) unilaterally into the basal forebrain at the onset of the active (dark) period, from 7 pm

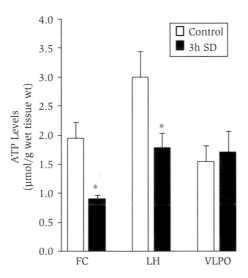

FIGURE 2.3 Effect of sleep deprivation (SD) on the levels of ATP in lateral hypothalamus (LH) and ventrolateral preoptic area (VLPO). Rats (N = 5/group), sleep deprived for 3 hours (7–10 am, black bar), showed significant decrease in ATP in frontal cortex (FC) (**$p < .01$) and LH (*$p < .05$), whereas no significant change was observed in VLPO ($p = .719$) when compared to undisturbed time of day matched sleeping controls (white bars). (Adapted from Dworak et al.[24])

to 10 pm, a procedure previously shown by us to increase non-REM delta.[14] Indeed, compared to the rats that were perfused with artificial cerebrospinal fluid (aCSF), adenosine perfused animals showed higher increases in percent time in non-REM sleep and non-REM delta activity when compared to the same time period on a baseline day with no perfusion. Moreover, there was a significant increase in ATP at the end of adenosine perfusion in all four brain regions compared with aCSF controls (Fig. 2.4). The hypothesis of a direct association between non-REM delta and ATP over the 3 hours of perfusion was most clearly illustrated by their strong correlation in both FC (*rho* = 0.83, *p* < .0006), the site of electroencephalographic (EEG) recording, and the BF (*rho* = 0.64, *p* < .04), a site known to be related to delta activity.[24]

Together, these data thus support our hypotheses that (1) non-REM delta-ATP levels are linked. The initial surge of ATP during spontaneous sleep is associated with non-REM delta and the associated reduced energy expenditure; (2) the ATP-delta association is not due to confounding diurnal factors; and (3) preventing sleep prevents ATP surge independent of the time of day.

Our data strongly support the hypothesis that ATP levels in the tissue can change with behavioral-state change; there are also complementary changes in the levels and activities of enzymes involved in ATP synthesis as well as breakdown. Reports on the protein and activity of ATP synthesizing enzymes of oxidative phosphorylation pathways, cytochrome oxidase c (COX), enzymes in rat and mouse brain, show an increase at the end of the wake period (7 am, time of lowest ATP) and a decrease at 10 am (time of highest ATP) [25,26] (see Fig. 2.5). Similarly, following 3 hours of SD from 7 am to 10 am the cytochrome c activity is higher at 10 am (and ATP is lower) when compared to undisturbed controls (Fig. 2.5). This reciprocity between ATP levels and

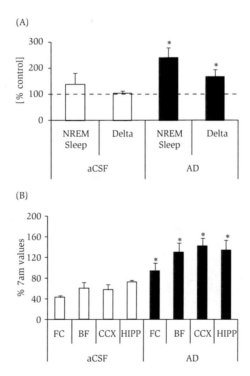

FIGURE 2.4 Unilateral adenosine (AD) perfusion into basal forebrain causes highly correlated delta and ATP increases. (*A*) Compared with no treatment (dotted line, 100%), unilateral AD perfusion into basal forebrain (black bars) during 3 hours (7–10 pm) in the dark period significantly increased both non-REM sleep duration and non-REM delta activity. (*B*) ATP concentrations measured in frontal cortex (FC), basal forebrain (BF), cingulate cortex (CCX), and hippocampus (HIPP) at the end of 3 hours of AD or artificial cerebrospinal fluid (aCSF) infusion into basal forebrain showed a significant increase in ATP concentrations in all brain regions in AD perfused rats when compared to aCSF perfused rats. (Adapted from Dworak et al.[24])

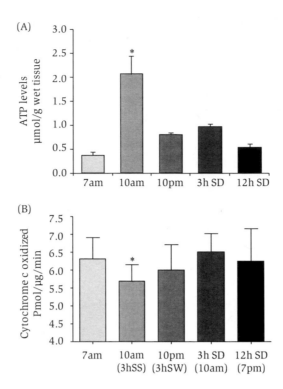

(A)

(B)

FIGURE 2.5   Reciprocal changes in the ATP levels and cytochrome oxidase c (COX) activity. (A) The ATP levels are significantly higher at 10 am in sleeping rats' cortex when compared to the end of wake period (7 am) and following sleep deprivation. (B) The COX enzyme activity in mouse brain shows trends opposite to that seen for ATP. (Adapted from Dworak et al.[24] and Nikonova et al.[26])

cytochrome c strongly suggests that the decline in ATP levels below critical levels needed to prevent an arrest of brain function is prevented by the simultaneous upregulation of ATP synthesis.

ATP LEVEL REGULATION BY AMPK

We next addressed the mechanism causing the sleep-associated initial surge in ATP to return to baseline levels during the later hours in the light (sleep) period. We investigated whether the "ATP sensor," the AMP (adenosine monophosphate)-activated protein kinase (AMPK),[27] has a role in detecting and responding to ATP changes during sleep and SD. This phylogenetically conserved kinase monitors changes in cellular concentrations of ATP and AMP. Increased ATP usage (higher AMP/ATP ratio) activates AMPK by phosphorylation. Phosphorylated AMPK (P-AMPK), in turn, phosphorylates many downstream target proteins, regulating cellular energy metabolism by inhibition of ATP-consuming anabolic

pathways and activation of ATP-generating catabolic pathways).[27] We hypothesized that at 7 am, when the AMP/ATP ratio is presumably high after 12 hours of waking, a more elevated level of P-AMPK would be detected than at 10 am, at the peak of the sleep-induced ATP surge, presumably accompanied by a decreased AMP/ATP ratio. In contrast, if sleep were to be prevented by 3 hours of SD between 7 am and 10 am, P-AMPK levels would be expected to remain high until recovery sleep is allowed.

To test this hypothesis, we compared the levels of P-AMPK in BF and FC at two diurnal time points, 7 am when ATP levels are the lowest, and 10 am when the ATP levels are the highest (see Fig. 2.1A). P-AMPK protein levels were detected using Western blots. As hypothesized, P-AMPK levels were significantly higher (at 7 am when compared to 10 am in BF; N = 4, $p < .02$) and showed a similar tendency in FC, although not statistically significant (N = 5, t-test, $p < .13$) (Fig. 2.6A, B, C, and D). Also in accord with this hypothesis, similar reciprocal relationships between P-AMPK and ATP levels

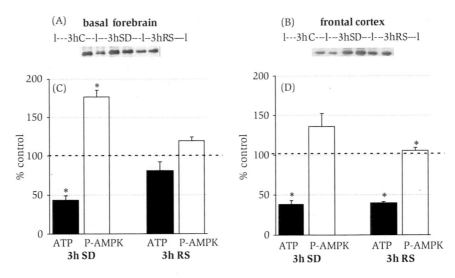

FIGURE 2.6   Sleep deprivation (SD)-induced reciprocal changes in ATP levels and in phosphorylated AMPK (P-AMPK). (*A* and *B*) Western blots showing P-AMPK protein (two represented from each group) changes after 3 and 6 hours of SD and 3 hours of recovery sleep (RS) in basal forebrain (BF) and frontal cortex (FC), respectively. (*C* and *D*) A graphical presentation of changes in basal forebrain in P-AMPK (N = 5) and ATP (N = 6) when compared to their respective diurnal (time of the day) controls. In BF, 3 hours of SD significantly decreased ATP levels ($p < .01$) while P-AMPK levels increased ($p < .01$). However, after 3 hours of RS both ATP and P-AMPK returned to control levels. Similar trends were seen in FC. However, after 6 hours of SD, although the ATP levels continued to decrease both in BF and FC, the reciprocal and significant increase was observed in FC only. * $p < .01$

were also observed when 3 hours of SD rats were compared with 10 am diurnal controls (N = 4, BF, $p < .02$; FC showed a similar trend, $p < .08$). Thus, our data suggest that the decrease in AMP/ATP ratio will decrease the levels of P-AMPK and favor anabolic enzyme activity; on the contrary, during SD when neuronal energy consumption is high, high AMP/ATP ratio will increase P-AMPK levels and favor catabolic processes to generate more ATP (see the model in Fig. 2.7).

DISCUSSION

In summary, our data showing an increase in ATP levels during sleep provide molecular evidence in support of the long-standing view that an important function of sleep is related to providing the brain with increased energy stores.[7,8] Our data, however, significantly recast the sleep and energy restoration hypothesis. Instead of speaking of energy "restoration," since ATP levels at the end of the wake period are not strikingly lower than at wake period onset, we restate the hypothesis as "sleep is

for an energy surge," a surge that permits energy-consuming processes, such as protein and fatty acid synthesis, to occur. Short-term SD delays and longer term SD delays and limits the extent of this ATP surge, a limitation that may impair energy-requiring biosynthetic processes. This view is in agreement with previous reports demonstrating an increase, during sleep, in the transcription of genes involved in protein synthesis and synaptic plasticity[28,29] and increased translation of proteins,[30] and, following SD, an overall decrease in protein synthesis.[31] High ATP levels are also needed for ribosome biosynthesis, which is linked to yet another energy-consuming process, protein synthesis.

The changes in AMPK reciprocal to those of ATP favor an anabolic state of the brain. Our data thus suggest that an initial ATP surge nourishes the anabolic, restorative biosynthetic processes occurring during sleep, in accord with Shakespeare's intuitive phrasing, "Sleep...great nature's second course, Chief nourisher in life's feast" (Macbeth, Act II, Scene II).

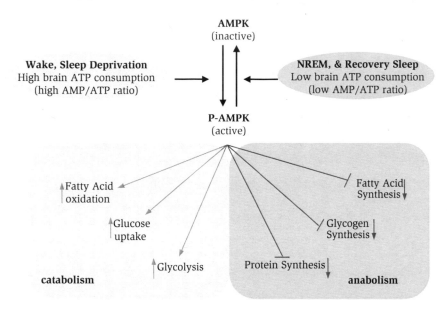

FIGURE 2.7 A model showing the two states of AMP-activated protein kinase (AMPK) and their functional role in the regulation of catabolic and anabolic pathways. (Adapted from Dworak et al.[24])

RESPONSE TO THIS HYPOTHESIS AND THESE DATA

In commentaries in the journal *Sleep*, two principal and related concerns were expressed.[32–35] The first major concern was whether ATP changed very much or at all, given the complex buffering systems within the cell. We believe there is now strong evidence indicating changes. The levels of intracellular ATP decrease during reticulocyte differentiation,[36] whereas severalfold increases are observed during ascorbate-induced differentiation of osteoblasts.[37] The ATP levels show circadian variations in liver and heart.[38] Induction of anorectic activity by steroidal glycoside causes a two-fold increase in hypothalamic ATP.[18] Intracellular ATP levels drop two- to three-fold during muscle fatigue.[39] Large changes in ATP are often accompanied by changes in other adenylate nucleotides in an attempt to maintain the energy charge above 0.519, since values < 0.5 are lethal. The energy charge of the adenylate system is defined as half the average number of anhydride-bound phosphate groups per adenine moiety and may assume a value between 1 (ATP only) and 0 (only AMP present).[40] The energy charge of the adenylate pool: ([ATP] + 1/2[ADP]/ ([ATP] + [ADP] + [AMP]) has been proposed as a control parameter in the regulatory interactions by which biological homeostasis is maintained.[40]

Decrease in ATP concentration results in increases in ADP and more so in AMP, but without drastic changes in the overall energy charge. In normal brain tissue the energy charge is closer to 0.85 [41] and is regulated by direct participation of adenine nucleotides in energy-converting processes such as glycolysis, oxidative phosphorylation, and in many energy-expending biosynthetic pathways, such as those of amino acids, nucleic acids, protein, fatty acids, and cholesterol synthesis.[42]

The second major concern was whether our methods were adequate to measure ATP. In part, this concern was driven by our failing to convert the molar values of ATP/μl of tissue extract to molality (μmol/g of wet tissue weight), leading to mislabeling of ATP values in molar units in the published manuscript in its figures 3 and 5. We note that, in the present chapter, the ATP values in the text and Table 2.1 are correctly expressed as micromoles per gram of wet tissue weight and Figure 2.3 and the new Figure 2.5 are correctly labeled, with ATP levels having units of molality. As shown in Table 2.1, these values obtained with our methods are similar to values obtained with other methods, including rapid freezing and microwave irradiation. It should be noted that the time of day of collection of the ATP measurements in this table is not known.

Table 2.1 ATP Levels (Molality)

BRAIN SAMPLE COLLECTION	METHODS OF ATP MEASUREMENT	ATP LEVELS	REFERENCE
Mice: decapitation + brain in liquid nitrogen	Homogenized in TCA, HPLC	2.1 μmol/g wet weight	Lin et al.[44]
Rats: decapitation + liquid nitrogen	99% methanol + HPLC	2.8 μmol/g wet weight	Yoshida et al.[45]
Mice: decapitation + brain frozen in Freon 12	PCA, spectrophotometry	2.01 μmol/g wet weight	Lowry et al.[46]
Rats: decapitation + liquid nitrogen	PCA, ^{31}P NMR spectroscopy	2.4 μmol/g wet weight	Kopp et al.[47]
Rats: decapitation + liquid nitrogen	PCA, 31P NMR spectroscopy	2.8 μmol/g wet weight	Aureli et al.[48]
Rats: decapitation + liquid nitrogen	PCA, firefly lantern extract assay	2.01 μmol/g wet weight	Ridge[49]
Rats: high energy focused microwave irradiation	TCA + HPLC	2.8 μmol/g wet weight	Delaney & Geiger[50]
Rats: basal forebrain dissected on dry ice	TCA + luciferin-luciferase bioluminescence	1.77 μmol/g wet weight	Dworak et al.[24]
Rats: frontal cortex dissected on dry ice	TCA + luciferin-luciferase bioluminescence	1.96 μmol/g wet weight	Dworak et al.[24]

HPLC, high-pressure liquid chromatography; NMR, nuclear magnetic resonance, PCA, perchloric acid; TCA, trichloroacetic acid.

Presuming that these samples were collected during the light period, the phase most convenient for the experimenter, we have used our 10 am light period values in the table. It also is clear that ATP measurements may differ according to brain region, as was seen in our data cited earlier.

As a final comment, we think that replication of these data by others will be most convincing to skeptics, as is generally true in science for new findings.

FUTURE DIRECTIONS

Future research will benefit from investigations on the changes in specific anabolic and catabolic pathways by examining the phosphorylated AMPK and its target enzymes. In addition to AMPK, many other proteins have been identified as sensors of intracellular ATP, such as the membrane ATP-sensitive potassium channels. It is also important to examine the changes in extracellular ATP and how it relates to intracellular levels of ATP and sleep wake behavior.

ACKNOWLEDGMENTS

This work was supported by the Department of Veterans Affairs Medical Research Service Awards to RWM and RB and by the National Institute of Mental Health (NIMH39683, RWM).

AUTHORS' NOTE

Much of the material in this essay was taken from our *Journal of Neuroscience* published paper and from our response to commentaries in the journal *Sleep*.[24,43] An important note is that the figures in this essay use corrected notation for ATP concentrations, μmol/gram wet tissue weight, compared with the *Journal of Neuroscience* paper.

REFERENCES

1. Walters AS. Clinical identification of the simple sleep-related movement disorders. *Chest* 2007;4:1260–6.
2. Merlino G, Gigli GL. Sleep -related movement disorders. *Neurol Sci* 2012;33(3):491–513.
3. Lavoie S, deBilbao F, Haba-Rubio J, et al. Influence of sleep stage and wakefulness on the spectral EEG activity and heart rate variations around periodic leg movements. *Clin Neurophysiol* 2004;115:2236–46.
4. Knutson KL. Impact of sleep and sleep loss on glucose homeostasis and appetite regulation. *Sleep Med Clin* 2007;2:187–97.
5. Haack M, Mullington JM. Sustained sleep restriction reduces emotional and physical well-being. *Pain* 2005;119:56–64.
6. Lim J, Dinges DF. Sleep deprivation and vigilant attention. *Ann NY Acad Sci* 2008;1129:305–22.
7. Benington JH, Heller HC. Restoration of brain energy metabolism as the function of sleep. *Prog Neurobiol* 1995;45:347–60.
8. Scharf MT, Naidoo N, Zimmerman JE, et al. The energy hypothesis of sleep revisited. *Prog Neurobiol* 2008;86:264–80.
9. Magistretti PJ. Brain energy metabolism. In: Zigmond M, Bloom FE, Landis S, Roberts J, Squire L, eds. *Fundamental Neuroscience*, Academic Press (San Diego), 1999:389–413.
10. Maquet P. Sleep function(s) and cerebral metabolism. *Behav Brain Res* 1995;69:75–83.
11. Madsen PL, Schmidt JF, Wildschiodtz G, et al. Cerebral O2 metabolism and cerebral blood flow in humans during deep and rapid-eye-movement sleep. *J Appl Physiol* 1991;70:2597–601.
12. Porkka-Heiskanen T, Strecker RE, Thakkar M, et al. Adenosine: a mediator of the sleep-inducing effects of prolonged wakefulness. *Science* 1997;276:1265–8.
13. McKenna JT, Dauphin LJ, Mulken KJ, et al. Nocturnal elevation of extracellular adenosine in the rat basal forebrain. *Sleep Res Online* 2003;5:155–60.
14. Basheer R, Porkka-Heiskanen T, Stenberg D, et al. Adenosine and behavioral state control: adenosine increases c-Fos protein and AP1 binding in basal forebrain of rats. *Brain Res Mol Brain Res* 1999;73:1–10.
15. Kalinchuk AV, Lu Y, Stenberg D, et al. Nitric oxide production in the basal forebrain is required for recovery sleep. *J Neurochem* 2006;99:483–98.
16. Christian SL, Ross AP, Zhao HW, et al. Arctic ground squirrel (Spermophilus parryii) hippocampal neurons tolerate prolonged oxygen-glucose deprivation and maintain baseline ERK1/2 and JNK activation despite drastic ATP loss. *J Cereb Blood Flow Metab* 2008;28:1307–19.
17. Bao L, Avshalumov MV, Rice ME. Partial mitochondrial inhibition causes striatal dopamine release suppression and medium spiny neuron depolarization via H2O2 elevation, not ATP depletion. *J Neurosci* 2005;25:10029–40.
18. MacLean DB, Luo LG. Increased ATP content/production in the hypothalamus may be a signal for energy-sensing of satiety: studies of the anorectic mechanism of a plant steroidal glycoside. *Brain Res* 2004;1020:1–11.
19. Peters A, Schweiger U, Pellerin L, et al. The selfish brain: competition for energy resources. *Neurosci Biobehav Rev* 2004;28:143–80.
20. Dash MB, Douglas CL, Vyazovskiy VV, et al. Long-term homeostasis of extracellular glutamate in the rat cerebral cortex across sleep and waking states. *J Neurosci* 2009;29:620–9.
21. Szymusiak R, McGinty D. Hypothalamic regulation of sleep and arousal. *Ann NY Acad Sci* 2008;1129:275–86.
22. Hassani OK, Lee MG, Jones BE. Melanin-concentrating hormone neurons discharge in a reciprocal manner to orexin neurons across the sleep-wake cycle. *Proc Natl Acad Sci USA* 2009;106:2418–22.
23. Sherin JE, Shiromani PJ, McCarley RW, et al. Activation of ventrolateral preoptic neurons during sleep. *Science* 1996;27:216–19.
24. Dworak M, McCarley RW, Kim T, et al. Sleep and brain energy levels: ATP changes during sleep. *J Neurosci* 2010;30:9007–16.
25. Nikonova EV, Vijayasarathy C, Zhang L, et al. Differences in activity of cytochrome C oxidase in brain between sleep and wakefulness. *Sleep* 2005;28:21–7.
26. Nikonova EV, Naidoo N, Zhang L, et al. Changes in components of energy regulation in mouse cortex with increase in wakefulness. *Sleep* 2010;33:889–900

27. Hardie DG. AMP-activated/SNF1 protein kinases: conserved guardians of cellular energy. *Nat Rev Mol Cell Biol* 2007;8:774–85.

28. Cirelli C, Gutierrez CM, Tononi G. Extensive and divergent effects of sleep and wakefulness on brain gene expression. *Neuron* 2004;41:35–43.

29. Mackiewicz M, Shockley KR, Romer MA, et al. Macromolecule biosynthesis: a key function of sleep. *Physiol Genomics* 2007;31:441–57.

30. Nakanishi H, Sun Y, Nakamura RK, et al. Positive correlations between cerebral protein synthesis rates and deep sleep in Macaca mulatta. *Eur J Neurosci* 1997;9:271–9.

31. O'Hara BF, Ding J, Bernat RL, et al. Genomic and proteomic approaches towards an understanding of sleep. *CNS Neurol Disord Drug Targets* 2007;6:71–81.

32. Haddad GG. Does the brain gain back energy during sleep? But what does it mean? *Sleep* 2011;34:835–6.

33. Heller HC. Repeatability is not the same as accuracy. *Sleep* 2011;34:839–40.

34. Wilson DF. Measuring in vivo metabolite levels in brain. *Sleep* 2011;34:837.

35. Wong-Riley M. What is the meaning of the ATP surge during sleep? *Sleep* 2011;34:833–4.

36. Kostic MM, Ziivkovic RV, Rapoport SM. Maturation-dependent changes of the rat reticulocyte energy metabolism and hormonal responsiveness. *Biomed Biochim Acta* 1990;49:S178–82.

37. Komarova SV, Ataullakhanov FI, Globus RK. Bioenergetics and mitochondrial transmembrane potential during differentiation of cultured osteoblasts. *Am J Physiol Cell Physiol* 2000;279:C1220–9.

38. Kaminsky YG, Kosenko EA, Kondrashova MN. Analysis of the circadian rhythm in energy metabolism of rat liver. *Int J Biochem* 1984;16:629–39.

39. Harris DA. Cellular ATP. In: Bittar EE, ed. *Principles of Medical Biology, Vol 4*. Connecticut: Elsevier; 1996:1–47.

40. Atkinson DE, Walton GM. Adenosine triphosphate conservation in metabolic regulation. *J Biol Chem* 1967;242:3239–41.

41. Derr RF, Zieve L. Adenylate energy charge: relation to guanylate energy charge and the adenylate kinase equilibrium constant. *Biochem Biophys Res Commun* 1972;49:1385–90.

42. Thompson FM, Atkinson DE. Response of nucleoside diphosphate kinase to the adenylate energy charge. *Biochem Biophys Res Commun* 1971;45:1581–5.

43. Dworak M, McCarley RW, Kim T, et al. Replies to commentaries on ATP changes during sleep. *Sleep* 2011;34:841–3.

44. Lin T-A, Zhang J-P, Sun GY. Metabolism of inositol-1,4,5-trisphosphate in mouse brain due to decapitation ischemic insult: effects of acute lithium administration and temporal relationship to diacylglycerols, free fatty acids and energy metabolites. *Brain Res* 1993;606:200–6.

45. Yoshida S, Harik SI, Busto R, et al. Free fatty acids and energy metabolites in ischemic cerebral cortex with noradrenaline depletion. *J Neurochem* 1984;42:711–17.

46. Lowry OH, Passonneau JV, Hasselberger FX, et al. Effect of ischemia on known substrates and cofactors of the glycolytic pathway in brain. *J Biol Chem* 1964;239:18–30.

47. Kopp SJ, Krieglstein J, Freidank A, et al. P-31 nuclear magnetic resonance analysis of brain: II. Effects of oxygen deprivation on isolated perfused and nonperfused rat brain. *J Neurochem* 1984;43:1716–31.

48. Aureli T, Miccheli A, Di Cocco ME, et al. Effect of acetyl-L-carnitine on recovery of brain phosphorus metabolites and lactic acid level during reperfusion after cerebral ischemia in the rat-study by 31P- and 1H-NMR spectroscopy. *Brain Res* 1994;643:92–9.

49. Ridge JW. Hypoxia and the energy charge of the cerebral adenylate pool. *Biochem J* 1972;127:351–5.

50. Delaney SM, Geiger JD. Brian regional levels of adenosine and adenosine nucleotides in rats killed by high-energy focused microwave irradiation. *J Neurosci Meth* 1996;64:151–6.

3

An Overview of Normal Sleep

SUDHANSU CHOKROVERTY

THE TWO major behavioral states in human wakefulness, non–rapid eye movement (non-REM) sleep and rapid eye movement (REM) sleep, are basic biologic processes that have independent functions and controls. Everyone on this planet, from invertebrates to vertebrates, mammals to nonmammals, sleeps because sleep is essential and one cannot live well without it. Sleep, however, remains the greatest mystery to neuroscientists. The two fundamental questions—What is sleep? and Why do we sleep?—have been raised repeatedly since antiquity by scientists, philosophers, writers, and religious scholars in all cultures and continents. Sleep is not simply an absence of wakefulness such as Lucretius postulated 2000 years ago.[1] Sleep is not just a suspension of sensorial processes but is the result of a combination of a passive withdrawal of afferent stimuli to the brain and functional activation of certain neurons in selective brain areas. Scientific progress in understanding sleep and its disorders has been rather slow, but great advances have been made in the last century. The driving forces in our understanding have been the discovery of electroencephalography (EEG) in 1929[2] and REM sleep in 1953,[3] as well as physiologic studies to elucidate consciousness and wakefulness in the 1930s and 1940s.[4–8] Observations of muscle atonia in cats by Jouvet and Michel[8a] in 1959 and in human laryngeal muscles by Berger[8b] in 1961 completed the discovery of all major components of REM sleep.

A general understanding of the nature of sleep and its alteration, functions, physiology, and neuroanatomic substrates is essential for a comprehensive evaluation of patients with abnormal movements during sleep. This chapter outlines a brief overview of sleep and uses the International Classification of Sleep Disorders (ICSD ed. 2) categorization to provide a basis for evaluating patients with movement disorders during sleep.

DEFINITION OF SLEEP AND SLEEP ONSET

Despite considerable progress in understanding the nature of sleep in the last century, a suitable scientific definition of sleep is still lacking. It is easy to comprehend what sleep is if one asks oneself that question as one is trying to get to sleep. Modern sleep researchers define sleep on the basis of behavior of the person while asleep and the related physiologic changes that occur to the waking brain's electrical rhythm in sleep.[9-13]

The behavioral criteria (Table 3.1) include lack of mobility or slight mobility, closed eyes, a characteristic species-specific sleeping posture, quiescence, increased reaction time, elevated arousal threshold with reduced response to external stimulation, impaired cognitive function, and a reversible state of unconsciousness.

The physiologic criteria (see the stages of sleep and architecture of sleep later in this chapter) are based on the findings from EEG, electrooculography (EOG), and electromyography (EMG), as well as other physiologic changes in ventilation, circulation, and heart rate.

While trying to define the process of falling asleep, we must differentiate sleepiness from fatigue or tiredness. Fatigue can be defined as a state of sustained lack of energy coupled with a lack of motivation and drive, but it does not require the behavioral criteria of sleepiness, such as heaviness and drooping of the eyelids, sagging or nodding of the head, and yawning. On the other hand, fatigue is often a secondary consequence of sleepiness. Another point of distinction is that given an opportunity to fall asleep a patient with excessive sleepiness (who is not simply fatigued) will fall asleep.

The Moment of Sleep Onset

There is no exact moment of sleep onset—there are gradual changes in behavior, reaction time, and cognitive function and physiologic changes.[13]

Sleepiness begins at sleep onset even before reaching stage N1 sleep (as defined later)—heaviness and drooping of the eyelids; clouding of the sensorium; and inability to see, hear, or perceive things in a rational or logical manner. At this point an individual trying to get to sleep is now entering into another world in which the person has no control and the brain cannot respond logically and adequately; this is the stage coined by Macdonald Critchley as the "pre-dormitum."[14]

Slow rolling eye movements (SEMs) begin at sleep onset and continue through stage N1 sleep. At sleep onset there is a progressive decline in thinking process and sometimes there may be hypnagogic imagery. In summary, at sleep onset there are gradual changes in many behavioral and physiologic characteristics (both somatic and autonomic), including EEG rhythms, cognition, and mental processing.

Table 3.1 Behavioral Criteria of Wakefulness and Sleep

CHARACTERISTICS	WAKEFULNESS	NON–RAPID EYE MOVEMENT SLEEP	RAPID EYE MOVEMENT SLEEP
Posture	Erect, sitting, or recumbent	Recumbent	Recumbent
Mobility	Normal	Mildly reduced to absent; postural shifts	Moderately reduced to absent; myoclonic jerks
Response to stimulation	Normal	Mildly to moderately reduced	Moderately reduced to absent
Level of alertness	Alert	Unconscious but reversible	Unconscious but reversible
Eye position	Open	Closed	Closed
Eye movements	Waking eye	Slow eye movements	Rapid eye movements

Similar to sleep onset, the moment of awakening or sleep offset is also a gradual process from the fully established sleep stages. This period is sometimes described as manifesting sleep inertia. There is a gradual return to state of alertness or wakefulness.

MACROSTRUCTURE AND MICROSTRUCTURE OF SLEEP

Based on three physiologic measurements (EEG, EOG, and EMG), sleep is divided into two states with independent controls and functions: non-REM and REM sleep. [11] Table 3.2 lists the physiologic criteria of wakefulness and sleep, and Table 3.3 summarizes non-REM and REM sleep states. In an ideal situation (which may not be seen in all normal individuals), non-REM and REM alternate in a cyclical manner, each cycle lasting on an average for about 90 to 110 minutes. During a normal sleep period in adults, four to six such cycles are noted. The first two cycles are dominated by slow-wave sleep (SWS) (stage N3 sleep); subsequent cycles contain less SWS, and sometimes SWS does not occur at all. In contrast, the REM sleep cycle increases from the first to the last cycle, and the longest REM sleep episode toward the end of the night may last for an hour. Thus, in human adult sleep the first third is dominated by the SWS and the last third is dominated by REM sleep. It is important to be aware of these facts because certain abnormal motor activities are characteristically associated with SWS and REM sleep.

Non–Rapid Eye Movement Sleep

Non–REM sleep is subdivided into three stages based mainly on EEG criteria (see Table 3.3). Non-REM sleep comprises 75% to 80% of sleep time in adult humans. Stage N1 sleep occupies 3% to 8% of sleep time, Stage N2 comprises 45% to 55%, and stage N3 (SWS) makes up 15% to 20% of total sleep time. The dominant rhythms during adult human wakefulness consist of the alpha rhythm (8 to 13 Hz) noted predominantly in the posterior region intermixed with a small amount of beta rhythm (>13 Hz) seen mainly in the anterior regions (Fig. 11.1). In stage N1 sleep, alpha rhythm diminishes to less than 50% in an epoch (i.e., a 30-second segment of a polysomnographic tracing with the monitor screen speed of 10 mm/second) intermixed with slower theta rhythms (4 to 7 Hz) and beta waves (Figs. 11.2a and 11.2b). EMG activity decreases slightly and SEMs appear. Toward the end of stage N1 sleep, vertex sharp waves are noted. Stage N2 sleep begins after approximately 10 to 12 minutes of stage N1 sleep. Sleep spindles (12 to 18 Hz, most often 14 Hz) and K-complexes intermixed with vertex sharp waves herald the onset of stage N2 sleep (Fig. 11.3). EEG at this stage also shows theta waves and delta waves (<4 Hz) that occupy less than 20% of the epoch. After about 30 to 60 minutes of stage N2 sleep,

Table 3.2 Physiologic Criteria of Wakefulness and Sleep

CHARACTERISTICS	WAKEFULNESS	NON–RAPID EYE MOVEMENT SLEEP	RAPID EYE MOVEMENT SLEEP
Electroencephalography	Parieto-occipital alpha waves (8–13 Hz) mixed with frontocentral beta rhythms (>13 Hz)	Theta (4–7 Hz) and delta (<4 Hz) waves, sleep spindles, vertex waves and K complexes	Theta or "sawtooth" waves, beta rhythms
Electromyography (muscle tone)	Normal	Mildly reduced	Markedly reduced to absent
Electrooculography	Waking eye movements	Slow eye movements	Rapid eye movements

Table 3.3 Summary of Non–Rapid Eye Movement (Non-REM) and Rapid Eye Movement (REM) Sleep States

Non-REM sleep: 75%–80% of sleep time
Stage N1: 3%–8% of sleep time
Stage N2: 45%–55% of sleep time
Stage N3: 15%–23% of sleep time

REM sleep: 20%–25% of sleep time
Tonic stage
Phasic stage

stage N3 sleep begins and delta waves now comprise 20% to 100% of the epoch (Fig. 11.4). Stage N3 sleep is also known as SWS. Body movements often are recorded as artifacts in polysomnography (PSG) recordings toward the end of SWS as sleep is lightening.

Rapid Eye Movement Sleep

Rapid eye movement (REM) sleep (or stage R) (Fig. 11.5) is subdivided into tonic and phasic stages. (This subdivision is not recognized in the latest AASM manual.[15a]) REM sleep accounts for 20% to 25% of sleep time. The first REM sleep episode occurs 60 to 90 minutes after sleep onset in a normal adult human. A desynchronized EEG, hypotonia or atonia of major muscle groups, and depression of monosynaptic and polysynaptic reflexes are characteristics of tonic REM stage. The tonic stage persists throughout the REM sleep, whereas the phasic stage is discontinuous and superimposed on the tonic stage. Phasic REM sleep is characterized by bursts of REMs in all directions, phasic swings in blood pressure and heart rate, irregular respiration, spontaneous middle ear muscle activity, myoclonic twitching of the facial and limb muscles, and

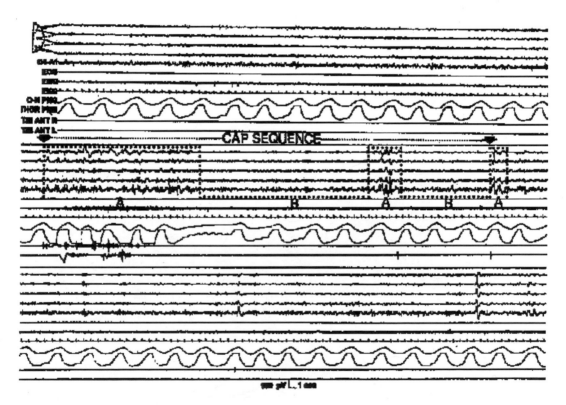

FIGURE 3.1 Polysomnographic recording showing consecutive stretches of non-cyclic alternating pattern (non-CAP) (*top*), cyclic alternating pattern (CAP) (*middle*), and non-CAP (*bottom*). The CAP sequence, confined between the two black arrows, shows three phase As and two phase Bs, which illustrate the minimal requirements for the definition of a CAP sequence (at least three phase A in succession). Electroencephalographic derivation (top five channels in top panel): FP2-F4, F4,-C4, C4-P4, P4–02, and C4-A1. Similar electroencephalographic derivation is used for the middle and lower panels. (Reproduced with permission.[20])

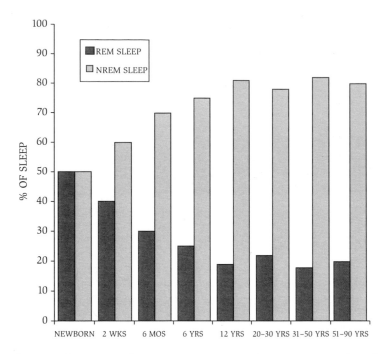

FIGURE 3.2   Schematic diagram to show percentages of rapid eye movement (REM) and non–rapid eye movement (NREM) sleep at different ages. Note the marked changes in REM sleep in the early years. (Modified and adapted from Roffwarg HP, Muzzio JN, Dement WC: Ontogenic development of the human sleep-dream cycle. Science 152:604, 1966. Reproduced with permission from Chokroverty S: Sleep Disorders Medicine: Basic Science Technical Consideration and Clinical Aspects. Philadelphia: Saunders/Elsevier, 2009.)

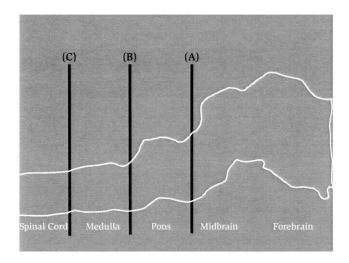

FIGURE 3.3   Schematic sagittal section of the brainstem of the cat. (A) Junction of midbrain and pons. (B) Junction of pons and medulla. (C) Junction of medulla and spinal cord. (Reproduced with permission.[95])

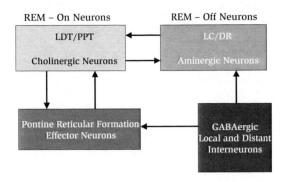

FIGURE 3.4   Schematic diagram of McCarley-Hobson model of REM sleep mechanism. DR, dorsal raphe; GABA, y-aminobutyric acid; LC, locus ceruleus; LDT, laterodorsal tegmental; PPT, pedunculopontine tegmental nuclei. (Reproduced with permission.[95])

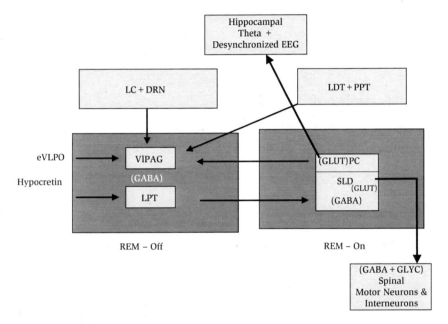

FIGURE 3.5   Lu-Saper "flip-flop" model to show schematically the REM sleep mechanism. eVLPO, extended region of ventrolateral preoptic nucleus; GABA, y-aminobutyric acid; GLUT, glutamatergic neurons; GLYC<, glycinergic neurons; LC + DRN, locus ceruleus + dorsal raphe nuclei; LDT + PPT, laterodorsal tegmental + pedunculopontine tegmental nuclei; LPT, lateral pontine tegmentum; PC, preceruleus; SLD, sublaterodorsal nucleus; VIPAG, ventrolateral periaqueductal gray. (Reproduced with permission.[95])

tongue movements. A few periods of apnea or hypopnea may occur during REM sleep. EEG tracing during REM sleep consists of low-amplitude fast pattern mixed with a small amount of theta rhythms, some of which may have a "sawtooth" appearance (see Fig. 11.5); sawtooth waves are thought to be the gateway to REM sleep. The first REM sleep lasts only a few minutes. Sleep then progresses to stage N2 followed by stage N3 before the second REM sleep begins.

In summary, during normal sleep in adults there is an orderly progression from wakefulness to sleep onset to non-REM sleep and then to REM sleep. Relaxed wakefulness is characterized by a behavioral state of quietness and physiologic state of alpha and beta frequency in the EEG, waking eye movements (WEMs), and increased muscle tone. Non-REM sleep is characterized by progressively decreased responsiveness to external stimulation accompanied by SEMs followed by EEG slow activity associated with sleep spindles and K-complexes and decreased muscle tone. REMs, further reduction of responsiveness to stimulation, absent muscle tone, and low-voltage fast EEG activity mixed with distinctive sawtooth waves (sharp-contoured waves of 2 to 7 Hz) characterize REM sleep.

The sleep stages and the method of scoring sleep stages in normal adult humans had been the gold standard in the past based on the system devised by Rechtschaffen and Kales (R-K) in 1968.[15] The R-K system addresses normal adult sleep and macrostructure of sleep. In patients with sleep disorders such as sleep apnea or parasomnias, it may be difficult to score sleep according to R-K criteria. Furthermore, the R-K staging system does not address the microstructure of sleep. The American Academy of Sleep Medicine (AASM) has now published the AASM Manual[15a] for the scoring of sleep and associated events which modified the R-K system and extended the scoring rules. The macrostructure of sleep is summarized in Table 3.4. There are several endogenous and exogenous factors, which will modify sleep macrostructure (Table 3.5).

Sleep microstructure includes momentary, dynamic phenomena such as arousals, which have been operationally defined by the Task Force of the American Sleep Disorders Association (now called American Academy of Sleep Medicine),[16] and the cyclic alternating pattern (CAP), which has been defined and described in various publications by Terzano and coinvestigators.[17–19]

Other components of microstructure include K-complexes and sleep spindles.

Arousals are transient phenomena resulting in fragmented sleep without behavioral awakening. According to the Task Force rules,[16] an arousal is an abrupt shift in EEG frequency lasting for 3 to 14 seconds (Fig. 11.6a) and including alpha, beta, or theta activities but not spindles or delta waves. Before an arousal can be scored, the subject must be asleep for 10 consecutive seconds. In REM sleep, arousals are scored only when accompanied by concurrent increase in submental EMG amplitude (Fig. 11.6b). K-complexes, delta waves, artifacts, and only increased submental EMG activities are not counted as arousals unless they are accompanied by EEG frequency shifts. Arousals can be expressed as number per hour of sleep or the arousal index. An arousal index up to 10 can be considered normal.

The CAP (Fig. 3.1) indicates sleep instability, whereas frequent arousals signify sleep fragmentation.[19] Sleep microstructure is best understood by the CAP, which is a repetitive EEG pattern in a cyclical manner noted mainly during non-REM sleep. This has not been widely known, but this is a promising technique in evaluating both normal and abnormal sleep, as well as in understanding the neurophysiologic and neurochemical basis of sleep. A CAP cycle consists of an unstable phase (phase A) and relatively stable phase (phase B), each lasting between 2 and 60 seconds.[20] Phase A of CAP is marked by an increase of EEG potentials with contributions from both synchronous high-amplitude (slow) and desynchronous (fast) waveforms in the EEG standing out from a relatively low-amplitude slow background. The A phase is associated with an increase in heart rate, respiration, blood pressure, and muscle tone. CAP rate (total CAP time during non-REM sleep) and arousals both increase in older individuals and in a variety of sleep disorders, including both diurnal and nocturnal movement disorders. A non-CAP (a sleep period without CAP) is thought to indicate a state of sustained stability.

In summary, sleep macrostructure is based on cyclic patterns of non-REM and REM states, whereas sleep microstructure mainly consists of arousals, periods of CAP, and periods without CAP. An understanding of sleep macrostructure and microstructures is important because

Table 3.4 Sleep Macrostructure

- Sleep states and stages
- Sleep cycles
- Sleep latency
- Sleep efficiency (the ratio of total sleep time to total time in bed expressed in percent)
- Wake after sleep onset

Table 3.5 Factors Modifying Sleep Macrostructure

- Exogenous
  - Noise
  - Exercise
  - Ambient temperature
  - Drugs and alcohol
- Endogenous
  - Age
  - Prior sleep-wakefulness
  - Circadian phase
  - Sleep pathologies

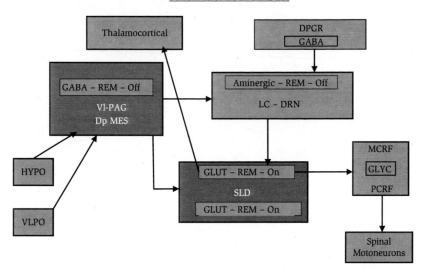

FIGURE 3.6 Schematic diagram of Boissard-Luppi model to explain the REM sleep mechanism. DPGR, dorsal paragigantocellular reticular nucleus; Dp-MES, deep mesencephalic; GABA, y-aminobutyric acid; GLUT, glutamatergic; GLYC, glycinergic neurons; HYPO, hypothalamus (hypocretinergic neurons in lateral hypothalamus); LC-DRN, locus ceruleus-dorsal raphe nuclei; MCRF, magnocellular reticular formation; PCRF, parvocellular reticular formation; SLD, sublaterodorsal nucleus; VI-PAG, ventrolateral periaqueductal gray; VLPO, ventrolateral preoptic region. (Reproduced with permission.[95])

emergence of abnormal motor activity during sleep may be related to disturbed macrostructure and microstructure of sleep.

EVOLUTION OF SLEEP PATTERNS FROM NEWBORN TO OLD AGE

Newborns have a polyphasic sleep pattern, sleeping approximately 16 hours per day.[11,21,22] The sleep requirement decreases to approximately 11 hours between the ages of 3 and 5 years, and the sleep requirement for adolescents (9–10 years) is about 10 hours per day. The biphasic sleep pattern of preschool children, which includes a midday nap, changes to a monophasic nap-free sleep pattern in adults with an average of 7.5 to 8 hours of consolidated sleep at night. Sleep pattern again reverts to biphasic pattern in old age.

In newborn infants about 50% of the time of sleep is spent in REM sleep, but this decreases to a normal adult pattern of 20% to 25% by the age of 6 years. At sleep onset, a newborn baby goes immediately into REM sleep or active sleep accompanied by restless movements of the arms, legs, and facial muscles. In premature babies it is often difficult to differentiate active sleep from wakefulness.

The non-REM–REM cyclic pattern of adult sleep is established by 3 months of age. The non-REM–REM cycle duration, however, is shorter in infants and lasts for about 45 to 50 minutes; by 5 to 10 years the cycle duration increases to 60 to 70 minutes, and by the age of 10 the normal adult cyclic pattern of 90 to 110 minutes is established. Between 8 and 12 weeks of age, sleep spindles[23] begin to appear and by about 6 months of age K-complexes[24] are seen in the EEG. Hypnagogic hypersynchrony characterized by transient bursts of high-amplitude waves in the slower frequencies appears at 5–6 months and is prominent at 1 year. A weak circadian rhythm is probably present at birth, but by 6–8 weeks it is established. The nighttime sleep gradually increases and daytime sleep decreases, and the number of naps decreases. There are two important changes that occur in the sleep pattern in old age: repeated awakenings throughout the night, including early morning awakenings that prematurely terminate the night's sleep, and a marked reduction of the amplitude of delta waves resulting in a decreased percentage of delta sleep in this age group. The percentage of REM sleep in normal adults remains relatively constant. Figure 3.2 schematically shows sleep stage distribution in different ages.

SLEEP NEED

Sleep need is defined as the optimal amount of sleep required to remain alert and fully awake and to function adequately throughout the day. Sleep debt is defined as the difference between the ideal sleep requirement and the actual duration of sleep obtained. There are two divergent views: Harrison and Horne[25] concluded that society is not sleep deprived, whereas Bonnet and Arand[26] stated that modern society is chronically sleep deprived. Between 1910 and 1963 there was a mean reduction of 1.5 hours of sleep in adolescents aged 8 to 17 years.[27] However, there may be a significant sampling error in this survey. A study by Bliwise, King, Harris, and Haskell[28] in healthy adults aged 50 to 65 years showed a reduction of about 1 hour of sleep between the 1959 and 1980 surveys.

It has been traditionally stated that women need more sleep than men, but this has been questioned in a recent field study.[29] There is also a general perception based on questionnaire, actigraphic, and PSG studies that sleep duration decreases with increasing age.[30,31] This relationship, however, remains controversial. Older adults take naps, and these naps may compensate for nighttime sleep duration curtailment. As I discuss later, sleep is regulated by homeostasis (increasing sleep drive during continued wakefulness) and circadian factors (the sleep drive varying with time of day). The influence of these factors is reduced in older adults but is still present. Older adults are also phase advanced (e.g., internal clock set earlier yielding early bedtime and early morning awakenings).

MORNING VERSUS EVENING TYPE

Two groups of individuals are recognized based on sleep habits: evening types and morning types. [11] There is a third group called the intermediate type not strictly conforming to evening and morning types. Evening types ("owls") have difficulty getting up early in the morning and they then feel tired; in contrast, they feel fresh and energetic toward the end of the day. These people perform best in the evening. If allowed their choice, they go to sleep late and wake up late. On the other hand, the morning types ("larks") wake up early, rested and refreshed, and work efficiently in the morning. Evening types are characterized by a delay

in markers of the internal clock: They have a later rise in melatonin and delayed core body temperature rhythms compared with morning types. Morningness and eveningness are most likely determined by a genetic component.

Long versus Short Sleepers

Sleep requirement for an average adult is approximately 7½–8 hours regardless of environmental or cultural differences.[11,32] It is likely that whether a person is a long or a short sleeper is determined by heredity rather than by different personality traits or other psychological factors.[11] Social (e.g., occupational factors) or biologic factors (e.g., illness) may also play a role. Long sleepers spend more time asleep but have less SWS and more stage N2 sleep than do short sleepers.[33] An early important epidemiologic study found that the chances of death from coronary arterial disease, cancer, or stroke are greater for adults who sleep less than 4 hours or more than 9 hours when compared with those who sleep an average number of 8 hours.[34] Later reports[34a] confirm this observation but remain controversial regarding cause and effect. There is some controversy whether a person can extend sleep beyond the average requirement. One study showed that sleep extension beyond the average hours may cause exhaustion and irritability with detriment of sleep efficiency,[35] and these symptoms have been dubbed as the "Rip Van Winkle"[36] effect. The overall conclusions, however, of all the studies involving sleep extension is that sleep extension has minimal effect on sleepiness and performance in absence of sleep debt.

CIRCADIAN RHYTHM AND CHRONOBIOLOGY OF SLEEP

The existence of a circadian rhythm was first suggested when the 18th-century French astronomer De Mairan noted that a heliotrope plant's leaves closed at sunset and opened at sunrise even when the plant was kept in darkness.[37] This observation suggests that an internal clock controls the 24-hour rhythm. The modern sleep scientists have confirmed the existence of a circadian rhythm in human beings and other animals.[38–41] The term *circadian rhythm* is derived from the Latin *circa*, which means "about," and *dien*, which means "day." It is generally accepted that the human circadian rhythm has a cycle length of just over 24 hours (24.3 hours).[42]

The experimental isolation of humans from all environmental time cues (the German term *zeitgeber* or "time giver"), as in a cave or underground bunker to study free-running rhythms, has demonstrated that circadian rhythms exist independently of environmental stimuli.[40,41] Environmental cues of light and darkness normally synchronize and entrain rhythms to the day-night cycle; however, the existence of environment-independent autonomous rhythms suggests that the human body also has an internal biologic clock.[40-44] The site of the clock has been located in the suprachiasmatic nuclei of the hypothalamus above the optic chiasm.[45-47] The master circadian clock in the suprachiasmatic nucleus (SCN) receives photic information from the retinohypothalamic tract and sends signals through multiple synaptic pathways to other parts of hypothalamus, the superior cervical ganglion, and the pineal gland where melatonin is released.[48-51] There is a feedback loop from the pineal gland to the SCN, which contains melatonin receptors. The neurons in the SCN are responsible for generating circadian rhythms, and time isolation experiments have clearly shown the presence of daily rhythms in many physiologic processes such as the sleep-wake cycle, body temperature, and neuroendocrine secretion.[41,52-54] The body temperature rhythm is closely synchronized with the circadian rhythm of sleep-wakefulness. During free-running experiments there is internal desynchronization and the body temperature rhythm dissociates from the sleep rhythm.[41-44] Several neurotransmitters have been located within terminals of the SCN afferents and inteneurons, including serotonin, neuropeptides Y, vasopressin, vasoactive intestinal peptides, and gamma-aminobutyric acid. The molecular basis of the mammalian circadian clock has been the focus of much recent circadian rhythm research.[54a] The paired SSCN are controlled by a total of at least seven genes (e.g., *clock, bmal1, per, cry, tim, cyc, frq*) and their protein products and regulatory enzymes (e.g., casein kinase 1 epsilon, and casein kinase 1 delta). There has been remarkable progress in a few years in identifying key components of the circadian clock in the fruit flies (Drosophila), bread molds (Neurospora), and mammals. There is clear anatomical and physiologic evidence to suggest a close interaction between the SCN and the regions regulating sleep-wake states. There are projections from SCN to wake-promoting hypocretin (orexin) neurons (indirectly via dorsomedial hypothalamus) and locus coeruleus as well as to sleep-promoting neurons in ventrolateral preoptic (VLPO) neurons. Based on the studies in mice (e.g., knockout mice lacking core clock genes and mice with mutant clock genes), it has been suggested also that circadian clock genes may affect sleep regulation and sleep homeostasis independent of circadian rhythm generation. Melatonin is secreted maximally during the night and is an important modulator of human circadian rhythm entrainment by the light-dark cycle. A circadian rhythm generated by the rhythmic SCN output is responsible for the melatonin circadian rhythm.[51,55-57] Melatonin has a fairly abrupt rise in the evening, then reaches a maximum value between 3 am and 5 am, after which it decreases to low levels during the daytime.[49,50,51,55]

Dysfunction of circadian rhythm results in some important human sleep disorders. Melatonin administration has been shown to have some beneficial effects on the symptoms of jet lag,[51,58] an improvement of the nighttime alertness and the daytime sleepiness of shift workers,[51,59] and the sleep disturbances in non–24-hour sleep-wake syndrome, which occurs in many individuals with total blindness.[60,61]

CIRCADIAN, HOMEOSTATIC, AND OTHER SLEEP FACTORS

Regulation of sleep and wakefulness is modulated by homeostatic and circadian factors. The homeostatic factor refers to the increased propensity for sleepiness with longer periods of prior wakefulness, whereas the circadian factor refers to variations in physiologic alertness and sleepiness (timing, duration, and characteristics) that vary cyclically with time of day. There are two highly vulnerable periods of sleepiness: 2 to 6 am, especially 3:00 to 5:00 am, and 2:00 to 6:00 pm; the former is stronger than the latter. The timing of this physiologic sleepiness (e.g., midafternoon and early morning hours) depends on circadian factors. The highest number of sleep-related accidents has been observed during these periods. The circadian pacemaker and homeostatic mechanism have a reciprocal relationship with bidirectional anatomical connections, but the neurologic basis for this interaction is unknown.

The role of various sleep factors in maintaining homeostasis has not been clearly established.[62] Several cytokines, including interleukin-1, interferon-alpha, and tumor necrosis factor, promote sleep. Other sleep-promoting substances called sleep factors increase in concentration during prolonged wakefulness or infection. It has been shown that adenosine can fulfill the major criteria for a neural sleep factor that mediates the somnogenic effects of prolonged wakefulness. Several additional endogenous compounds that are thought to enhance sleep include the following: delta sleep–inducing peptides, muramyl peptides, cholecystokinins, arginine vasotocin, vasoactive intestinal peptide, growth hormone–releasing factors, and somatostatin.

NEUROANATOMIC SUBSTRATES OF SLEEP AND WAKEFULNESS

Neuroanatomic and neurochemical substrates and physiologic mechanisms controlling wakefulness, non-REM, and REM sleep are located in separate parts of the central nervous system (CNS). There are no discrete sleep-wake promoting centers, but these states are produced by changes in the interconnecting neuronal systems modulated by neurotransmitters and neuromodulators. The methods employed to characterize sleep-wake generator sites included lesion, stimulation, ablation, intracellular recording, C-fos immunoreactivity (C-FOS or immediate early gene is a nuclear protein released during activation of neurons), and neuroimaging mapping of neuronal networks.

Neuroanatomical Substrates of Non-REM Sleep

In 1920 Von Economo[63] noted that patients with encephalitis lethargica with excessive sleepiness had pathologic alterations in the posterior hypothalamus, whereas those with severe insomnia had predominant lesions in the anterior hypothalamus. These findings immediately suggested the existence of sleep-wake centers in the hypothalamus. Sleep-promoting neurons are thought to reside in the preoptic area of the anterior hypothalamus (PAOH) and wake-promoting neurons in the posterior area.

Beginning in the late 1950s, emphasis was shifted toward active sleep mechanisms,[64–75] and the debate about active versus passive mechanisms of sleep continued throughout most of the 20th century. The passive theory originated with two classic preparations in cats by Bremer[76,77]: cerveau isole and encephale isole. Bremer found that in cerveau isole preparation

(e.g., midcollicular transection), all specific sensory stimuli were withdrawn and the animals were somnolent, whereas in encephale isole preparation (transection at C1 vertebral level to disconnect the entire brain from the spinal cord), these specific stimuli maintained activation of the brain and the animals were awake. Moruzzi and Magoun[78] postulated that withdrawal of generalized activation from the ascending reticular activating system (ARAS) is responsible for somnolence in cerveau isole preparation, whereas activation of the midbrain reticular neurons causing direct excitation of the thalamocortical projections results in EEG desynchronization and behavioral arousal. These observations have later been confirmed by experimental studies.[79] These observations support the later suggestion of Steriade, McCormick, and Sejnowski[80] that at the onset of non-REM sleep there is deafferentation of the brain because of blockage of afferent information, first at the thalamic level, causing the waking "open" brain to be converted into a "closed" brain resulting from thalamocortical inhibition. The reticular nucleus of the thalamus is responsible for the generation of sleep spindles.[79] Simulation of this nucleus produces spindle-like activity, whereas unilateral destruction of this nucleus abolishes the spindles ipsilaterally and bilateral destruction abolishes the spindles on both sides.

The experiments in cats by Batini, Moruzzi, and Palestini et al.[66,67] in 1959 challenged the passive theory. This preparation is only a few millimeters below the section that produces cerveau isole preparation. The midpontine pretrigeminal section produced persistent EEG and behavioral signs of alertness. These observations suggest that structures located in the brainstem between cerveau isole and midpontine pretrigeminal preparations are responsible for wakefulness. Experimental data have shown that cholinergic neurons in the pedunculopontine tegmental (PPT) and laterodorsal tegmental (LDT) nuclei in the pontomesencephalic region maintain activation and wakefulness through thalamocortical and basal forebrain projections to the cerebral cortex. The active hypnogenic neurons for non-REM sleep are located primarily in the PAOH and the basal forebrain area, as well as in the neurons in the region of the nucleus tractus solitarius in the medulla.[79] The evidence for this conclusion is based on stimulation, lesion, and ablation studies, as well as extracellular and intracellular recordings. The active inhibitory role of lower brainstem hypnogenic neurons on the upper brainstem ARAS was clearly demonstrated by Batini's, Moruzzi's, and Palestini's[66] and Batini's, Moruzzi's, and Palestini's[67] experiments of mid-pontine pretrigeminal section. Electrical stimulation of the preoptic area, which produces EEG synchronization and behavioral state of sleep, also supports the idea of the existence of active hypnogenic neurons in the preoptic area.[71,79] In addition, experiments showing insomnia after lesion of the preoptic region supported the hypothesis of active hypnogenic neurons in the forebrain preoptic area.[81] Insomnia induced by preoptic lesions is transiently reversed by injections of gamma-aminobutyric acid agonist, muscimol, in the posterior hypothalamus, suggesting that the sleep-promoting role of the anterior hypothalamus depends on inhibition of posterior hypothalamic histaminergic awaking neurons.[82] It is notable that in 1934 Dikshit[83] induced sleep by intrahypothalamic injection of acetylcholine, suggesting the presence of sleep center in the hypothalamus. The contemporary theory suggests that non-REM sleep-promoting neurons are found in the VLPO area of the anterior hypothalamus as well as in the region of the NTS in the medulla. VLPO neurons consist of two supgroups: "clustered" and "diffuse" or extended (eVLPO) depending on the distribution pattern.[84,85] The tightly clustered neurons project to the tuberomammilary nuclei, inhibiting them and promoting non-REM sleep, whereas diffusely distributed neurons project to and inhibit the aminergic nuclei in the locus coeruleus and the dorsal raphe region of the brainstem participating in REM sleep. The VLPO neurons fire actively during non-REM sleep, and their lesion induces insomnia. The GABA- and Galanin-containing VLPO neurons project to and inhibit locus coeruleus, dorsal raphe, and tuberomammillary aminergic nuclei, which in turn inhibit VLPO neurons. The contemporary theory for the mechanism of non-REM sleep thus suggests a reciprocal interaction between two antagonistic neurons in the VLPO of the anterior hypothalamus and wake-promoting neurons in the tuberomammillary nuclei of the posterior hypothalamus, as well as locus coeruleus, dorsal raphe, basal forebrain, and mesopontine tagementum.[79,85a] Reciprocal interaction between sleep-promoting neurons in the regions of the NTS and wake-promoting neurons within the ARAS of the brainstem independently of the reciprocal interaction of the neurons of the forebrain also plays a role in the generation of non-REM sleep as stated earlier. In summary, the active and passive theories of sleep may be viewed as complementary rather than mutually exclusive mechanisms.

Recent discovery of intrahypothalamic hypocretin neurons and their widespread CNS projections has directed attention to the role of the hypocretin system in mediating sleep-wake regulation.[86-90] Reduced activity of the hypocretin projections to the locus coeruleus noradrenergic, midline raphe serotonergic, hypothalamic and mesopontine dopaminergic, and tuberomammillary histaminergic cells may theoretically reduce the level of arousal causing sleepiness.

Neuroanatomic Substrates of REM Sleep

Transection experiments through different regions of the midbrain, pons, and medulla clearly show the existence of REM sleep–generating neurons in the pontine cat brain (Fig. 3.3).[79,91-94] A transection at the junction of pons and midbrain produced all the physiologic findings compatible with REM sleep in the section caudal to the transection, whereas in the forebrain region rostral to the section, the recording showed no signs of REM sleep. After a transection between the pons and medulla, structures rostral to the section showed signs of REM sleep, but, in structures caudal to the section, there were no signs of REM sleep. After a section at the junction of the spinal cord and medulla, REM sleep signs were noted in the rostral brain areas. Finally, transection at the pontomesencephalic and the pontomedullary junctions produced an isolated pons that showed all the signs of REM sleep. The pons is, therefore, sufficient and necessary to generate all the signs of REM sleep.

To explain the mechanism of REM sleep there are three animal models available.[95] The earliest and most generally well known is the McCarley-Hobson reciprocal interaction model (Fig. 3.4) based on reciprocal interaction of REM-on and REM-off neurons.[79,94] The cholinergic neurons in the PPT and LDT nuclei in the ponto-mesencephalic region are REM-on cells responsible for REM sleep and show the highest firing rates at this stage. The aminergic neurons located in the locus coeruleus (LC) and dorsal raphe nuclei (DRN) are REM-off cells and are inactive during REM sleep. Histaminergic neurons in the tuberomammillary region of the posterior hypothalamus can also be considered as REM-off cells. Thus, the cholinergic REM-on and aminergic REM-off cells are all located within the transections of the pons as described earlier. LDT-PPT cholinergic neurons promote REM sleep through pontine reticular formation (PRF) effector neurons, which in turn send feedback loops to LDT-PPT. Cholinergic neurons of the PPT and LDT project into the thalamus and basal forebrain regions as well as to the PRF and are responsible for activation and generation of REM sleep. Aminergic cells play a permissive role in maintenance of REM sleep state. In the latest modification of the reciprocal interaction model, MCCarley[85a] suggested that the gamma-aminobutyric acid (GABA) also plays a role in the REM sleep generation. At the onset of REM sleep, there is activation of GABA neurons in the pons, which causes inhibition of LC/DRN (REM-off neurons) as well as activation of (or disinhibition) of cholinergic neurons in the pons. The reason for GABA activation is not known and the source of GABA-ergic neurons is probably both local (e.g., a subgroup of PRF GABA-neurons) and distant (e.g., GABA-ergic neurons in the ventrolateral periaqueductal brain).

In the second model proposed by Lu and coworkers[96] (Fig. 3.5), there is a flip-flop switch interaction between GABA-ergic REM-off neurons in deep mesencephalatic (DM), ventrolateral peri-aqueductal gray (VLPAG) and lateral pontine tagmentum (LPT) and GABA-ergic REM-on neurons in sublaterodorsal nucleus (SLD), and a dorsal extension of SLD named the precoeruleus (PC). These mutually inhibitory neuronal populations (SLD GABA-ergic REM-on and GABA-ergic REM-off neurons in the DM-LPT) serve as a flip-flop switch. Ascending glutamatergic projections from PC neurons to medial septum are responsible for hippocampal EEG theta rhythm during REM sleep. Descending glutamatergic projections from ventral SLD directly to the spinal interneurons apparently without a relay in the medial medulla inhibit spinal ventral horn cells by both glycerinergic and GABA-ergic mechanisms. Cholinergic and aminergic neurons play a modulatory role and are not part of the flip-flop switch. McCarley[85a] suggested that this model is based on c-fos labeling only without electrophysiologic recordings. Furthermore, this model does not address how REM periodicity occurs in this flip-flop switch utilizing two mutually inhibitory neuronal populations. Finally, this model also does not explain the gradually increasing duration of REM sleep throughout the night and generally absent REM sleep during daytime naps. It should

be noted that in a recent paper, Brooks and Peever[97] challenged the glycinergic and GABA-ergic neurochemical mechanism of REM motor atonia based on experimental evidence in rats that REM atonia persists even when glycine and GABA receptors are blocked and after simultaneous application of glutamatergic agonists to trigeminal motor pool. Brooks and Peever concluded that multiple biochemical pathways are responsible for controlling muscle tone in REM sleep. In a later paper,[98] however, these authors agreed that both glycinergic and GABA-ergic mechanisms play a role.

In the third model proposed by Luppi's group[99] (Fig. 3.6), active neurons during REM sleep are identified in a small area in the dorsolateral pontine tagmentum called sublaterodorsal (SLD) nucleus in the rats (corresponding to dorsal sub-coeruleus in humans or perilocus coeruleus alpha region in the cats). The onset of REM sleep is thought to be due to activation of REM-on glutamatergic neurons from the SLD. During non-REM sleep and wakefulness these neurons in the SLD would be inhibited (hyperpolarized) by tonic GABA-ergic input from GABA-ergic REM-off neurons located in the deep mesencephalic and pontine reticular nuclei, and ventrolateral peri-aqueductal gray (V1PAG) as well as by monoaminergic neurons. Ascending REM-on glutametergic dorsal SLD neurons can cause cortical activation through projections to thalamocortical neurons along with REM-on cholinergic and glutamatergic neurons from the LDT/PPT mesencephalic and pontine reticular nuclei and basal forebrain regions. Descending REM-on glutamatergic ventral SLD neurons would cause muscle atonia through both direct projections to spinal motor neurons and indirect projections through the magnocellularis and parvocellularis reticular nuclei in the medulla, causing hyperporalization of the motor neurons utilizing glycinergic and GABAergic inhibitory premotor neurons. In the Luppi model,[99] therefore, glutamatergic neurons play a crucial role in REM generation. GABA-ergic neurons in addition to their role in motoneurons hyperpolarization are also responsible for inactivation of monoaminergic neurons during REM sleep, and cholinergic neurons do not play a crucial role in activating REM executive neurons in this model.

Muscle hypotonia or atonia during sleep is thought to depend on inhibitory postsynaptic potentials generated by dorsal pontine interneurons sending descending axons.[91,100,101] The pathway from the peri-locus coeruleus alpha region ventral to the locus coeruleus via the lateral

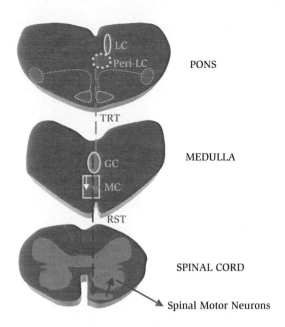

FIGURE 3.7   Schematic diagram to explain the mechanism of muscle atonia in REM sleep. GC, gigantocellularis; LC, locus ceruleus; MC, magnocellularis; Peri-LC: peri-locus ceruleus alpha; RST, reticulospinal tract; TRT, tegmentoreticular tract. (Reproduced with permission.[95])

tegmental reticular tract to the medial medullary region (e.g., nucleus magnocellularis and gigantocellularis) and then to the reticulospinal tract, projecting to the anterior horn cells of the spinal cord (Fig. 3.7) controls REM sleep-induced muscle atonia.[100] An experimental lesion in the perilocus coerulus alpha region, as well as in the medial medullary region, produced REM sleep without muscle atonia.[102] REM behavior disorder in humans includes dream-enacting behavior associated with REM sleep without muscle atonia.[103] A structural or functional alteration of the pathway maintaining muscle hypotonia or atonia during REM sleep is most likely responsible for REM behavior disorder. The most likely sites are ventral SLD and ventromedial medulla (see also Chapter 4).

Neurotransmitters and Neuromodulators Responsible for Maintaining Wakefulness

The major neurotransmitter pathways that regulate the wakefulness systems use the cholinergic, noradrenergic, dopaminergic, and histaminergic neurons.[104] The recently described hypocretin system in the lateral hypothalamus with its widespread projections also plays a role in maintaining wakefulness.[86–89] Cholinergic neurons in the LDT and PPT projecting to the thalamus,

posterior hypothalamus, and basal forebrain region fire at their highest rate during wakefulness and during REM sleep but decrease their rates of firing at the onset of non-REM sleep.[94] The role of dopamine is uncertain; however, pharmacologic, biochemical, and physiologic studies and recent immunocytochemical staining in the ventrolateral periaqueductal gray region suggest that dopamine may help maintain wakefulness, probably through D1 and possibly through D2 receptors.[105] The noradrenergic system promotes wakefulness. Norepinephrine-containing locus coerulus neurons show their highest firing rates during wakefulness, their lowest during REM sleep, and intermediate rate during non-REM sleep. Pharmacologic studies also suggest that posterior hypothalamic histaminergic neurons help maintain wakefulness. The excitatory amino acids, glutamate and aspartate, are intermingled within the ARAS and are present in many neurons projecting to the cerebral cortex, forebrain, and brainstem. These excitatory amino acids are released maximally during wakefulness.

SLEEP AND DREAMS

Sigmund Freud called dreams the "royal road to the unconscious," representing repressed feelings, which are psychologically suppressed in the unconscious mind.[106] Freudian theory has fallen in disrepute, and the modern sleep scientists interpret dreams in anatomic and physiologic terms. Dream research has taken a new direction since the existence of REM sleep was first observed by Aserinssy and Kleitman in 1953.[3] It is believed that approximately 80% of dreams occur during REM sleep, and 20% occur during non-REM sleep.[107] Highly emotionally charged, complex, and bizarre dreams occur during REM sleep; in contrast, non-REM dreams are more realistic and rational. People are generally oriented when awakened from REM sleep but are somewhat disoriented and confused on awakening from non-REM sleep. It is easier to recall REM dreams than non-REM dreams and also easier to recall dreams if the subject is awakened immediately after the onset of an REM dream.

During REM sleep, nerve cells, synapses, and nerve fibers connecting these nerve cells become activated first in the brainstem and then the signals are transmitted to the hemisphere, which synthesizes the signals, creating colorful (most of our dreams take place in natural color) or black-and-white images during dreams. In our dreams, we employ all five senses. In general, we use mostly our visual sensations, followed by auditory sensations, tactile, smell, and taste sensations, which are represented least. Dreams can be pleasant, unpleasant, frightening, or sad. They generally reflect one's day-to-day activities. Fear, anxiety, and apprehension are incorporated into our dreams. Additionally, stressful events of past or present may occupy our dreams. The dream scenes or events are rarely rational but often occur in an irrational manner with rapid change of scene, place, or people (or a bizarre mixture of these elements). Sometimes lucid dreams may arise in which the dreamer seems to realize vividly that he or she is actually dreaming and may actually control the content of dreams. Some people have frequent, frightening dreams called nightmares or dream anxiety attacks, which appear to arise from intense, anxiety-provoking incidents in the dreamer's life. Nightmares are very common in children, beginning around the age of 3 to 5 years. Nightmares decrease in old age. Sometimes in fearful dreams, the individual may enact past stressful events (for example, a scene in a battlefield or a car accident). The neurobiological significance of dreams remains unknown. Some suggestions include activation of the neural networks in the brain, restructuring and reinterpretation of data stored in memories and removal of unnecessary and useless information from the brain of a dreamer.[108] Some have also suggested that memory consolidation takes place during the dream stage of sleep. In addition, stories abound regarding artists, writers, and scientists who have developed innovative ideas about their art, literature, and scientific projects during dreams. Dream-enacting behavior associated with abnormal movements during sleep constitutes an important REM parasomnia called REM sleep behavior disorder (see also Chapter 29).[103]

SLEEP DEPRIVATION AND SLEEPINESS

Sleep deprivation causes excessive sleepiness, which results from circadian dysrhythmia and disruption of homeostasis of the body.[109] Experiments have been conducted to study the effects of total, partial, and selective sleep deprivation. These experiments in animals have clearly shown that sleep is necessary for survival,[110] but, from a practical point of view, complete sleep deprivation for prolonged periods cannot be conducted in humans. Experiments in rats by Rechtschaffen and coinvestigators using a carousel device provided clear evidence that sleep is essential for survival. All rats deprived of sleep for 10 to 30 days died after having lost weight despite increasing food intake. It took longer for rats deprived of REM sleep to die than those deprived of SWS.

Sleep deprivation studies in humans have shown an impairment of performance, which demonstrates the need for sleep. There is no permanent impairment of the nervous system following partial or total sleep deprivation; however, there is loss of performance after prolonged sleep deprivation as a result of decreased motivation and frequent "microsleeps."[11] Sleep deprivation increases daytime sleepiness as shown by decreased mean sleep latency in the multiple sleep latency tests. The percentage of SWS increases considerably during the recovery sleep following sleep deprivation. REM sleep percentage also increases during the recovery sleep following a prolonged period of sleep deprivation, but REM sleep percentage may not increase after a short period of sleep deprivation. Overall, human sleep deprivation experiments have proven that sleep deprivation causes sleepiness and impairment of performance, vigilance, attention, and concentration. In addition, sleep deprivation may also cause some metabolic, hormonal, and immunologic effects. However, sleep deprivation does not cause permanent memory or other CNS changes.[11] Sleep deprivation causes immune suppression.[111] Even partial sleep deprivation reduces cellular immune responses. Some important studies from Van Cauter's group have clearly documented an elevation of cortisol level following even partial sleep loss.[112] These findings suggest an alteration in the hypothalamo-pituitary-adrenal (HPA) axis function. This has been confirmed even in chronic sleep deprivation, which causes impairment of glucose tolerance. Glucose intolerance may contribute to memory impairment as a result of decreased hippocampal function. Chronic sleep deprivation may also cause a decrement of thyrotropin concentration, increased evening cortisol level, and sympathetic hyperactivity, which may serve as risk factors for obesity, hypertension, and diabetes mellitus.[112] Thus, sleep deprivation causes both short-term (e.g., sleepiness, impaired mood and performance) and long-term adverse health outcomes (e.g., obesity, type 2 diabetes mellitus, cardiovascular morbidity and mortality, memory impairment). It should be noted that it is very difficult to design human sleep deprivation experiments without eliminating the stress factor associated with acute or chronic sleep restriction experiments. It is possible that many of the long-term and short-term adverse consequences may have resulted from stress.

FUNCTIONS OF SLEEP

The exact biologic function of sleep is unknown, but several theories[11,113,114] of the function of sleep have been proposed (Table 3.6). In support of the theory of body and brain tissue restoration by sleep, the findings of increased secretion of anabolic hormone (e.g., growth hormone, prolactin, testosterone, and luteinizing hormone) and decreased levels of catabolic hormone (e.g., cortisol), as well as a subjective

Table 3.6 Theories of Sleep Functions

Body and brain tissue restoration
Energy conservation
Adaptation
Memory reinforcement and consolidation
Synaptic and neural network integrity
Thermoregulation

feeling of refreshment after sleep, may be cited. Increased SWS after sleep deprivation further suggests a role for non-REM sleep in restoring the body. The critical role of REM sleep for CNS development in young organisms and increased protein synthesis in the brain during REM sleep may be cited in support of the theory of restoration of brain function by REM sleep. An enhanced synthesis of brain macromolecules such as nucleic acids and proteins during sleep may also provide an argument in favor of the restorative theory of sleep.[115]

The fact that animals with high metabolic rates sleep longer than those with slower metabolism has been cited in support of energy conservation theory. The conservation of a mere 120 calories during 8 hours of sleep in humans, however, considerably weakens this theory.

Proponents of the adaptive theory suggest that sleep is an adaptive behavior that allows the creature to survive under a variety of environmental conditions.[116]

REM sleep and SWS deprivation experiments suggest that memory reinforcement and consolidation take place during REM sleep.[117] Furthermore, because REM sleep occurs in all mammals and because there is a large REM rebound following sleep deprivation, there is an indication that there are some important biologic functions of REM sleep.

The theory that memory reinforcement with consolidation during both REM and non-REM sleep has been strengthened by scientific data but remains a hotly debated issue with both proponents and opponents, with proponents outnumbering the opponents. The theory of memory consolidation during REM sleep has been strengthened by scientific data provided by Kearny and colleagues.[53] Recent studies by Stickgold and Walker,[54] and Walker and Stickgold[55] strongly supported the theory of sleep-memory consolidation. Several studies in the past decade have provided evidence to support the role of sleep in sleep-dependent memory processing, which includes memory encoding, memory consolidation and reconsolidation, and brain plasticity. Walker's group[55] concluded after sleep deprivation experiments that sleep before learning is critical for human memory consolidation. In contrast to all these studies, Vertes and Siegel[56] took the opposite position, contending that REM sleep is not involved in memory consolidation, at least not in humans, citing several lines of evidence. The strongest evidence cited by Vertes and Siegel[56] includes examples of individuals with brainstem lesions with elimination of REM sleep or those on antidepressant medications suppressing REM sleep and exhibiting no apparent cognitive deficits. Vertes and Siegel[56] concluded that REM sleep is not involved in declarative memory and REM sleep is not critical for cognitive processing and sleep. Whether non-REM sleep is important for declarative memory also remains somewhat contentious.

An emerging recent concept concerning the primary function of sleep is the theory of maintenance of synaptic and neuronal network integrity.[118-120] According to this theory, intermittent stimulation of neural networks and synapses is necessary to preserve CNS function.

The theory of thermoregulatory function of sleep[121] is based on the observation that thermoregulatory homeostasis is maintained during non-REM sleep, whereas severe thermoregulatory abnormality is observed during total sleep deprivation. The preoptic-anterior hypothalamic neurons participate in thermoregulation and non-REM sleep. These two processes are closely linked by preoptic-anterior hypothalamic neurons but are clearly separate. Thermoregulation is maintained during non-REM but suspended during REM sleep. During REM sleep there is impairment of thermoregulatory responses such as shivering, piloerection, panting, and sweating. There is loss of thermosensitivity in the preoptic-anterior hypothalamic neurons during REM sleep.

CLASSIFICATION OF SLEEP DISORDERS

The International Classification of Sleep Disorders (ICSD), described in 1990, slightly revised in 1997, and completely modified in the latest edition (ICSD-2),[122] is the system used by sleep specialists. The ICSD-2 lists eight broad categories of disorders of sleep along with several subcategories under each category as well as appendices A and B (Table 3.7). The eight broad categories consist of insomnia, sleep-related breathing disorders, hypersomnia of central origin not due to a circadian rhythm sleep disorder,

Table 3.7 International Classification of Sleep Disorders

I. Insomnia
  1. Acute insomnia
  2. Psychophysiologic insomnia
  3. Paradoxical insomnia (sleep state misperception)
  4. Idiopathic insomnia
  5. Insomnia due to mental disorder
  6. Inadequate sleep hygiene
  7. Behavioral insomnia of childhood
  8. Insomnia due to drug or substance
  9. Insomnia due to medical condition
  10. Insomnia not due to substance or known physiologic condition, unspecified (nonorganic)
  11. Physiologic insomnia, unspecified (organic)

II. Sleep-related breathing disorders
  A. Central sleep apnea syndromes
    1. Primary central sleep apnea
    2. Central sleep apnea due to Cheyne-Stokes breathing pattern
    3. Central sleep apnea due to high-altitude periodic breathing
    4. Central sleep apnea due to medical condition not Cheyne-Stokes
    5. Central sleep apnea due to drug or substance
    6. Primary sleep apnea of infancy (formerly primary sleep apnea of newborn)
  B. Obstructive sleep apnea syndromes
    7. Obstructive sleep apnea, adult
    8. Obstructive sleep apnea, pediatric
  C. Sleep-related hypoventilation/hypoxemic syndromes
    9. Sleep-related nonobstructive alveolar hypoventilation, idiopathic
    10. Congenital central alveolar hypoventilation syndrome

Table 3.7 International Classification of Sleep Disorders (*Continued*)

     D. Sleep-related hypoventilation/hypoxemia due to medical condition

        11. Sleep-related hypoventilation/hypoxemia due to pulmonary parenchymal or vascular pathology

        12. Sleep-related hypoventilation/hypoxemia due to lower airways obstruction

        13. Sleep-related hypoventilation/hypoxemia due to neuromuscular and chest wall disorders

     E. Other sleep-related breathing disorder

        14. Sleep apnea/sleep-related breathing disorder, unspecified

III. Hypersomnias of central origin not due to a circadian rhythm sleep disorder, sleep-related breathing disorder, or other cause of disturbed nocturnal sleep

     1. Narcolepsy with cataplexy

     2. Narcolepsy without cataplexy

     3. Narcolepsy due to medical condition

     4. Narcolepsy, unspecified

     5. Recurrent hypersomnia

        a. Kleine-Levin syndrome

        b. Menstrual-related hypersomnia

     6. Idiopathic hypersomnia with long sleep time

     7. Idiopathic hypersomnia without long sleep time

     8. Behaviorally induced insufficient sleep syndrome

     9. Hypersomnia due to medical condition

     10. Hypersomnia due to drug or substance

     11. Hypersomnia not due to substance or known physiologic condition (nonorganic hypersomnia, not otherwise specified [NOS])

     12. Physiological (organic) hypersomnia, unspecified (organic hypersomnia, NOS)

IV. Circadian rhythm sleep disorders

     1. Circadian rhythm sleep disorder, delayed sleep phase type (delayed sleep phase disorder)

     2. Circadian rhythm sleep disorder, advanced sleep phase type (advanced sleep-wake rhythm)

     3. Circadian rhythm sleep disorder, irregular sleep-wake type (irregular sleep-wake rhythm)

     4. Circadian rhythm sleep disorder, free-running type (nonentrained type)

     5. Circadian rhythm sleep disorder, jet lag type (jet lag disorder)

     6. Circadian rhythm sleep disorder, shift work type (shift work disorder)

     7. Circadian rhythm sleep disorder due to medical condition

     8. Other circadian rhythm sleep disorder (circadian rhythm disorder, NOS)

     9. Other circadian rhythm sleep disorder due to drug or substance

V. Parasomnias

     A. Disorders of arousal (from non-REM sleep)

        1. Confusional arousals

        2. Sleepwalking

        3. Sleep terrors

     B. Parasomnias usually associated with REM sleep

        4. REM sleep behavior disorder (including parasomnia overlap disorder and status dissociatus)

        5. Recurrent isolated sleep paralysis

        6. Nightmare disorder

     C. Other parasomnias

        7. Sleep-related dissociative disorders

        8. Sleep enuresis

        9. Sleep-related groaning (catathrenia)

        10. Exploding head syndrome

(Continued)

Table 3.7 International Classification of Sleep Disorders (*Continued*)

    11. Sleep-related hallucinations
    12. Sleep-related eating disorders
    13. Parasomnia, unspecified
    14. Parasomnia due to drug or substance
    15. Parasomnia due to medical condition

VI. Sleep related movement disorders
    1. Restless legs syndrome
    2. Periodic limb movement disorder
    3. Sleep-related leg cramps
    4. Sleep-related bruxism
    5. Sleep-related rhythmic movement disorder
    6. Sleep-related movement disorder, unspecified
    7. Sleep-related movement disorder due to drug or substance
    8. Sleep-related movement disorder due to medical condition

VII. Isolated symptoms, apparently normal variants and unresolved issues
    1. Long sleeper
    2. Short sleeper
    3. Snoring
    4. Sleep talking
    5. Sleep starts (hypnic jerks)
    6. Benign sleep myoclonus of infancy
    7. Hypnagogic foot tremor and alternating leg muscle activation during sleep
    8. Propriospinal myoclonus at sleep onset
    9. Excessive fragmentary myoclonus

VIII. Other sleep disorders
    1. Other physiologic (organic) sleep disorder
    2. Other sleep disorder not due to substance or known physiologic condition
    3. Environmental sleep disorder

Appendix A: Sleep disorder associated with conditions classifiable elsewhere
    1. Fatal familial insomnia
    2. Fibromyalgia
    3. Sleep-related epilepsy
    4. Sleep-related headaches
    5. Sleep-related gastroesophageal reflux disease
    6. Sleep-related coronary artery ischemia
    7. Sleep-related abnormal swallowing, choking, and laryngospasm

Appendix B: Other psychiatric and behavioral disorders frequently encountered in the differential diagnosis of sleep disorders
    1. Mood disorders
    2. Anxiety disorders
    3. Somatoform disorders
    4. Schizophrenia and other psychotic disorders
    5. Disorders usually first diagnosed in infancy, childhood, or adolescence
    6. Personality disorders

REM, rapid eye movement.

circadian rhythm sleep disorders, parasomnias, sleep-related movement disorders, isolated systems, apparently normal variant and unresolved issues, and other sleep disorders.

The category of insomnia includes acute insomnia; psychophysiologic insomnia; paradoxical insomnia (sleep-state misperception); idiopathic insomnia; insomnia due to mental disorder; inadequate sleep hygiene; behavioral insomnia of childhood; insomnia due to drug or substance; insomnia due to medical conditions; insomnia not due to substance; sleep-related breathing disorder or other nonphysiologic condition, unspecified (nonorganic); and physiologic insomnia, unspecified (organic).

The category of sleep-related breathing disorders (SRBDs) includes central sleep apnea syndromes, including primary central sleep apnea, central sleep apnea due to Cheyne-Stokes breathing pattern, central sleep apnea due to high-altitude periodic breathing, central sleep apnea due to medical condition not Cheyne-Stokes, central sleep apnea due to drug or substance and primary sleep apnea of infancy (formerly primary sleep apnea of newborns); obstructive sleep apnea syndromes (OSAS), including adult obstructive and pediatric obstructive sleep apnea; sleep-related hypoventilation/hypoxemia syndrome; sleep-related hypoventilation/hypoxemia due to medical condition; and other sleep-related breathing disorders (sleep apnea/sleep-related breathing disorders, unspecified).

Hypersomnias of central origin not due to a circadian rhythm sleep disorder, sleep-related breathing disorder, or other causes of disturbed nocturnal sleep include narcolepsy with cataplexy, narcolepsy without cataplexy, narcolepsy due to medical condition, narcolepsy unspecified, recurrent hypersomnia, Kleine-Levin syndrome, menstrual-related hypersomnia, behaviorally induced insufficient sleep syndrome, hypersomnia due to medical condition, hypersomnia due to drug or substance, hypersomnia not due to substance or known physiologic condition (nonorganic hypersomnia, not other otherwise specified, NOS), and physiologic (organic) hypersomnia unspecified (organic hypersomnia, NOS).

Circadian rhythm sleep disorders include delayed sleep phase type, advanced phase type, irregular sleep/wake type, free-running type, jet lag type, shift work type, circadian rhythm sleep disorder, circadian rhythm disorder (NOS), and other circadian rhythm due to drug or substance.

Parasomnias are characterized by abnormal movements and behavior during sleep but do not necessarily disrupt sleep architecture. Parasomnias include disorders of arousal from non-REM sleep (confusional arousals, sleepwalking, and sleep terrors); parasomnias usually associated with REM sleep (REM sleep behavior disorder, including parasomnia overlap disorder and status dissociatus, recurrent isolated sleep paralysis, and nightmare disorder); other parasomnias (sleep-related dissociated disorders, sleep enuresis, sleep-groaning or catathrenia, exploding head syndrome, sleep-related hallucinations, sleep-related eating disorders, parasomnia unspecified, parasomnia due to drug or substance, and parasomnia due to medical conditions).

Sleep-related movement disorders include restless legs syndrome, Periodic limb movement disorder, sleep-related leg cramps, sleep-related bruxism, sleep-related rhythmic movement disorder, sleep-related movement disorder due to drug or substance, and sleep-related movement disorder due to medical condition.

Isolated symptoms, apparently normal variants, and unresolved issues include long sleeper, short sleeper, snoring, sleep talking, sleep starts (hypnic jerks), benign sleep myoclonus of infancy, hypnagogic foot tremor and alternating leg muscle activation during sleep, propriospinal myoclonus at sleep onset, and excessive fragmentary myoclonus.

Other sleep disorder categories include other physiologic (organic) sleep disorders, other sleep disorders not due to substance or known physiologic condition, and environmental sleep disorder.

Appendix A includes sleep disorders associated with conditions classifiable elsewhere (fatal familial insomnia; fibromyalgia; sleep-related epilepsy; sleep-related headaches; sleep-related gastroesophageal reflux disease; sleep-related coronary artery ischemia; and sleep-related abnormal swallowing, choking, and laryngospasm).

Appendix B includes other psychiatric and behavioral disorders frequently encountered in the differential diagnosis of sleep disorders (mood disorders, anxiety disorders, somatoform disorders, schizophrenia, and other psychotic disorders); disorders usually first diagnosed in infancy, childhood, or adolescence; and personality disorders.

REFERENCES

1. Moruzzi G. The historical development of the deafferentation hypothesis of sleep. *Proc Am Philosoph Soc* 1964;108:19.

2. Berger H. Uber das Elektroenkephalogramm des Menschen. *Arch Psychiatry Nervenber* 1929;87:527.

3. Aserinsky E, Kleitman N. Regularly occurring periods of eye motility and concomitant phenomena during sleep. *Science* 1953;118:273.

4. Hess WR. Le sommeil. *C R Soc Biol (Paris)* 1931;107:1333.

5. Nauta WJH. Hypothalamic regulation of sleep in rats. An experimental study. *J Neurophysiol* 1946;9:285.

6. Bremer F. Cerveau "isole" et physiologie due sommeil. *C R Soc Biol (Paris)* 1935;118:1235.

7. Moruzzi G, Magoun HW. Brain stem reticular formation and activation of the EEG. *Electroencephalogr Clin Neurophysiol* 1949;1:455.

8. Moruzzi G. Active processes in the brain stem during sleep. *Harvey Lect* 1963;58:233.

8a. Jouvet M, Michel F. Correlatios electromyographique du sommeil chez le chat decortique et mesencephalique chronique. *C R Soc Bil (Paris)* 1959;153:422–5.

8b. Berger RJ. Tonus of extrinsic laryngeal muscles during sleep and dreaming. *Science* 1961;134:840.

9. Tobbler I. Is sleep fundamentally different between mammalian species? *Behav Brain Res* 1995;69:35.

10. Mahowald MW, Schenck CH. Status dissociatus: a perspective on states of being. *Sleep* 1991;14:69.

11. Chokroverty S. An overview of sleep. In Chokroverty S, ed: *Sleep Disorders Medicine: Basic Science, Technical Considerations and Clinical Aspects*. Philadelphia, PA: Saunders/Elsevier; 2009:5.

12. Ogilvie RD, Harsh JR, eds. *Sleep Onset: Normal and Abnormal Processes*. Washington, DC: American Psychological Association; 1995.

13. Ogilvie RD. The process of falling asleep: physiological review. *Sleep Med Rev* 2001;5:247.

14. Critchley M. The pre-dormitum. *Rev Neurol (Paris)* 1955;93:101.

15. Rechtschaffen A, Kales A. *A Manual of Standardized Terminology, Techniques and Scoring Systems for Sleep Stages of Human Subjects*. Los Angeles, CA: UCLA Brain Information Service/Brain Research Institute; 1968.

15a. Iber C, Ancoli-Israel S, Chesson A, and Quan SF for the American Academy of Sleep Medicine. *The AASM Manual for the Scoring of Sleep and Associated Events. Rules, Terminology and Technical Specifications*, 1st ed.: Westchester, IL: American Academy of Sleep Medicine,; 2007.

16. Sleep Disorders Atlas Task Force of the American Sleep Disorders Association (Preliminary Report). EEG arousals: Scoring rules and examples. *Sleep* 1992;15:174.

17. Terzano MG, Parrino L, Spaggiari MC. The cyclic alternating pattern sequences in the dynamic organization of sleep. *Electroencephalogr Clin Neurophysiol* 1988;69:437.

18. Terzano MG, Mancia D, Salati MR, et al. The cyclic alternating pattern as a physiologic component of normal NREM sleep. *Sleep* 1985;8:137.

19. Terzano MG, Parrino L. Origin and significance of the cyclic alternating pattern (CAP): review article. *Sleep Med Rev* 2000;4:101.

20. Terzano MG, Parrino L, Smeriari A, et al. Atlas, rules and recording techniques for the scoring of cyclic alternating pattern (CAP) in human sleep. *Sleep Med* 2002;3:187.

21. Roffwarg HP, Muzzio JN, Dement WC. Ontogenetic development of the human sleep-dream cycle. *Science* 1966;152:604.

22. Anders TF. Maturation of sleep patterns in the newborn infant. In: Weitzman ED, ed. *Advances in Sleep Research*. New York: Spectrum; 1975:43.

23. Metcalf DR. The effects of extrauterine experience on the ontogenesis of EEG sleep spindles. *Psychosom Med* 1969;31:393.

24. Metcalf DR, Mondale J, Burler FK. Ontogenesis of spontaneous K complexes. *Psychophysiology* 1971;8:340.

25. Harrison Y, Horne JA. Should we be taking more sleep? *Sleep* 1995;18:901.

26. Bonnet M, Arand D. We are chronically sleep deprived. *Sleep* 1995;18:908.

27. Webb WB, Agnew HW. Are we chronically sleep deprived? *Bull Psychom Soc* 1975;6:47.

28. Bliwise DL, King A, Harris R, et al. Prevalence of self-reported poor sleep in a healthy population aged 50–65. *Soc Sci Med* 1992;34:49.

29. Hume KI, Van F, Watson A. A field study of age and gender differences in habitual adult sleep. *J Sleep Res* 1998;7:85.

30. Reyner LA, Horne JA, Reyner A. Gender- and age-related differences in sleep determined by

home-recorded sleep logs and actimetry from 400 adults. *Sleep* 1995;18:127.

31. Ferrara M, Gennaro LD. How much sleep do we need? *Sleep Med Rev* 2001;5:155.

32. Kleitman N. *Sleep and Wakefulness*. Rev ed. Chicago, IL: University of Chicago Press; 1963.

33. Webb WB, Agnew HW. Sleep stage characteristics of long and short sleepers. *Science* 1970;168:146.

34. Kripke DF, Simons RN, Garfinkel L, et al. Short and long sleep and sleeping pills: is increased mortality associated? *Arch Gen Psychiatry* 1979;36:103.

34a. Kronholm E, Laatikainen T, Peltonen M, et al. Self-reported sleep duration, all-cause mortality, cardiovascular mortality and morbidity in Finland. *Sleep Med* 2011;12:215–21.

35. Taub JM, Berger RJ. Effects of acute sleep pattern alteration depend upon sleep duration. *Physiol Psychol* 1976;4:412.

36. Taub JM, Berger RJ. Extended sleep and performance: The Rip Van Winkle effect. *Psychonom Sci* 1969;16:204.

37. De Mairan JJ. *Observation Botanique. Histoire de l'Academie Royale des Sciences*. Paris: Imprimerie Royale; 1731:35.

38. Pittendrigh CS. Circadian rhythms and the circadian organization of living systems. *Cold Spring Harb Symp Quant Biol* 1960;25:159.

39. Aschoff J. Exogenous and endogenous components in circadian rhythms. *Cold Spring Harb Symp Quant Biol* 1960;25:11.

40. Aschoff J. Circadian rhythms in man. *Science* 1965;148:1427.

41. Miller JD, Morin LP, Schwartz WJ, et al. New insights into the mammalian circadian clock. *Sleep* 1996;19:641.

42. Czeisler CA, Duffy JF, Shanahan TL, et al. Stability, precision, and near 24-hour period of the human circadian pacemaker. *Science* 1999;284:2177.

43. Moore-Ede M, Sulzman FM, Fuller CA. *The Clocks that Time Us*. Cambridge, MA: Harvard University Press; 1982.

44. Wever RA. *The Circadian System of Man: Results of Experiments Under Temporal Isolation*. New York: Springer; 1979.

45. Stephan FK, Zucker I. Circadian rhythms in drinking behavior and locomotor activity of rats are eliminated by hypothalamic lesions. *Proc Natl Acad Sci USA* 1972;69:1583.

46. Moore RY, Eichler VB. Loss of a circadian adrenal corticosterone rhythm following suprachiasmatic lesion in the rat. *Brain Res* 1972;42:201.

47. Lydic R, Schoene WC, Czeisler CA, et al. Suprachiasmatic region of the human hypothalamus: homolog to the primate circadian pacemaker? *Sleep* 1980;2:355.

48. Moore RY, Lenn NJ. A retinohypothalamic projection in the rat. *J Comp Neurol* 1972;146:1.

49. Brzezinski A. Melatonin in humans. *N Engl J Med* 1997;336:186.

50. Penev PD, Zee PC. Melatonin: a clinical perspective. *Ann Neurol* 1997;42:545.

51. Arend TJ. *Melatonin and the Mammalian Pineal Gland*. London: Chapman & Hall; 1995.

52. Schwartz WJ. Understanding circadian clocks: from c-Fos to fly balls. *Ann Neurol* 1997;41:289.

53. Ralph MR, Joyner AL, Lehman MN. Culture and transplantation of the mammalian circadian pacemaker. *J Biol Rhythms* 1993;8:S83.

54. Murphy PJ, Campbell SS. Physiology of the circadian system in animals and humans. *J Clin Neurophysiol* 1996;13:2.

54a. Turek FW, Vitaterna MH. Molecular neurobiology of circadian rhythms. In: Montagna P, Chokroverty S, eds. *Handbook of Clinical Neurology: Sleep Disorders, Part 2*. Amsterdam, The Netherlands: Elsevier 2011;951–61.

55. Zhdanova IV, Lynch HJ, Wurtman RJ. Melatonin: a sleep-promoting hormone. *Sleep* 1997;20:899.

56. Sack RL, Hughes RJ, Edgar DM, et al. Sleep-promoting effects of melatonin: at what dose, under what conditions, and by what mechanisms? *Sleep* 1997;20:908.

57. Kennaway DJ, Goble FC, Stamp GE. Factors influencing the development of melatonin rhythmicity in humans. *J Clin Endocrinol Metab* 1996;81:1525.

58. Samel A, Wegmann HM, Vijvoda M, et al. Influence of melatonin treatment on human circadian rhythmicity before and after a simulated 9-hr time shift. *J Biot Rhythms* 1991;6:235.

59. Dawson D, Encel N, Lushington K. Improving adaption to simulated night shift: timed exposure to bright light versus daytime melatonin administration. *Sleep* 1995;18:11.

60. Sack RL, Lewy AJ, Blood ML, et al. Melatonin administration to blind people: phase advances and entrainment. *J Biol Rhythms* 1991;6:249.

61. McArthur AJ, Lewy AJ, Sack RL. Non-24-hour sleep/wake syndrome in a sighted man: circadian rhythm studies and efficacy of melatonin treatment. *Sleep* 1995;19:544.

62. Krueger JM, Obal F, Jr. Sleep factors. In: Saunders NA, Sullivan CE, eds. *Sleep and Breathing*. Philadelphia, PA: WB Saunders; 1994:79.

63. Von Economo C. *Encephalitis Lethargica. Its Sequelae and Treatment*. London: Oxford University Press; 1931.

64. Moruzzi G. The sleep waking cycle. *Ergeb Physiol* 1972;64:1.

65. Jouvet M. The role of monoamines and acetylcholine containing neurons in the regulation of the sleep-waking cycle. *Ergeb Physiol* 1972;64:166.

66. Batini C, Moruzzi G, Palestini M, et al. Persistent patterns of wakefulness in the pre-trigeminal mid-pontine preparation. *Science* 1958;128:30.

67. Batini C, Moruzzi G, Palestini M, et al. Effect of complete pontine transections on the sleep-wakefulness rhythm: the mid-pontine pre-trigeminal preparation. *Arch Ital Biol* 1959;97:1.

68. Jouvet M. Neurophysiology of the states of sleep. *Physiol Rev* 1967;47:117.

69. Magnes J, Moruzzi G, Pompeiano O. Synchronization of the EEG produced by low-frequency electrical stimulation of the region of the solitary tract. *Arch Ital Biol* 1961;99:33.

70. Sterman MB, Clemente CD. Forebrain inhibitory mechanisms: cortical synchronization induced by basal forebrain stimulation. *Exp Neurol* 1962;6:103.

71. Sterman MB, Clemente CD. Forebrain inhibitory mechanisms: sleep patterns induced by basal forebrain stimulation. *Exp Neurol* 1962;6:91.

72. Lucas EA, Sterman MB. Effect of a forebrain lesion on the polycyclic sleep-wake cycle and sleep-wake patterns in the cat. *Exp Neurol* 1975;46:368.

73. McGinty DJ, Sterman MB. Sleep suppression after basal forebrain lesions in the cat. *Science* 1968;160:1253.

74. Ricardo JA, Koh ET. Anatomical evidence of direct projections from the nucleus of the solitary tract to the hypothalamus, amygdala, and other forebrain structures in the rat. *Brain Res* 1978;153:1.

75. Jones BE. Basic mechanisms of sleep-wake states. In Kryger MH, Roth T, Dement WC, eds. *Principles and Practice of Sleep Medicine*. 3rd ed. Philadelphia, PA: Saunders; 2000:134.

76. Bremer F. Cerveau "isole" et physiologie du sommeil. *C R Soc Biol (Paris)* 1935;118:1235.

77. Bremer F. Cerebral hypnogenic centers. *Ann Neurol* 1977;2:1.

78. Moruzzi G, Magoun HW. Brain stem reticular formation and activation of the EEG. *Electroencephalogr Clin Neurophysiol* 1949;1:455.

79. Steriade M, McCarley RW. *Brainstem Control of Wakefulness and Sleep*. 2nd ed. New York: Kluwer Academic/Plenum Publishers; 2005.

80. Steriade M, McCormick DA, Sejnowski TJ. Thalamocortical oscillations in the sleeping and aroused brain. *Science* 1993;262:679.

81. Nauta WJH. Hypothalamic regulation of sleep in rats. An experimental study. *J Neurophysiol* 1946; 9:285.

82. Sallanon M, Denoyer M, Kitahama K, et al. Long-lasting insomnia induced by preoptic neuron lesions and its transient reversal by muscimol injection into the posterior hypothalamus in the cat. *Neuroscience* 1989;32:669.

83. Diskhit VV. Action of acetylcholine on the "sleep center." *J Physiol* 1934;83:42.

84. Saper CB, Chou T, Scammell TE. The sleep switch: hypothalamic control of sleep and wakefulness. *Trends Neurosci* 2001;24:726–31.

85. Scammell TE. The neurobiology, diagnosis and treatment of narcolepsy. *Ann Neurol* 2003;53:154–66.

85a. McCarley RW. Neurobiology of REM and NREM sleep. *Sleep Med* 2007;8:302–30.

86. De Lecea L, Kilduff TS, Peyron C, et al. The hypocretins: hypothalamus-specific peptides with neuroexcitatory activity. *Proc Natl Acad Sci USA* 1999;98:365.

87. Sakurai T, Amemiya A, Ishii M, et al. Orexins and orexin receptors: a family of hypothalamic neuropeptides and G protein-coupled receptors that regulate feeding behavior. *Cell* 1998;92:573.

88. Peyron C, Tighe DK, van den Pol AN, et al. Neurons containing hypocretin (orexin) project to multiple neuronal systems. *J Neurosci* 1998;18:9996.

89. Mignot E. Perspectives in narcolepsy and hypocretin (orexin) research. Editorial. *Sleep Med* 2000;1:87.

90. Overeem S, Mignot E, Van Dijk JG, et al. Narcolepsy: clinical features, new pathophysiologic insights, and future perspectives. *J Clin Neurophysiol* 2001;18:78.

91. Vertes RP. Brainstem control of the events of REM sleep. *Prog Neurobiol* 1984;22:241.

92. Jouvet M. The role of monoamines and acetylcholine containing neurons in the regulation of the sleep-waking cycle. *Ergeb Physiol* 1972;64:166.

93. Jouvet M. Neurophysiology of the states of sleep. *Physiol Rev* 1967;47:117.

94. McCarley RW. Sleep neurophysiology: basic mechanisms underlying control of wakefulness and sleep. In Chokroverty S, ed. *Sleep Disorders Medicine: Basic Science, Technical Considerations and Clinical Aspects.* Boston, MA: Butterworth-Heinemann; 2009:29–58.

95. Chokroverty S, Motagna P. Sleep, breathing and neurological disorders. In: Chokroverty S, ed. *Sleep Disorders Medicine: Basic Science, Technical Considerations and Clinical Aspects.* 3rd ed. Philadelphia, PA: Elsevier/Butterworth; 2009:436.

96. Lu J, Sherman D, Devor M, et al. A putative flip-flop switch for control of REM sleep. *Nature* 2006;441:589.

97. Brooks PL, Peever JH. Glycinergic and GABA a-mediated inhibition of somatic motoneurons does not mediate rapid eye movement sleep motor atonia. *J Neurosci* 2008;28:3535–45.

98. Brooks PL, Peever JH. Impaired GABA and glycine transmission triggers cardinal features of rapid eye movement sleep behavior disorder in mice. *J Neurosci* 2011;31:7111–21.

99. Luppi P-H, Clement O, Sapin E, et al. The neural network responsible for paradoxical sleep and its dysfunctions causing narcolepsy and rapid eye movement (REM) behavior disorder. *Sleep Med Rev* 2011;15:153–63.

100. Sakai K, Sastre JP, Salvert D, et al. Tegmentoreticular projections with special reference to the muscular atonia during paradoxical sleep in the cat. An HRP study. *Brain Res* 1979;176:233.

101. Chase MH, Morales FR, Boxer PA, et al. Effect of stimulation of the nucleus reticularis gigantocellularis on the membrane potential of cat lumbar motoneurons during sleep and wakefulness. *Brain Res* 1986;386:237.

102. Jouvet M. Locus coeruleus et sommeil paradoxal. *C R Soc Biol* 1965;159:895.

103. Schenck CH, Bundlie SR, Patterson AL, et al. Rapid eye movement sleep behavior disorder: a treatable parasomnia affecting older patients. *JAMA* 1987;257:1786.

104. Hirshkowitz M, Rose MW, Sharafkhaneh A. Neurotransmitters, neurochemistry, and the clinical pharmacology of sleep. In: Chokroverty S, ed. *Sleep Disorders Medicine: Basic Science, Technical Considerations and Clinical Aspects.* Philadelphia, PA: Saunders/Elsevier; 2009:67–79.

105. Fuller PM, Lu J. Dopamine. In: Stickgold R, Walker M, eds. *The Neuroscience of Sleep.* London: Academic Press/Elsevier; 2009:125–30.

106. Freud S. *The Interpretation of Dreams.* New York: Basic Books; 1955 (originally published in 1900).

107. Foulkes D. Dream research 1953–1993. *Sleep* 1996;19:609.

108. Crick F, Mitchison G. The function of dream sleep. *Nature* 1983;304:111.

109. Dinges DF, Broughton RJ. *Sleep and Alertness: Chronobiological, Behavioral and Medical Aspects of Napping.* New York: Raven; 1989.

110. Rechtschaffen A, Gilliland MA, Bergmann BM, et al. Physiological correlates of prolonged sleep deprivation in rats. *Science* 1983;221:182.

111. Moldofsky H. Sleep and the immune system. *Int J Immunopharmacol* 1995;17:649.

112. Spiegel K, Leproult R, Van Cauter E. Impact of sleep debt on metabolic and endocrine function. *Lancet* 1999;354:1435.

113. Horne J. *Why We Sleep.* New York: Oxford University Press; 1988.

114. Hartmann E. *The Functions of Sleep.* New Haven, CT: Yale University Press; 1973.

115. Maquet P. Sleep function (S and cerebral metabolism). *Behav Brain Res* 1995;69:75.

116. Webb WB. *Sleep: The Gentle Tyrant.* Bolton, MA: Anker; 1992.

117. Karni A, Tanne D, Rubenstein BS, et al. Dependence on REM sleep of overnight improvement of a perceptual skill. *Science* 1994;265:679.

118. Krueger JM, Obal F, Jr. Kapas L, et al. Brain organization and sleep function. *Behav Brain Res* 1995;69:177.

119. Kavanau JL. Memory, sleep and the evolution of mechanisms of synaptic efficacy maintenance. *Neuroscience* 1997;79:7.

120. Kavanau JL. Origin and evolution of sleep: roles of vision and endothermy. *Brain Res Bull* 1997;42:245.

121. Mahowald MW, Chokroverty S, Kader G, et al. *Sleep Disorders. Continuum Vol. 3, No. 4. A Program of the American Academy of Neurology.* Baltimore, MD: Williams & Wilkins; 1997.

122. American Academy of Sleep Medicine. *The International Classification of Sleep Disorders Diagnostic and Coding Manual.* 2nd ed. Westchester, IL: American Academy of Sleep Medicine; 2005.

4

Neurobiology of the REM–Non-REM Sleep Cycle

Md. NOOR ALAM AND RONALD SZYMUSIAK

MAMMALIAN SLEEP is a complex neurological state consisting of two alternating and distinct stages: non–rapid eye movement (non-REM) sleep and rapid eye movement (REM) sleep. Over the sleep period, an individual alternates between episodes of non-REM to REM sleep with a species-specific periodicity. The non-REM–REM sleep cycle length is approximately 90 minutes in humans, 22 minutes in cats, and 12 minutes in rats.[1] The duration of waking, non-REM, and REM sleep bouts within a species can also vary as a function of age, environmental factors (e.g., ambient temperature), and health condition.

Sleep onset in normal adult humans occurs invariably through non-REM sleep, which accounts for 75%–80% of sleep amount and dominates the first third of the nocturnal sleep period. Based on the degree of cortical electroencephalographic (EEG) synchronization, non-REM sleep is divided into three substages (N1, N2, and N3), roughly paralleling the depth of sleep continuum. Stage-N1 sleep is characterized by a reduction of rhythmic alpha activity (8–13 Hz) and onset of a relatively low-voltage and mixed-frequency (3–7 Hz) EEG activity. Eye movements become rolling and muscle tone diminishes. Stage-N2 sleep is characterized by sleep spindles and K-complexes, interspersed with less than 20% delta waves (0.1–4.0 Hz). Eye movements are absent and motor tone is further diminished. Stage-N3 sleep, also referred to as slow-wave sleep or delta sleep, is typified by the predominance of high-amplitude delta activity in the cortical EEG.

REM sleep occupies 20%–25% of sleep time and predominates during the last third of the night in humans. REM sleep, by contrast to non-REM sleep, is characterized primarily by EEG desynchronization, postural muscle atonia, and episodic bursts of eye movements, hence the name. REM sleep is often subdivided into tonic and phasic components. Tonic processes are reflected in generalized EEG desynchronization and muscle atonia that is present throughout REM sleep episodes. Phasic events include bursts of eye movements, somatic muscle twitches, and large electrical potentials that originate in the pons and are subsequently transmitted to the lateral geniculate nucleus and occipital cortex (PGO spikes). REM sleep is frequently associated with vivid dreams.

The conception of the neural basis of sleep control dates back to the early 20th century, when Von Economo[2] found that lesions in the preoptic area (POA) of the hypothalamus were associated with profound insomnia in victims of viral encephalitis. Since then, several structures in the mammalian central nervous system, including sites in the neocortex, basal forebrain (BF), preoptic/hypothalamic area, thalamus, brainstem, and medulla, have been shown to modulate amounts of waking and sleep. During the last two to three decades, our understanding about the cell types within those brain structures, the neurotransmitters, and synaptic interactions that influence non-REM–REM sleep cycling has progressed substantially. There are excellent reviews on various aspects of non-REM–REM sleep regulation.[3–8] This chapter summarizes our current understanding of the neuronal mechanisms underlying non-REM–REM sleep control, mainly based on the anatomy, physiology, and pharmacology of extensively studied structures. An emphasis is on circuits that have more direct sleep-regulatory actions, as opposed to modulatory effects.

MECHANISMS OF SLEEP ONSET

A critical task for brain mechanisms that generate sleep is to achieve a coordinated inhibition and/or disfacilitation of several arousal-regulatory neuronal groups located in the hypothalamus and brainstem. These include monoaminergic neurons in the rostral pons, midbrain and posterior hypothalamus, cholinergic neurons in the brainstem and the BF, dopaminergic neurons in the ventral tegmentum, and hypocretin- (orexin-) containing neurons in the perifornical-lateral hypothalamus.[4,7,9,10] Collective activity in these systems during waking imparts a tonic background level of activation that is reflected in low-voltage, fast-frequency cortical EEG patterns. Neuronal activity in these systems is characterized by high levels of tonic or phasic discharge during waking and quiescence during sleep. Some arousal systems (e.g., cholinergic) exhibit elevated discharge during waking and REM sleep and minimum

activity during non-REM sleep.[11–12] Others (e.g., monoaminergics) display discharge rates during REM sleep that are as low or lower than rates observed during non-REM sleep, that is, a "REM-off" discharge pattern.[13–15] What is common to all of the arousal systems is a rapid decline in neuronal activity just prior to or at the time of sleep onset.

Coordinated inhibition of these arousal systems is accomplished by three interrelated cellular and neurochemical mechanisms. First is a system of sleep-active, GABA-ergic neurons located in the preoptic area (POA) that project directly to several key arousal-promoting neuronal groups and exert monosynaptic sleep-related inhibition over these systems. A second mechanism entails regulation of the excitability of arousal systems by the circadian clock in the suprachiasmatic nucleus (SCN) of the hypothalamus. A third mechanism involves the wake-related production of endogenous sleep-regulatory substances or sleep factors. During sustained waking driven by the SCN, homeostatic pressure for sleep accumulates through increased expression of sleep factors, many of them being the by-products of waking brain activity. These factors act as sensors of prior waking time and exert inhibitory neuromodulatory effects on one or more arousal systems and may also activate sleep-regulatory neuronal systems to promote sleep onset and sleep maintenance.

NON-REM SLEEP REGULATION: THE PREOPTIC HYPOTHALAMUS

The discovery of the POA as a functionally important sleep-promoting region dates to studies of patients with encephalitis lethargica during the early 20th century.[2] Patients with insomnia as a prominent symptom before death had damage in the POA. Another group of patients with hypersomnia before death had lesions in the vicinity of the posterior hypothalamus. These observations led to the concept of opposing hypothalamic sleep- and wake-promoting systems. Later, Nauta[16], using brain transactions, experimentally confirmed the existence of hypnogenic substrates in the POA. Since then, a role of the POA in sleep regulation has been confirmed across species using multiple approaches.[4,7,9,10]

The POA is located in the rostral-most portion of the hypothalamus around the supraoptic recess of the third ventricle. It extends rostrally to the lamina terminalis and caudally to the anterior hypothalamic nuclei at the level of the optic chiasm. It extends ventrally to the base of the brain and dorsally to the anterior commissure and its bed nucleus. Medially, it is bordered by the periventricular nucleus and the third ventricle. Laterally, it merges with the magnocellular BF region.

Electrical or chemical stimulation of the POA evokes sleep onset, while its lesion yields profound and persistent insomnia.[17] Generally, the size of the lesion in this area determines the magnitude of sleep deficit, with larger lesions extending into the adjacent BF, producing total or near total insomnia. Neuronal recording studies confirmed the presence of sleep-active neurons in the POA and adjacent BF.[11,18,19] Collectively, findings such as insomnia caused by neuronal lesions of the POA, a suppression of EEG slow-wave activity in residual sleep after POA lesion, and presence of sleep-active neurons in this area support that a hypnogenic process originates in the POA neuronal tissue.

Non-REM-Sleep-Regulatory Preoptic Area Subregions: The Ventrolateral Preoptic Area and Median Preoptic Nucleus

A precise localization of hypnogenic subregions within the POA was realized in the 1990s with the introduction of c-Fos protein immunoreactivity (Fos-IR) as a marker of neuronal activation to the study of sleep mechanisms.[20] This technique, although limited by poor temporal resolution, helped determine the anatomical distribution of sleep- or wake-active neurons by comparing Fos-IR in the brain of animals that were predominately asleep or predominately awake during the 1–2 hours prior to sacrifice. This approach has identified two subregions of the POA that contain high densities of sleep-active neurons: the ventrolateral preoptic nucleus (VLPO) and the median preoptic nucleus (MnPN).[21,22]

Extracellular neuronal recording studies across spontaneous sleep-wake cycles further confirm that both VLPO and MnPN contain non-REM/REM-active neurons that are intermingled with relatively smaller populations of wake-active, state-indifferent, and REM-active neurons.[23,24] These neurons typically exhibit increasing discharge from waking to non-REM transition, to stable non-REM and to REM sleep. Combined staining for sleep-related Fos-IR and

neurotransmitter markers reveals that most sleep-active neurons in the MnPN synthesize the inhibitory neurotransmitter GABA[25] and that sleep-active neurons in the VLPO contain both GABA and the inhibitory neuropeptide galanin.[26]

The discharge activity of VLPO or MnPN neurons with increasing homeostatic sleep drive or diminishing homeostatic sleep pressure remains incompletely understood. However, evidence indicates that MnPN and VLPO may play complementary roles in regulating the homeostatic component of non-REM sleep.[27] A significantly higher number of MnPN GABA-ergic neurons exhibit Fos-IR during sleep deprivation (SD) as compared to spontaneous and recovery sleep. This suggests that MnPN neurons are strongly driven by increasing sleep pressure during waking and suggests a role for these neurons in promoting sleep onset. Fos-IR in VLPO GABA-ergic neurons is higher during spontaneous sleep and recovery sleep compared to SD, suggesting that these neurons are involved in consolidating sleep and promoting sleep maintenance.

VLPO neurons project extensively to major wake-promoting regions, including brainstem and hypothalamic nuclei with monoaminergic neurons, that is, locus coeruleus (LC), dorsal raphe nucleus (DRN), and tuberomammillary nucleus (TMN). Afferents to VLPO include the TMN, DRN, ventrolateral periaqueductal gray (VLPAG), and LC. Additional afferents arise from hypothalamic regions, including MnPN, perifornical-lateral hypothalamic area (PF-LHA), and dorsomedial hypothalamic nucleus (DMH).[7,8]

MnPN neurons send direct projections to major regions implicated in arousal, including PF-LHA, LC, DRN, and VLPAG.[17] MnPN is a source of major input to the VLPO as well. MnPN neurons that project to the VLPO include both sleep- and wake-active populations. An in vitro study indicates that VLPO neurons are subject to tonic, local GABA-ergic-mediated inhibition.[28] The subset of GABA-ergic, sleep-active neurons in the MnPN that project to VLPO may function to disinhibit VLPO neurons during non-REM and REM sleep.

The discharge profiles of both VLPO and MnPN neurons are reciprocal to those exhibited by wake-promoting monoaminergic and hypocretinergic neurons that are active during waking and quiescent during non-REM and REM sleep. Activation of GABA-ergic neurons in the MnPN and VLPO at the transitions from waking to sleep can simultaneously achieve inhibition of several key arousal systems in the posterior hypothalamus and brainstem, orchestrating a rapid transition to stable sleep. One mechanism contributing to stabilization of sleep-waking transitions arises from mutually inhibitory interactions between VLPO neurons and the monoaminergic arousal systems in the brainstem. VLPO neurons are inhibited by noradrenalin (NA); thus, waking-related monoaminergic activity prevents inappropriate activation of VLPO sleep-generating cells during an animal's active phase. During wake-to-sleep transitions, activation of VLPO neurons is reinforced by disinhibition as monoaminergic activity wanes. The mutual inhibitory interactions between sleep- and arousal-regulatory neurons function like a bistable switch (or flip-flop switch) and can help promote rapid and stable transitions between sleep and wakefulness.[7,8]

REM SLEEP-REGULATORY SYSTEMS

The classic transaction studies of Jouvet and others in cat concluded that the neural substrates critical for REM sleep generation reside in the pons and caudal midbrain.[6,29] While the isolated brainstem is capable of generating many features of the REM sleep state, in the intact brain, interactions among brainstem and forebrain neuronal systems are involved in the generation of the non-REM–REM sleep cycle.

Cholinergic-Monoaminergic Mechanisms

A role for brainstem cholinergic mechanisms in REM sleep generation was first indicated by the findings that microinjection of the muscarinic receptor agonist carbachol into the pontine reticular formation (PRF) of cats evoked prolonged episodes of a REM sleep-like state with short latency.[30] The critical site for carbachol-induced REM sleep was a region of the PRF ventral to the LC.[31] Microinjections of cholinergic antagonists into this area suppress REM sleep. Release of ACH in the PRF is elevated during REM sleep compared to both waking and non-REM sleep.[32] The importance of cholinergic neurons in the pedunculopontine and laterodorsal tegmentum (PPT and LDT) neurons in REM sleep generation is reflected in the ability of lesions in this area to suppress REM sleep in cats.[33] Recordings

of neuronal activity in the cholinergic PPT/LDT reveal neurons with a wake-REM active discharge pattern, as well as neurons with a more selective REM-on discharge profile.[4,34,35] REM-on neurons display low rates of discharge during waking and non-REM sleep and exhibit increased activity during non-REM–REM transitions and during REM sleep. REM-on cholinergic neurons project to neurons in the PRF. PRF neurons are cholinoceptive and many utilize glutamate as their neurotransmitter.[1] PRF neurons orchestrate the various components of the REM sleep state (bursts of eye movements, muscle atonia) via projections to other brainstem nuclei. LDT/PPT cholinergic REM-on neurons may be directly responsible for triggering some phasic events in REM sleep, as a subset of LDT/PPT neurons discharge high-frequency bursts just preceding the generation of PGO waves. Ascending projections of REM-on cholinergic neurons and wake-REM active cholinergic neurons in the LDT/PPT excite the thalamus and promote tonic neocortical EEG activation during REM sleep.

NA neurons in the LC, 5-HT neurons in the DRN, and TMN histaminergic neurons are continuously active during waking, decrease their activity during non-REM sleep, and further reduce or cease activity during REM sleep.[13–15] A critical regulator of LDT/PPT cholinergic REM-on neuronal activity is input from 5HT and NA neurons in the DRN and LC, respectively. Both 5HT and NA inhibit LDT/PPT REM-on neurons.[1] The cessation of neuronal activity in the DRN and LC that normally occurs at the time of transition between non-REM and REM sleep provides a critical step of disinhibition of cholinergic REM-on neurons that allows for the generation of the REM sleep state. Complex reciprocal interactions between cholinergic REM-on neurons and monoaminergic REM-off neurons are hypothesized to underlie the generation of the ultradian REM–non-REM sleep cycle.[1] Increased GABA-ergic release in the LC and DRN appears to be a major factor for the cessation of activity in these nuclei during REM sleep.[36–38] Blocking GABA receptors in the DRN or LC suppresses REM sleep, whereas pharmacological agents that increase monoaminergic signaling reduce the amount and delay the onset of REM sleep.[39] The various sources of GABA-ergic input to these nuclei that potentially contribute to REM sleep control include local interneurons, projections from the medial medulla, the PAG, and projections from the POA.[1,6]

Brainstem GABA-ergic–Glutamatergic Mechanisms

Studies done in rats, utilizing visualization of Fos-IR during augmented REM sleep have identified additional brainstem structures that contain REM-active neurons. These include the sublaterodorsal nucleus (SLD), precoeruleus region, and medial parabrachial nucleus.[40,41] These observations, along with anatomical, lesion, and pharmacological studies, have led to the development of a model of REM sleep generation that involves reciprocal inhibitory interactions among groups of brainstem GABA-ergic neurons.[8,41] In this model, GABA-ergic REM-on neurons localized in the SLD inhibit GABA-ergic wake-on/REM-off neurons, localized in the VLPAG and lateral pontine tegmentum (LPT). A subset of glutamatergic neurons that are intermingled with REM-on GABA-ergic neurons are REM-active projection neurons. One group of such glutamatergic neurons in the ventral SLD project to the ventromedial medulla and spinal cord and regulate muscle atonia of REM sleep. Another set of glutamatergic neurons from the precoeruleus and parabrachial regions project to the BF and regulate EEG phenomena of REM sleep. Cell-specific lesions or inhibition of the VLPAG/LPT increases the amount of REM sleep and produces cataplexy-like periods of atonia during wakefulness, whereas SLD lesions reduce REM sleep in rats and REM sleep without atonia in cats.[4,6,41,42]

Hypocretin Mechanisms of REM Sleep Control

Neurons containing the peptides hypocretins (HCRT-1 and HCRT-2, also called orexin-A and orexin-B) are localized within the hypothalamus, including the perifornical-lateral hypothalamic area (PF-LHA), dorsomedial hypothalamic nucleus (DMH), and posterior hypothalamic (PH) areas.[43,44] Activation of HCRT neurons is critical for the maintenance of waking, whereas inactivation or cessation of these neurons is necessary for maintaining consolidated sleep, including REM sleep and its muscle atonia.

Electrophysiological recordings of identified HCRT neurons across the sleep-waking cycle reveal that these neurons are active during waking, particularly during active waking, when postural muscle tone is high in association with movement. HCRT decrease discharge during quiet waking and virtually cease firing during non-REM and REM sleep.[45,46] HCRT neurons exhibit elevated discharge several seconds prior to the return to waking at the termination of REM sleep episodes. Consistent with these sleep-wake discharge profiles, higher levels of HCRT peptides in the cerebrospinal fluid (CSF) have been reported during active waking.[47] Optogenetic photostimulation of HCRT neurons increases the probability of transitioning to waking from either non-REM or REM sleep.[48] Deficiency of HCRT signaling is a key feature of the pathophysiology of narcolepsy. Patients with narcolepsy/cataplexy have severely reduced levels of HCRT in CSF.[49] The brains of narcoleptics display profound reductions in the numbers of HCRT neurons.[50,51] Genetic deletion of HCRT peptides or HCRT receptors in animal models produces a narcolepsy-like phenotype, including sudden episodes of cataplexy during waking, rapid state transitions and an impaired ability to sustain waking.[6,52,53] The ability of selective HCRT deficiency to have a significant impact on maintenance of wakefulness and intrusion of cataplexy during waking reflects the importance of the normal HCRT signaling in waking and suppression of REM sleep and muscle atonia.

The anatomical projections, receptor distribution, and pharmacological studies support that HCRT-induced arousal and suppression of REM sleep is predominantly mediated via its excitatory effects on multiple systems, including the cerebral cortex, nonspecific thalamocortical projection system, BF, hypothalamic, and brainstem arousal systems, as well as sympathetic and motor circuits in the spinal cord.[1,5,53-55] LDT/PPT and SLD also receive HCRT-ergic and monoaminergic inputs that can antagonize cholinergic action of eliciting REM sleep and its atonia.[1,5] Application of antisense oligonucleotides against HCRT receptor-2 mRNA in the PRF and adjoining SLD area increase REM sleep and induce cataplexy-like attacks.[56] Many neurons in this region bear HCRT-R2 receptor, which is mutated in narcoleptic dogs.[57] In this area some HCRT-R2 bearing neurons also bear M2 receptors, associated with hyperpolarizing responses to acetylcholine (ACH). Therefore, through effects on such neurons, HCRT facilitates and Ach suppresses muscle tone. It is proposed that by such opponent processes, HCRT overrides any inhibitory effects of ACH on muscle tone.[5] Thus, concurrent release of ACH in forebrain and brainstem during waking is associated with cortical activation and sustained muscle activity due to HCRT actions in the brainstem, but ACH release is associated with cortical activation and muscle atonia during REM sleep when HCRT signaling is absent.[5] GABA-ergic neurons in the VLPAG and LPT are innervated by HCRT neurons. Activation of HCRT neurons may inhibit atonia and REM sleep by activating VLPAG/LPT GABA-ergic wake-active/REM-off neurons and associated pathways.[42]

Melanin-Concentrating Hormone

Neurons containing the inhibitory peptide melanin-concentrating hormone (MCH) are localized in the hypothalamus, including the PF-LHA, zona incerta, and medial hypothalamic areas.[58] Within the PF-LHA, MCH and HCRT neurons are intermingled; however, the two neuronal types are distinct. MCH neurons project widely throughout the central nervous system, including dense innervation to regions with wake-promoting neuronal groups (e.g., LC, DRN, and VLPAG). Several observations suggest that MCH neurons play a role in the regulation of REM sleep. For example, electrophysiological recordings of identified MCH neurons across the sleep-wake cycle and Fos-IR studies suggest that MCH neurons are active during REM sleep.[59-61] MCH neurons seldom fire during waking, fire occasionally during non-REM sleep, and fire maximally during REM sleep, that is, in a manner reciprocal to HCRT and monoaminergic REM-off neurons. Intracerbroventricular (ICV) administration of MCH induces sleep, specifically REM sleep, whereas blockade of MCH transmission suppresses REM sleep.[59,62] Many of the MCH neurons also contain GABA. It is hypothesized that MCH neurons promote sleep, especially REM sleep via MCH-GABA inhibitory actions on multiple arousal systems, including HCRT-ergic and monoaminergic systems.[63] However, MCH knockout mice have essentially normal baseline REM sleep amounts and intact homeostatic responses to SD.[64] These findings indicate that the MCH system plays a modulatory role in REM sleep regulation.

THE SUPRACHIASMATIC NUCLEUS AND SLEEP GENERATION

As articulated 25 years ago by Borbely[65] in his two-process model, the generation of sleep is under both circadian and homeostatic control. Homeostatic pressure for sleep increases in proportion to prior time awake, but the circadian system regulates the timing of sleep, such that it is largely confined to the species-appropriate time of day.

The SCN is the master clock in the mammalian brain, responsible for regulating the timing of multiple physiological and behavioral events, including waking and sleep. The SCN is a paired structure, located in the ventromedial anterior hypothalamus, lateral to the third ventricle and dorsal to the optic chiasm. The SCN generates a self-sustaining rhythm of approximately 24 hours through auto-regulatory feedback loops in which protein products of circadian clock genes regulate their own expression through a sequence of transcription, translation, and posttranslation processes.[66] The SCN receives input from the retina directly through the retinohypothalamic tract and indirectly from the geniculohypothalamic tract.[67] Light is the most powerful stimulus that entrains the SCN and aligns the molecular clock with the environmental light/dark cycle, and through the outputs of the SCN, organizes the timing of wake and sleep. Melatonin secretion by the pineal gland is another synchronizer of the SCN that is important in generating the rhythms of wake and sleep. The SCN controls the secretion of melatonin through a complex pathway involving the paraventricular nucleus of the hypothalamus, preganglionic sympathetic neurons in the spinal cord, and the superior cervical ganglion.[67-69] The pineal gland secretes melatonin in a circadian pattern such that levels of melatonin are low during light exposure and high during the dark phase of the day. Once secreted melatonin can influence the timing of the circadian clock and the output of the SCN by its actions at MT1 and MT2 melatonin receptors that are present with high density in the SCN.[67,68]

The anatomical and neurochemical details of how the mammalian SCN interacts with sleep-generating mechanisms are far from completely understood. The SCN may regulate the timing of sleep primarily through modulating activity in one or more arousal systems, producing a clock-dependent drive for waking.[69-71] Ablation of the SCN in primates, while eliminating free running circadian rhythms in rest and activity, causes a significant increase in daily total sleep time, suggestive of an arousal deficit.[70] This suggests that the SCN actively promotes waking at the species-appropriate portion of the light-dark cycle. SCN modulation of arousal systems may involve neurohormones, since transplantation of SCN tissue can restore rest-activity rhythms in rats with SCN ablation.[69,72] Transforming growth factor-α (TGF-α) and prokinectin-2 are candidate molecules that are expressed in the SCN during the subjective day and bind to receptors in hypothalamic nuclei.[69,73] Central administration of TGF-α suppresses locomotor activity and disrupts the sleep-wake diurnal rhythm.[74]

The SCN has few direct efferent projections to hypothalamic or brainstem arousal systems. One of the densest targets of SCN neuronal output is the subparaventricular zone (SPZ) that is located immediately dorsal to the SCN.[75] A multisynaptic pathway, involving the hypothalamic SPZ and the dorsomedial hypothalamic nucleus (DMH), links the SCN with HCRT neurons in the PF-LHA and with brainstem arousal systems.[76] Glutamatergic projections from the DMH could convey excitatory influences from the SCN to arousal systems.[10] GABA-ergic projections from the DMH to the VLPO could convey inhibitory effects from the SCN.[10] A direct SCN to VLPO pathway may play a role in sleep-wake timing, as electrical or chemical activation of the SCN in a horizontal hypothalamic slice evokes inhibition in VLPO neurons.[77]

ENDOGENOUS SLEEP-REGULATORY SUBSTANCES

The attempts to identify the underlying mechanisms that regulate the waxing and waning of the sleep drive have led to the identification of a variety of factors/metabolites, including adenosine, interleukin 1ß, nitric oxide, prostaglandin-D2, and growth hormone-releasing hormone. Humoral theories of sleep generation have a long history and are appealing because the cycling between waking and sleep seems consistent with the waxing and waning of endogenous sleep-regulatory substances or sleep factors.[78–81] Generally, these factors are produced during waking, increase proportionately with increasing duration and intensity of arousal, and decline during sleep. It is hypothesized that the production of such factors during sustained waking provides a feedback signal, which either inhibits wake-promoting systems and/or activates sleep-promoting systems, to promote non-REM–REM sleep. Here, the experimental findings for some of the most extensively studied sleep factors are described.

Adenosine

Adenosine is the most extensively studied sleep factor.[1,4,78,79,81–83] Its production is coupled to the metabolic activity, which is higher during waking compared with sleep. Consequently, adenosine levels in some brain regions (e.g., BF) are higher during waking compared to sleep, rise during SD, and decline during recovery sleep.[84] Adenosine and its agonists promote sleep, whereas, its antagonists, for example, caffeine, suppress sleep. Of known adenosinergic receptors (R), A_1R and $A_{2A}R$ have been implicated in sleep regulation. The A_1R is inhibitory and seems to mediate the sleep-promoting actions of adenosine by (a) predominantly inhibiting wake-active neurons in multiple regions, including BF, PF-LHA, TMN, and LC, and (b) by disinhibiting sleep-active POA neurons.[80–88] The $A_{2A}R$ is excitatory and potentially contributes to the adenosinergic regulation of sleep via activation of sleep-active POA neurons. For example, (1) application of $A_{2A}R$ agonist into the POA increases sleep[89]; (2) adenosine excites a subset of VLPO neurons in vitro via $A_{2A}R$ [90]; (3) the wake-promoting ability of caffeine is attenuated in $A_{2A}R$ knockout mice [91]; and (4) $A_{2A}R$ agonist delivered into the subarachnoid space, underlying the VLPO/BF, induces sleep and Fos-IR in the POA.[92] Some recent studies indicate that waking-related release of ATP by astrocytes, a process known as gliotransmission, is an important source of adenosine that contributes to sleep homeostasis.[93] Collectively, these findings implicate adenosine in homeostatic sleep regulation.

Interleukin 1ß (IL-1)

Of a number of cytokines and chemokines that have been implicated in sleep regulation, IL-1 is possibly the most extensively studied.[79,94] The administration of this pro-inflammatory cytokine induces non-REM sleep in several species, irrespective of the route of administration.[95–98] Inhibition of endogenous IL-1 by IL-1-receptor antagonist (IL-1ra) or anti-IL-1 antibodies suppresses the occurrence of spontaneous non-REM sleep as well as sleep rebound subsequent to SD.[99–100] IL-1 type-1 receptor (IL-1R1) knockout mice are deficient in sleep.[101] Evidence indicates that IL-1 acts at multiple sites, including the cortex, DRN, and POA, to modulate non-REM sleep. Recent studies suggest that IL-1 in the POA/BF promotes sleep in part by inhibiting most of its wake-active neurons and activating a subpopulation of sleep-active neurons.[102] Although the mechanism that contributes to IL-1-induced suppression of POA wake-active neurons is not known, an in vitro study indicates that this could be due to IL-1-induced GABA release.[103] In addition to its direct action on specific brain circuits, IL-1 stimulates the synthesis and/or release of other neuromodulators, including adenosine, NO, PGD$_2$, and GHRH, all of which have been implicated in the regulation of sleep.

Nitric Oxide

Growing evidence supports a role of nitric oxide (NO) in the regulation of sleep. In the brain NO is mainly synthesized by inducible (i) and neuronal (n) NO synthases (NOS). Administration of NOS inhibitors, peripherally, centrally, or locally into various brain regions, including the BF, PPT, and DRN, decreases sleep, whereas NO donors promote sleep.[104-107] In the BF, infusion of an NO scavenger or NOS inhibitor attenuates recovery sleep subsequent to SD, whereas an NO donor increases sleep that closely resembles recovery sleep.[108] NO levels are higher in the cortex during spontaneous arousal and higher in the BF and the PF-LHA during SD.[109-112] Recent studies show that NO predominantly exerts inhibitory effects on the discharge of BF and PF-LHA neurons.[112,113] Such inhibition is hypothesized to induce recovery sleep after SD, since blockade of NO synthesis in the BF impairs recovery sleep.[108,110] Evidence suggests that in the BF, NO contributes to the production of adenosine during SD and that the inhibitory action of NO on BF neurons is mediated via A$_1$R-dependent adenosinergic mechanism.[113] Some evidence indicates a differential and localized role of iNOS and nNOS in sleep regulation. In the BF, iNOS has been implicated in SD-induced increases in NO levels.[110] A subset of cortical interneurons that express nNOS exhibit sleep-associated Fos-IR, and the activity of these neurons is correlated with homeostatic sleep pressure.[114] iNOS knockout mice are deficient in sleep, while no such effect is observed in nNOS knockout mice.[115]

Growth Hormone–Releasing Hormone

Growth hormone–releasing hormone (GHRH) is implicated in the regulation of spontaneous as well as in homeostatic aspects of sleep control.[4,7,116] GHRH neurons are localized in the arcuate nucleus and around the ventromedial and the periventricular nuclei. Exogenous GHRH has been shown to promote sleep in several species.[116-118] Inhibition of endogenous GHRH by its antagonist or anti-GHRH antibodies suppresses sleep. Hypothalamic GHRH mRNA levels in rats peak around the first part of the light period, when sleep amounts are highest.[119,120] Mutant mice with GHRH signaling abnormalities have reduced sleep.[121] Microinjection of GHRH into the POA promotes sleep, whereas its antagonist suppresses sleep, as well as recovery sleep after SD.[122] ICV administration of GHRH during the dark phase increases sleep as well as Fos-IR in GABA-ergic neurons in the MnPN and VLPO.[123] These findings indicate that GABA-ergic neurons in the MnPN and VLPO potentially mediate sleep-regulatory actions of GHRH.

Prostaglandin-D$_2$

Prostaglandin-D$_2$ (PGD$_2$) is the most abundant prostanoid in the mammalian brain. It is produced mainly by lipocalin-type PGD synthase (L-PGDS), which is localized in the leptomeninges, choroid plexus, and oligodendrocytes. Administration of PGD$_2$ via various routes, including ICV, directly into the POA, and into the subarachnoid space, promotes sleep, whereas administration of L-PGDS inhibitor suppresses sleep.[4,7,124,125] The most potent site for the sleep-promoting effects of PGD$_2$ is the subarachnoid space rostral and ventral to the POA. PGD$_2$ increases the discharge of sleep-active neurons in the POA.[126,127] ICV infusion of PGD$_2$ has no effect in DP$_1$-receptor knockout mice and infusion of DP$_1$ receptor antagonist in sleeping rats reduces the amounts of sleep.[128,129] Furthermore, PGD$_2$ levels in the brain increase during SD in wild-type mice but not in L-PGDS knockout mice, and sleep rebound is not observed in either L-PGDS knockout or DP$_1$R knockout mice.[125,129] Collectively, the aforementioned findings indicate that the L-PGDS/PGD$_2$/DP$_1$-receptor system plays a role in sleep regulation. Some evidence indicates that PGD$_2$-induced sleep is mediated via adenosine and the A$_{2A}$R system. Administration of A$_{2A}$R antagonist into the subarachnoid space blocks PGD$_2$-induced sleep. It is hypothesized that PGD$_2$ stimulates DP1-receptors on leptomeningeal cells to release adenosine, which in turn activates A$_{2A}$R-expressing sleep-active neurons in the POA/BF to promote sleep.[125]

MECHANISMS OF REM–NON-REM SLEEP CYCLE REGULATION

The two-process model of sleep control[65] continues to provide a useful framework for understanding many aspects of the cycling between waking and sleep, and the temporal organization of sleep-wake cycles. Output of the SCN actively promotes waking during certain times of the day. The mechanism of this clock-dependent alerting appears to be excitation of a subset of the arousal systems via secretion of neurohormones by the SCN and a multisynaptic pathway to arousal/sleep systems originating in the SCN and involving the SPZ and DMH. The SCN control of melatonin secretion is an additional factor in regulating the timing of sleep.

During waking, HCRT neurons are further activated in response to stress, hunger, and autonomic challenges and function to promote and consolidate waking. Activated HCRT neurons enhance arousal and motor activity predominantly by exciting and sustaining the activities of monoaminergic neurons in LC, DRN, and TMN; cholinergic neurons in the LDT/PPT and BF; and GABA-ergic wake-active neurons in the VLPAG/LPT. Activated NA and 5HT neurons may increase muscle tone by inhibiting atonia- and REM sleep-producing neurons of the SLD, reticular formation, and LDT/PPT. In addition, NA and 5HT increase muscle tone by directly exciting motor neurons. HCRT neurons also activate glutamatergic neurons in the PF-LHA and BF, which in turn further activates HCRT neurons. Activity of monoaminergic and cholinergic wake-promoting systems inhibit GABA-ergic sleep-promoting neurons in the POA region.[130] BF/POA sleep-active GABA-ergic neurons bearing α-2 receptors would be hyperpolarized by NA, whereas BF cholinergic neurons would be excited by NA via α-1 receptors.[9,131] Rapid state-transitions, including transitions into REM like states of muscle atonia directly from wakefulness in animals with loss of HCRT

signaling, suggest that HCRT neurons normally reinforce the waking side of the flip-flop switch, thus stabilizing it and preventing sudden and inappropriate transitions between wakefulness and sleep.[8]

During sustained waking driven by the SCN, homeostatic pressure for sleep (Process S in the two-process model) accumulates through increased expression of endogenous sleep factors that occur as a result of waking brain activity. Expression of several genes in cortical and subcortical areas (e.g., genes involved in neuronal plasticity; circadian clock genes) are elevated in response to sustained waking,[132,133] and the protein products of these genes may also contribute to homeostatic sleep drive. At the end of the active period, when SCN output begins to decline, activity in arousal systems declines due to diminution of SCN-dependent alerting and to increased arousal-suppressing effects of sleep factors. The increase in activity in GABA-ergic neurons in the MnPN and VLPO is a critical, short-latency event in switching from wakefulness to non-REM sleep, because these neurons can orchestrate rapid and powerful inhibition of several key arousal systems via their direct synaptic projections to multiple hypothalamic and brainstem sites. Sustained activity of POA neurons and high levels of sleep factors early in the rest phase reinforce sleep continuity. The termination of the rest phase arises from a combination of reduced levels of sleep factors as a result of sustained sleep and the re-emergence of SCN-dependent alerting. In humans, reinstatement of clock-dependent alerting emerges following the nadir of the circadian body temperature rhythm, in association with increasing cortisol levels.

Within the sleep period, cycling between non-REM and REM sleep involves interactions among forebrain/hypothalamic and brainstem circuits, although not all of the details are fully understood. Since the generation of REM sleep is normally dependent upon a prior period of non-REM sleep, one factor that may couple the occurrence of non-REM and REM sleep is the inhibition of brainstem monoaminergic neurons by MnPN and VLPO neurons during sleep. The majority of sleep-active neurons in these preoptic nuclei exhibit elevated discharge during both non-REM and REM sleep compared to waking. The extended VLPO also contains a less well-defined population of REM-active neurons.[134] Therefore, it is possible that the continued/progressive activation of preoptic GABA-ergic neurons during non-REM sleep contributes to the sustained cessation and ultimately silencing of HCRT and mono-amine neuronal activity at non-REM–REM transition, thereby promoting the disfacilitation/disinhibition of key brainstem REM sleep-generators, that is, cholinergic LDT/PPT REM-on neurons and GABA-ergic SLD REM-on neurons. Consistent with this idea, progressively increasing extracellular GABA levels (REM>non-REM>waking) have been reported in the LH, DRN, and LC.[6,7]

There continues to be disagreement in the literature about the brainstem cell types involved in the generation of the REM sleep state and its different components, and about which circuits are most important in regulating the cycling between non-REM and REM sleep.[1,3,6,41] A large body of evidence derived primarily from experiments in cats identifies LDT/PPT cholinergic neurons as the key elements in REM sleep induction. The timing of the non-REM–REM cycle is hypothesized to emerge from reciprocal inhibitory interactions between cholinergic REM-on and monoaminergic REM-off neurons.[1] A different perspective emerges from studies of REM sleep control in rats. In this species, cholinergic REM-generating mechanisms appear to be less potent.[3,8,41] Rather, the critical reciprocal interactions are hypothesized to be among GABA-ergic REM-on neurons in the SLD and GABA-ergic REM-off neurons in the VLPAG. It is possible that both mechanisms function in the cat and the rat but differ in relative importance.

Factors determining the duration of the REM sleep episode and the transition back to non-REM sleep are also incompletely understood. Again, the mechanism may involve interactions among hypothalamic and brainstem circuits. Tonic activity of REM-active MCH neurons in the PF-LHA and of non-REM–REM-on neurons in VLPO/extended VLPO during REM sleep potentially exert tonic inhibitory influences on key REM-off neuronal groups, namely, HCRT neurons in the PF-LHA, GABA-ergic neurons in the VLPAG, and monoaminergic neurons in the DRN and LC. These tonic processes during the REM episode maintain the activation of LDT/PPT and SLD REM generators. The critical role of the HCRT system in modulating REM generating circuits is evidenced by findings that HCRT deficiency in human narcolepsy and in knockout mice results in enhanced expression of REM sleep features during waking (cataplexy, sleep paralysis, sleep onset REM sleep). Re-emergence of HCRT activity may be one factor orchestrating the termination of REM sleep episodes, as unit recordings of HCRT neurons in rats demonstrate that these neurons become active several seconds prior to the spontaneous arousal from REM sleep. Understanding the mechanisms responsible for terminating REM sleep bouts will require a detailed accounting of the temporal changes in neuronal discharge occurring in hypothalamic and brainstem REM-on/REM-off neurons during spontaneous transitions from REM sleep to waking or non-REM sleep.

REFERENCES

1. McCarley RW. Neurobiology of REM and NREM sleep. *Sleep Med* 2007;8:302–30.
2. Von Economo C. Sleep as a problem of localization. *J Nerv Ment Dis* 1930;71:249–59.
3. Luppi PH, Gervasoni D, Verret L, et al. Paradoxical (REM) sleep genesis: the switch from an aminergic-cholinergic to a GABAergic-glutamatergic hypothesis. *J Physiol (Paris)* 2006;100:271–83.
4. Datta S, Maclean RR. Neurobiological mechanisms for the regulation of mammalian sleep-wake behavior: reinterpretation of historical evidence and inclusion of contemporary cellular and molecular evidence. *Neurosci Biobehav Rev* 2007;31:775–824.
5. Jones BE. Modulation of cortical activation and behavioral arousal by cholinergic and orexinergic systems. *Ann NY Acad Sci* 2008;1129:26–34.
6. Siegel JM. The neurobiology of sleep. *Semin Neurol* 2009;29:277–96.
7. McGinty D, Szymusiak R. NonREM sleep mechanisms. In: Kryger MH, Roth T, Dement WC, eds. *Principles and Practice of Sleep Medicine*, 5th ed. Philadelphia: W.B. Saunders Company; 2010:76–91.
8. Saper CB, Fuller PM, Pedersen NP, et al. Sleep state switching. *Neuron* 2011;68:1023–42.
9. Jones BE. From waking to sleeping: neuronal and chemical substrates. *Trends Pharmacol Sci* 2005;26:578–86.
10. Saper CB, Scammell TE, Lu J. Hypothalamic regulation of sleep and circadian rhythms. *Nature* 2005;437:1257–63.
11. Szymusiak R, McGinty D. Sleep-related neuronal discharge in the basal forebrain of cats. *Brain Res* 1986;370:82–92.

12. Lee MG, Hassani OK, Alonso A, et al. Cholinergic basal forebrain neurons burst with theta during waking and paradoxical sleep. *J Neurosci* 2005;25:4365–9.

13. Aston-Jones G, Chiang C, Alexinsky T. Discharge of noradrenergic locus coeruleus neurons in behaving rats and monkeys suggests a role in vigilance. *Prog Brain Res* 1991;88:501–20.

14. Guzman-Marin R, Alam MN, Szymusiak R, et al. Discharge modulation of rat dorsal raphe neurons during sleep and waking: effects of preoptic/basal forebrain warming. *Brain Res* 2000;875:23–34.

15. Vanni-Mercier G, Gigout S, Debilly G, et al. Waking selective neurons in the posterior hypothalamus and their response to histamine H3-receptor ligands: an electrophysiological study in freely moving cats. *Behav Brain Res* 2003;144:227–41.

16. Nauta WJ. Hypothalamic regulation of sleep in rats; an experimental study. *J Neurophysiol* 1946;9:285–316.

17. Szymusiak R, McGinty D. Hypothalamic regulation of sleep and arousal. *Ann NY Acad Sci* 2008;1129:275–86.

18. Kaitin KI. Preoptic area unit activity during sleep and wakefulness in the cat. *Exp Neurol* 1984;83:347–57.

19. Alam MN, McGinty D, Szymusiak R. Preoptic/anterior hypothalamic neurons: thermosensitivity in wakefulness and non rapid eye movement sleep. *Brain Res* 1996;718:76–82.

20. Morgan JI, Curran T. Stimulus-transcription coupling in the nervous system: involvement of the inducible proto-oncogenes fos and jun. *Annu Rev Neurosci* 1991;14:421–51.

21. Sherin JE, Shiromani PJ, McCarley RW, et al. Activation of ventrolateral preoptic neurons during sleep. *Science* 1996;271:216–19.

22. Gong H, Szymusiak R, King J, et al. Sleep-related c-Fos protein expression in the preoptic hypothalamus: effects of ambient warming. *Am J Physiol Regul Integr Comp Physiol* 2000;279:R2079–88.

23. Suntsova N, Szymusiak R, Alam MN, et al. Sleep-waking discharge patterns of median preoptic nucleus neurons in rats. *J Physiol* 2002;543:665–77.

24. Szymusiak R, Alam N, Steininger TL, et al. Sleep-waking discharge patterns of ventrolateral preoptic/anterior hypothalamic neurons in rats. *Brain Res* 1998;803:178–88.

25. Gong H, McGinty D, Guzman-Marin R, et al. Activation of c-fos in GABAergic neurones in the preoptic area during sleep and in response to sleep deprivation. *J Physiol* 2004;556:935–46.

26. Gaus SE, Strecker RE, Tate BA, et al. Ventrolateral preoptic nucleus contains sleep-active, galaninergic neurons in multiple mammalian species. *Neuroscience* 2002;115:285–94.

27. Gvilia I, Xu F, McGinty D, et al. Homeostatic regulation of sleep: a role for preoptic area neurons. *J Neurosci* 2006;26:9426–33.

28. Chamberlin NL, Arrigoni E, Chou TC, et al. Effects of adenosine on GABAergic inputs to identified ventrolateral preoptic neurons. *Neuroscience* 2003;119:913–18.

29. Jouvet M. [Research on the neural structures and responsible mechanisms in different phases of physiological sleep]. *Arch Ital Biol* 1962;100:125–206.

30. George R, Haslett WL, Jenden DJ. A cholinergic mechanism in the brainstem reticular formation: induction of paradoxical sleep. *Int J Neuropharmacol* 1964;3:541–52.

31. Baghdoyan HA, Lydic R, Callaway CW, et al. The carbachol-induced enhancement of desynchronized sleep signs is dose dependent and antagonized by centrally administered atropine. *Neuropsychopharmacology* 1989;2:67–79.

32. Kodama T, Takahashi Y, Honda Y. Enhancement of acetylcholine release during paradoxical sleep in the dorsal tegmental field of the cat brain stem. *Neurosci Lett* 1990;114:277–82.

33. Webster HH, Jones BE. Neurotoxic lesions of the dorsolateral pontomesencephalic tegmentum-cholinergic cell area in the cat. II. Effects upon sleep-waking states. *Brain Res* 1988;458:285–302.

34. Steriade M, Pare D, Datta S, et al. Different cellular types in mesopontine cholinergic nuclei related to ponto-geniculo-occipital waves. *J Neurosci* 1990;10:2560–79.

35. Datta S, Siwek DF. Single cell activity patterns of pedunculopontine tegmentum neurons across the sleep-wake cycle in the freely moving rats. *J Neurosci Res* 2002;70:611–21.

36. Nitz D, Siegel JM. GABA release in posterior hypothalamus across sleep-wake cycle. *Am J Physiol* 1996;271:R1707–12.

37. Nitz D, Siegel J. GABA release in the dorsal raphe nucleus: role in the control of REM sleep. *Am J Physiol* 1997;273:R451–5.

38. Gervasoni D, Darracq L, Fort P, et al. Electrophysiological evidence that noradrenergic neurons of the rat locus coeruleus are tonically inhibited by GABA during sleep. *Eur J Neurosci* 1998;10:964–70.

39. Wilson S, Argyropoulos S. Antidepressants and sleep: a qualitative review of the literature. Drugs 2005;65:927–47.

40. Boissard R, Gervasoni D, Schmidt MH, et al. The rat ponto-medullary network responsible for paradoxical sleep onset and maintenance: a combined microinjection and functional neuroanatomical study. *Eur J Neurosci* 2002;16:1959–73.

41. Lu J, Sherman D, Devor M, et al. A putative flip-flop switch for control of REM sleep. *Nature* 2006;441:589–94.

42. Kaur S, Thankachan S, Begum S, et al. Hypocretin-2 saporin lesions of the ventrolateral periaquaductal gray (vlPAG) increase REM sleep in hypocretin knockout mice. *PLoS One* 2009;4:e6346.

43. de Lecea L, Kilduff TS, Peyron C, et al. The hypocretins: hypothalamus-specific peptides with neuroexcitatory activity. *Proc Natl Acad Sci USA* 1998;95:322–7.

44. Peyron C, Tighe DK, van den Pol AN, et al. Neurons containing hypocretin (orexin) project to multiple neuronal systems. *J Neurosci* 1998;18:9996–10015.

45. Lee MG, Hassani OK, Jones BE. Discharge of identified orexin/hypocretin neurons across the sleep-waking cycle. *J Neurosci* 2005;25:6716–20.

46. Mileykovskiy BY, Kiyashchenko LI, Siegel JM. Behavioral correlates of activity in identified hypocretin/orexin neurons. Neuron 2005;46:787–98.

47. Nishino S, Okuro M, Kotorii N, et al. Hypocretin/orexin and narcolepsy: new basic and clinical insights. *Acta Physiol (Oxf)* 2010;198(3):209–22.

48. Adamantidis AR, Zhang F, Aravanis AM, et al. Neural substrates of awakening probed with optogenetic control of hypocretin neurons. *Nature* 2007;450:420–4.

49. Nishino S, Ripley B, Overeem S, et al. Low cerebrospinal fluid hypocretin (Orexin) and altered energy homeostasis in human narcolepsy. *Ann Neurol* 2001;50:381–8.

50. Peyron C, Faraco J, Rogers W, et al. A mutation in a case of early onset narcolepsy and a generalized absence of hypocretin peptides in human narcoleptic brains. *Nat Med* 2000;6:991–7.

51. Thannickal TC, Moore RY, Nienhuis R, et al. Reduced number of hypocretin neurons in human narcolepsy. *Neuron* 2000;27:469–74.

52. Chemelli RM, Willie JT, Sinton CM, et al. Narcolepsy in orexin knockout mice: molecular genetics of sleep regulation. *Cell* 1999;98:437–51.

53. Ohno K, Sakurai T. Orexin neuronal circuitry: role in the regulation of sleep and wakefulness. *Front Neuroendocrinol* 2008;29:70–87.

54. Siegel JM. Hypocretin (orexin): role in normal behavior and neuropathology. *Ann Rev Psychol* 2004;55:125–48.

55. Eriksson KS, Sergeeva OA, Haas HL, et al. Orexins/hypocretins and aminergic systems. *Acta Physiol (Oxf)* 2010;198(3):263–75.

56. Thakkar MM, Ramesh V, Cape EG, et al. REM sleep enhancement and behavioral cataplexy following orexin (hypocretin)-II receptor antisense perfusion in the pontine reticular formation. *Sleep Res Online* 1999;2:112–20.

57. Lin L, Faraco J, Li R, et al. The sleep disorder canine narcolepsy is caused by a mutation in the hypocretin (orexin) receptor 2 gene. *Cell* 1999;98:365–76.

58. Bittencourt JC, Presse F, Arias C, et al. The melanin-concentrating hormone system of the rat brain: an immuno- and hybridization histochemical characterization. *J Comp Neurol* 1992;319:218–45.

59. Verret L, Goutagny R, Fort P, et al. A role of melanin-concentrating hormone producing neurons in the central regulation of paradoxical sleep. *BMC Neurosci* 2003;4:19.

60. Modirrousta M, Mainville L, Jones BE. Orexin and MCH neurons express c-Fos differently after sleep deprivation vs. recovery and bear different adrenergic receptors. *Eur J Neurosci* 2005;21:2807–16.

61. Hassani OK, Lee MG, Jones BE. Melanin-concentrating hormone neurons discharge in a reciprocal manner to orexin neurons across the sleep-wake cycle. *Proc Natl Acad Sci USA* 2009;106:2418–22.

62. Ahnaou A, Drinkenburg WH, Bouwknecht JA, et al. Blocking melanin-concentrating hormone MCH1 receptor affects rat sleep-wake architecture. *Eur J Pharmacol* 2008;579:177–88.

63. Fort P, Bassetti CL, Luppi PH. Alternating vigilance states: new insights regarding neuronal networks and mechanisms. *Eur J Neurosci* 2009;29:1741–53.

64. Willie JT, Sinton CM, Maratos-Flier E, et al. Abnormal response of melanin-concentrating

hormone deficient mice to fasting: hyperactivity and rapid eye movement sleep suppression. *Neuroscience* 2008;156:819–29.

65. Borbely AA. A two process model of sleep regulation. *Hum Neurobiol* 1982;1:195–204.

66. Ko CH, Takahashi JS. Molecular components of the mammalian circadian clock. *Hum Mol Genet* 2006;15(Spec No 2):R271–7.

67. Moore RY. Suprachiasmatic nucleus in sleep-wake regulation. Sleep Med 2007;8(Suppl 3):27–33.

68. Turek FW, Gillette MU. Melatonin, sleep, and circadian rhythms: rationale for development of specific melatonin agonists. *Sleep Med* 2004;5:523–32.

69. Mistlberger RE. Circadian regulation of sleep in mammals: role of the suprachiasmatic nucleus. *Brain Res Brain Res Rev* 2005;49:429–54.

70. Edgar DM, Dement WC, Fuller CA. Effect of SCN lesions on sleep in squirrel monkeys: evidence for opponent processes in sleep-wake regulation. *J Neurosci* 1993;13:1065–79.

71. Fuller PM, Gooley JJ, Saper CB. Neurobiology of the sleep-wake cycle: sleep architecture, circadian regulation, and regulatory feedback. *J Biol Rhythms* 2006;21:482–93.

72. Lehman MN, Silver R, Gladstone WR, et al. Circadian rhythmicity restored by neural transplant. Immunocytochemical characterization of the graft and its integration with the host brain. *J Neurosci* 1987;7:1626–38.

73. Zhou QY, Cheng MY. Prokineticin 2 and circadian clock output. *Febs J* 2005;272:5703–9.

74. Kramer A, Yang FC, Snodgrass P, et al. Regulation of daily locomotor activity and sleep by hypothalamic EGF receptor signaling. *Science* 2001;294:2511–15.

75. Gooley JJ, Saper CB. Anatomy of the mammalian circadian system. In: Kryger MH, Roth T, Dement WC, eds. *Principles and Practice of Sleep Medicine*, 4th ed. New York: Elsevier Saunders; 2005:335–50.

76. Chou TC, Scammell TE, Gooley JJ, et al. Critical role of dorsomedial hypothalamic nucleus in a wide range of behavioral circadian rhythms. *J Neurosci* 2003;23:10691–702.

77. Saint-Mleux B, Bayer L, Eggermann E, et al. Suprachiasmatic modulation of noradrenaline release in the ventrolateral preoptic nucleus. *J Neurosci* 2007;27:6412–16.

78. Benington JH, Heller HC. Restoration of brain energy metabolism as the function of sleep. *Prog Neurobiol* 1995;45:347–60.

79. Obal F, Jr., Krueger JM. Biochemical regulation of non-rapid-eye-movement sleep. *Front Biosci* 2003;8:d520–50.

80. Blanco-Centurion C, Xu M, Murillo-Rodriguez E, et al. Adenosine and sleep homeostasis in the basal forebrain. *J Neurosci* 2007;26:8092–100.

81. Porkka-Heiskanen T, Kalinchuk AV. Adenosine, energy metabolism and sleep homeostasis. *Sleep Med Rev* 2011;15:123–35.

82. Basheer R, Strecker RE, Thakkar MM, et al. Adenosine and sleep-wake regulation. *Prog Neurobiol* 2004;73:379–96.

83. Landolt HP. Sleep homeostasis: a role for adenosine in humans? *Biochem Pharmacol* 2008;75:2070–9.

84. Porkka-Heiskanen T, Strecker RE, Thakkar M, et al. Adenosine: a mediator of the sleep-inducing effects of prolonged wakefulness. *Science* 1997;276:1265–8.

85. Alam MN, Szymusiak R, Gong H, et al. Adenosinergic modulation of rat basal forebrain neurons during sleep and waking: neuronal recording with microdialysis. *J Physiol* 1999;521(Pt 3):679–90.

86. Thakkar MM, Delgiacco RA, Strecker RE, et al. Adenosinergic inhibition of basal forebrain wakefulness-active neurons: a simultaneous unit recording and microdialysis study in freely behaving cats. *Neuroscience* 2003;122:1107–13.

87. Morairty S, Rainnie D, McCarley R, et al. Disinhibition of ventrolateral preoptic area sleep-active neurons by adenosine: a new mechanism for sleep promotion. *Neuroscience* 2004;123:451–7.

88. Rai S, Kumar S, Alam MA, et al. A(1) receptor mediated adenosinergic regulation of perifornical-lateral hypothalamic area neurons in freely behaving rats. *Neuroscience* 2010;167:40–8.

89. Methippara MM, Kumar S, Alam MN, et al. Effects on sleep of microdialysis of adenosine A1 and A2a receptor analogs into the lateral preoptic area of rats. *Am J Physiol Regul Integr Comp Physiol* 2005;289:R1715–23.

90. Gallopin T, Luppi PH, Cauli B, et al. The endogenous somnogen adenosine excites a subset of sleep-promoting neurons via A2A receptors in the ventrolateal preoptic nucleus. *Neuroscience* 2005;134:1377–90.

91. Huang ZL, Qu WM, Eguchi N, et al. Adenosine A2A, but not A1, receptors mediate the arousal effect of caffeine. *Nat Neurosci* 2005;8:858–9.

92. Scammell TE, Gerashchenko DY, Mochizuki T, et al. An adenosine A2a agonist increases sleep and induces Fos in ventrolateral preoptic neurons. *Neuroscience* 2001;107:653–63.

93. Halassa MM, Florian C, Fellin T, et al. Astrocytic modulation of sleep homeostasis and cognitive consequences of sleep loss. *Neuron* 2009;61:213–19.

94. Imeri L, Opp MR. How (and why) the immune system makes us sleep. *Nat Rev Neurosci* 2009;10:199–210.

95. Opp MR, Obal F, Jr., Krueger JM. Interleukin 1 alters rat sleep: temporal and dose-related effects. *Am J Physiol* 1991;260:R52–8.

96. Terao A, Matsumura H, Saito M. Interleukin-1 induces slow-wave sleep at the prostaglandin D2-sensitive sleep-promoting zone in the rat brain. *J Neurosci* 1998;18:6599–607.

97. Chang FC, Opp MR. IL-1 is a mediator of increases in slow-wave sleep induced by CRH receptor blockade. *Am J Physiol Regul Integr Comp Physiol* 2000;279:R793–802.

98. Opp MR, Imeri L. Rat strains that differ in corticotropin-releasing hormone production exhibit different sleep-wake responses to interleukin 1. *Neuroendocrinology* 2001;73:272–84.

99. Opp MR, Krueger JM. Anti-interleukin-1 beta reduces sleep and sleep rebound after sleep deprivation in rats. *Am J Physiol* 1994;266:R688–95.

100. Takahashi S, Fang J, Kapas L, et al. Inhibition of brain interleukin-1 attenuates sleep rebound after sleep deprivation in rabbits. *Am J Physiol* 1997;273:R677–82.

101. Fang J, Wang Y, Krueger JM. Effects of interleukin-1 beta on sleep are mediated by the type I receptor. *Am J Physiol* 1998;274:R655–60.

102. Alam MN, McGinty D, Bashir T, et al. Interleukin-1beta modulates state-dependent discharge activity of preoptic area and basal forebrain neurons: role in sleep regulation. *Eur J Neurosci* 2004;20:207–16.

103. Tabarean IV, Korn H, Bartfai T. Interleukin-1beta induces hyperpolarization and modulates synaptic inhibition in preoptic and anterior hypothalamic neurons. *Neuroscience* 2006;141:1685–95.

104. Kapas L, Fang J, Krueger JM. Inhibition of nitric oxide synthesis inhibits rat sleep. *Brain Res* 1994;664:189–96.

105. Datta S, Patterson EH, Siwek DF. Endogenous and exogenous nitric oxide in the pedunculopontine tegmentum induces sleep. *Synapse* 1997;27:69–78.

106. Monti JM, Jantos H, Monti D. Increase of waking and reduction of NREM and REM sleep after nitric oxide synthase inhibition: prevention with GABA(A) or adenosine A(1) receptor agonists. *Behav Brain Res* 2001;123:23–35.

107. Monti JM, Jantos H. Effects of L-arginine and SIN-1 on sleep and waking in the rat during both phases of the light-dark cycle. *Life Sci* 2004;75:2027–34.

108. Kalinchuk AV, Stenberg D, Rosenberg PA, et al. Inducible and neuronal nitric oxide synthases (NOS) have complementary roles in recovery sleep induction. *Eur J Neurosci* 2006;24:1443–56.

109. Burlet S, Cespuglio R. Voltammetric detection of nitric oxide (NO) in the rat brain: its variations throughout the sleep-wake cycle. *Neurosci Lett* 1997;226:131–5.

110. Kalinchuk AV, Lu Y, Stenberg D, et al. Nitric oxide production in the basal forebrain is required for recovery sleep. *J Neurochem* 2006;99:483–98.

111. Kalinchuk AV, McCarley RW, Porkka-Heiskanen T, et al. Sleep deprivation triggers inducible nitric oxide-dependent nitric oxide production in wake-active basal forebrain neurons. *J Neurosci* 2010;30:13254–64.

112. Kostin A, Rai S, Kumar S, et al. Nitric oxide production in the perifornical-lateral hypothalamic area and its influences on the modulation of perifornical-lateral hypothalamic area neurons. *Neuroscience* 2011;179:159–69.

113. Kostin A, Stenberg D, Kalinchuk AV, et al. Nitric oxide modulates the discharge rate of basal forebrain neurons. *Psychopharmacology (Berl)* 2008;201:147–60.

114. Kilduff TS, Cauli, B, Geraschenko D. Activation of cortical interneurons during sleep: an anatomical link to homeostatic sleep regulation? *Trends Neurosci* 2011;34:10–20.

115. Chen L, Majde JA, Krueger JM. Spontaneous sleep in mice with targeted disruptions of neuronal or inducible nitric oxide synthase genes. *Brain Res* 2003;973:214–22.

116. Obal F, Jr., Krueger JM. GHRH and sleep. *Sleep Med Rev* 2004;8:367–77.

117. Nistico G, De Sarro GB, Bagetta G, et al. Behavioural and electrocortical spectrum power effects of growth hormone releasing factor in rats. *Neuropharmacology* 1987;26:75–8.

118. Marshall L, Derad I, Strasburger CJ, et al. A determinant factor in the efficacy of GHRH administration in promoting sleep: high peak concentration versus recurrent increasing slopes. *Psychoneuroendocrinology* 1999;24:363–70.

119. Bredow S, Taishi P, Obel F, Jr., et al. Hypothalamic growth hormone-releasing hormone mRNA varies across the day in rats. *Neuroreport* 1996;7:2501–5.

120. Toppila J, Alanko L, Asikainen M, et al. Sleep deprivation increases somatostatin and growth hormone-releasing hormone messenger RNA in the rat hypothalamus. *J Sleep Res* 1997;6:171–8.

121. Obal F, Jr., Alt J, Taishi P, et al. Sleep in mice with nonfunctional growth hormone-releasing hormone receptors. *Am J Physiol Regul Integr Comp Physiol* 2003;284:R131–9.

122. Zhang J, Obal F, Jr., Zheng T, et al. Intrapreoptic microinjection of GHRH or its antagonist alters sleep in rats. *J Neurosci* 1999;19:2187–94.

123. Peterfi Z, McGinty D, Sarai E, et al. Growth hormone-releasing hormone activates sleep regulatory neurons of the rat preoptic hypothalamus. *Am J Physiol Regul Integr Comp Physiol* 2011;298:R147–56.

124. Hayaishi O, Urade Y. Prostaglandin D2 in sleep-wake regulation: recent progress and perspectives. *Neuroscientist* 2002;8:12–15.

125. Huang ZL, Urade Y, Hayaishi O. Prostaglandins and adenosine in the regulation of sleep and wakefulness. *Curr Opin Pharmacol* 2007;7:33–8.

126. Koyama Y, Hayaishi O. Modulation by prostaglandins of activity of sleep-related neurons in the preoptic/anterior hypothalamic areas in rats. *Brain Res Bull* 1994;33:367–72.

127. Scammell T, Gerashchenko D, Urade Y, et al. Activation of ventrolateral preoptic neurons by the somnogen prostaglandin D2. *Proc Natl Acad Sci USA* 1998;95:7754–9.

128. Mizoguchi A, Eguchi N, Kimura K, et al. Dominant localization of prostaglandin D receptors on arachnoid trabecular cells in mouse basal forebrain and their involvement in the regulation of non-rapid eye movement sleep. Proc Natl Acad Sci USA 2001;98:11674–9.

129. Hayaishi O, Urade Y, Eguchi N, et al. Genes for prostaglandin d synthase and receptor as well as adenosine A2A receptor are involved in the homeostatic regulation of nrem sleep. *Arch Ital Biol* 2004;142:533–9.

130. Gallopin T, Fort P, Eggermann E, et al. Identification of sleep-promoting neurons in vitro. *Nature* 2000;404:992–5.

131. Modirrousta M, Mainville L, Jones BE. Gabaergic neurons with alpha2-adrenergic receptors in basal forebrain and preoptic area express c-Fos during sleep. *Neuroscience* 2004;129:803–10.

132. Cirelli C, Tononi G. Differential expression of plasticity-related genes in waking and sleep and their regulation by the noradrenergic system. *J Neurosci* 2000;20:9187–94.

133. Franken P, Dijk DJ. Circadian clock genes and sleep homeostasis. *Eur J Neurosci* 2009;29:1820–9.

134. Lu J, Bjorkum AA, Xu M, et al. Selective activation of the extended ventrolateral preoptic nucleus during rapid eye movement sleep. *J Neurosci* 2002;22:4568–76.

5

The Control of Motoneurons during Sleep

MICHAEL H. CHASE, SIMON J. FUNG, JACK YAMUY,
AND MING-CHU XI

WE FIRST present a discussion of the cellular mechanisms that result in an increase (hypertonia) or decrease (hypotonia or atonia) in muscle tone during states of sleep and wakefulness.[1,2] Subsequently, the brainstem sites, circuitry, and neurotransmitters that control the state-dependent patterns of motoneuron excitability during sleep and wakefulness are presented. Unless otherwise specified, the information presented in this chapter is based on data that are presented in the References.[3–9]

MOTONEURON EXCITABILITY DURING SLEEP AND WAKEFULNESS

One reflection of the excitability of motoneurons is the degree of polarization of their membrane potential.[5] Generally, when a motoneuron is hyperpolarized, it is relatively less excitable; when it is depolarized, it is more excitable. When depolarization of a motoneuron reaches a certain "threshold" level, the motoneuron discharges, that is, a spike potential is initiated at the axon hillock of the cell's soma, which results in contraction of the muscle fibers that are innervated by the motoneuron. Thus, there is a direct positive correlation between the degree of polarization of a motoneuron's membrane potential, the discharge of the motoneuron, and the contraction of the innervated musculature.

During wakefulness, in the absence of movements, most somatic muscles exhibit a low level of activity or tone. The passage from quiet wakefulness to quiet sleep is accompanied by a slight reduction in muscle tone, that is, hypotonia.[7,8,10–12]* Atonia (i.e., an absence of muscle contraction or tone) occurs during active sleep.[7,8,10–12] However, during active sleep

---

*In the animal literature, non-REM sleep is often referred to as quiet sleep, and REM sleep is called active sleep.[8]

there are also brief periods of muscle twitches and jerks that occur against a background of atonia.[7,8,10–12] On the basis of these patterns of decreased and increased motor activity, active sleep is divided into sustained "tonic" periods of atonia and brief phasic periods of motor activation.

Practically all somatic muscles exhibit the preceding pattern of control during active sleep. Thus, muscles that are innervated by motoneurons that are located throughout the neuraxis are tonically suppressed, to greater (atonia) or lesser (hypotonia) degrees, and phasically excited, during active sleep. This pattern of control has been documented for muscles innervated by ventral horn neurons throughout the spinal cord, as well as the masseter, digastric and diaphragmatic muscles, the extrinsic and intrinsic muscles of the larynx, the submental muscle, and various pharyngeal muscles, among others.[13,14] Even ocular muscles are inhibited and phasically excited during active sleep, which results in brief intermittent bursts of rapid eye movement.[15–18]

The muscles of the middle ear, however, are not subjected to motor suppression for they exhibit an increase in activity during active sleep.[19] This idiosyncratic pattern of motor control may reflect the function of middle ear muscles, which is to reduce the transmission of auditory information. Consequently, activation of the middle ear musculature can be viewed as being congruent with the general inhibition of motor activity during active sleep, since both patterns of control result in reduced responsiveness to external or intrinsic (internal) excitatory stimuli during this state (see section on "Reticular Response-Reversal and Motor Control").

Transitions between Wakefulness and Quiet (Non-REM) Sleep

When animals (and humans) are awake and resting quietly, passage into quiet sleep from wakefulness is accompanied by either a slight increase or no discernible change in the degree of motoneuron hyperpolarization. When an animal is alert or actively moving immediately before entering into quiet sleep, the subsequent transition to quiet sleep is accompanied by a relatively greater increase in the degree of hyperpolarization. In most cases, the membrane potential of motoneurons is slightly hyperpolarized during the transition from wakefulness to quiet sleep.

The transition from quiet sleep to aroused wakefulness is accompanied by membrane depolarization (Fig. 5.1). The degree of depolarization is usually correlated with the level of arousal, as indicated in the initial 15-second period of wakefulness in Figure 5.1 and the subsequent 15-second epoch, in which there occurs an increase in neck muscle activity and membrane depolarization.

Transition from Quiet (Non-REM) Sleep to Active (REM) Sleep

Motoneurons are significantly hyperpolarized during active sleep compared with quiet sleep (Fig. 5.2). The development of hyperpolarization parallels the various ways in which the transition occurs from quiet sleep to active sleep. For example, although the onset of active sleep is demarcated by electroencephalographic desynchronization and a reduction in muscle tone, these indices do not always appear at the same time and either may precede the other as the animal enters the active sleep state. However, electroencephalographic desynchronization and electromyographic suppression (see Fig. 5.2, 3- to 4-minute time marks) usually are correlated with each other and with membrane hyperpolarization.

Transition from Active (REM) Sleep to Wakefulness

The membrane potential of motoneurons rapidly depolarizes when wakefulness occurs following active sleep (see Fig. 5–2, 12- to 13-minute marks). The degree of depolarization almost always exceeds the level maintained during the preceding episode of quiet sleep.

In summary, the membrane potential of motoneurons is only slightly hyperpolarized or remains at the same potential level when quiet wakefulness precedes quiet sleep. However, motoneurons are strongly hyperpolarized during active sleep compared with any other state; that is, motoneurons are less excitable during active sleep compared with quiet sleep and wakefulness.

SYNAPTIC CONTROL OF MOTONEURONS DURING SLEEP AND WAKEFULNESS

The synapse is the site at which the state-dependent control of motoneurons takes place.

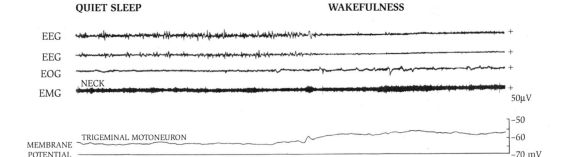

QUIET SLEEP   **WAKEFULNESS**

FIGURE 5.1   Intracellular recording from a trigeminal jaw-closer motoneuron: change in membrane potential during quiet sleep compared with wakefulness. When quiet sleep was followed by sustained wakefulness, membrane depolarization occurred. The degree of depolarization was positively correlated with the level of arousal and muscular activity during wakefulness, as shown in the middle of the figure when a brief increase in neck electromyogram (EMG) activity was correlated with a time-locked decrease in membrane polarization. Membrane potential band pass on polygraphic record: DC to 0.1 Hz. Other polygraphic traces are the same as in Figure 5.2: EEG, electroencephalogram; EMG, electromyogram; EOG, electro-oculogram. (From Chase MH: The motor functions of the reticular formation are multifaceted and state-determined. In Hobson JM, Brazier MAB [eds]: Reticular Formation Revisited. New York, Raven Press, 1980, p. 449.)

This control is evidenced by the presence of synaptic potentials. Consequently, an examination of the synaptic control of motoneurons is central to understanding motor control during sleep as well as wakefulness.

The synaptic control of motoneurons during quiet sleep compared with active wakefulness is reflected primarily by a decrease in the degree of motor activation. Thus, disfacilitation, or the withdrawal of excitatory synaptic potentials that impinge on motoneurons, is the principal control mechanism that is responsible for the decrease in motor activity during quiet sleep compared with the waking state. In contrast to the withdrawal of excitatory synaptic drives during quiet sleep, active sleep is characterized by complex patterns of synaptic control that entail the generation of inhibitory as well as excitatory postsynaptic potentials that are directed to motoneurons.

Inhibitory Postsynaptic Potentials during the Tonic and Phasic Periods of Active (REM) Sleep

During the tonic periods of active sleep, motoneurons are bombarded by an enormous number of inhibitory postsynaptic potentials (IPSPs)

(Fig. 5.3A). These are large-amplitude, high-frequency IPSPs that are unique to this state. These active sleep-specific IPSPs (AS-IPSPs) are readily reversed by the intracellular iontophoretic injection of chloride ions (see Fig. 5.3B), a finding that indicates that the responsible synapses are situated close to the soma region; therefore, they are strategically located to exert a potent pattern of suppression of motoneuron activity.

Since there is a unique set of inhibitory synapses that generate these large-amplitude IPSPs which are activated only during active sleep, there must exist a group of inhibitory interneurons that are driven to discharge, selectively, during this state. Evidence developed with immunohistochemical techniques supports the conclusion that the active sleep-specific inhibitory premotor neurons, rather than being located in the spinal cord, are situated in the brainstem; their axons end directly on spinal cord and brainstem (e.g., masseter, hypoglossal) motoneurons.[4,20] These active sleep-specific IPSPs represent the direct synaptic expression of a supraspinal inhibitory system that is responsible for promoting the suppression of motoneuron activity and the generation of atonia during active sleep.

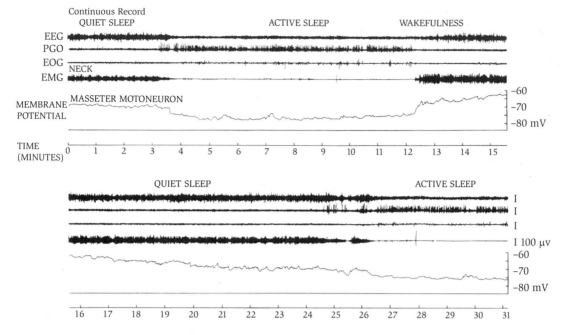

FIGURE 5.2 Intracellular recording from a trigeminal jaw-closer motoneuron: correlation of membrane potential and state changes. The membrane potential increased rather abruptly at 3.5 minutes in conjunction with the decrease in neck muscle tone and transition from quiet to active sleep. At 12.5 minutes the membrane depolarized and the animal awakened. After the animal passed into quiet sleep again, a brief, aborted episode of active sleep occurred at 25.5 minutes that was accompanied by a phasic period of hyperpolarization. A minute later the animal once again entered active sleep, and the membrane potential increased. Electroencephalogram (EEG) trace; marginal cortex, membrane potential bandpass on polygraphic record, DC to 0.1 Hz. EMG, electromyogram; EOG, electro-oculogram; PGO, ponto-geniculo-occipital potential. (From Chase MH: The motor functions of the reticular formation are multifaceted and state-determined. In Hobson JM, Brazier MAB (eds): Reticular Formation Revisited. New York, Raven Press, 1980, p. 449.)

The phasic periods of active sleep are characterized by brief episodes of rapid eye movements and twitches and jerks of the somatic musculature. During these periods, there are also phasic enhancements of postsynaptic inhibition, as evidenced by an increase in the number and amplitude of the AS-IPSPs.[3,6] In addition, when ponto-geniculo-occipital (PGO) waves occur during active sleep, enhanced inhibitory postsynaptic potentials are also directed to motoneurons; these inhibitory potentials are reflected by the appearance of a complex pattern of motoneuron hyperpolarization that is centered around PGO waves (see Fig. 5.3C and D). Thus, it is clear that the postsynaptic inhibitory process that suppresses motoneuron excitability tonically during active sleep continues, and is enhanced, during the phasic periods. The result is a further reduction in the excitability of motoneurons during the phasic periods that occurs even in the presence of excitatory drives that are simultaneously directed to motoneurons.

Neurotransmitter Responsible for the Inhibitory Synaptic Control of Motoneurons during Active (REM) Sleep

It is generally accepted that glycine, rather than gamma-aminobutyric acid (GABA), is the major inhibitory neurotransmitter that is involved in the control of motoneurons in the spinal cord.[21–23] Strychnine is an antagonist of glycine; picrotoxin and bicuculline are effective antagonists for the actions of GABA$_A$.[7,22,24,25] On the basis of the preceding, the neurotransmitter antagonists strychnine, picrotoxin, and

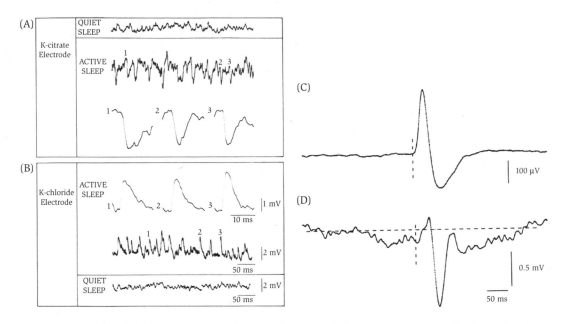

FIGURE 5.3 (A and B) Representative recording from two different motoneurons during quiet sleep and active sleep using microelectrodes filled with two different electrolyte solutions. (A) K-citrate electrode. During active sleep, hyperpolarizing potentials were easily distinguishable. Potentials labeled 1 to 3 are shown in an expanded format. Their 10% to 90% amplitude rise times, measured from the digitized record, were 1.4, 1.6, and 1 msec, respectively. B, K-chloride electrode. Recordings were maintained for 6 minutes during quiet sleep without any retention current. A hyperpolarizing current of 10 nA was passed for 45 seconds during quiet sleep approximately 1 minute before the animal entered into active sleep. The quiet sleep recording of the membrane potential was obtained after current injection had ceased. The active sleep record of the membrane potential revealed the advent of high-frequency depolarizing potentials. The potentials labeled 1 to 3 are shown in greater detail; their 10% to 90% rise times were 0.95, 1.05, and 1 msec, respectively. Depolarizing potentials like these were never observed during recording with K-citrate electrodes; they are interpreted as being reversed inhibitory potentials. Calibration signals are identical for the two cells. Both records are from sciatic motoneurons. Antidromic action potentials: A, 72 mV; B, 75 mV. (C and D) Changes in motoneuron membrane potential in conjunction with ipsilateral primary ponto-geniculo-occipital (PGO) waves. C and D are averages of 50 PGO waves and the corresponding motoneuron membrane potential. In this example, the changes in motoneuron membrane potential that were present in conjunction with PGO waves were PGO inhibitory postsynaptic potential (PGO-IPSP), the pre-PGO hyperpolarization, and a succession of IPSPs that followed the PGO-IPSP. The vertical dotted line marks the foot of the PGO wave, and the horizontal dotted line in D marks the baseline of the motoneuron membrane potential. (A and B from Chase MH, Morales FR: Phasic changes in motoneuron membrane potential during REM periods of active sleep. Neurosci Lett 34:177, 1982; C and D from Lopez-Rodriguez, et al., 1992.)

bicuculline were microiontophoretically administered adjacent to the cell bodies of motoneurons while intracellular records were obtained during naturally occurring episodes of sleep and wakefulness.[26–29]

The AS-IPSPs were found to be completely abolished by the juxtacellular microiontophoretic application of strychnine (Fig. 5.4A). This finding demonstrates that the neurotransmitter mediating these IPSPs is glycine. Neither picrotoxin nor bicuculline were effective in either suppressing the large-amplitude IPSPs of active sleep or in producing membrane depolarization. Since $GABA_A$ receptors produce IPSPs and $GABA_B$ receptors are associated with the generation of slow potential changes, it is evident that neither set of GABAergic receptors plays a role in the generation of the AS-IPSPs that are responsible for producing atonia during active sleep. Thus, glycine, but not GABA,

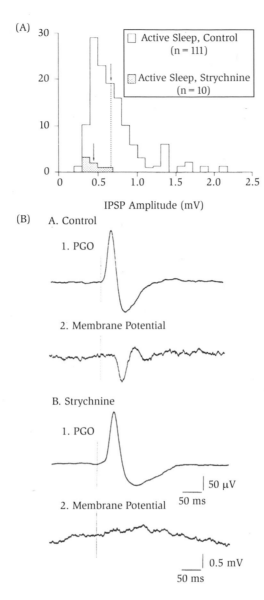

FIGURE 5.4 (*A*) Distribution of the amplitudes of spontaneous inhibitory postsynaptic potentials (IPSPs) recorded during active sleep from the same lumbar motoneuron before (open histogram) and after the microiontophoretic ejection of strychnine (dotted histogram). Arrows indicate the median value of each IPSP population. Note that before the application of strychnine, 50% of the potentials were larger in amplitude than the largest potential that was detected following the microiontophoretic ejection of strychnine (10 mM, 250 nA, 2.75 minutes). (*B*) Averaged ponto-geniculo-occipital (PGO) waves and the membrane potential in lumbar motoneurons recorded in two different cats before (control) (*A*) and following strychnine injection (*B*). The vertical bars are positioned at the foot of the averaged PGO waves. After the injection of strychnine, the PGO-related IPSP was no longer present; instead, a long depolarizing potential occurred. (*A* from Chase MH, Soja PJ, Morales FR: Evidence that glycine mediates the postsynaptic potentials that inhibit lumbar motoneurons during the atonia of active sleep. J Neurosci 9:743, 1989; *B* from Lopez-Rodriguez F, Morales FR, Soja PJ, Chase MH: Suppression of the PGO-related lumbar motoneuron IPSP by strychnine. Brain Res 535:331, 1990.)

is the postsynaptic inhibitory neurotransmitter that is responsible for muscle atonia during active sleep.

By applying strychnine juxtacellularly by microiontophoresis, it was also determined that PGO-related IPSPs in motoneurons during active sleep are also mediated by glycinergic synapses (see Fig. 5.4B). Therefore, the same inhibitory neurons that tonically inhibit motoneurons during active sleep are phasically activated during PGO waves. In addition, these potentials, and the neurotransmitter glycine, are responsible for the phasic enhancement of postsynaptic inhibition that occurs during the phasic periods of active sleep. In summary, the preceding data involve changes in hypoglossal, trigeminal, and spinal cord motoneuron activity during naturally occurring states of sleep and wakefulness. The data from these intracellular studies are consistent and reveal that glycinergic postsynaptic inhibition accounts for the atonia that occurs during active sleep.

There are only a few reports that have challenged the preceding body of data demonstrating that glycinergic postsynaptic inhibition accounts fully for the suppression of motoneuron activity during the tonic and phasic periods of active sleep. A critical review of these studies was conducted by a group of independent, knowledgeable researchers (see Critical Topics Forum in *Sleep*; Lydic, 2008[30]). They concluded that there was no credible reason to challenge the long-standing consensus that "glycinergic inhibition is the mechanisms controlling REM-sleep atonia" (Funk, 2008[31]), although under certain circumstances other mechanisms, for specific groups of motoneurons, may also influence motor excitability during active sleep.

EXCITATORY CONTROL OF MOTONEURONS DURING REM (ACTIVE) SLEEP

Postsynaptic inhibition is the principal synaptic process affecting motoneurons during the phasic periods of active sleep. In fact, all of the inhibitory phenomena that are described in the previous section are not only present but are also enhanced during the phasic periods of active sleep, including the frequency of the active sleep-specific IPSPs (Fig. 5.5A and B). How then could twitches and jerks of the eyes, limbs, diaphragm, and so on occur in the presence of enhanced inhibitory input to motoneurons? The answer is simple: the phasic periods

of active sleep are accompanied not only by increased motoneuron inhibition but also by the advent of strikingly potent motor excitatory drives (Figs. 5.6A to D).

The excitatory drives that impinge on motoneurons during the phasic periods of active sleep are revealed by the presence of motoneuron depolarization and spike potentials. This activity is illustrated in Figure 5.6A. During the second cluster of eye movements during this episode of active sleep, as shown in Figure 5.6B to D, there are depolarizing shifts in the membrane potential; subthreshold depolarizing potentials and action potentials are also present. These patterns of activation reflect descending excitatory activity emanating from supraspinal nuclei.[10,32]

To further understand the neurophysiologic basis for the excitatory drives that occur during the phasic periods of active sleep, antagonists of excitatory amino acids were individually applied, juxtacellularly, to motoneurons.[33] The broad-spectrum glutamatergic antagonist, kynurenic acid, completely abolished the phasic depolarizing events that occur during the phasic periods of active sleep. However, the N-methyl-D-aspartate (NMDA) blocker, aminophosphonovaleric acid (APV), did not have an effect. Therefore, we conclude that the excitatory motor events during phasic periods of active sleep are mediated by pathways that employ an amino acid such as glutamate as their neurotransmitter, and that its actions are mediated by non-NMDA receptors.[33,34]

Thus, from time to time, for reasons as yet unknown, during the phasic periods of active sleep, excitatory drives overpower inhibitory drives; motoneurons discharge and the muscle fibers that they innervate contract. These excitatory drives are accompanied by an increase in inhibitory drives; momentarily, the excitatory inputs predominate and motoneurons discharge (see Fig. 5.6). When motoneurons do discharge during the phasic periods of active sleep, their activity, as well as the resultant contraction of the muscles that they innervate, are unlike the pattern of motoneuron discharge that occurs during any other state; the resultant movements are abrupt, twitchy, and jerky; they are also without apparent purpose.

The coactivation of synaptic drives with opposite functions (inhibitory and excitatory) may appear, from a functional perspective, to be paradoxical. However, some rationality may be ascribed to each of these processes when

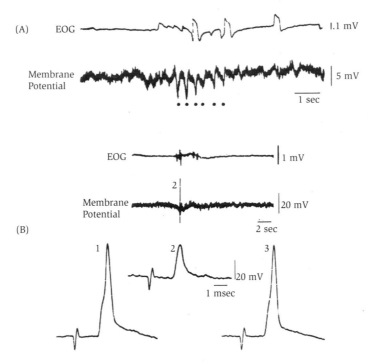

FIGURE 5.5 Summated hyperpolarizing membrane potentials (*A*) and blockade of antidromic action potentials (*B*) during active sleep accompanied by periods of rapid eye movements (REMs). In *A*, hyperpolarizing events arise (the most evident indicated by dots) that are composed of repetitively occurring inhibitory synaptic potentials. In *B*, an antidromic spike was induced immediately before (1) and after (3) a burst of REMs. When the antidromic action potential coincided with the period of hyperpolarizing potentials, the soma-dendritic spike was blocked and only the initial segment spike was present (2). Data are unfiltered; records were obtained from a peroneal motoneuron in *A* (resting membrane potential: −65mV) and from a tibial motoneuron in *B* (resting membrane potential: −72 mV). EOG, electro-oculogram. (From Chase MH, Morales FR: Phasic changes in motoneuron membrane potential during REM periods of active sleep. Neurosci Lett 34:177, 1982.)

they are examined individually. Although we do not understand the function of the phasic periods of active sleep (and perhaps rapid eye movements are only an easily observable indicator of a more basic process), we do know that during these periods most populations of cortical and subcortical cells discharge at rates that often exceed those that occur during wakefulness.[35] In fact, the activity of practically all motor pathways, including those whose discharge results in movements during wakefulness, is greatly enhanced during the phasic periods of active sleep.[32,35,36] The increase in inhibitory input that is present throughout active sleep may reflect a need to suppress contractions of the somatic musculature, thus protecting the organism from moving at a time when it is blind and unconscious.

In summary, postsynaptic inhibition is the principal process that is responsible not only for atonia of the somatic musculature during the tonic periods of active sleep but also for the phasic episodes of decreased motoneuron excitability that accompany bursts of rapid eye movements during this state. These postsynaptic processes depend on the presence of active sleep-specific IPSPs, which are mediated by glycine. The phasic excitation of motoneurons during active sleep is due to EPSPs which encounter motoneurons that are already subjected to enhanced postsynaptic inhibition via active sleep-specific IPSPs. As described in the following sections, there is a consensus that the preceding inhibitory drives originate in the ventromedial medulla and that cell groups in this region are activated by a more rostrally located nucleus, the nucleus

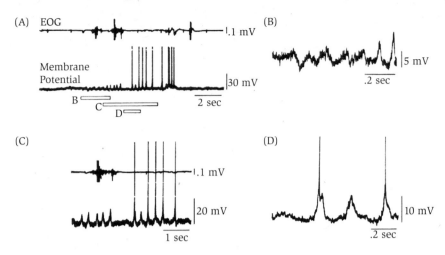

FIGURE 5.6 (A) Summated depolarizing potentials and spike activity in conjunction with active sleep periods of rapid eye movements (REMs). During the first burst of eye movements, phasic hyperpolarizing events arose (B). In conjunction with the second burst of eye movements, there was a series of rhythmic depolarizing shifts (C). Action potentials occurred during the third episode of eye movements; they were also present during the interval between the second and third bursts of ocular activity. The recordings over the bars in A are presented at a faster sweep speed and greater magnification in B, C, and D. In D, note that spikes arise from the first and third depolarizing shifts, whereas the second does not reach threshold. The action potentials in C and D are truncated because of the high gain of the records. Data are unfiltered; records were obtained from a tibial motoneuron (resting membrane potential: −70 mV). (From Chase MH, Morales FR: Phasic changes in motoneuron membrane potential during REM periods of active sleep. Neurosci Lett 34:177, 1982.)

pontis oralis, which is located in the pontine tegmentum.

BRAINSTEM CONTROL OF MOTONEURON INHIBITION DURING ACTIVE (REM) SLEEP

After a transection caudal to the medulla, facial muscles continue to be subjected to inhibition during active sleep, whereas the limb and trunk musculature are unaffected by changes in the animal's state of sleep and wakefulness.[37] A brainstem transection caudal to the mesencephalon does not significantly affect motor control during sleep and wakefulness.[37] Therefore, the neuronal elements that control motor inhibition during active sleep are situated caudal to the mesencephalon and rostral to the spinal cord. Consequently, the existence of active sleep-specific IPSPs (AS-IPSPs) reflects the activity of a supraspinal center that is located in the brainstem that activates inhibitory premotor neurons that discharge, selectively, during active sleep.

A coherent literature indicates that during active sleep, neurons within the nucleus pontis oralis (NPO), also called the sublateral dorsal nucleus, perilocus coeruleus alpha, and so on, which are activated by cholinergic projections from the LDT/PPT as well as glutamatergic projections from the amygdala and a number of substances, such as NGF, excite neurons in the NPO that send excitatory projections to the inhibitory region of Magoun and Rhines,[38] which in turn promote motor inhibition during active sleep.[13,20,39–42] Additional supporting data have emanated from immunocytochemical experiments that are based on the detection of the nuclear protein Fos, which is synthesized during neuronal activity.[43,44] In the ventral region of the medial medullary reticular formation, medial to the seventh nucleus and lateral to the inferior olive, during a pharmacologic state (AS-carbachol) that has been used successfully as a model of active sleep, there are, bilaterally, a great number of Fos-labeled cells (Fig. 5.7).[44] The region occupied by these cells corresponds to the inhibitory region of Magoun and Rhines.[38] Retrograde labeling, which was

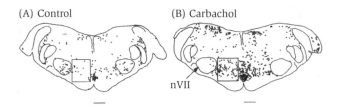

(A) Control   (B) Carbachol

nVII

FIGURE 5.7   Distribution of Fos + neurons in the medulla at the level of the facial nucleus of a control (*left*) and an AS-carbachol (*right*) cat. Each dot represents one Fos-labeled neuron. The region that contains double-labeled, Fos +, and cholera toxin + neurons is indicated by the squares. (Modified from Yamuy J, Mancillas JR, Morales FR, Chase MH: c-fos expression in the pons and medulla of the cat during carbachol-induced active sleep. J Neurosci 13:2703, 1993.)

achieved by injecting the subunit B of cholera toxin (Ctb), permitted the identification of neurons in this region that directly innervate motor nuclei.[4,20]

The most salient result of the combined use of the aforementioned techniques was the discovery of a subset of neurons in the ventral medulla that are not only activated during active sleep but that also innervate, monosynaptically, motor nuclei.[4] These premotor glycinergic neurons produce the postsynaptic inhibition of motoneurons, which results in the atonia of active sleep. Thus, a cascade of excitatory activity that originates in the nucleus pontis oralis activates medullary inhibitory premotor neurons, whose discharge results in motoneuron inhibition and muscle atonia during active sleep. This brainstem–spinal cord inhibitory system also encompasses the circuitry underlying the phenomenon of reticular response-reversal, which is described in the following section.

Reticular Response-Reversal and Motoneuron Control

Reticular response-reversal was discovered during the course of experiments investigating the control of motor activity by the nucleus pontis oralis, which is the executive pontine site that initiates active sleep as well as wakefulness (see Chase and Morales, 2005[13]; Chase et al., 1976,[45] Figs. 5.8 and 5.9). For these studies, chronically instrumented cats were implanted with electrodes to monitor sleep and waking states and to record the jaw-closing (masseteric) reflex. Sensory afferents in the masseter nerve were stimulated in order to induce the masseteric (jaw-closing) reflex whose amplitude was recorded, online, on an oscilloscope.

These experiments were designed to document the fact that reflex activity is enhanced when its induction is preceded by stimulation of the nucleus pontis oralis. This was the response that we expected, since the nucleus pontis oralis not only initiates active sleep but is also the heart of the reticular activating system, which generates arousal and promotes motor activities.[42]

However, during the course of these experiments, suddenly the reflex disappeared from the oscilloscopic screen. We thought that either the stimulator had failed or a recording lead had broken, but no equipment failure could be detected. So we continued the study and again observed an increase in reflex amplitude following stimulation of the nucleus pontis oralis, but after a few minutes, the reflex once more completely disappeared. The equipment was reexamined and confirmed to be working perfectly. At that moment the cat, which had been sleeping, awoke and began walking around in the experimental chamber. And when we glanced at the oscilloscopic screen, we saw that the reflex had reappeared. Instantly, there was a serendipitous scientific "Aha" moment when it dawned on us that the reflex might be disappearing only when the cat was asleep. And we were right. We then confirmed that the reflex response was absent whenever the animal was in active sleep, only to reappear at the exact moment that the animal either awoke or returned to quiet sleep. Subsequently, after a great number of studies, we were able to determine that it was the state of the animal—wakefulness, quiet sleep, or active sleep—and not any other factor that was determining whether motor activation or motor suppression resulted from stimulation of the nucleus pontis oralis. Thus was born the phenomenon of reticular response-reversal. This discovery led to the formulation of the concept

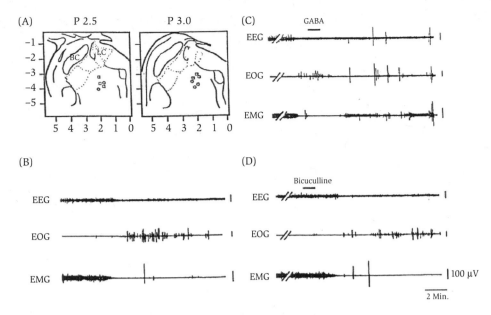

FIGURE 5.8   (A) The anatomic location of effective injection sites ($n = 11$) in the rostral pons of six cats. Schematic frontal planes of the cat brainstem are illustrated at levels P 2.5 and P 3.0. Sites where injections were delivered to the left and right side are indicated by circles and squares, respectively. Representative polygraphic recordings of an episode of spontaneous active sleep (B), an episode of wakefulness that occurred following the injection of gamma-aminobutyric acid (GABA) (C), and an active sleep episode that was induced following an injection of bicuculline, a GABA$_A$ receptor antagonist (D). The injection of GABA was performed during a spontaneous active sleep episode. Note that the bicuculline-induced state appears indistinguishable from a spontaneous episode of active sleep; however, the former lasted 52 minutes, almost eight times longer than the mean time of spontaneous episodes of active sleep. BC, brachium conjunctivum; EEG, electroencephalogram; EMG, electromyogram; EOG, electro-oculogram; LC, locus coeruleus. All vertical bars: 100μV. (From Xi MC, Morales FR, Chase MH: Evidence that wakefulness and REM sleep are controlled by a GABAergic pontine mechanism. J Neurophysiol 82:2015, 1999.)

underlying reticular-response reversal, which is that all activating or arousal-promoting stimuli, when present during wakefulness or quiet sleep, lead to enhanced motor activity, but when they occur during active sleep, they result in motor inhibition (Figs. 5.9 and 5.10).

The neuronal control exercised by reticular response-reversal is extraordinarily potent. It is consistently and dramatically evident in unanesthetized, undrugged chronic animals during spontaneously occurring states of sleep and wakefulness; in fact, it even persists during anesthesia (Fig. 5.10). Basically, all extrinsically generated or internally developed processes that are arousal promoting, which result in a general increase in motor activity during wakefulness, suppress somatomotor activity at all levels of the neuraxis when they occur during active sleep.

The basis for the functional reorganization of neuronal circuitry, which is reflected by reticular response-reversal, was determined by recording intracellularly from brainstem and spinal cord motoneurons. We found that prominent EPSPs are induced in motoneurons in conjunction with stimulation of the nucleus pontis oralis during wakefulness and quiet sleep (Fig. 5.9; Chandler et al.[46]). In contrast, during active sleep, following the excitation of the nucleus pontis oralis and its activation of premotor glycinergic cells in the medulla, potent glycinergically mediated IPSPs arise in motoneurons (Figs. 5.9 and 5.10).[13] Thus, we determined that motor suppression during active sleep, vis-à-vis reticular response-reversal, is mediated by glycinergic IPSPs.[13] In addition, during active sleep, depolarizing potentials were unmasked after stimuli-elicited IPSPs were abolished by

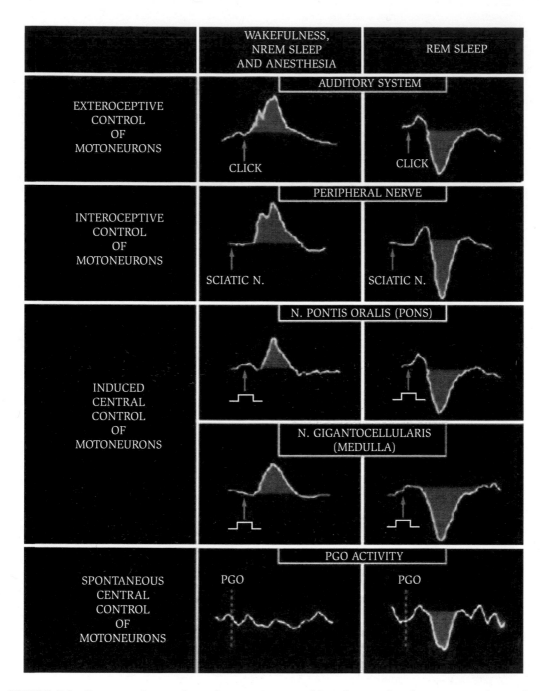

FIGURE 5.9 Patterns of state-dependent motor control based upon the phenomenon of reticular response-reversal. Motor inhibition during REM sleep replaces motor excitation during either wakefulness or non-REM sleep. Various excitatory stimuli that are accompanied by arousal or enhanced wakefulness result in the generation of depolarizing (i.e., excitation; upward cross-hatched deflection) postsynaptic activity in motoneurons during wakefulness, non-REM sleep, or anesthesia. On the other hand, when identical stimuli are present during REM sleep, motoneurons exhibit prominent hyperpolarizing (i.e., inhibitory; downward cross-hatched deflection) postsynaptic activity. However, the depolarizing drives that characterize the periods of wakefulness or NREM sleep are still present during REM sleep, as evidenced by the depolarizing potentials that immediately precede the onset of the more dominant hyperpolarizing potentials. (*See* color insert.)

the application of strychnine. Consequently, motor excitatory systems that are activated during wakefulness continue to exert their effects during active sleep, although functionally the excitatory drives are masked by more potent inhibitory inputs. The superimposition of inhibitory drives on excitatory inputs mirrors the motor control processes that occur spontaneously during the rapid eye movement periods of active sleep when, in a similar fashion, potent glycinergic inhibition takes place concurrently with excitatory postsynaptic potentials that are directed to the same motoneuron. This pattern of membrane potential modulation during the phasic periods of active sleep mirrors the phenomenon of reticular response-reversal.

The directives encompassed by reticular-response reversal extend far beyond the control of brainstem and spinal cord motoneuron activity by the nucleus pontis oralis, for they include other sites and systems that promote wakefulness and arousal by intrinsically or extrinsically generated inputs (Fig. 5.10). Thus, stimuli or conditions that promote arousal and/or an increase in motor activity during wakefulness and quiet sleep result in the suppression of motor activity

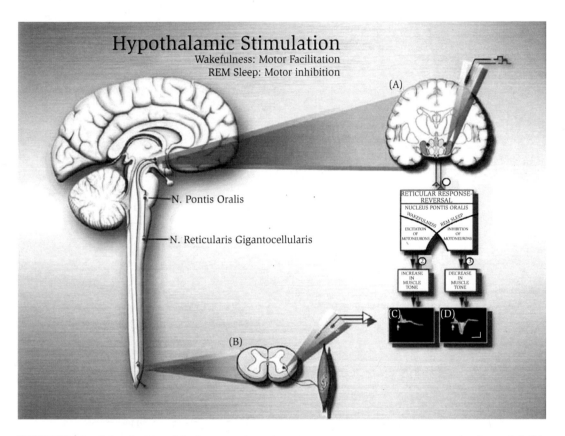

FIGURE 5.10 Stimulation of the hypocretinergic system promotes motoneuron excitation or inhibition according to the behavioral state of the individual. During wakefulness, intracellular recordings reveal that an excitatory potential (upward cross-hatched deflection) is induced in lumbar motoneurons. During carbachol-induced REM sleep, the same hypothalamic stimulus produces a large amplitude inhibitory (i.e., downward cross-hatched deflection) response (D). Note, however, that a short-latency depolarizing (excitatory) potential is still present during REM sleep, which is typical of reticular response-reversal. During wakefulness, the hypocretinergic system promotes an increase in motor activity by direct projections to brainstem nuclei such as the NPO and also to motoneurons. During REM sleep, these excitatory actions are superseded by hypocretinergically induced inhibitory drives. Cataplexy may be due to the absence of hypocretinergic directives, which would result in a decrease in motor activity during wakefulness and an increase during REM sleep. (See Yamuy et al., 2010.) (*See* color insert.)

when they occur during active sleep.[13] For example, auditory (e.g., clicks) and somatosensory stimuli (e.g., excitation of peripheral sensory nerves) result in the facilitation of motor activity during wakefulness and quiet sleep.[47] However, as soon as the animal enters active sleep, large amplitude IPSPs arise in response to the identical inputs.[47]

Reticular response-reversal is also part of the circuitry involved in the mechanisms of alerting during wakefulness as well as active sleep. PGO waves during wakefulness are associated with brief periods of intense arousal and motor activity, such as those which take place in conjunction with the startle reflex.[48] During active sleep, PGO waves also arise in conjunction with rapid eye movements during the phasic periods of this state. Each individual PGO wave as well as trains of PGO waves are time-locked to the generation of glycinergic postsynaptic potential motoneurons during active sleep, whereas EPSP activity and spike discharges are present when PGO waves occur during wakefulness.[29,49] This time-locked relationship between PGO waves and motoneuron IPSPs during active sleep suggests that both phenomena share common mechanisms of generation. Thus, the IPSPs of reticular response-reversal are likely generated by cells in the medulla (in and in the vicinity of the nucleus reticularis gigantocellularis) that are activated in response to stimulation of the nucleus pontis oralis. These glycinergic cells in the medulla produce atonia during active sleep.[13] Therefore, the premotor inhibitory neurons in the medulla that promote atonia during active sleep are also responsible for PGO-IPSPs, the IPSPs of reticular response-reversal, and the active-specific IPSPs that arise during the tonic and phasic periods of active sleep.

There are also important interactions between reticular-response reversal and the hypocretinergic system (Fig. 5.10). For example, one of the most prominent functional responses to activation of hypocretinergic neurons during wakefulness is arousal and motor activation.[50,51] Hypocretinergic axons project to the nucleus pontis oralis (NPO) as well as the nucleus reticularis gigantocellularis (including adjacent portions of the ventromedial medullary reticular formation).[52] These regions not only correspond to the brainstem-spinal cord system responsible for promoting arousal and somatomotor activation, but they are also responsible for producing active sleep and its accompanying patterns of physiological activity, including atonia

during this state.[13,53,54] Although not entirely unexpected, it was nevertheless surprising to find that the same hypocretinergic drives that produce arousal and motor activation yield, when an animal is in active sleep, postsynaptic glycine-mediated IPSPs in motoneurons, thus further confirming the ubiquitous role and importance of reticular response-reversal.

A number of extracellular recording studies demonstrate that hypocretinergic neurons are active during wakefulness; however, they also contain data which reveal that hypocretinergic cells discharge during active sleep.[55-57] In addition, studies of the expression of fos, which is an immediate early gene that is employed to detect cellular discharge, demonstrate that there is a population of hypocretinergic neurons that discharge during active sleep.[50] The preceding data confirm that hypocretin plays a role in active sleep in addition to promoting waking functions.

Participation of the hypocretinergic system in reticular response-reversal extends beyond the transformation of motor excitatory drives during wakefulness to motor inhibition during active sleep, for they also include mechanisms that control the states of wakefulness and active sleep. For example, when an animal is awake, the microinjection of hypocretin into the nucleus pontis oralis enhances wakefulness.[58] However, Xi et al.[58] have shown that when hypocretin is injected into the identical site during quiet sleep, active sleep is induced. Thus, the state of the animal at the time of the injection of hypocretin dictates whether the induced state is wakefulness or active sleep. Furthermore, as described earlier, reticular response-reversal involves, to a significant extent, hypocretin as a critical mediating neurotransmitter that is capable of promulgating dual directives which consist of the induction of wakefulness and somatomotor excitation as well as active sleep and motor inhibition.

PATHOLOGIC PATTERNS OF MOTONEURON CONTROL DURING ACTIVE (REM) SLEEP

The motor inhibition that normally occurs during active sleep, in conjunction with reticular response-reversal, functions to prevent the "alerting" consequences of a variety of excitatory stimuli by suppressing motor activities that would otherwise disrupt this sleep state.

From an evolutionary perspective, there are obvious advantages for an animal to remain quiescent during sleep, especially when its ability to process exteroceptive information is compromised, and its capabilities for responding are severely curtailed. The importance of these inhibitory processes is dramatically underscored when there is a deficiency in hypocretin, as discussed in the following section.

Thus, the suppression of movements during active sleep is necessary for an animal to maintain in this state and prevent it from moving when it is "functionally unconscious." Consequently, the release of glycine onto motoneurons during active sleep, which results in atonia, has implications of far-reaching and widespread importance. For example, abnormal patterns of motor behavior are evidenced by an abrupt and potent reduction in motor activity that occurs in disorders such as REM sleep behavior disorder (RBD). These and other sleep disorders that involve disrupted motor control during active sleep are the clinical reflections of the abnormal expression of the paradoxical phenomenon of reticular response-reversal.

Recent developments in the field of sleep medicine have resulted in a greater understanding of a variety of pathologic patterns of active sleep-related disorders (see Kryger, Roth, and Dement[59] for details of data referenced in this section). The following sections describe the disruption of inhibitory motor processes that occurs during pathologic conditions of active sleep and the abnormalities of motor control that ensue during this state.

PATHOLOGIC CONDITIONS INVOLVING AN INCREASE IN MOTOR ACTIVATION DURING REM (ACTIVE) SLEEP

REM behavior disorder (RBD) is a complex, vigorous, and often violent behavior that takes place during REM (active) sleep. Patients with RBD complain of sleep disruption; violent movements with injuries to themselves or to their bed partner; and unpleasant, vivid dreams. In these patients there is not only an abnormal preservation of muscle tone during some or all of active sleep, but there are also large-amplitude contractions of the peripheral musculature.

Numerous lines of evidence and a significant body of data that demonstrate that cataplexy is not only manifest by a decrease in muscle activity during wakefulness, but that it is also often accompanied by reduced motor suppression (i.e., hypotonia rather than atonia) during active sleep.[60,61] For example, close inspection of the records of narcoleptic dogs reveals a relative lack of muscle inhibition during cataplectic attacks in these animals (see Figure 1D in Mitler and Dement).[61] In addition, according to Jerome Siegel (personal communication), there is very poor motor suppression during active sleep in cataplectic canines. Thus, it is hypothesized that the mechanisms responsible for the preceding motor disorders that occur during wakefulness and active (REM) sleep in cataplexy are the result of a deficiency of hypocretin and the consequences of the resultant abnormal motor control that occurs due to processes that involve reticular-response reversal, as described in the following section.[62-64]

MECHANISMS RESPONSIBLE FOR PATHOLOGIC PATTERNS OF DECREASE IN MOTOR ACTIVITY DURING WAKEFULNESS—A PUTATIVE ROLE FOR HYPOCRETIN

At present, it is not clear how a lack of hypocretinergic functioning may be involved in cataplexy. One possibility is that hypocretin acts by modulating the activity of neurotransmitter cell groups that mediate sleep and wakefulness, for example, histaminergic neurons in the tuberomammillary nucleus, serotonergic neurons in the dorsal raphe, cholinergic neurons in the laterodorsal tegmental nucleus and the pedunculopontine tegmental nucleus, noradrenergic neurons in the locus coeruleus, and so on; all of these neuronal phenotypes are densely innervated by hypocretin terminals and contain their receptors.[52,63,65-68] Thakkar, Strecker, and McCarley (1998)[69] reported that the microdialysis of antisense to hypocretin-2 receptor into the rat pontine reticular formation increases active sleep and produces behavioral cataplexy, which indicates that the pons may be one of the sites of action of the hypocretinergic system vis-à-vis active sleep-related phenomena.

We have also obtained data that indicate that hypocretinergic axons project to the nucleus pontis oralis, as well as the nucleus reticularis gigantocellularis (including adjacent portions of the ventromedial medullary reticular formation) and to lamina 9 of the lumbar spinal cord, where spinal cord motoneurons are located.[70,71] These regions correspond to the brainstem-spinal cord system responsible for the suppression of motor activity that occurs during active sleep.[26,40,41,72] The microinjection of hypocretin into the NPO induces active sleep with a very short latency.[58] These findings have led us to hypothesize that the hypocretinergic system acts by modulating, through hypocretinergic synaptic contacts, the excitability of motoneurons, as well as the nuclei and circuitry that comprise the inhibitory system that controls motor excitability during active sleep.

Our working hypothesis is that the hypocretinergic system acts at various levels of the neuraxis to promote somatomotor activation during periods of arousal that occur during the waking state. We also suggest that hypocretin functions during active sleep to enhance/promote motor suppression during this state. This pattern of motor modulation mirrors precisely the control that we have described with respect to the phenomena of reticular response-reversal (see the section on "Reticular Response-Reversal and Motoneuron Control").

Consequently, in conjunction with certain behaviors during aroused wakefulness, when hypocretin is not present (or is present in a greatly reduced concentration), there is a reduction or absence of muscle activation; one consequence is cataplexy.[13,73–78] There are, however, other data which suggest that motor suppression during a cataplectic attack is due to the activation of motor inhibitory processes that are normally confined to active sleep.[79–83]

Clearly, there are paradoxical actions of hypocretin that are state dependent; namely, motoneuron excitation during wakefulness and motoneuron inhibition during active sleep on one hand, and the induction of arousal during wakefulness and the induction of active sleep during quiet sleep on the other. When there is a reduction in available hypocretin, pathological state-dependent patterns of motor control predominate during wakefulness as well as active sleep.

These dual actions of hypocretin mirror the phenomenon of reticular response-reversal. Thus, we believe that hypocretinergic neurons function within the context of reticular-response reversal to act at various levels of the neuraxis to enhance the nonreciprocal facilitation of motor activity during wakefulness and the nonreciprocal inhibition of motor activity during active (REM) sleep.

Pathologic circumstances arise and motor disorders of active sleep occur when there is an absence or deficiency of hypocretinergic actions. During wakefulness, there is an increase in motor suppression due to disruption of the circuitry of reticular-response reversal, which occurs as a result of a deficiency of hypocretin, whereas during active sleep, there is a decrease in the degree of atonia. Detailed knowledge of the role of the hypocretinergic system in mediating pathological patterns of motor control during sleep as well as wakefulness represents an important target for future research.

REFERENCES

1. Burke RE. Motor units: anatomy, physiology, and functional organization. In: *Handbook of Physiology. The Nervous System. Motor Control.* Bethesda, MD: American Physiology Society; 1981:345–422.
2. Hennemen E, Somjen G, Carpenter DO. Functional significance of cell size in spinal motoneurons. *J Neurophysiol* 1965;28:560–80.
3. Chase MH, Morales FR. Postsynaptic mechanisms responsible for motor inhibition during active sleep. In: Chase MH, Weitzman W, eds. *Sleep Disorders: Basic and Clinical Research.* New York: Spectrum; 1983:71.
4. Morales FR, Sampogna S, Yamuy J, et al. C-fos expression in brainstem premotor interneurons during cholinergically induced active sleep in the cat. *J Neurosci* 1999;19:9508.
5. Morales FR, Boxer P, Chase MH. Behavioral state-specific inhibitory postsynaptic potentials impinge on cat lumbar motoneurons during active sleep. *Exp Neurol* 1987;98:418–35.
6. Chase MH, Morales FR. Subthreshold excitatory activity and motoneuron discharge during REM periods of active sleep. *Science* 1983;221:1195.
7. Chase MH. Synaptic mechanisms and circuitry involved in motoneuron control during sleep. *Int Rev Neurobiol* 1983;24:213–58.
8. Chase, M.H. (Ed.). *The Sleeping Brain. Perspectives in the Brain Sciences*, Vol. 1. Los Angeles: Brain Information Service/Brain Research Institute, UCLA; 1972, 537.
9. Chase MH, Morales FR. Phasic changes in motoneuron membrane potential during REM periods of active sleep. *Neurosci Lett* 1982;34:177–82.

10. Pompeiano O. The neurophysiological mechanisms of the postural and motor events during desynchronized sleep. *Res Publ Assoc Res Nerv Ment Dis* 1967;45:351.

11. Kleitman N. *Sleep and Wakefulness*. Chicago, IL: University of Chicago Press; 1963.

12. Chase MH. The motor functions of the reticular formation are multifaceted and state-determined. In: Hobson JM, Brazier MAB, eds. *Reticular Formation Revisited*. New York: Press; 1980:449.

13. Chase MH, Morales FR. Control of motoneurons during sleep. In: Kryger MH, Roth T, Dement WC, eds. *Principles and Practice of Sleep Medicine*. 4th ed. Philadelphia, PA: WB Saunders; 2005:xx–xx .

14. Orem J, Anderson CA. Diaphragmatic activity during REM sleep in the adult cat. *J Appl Physiol* 1996;81:751–60.

15. Sieck GC, Trelease RB, Harper RM. Sleep influences on diaphragmatic motor unit discharge. *Exp Neurol* 1984;85:316–35.

16. Megirian D, Hinrichsen CF, Sherrey JH. Respiratory roles of genioglossus, sternothyroid, and sternohyoid muscles during sleep. *Exp Neurol* 1985;90:118–28.

17. Escudero M, Marquez-Ruiz J. Tonic inhibition and ponto-geniculo-occipital-related activities shape abducens motoneuron discharge during REM sleep. *J Physiol* 2008;586:3479–91.

18. Ferri R, Manconi M, Plazzi G, et al. A quantitative statistical analysis of the submentalis muscle EMG amplitude during sleep in normal controls and patients with REM sleep behavior disorder. *J Sleep Res* 2008;17:89–100.

19. Pessah MA, Roffwarg HP. Spontaneous middle ear muscle activity in man: a rapid eye movement sleep phenomenon. *Science* 1972;178:773–6.

20. Morales FR, Sampogna S, Rampon C, et al. Brainstem glycinergic neurons and their activation during active (rapid eye movement) sleep in the cat. *Neuroscience* 2006;142:37–47.

21. Curtis DR, Johnston GAR. Amino acid transmitters in the mammalian central nervous system. *Ergeb Physiol* 1974;69:97.

22. Davidoff RA, Hackmann JE. GABA presynaptic actions. In: Rogawshi MA, Barker JL, eds. *Neurotransmitter Action in the Vertebrate Nervous System*. New York: Plenum; 1985:3.

23. Young AB, McDonald RL. Glycine as a spinal neurotransmitter. In: Davidoff RA, ed. *Handbook of the Spinal Cord*. New York: Marcel Dekker; 1983:1.

24. Krnjevic K, Puil E, Werman R. Bicuculline, benzyl penicillin and inhibitory amino acids in the spinal cord of the cat. *Can J Physiol Pharmacol* 1976;55:670.

25. Nistri A. Spinal cord pharmacology of GABA and chemically related amino acids. In: Davidoff RA, ed. *Handbook of the Spinal Cord*. New York: Marcel Dekker; 1983:45.

26. Chase MH, Soja PJ, Finch DM. Pharmacological evidence of postsynaptic factors involved in the suppression of the masseteric reflex during active sleep. In: Chase MH, McGinty DJ, Crane G, eds. *Sleep Research*. Los Angeles, CA: Brain Information Service/Brain Research Institute; 1986: 3.

27. Chase MH, Soja PJ, Morales FR. Evidence that glycine mediates the postsynaptic potentials that inhibit lumbar motoneurons during the atonia of active sleep. *J Neurosci* 1989;9:743–51.

28. Soja PJ, López-Rodríguez F, Morales FR, et al. The postsynaptic inhibitory control of lumbar motoneurons during the atonia of active sleep: effect of strychnine on motoneuron properties. *J Neurosci* 1991;9:2804–11.

29. López-Rodríguez F, Morales FR, Soja PJ, et al. Suppression of the PGO-related lumbar motoneuron IPSP by strychnine. *Brain Res* 1990;535:331–4.

30. Lydic R. The motor atonia of REM sleep: a critical topics forum. *Sleep* 2008;31:1471–2.

31. Funk GD. Are all motoneurons created equal in the eyes of REM sleep and the mechanisms of muscle atonia? *Sleep* 2008;31:1479–82.

32. Marchiafava PL, Pompeiano O. Pyramidal influences on spinal cord during desynchronized sleep. *Arch Ital Biol* 1964;102:500.

33. Soja PJ, Lopez-Rodriguez F, Morales FR, et al. A non NMDA excitatory amino acid mediates subthreshold synaptic activity influencing cat lumbar motoneurons during quiet and active sleep. *Physiologist* 1988;31:A26.

34. Soja PJ, Lopez-Rodriguez F, Morales FR, et al. Depolarizing synaptic events influencing cat lumbar motoneurons during rapid eye movement episodes of active sleep are blocked by kyurenic acid. *Soc Neurosci Abstr* 1988;14:941.

35. Steriade M, Hobson J. Neuronal activity during the sleep-waking cycle. *Prog Neurobiol* 1976;6:155.

36. Evarts E. Temporal patterns of discharge of pyramidal tract neurons during sleep and waking in the monkey. *J Neurophysiol* 1964;27:152.

37. Siegel JM. Brainstem mechanisms generating REM sleep. In: Kryger MH, Roth T, Dement WC, eds. *Principles and Practice of Sleep Medicine*. 3rd ed. Philadelphia, PA: WB Saunders; 2000:112–133.

38. Magoun HW, Rhines R. An inhibitory mechanism in the bulbar reticular formation. *J Neurophysiol* 1946;9:165.

39. Chase MH, Morales FR, Boxer PA, et al. Effect of stimulation of the nucleus reticularis gigantocelluaris on the membrane potential of cat lumbar motoneurons during sleep and wakefulness. *Brain Res* 1986;386:237–44.

40. Fung SJ, Boxer PA, Morales FR, et al. Hyperpolarizing membrane responses induced in lumbar motoneurons by stimulation of the nucleus reticularis pontis oralis during active sleep. *Brain Res* 1982;248:267.

41. Yamuy J, Jimenez I, Morales FR, et al. Population synaptic potentials evoked in lumbar motoneurons following stimulation of the nucleus reticularis gigantocellularis during carbachol-induced atonia. *Brain Res* 1994;639:313.

42. Jones BE. Basic mechanisms of sleep-wake states. In: Kryger M, Roth T, Dement C, eds. *Principles and Practice of Sleep Medicine*. 5th ed. St Louis, MO: Elsevier Saunders; 2011:134–53.

43. Dragunow M, Faull R. The use of c-fos as a metabolic marker in neuronal pathway tracing. *J Neurosci Methods* 1989;29:261.

44. Yamuy J, Mancillas JR, Morales FR, et al. C-fos expression in the pons and medulla of the cat during carbachol-induced active sleep. *J Neurosci* 1993;13:2703.

45. Chase MH, Monoson R, Watanabe K, et al. Somatic reflex response-reversal of reticular origin. *Exp Neurol* 1976;50:561–7.

46. Chandler SH, Nakamura Y, Chase MH. Intracellular analysis of synaptic potentials induced in trigeminal jaw-closer motoneurons by pontomesencephalic reticular stimulation during sleep and wakefulness. *J Neurophysiol* 1980;44:372–82.

47. Kohlmeier KA, López-Rodríguez F, Morales FR, et al. Effects of excitation of sensory pathways on the membrane potential of cat masseter motoneurons before and during cholinergically induced motor atonia. *Neuroscience* 1998;86:557–69.

48. Bowker RM, Morrison AR. The startle reflex and PGO spikes. *Brain Res* 1976;102:185–90.

49. López-Rodriguez F, Chase MH, Morales FR. PGO-related potentials in lumbar motoneurons during active sleep. *J Neurophysiol* 1992;68:109–16.

50. Torterolo P, Yamuy J, Sampogna S, et al. Hypocretinergic neurons are primarily involved in activation of the somatomotor system. *Sleep* 2003;26:25–8.

51. Mieda M, Sakurai T. Integrative physiology of orexins and orexin receptors. *CNS Neurol Disord Drug Targets* 2009;8:281–95.

52. Peyron C, Tighe DK, van den Pol AN, et al. Neurons containing hypocretin (orexin) project to multiple neuronal systems. *J Neurosci* 1998;18:9996–10015.

53. Siegel JM. The neurotransmitters of sleep. *J Clin Psychiatry* 2004;65(Suppl 16):4–7.

54. España RA, Reis KM, Valentino RJ, et al. Organization of hypocretin/orexin efferents to locus coeruleus and basal forebrain arousal-related structures. *J Comp Neurol* 2005;481:160–78.

55. Takahashi K, Lin JS, Sakai K. Neuronal activity of orexin and non-orexin waking-active neurons during wake-sleep states in the mouse. *Neuroscience* 2008;153:860–70.

56. Mileykovskiy BY, Kiyashchenko LI, Siegel JM. Behavioral correlates of activity in identified hypocretin/orexin neurons. *Neuron* 2005;46:787–98.

57. Lee MG, Hassani OK, Jones BE. Discharge of identified orexin/hypocretin neurons across the sleep-waking cycle. *J Neurosci* 2005;25:6716–20.

58. Xi MC, Chase MH. The injection of hypocretin-1 into the nucleus pontis oralis induces either active sleep or wakefulness depending on the behavioral state when it is administered. *Sleep* 2010;33(9):1236–43.

59. Kryger MH, Roth T, Dement WC. *Principles and Practice of Sleep Medicine*. 3rd ed. Philadelphia, PA: WB Saunders; 2000.

60. Kaitin KI, Kilduff TS, Dement WC. Sleep fragmentation in canine narcolepsy. *Sleep* 1986;9:116.

61. Mitler MM, Dement WC. Sleep studies on canine narcolepsy: Pattern and cycle comparisons between affected and normal dogs. *Electroencephalogr Clin Neurophysiol* 1977;43:691.

62. Siegel JM. REM Sleep. In: Kryger MH, Roth T, Dement WC, eds. *Principles and Practices of Sleep Medicine*. 5th ed. Philadelphia, PA: Saunders/Elsevier; 2011:90–111.

63. Chemelli RM, Willie JT, Sinton CM, et al. Narcolepsy in orexin knockout

mice: Molecular genetics of sleep regulation. *Cell* 1999;98:437.

64. Lin L, Faraco J, Li R, et al. The sleep disorder canine narcolepsy is caused by a mutation in the hypocretin (orexin) receptor 2 gene. *Cell* 1999;98:365.

65. Date Y, Ueta Y, Yamashita H, et al. Orexins, orexigenic hypothalamic peptides, interact with autonomic, neuroendocrine and neuroregulatory systems. *Proc Natl Acad Sci USA* 1999;96:748.

66. Hagan JJ, Leslie RA, Patel S, et al. Orexin A activates locus coeruleus cell firing and increases arousal in the rat. *Proc Natl Acad Sci USA* 1999;96:10911.

67. Nambu T, Sakura T, Mizukami K, et al. Distribution of orexin neurons in the adult rat brain. *Brain Res* 1999;827:243.

68. van den Pol A. Hypothalamic hypocretin (orexin): Robust innervation of the spinal cord. *J Neurosci* 1999;19:3171.

69. Thakkar MM, Strecker RE, McCarley RW. Behavioral state control through differential serotonergic inhibition in the mesopontine cholinergic nuclei: a simultaneous unit recording and microdialysis study. *J Neurosci* 1998;18:5490.

70. Yamuy J, Fung SJ, Sampogna S, et al. Orexin (hypocretin)-A and orexin type 1 receptor immunoreactivity in the ventral horn of the cat spinal cord. *Soc Neurosci Abstr* 2000;26:2040.

71. Zhang JH, Sampogna S, Morales FR, et al. Distribution of hypocretin (orexin) immunoreactivity in the feline pons and medulla. *Brain Res* 2004;995:205–17.

72. Chase MH, Babb M. Masseteric reflex response to reticular stimulation reverses during active sleep compared with wakefulness or quiet sleep. *Brain Res* 1973;59:421–6.

73. Morales FR, Chase MH. Intracellular recording of lumbar motoneuron membrane potential during sleep and wakefulness. *Exp Neurol* 1978;62:821–7.

74. Nishino S, Ripley B, Overeem S, et al. Hypocretin (orexin) deficiency in human narcolepsy. *Lancet* 2000;355:39–40.

75. Overeem S, Lammers GJ, van Dijk JG. Cataplexy: "tonic immobility" rather than "REM-sleep atonia"? *Sleep Med* 2002;3:471–7.

76. Bassetti C. Cataplexy: "REM-atonia or tonic immobility"? *Sleep Med* 2002;3:465–6.

77. Overeem S, Lammers GJ, van Dijk JG. Weak with laughter. *Lancet* 1999;354:838.

78. Castillo P, Pedroarena C, Chase MH, et al. A medullary inhibitory region for trigeminal motoneurons in the cat. *Brain Res* 1991;549:346–9.

79. Siegel JM, Nienhuis R, Fahringer HM, et al. Activity of medial mesopontine units during cataplexy and sleep-waking states in the narcoleptic dog. *J Neurosci* 1992;12:1640–6.

80. Siegel JM, Nienhuis R, Fahringer HM, et al. Neuronal activity in narcolepsy: identification of cataplexy-related cells in the medial medulla. *Science* 1991;252:1315–18.

81. Wu MF, Gulyani SA, Yau E, et al. Locus coeruleus neurons: cessation of activity during cataplexy. *Neuroscience* 1999;91:1389–99.

82. John J, Wu MF, Maidment NT, et al. Developmental changes in CSF hypocretin-1 (orexin-A) levels in normal and genetically narcoleptic Doberman pinschers. *J Physiol* 2004;560:587–92.

83. Thannickal TC, Nienhuis R, Siegel JM. Localized loss of hypocretin (orexin) cells in narcolepsy without cataplexy. *Sleep* 2009;32:993–8.

6

Circadian Neurobiology

ALEKSANDAR VIDENOVIC, SUSAN BENLOUCIF,
AND PHYLLIS C. ZEE

IN ALL living organisms, including humans, daily rhythms exist in nearly all physiologic and behavioral parameters. These rhythms are regulated by an endogenous circadian timing system and are synchronized to the rotation of the earth and other external and internal time cues. Internal temporal organization insures that there is synchronization between the organism and the external environment, whereas lack of synchrony may lead to negative consequences for the health and survival of the organism.

The Circadian Timing System

The circadian timing system is conceptualized as three distinct components: a circadian oscillator that generates a rhythm approximating 24 hours, input pathways for light and other stimuli that synchronize the pacemaker to the environment, and output rhythms that are regulated by the pacemaker. An important property of circadian rhythms is that they persist in the absence of environmental synchronizing stimuli and are therefore endogenous.

An abundance of evidence indicates that the suprachiasmatic nucleus (SCN), located in the hypothalamus, is a circadian pacemaker. Hypothalamic lesions lead to severe disruption of the sleep-wake cycle, locomotor activity, drinking, temperature, and hormonal rhythms.[1-3] Surgical isolation of the SCN results in a loss of circadian electrical activity in areas outside of the SCN, whereas the island containing the SCN retains rhythmicity.[4] In addition, this is the only area of the brain that exhibits an endogenous rhythm of metabolism.[5,6]

The finding that fetal SCN tissue restores circadian rhythmicity with a period characteristic of the donor animal provides further evidence that the period of circadian rhythms is generated by the SCN.[7,8] In vitro studies support the view that the SCN contains one or more self-sustaining circadian oscillators. In hypothalamic tissue containing the SCN, stable rhythms of neuronal firing rate and vasopressin release continue for several days,[9,10] and pacemaker activity persists in single SCN cells.[11,12]

These data suggest that pacemaker activity in the SCN is generated by the synchronized activity of single-cell circadian oscillators.

FUNCTIONAL NEUROANATOMY AND NEUROCHEMISTRY OF THE SUPRACHIASMATIC NUCLEUS

The SCN has been traditionally divided into ventrolateral and dorsomedial subdivisions. More recently this classification has been revised and the SCN divided into SCN "core" and "shell" subnuclei. More than 25 neurochemicals of endogenous and exogenous origin have been identified in the SCN; only those of the highest density are discussed here.[13] The most prevalent neurotransmitter in the SCN is gamma-aminobutyric acid (GABA). GABA is located throughout the nucleus and has been identified in nearly all the neurons in the SCN.[14] In contrast, all of the neuropeptides are highly localized within either the core or shell nuclei. It has been suggested that the flow of information within the SCN usually occurs from core to shell. SCN core neurons project to other core neurons, to SCN shell neurons, and to extra SCN targets. SCN shell neurons project to other shell neurons, to extra-SCN targets, but not to SCN core neurons.[15] The SCN receives photic information from the retina via direct (retinohypothalamic) and indirect (retinogeniculate) pathways (Fig. 6.1).[16,17] Glutamate is the main neurotransmitter released from retinohypothalamic terminals, and stimulation of hypothalamic slices with glutamate mimics the effects of light on the circadian clock.[18,19] The retinohypothalamic tract terminates in the SCN core, an area containing a high density of

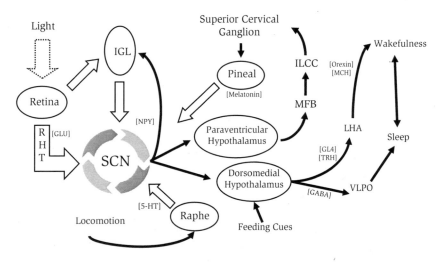

FIGURE 6.1 Components of the circadian timing system. The circadian timing system is composed of a circadian pacemaker in the suprachiasmatic nucleus (SCN), input pathways for light and other entraining stimuli (open arrow), and efferents that regulate behavioral and physiologic rhythms (closed arrows). Photic information is carried directly to the SCN via the retinohypothalamic tract (RHT) and indirectly from the intergeniculate leaflet (IGL) of the lateral geniculate nucleus via the geniculohypothalamic tract. Glutamate (GLU) and neuropeptide Y (NPY) are the predominate neurotransmitters carrying photic signals. Serotonin (5-HT) from the raphe nucleus and melatonin from the pineal gland can also modulate the timing of the clock. Numerous efferents arise from the dorsal SCN. The multisynaptic pathway involved in the regulation of melatonin synthesis traverses the paraventricular nucleus of the hypothalamus, the medial forebrain bundle (MFB), the intermediolateral cell column (ILCC), and the superior cervical ganglion, terminating at the pineal gland. This hormone influences circadian rhythmicity via highly localized receptors in the SCN. The circadian clock regulates sleep behavior through multisynaptic projections to the dorsomedial nucleus of hypothalamus (DMH), which has a critical role in the circadian regulation of sleep-wake cycles. Dense GABA-ergic projections from the DMH terminate in the ventrolateral preoptic nucleus (VLPO) and lateral hypothalamus.

VIP-producing neurons.[13,20,21] Gastrin-releasing peptide (GRP) and bombesin-containing neurons are found in the same region of the SCN as VIP.[13] Neuropeptide Y (NPY) is the neurotransmitter released from the terminals of the geniculohypothalamic tract. This tract originates in the lateral geniculate nucleus and terminates in the SCN core.[22,23] The core also receives nonphotic information via serotonin from the raphe nuclei.[13,24] Several less characterized afferents converge in the SCN shell, including projections form basal forebrain, pons, medulla, and posterior hypothalamus.[15]

Anatomic tracing has identified numerous efferent pathways from the SCN. The major efferents from the SCN project dorsally to the subparaventricular zone and the paraventricular nucleus of the hypothalamus, the dorsomedial hypothalamus, and the thalamus.[25-27] Somatostatin, neurophysin, and arginine vasopress in AVP containing cell bodies are found in the SCN shell.[13] Numerous smaller pathways from the SCN include projections to the preoptic and retrochiasmatic areas, the stria terminalis, the lateral septum, and the intergeniculate nucleus.[25-27] In addition to these neural pathways, there is evidence that the SCN communicates via humoral signals to the rest of the brain.[28] The most likely candidates for these diffusible SCN outputs include transforming growth factor (TGF)-α,[29] cardiotrophin-like cytokine (CLC),[30] and prokineticin 2 (PK2).[31] These substances exhibit a circadian rhythm of expression in the SCN and may function as the SCN output factors modulating rest-activity cycles. A major development in chronobiology research has been the discovery of circadian clocks in non-SCN brain regions and almost all peripheral tissues.[32] These peripheral clocks relay on feedback loops of clock genes, similarly to the SCN. While the signals mediating communication between the SCN and peripheral oscillators remain under extensive investigation, it is clear that the central clock (SCN) and peripheral clocks may have distinct circadian synchronizers.[33,34] The SCN, however, is most likely dominant in maintaining circadian rhythmicity of peripheral clocks.

GENETIC REGULATION OF THE CIRCADIAN SYSTEM

Studies in *Drosophila* and *Neurospora* in the 1970s provided clear evidence that circadian timing is under genetic control.[35-37] In 1988 the discovery of the Tau mutation in the hamster, which results in a shortened circadian period, indicated a genetic basis for the regulation of circadian rhythms in mammals.[38] However, a major breakthrough leading to an understanding of the genetic regulation of circadian rhythms in mammals did not occur until almost a decade later with identification of the *Clock* gene in mice.[39-41] Subsequently, several core circadian clock genes have been identified in mammals: Clock; Bmal1; casein kinase 1ε (CK1ε); cryptochromes 1 and 2 (Cry1, Cry2); Period 1, 2, and 3 (Per1, Per2, Per3); and Rev-erb-α.[42-47] There is significant homology in the genetic mechanisms responsible for the generation of circadian cycles between mammalian and nonmammalian systems.[48] This section is limited to a discussion of the mammalian system.

In its simplest form, the molecular clockwork consists of an autoregulatory transcriptional-translational feedback loop.[49] Central in this process, *Per* is rhythmically transcribed and translated, and as it accumulates, inhibits its own transcription. Binding of the CLOCK-B-MAL1 heterodimer is necessary to initiate transcription of *Per* genes. CLOCK and B-MAL1 proteins contain PAS regions, which form protein-protein heterodimers that contain a beta helix-loop-helix (bHLH) structure. The bHLH allows the protein heterodimers to bind DNA segments with specific sequences known as E-box elements (CACGTG) present within in the promoter sites for *Per1*, *Per2*, *Per3*, *Cry1*, and *Cry2*.[50-53] During the day, the bHLH containing transcription factor CLOCK interacts with B-MAL1 to activate transcription of the Per and Cry genes, resulting in high levels of these transcripts. Heterodimers of PER and CRY proteins translocate to the nucleus and inhibit CLOCK-B-MAL1-mediated transcription.[52-54] During the night, the PER-CRY repressor complex is degraded, and the cycle starts again. There are two main mechanisms that reduce the total amount of PER protein available in the cell. In the cytoplasm PER protein can be degraded, as following phosphorylation by CK1ε.[55] Alternatively, as a part of the feedback loop, PER protein in the cytoplasm may dimerize with binding partners, including PER3, CRY1, or CRY2, facilitating re-entry into the nucleus.[56,57] Once in the nucleus, PER1, PER2, CRY1, CRY2, and TIM are able to liberate CLOCK-B-MAL1 heterodimers from their DNA promoter sites. This stops the transcription and subsequent elaboration of PER protein.[57]

Circadian clock genes control a significant proportion of the genome. It is estimated that approximately 10% of all expressed genes are under regulation of the clock genes.[58-60] Furthermore, peripheral tissues contain independent clocks.[60,61] Several studies have demonstrated strong oscillatory expression patterns of core clock genes in human whole blood cells.[62-64] These studies demonstrate the feasibility of using clock gene expression in whole blood as a circadian marker. It is likely that peripheral clocks are synchronized by an input directly from the SCN or SCN-mediated messages. Several excellent reviews are available for more detailed overview of the molecular regulation of the circadian system.[65-69] Ultimately, physiologic and behavioral markers of circadian rhythms must be linked to the outputs of the central circadian clock. There is growing evidence that circadian genes act as gating mechanisms for production of factors involved in the expression of physiologic and behavioral processes in peripheral tissues.[49,70,71] Accumulating evidence in experimental models suggests tight connections between circadian and metabolic cycles. Mutation of the *Clock* gene in mice has been shown to alter metabolism.[72] Similar metabolic defects have also been associated with mutations in other core circadian genes, including *Bmal1*, *Per2*, *Cry1*, and *Cry2*.[73-75] Alterations in metabolism itself may lead to disruption of circadian rhythms and sleep-wake cycles. High-fat-diet-induced changes of animal circadian rhythmicity manifest as disrupted locomotor activity, changes in rhythmicity of clock genes, increased total sleep time, and increased sleep fragmentation.[76-78] Emerging studies in humans suggest associations between sleep disruption and obesity, diabetes, and cardiovascular disease.[79-82] These data support a model of reciprocal relationships between the metabolic and circadian system, where disruptions of molecular clock network impact metabolic homeostasis, and changes in metabolism alter the circadian rhythmicity and sleep-wake cycles.

Circadian Entrainment

Circadian rhythms are synchronized, or entrained, to the environmental light-dark cycle by daily adjustments in the timing of the pacemaker.[83] Circadian output rhythms are used to estimate the time (the phase) of the clock.[84] In humans, timing of the circadian core body temperature and hormonal rhythms are the most commonly used phase markers. Changes in phase occur following exposure to stimuli that signal the time of day or state of the animal. These stimuli are known as *zeitgebers*, a German word meaning "time givers." Light is the primary and most effective zeitgeber, and stable entrainment to the light-dark cycle is the result of daily light-induced shifts in the phase of the clock.[83] The magnitude and direction of the change in phase depend on when within the circadian system the light pulse is presented. A plot of phase changes according to the time of light stimulus presentation provides a phase response curve (PRC) (Fig. 6.2).

The PRCs to light for both nocturnal and diurnal mammals are similar, with phase shifts occurring only during the subjective night.[85,86] Exposure to light results in a PRC with delays in the early subjective night and advances in the late subjective night. Subjective night is defined as the active period for nocturnal animals and the sleep-rest period for diurnal animals. In humans, the transition point from delays to advances occurs near the temperature minimum, which averages 4:00 am to 5:00 am in young adults and somewhat earlier in older adults.[85-88] During most of the subjective day, light stimulus has relatively little effect, corresponding with the so-called *dead zone* on the PRC. In addition to well-established effects of light on circadian period, it is possible that extended daily light exposure in diurnal organisms may affect the amplitude of the circadian clock.[89]

Photic stimuli also induce the expression of a specific set of immediate early genes and their protein products in the mammalian SCN.[90-92] The most widely studied of the immediate early genes are c-*fos* and *jun*-B.[90,93,94] Under most conditions, the light-induced expression of c-*fos* correlates with the regulation of light-induced phase shifts of circadian activity rhythms.[90,95] In contrast, c-*fos* expression in the SCN is not induced by nonphotic zeitgebers such as activity or melatonin.[96-98] In addition to light, feeding schedules, activity, and the hormone melatonin can also affect the circadian timing. Presentation of these zeitgebers results in distinct PRCs (Fig. 6.3). The phase-shifting responses to nonphotic zeitgebers such as activity-inducing stimuli or melatonin are generally in the opposite direction to those produced by light, resulting in complementary PRCs.[99-103] Activity-inducing stimuli are maximally effective during periods

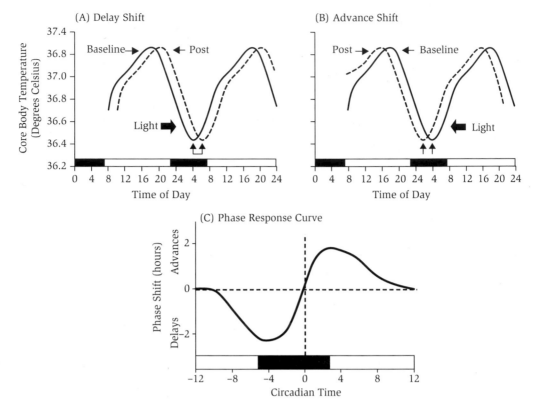

FIGURE 6.2   Generalized phase response curve (PRC) to light in humans. (*A*) Light administered before the nadir of the circadian core body temperature rhythm (approximately 4 am to 5 am in young adults) induces a delay in the rhythm. (*B*) Light administered after the nadir of the circadian core body temperature rhythm induces an advance in the rhythm. Phase shifts are calculated as the difference between the baseline and posttreatment phase markers (nadir of the circadian core body temperature rhythm, indicated by the double arrows). (*C*) The magnitude of the phase shift (advance, delay, or no shift) is plotted by the circadian time of treatment, resulting in a PRC. The crossover point between delay and advances occurs around the time of the nadir of the core body temperature rhythm. Note that exposure to light in the middle of the day does not induce shifts in phase. Circadian time (CT) 0 is defined as the time of the nadir of the core body temperature rhythm at baseline. The black bars denote a sleep period of 11:00 pm to 7:00 am (CT -5 to CT 3 with a temperature nadir of 4:00 am).

of usual inactivity, whereas the peak periods of sensitivity for melatonin occur at the light-dark transitions. The benzodiazepine triazolam alters clock timing and facilitates adjustment to changes in the light-dark cycle (a model of jet lag) in hamsters.[104] In hamsters the phase-shifting effects of triazolam are mediated by an increase in locomotor activity.[103] The similarity in the PRCs elicited by activity, serotonin, and NPY suggests that these two neurochemicals may mediate activity-induced phase shifts.[102,105–107]

The competing photic and nonphotic zeitgebers can antagonize each other even when one of the stimuli is applied during a normally inactive period. Administration of serotonin agonists inhibits light-induced phase shifts and *c-fos* expression during the subjective night, whereas light antagonizes serotonin agonist-induced phase advances during the subjective day.[108–110] Similarly, melatonin administered in combination with light results in phase shifts that could not be predicted based on the individual PRCs to either light or melatonin.[99,111]

MELATONIN

One of the most clearly understood output rhythms of the SCN is the hormone melatonin. The main source of circulating melatonin is the pineal gland.[112] Besides the pineal

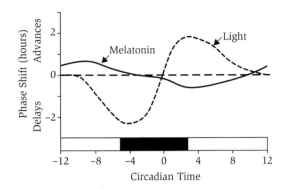

FIGURE 6.3   Generalized phase response curves (PRCs) following exposure to a photic (light) and a nonphotic (melatonin) zeitgeber in humans. Exposure to light (dashed line) in the first half of the night induces delays in phase, whereas exposure to light in the second half of the night advances phase. Exposure to light in the middle of the day does not affect the timing of the clock. The clock is maximally sensitive to melatonin administration at the day-night and night-day transitions. Exogenous melatonin (solid line) induces advances when administered before subjective night and delays when administered at the end of the night or beginning of the day. Melatonin administered in the middle of the subjective night does not affect the phase of the clock. Circadian time (CT) 0 is defined as the time of the nadir of the core body temperature rhythm at baseline. The black bars denote a sleep period of 11:00 pm to 7:00 am (CT -5 to CT 3 with a temperature nadir of 4:00 am).

gland, several other tissues have the capability of producing melatonin, including eye (retina) and the gastrointestinal tract.[113] Melatonin (N-acetyl-5-methoxytryptamine) is synthesized from the neurotransmitter serotonin (5-hydroxytryptamine) in two steps by the enzymes pineal arylalkylamine N-acetyltransferase (AANAT) and hydroxyindole-O-methyltransferase (HIOMT).[114,115] AANAT is the rate-limiting step in the synthesis of melatonin, and its activity is regulated both by the circadian timing system and by light.[116,117] The pathway through which the clock regulates melatonin synthesis is multisynaptic. This pathway begins in the SCN and traverses the paraventricular nucleus of the hypothalamus, the medial forebrain bundle, the intermediolateral cell column, and the superior cervical ganglion, which then provides sympathetic input to the pineal gland (see Fig. 6.1).[118,119] Sympathetic stimulation of the pineal gland increases pineal AANAT activity, and nocturnal melatonin levels are reduced by treatment with beta-adrenergic receptor antagonists.[120–122] Because the regulation of melatonin synthesis is so tightly controlled by the circadian pacemaker and because melatonin can be detected in human plasma and saliva by radioimmunoassay, the dim light melatonin onset (DLMO) is a reliable phase marker of the circadian timing system.[123] Some studies reported a decline in melatonin production with aging.[124]

A decreased number of beta-adrenergic receptors in the pinealocytes, decreased activity of AANAT, and increased clearance of plasma melatonin have been associated with aging.[125]

Levels of melatonin in plasma are at a minimum during the daytime, then rise in the evening, and remain high throughout the night, declining near dawn. In addition to its circadian regulation, presentation of light during the night results in a direct and rapid inhibition of melatonin synthesis.[126–128] Retinal ganglion cells mediate detection and transduction of critical wavelengths (460–480 nm) that inhibit pineal melatonin secretion.[129] The onset and the offset of melatonin production are differentially affected by light exposure in the morning and the evening, which allows compression and expansion of the nocturnal melatonin profile.[130,131] Thus, melatonin production parallels the duration of the dark period, expanding during long winter nights and contracting during long summer days.[132,133] In photoperiodic animals the duration of nocturnal melatonin synthesis is critical for seasonal changes such as reproductive status, weight, and coat color.[134,135] As a result, melatonin is thought of as a chemical transducer of darkness.

Acute melatonin administration can alter the phase of behavioral and physiologic rhythms, whereas daily administration entrains circadian activity rhythms.[99,136-138] Primary mediators of the chronobiotic activity of melatonin are via its activation of G_i protein–coupled melatonin receptors (MT). Binding of melatonin to two primary receptors, MT1 and MT2, induces changes in the timing and firing rate of SCN neurons.[139-144]

In addition to its receptor-mediated activity in the SCN, melatonin has been shown to influence cell physiology through nuclear binding sites and interactions with cytosolic molecules.[145] Thus, melatonin has been reported to have other physiologic effects, including vasoactive, antioxidant, and analgesic properties.[146,147]

ONTOGENY

Circadian rhythms of various behavioral and physiologic functions are initially evident prenatally and become entrained to light-dark cycles within the first few months of life. These rhythms may undergo changes in phase, period, amplitude, and responsiveness to zeitgebers throughout the lifetime. During fetal development, the SCN exhibits circadian rhythmicity even before synaptogenesis.[148-152] Fetal movements, heart rate, and other variables start to exhibit daily variations by 22 weeks of gestation.[153,154] Endogenous dopamine and maternal melatonin are in large part responsible for entrainment of the fetal SCN.[155,156] Initial sensitization of the SCN to photic stimuli occurs during the first week of life. In humans, circadian rhythms of core body temperature can be observed at birth; however, output rhythms of activity, melatonin, cortisol, and heart rate develop gradually over a period of several weeks to months after birth.[157-160] These data suggest that development of pacemaker control over the sleep-wake cycle, rather than development of the pacemaker itself, accounts for the gradual nocturnal consolidation of sleep that occurs in humans during the first months after birth.

At the other end of the life span there is a reduction in amplitude, increased fragmentation, and an advance in the phase of circadian rhythms. These changes may reflect modifications of the pacemaker itself or be result of changes upstream or downstream from the circadian clock. Age-related reductions in amplitude have been observed for a wide variety of clock-regulated functions, ranging from temperature and endocrine rhythms to cycles of subjective alertness and mood.[87,161-163] Habitual wake time, the rise of hormone secretion, and the core body temperature nadir of older subjects occur at an earlier time, suggesting an advance of the circadian clock.[87,163-165] This may be explained by a shortening of the period of the clock or by alterations of entrainment mechanisms.[165-167] Data from rodent models of aging support an age-related decrease in the response of the circadian clock to entraining agents such as light and activity.[168-171] In older adults, these changes in clock function are compounded by decreased exposure to these entraining agents.[172,173]

Aging is associated with morphologic changes within the SCN. Subtle dendritic changes and a loss of AVP- and VIP-containing neurons are observed.[174-176] There does not appear to be any correlation between age-related changes in clock function and total cell number.[177,178] Functional changes such as a decrease in metabolic activity, reduced amplitude of the firing rate rhythm, and a decrease in light-induced immediate-early gene expression are also seen.[168,171,179-181] Thus, changes in the morphology and physiology of the SCN, as well as substantial reductions in the daily exposure and/or sensitivity to bright light or other synchronizing agents, may affect the integrity of circadian rhythms with advanced age.

CIRCADIAN REGULATION OF SLEEP AND WAKEFULNESS

The daily cycle of sleep and wake is the most notable human behavior that is regulated by the circadian system. Although the precise mechanisms underlying the circadian regulation of sleep and wakefulness are not known, it is clear that the circadian timing system is important for the temporal distribution of sleep and wakefulness. Temporal isolation studies conducted by Aschoff[182] were the first to suggest a circadian influence on spontaneous sleep initiation and sleep duration. Based on the results of these and other studies, it has been suggested that a primary role of the human circadian pacemaker is to facilitate the consolidation of sleep and wakefulness.[183-186] More recent data indicate that in humans, sleep onset is most likely to occur during the declining phase of the core body temperature rhythm and that prolonged sleep episodes are possible only near the core body temperature minimum.[186,187] These findings correspond with earlier studies showing that the wake-promoting signal issued from the circadian pacemaker becomes stronger as the core body temperature rises and reaches a maximum in the evening or the "forbidden zone" for sleep.[188,189] Therefore, it appears that the circadian pacemaker functions to consolidate wakefulness and regulate the timing of sleep in humans. In humans, there is a biphasic circadian rhythm of alertness: there is a dip in alertness occurring at approximately 2–4 pm, followed by a robust increase in alertness lasting through the early to mid-morning hours, and subsequent decline to lowest levels of alertness between 4 and 6 am.[190]

The two-process model of sleep regulation has been proposed to explain the relationship between the circadian system and sleep. This model proposes a sleep homeostatic process (process S) that interacts with the circadian process (process C), which is independent of sleep.[191–194] Support for this model comes from findings that the time course of the buildup and decay of process S can be quantified using electroencephalographic (EEG) slow-wave activity (SWA) that reflects the duration of prior waking.[195,196] Sleep deprivation increases SWA, resulting in a buildup of "sleep pressure" as a result of the length of the previous wake period.[195] Thus, process S represents an internal, homeostatic requirement for sleep that increases during wakefulness and decreases with sleep. The sleep homeostatic process regulates the amount and depth of sleep. The circadian process (C) promotes wakefulness during the day and facilitates consolidation of sleep during the night.[191] The contributions of the sleep homeostatic and circadian components in sleep regulation can be estimated applying the forced desynchrony experimental paradigm in which the imposed sleep-waking cycles lies outside the range of circadian entrainment. Variation in SWA is accounted for mainly by homeostatic factors, while the percentage of REM sleep, NREM sleep, and sleep consolidation are determined by both homeostatic and circadian factors.[187]

Animal research has also provided important information on the role of the SCN in the regulation of sleep and wakefulness. In rats, SCN lesion fragments sleep onset and timing but has no significant effect on either the total amount of sleep or the amount of recovery sleep following sleep deprivation.[197–201] In contrast, SCN lesion in the squirrel monkey results not only in increased sleep fragmentation but also a 4-hour increase in the amount of non–rapid eye movement (non-REM) sleep, leading to the hypothesis that the SCN sends a signal that enhances waking, actively opposing the sleep process.[202] Our understanding of the role of the circadian clock in sleep-wake regulation has been greatly advanced during the past decade. The SCN has minimal monosynaptic outputs to sleep-regulatory centers such as the ventrolateral preoptic nucleus (VLPO) and lateral hypothalamus, and none at all to brainstem arousal centers.[203] Instead, the circadian clock regulates sleep behavior through multisynaptic projections to the ventral segment of the subparaventricular zone (vSPZ).[204] Secondary dense projections connect the SCN and vSPZ with the dorsomedial nucleus of hypothalamus (DMH), which has a critical role in the circadian regulation of sleep-wake cycles. Dense GABA-ergic projections from the DMH terminate in the VLPO and lateral hypothalamus.[205] The VLPO and components of the arousal system have mutually inhibitory connections and function similarly to an electronic "flip-flop" switch.[206] Lateral hypothalamus most likely plays a stabilizing role for this flip-flop switch. Circadian and homeostatic processes influence both sides of the switch to assure consolidation of sleep and wake.

SLEEP-WAKE CYCLE DISORDERS

Changes in the circadian regulation of sleep and wake have been implicated in the pathophysiology of several sleep disorders. Alterations in the length of circadian period, entraining pathways, or in the interaction between homeostatic and circadian processes can result in circadian rhythm sleep disorders (CRSDs). Of the CRSDs, advanced and delayed sleep phase disorders are the most common types of sleep phase disorders seen in clinical practice (Fig. 6.4). Advanced sleep phase disorder (ASPD) is defined as a disorder in which the major sleep episode is advanced in relation to the desired clock time, resulting in symptoms of compelling evening sleepiness, early sleep onset, and awakening that is earlier than desired.[207] Delayed sleep phase disorder (DSPD) is a disorder in which the major sleep episode is delayed in relation to the desired clock time, resulting in symptoms of sleep-onset insomnia or difficulty in awakening at the desired time.[207] Reports of polymorphisms in the circadian clock genes *Per2*, *Per3*, *Clock*, *casein kinase I-δ*, and *casein kinase I-ε* have been found to correlate with the propensity for "eveningness" or "morningness"[208] and suggest a genetic

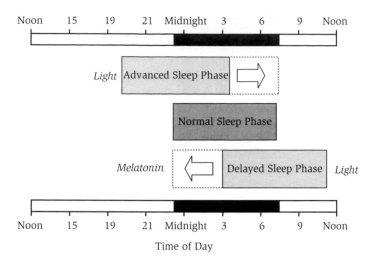

FIGURE 6.4   Schematic representation of circadian sleep-wake disorders and treatment strategies. The gray bars indicate typical sleep periods in individuals exhibiting usual sleep time, advanced sleep phase syndrome (ASPS), and delayed sleep phase syndrome (DSPS). Exposure to light in the evening induces delays in the phase of the clock and normalizes sleep timing in individuals with ASPS (arrow). Exposure to light in the morning, or melatonin in the evening, advances the phase of the clock and normalizes sleep timing in individuals with DSPS (arrow). The black bars indicate a usual sleep period.

basis for ASPD and DSPD.[209-217] A less common circadian rhythm disorder is the non–24-hour sleep-wake disorder, characterized by lack of entrainment of circadian rhythms to the usual 24-hour light-dark cycle.[207] Circadian rhythms are free-running, characterized by a consistent delay in the timing of the circadian cycle by as much as 60 to 70 minutes per day.[218] This condition is reported in the 50% of blind individuals who have no conscious light perception and is rare in sighted individuals.[219,220] In sighted individuals, there is often an overlap with delayed DSPD. Reduced responsiveness to ambient light has been postulated as the mechanism.[219,221] Irregular sleep-wake disorder is characterized by the absence of a clear circadian rhythm of sleep and wake. At least three sleep periods are interspersed throughout the 24-hour cycle, but the total sleep time is usually within normal limits. This disorder has been associated with dementia, mental retardation, and traumatic brain injury.[222-226]

Treatment with synchronizing agents for the circadian clock, such as bright light therapy and melatonin, can realign advanced and delayed sleep-wake rhythms to the desired schedule (see Figs. 6.3 and 6.4).[227,228] Light in the first half of the sleep period induces delays in circadian phase, whereas light in the second half of the sleep period advances circadian phase. Melatonin administration has been recommended as a treatment option for DSPD by the American Academy of Sleep Medicine (AASM).[229] Melatonin can improve the timing of sleep and circadian rhythms in subjects with DSPD.[227,230,231] Melatonin is most effective to advance circadian rhythms when administered relative to the dim light melatonin onset, approximately 3 to 6 hours before habitual sleep time (see Fig. 6.4).[100] The dim light melatonin onset usually rises 2 to 3 hours prior to habitual sleep time. Although large-scale controlled studies have not been conducted to determine the efficacy and safety of this compound in humans, results to date are promising.[232-237] The most common approach to treatment of ASPD is bright light therapy in the evening[229,238-240] In individuals with non–24-hour sleep-wake disorder, daily administration of melatonin, planned sleep schedules, and timed bright light have been shown to effectively stabilize sleep and circadian rhythms, and they are recommended as treatment approaches in the AASSM practice parameters.[218,229,241] Treatment approaches for the irregular sleep-wake disorder typically employ a combination of the following interventions: increased light exposure during the day, alone or in combination with evening melatonin administration, structured physical activity, measures to reduce nighttime noise and light exposure levels, and developing a bedtime routine.[242-245] The effectiveness of these approaches varies widely, and sustained benefit may be challenging to achieve. The ability of melatonin to modify the timing of the biologic clock also indicates a potential beneficial use for shift workers and travelers suffering from jet lag.[246-251]

RELATION OF MOVEMENT DISORDERS TO CIRCADIAN RHYTHMS

Abnormalities in nocturnal sleep and daytime alertness are recognized as common comorbidities in movement disorders. Disruption of the sleep-wake cycle is one of the most striking nonmotor symptoms of Parkinson's disease (PD), affecting up to 90% of patients. Several studies reported daily fluctuations of clinical and biologic factors in PD. These include changes in daily motor activity[252-255]; loss of normal circadian rhythm of blood pressure and heart rate[256-261]; impaired nocturnal sleep and daytime alertness[262-266]; and fluctuations in catecholamines,[267] cortisol,[267-269] and melatonin levels.[267-272] These investigations suggest modifications of circadian rhythmicity in PD. Increasing evidence indicates that dopamine (DA) is involved in the regulation of the circadian system. Activation of D_2 DA receptors modulates circadian effects of light on locomotion activity in mice[273] and regulates the expression of clock genes in retina[274,275] and striatum.[273,276] Depletion of striatal DA by 6-hydroxydopamine or blockade of D_2 DA receptors by raclopride abolishes the circadian rhythm of the PER2 gene, one of the key regulators of circadian timekeeping.[277] Furthermore, activation of D_2 DA receptors restores and entrains the PER2 rhythm in the DA-depleted striatum of mice.[277] Expression levels of the clock gene BMAL1 are dampened in total leukocytes of PD patients and correlate positively with PD severity.[278] These novel and exciting observations suggest that the loss of circadian rhythms after DA depletion may be linked to disruption of daily behavioral and physiologic rhythms frequently reported in PD.

Huntington's disease (HD), an autosomal neurodegenerative disorder characterized by abnormal involuntary movement, cognitive decline, and behavioral disturbances, is associated with progressive deterioration of the sleep-wake cycle. The neuroanatomic substrate of these abnormalities is likely to be a progressive neurodegeneration of brainstem nuclei and lateral hypothalamus. Disruption of rest-activity cycles and expression of the circadian clock genes worsen with the progression of HD.[279] Furthermore, there is a positive correlation between circadian rhythm disturbances and the degree of dementia in HD.[279-281] In the transgenic R6/2 model of HD, pharmacologic restoration of rest-activity cycles correlates with normalization of circadian clock gene expression in the SCN and a marked improvement in the cognitive deficits seen in this animal model of HD.

Circadian rhythms influence the timing of symptoms throughout the 24-hour day/night in several other movement disorders. Individuals with restless legs syndrome (RLS) consistently show a variation in subjective complaints and periodic limb movements over the course of the day.[282,283] Circadian melatonin secretion and body core temperature are normal in RLS patients.[283,284] The melatonin peak coincides with the maximum of RLS symptoms.[283] It is likely that factors such as vigilance or activity state together with increased homeostatic sleep drive contribute to the worsening of RLS symptoms at night.[284] Hereditary progressive dystonia with marked diurnal fluctuation (Segawa disease) is an autosomally dominantly inherited postural dystonia that is characterized by marked diurnal fluctuation of symptoms.[285,286] Dystonic symptoms are aggravated from afternoon toward the evening and alleviated markedly, rather completely in the morning after sleep. The diurnal fluctuation or aggravation toward the evening is mainly dependent on the longevity of the wakening time. This evidence for circadian rhythmicity of symptoms may have implications for treatment, and it provides direction for future studies of the pathophysiology of these movement disorders.

CONCLUSION

Circadian timing is ubiquitous and synchronizes living organisms with the environment. The rapid advancement in basic research in circadian neurobiology has vastly increased the understanding of the molecular, cellular, and physiologic mechanisms that regulate circadian timing in humans. In addition, circadian studies in humans suggest that the diurnal sleep-wake cycle is the result of complex interactions between the circadian clock, sleep homeostasis, and the environment. Disturbed circadian rhythmicity, whether extrinsic (e.g., jet lag and shift work) or intrinsic (e.g., sleep-wake cycle disorders), is often accompanied by disturbances of sleep and wakefulness that can severely affect the health, safety, and performance of humans. Furthermore, there is emerging evidence that circadian rhythm disturbances may be involved in the pathophysiology of sleep disorders in patients with movement disorders. Circadian-based treatment approaches may prove to be useful in the treatment of the circadian rhythm sleep disorders, as well as in the management of sleep disorders comorbid with medical and neurologic disorders.

REFERENCES

1. Moore RY, Eichler VB. Loss of a circadian adrenal corticosterone rhythm following suprachiasmatic lesions in the rat. *Brain Res* 1972;42:201–6.
2. Rusak B, Zucker I. Neural regulation of circadian rhythms. *Physiol Rev* 1979;59:449–526.
3. Stephan FK, Zucker I. Circadian rhythms in drinking behavior and locomotor activity of rats are eliminated by hypothalamic lesions. *Proc Natl Acad Sci USA* 1972;69:1583–6.
4. Inouye ST, Kawamura H. Persistence of circadian rhythmicity in a mammalian hypothalamic "island" containing the suprachiasmatic nucleus. *Proc Natl Acad Sci USA* 1979;76:5962–6.
5. Schwartz WJ, Davidsen LC, Smith CB. In vivo metabolic activity of a putative circadian oscillator, the rat suprachiasmatic nucleus. *J Comp Neurol* 1980;189:157–67.
6. Schwartz WJ, Gainer H. Suprachiasmatic nucleus: use of 14C-labeled deoxyglucose uptake as a functional marker. *Science* 1977;197:1089–91.
7. Lehman MN, Silver R, Gladstone WR, et al. Circadian rhythmicity restored by neural transplant. Immunocytochemical characterization of the graft and its integration with the host brain. *J Neurosci* 1987;7:1626–38.
8. Ralph MR, Foster RG, Davis FC, et al. Transplanted suprachiasmatic nucleus determines circadian period. *Science* 1990;247:975–8.
9. Earnest DJ, Sladek CD. Circadian rhythms of vasopressin release from individual rat suprachiasmatic explants in vitro. *Brain Res* 1986;382:129–33.
10. Green DJ, Gillette R. Circadian rhythm of firing rate recorded from single cells in the rat suprachiasmatic brain slice. *Brain Res* 1982;245:198–200.
11. Earnest DJ, Liang FQ, Ratcliff M, et al. Immortal time: circadian clock properties of rat suprachiasmatic cell lines. *Science* 1999;283:693–5.
12. Welsh DK, Logothetis DE, Meister M, et al. Individual neurons dissociated from rat suprachiasmatic nucleus express independently phased circadian firing rhythms. *Neuron* 1995;14:697–706.
13. van den Pol AN, Tsujimoto KL. Neurotransmitters of the hypothalamic suprachiasmatic nucleus: immunocytochemical analysis of 25 neuronal antigens. *Neuroscience* 1985;15:1049–86.
14. Moore RY, Speh JC. GABA is the principal neurotransmitter of the circadian system. *Neurosci Lett* 1993;150:112–16.
15. Rosenwasser AM, Turek FW. Phisiology of the mamalian circadian system. In: Kryger MH, Roth T, Dement WC, eds. *Priciples and Pratice of Sleep Medicine*. St. Louis, MO: Elsevier Saunders; 2010:390–401.
16. Hendrickson AE, Wagoner N, Cowan WM. An autoradiographic and electron microscopic study of retino-hypothalamic connections. *Z Zellforsch Mikrosk Anat* 1972;135:1–26.
17. Moore RY, Lenn NJ. A retinohypothalamic projection in the rat. *J Comp Neurol* 1972;146:1–14.
18. Gillette MU, Tischkau SA. Suprachiasmatic nucleus: the brain's circadian clock. *Recent Prog Horm Res* 1999;54:33–58; discussion -9.
19. Meijer JH, Rietveld WJ. Neurophysiology of the suprachiasmatic circadian pacemaker in rodents. *Physiol Rev* 1989;69:671–707.
20. Card JP, Brecha N, Karten HJ, et al. Immunocytochemical localization of vasoactive intestinal polypeptide-containing cells and processes in the suprachiasmatic nucleus of the rat: light and electron microscopic analysis. *J Neurosci* 1981;1:1289–303.
21. Card JP, Moore RY. The suprachiasmatic nucleus of the golden hamster: immunohistochemical analysis of cell and fiber distribution. *Neuroscience* 1984;13:415–31.

22. Card JP, Moore RY. Ventral lateral genicu-late nucleus efferents to the rat suprachi-asmatic nucleus exhibit avian pancreatic polypeptide-like immunoreactivity. *J Comp Neurol* 1982;206:390–6.

23. Card JP, Moore RY. Organization of lateral geniculate-hypothalamic connections in the rat. *J Comp Neurol* 1989;284:135–47.

24. Meyer-Bernstein EL, Morin LP. Differential serotonergic innervation of the suprachias-matic nucleus and the intergeniculate leaflet and its role in circadian rhythm modulation. *J Neurosci* 1996;16:2097–111.

25. Morin LP, Goodless-Sanchez N, Smale L, et al. Projections of the suprachiasmatic nuclei, subparaventricular zone and retrochiasmatic area in the golden hamster. *Neuroscience* 1994;61:391–410.

26. Watts AG, Swanson LW. Efferent projections of the suprachiasmatic nucleus: II. Studies using retrograde transport of fluorescent dyes and simultaneous peptide immuno-histochemistry in the rat. *J Comp Neurol* 1987;258:230–52.

27. Watts AG, Swanson LW, Sanchez-Watts G. Efferent projections of the suprachiasmatic nucleus: I. Studies using anterograde trans-port of Phaseolus vulgaris leucoagglutinin in the rat. *J Comp Neurol* 1987;258:204–29.

28. Silver R, LeSauter J, Tresco PA, et al. A diffusible coupling signal from the trans-planted suprachiasmatic nucleus control-ling circadian locomotor rhythms. *Nature* 1996;382:810–13.

29. Kramer A, Yang FC, Snodgrass P, et al. Regulation of daily locomotor activity and sleep by hypothalamic EGF receptor signaling. *Science* 2001;294:2511–15.

30. Kraves S, Weitz CJ. A role for cardiotrophin-like cytokine in the circadian control of mammalian locomotor activity. *Nat Neurosci* 2006;9:212–19.

31. Cheng MY, Bullock CM, Li C, et al. Prokineticin 2 transmits the behavioural circadian rhythm of the suprachiasmatic nucleus. *Nature* 2002;417:405–10.

32. Cermakian N, Boivin DB. The regulation of central and peripheral circadian clocks in humans. *Obes Rev* 2009;10(Suppl 2):25–36.

33. Cermakian N, Sassone-Corsi P. Environ-mental stimulus perception and control of circadian clocks. *Curr Opin Neurobiol* 2002;12:359–65.

34. Hara R, Wan K, Wakamatsu H, et al. Restricted feeding entrains liver clock without participation of the suprachiasmatic nucleus. *Genes Cells* 2001;6:269–78.

35. Benzer S. From the gene to behavior. *JAMA* 1971;218:1015–22.

36. Feldman JF, Hoyle MN. Isolation of circadian clock mutants of Neurospora crassa. *Genetics* 1973;75:605–13.

37. Konopka RJ, Benzer S. Clock mutants of Drosophila melanogaster. *Proc Natl Acad Sci USA* 1971;68:2112–16.

38. Ralph MR, Menaker M. A mutation of the circadian system in golden hamsters. *Science* 1988;241:1225–7.

39. Antoch MP, Song EJ, Chang AM, et al. Functional identification of the mouse circa-dian Clock gene by transgenic BAC rescue. *Cell* 1997;89:655–67.

40. King DP, Zhao Y, Sangoram AM, et al. Positional cloning of the mouse circadian clock gene. *Cell* 1997;89:641–53.

41. Vitaterna MH, King DP, Chang AM, et al. Mutagenesis and mapping of a mouse gene, Clock, essential for circadian behavior. *Science* 1994;264:719–25.

42. Lowrey PL, Shimomura K, Antoch MP, et al. Positional syntenic cloning and functional characterization of the mammalian circadian mutation tau. *Science* 2000;288:483–92.

43. Shearman LP, Zylka MJ, Weaver DR, et al. Two period homologs: circadian expression and photic regulation in the suprachiasmatic nuclei. *Neuron* 1997;19:1261–9.

44. Takumi T, Taguchi K, Miyake S, et al. A light-independent oscillatory gene mPer3 in mouse SCN and OVLT. *EMBO J* 1998;17:4753–9.

45. Tei H, Okamura H, Shigeyoshi Y, et al. Circadian oscillation of a mammalian homo-logue of the Drosophila period gene. *Nature* 1997;389:512–16.

46. Vitaterna MH, Selby CP, Todo T, et al. Differential regulation of mammalian period genes and circadian rhythmicity by cryp-tochromes 1 and 2. *Proc Natl Acad Sci USA* 1999;96:12114–19.

47. Zylka MJ, Shearman LP, Levine JD, et al. Molecular analysis of mammalian timeless. *Neuron* 1998;21:1115–22.

48. Young MW. Circadian rhythms. Marking time for a kingdom. *Science* 2000;288:451–3.

49. Dunlap JC. Molecular basis for circadian clocks. *Cell* 1999;96:271–90.

50. Cermakian N, Sassone-Corsi P. Multilevel regulation of the circadian clock. *Nat Rev Mol Cell Biol* 2000;1:59–67.

51. Dunlap JC, Loros JJ, Liu Y, et al. Eukaryotic circadian systems: cycles in common. *Genes Cells* 1999;4:1–10.
52. Reppert SM, Weaver DR. Molecular analysis of mammalian circadian rhythms. *Ann Rev Physiol* 2001;63:647–76.
53. Young MW, Kay SA. Time zones: a comparative genetics of circadian clocks. *Nat Rev Genet* 2001;2:702–15.
54. Bell-Pedersen D, Cassone VM, Earnest DJ, et al. Circadian rhythms from multiple oscillators: lessons from diverse organisms. *Nat Rev Genet* 2005;6:544–56.
55. Keesler GA, Camacho F, Guo Y, et al. Phosphorylation and destabilization of human period I clock protein by human casein kinase I epsilon. *NeuroReport* 2000;11:951–5.
56. Griffin EA, Staknis D, Weitz CJ. Light-independent role of CRY1 and CRY2 in the mammalian circadian clock. *Science* 1999;286:768–71.
57. Yagita K, Yamaguchi S, Tamanini F, et al. Dimerization and nuclear entry of mPER proteins in mammalian cells. *Genes Dev* 2000;14:1353–63.
58. Akhtar RA. Circadian cycling of the mouse liver transcriptome, as revealed by cDNA microarray, is driven by the suprachiasmatic nucleus. *Curr Biol* 2001;12:540–50.
59. Duffield GE. Circadian programs of transcriptional activation, signaling, and protein turnover revealed by microarray analysis of mammalian cells. *Curr Biol* 2002;12:551–7.
60. Panda S, Antoch MP, Miller BH, et al. Coordinated transcription of key pathways in the mouse by the circadian clock. *Cell* 2002;109:307–20.
61. Brown SA, Zumbrunn G, Fleury-Olela F, et al. Rhythms of mammalian body temperature can sustain peripheral circadian clocks. *Curr Biol* 2002;12:1574–83.
62. Boivin DB, James FO, Wu A, et al. Circadian clock genes oscillate in human peripheral blood mononuclear cells. *Blood* 2003;102:4143–5.
63. Takimoto M, Hamada A, Tomoda A, et al. Daily expression of clock genes in whole blood cells in healthy subjects and a patient with circadian rhythm sleep disorder. *Am J Physiol* 2005;289:R1273–9.
64. Teboul M, Barrat-Petit MA, Li XM, et al. Atypical patterns of circadian clock gene expression in human peripheral blood mononuclear cells. *J Mol Med* (Berlin) 2005;83:693–9.
65. Dardente H, Cermakian N. Molecular circadian rhythms in central and peripheral clocks in mammals. *Chronobiol Intl* 2007;24:195–213.
66. King DP, Takahashi JS. Molecular genetics of circadian rhythms in mammals. *Ann Rev Neurosci* 2000;23:713–42.
67. Ko CH, Takahashi JS. Molecular components of the mammalian circadian clock. *Human Mol Genet* 2006;15:R271-R7.
68. Lowrey PL. Positional syntenic cloning and functional characterization of a mammalian circadian mutation tau. *Science* 2000;288:483–91.
69. Lowrey PL, Takahashi JS. Mammalian circadian biology: elucidating genome-wide levels of temporal organization. *Ann Rev Genomics Human Genet* 2004;5:407–41.
70. Chong NW, Bernard M, Klein DC. Characterization of the chicken serotonin N-acetyltransferase gene. Activation via clock gene heterodimer/E box interaction. *J Biol Chem* 2000;275:32991–8.
71. Maemura K, de la Monte SM, Chin MT, et al. CLIF, a novel cycle-like factor, regulates the circadian oscillation of plasminogen activator inhibitor-1 gene expression. *J Biol Chem* 2000;275:36847–51.
72. Turek FW, Joshu C, Kohsaka A, et al. Obesity and metabolic syndrome in circadian Clock mutant mice. *Science* 2005;308:1043–5.
73. Bur IM, Cohen-Solal AM, Carmignac D, et al. The circadian clock components CRY1 and CRY2 are necessary to sustain sex dimorphism in mouse liver metabolism. *J Biol Chem* 2009;284:9066–73.
74. Shimba S, Ishii N, Ohta Y, et al. Brain and muscle Arnt-like protein-1 (BMAL1), a component of the molecular clock, regulates adipogenesis. *Proc Natl Acad Sci USA* 2005;102:12071–6.
75. Yang S, Liu A, Weidenhammer A, et al. The role of mPer2 clock gene in glucocorticoid and feeding rhythms. *Endocrinology* 2009;150:2153–60.
76. Danguir J, Nicolaidis S. Dependence of sleep on nutrients' availability. *Physiol Behav* 1979;22:735–40.
77. Jenkins JB, Omori T, Guan Z, et al. Sleep is increased in mice with obesity induced by high-fat food. *Physiol Behav* 2006;87:255–62.
78. Kohsaka A, Laposky AD, Ramsey KM, et al. High-fat diet disrupts behavioral and molecular circadian rhythms in mice. *Cell Metab* 2007;6:414–21.

79. Spiegel K, Knutson K, Leproult R, et al. Sleep loss: a novel risk factor for insulin resistance and Type 2 diabetes. *J Appl Physiol* 2005;99:2008–19.

80. Tasali E, Leproult R, Ehrmann DA, Van Cauter E. Slow-wave sleep and the risk of type 2 diabetes in humans. *Proc Natl Acad Sci USA* 2008;105:1044–9.

81. Van Cauter E, Spiegel K, Tasali E, et al. Metabolic consequences of sleep and sleep loss. *Sleep Med* 2008;9(Suppl 1):S23–8.

82. Tasali E, Leproult R, Spiegel K. Reduced sleep duration or quality: relationships with insulin resistance and type 2 diabetes. *Prog Cardiovasc Dis* 2009;51:381–91.

83. Moore-Ede MC, Sulzman FM, Fuller CA. *The Clocks That Time Us*. Cambridge, MA: Harvard Univeristy Press; 1982.

84. Daan S, Pittendrigh CS. A functuional analysis of circadian pacemakers in nocturnal rodents. II. The variability of phase response curve. *J Comp Physiol* 1976;106:253.

85. Czeisler CA, Kronauer RE, Allan JS, et al. Bright light induction of strong (type 0) resetting of the human circadian pacemaker. *Science* 1989;244:1328–33.

86. Minors DS, Waterhouse JM, Wirz-Justice A. A human phase-response curve to light. *Neurosci Lett* 1991;133:36–40.

87. Czeisler CA, Dumont M, Duffy JF, et al. Association of sleep-wake habits in older people with changes in output of circadian pacemaker. *Lancet* 1992;340:933–6.

88. Monk TH, Buysse DJ, Reynolds CF, 3rd, et al. Circadian temperature rhythms of older people. *Exp Gerontol* 1995;30:455–74.

89. Johnosn CH, Elliott J, Foster R. Fundamental properties of circadian rhythms. In: Dunlap JC, Loros J, DeCoursey PJ, eds. *Chronobiology: Biological Timekeeping*. Sunderland, England: Sinauer; 2004:67–106.

90. Kornhauser JM, Mayo KE, Takahashi JS. Light, immediate-early genes, and circadian rhythms. *Behav Genet* 1996;26:221–40.

91. Rusak B, McNaughton L, Robertson HA, et al. Circadian variation in photic regulation of immediate-early gene mRNAs in rat suprachiasmatic nucleus cells. *Brain Res Mol Brain Res* 1992; 14:124–30.

92. Sutin EL, Kilduff TS. Circadian and light-induced expression of immediate early gene mRNAs in the rat suprachiasmatic nucleus. *Brain Res Mol Brain Res* 1992;15:281–90.

93. Aronin N, Sagar SM, Sharp FR, Schwartz WJ. Light regulates expression of a Fos-related protein in rat suprachiasmatic nuclei. *Proc Natl Acad Sci USA* 1990;87:5959–62.

94. Kornhauser JM, Nelson DE, Mayo KE, et al. Photic and circadian regulation of c-fos gene expression in the hamster suprachiasmatic nucleus. *Neuron* 1990;5:127–34.

95. Rea MA, Michel AM, Lutton LM. Is fos expression necessary and sufficient to mediate light-induced phase advances of the suprachiasmatic circadian oscillator? *J Biol Rhythms* 1993;8(Suppl):S59–64.

96. Kumar V, Goguen DM, Guido ME, et al. Melatonin does not influence the expression of c-fos in the suprachiasmatic nucleus of rats and hamsters. *Brain Res Mol Brain Res* 1997;52:242–8.

97. Mead S, Ebling FJ, Maywood ES, et al. A non-photic stimulus causes instantaneous phase advances of the light-entrainable circadian oscillator of the Syrian hamster but does not induce the expression of c-fos in the suprachiasmatic nuclei. *J Neurosci* 1992;12:2516–22.

98. Zhang Y, Van Reeth O, Zee PC, et al. Fos protein expression in the circadian clock is not associated with phase shifts induced by a nonphotic stimulus, triazolam. *Neurosci Lett* 1993;164:203–8.

99. Benloucif S, Dubocovich ML. Melatonin and light induce phase shifts of circadian activity rhythms in the C3H/HeN mouse. *J Biol Rhythms* 1996;11:113–25.

100. Lewy AJ, Bauer VK, Ahmed S, et al. The human phase response curve (PRC) to melatonin is about 12 hours out of phase with the PRC to light. *Chronobiol Int* 1998;15:71–83.

101. Mrosovsky N, Reebs SG, Honrado GI, et al. Behavioural entrainment of circadian rhythms. *Experientia* 1989;45:696–702.

102. Smith RD, Turek FW, Takahashi JS. Two families of phase-response curves characterize the resetting of the hamster circadian clock. *Am J Physiol* 1992;262:R1149–53.

103. Van Reeth O, Turek FW. Stimulated activity mediates phase shifts in the hamster circadian clock induced by dark pulses or benzodiazepines. *Nature* 1989;339:49–51.

104. van Reeth O, Turek FW. Adaptation of circadian rhythmicity to shift in light-dark cycle accelerated by a benzodiazepine. *Am J Physiol* 1987;253:R204–7.

105. Albers HE, Ferris CF. Neuropeptide Y: role in light-dark cycle entrainment of

hamster circadian rhythms. *Neurosci Lett* 1984;50:163–8.

106. Gillette MU, DeMarco SJ, Ding JM, et al. The organization of the suprachiasmatic circadian pacemaker of the rat and its regulation by neurotransmitters and modulators. *J Biol Rhythms* 1993;8(Suppl):S53–8.

107. Medanic M, Gillette MU. Serotonin regulates the phase of the rat suprachiasmatic circadian pacemaker in vitro only during the subjective day. *J Physiol* 1992;450:629–42.

108. Glass JD, Selim M, Srkalovic G, et al. Tryptophan loading modulates light-induced responses in the mammalian circadian system. *J Biol Rhythms* 1995;10:80–90.

109. Penev PD, Zee PC, Turek FW. Serotonin in the spotlight. *Nature* 1997;385:123.

110. Ralph MR, Mrosovsky N. Behavioral inhibition of circadian responses to light. *J Biol Rhythms* 1992;7:353–9.

111. Benloucif S, Masana MI, Yun K, et al. Interactions between light and melatonin on the circadian clock of mice. *J Biol Rhythms* 1999;14:281–9.

112. Lewy AJ, Tetsuo M, Markey SP, et al. Pinealectomy abolishes plasma melatonin in the rat. *J Clin Endocrinol Metab* 1980;50:204–5.

113. Hardeland R. Melatonin: signaling mechanisms of a pleiotropic agent. *BioFactors* 2009;35:183–92.

114. Foley PB, Cairncross KD, Foldes A. Pineal indoles: significance and measurement. *Neurosci Biobehav Rev* 1986;10:273–93.

115. Reiter RJ. Pineal melatonin: cell biology of its synthesis and of its physiological interactions. *Endocr Rev* 1991;12:151–80.

116. Klein DC, Moore RY. Pineal N-acetyltransferase and hydroxyindole-O-methyltransferase: control by the retinohypothalamic tract and the suprachiasmatic nucleus. *Brain Res* 1979;174:245–62.

117. Vanecek J, Illnerova H. Effect of light at night on the pineal rhythm in N-acetyltransferase activity in the Syrian hamster Mesocricetus auratus. *Experientia* 1982;38:513–14.

118. Klein DC, Smoot R, Weller JL, et al. Lesions of the paraventricular nucleus area of the hypothalamus disrupt the suprachiasmatic leads to spinal cord circuit in the melatonin rhythm generating system. *Brain Res Bull* 1983;10:647–52.

119. Moore RY. Neural control of the pineal gland. *Behav Brain Res* 1996;73:125–30.

120. Cowen PJ, Bevan JS, Gosden B, et al. Treatment with beta-adrenoceptor blockers reduces plasma melatonin concentration. *Br J Clin Pharmacol* 1985;19:258–60.

121. Klein DC, Sugden D, Weller JL. Postsynaptic alpha-adrenergic receptors potentiate the beta-adrenergic stimulation of pineal serotonin N-acetyltransferase. *Proc Natl Acad Sci USA* 1983;80:599–603.

122. Nathan PJ, Maguire KP, Burrows GD, et al. The effect of atenolol, a beta1-adrenergic antagonist, on nocturnal plasma melatonin secretion: evidence for a dose-response relationship in humans. *J Pineal Res* 1997;23:131–5.

123. Lewy AJ, Cutler NL, Sack RL. The endogenous melatonin profile as a marker for circadian phase position. *J Biol Rhythms* 1999;14:227–36.

124. Pandi-Perumal SR, Zisapel N, Srinivasan V, et al. Melatonin and sleep in aging population. *Exp Gerontol* 2005;40:911–25.

125. Rios ERV, Venâncio ET, Rocha NFM, et al. Melatonin: pharmacological aspects and clinical trends. *Intl J Neurosci* 2010;120:583–90.

126. Illnerova H, Vanecek J, Krecek J, et al. Effect of one minute exposure to light at night on rat pineal serotonin N-acetyltransferase and melatonin. *J Neurochem* 1979;32:673–5.

127. Lewy AJ, Wehr TA, Goodwin FK, et al. Light suppresses melatonin secretion in humans. *Science* 1980;210:1267–9.

128. McIntyre IM, Norman TR, Burrows GD, et al. Human melatonin suppression by light is intensity dependent. *J Pineal Res* 1989;6:149–56.

129. Brainard GC, Sliney D, Hanifin JP, et al. Sensitivity of the human circadian system to short-wavelength (420-nm) light. *J Biol Rhythms* 2008;23:379–86.

130. Illnerova H, Vanecek J. Response of rat pineal serotonin N-acetyltransferase to one min light pulse at different night times. *Brain Res* 1979;167:431–4.

131. Yellon SM, Tamarkin L, Pratt BL, et al. Pineal melatonin in the Djungarian hamster: photoperiodic regulation of a circadian rhythm. *Endocrinology* 1982;111:488–92.

132. Maywood ES, Hastings MH, Max M, et al. Circadian and daily rhythms of melatonin in the blood and pineal gland of free-running and entrained Syrian hamsters. *J Endocrinol* 1993;136:65–73.

133. Wehr TA. The durations of human melatonin secretion and sleep respond to changes in

daylength (photoperiod). *J Clin Endocrinol Metab* 1991;73:1276–80.

134. Bartness TJ, Powers JB, Hastings MH, et al. The timed infusion paradigm for melatonin delivery: what has it taught us about the melatonin signal, its reception, and the photoperiodic control of seasonal responses? *J Pineal Res* 1993;15:161–90.

135. Underwood H, Goldman BD. Vertebrate circadian and photoperiodic systems: role of the pineal gland and melatonin. *J Biol Rhythms* 1987;2:279–315.

136. Cassone VM, Chesworth MJ, Armstrong SM. Dose-dependent entrainment of rat circadian rhythms by daily injection of melatonin. *J Biol Rhythms* 1986;1:219–29.

137. Lewy AJ, Ahmed S, Jackson JM, et al. Melatonin shifts human circadian rhythms according to a phase-response curve. *Chronobiol Int* 1992;9:380–92.

138. Redman J, Armstrong S, Ng KT. Free-running activity rhythms in the rat: entrainment by melatonin. *Science* 1983;219:1089–91.

139. Cassone VM, Roberts MH, Moore RY. Effects of melatonin on 2-deoxy-[1–14C]glucose uptake within rat suprachiasmatic nucleus. *Am J Physiol* 1988;255:R332–7.

140. Liu C, Weaver DR, Jin X, et al. Molecular dissection of two distinct actions of melatonin on the suprachiasmatic circadian clock. *Neuron* 1997;19:91–102.

141. Shibata S, Cassone VM, Moore RY. Effects of melatonin on neuronal activity in the rat suprachiasmatic nucleus in vitro. *Neurosci Lett* 1989;97:140–4.

142. Stehle J, Vanecek J, Vollrath L. Effects of melatonin on spontaneous electrical activity of neurons in rat suprachiasmatic nuclei: an in vitro iontophoretic study. *J Neural Transm* 1989;78:173–7.

143. Vanecek J, Pavlik A, Illnerova H. Hypothalamic melatonin receptor sites revealed by autoradiography. *Brain Res* 1987;435:359–62.

144. Weaver DR, Rivkees SA, Reppert SM. Localization and characterization of melatonin receptors in rodent brain by in vitro autoradiography. *J Neurosci* 1989;9:2581–90.

145. Reiter RJ, Tan DX, Fuentes-Broto L. Melatonin: a multitasking molecule. *Prog Brain Res* 2010;181:127–51.

146. Ergun Y, Ergun UG, Orhan FO, et al. Co-administration of a nitric oxide synthase inhibitor and melatonin exerts an additive antidepressant-like effect in the mouse forced swim test. *Med Sci Monit* 2006;12:BR307–12.

147. Mantovani M, Kaster MP, Pertile R, et al. Mechanisms involved in the antinociception caused by melatonin in mice. *J Pineal Res* 2006;41:382–9.

148. Campbell CB, Ramaley JA. Retinohypothalamic projections: correlations with onset of the adrenal rhythm in infant rats. *Endocrinology* 1974;94:1201–4.

149. Fuchs JL, Moore RY. Development of circadian rhythmicity and light responsiveness in the rat suprachiasmatic nucleus: a study using the 2-deoxy[1–14C]glucose method. *Proc Natl Acad Sci USA* 1980;77:1204–8.

150. Moore RY, Bernstein ME. Synaptogenesis in the rat suprachiasmatic nucleus demonstrated by electron microscopy and synapsin I immunoreactivity. *J Neurosci* 1989;9:2151–62.

151. Reppert SM, Schwartz WJ. The suprachiasmatic nuclei of the fetal rat: characterization of a functional circadian clock using 14C labeled deoxyglucose. *J Neurosci* 1984;4:1677–82.

152. Reppert SM, Schwartz WJ. Functional activity of the suprachiasmatic nuclei in the fetal primate. *Neurosci Lett* 1984;46:145–9.

153. Rivkees SA. Emergence and influences of circadian rhythmicity in infants. *Clin Perinatol* 2004;31:217–28, v–vi.

154. Rivkees SA. The development of circadian rhythms: from animals to humans. *Sleep Med Clin* 2007;2:331–41.

155. Reppert SM, Weaver DR. Coordination of circadian timing in mammals. *Nature* 2002;418:935–41.

156. Reppert SM. Interaction between the circadian clocks of mother and fetus. *Ciba Found Symp* 1995;183:198–207; discussion -11.

157. Kennaway DJ, Goble FC, Stamp GE. Factors influencing the development of melatonin rhythmicity in humans. *J Clin Endocrinol Metab* 1996;81:1525–32.

158. Mirmiran M, Kok JH. Circadian rhythms in early human development. *Early Hum Dev* 1991;26:121–8.

159. Spangler G. The emergence of adrenocortical circadian function in newborns and infants and its relationship to sleep, feeding and maternal adrenocortical activity. *Early Hum Dev* 1991;25:197–208.

160. Weinert D, Sitka U, Minors DS, et al. The development of circadian rhythmicity in neonates. *Early Hum Dev* 1994; 36:117–26.

161. Monk TH, Buysse DJ, Reynolds CF, 3rd, et al. Subjective alertness rhythms in elderly people. *J Biol Rhythms* 1996;11:268–76.

162. Touitou Y, Reinberg A, Bogdan A, et al. Age-related changes in both circadian and seasonal rhythms of rectal temperature with special reference to senile dementia of Alzheimer type. *Gerontology* 1986;32:110–18.

163. van Coevorden A, Stolear JC, Dhaene M, et al. Effect of chronic oral testosterone undecanoate administration on the pituitary-testicular axes of hemodialyzed male patients. *Clin Nephrol* 1986;26:48–54.

164. Miles LE, Dement WC. Sleep and aging. *Sleep* 1980;3:1–220.

165. Weitzman ED, Moline ML, Czeisler CA, et al. Chronobiology of aging: temperature, sleep-wake rhythms and entrainment. *Neurobiol Aging* 1982;3:299–309.

166. Czeisler CA, Duffy JF, Shanahan TL, et al. Stability, precision, and near-24-hour period of the human circadian pacemaker. *Science* 1999;284:2177–81.

167. Moore RY. A clock for the ages. *Science* 1999;284:2102–3.

168. Benloucif S, Masana MI, Dubocovich ML. Light-induced phase shifts of circadian activity rhythms and immediate early gene expression in the suprachiasmatic nucleus are attenuated in old C3H/HeN mice. *Brain Res* 1997;747:34–42.

169. Campbell SS, Kripke DF, Gillin JC, et al. Exposure to light in healthy elderly subjects and Alzheimer's patients. *Physiol Behav* 1988;42:141–4.

170. Van Reeth O, Zhang Y, Reddy A, et al. Aging alters the entraining effects of an activity-inducing stimulus on the circadian clock. *Brain Res* 1993;607:286–92.

171. Zhang Y, Kornhauser JM, Zee PC, et al. Effects of aging on light-induced phase-shifting of circadian behavioral rhythms, fos expression and CREB phosphorylation in the hamster suprachiasmatic nucleus. *Neuroscience* 1996;70:951–61.

172. Ancoli-Israel S, Klauber MR, Jones DW, et al. Variations in circadian rhythms of activity, sleep, and light exposure related to dementia in nursing-home patients. *Sleep* 1997;20:18–23.

173. Ancoli-Israel S, Martin JL, Kripke DF, et al. Effect of light treatment on sleep and circadian rhythms in demented nursing home patients. *J Am Geriatr Soc* 2002;50:282–9.

174. Machado-Salas J, Scheibel ME, Scheibel AB. Morphologic changes in the hypothalamus of the old mouse. *Exp Neurol* 1977;57:102–11.

175. Roozendaal B, van Gool WA, Swaab DF, et al. Changes in vasopressin cells of the rat suprachiasmatic nucleus with aging. *Brain Res* 1987;409:259–64.

176. Swaab DF, Fliers E, Partiman TS. The suprachiasmatic nucleus of the human brain in relation to sex, age and senile dementia. *Brain Res* 1985;342:37–44.

177. Madeira MD, Sousa N, Santer RM, et al. Age and sex do not affect the volume, cell numbers, or cell size of the suprachiasmatic nucleus of the rat: an unbiased stereological study. *J Comp Neurol* 1995;361:585–601.

178. Peng MT, Jiang MJ, Hsu HK. Changes in running-wheel activity, eating and drinking and their day/night distributions throughout the life span of the rat. *J Gerontol* 1980;35:339–47.

179. Sutin EL, Dement WC, Heller HC, et al. Light-induced gene expression in the suprachiasmatic nucleus of young and aging rats. *Neurobiol Aging* 1993;14:441–6.

180. Satinoff E, Li H, Tcheng TK, et al. Do the suprachiasmatic nuclei oscillate in old rats as they do in young ones? *Am J Physiol* 1993;265:R1216–22.

181. Wise PM, Cohen IR, Weiland NG, et al. Aging alters the circadian rhythm of glucose utilization in the suprachiasmatic nucleus. *Proc Natl Acad Sci USA* 1988;85:5305–9.

182. Aschoff J. Circadian rhythms in man. *Science* 1965;148:1427–32.

183. Akerstedt T, Gillberg M. The circadian variation of experimentally displaced sleep. *Sleep* 1981;4:159–69.

184. Czeisler CA, Weitzman E, Moore-Ede MC, et al. Human sleep: its duration and organization depend on its circadian phase. *Science* 1980;210:1264–7.

185. Dijk DJ, Czeisler CA. Paradoxical timing of the circadian rhythm of sleep propensity serves to consolidate sleep and wakefulness in humans. *Neurosci Lett* 1994;166:63–8.

186. Zulley J, Wever R, Aschoff J. The dependence of onset and duration of sleep on th circadian rhythm of rectal temperature. *Pflugers Arch* 1981;391:314–18.

187. Dijk DJ, Czeisler CA. Contribution of the circadian pacemaker and the sleep homeostat to sleep propensity, sleep structure, electroencephalographic slow waves, and sleep spindle activity in humans. *J Neurosci* 1995;15:3526–38.

188. Lavie P. Ultrashort sleep-waking schedule. III. "Gates" and "forbidden zones" for sleep. *Electroencephalogr Clin Neurophysiol* 1986;63:414–25.

189. Strogatz SH, Kronauer RE, Czeisler CA. Circadian pacemaker interferes with sleep onset at specific times each day: role in insomnia. *Am J Physiol* 1987;253:R172–8.

190. Reid KJ, Zee PC. Circadian rhythm sleep disorders. *Handb Clin Neurol* 2011;99:963–77.

191. Borbely AA. A two process model of sleep regulation. *Hum Neurobiol* 1982;1:195–204.

192. Borbely AA, Achermann P. Concepts and models of sleep regulation: an overview. *J Sleep Res* 1992;1:63–79.

193. Borbely AA, Achermann P. Sleep homeostasis and models of sleep regulation. *J Biol Rhythms* 1999;14:557–68.

194. Daan S, Beersma DG, Borbely AA. Timing of human sleep: recovery process gated by a circadian pacemaker. *Am J Physiol* 1984;246:R161–83.

195. Dijk DJ, Brunner DP, Beersma DG, et al. Electroencephalogram power density and slow wave sleep as a function of prior waking and circadian phase. *Sleep* 1990;13:430–40.

196. Dijk DJ, Brunner DP, Borbely AA. Time course of EEG power density during long sleep in humans. *Am J Physiol* 1990;258:R650–61.

197. Ibuka N, Inouye SI, Kawamura H. Analysis of sleep-wakefulness rhythms in male rats after suprachiasmatic nucleus lesions and ocular enucleation. *Brain Res* 1977;122:33–47.

198. Mistlberger RE, Bergmann BM, Waldenar W, et al. Recovery sleep following sleep deprivation in intact and suprachiasmatic nuclei-lesioned rats. *Sleep* 1983;6:217–33.

199. Mouret J, Coindet J, Debilly G, et al. Suprachiasmatic nuclei lesions in the rat: alterations in sleep circadian rhythms. *Electroencephalogr Clin Neurophysiol* 1978;45:402–8.

200. Tobler I, Borbely AA, Groos G. The effect of sleep deprivation on sleep in rats with suprachiasmatic lesions. *Neurosci Lett* 1983;42:49–54.

201. Trachsel L, Edgar DM, Seidel WF, et al. Sleep homeostasis in suprachiasmatic nuclei-lesioned rats: effects of sleep deprivation and triazolam administration. *Brain Res* 1992;589:253–61.

202. Edgar DM, Dement WC, Fuller CA. Effect of SCN lesions on sleep in squirrel monkeys: evidence for opponent processes in sleep-wake regulation. *J Neurosci* 1993;13:1065–79.

203. Fuller PM, Gooley JJ, Saper CB. Neurobiology of the sleep-wake cycle: sleep architecture, circadian regulation, and regulatory feedback. *J Biol Rhythms* 2006;21:482–93.

204. Saper CB, Lu J, Chou TC, et al. The hypothalamic integrator for circadian rhythms. *Trends Neurosci* 2005;28:152–7.

205. Chou TC, Scammell TE, Gooley JJ, et al. Critical role of dorsomedial hypothalamic nucleus in a wide range of behavioral circadian rhythms. *J Neurosci* 2003;23:10691–702.

206. Saper CB, Chou TC, Scammell TE. The sleep switch: hypothalamic control of sleep and wakefulness. *Trends Neurosci* 2001;24:726–31.

207. AASM. *The International Classification of Sleep Disorders.* 2nd ed. Westchester, IL: American Academy of Sleep Medicne; 2005.

208. Katzenberg D, Young T, Finn L, et al. A CLOCK polymorphism associated with human diurnal preference. *Sleep* 1998;21:569–76.

209. Toh KL. An hPer2 phosphorylation site mutation in familial advanced sleep phase syndrome. *Science* 2001;291:1040–3.

210. Xu Y, Padiath QS, Shapiro RE, et al. Functional consequences of a CKIdelta mutation causing familial advanced sleep phase syndrome. *Nature* 2005;434:640–4.

211. Archer SN, Robilliard DL, Skene DJ. A length polymorphism in the circadian clock gene Per3 is linked to delayed sleep phase syndrome and extreme diurnal preference. *Sleep* 2003;26(4):413–5.

212. Ebisawa T, Uchiyama M, Kajimura N. Association of structural polymorphisms in the human period3 gene with delayed sleep phase syndrome. *EMBO Rep* 2001;2(4):342,6.

213. Iwase T, Kajimura N, Uchiyama M. Mutation screening of the human Clock gene in circadian rhythm sleep disorders. *Psychiatry Res* 2002;109(2):121,8.

214. Toh KL, Jones CR, He Y. An hPer2 phosphorylation site mutation in familial advanced sleep phase syndrome. *Science* 2001;291(5506):1040,3.

215. Hohjoh H, Takahashi Y, Hatta Y, et al. Possible association of human leucocyte antigen DR1 with delayed sleep phase syndrome. *Psychiatry Clin Neurosci* 1999;53:527–9.

216. Jones CR, Campbell SS, Zone SE, et al. Familial advanced sleep-phase syndrome: a short-period circadian rhythm variant in humans. *Nat Med* 1999;5:1062–5.

217. Reid KJ, Chang AM, Dubocovich ML, et al. Familial advanced sleep phase syndrome. *Arch Neurol* 2001;58:1089–94.

218. Sack RL, Brandes RW, Kendall AR, et al. Entrainment of free-running circadian rhythms by melatonin in blind people. *N Engl J Med* 2000;343:1070–7.

219. McArthur AJ, Lewy AJ, Sack RL. Non-24-hour sleep-wake syndrome in a sighted man: circadian rhythm studies and efficacy of melatonin treatment. *Sleep* 1996;19:544–53.

220. Sack RL, Lewy AJ, Blood ML, et al. Circadian rhythm abnormalities in totally blind people: incidence and clinical significance. *J Clin Endocrinol Metab* 1992;75:127–34.

221. Nakamura K, Hashimoto S, Honma S, et al. Daily melatonin intake resets circadian rhythms of a sighted man with non-24-hour sleep-wake syndrome who lacks the nocturnal melatonin rise. *Psychiatry Clin Neurosci* 1997;51:121–7.

222. Ayalon L, Borodkin K, Dishon L, et al. Circadian rhythm sleep disorders following mild traumatic brain injury. *Neurology* 2007;68:1136–40.

223. Bombois S, Derambure P, Pasquier F, et al. Sleep disorders in aging and dementia. *J Nutr Health Aging* 2010;14:212–17.

224. Neikrug AB, Ancoli-Israel S. Sleep disturbances in nursing homes. *J Nutr Health Aging* 2010;14:207–11.

225. Pillar G, Etzioni A, Shahar E, et al. Melatonin treatment in an institutionalised child with psychomotor retardation and an irregular sleep-wake pattern. *Arch Dis Child* 1998;79:63–4.

226. Pillar G, Shahar E, Peled N, et al. Melatonin improves sleep-wake patterns in psychomotor retarded children. *Pediatr Neurol* 2000;23:225–8.

227. Nagtegaal JE, Kerkhof GA, Smits MG, et al. Delayed sleep phase syndrome: a placebo-controlled cross-over study on the effects of melatonin administered five hours before the individual dim light melatonin onset. *J Sleep Res* 1998;7:135–43.

228. Rosenthal NE, Joseph-Vanderpool JR, Levendosky AA, et al. Phase-shifting effects of bright morning light as treatment for delayed sleep phase syndrome. *Sleep* 1990;13:354–61.

229. Morgenthaler TI, Lee-Chiong T, Alessi C, et al. Practice parameters for the clinical evaluation and treatment of circadian rhythm sleep disorders. An American Academy of Sleep Medicine report. *Sleep* 2007;30:1445–59.

230. Dahlitz M, Alvarez B, Vignau J, et al. Delayed sleep phase syndrome response to melatonin. *Lancet* 1991;337:1121–4.

231. Oldani A, Ferini-Strambi L, Zucconi M, et al. Melatonin and delayed sleep phase syndrome: ambulatory polygraphic evaluation. *NeuroReport* 1994;6:132–4.

232. Brzezinski A, Vangel MG, Wurtman RJ, et al. Effects of exogenous melatonin on sleep: a meta-analysis. *Sleep Med Rev* 2005;9:41–50.

233. Lockley SW. Timed melatonin treatment for delayed sleep phase syndrome: the importance of knowing circadian phase. *Sleep* 2005;28:1214–16.

234. van Geijlswijk IM, Korzilius HP, Smits MG. The use of exogenous melatonin in delayed sleep phase disorder: a meta-analysis. *Sleep* 2010;33:1605–14.

235. Zee PC. Melantonin for the treatment of advanced sleep phase disorder. *Sleep* 2008;31:923; author reply 5.

236. Zee PC. Shedding light on the effectiveness of melatonin for circadian rhythm sleep disorders. *Sleep* 2010;33:1581–2.

237. Penev PD, Zee PC. Melatonin: a clinical perspective. *Ann Neurol* 1997;42:545–53.

238. Lack L, Wright H. The effect of evening bright light in delaying the circadian rhythms and lengthening the sleep of early morning awakening insomniacs. *Sleep* 1993;16:436–43.

239. Lack L, Wright H, Kemp K, et al. The treatment of early-morning awakening insomnia with 2 evenings of bright light. *Sleep* 2005;28:616–23.

240. Terman M, Lewy AJ, Dijk DJ, et al. Light treatment for sleep disorders: consensus report. IV. Sleep phase and duration disturbances. *J Biol Rhythms* 1995;10:135–47.

241. Lockley SW, Skene DJ, James K, et al. Melatonin administration can entrain the free-running circadian system of blind subjects. *J Endocrinol* 2000;164:R1–6.

242. Dowling GA, Mastick J, Hubbard EM, et al. Effect of timed bright light treatment for rest-activity disruption in institutionalized patients with Alzheimer's disease. *Int J Geriatr Psychiatry* 2005;20:738–43.

243. Dowling GA, Hubbard EM, Mastick J, et al. Effect of morning bright light treatment for rest-activity disruption in institutionalized patients with severe Alzheimer's disease. *Int Psychogeriatr* 2005;17:221–36.

244. Dowling GA, Burr RL, Van Someren EJ, et al. Melatonin and bright-light treatment for rest-activity disruption in institutionalized patients with Alzheimer's disease. *J Am Geriatr Soc* 2008;56:239–46.

245. Alessi CA, Martin JL, Webber AP, et al. Randomized, controlled trial of a nonpharmacological intervention to improve abnormal sleep/wake patterns in nursing home residents. *J Am Geriatr Soc* 2005;53:803–10.

246. Srinivasan V, Singh J, Pandi-Perumal SR, et al. Jet lag, circadian rhythm sleep disturbances, and depression: the role of melatonin and its analogs. *Adv Ther* 2010;27:796–813.

247. Jackson G. Come fly with me: jet lag and melatonin. *Int J Clin Pract* 2010;64:135.

248. Srinivasan V, Spence DW, Pandi-Perumal SR, et al. Jet lag: therapeutic use of melatonin and possible application of melatonin analogs. *Travel Med Infect Dis* 2008;6:17–28.

249. Sadeghniiat-Haghighi K, Aminian O, Pouryaghoub G, et al. Efficacy and hypnotic effects of melatonin in shift-work nurses: double-blind, placebo-controlled crossover trial. *J Circadian Rhythms* 2008;6:10.

250. Petrie K, Conaglen JV, Thompson L, et al. Effect of melatonin on jet lag after long haul flights. *BMJ* 1989;298:705–7.

251. Sack RL, Lewy AJ. Melatonin as a chronobiotic: treatment of circadian desynchrony in night workers and the blind. *J Biol Rhythms* 1997;12:595–603.

252. Bonuccelli U, Del Dotto P, Lucetti C, et al. Diurnal motor variations to repeated doses of levodopa in Parkinson's disease. *Clinical Neuropharmacol* 2000;23:28–33.

253. Nutt JG, Woodward WR, Carter JH, et al. Influence of fluctuations of plasma large neutral amino acids with normal diets on the clinical response to levodopa. *J Neurol Neurosurg Psychiatry* 1989;52:481–7.

254. van Hilten JJ, Kabel JF, Middelkoop HA, et al. Assessment of response fluctuations in Parkinson's disease by ambulatory wrist activity monitoring. *Acta Neurol Scand* 1993;87:171–7.

255. van Hilten JJ, Middelkoop HA, Kerkhof GA, et al. A new approach in the assessment of motor activity in Parkinson's disease. *J Neurol Neurosurg Psychiatry* 1991;54:976–9.

256. Arias-Vera JR, Mansoor GA, White WB. Abnormalities in blood pressure regulation in a patient with Parkinson's disease. *Am J Hypertension* 2003;16:612–13.

257. Devos D, Kroumova M, Bordet R, et al. Heart rate variability and Parkinson's disease severity. *J Neural Transm* 2003;110:997–1011.

258. Ejaz AA, Sekhon IS, Munjal S. Characteristic findings on 24-h ambulatory blood pressure monitoring in a series of patients with Parkinson's disease. *European J Int Med* 2006;17:417–20.

259. Mihci E, Kardelen F, Dora B, et al. Orthostatic heart rate variability analysis in idiopathic Parkinson's disease. *Acta Neurol Scand* 2006;113:288–93.

260. Pathak A, Senard JM. Blood pressure disorders during Parkinson's disease: epidemiology, pathophysiology and management. *Exp Rev Neurotherap* 2006;6:1173–80.

261. Pursiainen V, Haapaniemi TH, Korpelainen JT, et al. Circadian heart rate variability in Parkinson's disease. *J Neurol* 2002;249:1535–40.

262. Comella CL. Sleep disorders in Parkinson's disease: an overview. *Mov Disord* 2007;22:S367-S73.

263. Placidi F, Izzi F, Romigi A, et al. Sleep-wake cycle and effects of cabergoline monotherapy in de novo Parkinson's disease patients. An ambulatory polysomnographic study. *J Neurol* 2008;255:1032–7.

264. Porter B, Macfarlane R, Walker R. The frequency and nature of sleep disorders in a community-based population of patients with Parkinson's disease. *Eur J Neurol* 2008;15:50–4.

265. van Hilten JJ, Weggeman M, van der Velde EA, et al. Sleep, excessive daytime sleepiness and fatigue in Parkinson's disease. *J Neural Transm* 1993;5:235–44.

266. Verbaan D, van Rooden SM, Visser M, et al. Nighttime sleep problems and daytime sleepiness in Parkinson's disease. *Mov Disord* 2008;23:35–41.

267. Sowers JR, Vlachakis N. Circadian variation in plasma dopamine levels in man. *J Endocrinol Invest* 1984;7:341–5.

268. Hakamaki T, Rajala T, Lehtonen A. Ambulatory 24-hour blood pressure recordings in patients with Parkinson's disease with or without fludrocortisone. *Intl J Clin Pharmacol Therap* 1998;36:367–9.

269. Hartmann A, Veldhuis JD, Deuschle M, et al. Twenty-four hour cortisol release profiles in patients with Alzheimer's and Parkinson's disease compared to normal controls: ultradian secretory pulsatility and diurnal variation. *Neurobiol Aging* 1997;18:285–9.

270. Bordet R, Devos D, Brique S, et al. Study of circadian melatonin secretion pattern at different stages of Parkinson's disease. *Clinical Neuropharmacol* 2003;26:65–72.

271. Fertl E, Auff E, Doppelbauer A, et al. Circadian secretion pattern of melatonin in Parkinson's disease. *J Neural Transm* 1991;3:41–7.

272. Fertl E, Auff E, Doppelbauer A, et al. Circadian secretion pattern of melatonin in de novo parkinsonian patients: evidence for phase-shifting properties of l-dopa. *J Neural Transm* 1993;5:227–34.

273. Imbesi M, Yildiz S, Dirim Arslan A, et al. Dopamine receptor-mediated regulation of neuronal "clock" gene expression. *Neuroscience* 2009;158:537–44.

274. Besharse JC, Zhuang M, Freeman K, et al. Regulation of photoreceptor Per1 and Per2 by light, dopamine and a circadian clock. *Eur J Neurosci* 2004;20:167–74.

275. Yujnovsky I, Hirayama J, Doi M, et al. Signaling mediated by the dopamine D2 receptor potentiates circadian regulation by CLOCK:BMAL1. *Proc Nat Acad Sci USA* 2006;103:6386–91.

276. Sahar S, Zocchi L, Kinoshita C, et al. Regulation of BMAL1 protein stability and circadian function by GSK3beta-mediated phosphorylation. *PLoS One* 2010;5:e8561.

277. Hood S, Cassidy P, Cossette MP, et al. Endogenous dopamine regulates the rhythm of expression of the clock protein PER2 in the rat dorsal striatum via daily activation of D2 dopamine receptors. *J Neurosci* 2010;30:14046–58.

278. Cai Y, Liu S, Sothern RB, et al. Expression of clock genes Per1 and Bmal1 in total leukocytes in health and Parkinson's disease. *Eur J Neurol* 2010;17(4):550–4.

279. Morton AJ, Wood NI, Hastings MH, et al. Disintegration of the sleep-wake cycle and circadian timing in Huntington's disease. *J Neurosci* 2005;25:157–63.

280. Pallier PN, Maywood ES, Zheng Z, et al. Pharmacological imposition of sleep slows cognitive decline and reverses dysregulation of circadian gene expression in a transgenic mouse model of Huntington's disease. *J Neurosci* 2007;27:7869–78.

281. Witting W, Kwa IH, Eikelenboom P, et al. Alterations in the circadian rest-activity rhythm in aging and Alzheimer's disease. *Biol Psychiatry* 1990;27:563–72.

282. Baier PC, Trenkwalder C. Circadian variation in restless legs syndrome. *Sleep Med* 2007;8:645–50.

283. Michaud M, Dumont M, Selmaoui B, et al. Circadian rhythm of restless legs syndrome: relationship with biological markers. *Ann Neurol* 2004;55:372–80.

284. Trenkwalder C, Hening WA, Walters AS, et al. Circadian rhythm of periodic limb movements and sensory symptoms of restless legs syndrome. *Mov Disord* 1999;14:102–10.

285. Phanthumchinda K, Vichichanyakul M, Yodnophaklao P. Segawa disease. *J Med Assoc Thai* 1996;79:473–6.

286. Segawa M. Autosomal dominant GTP cyclohydrolase I (AD GCH 1) deficiency (Segawa disease, dystonia 5; DYT 5). *Chang Gung Med J* 2009;32:1–11.

7

The Normal Motor System

Sleep/Wake States, Circadian Rhythms, and Ontogeny[*]

ARTHUR S. WALTERS

THE MOTOR system is highly modulated by the changes in state from wake to drowsiness to slow-wave sleep (SWS) and then to rapid eye movement (REM) sleep. Indeed, so significant are the changes in motor activity depending on state that various researchers have used quantitative recordings of motor activity, known as actigraphy, as a basis for determining sleep and wake states.[1] The importance of measuring such activity is growing and is reflected throughout this volume, as well as in the specific chapter on actigraphy, a primary technique for assessing bodily movement (see Chapter 12).[1]

The normal motor system shows marked variations in activity and responsiveness as a function of both sleep-wake state and time of day (based on circadian rhythm as well as sleep history). Age is also an important factor because the relation of the motor system to sleep changes throughout the life span. However, there are many other influences that can modulate motor activity during sleep. It is also important to recognize that movements themselves can affect sleep and other bodily functions such as sympathetic nervous system activity.[2]

This body of the chapter is divided into five sections: the first section briefly introduces the various techniques for observing movement during sleep; the second section examines the relationship of the sleep/wake states to movement and the various "normal" motor phenomena that are associated with the various sleep states; the third section briefly introduces the issue of the circadian control of motor activity; the fourth section examines the changes in motor activity related to sleep during the life span; and the final section examines the question of changes in the

* This chapter is a revised, updated version of a previous chapter for the first edition of our book written by our good friend and colleague, Wayne Alfred Hening, MD, PhD.

normal pattern that are associated with a variety of other conditions.

TECHNIQUES FOR EVALUATING MOTOR ACTIVITY

Activity Monitoring

The simplest means of measuring movement is through activity monitoring, or actigraphy.[3-9] This is the most direct and specific technique for quantifying and recording movements. A value for movement is determined and assigned to a sample period that can range from a few milliseconds up to many hours. Actigraphy can be used for various purposes: to measure the degree of movement, to demonstrate circadian or other cyclical patterns of movement, and to discriminate wake from sleep.[3-9] These uses vary in their success. Typically, these activity-monitoring devices use accelerometry to quantify movement, so that, to be accurate, they measure acceleration, not movement, but movement can be derived from acceleration. Direction can also be derived if three-dimensional (3D) acceleration is measured. Several small self-contained devices currently available provide a direct assessment of the amount of activity or body movement at the point of the body where they are attached. They now come with a variety of different types of software for processing the movement signal and can be combined with light detectors[3-9] or positional detectors to determine whether the subject is sitting, lying, or upright.[3-9] The technology is constantly improving, permitting faster sampling rates and more extended durations of data collection.

Activity monitoring has a number of advantages over sleep lab polysomnography (PSG) or even ambulatory PSG monitoring. First, it can be efficiently and inexpensively used for extended periods. Depending on the equipment and technique used, recordings can be made for many days or even months. This extended recording can allow for the capture of rare events, overcoming the problem of variability that can limit the accuracy of more abbreviated studies and repeated measurement under different conditions. Second, because the activity monitors are usually small, lightweight, and self-contained, activity monitoring can occur in multiple settings, including the home, and in varied activity states. The activity monitors can be taken out of the laboratory, self-applied, and even transmitted by mail. They may be useful in uncooperative patient groups with degenerative disease who would not tolerate a laboratory sleep study[3-9] and may simplify large studies of therapeutic interventions in insomnia or other sleep disturbances. Third, some PMG channels, such as electromyographic (EMG), may indicate activity that is not, in fact, significant for the patient. Activity monitoring can discriminate actual movement from EMG potentials, which may occur without any significant displacement of a limb.

The limitations on activity monitoring result from the relatively nonspecific results and the limited information monitored. The results are generally nonspecific because all movement, even transmitted movement, is recorded. Therefore, the exact nature of a movement, its distribution, and even its speed may not be reflected in the recording. It cannot be described or, in many instances, meaningfully categorized. Certain nonspecific movements such as gravity or almost constant velocity movement (e.g., car on highway) can be largely eliminated by filtering, but activity monitors may not discriminate between normal or abnormal movements or even active and passive movements. The information obtained by activity monitoring is also limited because there may be no information about cerebral state (electroencephalogram [EEG]), eye movements (too small to be reflected in a limb monitor), or breathing. Therefore, they do not provide much useful information about physiologic state or crucial information about exact sleep stages.

To examine specific movements, the activity monitor is placed at the site of the movement.[3-9] This may mean placing the monitor at multiple sites to monitor a variety of different movements,[3-9] which may show dramatically different variations with sleep state and stages. In general, the goal of such recording is to count and quantify such movements, not merely to indicate when movement occurs.

Activity meters that measure specific types of movements such as periodic limb movements in sleep (PLMS) have been designed.[10,11] Two of these devices, the Actiwatch and the PAM-RL, have undergone validation studies and show a reasonable correlation with PLMS obtained by PMG.[10,11]

Sleep Studies

Standard sleep studies are of established worth in evaluating motor activity in sleep. A standard PSG, with at least one EMG lead for the legs, provides a fair amount of information about motor activity. This can be supplemented by technician observations, wherever feasible, to explain and better characterize motor events on the record. Standard sleep recording uses the chin EMG lead to record branchial muscle tone and EMG leads on one or both legs for evaluation of possible PLMS. Where a specific motor complaint is noted that involves movement of other body parts—arms, trunk, abdomen, neck, or face—additional leads can be applied. Most laboratories perform EMGs with a standard EEG filter setting (bandpass of 5 to 70 Hz), but a more artifact-free recording of muscle potentials can be obtained if a higher bandpass (e.g., 50 to 1500 Hz) is employed. These frequencies better match the frequency of actual muscle potentials. It is also useful to set the amplitude before the study so that a maximal voluntary contraction is near or slightly above the full pen excursion for a polygraphic recorder.

Videotape studies can be extremely helpful in sorting out different movements. This can permit correlation of computer-generated records of movement or EMG potentials with actual movements and allow, in some cases, distinguishing further the character of the movements. In-laboratory sleep studies with associated videotape are often critical in making the diagnosis of REM sleep behavior disorder, disorders of partial arousal (sleep walking, sleep terrors, confusional arousals), or sleep-related epilepsy and in being able to discriminate these disorders from each other. Accompanying audio is often critical in diagnosing sleep-related bruxism or tooth grinding.[12] Split-screen studies, with polygraphic montages correlated directly with videotaping of the associated behavior, are especially helpful in this regard. To provide the best natural conditions, infrared cameras are optimal, although many modern color video cameras can perform under relatively low-light conditions. If possible, subjects should sleep with minimal covers because this makes visualization of movements much easier. To do this, carefully temperature-controlled rooms, especially warmer ones, are helpful. Time bases, including those added by special-effects generators or an onscreen clock, can facilitate search and retrieval of movements. Long-term monitoring may also help understand less common motor activity, as well as the day-to-day variation of motor activity.[13]

HOME-BASED POLYSOMNOGRAPHY

A variety of systems (e.g., the Nightcap system[14]) are available for home or ambulatory monitoring of sleep,[15-17] with capacity that can now include 16 or more channels. Most of the customary sleep-recording channels can be used in the ambulatory setting. Generally, technicians prepare the patient for study either in the laboratory or at home. The various channels are recorded on tape for later display and analysis with computer systems. The advantage of these systems is that they reduce the personnel required and can reduce cost. This may permit analysis of less frequent phenomena than those profitably studied in the laboratory or permit repeated studies. In addition, the subject is studied under his or her normal conditions in the more relevant home environment. However, because these systems lack supervision, clear identification of events may not be feasible. At the current juncture the American Academy of Sleep Medicine (AASM) only recommends standard in-home PSG for uncomplicated sleep apnea.[18]

OTHER RECORDING SYSTEMS

In recent years, a number of other movement-detecting systems have been proposed.[19] The static charge-sensitive bed is a device,[20-23] suitable for adult and pediatric[20] recordings, which is highly sensitive to movements, including such physiologic movements as those associated with breathing or the heartbeat. Different kinds of movement, such as body movements or respiratory pauses, can be differentiated by selective filtration of the potentials transmitted by the bed.[20-23] This can allow for quantification of sleep states for counting of movements. Because the bed is rather simple and not particularly expensive, it may offer an alternative to some PSG in the future, although, like other simplified recording systems, it is not as yet as accurate as PSG in detailing sleep states and associated movements.[20-23] Recently, it has been reported to have good accuracy in quantifying PLMS.[23] An alternate system measures temperature relations as a means of determining movement[24,25] and has been validated against video-PSG.[26] Ultrasound has been used to record prenatal movement,[27,28] including those believed to be related to specific sleep stages.[27,28]

Basic Studies of the Motor System and Sleep

A variety of techniques have been used to examine the activity of the brain and nervous system during sleep in ways relevant to motor activity.

Although most of these techniques have been applied to animals or even in vitro preparations, some of them, especially a range of imaging techniques,[29-32] have been applied to humans. Neurophysiologic techniques applied to humans include studies of a variety of reflexes[33-35] and evoked potentials,[36,37] and magnetic stimulation[38] or electric stimulation over the brain. It is even possible to combine techniques such as functional magnetic resonance imaging (fMRI) and evoked potential studies by EEG.[39]

Changes include alterations of the level or pattern of neuronal activity, changes in the connectivity of specific circuits, and shifts in the degree of overall activity in different brain regions. The pattern that emerges suggests that the various wake and sleep states should be regarded as systematic regimens of altered functional organization. Not only is the activity of specific cells shifted up or down, but the signs of specific relationships are changed: a sensory input that can cause excitation in wake may cause inhibition in sleep.[40,41] This can include conditioned responses.[40,41]

Basic discoveries in animal models and pathologic cases can also be applied to understanding human sleep movement control. For instance, strong evidence has developed that hypocretins can help stimulate wake and motor activity. Information about the presence of both tonic and phasic inhibition during REM has been extended to measurements of the degree of chin muscle inhibition both tonically and phasically (associated with REMS).[12,42]

Analysis of Movements

Besides association of movements with macro-structural and microstructural sleep features, movements can be examined with statistical techniques that can analyze the distribution of movements. The parameters that define the statistical distribution can then be used to characterize the relation of movements to sleep, specifying the frequency and intensity of movements.[43]

THE NORMAL MOTOR SYSTEM AND SLEEP

During the night, a major change in motor activity depends on the sleep state (wake, REM, non–rapid eye movement [non-REM] sleep stages). For example, one commonly used sleep/wake state monitor, the chin EMG, is an indicator of branchial (brainstem) muscle tone. During wake, chin muscle tone is high and a tonically active chin EMG is interrupted by phasic contractions (e.g., facial expressions, tension, chewing). With relaxation and drowsiness, the level of EMG activity decreases. It further decreases as non-REM sleep is achieved and deepens to SWS levels. Then, during REM sleep, EMG activity becomes minimal or even inapparent, although it may be occasionally interrupted with brief, irregular bursts of activity. These changes mirror, to a fair degree, the changes undergone by much of the motor system during sleep. Much of this variability can be understood on the basis of the altered activity of different levels of the motor system, as well as their interaction, during different sleep stages.

However, the relationship between motor activity and sleep stage may need to be qualified in various contexts. First, at a technical level, sleep scoring may not adequately reflect the underlying brain processes at the time of a given event, such as a movement. Sleep is generally scored as arbitrary epochs of fixed length, usually 30 seconds, whereas physiologic processes may occur on a whole variety of time scales. This has led some investigators to examine microepochs of a few seconds for momentary state.[44] Second, some sleep may not be adequately scorable according to the current rules. This has led to various proposals to revise the scoring system or even to use very different methods of scoring. Terzano, Mancia, Salati, et al.[45,46] have defined a pattern seen in non-REM sleep, the cyclic alternating pattern (CAP). This pattern, normally appearing only in non-REM sleep, demonstrates an alternation between two periods (each lasting 2 to 60 seconds) called phase A (higher amplitude, activated rhythms) and phase B (lower amplitude, background), respectively. This pattern is often associated in a time-locked fashion with sleep disorders such as sleep apnea or PLMS. The description of phase A is inclusive of the AASM definition of an arousal but is more inclusive.[47] Third, the sleep stages are not fully discrete or comprehensive. Fragments of a stage, such as REM-related atonia, may occur during other states such as wake, even in fully normal individuals. For example, Mahowald and Schenck[48] reported on six patients with marked admixture of features from the different sleep/wake states (wake, non-REM sleep, REM sleep). These patients showed abnormal distribution of motor activity with relation to sleep features. Fourth, motor events, although typical of one sleep stage or state, may less commonly occur in other stages. Although PLMS occur primarily in non-REM sleep, they may occur in REM sleep.[49,50] Similar movements may occur during arousals or wake periods[49,50] after sleep onset, usually as part of a periodic sequence of movements that span the sleep-wake divide.

Table 7.1 presents a summary of the frequency of normal motor activities that occur during the various phases of sleep and waking. Because many of these movements have not been fully and exhaustively studied, this table is a preliminary guide rather than a definitive pronouncement.

Drowsiness, Sleep Onset, and Arousals

In the period before sleep begins, humans, as well as other animals, enter a period of relative repose. The transition to sleep is signaled by a variety of behavioral and EEG features.[51] Even before actual sleep onset, the motor system reduces its level of activity. It is during this period that the symptoms of the restless legs syndrome (RLS) become prominent. RLS is relatively distinctive in that, unlike almost all other movement disorders, it is activated by relaxation. The eye movement system goes from a pattern of saccadic and pursuit movements to slow rolling eye movements.[52] Rectal motor activity decreases.[53]

The transition to sleep features a very common sleep-related movement, the sleep start or hypnic jerk.[54] This is an abrupt, myoclonic flexion movement, generalized or partial, often asymmetric, which may be accompanied by a sensation. There is often an illusion of falling. Unless very frequent, which does rarely occur,[55] this is a benign movement that has little effect on sleep and carries no negative prognosis. It probably occurs in most people. When it occurs, it is usually a single event, which causes a brief arousal. EMG records show relatively brief EMG complexes (less than 250 msec in duration) that may be simultaneous or sequential in various muscles. Less commonly, normals show rhythmic foot movements when falling asleep that cannot be considered a form of rhythmic movement disorder.[56] Currently these types of movements are classified by the AASM as either hypnogogic foot tremor or alternating leg muscle activation (ALMA) based upon whether one leg is involved or whether leg movements alternate from one leg to another.[57]

Arousals, brief periods of interrupted, lighter sleep that may lead to full awakening, are often associated with movements. Arousals may both follow and lead movements such as body shifts. Abnormal movements, such as parkinsonian tremor, may recur during arousals. Sleep-related movements, such as PLMS, may provoke frequent arousals or even awakenings and may also continue during periods of waking during sleep. In the period of sleep inertia after waking, there can also be a distinct arousal state.[58] Arousals are associated with the activated phases of the CAP, especially those that are dominated by more rapid, desynchronized rhythms.[59]

Transitions into and out of sleep may also be associated with sleep paralysis. In this condition, an individual is unable to move, although awake. Breathing and eye movements are usually preserved. This condition is thought to represent a variety of REM sleep tonic motor inhibition; recordings of the state can show REMs together with an electrophysiologic pattern consistent with REM sleep.[60-63] The state transition may be associated with arousal from an REM period or, less commonly except in narcolepsy, progress into REM sleep from wake. Although most frequent in narcolepsy, sleep paralysis also occurs in many nonnarcoleptic individuals, sometimes with a familial pattern. Recent studies suggest that, at least in some populations, sleep paralysis may be common.[60-63] It has been suggested that sleep paralysis may occur when there is an early-onset REM period, for example, after an awakening from non-REM.[60-63] In normal individuals, it is generally infrequent, but it may cause significant anxiety, especially the first time that it occurs. In the absence of other narcoleptic phenomena or abnormal neurologic findings, someone with occasional sleep paralysis may be reassured that it is almost certainly benign. A somewhat similar condition, nocturnal alternating hemiplegia, involves selective paralysis limited to one side arising out of sleep.[64] This may be a variant of hemiplegic migraine, a complicated headache disorder with paralysis resulting from suppressed activity in select brain regions.

Non-REM Sleep

In non-REM sleep, motor activity is less than in the waking or resting state. Postural shifts, which may signal stage changes (into or out

Table 7.1 Occurrence of Movements during Sleep

MOTOR ACTIVITY	AWAKE/ ACTIVE	DROWSINESS/ SLEEP ONSET	AROUSAL/ AWAKENING	STAGE I NON-REM	STAGE II NON-REM	STAGE I AND II NON-REM	REM SLEEP
Postural shifts	Very frequent	Frequent	Frequent	Common	Occasional	Rare	Occasional
Sleep myoclonus	Unreported	Rare	Rare	Common	Occasional	Rare	Frequent
Hypnic jerk	Unreported	Frequent	Occasional	Occasional	Rare	Unreported	Unreported
Sleep paralysis*	NA	Common	Common	Rare	Unreported	Unreported	Frequent
Periodic limb movements	NA	Occasional	Occasional	Frequent	Common	Rare	Occasional

*In narcolepsy, presents as cataplexy in wake state.
NA, not applicable; non-REM, non–rapid eye movement; REM, rapid eye movement.

from wake or REM), occur. There are also small flickering movements, called sleep myoclonus, which may cause no apparent movement and are associated with very brief, highly localized EMG potentials.[65,66] In some cases, these movements may have a greater amplitude and increased frequency, at which point they are called excessive fragmentary myoclonus, a possible sleep disorder.[57,67] Some normal or abnormal waking movements may persist into non-REM sleep. For example, voluntary scratching may persist during sleep in patients with atopic dermatitis, and rhythmic movement disorder can advance from drowsiness into well-defined non-REM sleep. The frequency of all movements decreases with depth of sleep; they are least in SWS (non-REM stages III and IV).[68,69] Postural shifts rarely occur before SWS; this period, associated with the descent to SWS, may have even fewer movements than stable SWS. This period is often associated with CAP in which the activated phases are dominated by slow, synchronized activity.[70] Such CAP periods are thought to facilitate the descent into stable SWS.

PLMS are most often observed during non-REM sleep in those without other sleep or neurologic disorders. Recent studies have supported the presence of large numbers of these movements both in older adults and, more recently, in adults of all ages. Given the high prevalence observed, approaching 50% in older adults,[71–75] and the difficulty of establishing any specific impact or morbidity associated with these movements,[71–75] one can ask whether they should not at least be called a normal variant of sleep-related movements. On the other hand, PLMS can occur in wakefulness in RLS patients and disrupt sleep, and occasional patients who do not have RLS may have sleep disruption from PLMS and, in this latter case, the term periodic limb movement disorder (PLMD) is invoked.[57] In addition, recent research has investigated the relationship between PLMS and attention-deficit/hyperactivity disorder (ADHD) and between PLMS and hypertension, heart disease, and stroke.[76,77] Whether there is a causal relationship between these other disorders and PLMS is the subject of ongoing investigation. Similarly, common movements that would be regarded as normal variants can, if accentuated, present as a clinical disorder. One example of such a movement is the presence of rhythmic masticatory muscle activity (RMNIA) in sleep. This is a characteristic pathologic movement seen in bruxism, but RMNIA also occurs at a lower frequency and intensity within the normal population.[78] Such conditions as excessive fragmentary myoclonus, PLMD, and bruxism may be disorders based on exaggerations of selected elements of the normal sleep-related movement repertoire.

REM Sleep

REM sleep is dramatically different from non-REM. The motor system is dominated by central activation and peripheral inhibition, so that muscle tone is tonically reduced, even below that of SWS, but bursts of small movements (sleep myoclonus), similar to those seen in non-REM sleep, but more clustered, occur phasically in association with REMs. Studies have shown a relative sequence of aspects of REM sleep with muscle tone reduction followed by EEG changes (sawtooth waves) and then the emergence of REMs.[79]

REMs are an interesting aspect of altered motor behavior in sleep. In general, REMs are saccade-like, but they have different properties from normal saccades: They are slower or more slowly accelerated or jerked,[79–84] they have a predominance of horizontal movements, and they are much less conjugate than normal saccades that are made in waking life to a real-world target.[79–84] Are these differences caused by differences in higher control? With targets selected not by a compelling external input but some vaguely described internal target? Are they caused by changes in the level of activation and availability of different brain systems controlling eye movement that may be differentially depressed by REM sleep? These questions remain. The parameters of REMs can also change during the course of successive REM episodes.[79–84]

During REM there is increased nervous system activity and a close balance between strong upper motor center excitation and inhibition at the level of the motor effector. When the inhibitory influences break down, significant motor activity may be released. The resulting movements may represent an "acting out" of dreams, which characteristically have a motoric component.[79–84]

In an opposite direction, sleep paralysis can occur outside the REM period as a generalized motor inhibition without dreaming sleep. This can occur at all ages[85] and, at low frequencies of occurrence, is essentially benign.

Sleep Deprivation

By altering sleep macrostructure (more SWS and REM sleep) and microstructure (fewer CAP and a shift in the CAP type),[86] sleep deprivation at least indirectly alters motor activity in sleep. Recuperative sleep has fewer movements.[86]

CIRCADIAN ACTIVITY CYCLES

In many, if not most, animal species, the motor system's level of activity depends on the time of day. Even in the absence of a day/night light cycle (i.e., under constant conditions), such activity cycling persists in a "free running state" with a circadian period. These cycles are regulated by a complex set of interrelated biochemical processes in the suprachiasmatic nucleus that ultimately control activity as well as many other important physiologic variables, such as temperature, which also show circadian periods. In humans, of course, sleep usually occurs at night, so that activity is concentrated during the daytime hours. This basic pattern, however, can be disturbed in a number of different settings, for example, among shift workers or those with unusual schedules or in patients who have a variety of sleep disorders or degenerative neurologic conditions. Shifts in the pattern of circadian motor activity can thereby be a marker for a sleep/wake motor disorder such as RLS.[87-89]

Circadian influences may appear more directly on sleep macrostructure or microstructure, but they can also influence movements. PLMS in RLS have been shown to follow a circadian pattern, independent of sleep state.[87-89] This may be true of PLMS in otherwise normal individuals. The frequency of REMs in REM sleep, as well as those associated with sleep history, also depends on circadian factors.[90] The circadian influence on PLMS and REM is opposite with "morning" by internal time associated with decreased PLMS and increased REM density. During waking, eye blink rate varies with time of day with an increase in the evening.[91] Even fetal movements may increase in the evening.[92]

Ontogeny of the Motor System during Sleep

In addition to sleep stage or circadian factors, normal sleep movements are also affected by age. The number of movements during sleep is greatest in infants, then decreases with age.[93,94]

This difference may extend back into prenatal life. One study examining fetuses in vitro and the resulting babies early in life found consistent relative movement activity before and after birth. Over a wider span of ages, De Koninck, Lorrain, and Gagnon found that position shifts during sleep decreased from 4.7 per hour in 8- to 12-year-old sleepers to 2.1 per hour in those 65 to 80 years old.[94]

Children are also thought to lack a fully "mature" sleep-regulatory system. For instance, in one recent study, Kohyame found that younger infants appear to lack the profound motor inhibition during phasic REMs that is seen in older children and adults. Similarly, tonic inhibition of chin muscle tone during REM sleep increases during childhood to reach adult values.[95] Perhaps as a result of such immaturity, parasomnias such as bruxism, somnambulism, or somniloquy are present with a greater prevalence during childhood, tending to decrease with age from early childhood on. Similarly, toward the end of life, as neural and other bodily systems age and perhaps deteriorate, some forms of excessive motor activity may emerge again, including PLMS or REM sleep behavior disorder. Similarly, in at least one study, movements were increased in older adults compared with younger adults.[96] Reconciliation of this finding with other findings showing decreased movements with age requires further study. Other movements in the oldest subjects show subtle changes, with the duration of REMs found to decrease, although frequency of REMs remained constant in REM sleep.[97]

OTHER FACTORS GOVERNING THE MOTOR SYSTEM IN SLEEP

A wide range of factors can influence sleep. In this chapter, these are just listed and representative examples given. However, the totality of the individual and the environment's characteristics can impact on sleep and associated movements. We have only begun to probe a few of these factors.

Physical, Biologic, and Social Influences

A major influence on movement during sleep may be sensory input, which can elicit a wide range of responses. Progressively more intrusive stimuli may lead to recruitment of progressively more extensive movement sequences.[98] Stimulus properties (e.g., infrequent tones or real words compared with nonsense syllables) can be analyzed during sleep,[99-103] and those stimuli of specific significance (e.g., the sleeper's name[104]) may cause differential responsiveness. As a result, the brain appears to perform a complex set of discriminations that can lead, under specific situations (stimulus intensity or meaning), to movement, arousal, and waking.

Previous activity has been found to alter the nature of motor activity during sleep. Presleep repeated saccades can suppress REMs and alter the amplitude and direction of REMs.[105] Similar effects can be seen with middle ear muscle activity.[106] Increased movement during the day is associated with decreased movement at night in older adults.[107] Specific environmental conditions can also influence movement. Bright light in the morning can decrease generalized movement at night.[108]

Ethnicity may influence motor activity in sleep, especially phasic REM parameters.[109] Ethnicity may also be associated with a differential amount of abnormal motor activity, such as RLS. Other influences include the presence or absence of a bed partner.[110]

Anatomic and physiologic factors can influence motor activity during sleep. Relative changes in jaw position can influence the muscular dynamics of the jaw muscles during sleep, leading to distinctive patterns of activity not seen in normal, waking jaw clenching.[111] Laterality also matters. There is a significant phase gap between the circadian activity pattern of the dominant and nondominant hands with the nondominant hand's activity relatively phase delayed. Mean activity of the nondominant hand is higher during the middle of the night (midnight to 4:00 am).[112] Hormonal abnormalities can also cause changes. Hypothyroidism in children is associated with decreased movements during sleep.[113]

Bed partners can also influence motor activity. Both mothers of infants[114] and caretakers of sleep-disordered older adults[114] may show associated changes of motor activity. This can extend to bed partners of patients with motor sleep disorders, such as PLMD.

Neuropsychiatric Disorders

One of the more important influences on the motor system during sleep is the presence of neurologic or psychiatric disorders. Alteration of the pattern or amount of normal activity can also be a disease marker or associated finding. In attention-deficit/hyperactivity disorder (ADHD), sleep is often disrupted and motor activity is increased. ADHD children more commonly demonstrate a significant number of PLMS[76,115,116] and also show increases in generalized motor activity.[116] Excessive movements can be subsequently reduced by treatment.[117] Patients with tics not only have tics during sleep but also increased normal movements.[118] In sleep bruxism, general body movements (not PLMS) are increased over matched controls.[119] Patients with depression[120] or a history of child abuse[121] may also show increased motor activity at night, associated with sleep disruption.

Even pervasive cerebral damage leading to a vegetative state does not completely abolish movement but may alter the characteristics of movements, including REMs and associated hypnic myoclonus.[122]

DISCUSSION AND CONCLUSIONS

Recent decades have seen a major increase in interest in and knowledge about the brain, its motor system, sleep, and the resulting movements of the sleeping human. However, despite the great advances we have made, the results have been fragmentary and there remain many challenges for the coming generations of sleep and movement professionals. For one thing, we do not have a complete inventory or even, in some cases, a good description (phenomenology) of those motor activities that occur during sleep. (Of course, this is also true of waking motor behavior.) We cannot yet trace out the pathways that bring about bodily shifts, REMs, or PLMS during sleep or indicate how their pathways differ from those used during more or less conscious motor activity during waking. For another thing, we do not understand the varying influences that change the amount or kind of motor activity during sleep or those alterations of brain function that permit the emergence of abnormal motor activity during sleep. In many cases, we can suspect that the abnormal motor activities we observe must also use parts of the brain that are employed for normal motor activity. Motor activity during sleep varies from complex, purposeful activity[123] to simple movements that are dyskinetic or primitive in character. Each of these different kinds of motor activity may be associated with distinctive constellations of neural circuits that may more or less overlap with those used for normal motor control. All in all, it is as if we have caught some fascinated glimpses of a very complex and multifunctional device, but we still need to find out what its parts are, how they are assembled, and how they are made to work in different modes. Fortunately, we are now better placed than ever, with new physiologic, imaging, and molecular biologic techniques, to begin to address such questions.

AUTHOR'S NOTE

This chapter is a revised, updated version of a previous chapter for the first edition of this book written by our good friend and colleague Wayne Alfred Hening, MD, PhD.

REFERENCES

1. Tryon WW. *Activity Measurement in Psychology and Medicine*. New York: Plenum; 1991.
2. Curzi-Dascalova L, Kauffinann F, Gaultier C, et al. Heart rate modifications related to spontaneous body movements in sleeping premature and full-term newborns. *Pediatr Res* 1999;45:515.
3. Jean-Louis G, Kripke DF, Cole RJ, et al. Sleep detection with an accelerometer actigraph: comparisons with polysomnography. *Physiol Behav* 2001;72:21.
4. Ancoli-Israel S, Clopton P, Klauber MR, et al. Use of wrist activity for monitoring sleep/wake in demented nursing-home patients. *Sleep* 1997;20:24.
5. Ancoli-Israel S, Klauber MR, Jones DW, et al. Variations in circadian rhythms of activity, sleep, and light exposure related to dementia in nursing-home patients. *Sleep* 1997;20:18.
6. Gorny SW, Allen RP, Krausman DT, et al. Initial demonstration of the accuracy and utility of an ambulatory, three-dimensional body position monitor with normals, sleepwalkers and restless legs patients. *Sleep Med* 2001;2:135.
7. Van Someren EJ. Actigraphic monitoring of movement and rest-activity rhythms in aging, Alzheimer's disease, and Parkinson's disease. *IEEE Trans Rehabil Eng* 1997;5:394.
8. Ebata T, Iwasaki S, Kamide R, et al. Use of a wrist activity monitor for the measurement of nocturnal scratching in patients with atopic dermatitis. *Br J Dermatol* 2001;144:305.
9. Middelkoop HA, van Dam EM, Smilde-van den Doel DA, et al. 45-hour continuous quintuple-site actimetry: relations between trunk and limb movements and effects of circadian sleep-wake rhythmicity. *Psychophysiology* 1997;34:199.
10. Gschliesser V, Frauscher B, Brandauer E, et al. PLM detection by actigraphy compared to polysomnography: a validation and comparison of two actigraphs. *Sleep Med* 2009;10:306–11.
11. Sforza E, Johannes M, Claudio B. The PAM-RL ambulatory device for detection of periodic leg movements: a validation study. *Sleep Med* 2005;6:407–13.
12. Iber C, Ancoli-Israel S, Chesson, AL Jr., et al., eds. *The AASM Manual for the Scoring of Sleep and Associated Events: Rules, Technology and Technical Specifications*. Westchester, IL:The American Academy of Sleep Medicine;2007:1–59.
13. Tatum WI. Long-term EEG monitoring: a clini- cal approach to electrophysiology. *J Clin Neurophysiol* 2001;18:442.
14. Cantero JL, Atienza M, Stickgold R, et al. Nightcap: a reliable system for determining sleep onset latency. *Sleep* 2002;25:238.
15. Broughton R, Fleming J, Fleetham J. Home assessment of sleep disorders by portable moni- toring. *J Clin Neurophysiol* 1996; 13:272.
16. Edinger JD, Fins AI, Sullivan RJ, Jr, et al. Sleep in the laboratory and sleep at home: comparisons of older insomniacs and normal sleepers. *Sleep* 1997;20:1119.
17. Mykytyn IJ, Sajkov D, Neill AM, et al. Portable computerized polysomnography in attended and unattended settings [see comments]. *Chest* 1999;115:114.
18. Collop NA, Anderson WM, Boehlecke B, et al, Clinical guidelines for the use of unattended portable monitors in the diagnosis of obstructive sleep apnea in adult patients. Portable Monitoring Task Force of the American Academy of sleep Medicine. *J Clin Sleep Med* 2007;3:737–47.
19. Alihaka J, Vaahtoranta K, Saarikivi J. A new method of long-term monitoring of the ballisto- cardiogram, heart rate and respiration. *Am J Physiol* 1981;240:384.
20. Erkinjuntti M, Vaahtoranta K, Alihanka J, et al. Use of the SCSB method for monitoring of the respiration, body movements, and

ballisto- cardiogram in infants. *Early Hum Dev* 1984;9:119.

21. Salmi T, Leinonen L. Automatic analysis of sleep records with static charge sensitive bed. *Electroencephalogr Clin Neurophysiol* 1986;64:84.

22. Salmi T, Telakivi T, Partinen M. Evaluation of automatic analysis of SCSB airflow and oxygen saturation signals in patients with sleep related apneas. *Chest* 1989;96:255.

23. Rauhala E, Erkinjuntti M, Polo O. Detection of periodic leg movements with a static-charge-sensitive bed. *J Sleep Res* 1996;5:246.

24. Tamura T, Zhou J, Mizukami H, et al. A system for monitoring temperature distribution in bed and its application to the assessment of body movement. *Physiol Meas* 1993;14:33.

25. Lu L, Tamura T, Togawa T. Detection of body movements during sleep by monitoring of bed temperature. *Physiol Meas* 1999;20:137.

26. Tamura T, Miyasako S, Ogawa M, et al. Assessment of bed temperature monitoring for detecting body movement during sleep: comparison with simultaneous video image recording and actigraphy. *Med Eng Phys* 1999;21:1.

27. Almli CR, Ball RH, Wheeler ME. Human fetal and neonatal movement patterns: gender differences and fetal-to-neonatal continuity. *Dev Psychobiol* 2001;38:252.

28. Groome LJ, Swiber MJ, Holland SB, et al. Spontaneous motor activity in the perinatal infant before and after birth: stability in individual differences. *Dev Psychobiol* 1999;35:15.

29. Andersson JL, Onoe H, Hetta J, et al. Brain networks affected by synchronized sleep visualized by positron emission tomography. *J Cereb Blood Flow Metab* 1998;18:701.

30. Shiotsuka S, Atsumi Y, Ogata S, et al. Cerebral blood volume in the sleep measured by near-infrared spectroscopy. *Psychiatry Clin Neurosci* 1998;52:172.

31. Buchsbaum MS, Hazlett EA, Wu J, et al. Positron emission tomography with deoxyglucose-fl8 imaging of sleep. *Neuropsychopharmacology* 2001;25 (5 Suppl 1):550.

32. Lovblad KO, Thomas R, Jakob PM, et al. Silent functional magnetic resonance imaging demonstrates focal activation in rapid eye movement sleep. *Neurology* 1999;53:2193.

33. Hening WA, Allen R, Walters AS, et al. Motor functions and dysfunctions of sleep. In: Chokroverty S, ed. *Sleep Disorders Medicine*. 2nd ed. Boston, MA: Butterworth-Heinemann; 1999:441.

34. Manganotti P, Palermo A, Patuzzo S, et al. Decrease in motor cortical excitability in human subjects after sleep deprivation. *Neurosci Lett* 2001;304:153.

35. Sandrini G, Milanov I, Rossi B, et al. Effects of sleep on spinal nociceptive reflexes in humans. *Sleep* 2001;24:13.

36. Atienza M, Cantero JL, Gomez CM. The mismatch negativity component reveals the sensory memory during REM sleep in humans. *Neurosci Lett* 1997;237:21.

37. Atienza M, Cantero JL, Gomez CM. Decay time of the auditory sensory memory trace during wakefulness and REM sleep. *Psychophysiology* 2000;37:485.

38. Civardi C, Boccagni C, Vicentini R, et al. Cortical excitability and sleep deprivation: a tanscranial magnetic stimulation study. *J Neurol Neurosurg Psychiatry* 2001;71:809.

39. Portas CM, Krakow K, Allen P, et al. Auditory processing across the sleep-wake cycle: simultaneous EEG and fMRI monitoring in humans. *Neuron* 2000;28:991.

40. Kohlmeier KA, Lopez-Rodriguez F, Morales FR, Chase MH. Relationship between sensory stimuli-elicited IPSPs in motoneurons and PGO waves during cholinergically induced muscle atonia. *J Neurophysiol* 1997;78:2145.

41. Ikeda K, Morotomi T. Reversed discriminatory responses of heart rate during human REM sleep. *Sleep* 1997;20:942.

42. Kohyama J. REM sleep atonia: responsible brain regions, quantification, and clinical impli- cation. *Brain Dev* 2000;22(Suppl 1):5136.

43. Gimeno V, Sagaies T, Miguel L, et al. The statistical distribution of wrist movements during sleep. *Neuropsychobiology* 1998;38:108.

44. Fish DR, Sawyers D, Allen PJ, et al. The effect of sleep on the dyskinetic movements of Parkinson's disease, Gilles de la Tourette syndrome, Huntington's disease, and torsion dystonia. *Arch Neurol* 1991;48:210.

45. Terzano MG, Mancia D, Salati MR, et al. The cyclic alternating pattern as a physiological component of normal NREM sleep. *Sleep* 1985;8:137.

46. Terzano MG, Parrino L. Clinical applications of cyclic alternating pattern [published erratum appears in Physiol Behav 1994;55:199]. *Physiol Behav* 1993;54:807.

47. Bonnet MH, Doghramji K, Roehrs T, et al. The scoring of arousal in sleep: Reliability,

validity, and alternatives. *J Clin Sleep Med* 2007;3:133–146.

48. Mahowald MW, Schenck CH. Status dissociatus a perspective on states of being. *Sleep* 1991;14:69.

49. Lugaresi E, Cirignotta F, Coccagna G, et al. Nocturnal myoclonus and restless legs syndrome. In: Faim S, Marsden CD, Van Woert M, eds. *Myoclonus. Advances in Neurology*. Vol 43. New York: Raven Press; 1986:295.

50. Pollmacher T, Schulz H. Periodic leg movements (PLM): their relationship to sleep stages. *Sleep* 1993;16:572.

51. Santamaria J, Chiappa KH. The EEG of drowsiness in normal adults. *J Clin Neurophysiol* 1987;4:327.

52. Hiroshige Y. Linear automatic detection of eye movements during the transition between wake and sleep. *Psychiatry Clin Neurosci* 1999;53:179.

53. Auwerda JJ, Bac DJ, Schouten WR. Circadian rhythm of rectal motor complexes. *Dis Colon Rectum* 2001;44:1328.

54. Oswald I. Sudden bodily jerks on falling asleep. *Brain* 1959;82:92.

55. Broughton R. Pathological fragmentary myoclonus, intensified sleep starts and hypna- gogic foot tremor: three unusual sleep related disorders. In Koella WP, ed. *Sleep 1986*. New York: Fischer-Verlag; 1988:240.

56. Wichniak A, Tracik F, Geisler P, et al. Rhythmic feet movements while falling asleep. *Mov Disord* 2001;16:1164.

57. AASM. *The International Classification of Sleep Disorders. Diagnostic and Coding Manual*. 2nd ed. Westchester, IL: *The American Academy of Sleep Medicine*; 2005:1–297.

58. Homer RL, Sanford LD, Pack AI, et al. Activation of a distinct arousal state immediately after spontaneous awakening from sleep. *Brain Res* 1997;778:127.

59. Parrino L, Smerieri A, Rossi M, et al. Relationship of slow and rapid EEG components of CAP to ASDA arousals in normal sleep. *Sleep* 2001;24:881.

60. Dyken ME, Yamada T, Lin-Dyken DC, et al. Diagnosing narcolepsy through the simultaneous clinical and electrophysiologic analysis of cataplexy. *Arch Neurol* 1996;53:456.

61. Bell CC, Dixie-Bell DD, Thompson B. Further studies on the prevalence of isolated sleep paralysis in black subjects. *J Nat Med Assoc* 1986;78:649.

62. Fukuda K, Miyasita A, Inugami M, et al. High prevalence of isolated sleep paralysis: *kanashibari* phenomenon in Japan. *Sleep* 1987;10:279.

63. Takeuchi T, Miyasita A, Sasaki Y, et al. Isolated sleep paralysis elicited by sleep interruption. *Sleep* 1992;15:217.

64. Andermann E, Andermann F, Silver K, et al. Benign familial nocturnal alternating hemiplegia of childhood. *Neurology* 1994;44:1812.

65. Dagnino N, Loeb C, Massazza G, et al. Hypnic physiological myoclonus in man: an EEG-EMG study in normals and neurological patients. *Eur Neurol* 1969;2:47.

66. Montagna P, Liguori R, Zucconi M, et al. Physiological hypnic myoclonus. *Electroencephalogr Clin Neurophysiol* 1988;70:172.

67. Broughton R, Tolentino MA, Krelina M. Excessive fragmentary myoclonus in NREM sleep: a report of 38 cases. *Electroencephalogr Clin Neurophysiol* 1985;61:121.

68. Gardner R, Jr., Grossman WI. Normal motor patterns in sleep in man In: Weitzman E, ed. *Advances in Sleep Research*. Vol. 2. New York: Spectrum; 1975:67.

69. Wilde-Frenz J, Schulz H. Rate and distribution of body movements during sleep in humans. *Percept Mot Skills* 1983;56:2751.

70. Terzano MG, Parrino L, Boselli M, et al. CAP components and EEG synchronization in the first 3 sleep cycles. *Clin Neurophysiol* 2000;111:283.

71. Ancoli-Israel S, Kripke DF, Mason W, et al. Sleep apnea and periodic movements in an aging sample. *J Gerontol* 1985;40:419.

72. Mosko SS, Dickel MJ, Paul T, et al. Sleep apnea and sleep-related periodic leg movements in community resident seniors. *J Am Geriatr Soc* 1988;36:502.

73. Mendelson WB. Are periodic leg movements associated with clinical sleep disturbance? *Sleep* 1996;19:219.

74. Karadeniz D, Ondze B, Besset A, et al. Are periodic leg movements during sleep (PLMS) responsible for sleep disruption in insomnia patients? *Eur J Neurol* 2000;7:331.

75. Montplaisir J, Michaud M, Denesle R, et al. Periodic leg movements are not more prevalent in insomnia or hypersomnia but are specifically associated with sleep disorders involving a dopaminergic impairment. *Sleep Med* 2000;1:163.

76. Walters AS, Silvestri R, Zucconi M, et al. Review of the possible relationship and hypothetical links between attention

deficit hyperactivity disorder (ADHD) and the simple sleep related movement disorders, Parasomnias, hypersomnias and circadian rhythm disorders. *J Clin Sleep Med* 2008;4:591–600.

77. Walters AS, Rye DB. Review of the relationship of restless legs syndrome/periodic limb movements in sleep to hypertension, *Heart Dis Stroke Sleep* 2009;32:589–97.

78. Lavigne GJ, Rompre PH, Poirier G, et al. Rhythmic masticatory muscle activity during sleep in humans. *J Dent Res* 2001;80:443.

79. Sato S, McCutchen C, Graham B, et al. Relationship between muscle tone changes, sawtooth waves and rapid eye movements during sleep. *Electroencephalogr Clin Neurophysiol* 1997;103:627.

80. Aserinsky E. The discovery of REM sleep. *J Hist Neurosci* 1996;5:213.

81. Zhou W, King WM. Binocular eye movements not coordinated during REM sleep. *Exp Brain Res* 1997;117:153.

82. Takahashi K, Atsumi Y. Precise measurement of individual rapid eye movements in REM sleep of humans. *Sleep* 1997;20:743.

83. Hong CC, Potkin SG, Antrobus JS, et al. REM sleep eye movement counts correlate with visual imagery in dreaming: a pilot study. *Psychophysiology* 1997;34:377.

84. McCarley RW. The biology of dreaming sleep. In: Kryger MH, Roth T, Dement WC, eds. *Principles and Practice of Sleep Medicine*. 2nd ed. Philadelphia, PA: WB Saunders; 1994:373.

85. Wing YK, Chiu H, Leung T, et al. Sleep paralysis in the elderly. *J Sleep Res* 1999;8:151.

86. De Gennaro L, Ferrara M, Spadini V, et al. The cyclic alternating pattern decreases as a conse- quence of total sleep deprivation and correlates with EEG arousals. Neuropsychobiology 2002;45:95.

87. Blagrove M, Owens DS, MacDonald I, et al. Time of day effects in, and the relationship between, sleep quality and movement. *J Sleep Res* 1998;7:233.

88. Hening WA, Youssef E, Wagner ML, et al. The use of actigraphically determined activity ratios to measure the presence of excessive motor activity in the restless legs syndrome. *Sleep* 2001;24(Suppl):A354.

89. Trenkwalder C, Hening WA, Walters AS, et al. Circadian rhythm of periodic limb movements and sensory symptoms of restless legs syndrome. *Mov Disord* 1999;14:102.

90. Khalsa SB, Conroy DA, Duffy JF, et al. Sleep- and circadian-dependent modulation of REM density. *J Sleep Res* 2002;11:53.

91. Barbato G, Ficca G, Muscettola G, et al. Diurnal variation in spontaneous eye-blink rate. *Psychiatry Res* 2000;93:145.

92. St James-Roberts I, Menon-Johansson P. Predicting infant crying from fetal movement data: an exploratory study. *Early Hum Dev* 54:55, 1999.

93. Hume M, Van F, Watson A. A field study of age and gender differences in habitual adult sleep. *J Sleep Res* 1998;7:85.

94. De Koninck J, Lorrain D, Gagnon P. Sleep positions and position shifts in five age groups: an ontogenetic picture. *Sleep* 1992;15:143.

95. Kohyama J. A quantitative assessment of the maturation of phasic motor inhibition during REM sleep. *J Neurol Sci* 1996;143:150.

96. Ohnaka T, Tochihara Y, Kanda K. Body movements of the elderly during sleep and thermal conditions in bedrooms in summer. *Appl Human Sci* 1995;14:89.

97. Vegni C, Ktonas P, Giganti F, et al. The organization of rapid eye movement activity during rapid eye movement sleep is further impaired in very old human subjects. *Neurosci Lett* 2001;297:58.

98. McNamara F, Wulbrand H, Thach BT. Characteristics of the infant arousal response. *J Appl Physiol* 1998;85:2314.

99. Brualla J, Romero MF, Serrano M, et al. Auditory event-related potentials to semantic priming during sleep. *Electroencephalogr Clin Neurophysiol* 1998;108:283.

100. Voss U, Harsh J. Information processing and coping style during the wake/sleep transition. *J Sleep Res* 1998;7:225.

101. Pratt H, Berlad I, Lavie P. "Oddball" event-related potentials and information processing during REM and non-REM sleep. *Clin Neurophysiol* 1999;110:53.

102. Campbell KB. Information processing during sleep onset and sleep. *Can J Exp Psychol* 2000;54:209.

103. Sabri M, De Lugt DR, Campbell KB. The mismatch negativity to frequency deviants during the transition from wakefulness to sleep. *Can J Exp Psychol* 54:230, 2000.

104. Perrin F, Garcia-Larrea L, Mauguiere F, et al. A differential brain response to the subject's own name persists during sleep. *Clin Neurophysiol* 1999;110:2153.

105. De Gennaro L, Ferrara M. Effect of a presleep optokinetic stimulation on rapid eye movements during REM sleep. *Physiol Behav* 2000;69:471.

106. De Gennaro L, Ferrara M, Urbani L, et al. A complementary relationship between wake and REM sleep in the auditory system: a presleep increase of middle-ear muscle activity (MEMA) causes a decrease of MEMA during sleep. *Exp Brain Res* 2000;130:105.

107. Shirota A, Tamaki M, Hayashi M, et al. Effects of daytime activity on nocturnal sleep in the elderly. *Psychiatry Clin Neurosci* 2000;54:309.

108. Sakakibara S, Kohsaka M, Kobayashi R, et al. Effects of morning bright light in healthy elderly women: effects on wrist activity. *Psychiatry Clin Neurosci* 1999;53:235.

109. Rao U, Poland RE, Lutchmansingh P, et al. Relationship between ethnicity and sleep patterns in normal controls: implications for psychopathology and treatment. *J Psychiatr Res* 1999;33:419.

110. Nishihara K, Horiuchi S. Changes in sleep patterns of young women from late pregnancy to postpartum: relationships to their infants' movements. *Percept Mot Skills* 1998;87:1043.

111. Minagi S, Akamatsu Y, Matsunaga T, et al. Relationship between mandibular position and the coordination of masseter muscle activity during sleep in humans. *J Oral Rehabil* 1998;25:902.

112. Natale V. Circadian motor asymmetries in humans. *Neurosci Lett* 2002;320:102.

113. Hayashi M, Araki S, Kohyama J, et al. Sleep development in children with congenital and acquired hypothyroidism. *Brain Dev* 1997;19:43.

114. Pollak CP, Stokes PE, Wagner DR. Nocturnal interactions between community elders and caregivers, as measured by cross-correlation of their motor activity. *J Geriatr Psychiatry Neurol* 1997;10:168.

115. Picchietti DL, Underwood DJ, Farris WA, et al. Further studies on periodic limb movement disorder and restless legs syndrome in children with attention-deficit hyperactivity disorder. *Mov Disord* 1999;14:1000.

116. Konofal E, Lecendreux M, Bouvard MP, et al. High levels of nocturnal activity in children with attention-deficit hyper- activity disorder: a video analysis. *Psychiatry Clin Neurosci* 2001;55:97.

117. Kooij JJ, Middelkoop HA, van Gils K, et al. The effect of stimulants on nocturnal motor activity and sleep quality in adults with ADHD: an open-label case-control study. *J Clin Psychiatry* 2001;62:952.

118. Cohrs S, Rasch T, Altmeyer S, et al. Decreased sleep quality and increased sleep related movements in patients with Tourette's syndrome. *J Neurol Neurosurg Psychiatry* 2001;70:192.

119. Bader G, Kampe T, Tagdae T. Body movement during sleep in subjects with long-standing bruxing behavior. *Int J Prosthodont* 2000;13:327.

120. Lemke MR, Puhl P, Broderick A. Motor activity and perception of sleep in depressed patients. *J Psychiatr Res* 1999;33:215.

121. Glod CA, Teicher MH, Hartman CR, et al. Increased nocturnal activity and impaired sleep maintenance in abused children. *J Am Acad Child Adolesc Psychiatry* 1997;36:1236.

122. Oksenberg A, Gordon C, Arons E, et al. Phasic activities of rapid eye movement sleep in vegetative state patients. *Sleep* 2001;24:703.

123. Manni R, Ratti MT, Tartara A. Nocturnal eating: prevalence and features in 120 insomniac referrals. *Sleep* 1997;20:734.

8

Genetics of Sleep and Sleep Disorders

BARBARA SCHORMAIR AND JULIANE WINKELMANN

SLEEP IS a complex behavioral state that is conserved across highly diverse species ranging from arthropods to mammals. That it is a highly genetically determined trait has been known since the 1930s when twin studies showed exceptional concordance for sleep patterns in monozygotic twins.[1] This was confirmed in the ensuing electroencephalogram (EEG)-based studies of sleep, where several EEG traits showed heritabilities above 80%.[1] However, its function and regulation still are only partly understood. Pharmacological studies and lesion models in animals were the first tools used to study sleep and have uncovered anatomical structures and neurotransmitter signaling pathways in the central nervous system that play a role in sleep. Another, more recent and very successful approach is studying the genetic basis of sleep phenotypes and sleep disorders. Finding genes and thus molecular processes that govern different aspects of sleep significantly increases our understanding of sleep regulation and sleep function. Basically, two different approaches are being explored: the study of sleep- and

wakefulness-related molecular changes in animals under a variety of experimental conditions and the investigation of molecular mechanisms underlying human sleep disorders. Both, technological innovations such as high-throughput genotyping and sequencing, and extending the array of animal models for sleep to simpler organisms such as fly, worm, and zebrafish, have greatly advanced the field. The most important advances are reviewed here.

MOLECULAR MECHANISMS OF SLEEP AND WAKEFULNESS IN ANIMAL MODELS

Initially, the definition of sleep and wake state based on EEG activity limited the animal models for sleep research to mammals (mainly mice and rats) and birds. When the definition was adapted to a behaviorally oriented description, fruit fly (*Drosophila melanogaster*), worm (*Caenorhabditis elegans*), and zebrafish (*Danio rerio*) became frequently used models.[2] These simpler animals offer the advantage of easier genetic manipulation and fast and large-scale breeding, but they are more distant to humans in terms of evolution. Thus, some of the less conserved mechanisms underlying sleep might not be present in these animals.

Three different aspects are briefly discussed to demonstrate the impact of animal models on sleep research. First, we consider how animal models have been used to study neurotransmitter systems involved in sleep/wake regulation exemplified by the animal models for narcolepsy. Second, we discuss how they have advanced the understanding of the circadian rhythm and its influence on the timing and duration of sleep in humans. Third, we discuss how global gene expression analysis in animal models yields information on regulation and function of sleep.

Neurotransmitters in Sleep: Animal Model of Narcolepsy

Genetic studies of animal models, especially gene knockouts in mice, have confirmed and extended the results of earlier pharmacological and lesion studies of the major neurotransmitter systems.[3,4] Perhaps the most fascinating neurotransmitter system implicated in sleep is the hypocretin (also known as orexin) system, because loss of this neurotransmitter results in the sleep disorder narcolepsy. In narcolepsy, sleep/wake regulation is disrupted and rapid eye movement (REM) sleep features intrude in the wake state, causing excessive daytime sleepiness and episodes of skeletal muscle paralysis and atonia. Hereditary narcolepsy has been also described in several animal species. As in the human disorder, affected animals are excessively drowsy; have short sleep latency during the day and fragmented sleep during the night; and display the disease hallmark, cataplexy (episodes of muscle weakness induced by emotions). These models were key to understanding the pathophysiology of the disorder. Both a canine and a mouse model showed that defects in orexin neurotransmission were the cause of animal narcolepsy.[5,6] After establishing narcolepsy as an autosomal recessive trait with full penetrance in several dog breeds,[7-9] the group led by Mignot in Stanford was finally able to map a candidate locus to chromosome 12, then designated canarc-1.[7] With a positional cloning approach, the Stanford group demonstrated that the carnac-1 gene codes for a receptor for the neuropeptide *hypocretin*.[6] The name *hypocretin* indicates that this peptide is predominantly localized to the hypothalamus and that it shares homologies with another peptide-signaling molecule, secretin. The mutated gene in canine narcolepsy is the hypocretin type 2 receptor (*HCRTR2*).

The two neuropeptides (orexin-A and orexin-B or hypocretin-1 and hypocretin-2) that bind to orexin/hypocretin receptors are produced by a well-defined group of cells lateral in the hypothalamus sending axons to numerous regions throughout the central nervous system, including the major nuclei implicated in sleep regulation like locus coeruleus, raphe nuclei, medullary reticular formation, and paraventricular thalamic nuclei, as well as hypothalamus and brainstem.[10] The group led by Yanagisawa[5] engineered a knockout mouse for orexin/hypocretin. These animals share many behavioral and physiologic features with narcoleptic dogs and with narcolepsy patients, thus representing a model for narcolepsy that independently implicates the same molecular pathway. Orexin knockout mice show unexpected brief episodes of behavioral arrest that occur exclusively in the homozygous animals. Throughout the dark and light periods, the orexin null mice showed sleep-onset REM episodes, hypersomnia, and more rapid cycling between sleep and wakefulness during the dark phase. Moreover, modafinil, an antinarcoleptic drug, activates orexin-containing neurons.[5] Subsequent studies of human narcoleptic patients confirmed the importance of the orexin/hypocretin system in narcolepsy. Orexin/hypocretin was not detected or only at low levels in the cerebrospinal fluid, and postmortem studies showed loss of orexin neurons in the hypothalamus of these patients.[11-15]

Genes Involved in the Regulation of Circadian Rhythms

The clock that generates circadian rhythms is highly conserved and its molecular mechanisms are well understood by now. The core components that regulate circadian locomotor activity and other internally timed behavior were initially isolated and functionally characterized in the fruit fly.[16,17] The first gene controlling circadian behavior, *period*, was identified in a mutagenesis screen in flies where differences in the timing of eclosion (when adult flies hatch from the pupal cases) could be attributed to this genetic locus.[18] Subsequently, mammalian homologues identified in the mouse and mouse knockout models showed similar functions as observed in the fruit fly. In a simplified and shortened description, circadian rhythms are created and maintained by negative feedback loops driven mainly by transcription factors. In the mammalian main loop, the transcription factors Bmal1/Bmal2 and Clock/Npas2 heterodimerize and turn on the expression of negative regulators, the Period Per1-3 and Cryptochrome Cry1-2 proteins. These, in turn, then repress the transcription of Bmal1/Bmal2 and Clock/Npas2, thereby creating the feedback loop.[19] Many general functions and components of the circadian clock are conserved from fly to mammal, but there is substantial diversification of gene functions, molecular mechanisms, and regulatory pathways.

The identification and functional characterization of the molecular players of circadian rhythms in animal models have provided the necessary starting points for research in humans. Consequently, naturally occurring polymorphisms in "circadian" genes in humans have been associated with diurnal preferences and changes in sleep timing and duration, thus broadening our understanding of sleep regulation.[20] The PER3 gene is an especially interesting example because here the length of a common variable number tandem repeat (VNTR) polymorphism in the coding region is associated with both sleep timing and duration/quality. Carriers of the long allele (five repetitions of the VNTR) were shown to have an extreme morning preference ("larks"), whereas carriers of the short allele (four repetitions) prefer the evening ("owls").[21] At the same time, these variants also affect sleep structure and homeostasis.[22] Carriers of the long allele showed increased slow-wave sleep (SWS), EEG slow-wave activity in non–rapid eye movement (non-REM) sleep, and theta and alpha activity during wakefulness and REM sleep. In addition, their cognitive performance in response to sleep loss was significantly impaired compared to carriers of the short allele.[22]

Differential Gene Expression in Sleep and Wakefulness

Alterations in gene expression associated with sleep and wakefulness have been studied since the 1970s to better understand the restorative function of sleep and the molecular mechanisms of sleep regulation. Studies measuring and comparing rates of RNA and protein synthesis in sleep, spontaneous wakefulness, and sleep deprivation generally indicated an increased biosynthetic activity in the brain associated with sleep,[23] particularly SWS.[24] Technological advances have enabled the global, genome-wide analysis of gene expression changes related to sleep and wakefulness. These studies were conducted in mice, rats, and flies under various different experimental conditions, e.g., sleep-deprived or spontaneously awake animals, and different durations of sleep or wakefulness.[3,25-27] Despite the different designs, the results were highly concordant and showed that the states of sleep and wakefulness are associated with changes in expression of specific functional groups of genes.[3] Genes upregulated during wakefulness encode molecules that play a role in energy metabolism,[28,29] cellular stress response,[30,31] or synaptic plasticity.[32] In contrast, sleep leads to increased expression of genes involved in protein synthesis,[33] synaptic downscaling,[34] and cell membrane dynamics.[31,32] These observations have fueled theories on the function of sleep, such as synaptic homeostasis, memory consolidation or replenishment of energy, and signaling molecule stores.[3,4,34] However, the question of what purpose sleep serves is not conclusively answered at present.

GENETICS OF SLEEP DISORDERS

Another possible approach to the elucidation of the molecular regulation of the sleep-wake cycle is the study of its pathologic alterations in humans. Genes that cause sleep disturbances when mutated may code for gene products that are involved in the regulation of sleep and wakefulness. In addition, the analysis of genetic sleep disorders may provide important novel clues to diagnosis and treatment. Sleep disorders are reviewed, where causal mutations or susceptibility variants have been found.

Restless Legs Syndrome

Restless legs syndrome (RLS) is a major cause of disturbed sleep. It has been recognized for centuries and has been first described in great detail by Ekbom in 1945.[35] The hallmark symptom of RLS is an intense and unappeasable urge to move the legs at rest. Patients experience strong discomfort and uncomfortable or even painful sensations deep inside their legs. These symptoms are worse in the evening or at night and are abolished or at least alleviated by moving the extremities, that is, walking around.[36] Frequently, patients also report periodic limb movements in sleep (PLMS). The introduction of standardized diagnostic criteria based on these key symptoms in 1995[37] and their refinement in 2003[36] provided the necessary basis for large-scale comparative epidemiologic and genetic studies. RLS presents as either idiopathic (primary) RLS or as symptomatic (secondary) RLS, which develops as a consequence of other medical conditions.[36] It is a common complex disorder, where both genetic and nongenetic factors contribute to disease susceptibility.

EPIDEMIOLOGY OF RESTLESS LEGS SYNDROME

A number of studies assessed the prevalence of RLS in the general population mainly in Europe, North America, and Asia. Obtaining exact and reproducible prevalence estimates has been hampered by the lack of uniform diagnostic criteria before 1995. Even after the introduction of these criteria, differences in study design, study population characteristics, and the exact diagnostic procedures led to large discrepancies in prevalence estimates between individual studies, for example, estimates of 4.2%–15% in Caucasian populations.[38,39] Nevertheless, a general idea of the frequency of RLS has emerged from these studies. It is very common in the Caucasian populations of Europe and North America with an overall prevalence of approximately 10% and less common in South East Europe (~3.5%) and in Asian populations (1% to 2%).[38] These estimates refer to RLS of any symptom frequency and severity. For severe and thus clinically relevant RLS a prevalence of 2% is reported in Caucasian populations.[40-42] Ethnicity might influence the prevalence of RLS as suggested by the lower prevalence in Asian and East European countries. However, differences in study design and case classification or the varying sociocultural background could cause this difference.[39] There is only one study that assessed the prevalence of RLS in people of African descent.[43] This study found similar prevalence in African Americans and Caucasian Americans, thus arguing against an influence of ethnicity on the prevalence of RLS.[39] Female gender and age are established

risk factors for RLS. Women have been shown to be affected twice as often as men and prevalence was found to increase in an age-dependent manner in the majority of studies.[38,40,42,44,45] The prevalence of symptomatic RLS is even higher: 19% to 26% of pregnant women were shown to suffer from RLS, usually in the third trimester,[46-48] and 11% to 70% of end-stage renal disease patients, with most studies reporting a prevalence of around 30%.[38,49-51] Restless legs are also observed with a significantly increased prevalence in patients with different forms of anemia and iron deficiency.[52]

GENETICS OF RESTLESS LEGS SYNDROME

A strong hereditary component for RLS was already suspected by Ekbom in his seminal papers on the syndrome in 1944 and 1945, in which he described families with apparent autosomal-dominant inheritance, as well as concordant monozygotic (MZ) twins.[35] Since then, systematic genetic studies in families, twins, and unrelated individuals from the general population have confirmed a substantial genetic contribution to disease susceptibility and have led to a first understanding of the genetic architecture of RLS. Several aspects complicate the systematic genetic analysis of RLS. First, it is a common condition and thus secondary cases of RLS are observed by chance alone in a proportion of the families of patients, with their number depending on the number of first-degree family members questioned or examined. In addition, phenocopies, that is, the same phenotype is observed but it is present due to a different cause, can occur within families, thus obscuring the true mode of inheritance in the family. Second, no objective diagnostic test is available and the diagnosis is based on the description of symptoms by the patient. Consequently, depending on the modality of diagnosis (face-to-face interview, telephone interview, or self-administered questionnaire) and applied diagnostic criteria, misclassifications can occur. Third, the clinical picture and particularly the severity of RLS may be extremely variable.[36] Onset of symptoms may be in childhood, but the disease can also manifest in older adults. Initially, only mild symptoms may occur intermittently on no more than a few days of the year, and detailed questioning of members of RLS families demonstrated that a few affected individuals report classic

RLS symptoms for only a few days in their life (unpublished observations). Moreover, patients may report only or predominantly motor or sensory symptoms. Consequently, in addition to using strict diagnostic criteria in the selection of the index patients, it is crucial for all studies of the genetic epidemiology of RLS to personally interview as many first-degree relatives as possible, both reportedly affected and unaffected.

HERITABILITY AND MODE OF INHERITANCE OF RESTLESS LEGS SYNDROME

More than 50% of the phenotypic variance of RLS is due to genetic influences as heritability estimates of 54% to 69.4% from twin studies and familial aggregation analysis indicate.[53–55] This finding is corroborated by the observed increased risk for RLS in relatives of RLS patients. For first-degree relatives of RLS patients, a recurrence risk of 5.6 was found,[56] and a more specific analysis found a recurrence risk of 10.25 for parent-offspring pairs and a recurrence risk of 16.23 for siblings.[55] These systematic approaches are in concordance with the earlier observations of a strong familial aggregation of RLS. Several studies in RLS patient populations showed that between 40% and 65% reported a positive family history.[57–60] The exact estimates vary from 36.4%[35] to up to 92%,[60] probably due to differing methods of ascertaining affection status of further relatives, that is, contacting relatives personally or relying only on information given by the patient.

Starting with the first descriptions of RLS by Ekbom, studies of individual families suggested an autosomal-dominant mode of inheritance with high penetrance and variable expressivity of the underlying gene.[35,61–64] The variable expressivity manifested in differences in age of onset, progress of disease, or frequency and severity of symptoms. The phenomenon of anticipation has also been discussed in relation to familial RLS, and evidence for an earlier age of onset in later generations has been found in a subset of families.[63,64] However, as the awareness of the disease is likely to be higher in RLS families, this observation could also simply be an artifact. Anticipation is a phenomenon that has been described in several inherited neurologic disorders and has in many cases been found to be caused by "unstable" mutations in the form of expanded trinucleotide repeat sequences. Classic examples are Huntington's disease or the group of spinocerebellar ataxias. RLS was also described in patients with spinocerebellar ataxia, but the length of the repeat and the age of onset were not correlated.[65,66] Therefore, and because all of the expanded trinucleotide repeat disorders known so far are associated with neurodegeneration and RLS patients show no degenerative changes, it is rather unlikely that expanded trinucleotide repeats play a role in RLS.

Estimation of genetic parameters from single families is always limited by selection bias (families are ascertained because they suggest a certain genetic mechanism). This problem can be overcome by performing a segregation analysis in a large number of unselected index patients and their families. Two such studies have been performed for RLS. One study in German families included 196 participants. Only first-degree relatives were recruited and stratified according to age of onset of RLS symptoms.[67] For the group with an early onset of symptoms (≤30 years), results indicated an autosomal-dominant model with a single major gene and a significant multifactorial component. For the group with late onset of symptoms (>30 years), an oligogenic mode of inheritance with several major genes or substantial environmental influences was proposed.[67] The same model was suggested when analyzing the entire study population. The second study in 77 families from the United States included first- and second-degree relatives and analyzed the whole sample using gender as a covariate.[68] Here, an autosomal-dominant model with a single gene and complete penetrance was proposed. These studies indicated that there is a group of RLS cases, those with an earlier age of onset, where a single major gene may be mainly responsible for the disease, whereas in other cases, preferably those with a later age of onset, the genetic basis is more complex with at least several or even a large number of genetic contributors. Further support for the significant role of genetics and an autosomal-dominant mode of inheritance can be found in three twin studies conducted for RLS. A small study of 12 monozygotic twin pairs found a high concordance rate of 83.3% and the pedigree structures were in accordance with an autosomal-dominant mode of inheritance.[69] Two larger studies included monozygotic and dizygotic twins and found higher concordance rates in monozygotic compared to dizygotic twins.[53,54] However, there are certain limitations to these twin studies. The first study has a very small sample size, whereas the two larger studies recruited patients based on questionnaire-reported symptoms and use of self-defined diagnostic criteria, which increased the potential for misdiagnosis.

LINKAGE STUDIES IN RESTLESS LEGS SYNDROME

After establishing an autosomal-dominant mode of inheritance for RLS in families, parametric and nonparametric genome-wide linkage studies were conducted to identify genomic regions containing the causal genes. A total of six linkage regions and three loci with suggestive linkage have been identified, but not the causal genes or genetic variants in these regions.

A parametric linkage study in a large French-Canadian family identified a region on chromosome 12q22-23.3, named RLS-1, with a maximum two-point LOD score of 3.42 and a multipoint logarithm of the odds (LOD) score of 3.59.[70] The underlying genetic model was autosomal-recessive with a high disease allele frequency and a reduced penetrance, thereby modeling a pseudodominant mode of inheritance and suggesting a founder effect in the French-Canadian population leading to the high disease allele frequency. Linkage analyses in five further French-Canadian families,[71] in 12 German families by means of the nonparametric transmission disequilibrium test (TDT),[72] and in an Icelandic population[73] confirmed this locus.

The second locus, RLS-2 on chromosome 14q13-22, was found in a family from Northern Italy.[74] Using an autosomal-dominant mode of inheritance with a disease allele frequency of 0.003, they showed linkage with a maximum nonparametric LOD score of 3.47. Suggestive evidence for linkage to this locus found in a French-Canadian family[75] and a significant association detected in a family-based TDT association study of 159 European RLS trios[76] support this locus.

The third locus, RLS-3 on chromosome 9p24-22, was linked to RLS with a nonparametric linkage score of 3.22 in a study of 15 large families originating from North America.[55] Parametric linkage analysis confirmed this linkage in two of the families

based on an autosomal-dominant model with a disease allele frequency of 0.001. The results of this study have been contested,[77] but confirmation of this locus by several independent subsequent studies has dispelled the doubts. Parametric linkage analysis in a German family, classifying only early-onset RLS cases (≤32 years) as affected, resulted in a maximum multipoint LOD score of 3.78.[78] In addition, association to RLS-3 was found in European RLS trios by means of a TDT.[76] Another parametric linkage analysis of an extended German family also using an autosomal-dominant model yielded a maximum multipoint LOD score of 3.6 for a region centromeric of the original RLS-3 locus.[79] This region was termed RLS-3* and still awaits confirmation in other families.

The fourth locus, RLS-4 on chromosome 2q33, was identified in an isolated population in South Tyrol, Italy.[80] Parametric linkage analysis in three families assuming an autosomal-dominant mode of inheritance resulted in a maximum parametric two-point LOD score of 5.1 for this region.

The fifth locus, RLS-5 on chromosome 20p13, was revealed in a French-Canadian family also under an autosomal-dominant model with a maximum multipoint LOD score of 3.86.[81] It was confirmed in a Dutch kindred where the authors stratified affection status according to symptom severity and included only severely affected individuals.[82]

The sixth locus on chromosome 16p12.1 was identified in a French-Canadian family by parametric linkage analysis, again.[83] Assuming an autosomal-dominant mode of inheritance, a maximum multipoint LOD score of 3.5 for a candidate region of 1.18 Mb was found.

Three further loci with suggestive evidence for linkage (LOD score <3.3) have been identified. Two were found in one large German family using an autosomal-dominant model in a parametric linkage analysis, on chromosome 4q25-26 with a maximum multipoint LOD score of 2.92, and on 17p11-13 with a maximum multipoint LOD score of 2.83.[84] The third locus is located on chromosome 19p13 and was found in an Italian family with a maximum parametric LOD score of 2.61, also under an autosomal-dominant model.[85]

These linkage studies suggest monogenic forms of RLS, mainly following an autosomal-dominant mode of inheritance. However, the many different loci indicate substantial locus heterogeneity for RLS. In addition, the LOD scores found are lower than could be expected based on simulations.[78,86] Combined with the variable penetrance and expressivity observed within and between families, this points to a more complex genetic basis of RLS even in such "mendelian" pedigrees. Concerning the search for causal genes or genetic variants in these linkage regions, only a selection of the genes contained within them have been screened in the respective linked families. These were selected as plausible candidate genes based on knowledge of pathologic, pathophysiologic, or pharmacologic mechanisms in RLS. Therefore, the selection included mainly central nervous system (CNS) ion channels, neuronal transcription factors, and genes involved in iron and dopamine metabolism. However, no causal mutations were found when sequencing the coding exons of these genes.

ASSOCIATION STUDIES IN RESTLESS LEGS SYNDROME

Association Studies of Candidate Genes and Linkage Regions. Association studies of candidate genes have been focused on genes involved in dopaminergic neurotransmission system and iron metabolism, which are both implicated in RLS pathophysiology. A study in 92 RLS cases and 182 controls of French-Canadian ancestry tested eight functional polymorphisms in the dopamine receptors 1–5, the dopamine transporter, and the enzymes tyrosine hydroxylase and dopamine β-hydroxylase, but they did not detect any significant associations.[87] The same authors also performed an association study for the monoamine oxidase isoenzymes MAOA and MAOB, which degrade dopamine and other neuroactive amines.[88] A variable number of tandem repeats (VNTR) polymorphism in the MAOA and a dinucleotide repeat in the MAOB gene were genotyped in a French-Canadian population of 96 cases and 200 controls. The high transcription activity MAOA allele was found to be associated with RLS only in females (odds ratio [OR] = 2, 95% confidence interval [CI] = 1.06–3.77).[88] This result still needs to be confirmed by replication in independent case-control populations. Another study in 298 cases and 135 controls of German ancestry looked at a known functional polymorphism in the gene encoding catechol-O-methyltransferase, an enzyme involved in the degradation of catecholamines such as dopamine. There was no association

of the variant with RLS.[89] With regard to iron metabolism, the divalent metal transporter DMT1, important in cellular iron absorption, was analyzed in 179 cases and 180 controls, also of French-Canadian ancestry, by genotyping a total of 10 single nucleotide polymorphisms (SNPs).[90] Again, no association to RLS was found.

Larger scale association studies were conducted for two linkage regions, RLS-1 on chromosome 12 and RLS-3 on chromosome 9. RLS-1 was analyzed in cases and controls of German ancestry.[91] In the first stage, 1,536 tagging SNPs and nonsynonymous and synonymous coding and splice-site SNPs distributed over 366 genes in the RLS1 region were genotyped in 367 cases and 367 controls. The most significant SNPs were then genotyped in an independent sample consisting of 551 cases and 551 controls. The SNP rs7977109, located in the NOS1 (nNOS) gene, was the only SNP associated in this sample (P value = 0.049, OR = 0.76 with 95% CI = 0.64–0.9). Subsequent fine mapping of *NOS1* showed significant association for three SNPs in the first-stage sample (rs4766836, rs2293054, rs6490121), and for three different SNPs in second-stage sample (rs7977109, rs530393, rs816292) after correction for multiple testing (P ≤ 0.05).[91] Two SNPs (rs7977109 and rs693534) showed association in both samples: in one sample as a risk allele and in the other as a protective allele. This further complicates the interpretation of the results. Thus, for confirmation and further analysis, replication in independent population is needed. Nevertheless, NOS1 is an interesting candidate for RLS since it catalyzes the synthesis of nitric oxide, a signaling molecule implicated in pain perception, the control of sleep/wake regulation, and the modulation of the dopaminergic transmission.[92-94]

For RLS-3, a total of 3270 SNPs located in the region between 0.5 and 31.5 Mb on chromosome 9p were tested in a two-stage case-control association study.[95] In the explorative stage, 628 cases and 1,644 controls recruited in Germany were genotyped on commodity SNP arrays and eight SNPs with a P value of ≤ 10⁻³ were selected for replication in three independent case-control populations from Germany/Austria (1271 cases/1901 controls), Czech Republic (279/368), and Canada (285/842). In the combined analysis of all samples, two SNPs, rs1975197 and rs4626664, were associated with RLS after correction for multiple testing (rs4626664: P = 0.00012, OR = 1.44; rs1975197: P = 0.0012, OR = 1.31). The SNPs map to two different introns of the gene encoding protein tyrosine phosphatase receptor type delta (PTPRD) and represent two independent association signals in located in the same gene.[95] Known functions of PTPRD include long-term potentiation in memory and axon guidance and termination of mammalian motorneurons during embryonic development.[96,97] Its role in RLS is still unknown. The association of rs1975197 was confirmed in a set of 15 families and a sample of 189 cases and 560 controls from the US (P = 0.0004, OR = 1.68).[98]

These studies have identified genetic risk variants for RLS, but these are not the variants underlying the linkage signals found in families. To result in a linkage peak, a variant has to have a much bigger effect on disease risk than the associated SNPs have. Sequencing of the respective genes NOS1 and PTPRD in individuals from families with linkage to either RLS-1 or RLS-3 did not yield any such strong effect variants.[91,95]

Genome-Wide Association Studies. With the advent of high-throughput genotyping technologies for SNPs, genome-wide association studies (GWAS) assessing up to 1,000,000 SNPs have allowed hypothesis-free screening of the entire genome. Two such studies have been performed for RLS, one in German and French-Canadian cases and the other in Icelandic and US cases. The German study analyzed a total of 236,758 SNPs in 401 cases and 1644 population-based controls.[99] A total of 13 SNPs with a P value $\leq$ 10^{-5} were selected for replication and genotyped in two independent samples, a further German (903 cases/891 controls) and a French-Canadian sample (255/287). Three loci were significantly associated with RLS after correction for multiple testing: two intronic SNPs in MEIS1 on chromosome 2p (best-associated SNP rs2300478: P = 8.1×10^{-23}, OR = 1.74, 95% CI = 1.57–1.92), five intronic SNPs in BTBD9 on chromosome 6p (best-associated SNP rs9296249: P = 9.4×10^{-13}, OR = 1.67, 95% CI = 1.49–1.89), and seven intronic or intergenic SNPs in a region on chromosome 15q containing the 3′ end of the MAP2K5 gene and the adjacent SKOR1 (formerly LBXCOR1) gene (best-associated SNP rs1026732: P = 1.44×10^{-11}, OR = 1.53, 95% CI = 1.39–1.70). For MEIS1, a high-risk haplotype was identified, which had a larger effect than any individual

SNPs (OR = 2.7), suggesting the existence of more than one risk variant in this locus.[99] With the exception of BTBD9, for which no information on function exists, these genes have been implicated in developmental processes such as limb axis formation (MEIS1),[100] neuronal differentiation (MEIS1, SKOR1),[101,102] and muscle cell differentiation (MAP2K5).[103] The association to BTBD9 was also found in the other GWAS conducted in a sample of Icelandic ancestry consisting of 306 cases and 15,664 controls.[104] The only significant association was with SNPs in the BTBD9 gene (rs3923809, P = 2×10^{-9}, OR = 1.8, 95% CI = 1.5–2.2). This association was replicated in a second Icelandic sample (123 cases/1233 controls) and a US sample (188/662). In an additional analysis, the sample was stratified in cases with RLS with PLMS and RLS without PLMS. The association of rs3923809 was only found in RLS with PLMS (P = 2×10^{-12}) and not in RLS without PLMS (P = 0.81), suggesting an involvement of this locus in the genesis of PLMS. In addition, this SNP was associated with the serum ferritin levels in RLS patients. These levels were found to decrease by 13% per risk allele present (P = 0.002), suggesting a function in iron storage.[104] Defects in iron metabolism are also discussed as a possible cause of RLS, especially because RLS is frequent in conditions with iron deficiency.[36,105] One important difference between both GWAS are the diagnostic procedures. In the German study, all patients were diagnosed in a face-to-face interview by neurologists specialized in RLS, whereas the Icelandic study used a self-administered questionnaire incorporating the essential diagnostic criteria. This might have led to the inclusion of a significant proportion of misdiagnosed individuals and could explain why the association to BTBD9 was only present in cases with RLS with PLMS since PLMS are supportive for the diagnosis of RLS. The problem of misclassification is also indicated by the false-positive rate of 22.7% for RLS diagnosis found by the authors when they reassessed a subset of their cases in face-to-face interviews.[104] The associations found in these GWAS have been confirmed by additional, independent follow-up studies: The association of MEIS1 and BTBD9 was confirmed in an US case-control sample[106] and all three loci in a mixed sample of European descent,[107] including Czech, Austrian, and Finnish cases and controls and in another independent US sample.[108] Both MEIS1 and BTBD9 were also shown to be associated with RLS in end-stage renal disease, one of the most common forms of symptomatic RLS.[109] This indicates that the pathophysiological mechanisms in idiopathic and symptomatic RLS could overlap or even be the same.

In an extension of the initial GWAS in German samples, including a total of 4857 cases and 7280 controls of European ancestry, the known risk loci were confirmed and two further loci identified. First, an intergenic region on chromosome 2p14, 1.3Mb downstream of MEIS1 was found, suggesting a possible regulatory function of this locus for MEIS1 expression (rs6747972, $P = 9.03 \times 10^{-11}$, OR = 1.23). Second, a locus on chromosome 16q12.1 was found in a linkage disequilibrium block of 140 kb containing the 5'-end of TOX3 and the adjacent noncoding RNA BC034767. (rs3104767, $P = 9.4 \times 10^{-19}$, OR = 1.35). TOX3 is a transcription factor and plays an important role in mediating calcium-dependent transcription in neurons.[110]

Although several risk loci and genetic risk variants have been identified, the pathophysiology of RLS and the role of these genes and variants in it are still unknown. However, a first hypothesis can be generated and tested based on the genetic data. One hypothesis for RLS suggests a deregulation of spinal and cortical excitability.[105] In view of the established functions of some of the RLS-associated genes in neuronal specification and circuitry of neuron types during early development, defects in these processes could play a role in RLS pathophysiology. With regard to the question whether a specific RLS-associated SNP plays a causal role, two studies have been published so far. They assessed the role of the MEIS1 risk haplotype identified in the German GWAS[99] and suggest a function of the haplotype in the regulation of MEIS1 expression and in iron metabolism by upregulating ferritin and DMT1 expression.[111,112]

Narcolepsy

Narcolepsy is a sleep disorder characterized by attacks of disabling daytime drowsiness, episodes of skeletal muscle paralysis and atonia (cataplexy and sleep paralysis), and sleep-onset rapid eye movement (REM) phases, which can cause hypnagogic hallucinations. Sleep paralysis and cataplexy are pathologic manifestations of REM-sleep atonia, but only cataplexy is specific for narcolepsy. The normal physiologic components of REM sleep, dreaming and loss of muscle tone, become disconnected and also occur while the subject is awake. Unlike normal sleep, that of narcolepsy often begins with REM activity and the time taken to fall asleep is shorter than normal.

EPIDEMIOLOGY AND GENETICS OF NARCOLEPSY

Narcolepsy is a relatively rare disorder with an estimated prevalence in the range of 0.05% to 0.2%. Estimates of the frequency of a familial occurrence of narcolepsy are variable, ranging between 1% and 10%, possibly because of differing diagnostic criteria or because of different prevalence rates in different genetic populations studied.[113] In a study of 50 persons with narcolepsy-cataplexy, Baraitser and Parkes[114] found that 52% had an affected first-degree relative and that 41.9% of the sibs of those probands with an affected parent were similarly affected. In one third of instances in which two sibs were affected, a parent also showed symptoms of the disorder. After correction for age, 41.2% of children were affected. On the other hand, in a clinic population of 334 unrelated narcoleptic patients, Guilleminault, Mignot, and Grumet[115] found a much lower proportion of secondary cases. In their series, 40% of probands had at least one family member complaining of isolated daytime sleepiness, but only 6% had a positive family history of full-blown narcolepsy.[115] Multicase families were rare, because only two families were found with three or more relatives affected. However, the risk of disease for first-degree relatives was 6 to 18 times greater than that for unrelated individuals. In accordance with the latter findings, another study estimated the risk to first-degree relatives at 1% to 2%.[113] Twin studies demonstrated that only 25% to 31% of MZ twins are concordant for narcolepsy.[113,116] All these studies suggest that narcolepsy, except for the rare familial forms, is not a monogenically inherited disorder, but that one or several environmental factors are acting on a susceptible genetic background.

Looking for the causal genes, the animal models and the observed loss of hypocretin neurotransmitter and hypocretin neurons in humans suggested this neurotransmitter and its receptor as prime candidates. Genomic sequencing of the HCRTR2 gene in the narcoleptic Labradors and Dobermans identified two different mutations that both affect splicing and result in truncated transcripts. In Dobermans, a 226bp retrotransposon insertion caused skipping of the fourth exon, whereas in Labradors a G to A transition in a splice site led to loss of the sixth exon.[7] Sequencing of additional narcoleptic dogs identified only one further mutation, a missense mutation.[117] Functional analysis of these mutations confirmed the hypothesis that the exon-skipping mutations disrupt proper membrane localization and abolish binding to the receptor and thus block neurotransmission.[6,117] In human narcolepsy, orexin was not detected or only at low levels in the cerebrospinal fluid, and postmortem studies showed loss of orexin neurons in the hypothalamus of these patients.[11–15] However, this is not due to mutations in the orexin or orexin receptor genes in the great majority of cases. So far, only a single mutation in the orexin gene has been identified in an atypical narcolepsy with cataplexy patient, who presented with a very early age of onset and a very rapid disease progression.[13]

Due to the lack of multiplex families, genetic analysis of the familial form of narcolepsy has been limited. Three linkage studies have been conducted, but only one candidate causal mutation was identified. Nakayama et al. studied eight Japanese families, including 14 narcoleptic cases with cataplexy and seven cases with an incomplete form of narcolepsy and found suggestive evidence for linkage to chromosome 4p13-q21 with an LOD score of 3.09.[118] Dauvilliers et al. performed a genome-wide linkage analysis in a large family with four cases of narcolepsy-cataplexy, originating from France.[119] They found linkage to chromosome 21 with a maximum two-point LOD score of 3.36. All affected individuals shared a haplotype covering 5.15 Mb on chromosome 21q.[119] However, for both regions, no causal mutation was found. The third study was performed in a very large family from Spain with 12 affected individuals using an autosomal-dominant model and detected linkage to chromosome 6p22.1-6p22.3 with a maximum LOD score of 3.85.[120] The authors then employed next-generation sequencing and sequenced the complete exomes (the entire coding sequence of the genome) in three affected individuals. This led to the identification of a single missense mutation located in the linkage region and shared by all affected individuals in the family, in the gene encoding myelin oligodendrocyte glycoprotein (MOG). MOG is a component of the myelin sheath in the CNS, is present in oligodendrocytes, and is known as an autoimmune antigen, for example, in multiple sclerosis.[121,122] The function of MOG in narcolepsy and the causality of the detected mutation still remain to be established.

The majority of narcolepsy cases are sporadic cases. Here, genetic data suggest an autoimmune process that specifically targets the orexin neurons as the pathomechanism. The exact molecular and cellular processes, however, are still not known. Two major players in the immune system, the human leukocyte antigens (HLA) and the T cell receptor (TCR), have been implicated in narcolepsy. HLA molecules present antigens that are then recognized by the T cells via their receptors, thus inducing an immune reaction against the antigens. Many studies have demonstrated and confirmed a strong association of narcolepsy with a specific HLA class II haplotype. Ninety percent to almost 100% of narcoleptic patients with definite cataplexy share the HLA DQA1*0102-DQB1*0602 haplotype, as opposed to 12% to 38% of the general population in various ethnic groups.[123–126] Obviously, the presence of this HLA haplotype is frequently necessary but not sufficient to cause narcolepsy, both because family members often share the same HLA-DR2 haplotype with a proband but do not have narcolepsy and also the observed occurrence in a substantial proportion of nonnarcoleptic individuals. In addition, further HLA class II alleles have been shown to be either risk-increasing (DQB1*0301, DQA1*06, DRB1*04, DRB1*08, DRB1*11, and DRB1*12) or protective (DQB1*0601, DQB1*0501, and DQA1*01) in narcolepsy when present in trans with DQB1*0602. A GWAS in narcolepsy cases of European ancestry and heterozygous for the DQA1*0102-DQB1*0602 haplotype identified a strong protective haplotype DRB1*1301-DQB1*0603 (OR = 0.02).[127] For the TCR, a GWAS in DQB1*0602-positive cases and controls of European ancestry demonstrated strong association of a SNP (rs1154155) in the TCR alpha (TCRα) gene, encoding the alpha chain of the TCR, with narcolepsy (OR = 1.69, P < 10^{-21}).[128] This association was replicated in an independent European sample and in an Asian sample.[128] It is hypothesized that a specific interaction between these predisposing HLA class II and TCR alleles contributes to an autoimmune reaction targeting the hypocretin neurons. However, direct evidence for the postulated systemic or localized autoimmune process is still lacking.[129]

A further GWAS with replication in three ethnic groups (Europeans, Asians, and African Americans) found association of the purinergic receptor subtype 2Y11 (P2RY11) gene to narcolepsy (rs2305795, located in the 3'UTR of P2RY11, OR = 1.28, P = 6.1 × 10⁻¹⁰).[130] Purinergic signaling has previously been implicated in proliferation, apoptosis, and chemotaxis of immune system cells such as lymphocytes[131]; thus, these results strengthen the autoimmune hypothesis for narcolepsy. Further susceptibility variants for narcolepsy have been found in Asian populations. A polymorphism in the TNFα gene was associated with narcolepsy in a Japanese sample,[132] but this association could not be confirmed in a study of German narcoleptic samples.[133] Another GWAS identified a risk variant located between carnitine palmitoyltransferase 1B (CPT1B) and choline kinase B (CHKB) in a Japanese population.[134] This was confirmed in another Japanese sample but not in samples of European or African American descent.[134] Both genes encode molecules involved in metabolic pathways that regulate REM sleep and thus are interesting candidate genes for narcolepsy.[135]

FAMILIAL ADVANCED SLEEP-PHASE SYNDROME

Familial advanced sleep-phase syndrome (FASPS) is a rare, highly penetrant autosomal-dominant disease characterized by a chronically 4–5 hours advanced sleep phase, resulting in early sleep onset and premature awakening in the morning.[136] Causal mutations in families have been found in two genes so far: Period 2 (PER2) and Casein Kinase Delta (CK1δ), both components of the circadian clock.[137,138] PER2 is a known key player in circadian rhythm regulation, and its stability is regulated by phosphorylation status. A genome-wide linkage study identified a missense mutation (Serine662Glycine), affecting a phosphorylation site of the protein, segregating with FASPS in a multigeneration kindred.[137] Several studies have confirmed the negative effect of this mutation on PER2 phosphorylation and the interrelation between PER2 phosphorylation status and period length regulation.[139,140] However, genetic heterogeneity is present in FASPS because most cases do not have mutations in PER2. CK1δ was implicated in FASPS by a candidate gene study that found a missense mutation (Threonine44Alanine) in this gene segregating with FASPS in an affected family.[138] CK1δ encodes a kinase that phosphorylates PER proteins and this specific mutant protein showed reduced enzymatic activity in vitro. Transgenic mice carrying the mutation were found to have a shorter circadian period, whereas transgenic flies displayed the exact opposite.[138]

Fatal Familial Insomnia

Fatal familial insomnia (FFI) is an autosomal-dominant, inherited prion disease clinically characterized by inattention, sleep loss, dysautonomia, and motor signs. Pathologically, there is a preferential degeneration of the thalamus. FFI is caused by a missense mutation in codon 178 of the prion protein gene, PRNP, coupled with the presence of methionine at position 129 of the protein.[141] Coupled with valine at position 129 of PRNP, the missense mutation in codon 178 results in a form of Creutzfeld-Jakob disease. FFI is characterized by a progressive inability to sleep, accompanied by hypersomnolence while awake; a progressive sympathetic activation; and alterations in circadian hormonal secretions. The classic phenotype is found in individuals with the missense mutation in codon 178 of the prion protein, who are homozygous for methionine at the methionine/valine polymorphism at position 129 of the gene.[142,143] Heterozygotes have a longer disease duration (often longer than 1 year) and ataxia and dysarthria at disease onset (as opposed to the prominent sleep and autonomic disturbances even at onset in methionine homozygotes).[144] In transgenic mice expressing chimeric human-mouse PrPc, inoculation of brain tissue from FFI patients gives rise to a form of prion disorder in the recipient animal that resembles FFI pathologically because of predominant involvement of the thalamus. The protease-resistant prion protein (PrPSc) that accumulates in these animals is identical in its migratory pattern on Western blots to the human PrPSc isolated from patients with FFI but differs from the PrPSc isolated from patients with Creutzfeldt-Jakob disease, supporting the hypothesis that the conformation of the PrPSc protein determines the phenotype in the recipient after intracerebral inoculation.

It is hypothesized that the prion protein, which is a protein found on the cell surface and is widely expressed in the brain, may be involved in sleep regulation, more specifically in sleep consolidation. PrP knockout animals do not present obvious pathologic changes, but compared with controls they have longer circadian periods and a stronger reaction to sleep deprivation.[145,146]

CONCLUSION

Considerable progress has been made in recent years in the elucidation of the genetic basis of sleep, regulation of circadian rhythms, and sleep disorders. Based on animal experiments and on the study of familial sleep disorders, genes that are involved in sleep-wake cycle regulation are being identified and further complete our understanding of the underlying molecular processes. Genotype-phenotype correlations in patients and the construction of animal models by knockout or transgenic approaches are useful in studying the function of the encoded gene products on a molecular, cellular, and systemic level. High-throughput technologies allow the rapid screening for genetic variation and the subsequent functional characterization. This is exemplified by the huge progress made in deciphering the genetic underpinnings of such important sleep disorders as RLS and narcolepsy.

REFERENCES

1. Tafti M. Genetic aspects of normal and disturbed sleep. *Sleep Med* 2009;10(Suppl 1):S17–21.
2. Allada R, Siegel JM. Unearthing the phylogenetic roots of sleep. *Curr Biol* 2008;18(15):R670–R679.
3. Cirelli C. The genetic and molecular regulation of sleep: from fruit flies to humans. *Nat Rev Neurosci* 2009;10(8):549–60.
4. Crocker A, Sehgal A. Genetic analysis of sleep. *Genes Dev* 2010;24(12):1220–35.
5. Chemelli RM, Willie JT, Sinton CM, et al. Narcolepsy in orexin knockout mice: molecular genetics of sleep regulation. *Cell* 1999;98(4):437–51.
6. Lin L, Faraco J, Li R, et al. The sleep disorder canine narcolepsy is caused by a mutation in the hypocretin (orexin) receptor 2 gene. *Cell* 1999;98(3):365–76.
7. Mignot E, Wang C, Rattazzi C, et al. Genetic linkage of autosomal recessive canine narcolepsy with a mu immunoglobulin heavy-chain switch-like segment. *Proc Natl Acad Sci USA* 1991;88(8):3475–8.
8. Baker TL, Foutz AS, McNerney V, et al. Canine model of narcolepsy: genetic and developmental determinants. *Exp Neurol* 1982;75(3):729–42.
9. Foutz AS, Mitler MM, Cavalli-Sforza LL, et al. Genetic factors in canine narcolepsy. *Sleep* 1979;1(4):413–21.
10. van den Pol AN. Hypothalamic hypocretin (orexin): robust innervation of the spinal cord. *J Neurosci* 1999;19(8):3171–82.
11. Mignot E, Lammers GJ, Ripley B, et al. The role of cerebrospinal fluid hypocretin measurement in the diagnosis of narcolepsy and other hypersomnias. *Arch Neurol* 2002;59(10):1553–62.
12. Nishino S, Ripley B, Overeem S, et al. Low cerebrospinal fluid hypocretin (Orexin) and altered energy homeostasis in human narcolepsy. *Ann Neurol* 2001;50(3):381–8.
13. Peyron C, Faraco J, Rogers W, et al. A mutation in a case of early onset narcolepsy and a generalized absence of hypocretin peptides in human narcoleptic brains. *Nat Med* 2000;6(9):991–7.
14. Ripley B, Overeem S, Fujiki N, et al. CSF hypocretin/orexin levels in narcolepsy and other neurological conditions. *Neurology* 2001;57(12):2253–8.
15. Thannickal TC, Moore RY, Nienhuis R, et al. Reduced number of hypocretin neurons in human narcolepsy. *Neuron* 2000;27(3):469–74.
16. Schibler U. Circadian rhythms. New cogwheels in the clockworks. *Nature* 1998;393(6686):620–1.
17. Williams JA, Sehgal A. Molecular components of the circadian system in Drosophila. *Annu Rev Physiol* 2001;63:729–55.
18. Konopka RJ, Benzer S. Clock mutants of Drosophila melanogaster. *Proc Natl Acad Sci USA* 1971;68(9):2112–6.
19. Ko CH, Takahashi JS. Molecular components of the mammalian circadian clock. *Hum Mol Genet* 2006;15(Spec No 2):R271–7.
20. Wulff K, Porcheret K, Cussans E, et al. Sleep and circadian rhythm disturbances: multiple genes and multiple phenotypes. *Curr Opin Genet Dev* 2009;19(3):237–46.
21. Archer SN, Robilliard DL, Skene DJ, et al. A length polymorphism in the circadian clock gene Per3 is linked to delayed sleep phase syndrome and extreme diurnal preference. *Sleep* 2003;26(4):413–5.
22. Viola AU, Archer SN, James LM, et al. PER3 polymorphism predicts sleep structure and waking performance. *Curr Biol* 2007;17(7):613–8.

23. Bobillier P, Sakai K, Seguin S, et al. [Effects of sleep deprivation on the incorporation of labelled amino acids into cerebral proteins in rats]. *C R Seances Soc Biol Fil* 1971;165(1):118–23.

24. Ramm P, Smith CT. Rates of cerebral protein synthesis are linked to slow wave sleep in the rat. *Physiol Behav* 1990;48(5):749–53.

25. Cirelli C, Faraguna U, Tononi G. Changes in brain gene expression after long-term sleep deprivation. *J Neurochem* 2006;98(5):1632–45.

26. Cirelli C, Tononi G. Gene expression in the brain across the sleep-waking cycle. *Brain Res* 2000;885(2):303–21.

27. Terao A, Wisor JP, Peyron C, et al. Gene expression in the rat brain during sleep deprivation and recovery sleep: an Affymetrix GeneChip study. *Neuroscience* 2006;137(2):593–605.

28. Cirelli C, Tononi G. Differences in gene expression between sleep and waking as revealed by mRNA differential display. *Brain Res Mol Brain Res* 1998;56(1–2):293–305.

29. Petit JM, Tobler I, Allaman I, et al. Sleep deprivation modulates brain mRNAs encoding genes of glycogen metabolism. *Eur J Neurosci* 2002;16(6):1163–7.

30. Terao A, Steininger TL, Hyder K, et al. Differential increase in the expression of heat shock protein family members during sleep deprivation and during sleep. *Neuroscience* 2003;116(1):187–200.

31. Zimmerman JE, Rizzo W, Shockley KR, et al. Multiple mechanisms limit the duration of wakefulness in Drosophila brain. *Physiol Genomics* 2006;27(3):337–50.

32. Cirelli C, Gutierrez CM, Tononi G. Extensive and divergent effects of sleep and wakefulness on brain gene expression. *Neuron* 2004;41(1):35–43.

33. Mackiewicz M, Shockley KR, Romer MA, et al. Macromolecule biosynthesis: a key function of sleep. *Physiol Genomics* 2007;31(3):441–57.

34. Tononi G, Cirelli C. Sleep function and synaptic homeostasis. *Sleep Med Rev* 2006;10(1):49–62.

35. Ekbom K. Restless legs: a clinical study. *Acta Med Scand* 1945;158(Suppl):1–123.

36. Allen RP, Picchietti D, Hening WA, et al. Restless legs syndrome: diagnostic criteria, special considerations, and epidemiology. A report from the restless legs syndrome diagnosis and epidemiology workshop at the National Institutes of Health. *Sleep Med* 2003;4(2):101–19.

37. Walters AS. Toward a better definition of the restless legs syndrome. The International Restless Legs Syndrome Study Group. *Mov Disord* 1995;10(5):634–42.

38. Garcia-Borreguero D, Egatz R, Winkelmann J, et al. Epidemiology of restless legs syndrome: the current status. *Sleep Med Rev* 2006;10(3):153–67.

39. Berger K, Kurth T. RLS epidemiology—frequencies, risk factors and methods in population studies. *Mov Disord* 2007;22 (Suppl 18):S420–3.

40. Allen RP, Walters AS, Montplaisir J, et al. Restless legs syndrome prevalence and impact: REST general population study. *Arch Intern Med* 2005;165(11):1286–92.

41. Hogl B, Kiechl S, Willeit J, et al. Restless legs syndrome: a community-based study of prevalence, severity, and risk factors. *Neurology* 2005;64(11):1920–4.

42. Tison F, Crochard A, Leger D, et al. Epidemiology of restless legs syndrome in French adults: a nationwide survey: the INSTANT Study. *Neurology* 2005;65(2):239–46.

43. Lee HB, Hening WA, Allen RP, et al. Race and restless legs syndrome symptoms in an adult community sample in east Baltimore. *Sleep Med* 2006;7(8):642–5.

44. Berger K, Luedemann J, Trenkwalder C, et al. Sex and the risk of restless legs syndrome in the general population. *Arch Intern Med* 2004;164(2):196–202.

45. Bjorvatn B, Leissner L, Ulfberg J, et al. Prevalence, severity and risk factors of restless legs syndrome in the general adult population in two Scandinavian countries. *Sleep Med* 2005;6(4):307–12.

46. Manconi M, Govoni V, De Vito A, et al. Restless legs syndrome and pregnancy. *Neurology* 2004;63(6):1065–9.

47. Goodman JD, Brodie C, Ayida GA. Restless leg syndrome in pregnancy. *BMJ* 1988;297(6656):1101–2.

48. Manconi M, Govoni V, De Vito A, et al. Pregnancy as a risk factor for restless legs syndrome. *Sleep Med* 2004;5(3):305–8.

49. Collado-Seidel V, Kohnen R, Samtleben W, et al. Clinical and biochemical findings in uremic patients with and without restless legs syndrome. *Am J Kidney Dis* 1998;31(2):324–8.

50. Gigli GL, Adorati M, Dolso P, et al. Restless legs syndrome in end-stage renal disease. *Sleep Med* 2004;5(3):309–15.

51. Huiqi Q, Shan L, Mingcai Q. Restless legs syndrome (RLS) in uremic patients is related to the frequency of hemodialysis sessions. *Nephron* 2000;86(4):540.

52. Ekbom KA. Restless legs syndrome. *Neurology* 1960;10:868–73.

53. Desai AV, Cherkas LF, Spector TD, et al. Genetic influences in self-reported symptoms of obstructive sleep apnoea and restless legs: a twin study. *Twin Res* 2004;7(6):589–95.

54. Xiong L, Jang K, Montplaisir J, et al. Canadian restless legs syndrome twin study. *Neurology* 2007;68(19):1631–3.

55. Chen S, Ondo WG, Rao S, et al. Genomewide linkage scan identifies a novel susceptibility locus for restless legs syndrome on chromosome 9p. *Am J Hum Genet* 2004;74(5):876–85.

56. Allen RP, La Buda MC, Becker P, et al. Family history study of the restless legs syndrome. *Sleep Med* 2002;3(Suppl 7):S3–7.

57. Winkelmann J, Wetter TC, Collado-Seidel V, et al. Clinical characteristics and frequency of the hereditary restless legs syndrome in a population of 300 patients. *Sleep* 2000;23(5):597–602.

58. Montplaisir J, Boucher S, Poirier G, et al. Clinical, polysomnographic, and genetic characteristics of restless legs syndrome: a study of 133 patients diagnosed with new standard criteria. *Mov Disord* 1997;12(1):61–5.

59. Walters AS, Hickey K, Maltzman J, et al. A questionnaire study of 138 patients with restless legs syndrome: the "Night-Walkers" survey. *Neurology* 1996;46(1):92–5.

60. Ondo W, Jankovic J. Restless legs syndrome: clinicoetiologic correlates. *Neurology* 1996;47(6):1435–41.

61. Walters AS, Picchietti D, Hening W, et al. Variable expressivity in familial restless legs syndrome. *Arch Neurol* 1990;47(11):1219–20.

62. Montplaisir J, Godbout R, Boghen D, et al. Familial restless legs with periodic movements in sleep: electrophysiologic, biochemical, and pharmacologic study. *Neurology* 1985;35(1):130–4.

63. Trenkwalder C, Seidel VC, Gasser T, et al. Clinical symptoms and possible anticipation in a large kindred of familial restless legs syndrome. *Mov Disord* 1996;11(4):389–94.

64. Lazzarini A, Walters AS, Hickey K, et al. Studies of penetrance and anticipation in five autosomal-dominant restless legs syndrome pedigrees. *Mov Disord* 1999;14(1):111–6.

65. Desautels A, Turecki G, Montplaisir J, et al. Analysis of CAG repeat expansions in restless legs syndrome. *Sleep* 2003;26(8):1055–7.

66. Konieczny M, Bauer P, Tomiuk J, et al. CAG repeats in restless legs syndrome. *Am J Med Genet B Neuropsychiatr Genet* 2006;141B(2):173–6.

67. Winkelmann J, Muller-Myhsok B, Wittchen HU, et al. Complex segregation analysis of restless legs syndrome provides evidence for an autosomal dominant mode of inheritance in early age at onset families. *Ann Neurol* 2002;52(3):297–302.

68. Mathias RA, Hening W, Washburn M, et al. Segregation analysis of restless legs syndrome: possible evidence for a major gene in a family study using blinded diagnoses. *Hum Hered* 2006;62(3):157–64.

69. Ondo WG, Vuong KD, Wang Q. Restless legs syndrome in monozygotic twins: clinical correlates. *Neurology* 2000;55(9):1404–6.

70. Desautels A, Turecki G, Montplaisir J, et al. Identification of a major susceptibility locus for restless legs syndrome on chromosome 12q. *Am J Hum Genet* 2001;69(6):1266–70.

71. Desautels A, Turecki G, Montplaisir J, et al. Restless legs syndrome: confirmation of linkage to chromosome 12q, genetic heterogeneity, and evidence of complexity. *Arch Neurol* 2005;62(4):591–6.

72. Winkelmann J, Lichtner P, Putz B, et al. Evidence for further genetic locus heterogeneity and confirmation of RLS-1 in restless legs syndrome. *Mov Disord* 2006;21(1):28–33.

73. Hicks A, Rye D, Kristjansson K, et al. Population-based confirmation of the 12q RLS locus in Iceland. *Mov Disord* 2005;20(Suppl 10):S34.

74. Bonati MT, Ferini-Strambi L, Aridon P, et al. Autosomal dominant restless legs syndrome maps on chromosome 14q. *Brain* 2003;126(Pt 6):1485–92.

75. Levchenko A, Montplaisir JY, Dube MP, et al. The 14q restless legs syndrome locus in the French Canadian population. *Ann Neurol* 2004;55(6):887–91.

76. Kemlink D, Polo O, Montagna P, et al. Family-based association study of the restless legs syndrome loci 2 and 3 in a European population. *Mov Disord* 2007;22(2):207–12.

77. Ray A, Weeks DE. No convincing evidence of linkage for restless legs syndrome on chromosome 9p. *Am J Hum Genet* 2005;76(4):705–7.

78. Liebetanz KM, Winkelmann J, Trenkwalder C, et al. RLS3: fine-mapping of an autosomal dominant locus in a family with intrafamilial heterogeneity. *Neurology* 2006;67(2):320–1.

79. Lohmann-Hedrich K, Neumann A, Kleensang A, et al. Evidence for linkage of restless legs syndrome to chromosome 9p: are there two distinct loci? *Neurology* 2008;70(9):686–94.

80. Pichler I, Marroni F, Volpato CB, et al. Linkage analysis identifies a novel locus for restless legs syndrome on chromosome 2q in a South Tyrolean population isolate. *Am J Hum Genet* 2006;79(4):716–23.

81. Levchenko A, Provost S, Montplaisir JY, et al. A novel autosomal dominant restless legs syndrome locus maps to chromosome 20p13. *Neurology* 2006;67(5):900–1.

82. Sas AM, Di Fonzo A, Bakker SL, et al. Autosomal dominant restless legs syndrome maps to chromosome 20p13 (RLS-5) in a Dutch kindred. *Mov Disord* 25(11):1715–22.

83. Levchenko A, Montplaisir JY, Asselin G, et al. Autosomal-dominant locus for restless legs syndrome in French-Canadians on chromosome 16p12.1. *Mov Disord* 2009;24(1):40–50.

84. Winkelmann J, Lichtner P, Kemlink D, et al. New loci for restless legs syndrome map to chromosome 4q and 17p. *Mov Disord* 2006;21(Suppl 15):S412.

85. Kemlink D, Plazzi G, Vetrugno R, et al. Suggestive evidence for linkage for restless legs syndrome on chromosome 19p13. *Neurogenetics* 2008;9(2):75–82.

86. Winkelmann J, Polo O, Provini F, et al. Genetics of restless legs syndrome (RLS): state-of-the-art and future directions. *Mov Disord* 2007;22(Suppl 18):S449–58.

87. Desautels A, Turecki G, Montplaisir J, et al. Dopaminergic neurotransmission and restless legs syndrome: a genetic association analysis. *Neurology* 2001;57(7):1304–6.

88. Desautels A, Turecki G, Montplaisir J, et al. Evidence for a genetic association between monoamine oxidase A and restless legs syndrome. *Neurology* 2002;59(2):215–9.

89. Mylius V, Moller JC, Strauch K, et al. No significance of the COMT val158met polymorphism in restless legs syndrome. *Neurosci Lett* 2010;473(2):151–4.

90. Xiong L, Dion P, Montplaisir J, et al. Molecular genetic studies of DMT1 on 12q in French-Canadian restless legs syndrome patients and families. *Am J Med Genet B Neuropsychiatr Genet* 2007;144B(7):911–7.

91. Winkelmann J, Lichtner P, Schormair B, et al. Variants in the neuronal nitric oxide synthase (nNOS, NOS1) gene are associated with restless legs syndrome. *Mov Disord* 2008;23(3):350–8.

92. Gautier-Sauvigne S, Colas D, Parmantier P, et al. Nitric oxide and sleep. *Sleep Med Rev* 2005;9(2):101–13.

93. West AR, Galloway MP. Endogenous nitric oxide facilitates striatal dopamine and glutamate efflux in vivo: role of ionotropic glutamate receptor-dependent mechanisms. *Neuropharmacology* 1997;36(11–12):1571–81.

94. West AR, Galloway MP, Grace AA. Regulation of striatal dopamine neurotransmission by nitric oxide: effector pathways and signaling mechanisms. *Synapse* 2002;44(4):227–45.

95. Schormair B, Kemlink D, Roeske D, et al. PTPRD (protein tyrosine phosphatase receptor type delta) is associated with restless legs syndrome. *Nat Genet* 2008;40(8):946–8.

96. Uetani N, Chagnon MJ, Kennedy TE, et al. Mammalian motoneuron axon targeting requires receptor protein tyrosine phosphatases sigma and delta. *J Neurosci* 2006;26(22):5872–80.

97. Uetani N, Kato K, Ogura H, et al. Impaired learning with enhanced hippocampal long-term potentiation in PTPdelta-deficient mice. *Embo J* 2000;19(12):2775–85.

98. Yang Q, Li L, Yang R, et al. Family-based and population-based association studies validate PTPRD as a risk factor for restless legs syndrome. *Mov Disord* 2011;26(3):516–9.

99. Winkelmann J, Schormair B, Lichtner P, et al. Genome-wide association study of restless legs syndrome identifies common variants in three genomic regions. *Nat Genet* 2007;39(8):1000–6.

100. Mercader N, Leonardo E, Azpiazu N, et al. Conserved regulation of proximodistal limb axis development by Meis1/Hth. *Nature* 1999;402(6760):425–9.

101. Maeda R, Mood K, Jones TL, et al. Xmeis1, a protooncogene involved in specifying neural crest cell fate in Xenopus embryos. *Oncogene* 2001;20(11):1329–42.

102. Mizuhara E, Nakatani T, Minaki Y, et al. Corl1, a novel neuronal lineage-specific transcriptional corepressor for the homeodomain transcription factor Lbx1. *J Biol Chem* 2005;280(5):3645–55.

103. Dinev D, Jordan BW, Neufeld B, et al. Extracellular signal regulated kinase 5

(ERK5) is required for the differentiation of muscle cells. *EMBO Rep* 2001;2(9):829–34.

104. Stefansson H, Rye DB, Hicks A, et al. A genetic risk factor for periodic limb movements in sleep. *N Engl J Med* 2007;357(7):639–47.

105. Winkelman JW: Considering the causes of RLS. *Eur J Neurol* 2006;13(Suppl 3):8–14.

106. Vilarino-Guell C, Farrer MJ, Lin SC. A genetic risk factor for periodic limb movements in sleep. *N Engl J Med* 2008;358(4):425–7.

107. Kemlink D, Polo O, Frauscher B, et al. Replication of restless legs syndrome loci in three European populations. *J Med Genet* 2009;46(5):315–8.

108. Yang Q, Li L, Chen Q, et al. Association studies of variants in MEIS1, BTBD9, and MAP2K5/SKOR1 with restless legs syndrome in a US population. *Sleep Med* 2011;12(8):800–4.

109. Schormair B, Plag J, Kaffe M, et al. MEIS1 and BTBD9: genetic association with restless leg syndrome in end stage renal disease. *J Med Genet* 2011;48(7):462–6.

110. Yuan SH, Qiu Z, Ghosh A. TOX3 regulates calcium-dependent transcription in neurons. *Proc Natl Acad Sci USA* 2009;106(8):2909–14.

111. Xiong L, Catoire H, Dion P, et al. MEIS1 intronic risk haplotype associated with restless legs syndrome affects its mRNA and protein expression levels. *Hum Mol Genet* 2009;18(6):1065–74.

112. Catoire H, Dion PA, Xiong L, et al. Restless legs syndrome-associated MEIS1 risk variant influences iron homeostasis. *Ann Neurol* 2011;70(1):170–5.

113. Mignot E. Genetic and familial aspects of narcolepsy. *Neurology* 1998;50(2 Suppl 1):S16–22.

114. Baraitser M, Parkes JD. Genetic study of narcoleptic syndrome. *J Med Genet* 1978;15(4):254–9.

115. Guilleminault C, Mignot E, Grumet FC. Familial patterns of narcolepsy. *Lancet* 1989;2(8676):1376–9.

116. Dauvilliers Y, Maret S, Bassetti C, et al. A monozygotic twin pair discordant for narcolepsy and CSF hypocretin-1. *Neurology* 2004;62(11):2137–8.

117. Hungs M, Fan J, Lin L, et al. Identification and functional analysis of mutations in the hypocretin (orexin) genes of narcoleptic canines. *Genome Res* 2001;11(4):531–9.

118. Nakayama J, Miura M, Honda M, et al. Linkage of human narcolepsy with HLA association to chromosome 4p13-q21. *Genomics* 2000;65(1):84–6.

119. Dauvilliers Y, Blouin JL, Neidhart E, et al. A narcolepsy susceptibility locus maps to a 5 Mb region of chromosome 21q. *Ann Neurol* 2004;56(3):382–8.

120. Hor H, Bartesaghi L, Kutalik Z, et al. A missense mutation in myelin oligodendrocyte glycoprotein as a cause of familial narcolepsy with cataplexy. *Am J Hum Genet* 2011;89(3):474–9.

121. Reindl M, Linington C, Brehm U, et al. Antibodies against the myelin oligodendrocyte glycoprotein and the myelin basic protein in multiple sclerosis and other neurological diseases: a comparative study. *Brain* 1999;122(Pt 11):2047–56.

122. Menge T, Lalive PH, von Budingen HC, et al. Conformational epitopes of myelin oligodendrocyte glycoprotein are targets of potentially pathogenic antibody responses in multiple sclerosis. *J Neuroinflammation* 2011;8(161):161.

123. Matsuki K, Honda Y, Juji T. Diagnostic criteria for narcolepsy and HLA-DR2 frequencies. *Tissue Antigens* 1987;30(4):155–60.

124. Rogers AE, Meehan J, Guilleminault C, et al. HLA DR15 (DR2) and DQB1*0602 typing studies in 188 narcoleptic patients with cataplexy. *Neurology* 1997;48(6):1550–6.

125. Mignot E, Hayduk R, Black J, et al. HLA DQB1*0602 is associated with cataplexy in 509 narcoleptic patients. *Sleep* 1997;20(11):1012–20.

126. Mignot E, Lin L, Rogers W, et al. Complex HLA-DR and -DQ interactions confer risk of narcolepsy-cataplexy in three ethnic groups. *Am J Hum Genet* 2001;68(3):686–99.

127. Hor H, Kutalik Z, Dauvilliers Y, et al. Genome-wide association study identifies new HLA class II haplotypes strongly protective against narcolepsy. *Nat Genet* 2010;42(9):786–9.

128. Hallmayer J, Faraco J, Lin L, et al. Narcolepsy is strongly associated with the T-cell receptor alpha locus. *Nat Genet* 2009;41(6):708–11.

129. Overeem S, Black JL, 3rd, Lammers GJ. Narcolepsy: immunological aspects. *Sleep Med Rev* 2008;12(2):95–107.

130. Kornum BR, Kawashima M, Faraco J, et al. Common variants in P2RY11 are associated with narcolepsy. *Nat Genet* 2011;43(1):66–71.

131. Bours MJ, Swennen EL, Di Virgilio F, et al. Adenosine 5'-triphosphate and adenosine as endogenous signaling molecules in immunity and inflammation. *Pharmacol Ther* 2006;112(2):358–404.

132. Hohjoh H, Nakayama T, Ohashi J, et al. Significant association of a single nucleotide polymorphism in the tumor necrosis factor-alpha (TNF-alpha) gene promoter with human narcolepsy. *Tissue Antigens* 1999;54(2):138–45.

133. Wieczorek S, Dahmen N, Jagiello P, et al. Polymorphisms of the tumor necrosis factor receptors: no association with narcolepsy in German patients. *J Mol Med (Berl)* 2003;81(2):87–90.

134. Miyagawa T, Kawashima M, Nishida N, et al. Variant between CPT1B and CHKB associated with susceptibility to narcolepsy. *Nat Genet* 2008;40(11):1324–8.

135. Sehgal A, Mignot E: Genetics of sleep and sleep disorders. *Cell* 2011;146(2):194–207.

136. Jones CR, Campbell SS, Zone SE, et al. Familial advanced sleep-phase syndrome: a short-period circadian rhythm variant in humans. *Nat Med* 1999;5(9):1062–5.

137. Toh KL, Jones CR, He Y, et al. An hPer2 phosphorylation site mutation in familial advanced sleep phase syndrome. *Science* 2001;291(5506):1040–3.

138. Xu Y, Padiath QS, Shapiro RE, et al. Functional consequences of a CKIdelta mutation causing familial advanced sleep phase syndrome. *Nature* 2005;434(7033):640–4.

139. Shanware NP, Hutchinson JA, Kim SH, et al. Casein kinase 1-dependent phosphorylation of familial advanced sleep phase syndrome-associated residues controls PERIOD 2 stability. *J Biol Chem* 2011;286(14):12766–74.

140. Vanselow K, Vanselow JT, Westermark PO, et al. Differential effects of PER2 phosphorylation: molecular basis for the human familial advanced sleep phase syndrome (FASPS). *Genes Dev* 2006;20(19):2660–72.

141. Cortelli P, Gambetti P, Montagna P, et al. Fatal familial insomnia: clinical features and molecular genetics. *J Sleep Res* 1999;8(Suppl 1):23–9.

142. Goldfarb LG, Petersen RB, Tabaton M, et al. Fatal familial insomnia and familial Creutzfeldt-Jakob disease: disease phenotype determined by a DNA polymorphism. *Science* 1992;258(5083):806–8.

143. Medori R, Tritschler HJ, LeBlanc A, et al. Fatal familial insomnia, a prion disease with a mutation at codon 178 of the prion protein gene. *N Engl J Med* 1992;326(7):444–9.

144. Montagna P, Cortelli P, Avoni P, et al. Clinical features of fatal familial insomnia: phenotypic variability in relation to a polymorphism at codon 129 of the prion protein gene. *Brain Pathol* 1998;8(3):515–20.

145. Tobler I, Deboer T, Fischer M. Sleep and sleep regulation in normal and prion protein-deficient mice. *J Neurosci* 1997;17(5):1869–79.

146. Tobler I, Gaus SE, Deboer T, et al. Altered circadian activity rhythms and sleep in mice devoid of prion protein. *Nature* 1996;380(6575):639–42.

PART THREE

Laboratory Evaluation of Motor Disturbances During Sleep

9

An Introduction

MARK HALLETT AND SUDHANSU CHOKROVERTY

THE PHYSICIAN facing a patient with a complaint of a possible movement disorder during sleep is in a somewhat difficult position because typically it is not immediately possible to observe the problem in the office or in the clinic. This is only the beginning of the difficulties, however, because the patient may be asleep at the time or not fully aware of the disturbance, or the patient may not show the abnormal movement at that time. Family members who attempt to convey the correct information are not always reliable. Spending all night watching the patient is not a great option, either, and there is typically insufficient light for the usual home video recorder. Some disorders, however, may be present during the day, as well as the night, and the history may be clear enough by itself. Some elements of the physical examination might be helpful. There is, however, a significant role for the laboratory evaluation.

There are a variety of abnormal movements (dyskinesias) observed during sleep at night—some are clinically defined, but some remain undefined and unrecognized. How does the nervous system generate these abnormal movements during sleep? Sleep may release both the inhibitory and excitatory pathways, mostly inhibitory. Sophisticated studies involving functional magnetic resonance imaging (fMRI) and positron emission tomography (PET) scan during different sleep stages are needed to unravel our ignorance. We are recognizing new entities during sleep—some may be inherited and may need molecular neurobiology to uncover the mystery.

The most helpful laboratory examination to understand sleep-related movement disorders is typically the overnight polysomnogram (PSG), with associated audio-video recording. This allows a full evaluation of the sleep-wake states and different stages of sleep, the evolution of sleep through the night, and a clinical-physiologic assessment of the movement disorder. When in sleep does it occur? What is the electromyographic (EMG) pattern, and what, if any, is the electroencephalographic (EEG) correlate? What is the role of multiple muscle recordings during PSG?

One of the most difficult conditions to differentiate is a nocturnal seizure from a sleep-induced or a sleep-activated movement disorder. Video-PSG studies have been able to make clear diagnoses and even clear up clinical confusion in situations in which laboratory investigations were not undertaken. A case in point is nocturnal paroxysmal dystonia. The syndrome was confused for some time; the original article title by Lugaresi and Cirignotta was "Hypnogenic Paroxysmal Dystonia: Epileptic Seizure or a New Entity?" Is it a seizure disorder? Is it a parasomnia? Is it an unusual movement disorder occurring exclusively in sleep? In the *International Classification of Sleep Disorders*, edition 2, this was classified in Appendix A under "sleep-related epilepsy," as it is now recognized that almost all cases are due to nocturnal frontal lobe epilepsy. Laboratory evaluation, including video-PSG recordings, has played an important role in resolving this controversy. More recent careful studies now show that nocturnal paroxysmal dystonia, paroxysmal arousals or awakenings, and episodic nocturnal wandering are all related and part of the spectrum of nocturnal frontal lobe epilepsy.

There is still considerable ignorance in understanding hypnic jerks. Intensified hypnic jerks are still misdiagnosed as myoclonic seizures. Clinical and laboratory evaluations are important to differentiate this benign physiologic condition from more malignant myoclonic seizure. Furthermore, PSG recordings in these patients may help clarify different physiologic types based on propagation of the muscles and the muscle burst duration.

Rapid eye movement (REM) sleep behavior disorder, periodic limb movements in sleep (PLMS), and partial arousal disorders are some of the other conditions that may be mistaken for seizures. The question is often asked, "Is the seizure triggered by arousal or is the arousal triggered by the seizure?" Which comes first? Again laboratory evaluations go a long way toward resolving these issues.

Other laboratory evaluations carried on during the day may produce useful information. In patients with the complaint of excessive daytime sleepiness, special testing such as the multiple sleep latency tests (MSLTs) can formally assess daytime sleepiness and the tendency to go into REM sleep shortly after sleep onset. This is particularly valuable for assessment of narcolepsy-cataplexy syndrome. In a patient with a complaint of episodic weakness of the knees and occasional falls, so-called limping man or woman syndrome, an overnight PSG followed by an MSLT may confirm the diagnosis of narcolepsy-cataplexy syndrome in the context of appropriate history. In such a patient an MRI of the brain may show a mesencephalic or a diencephalecic tumor causing secondary narcolepsy-cataplexy.

Another important laboratory contribution is actigraphic recording. Actigraphy is a technique of motion detection ("acceleration" or "deceleration") that records activities during sleep and waking for days and weeks. It complements sleep log or sleep diary data and may be useful in diagnosing circadian rhythm sleep disorders, paradoxical insomnia, or assessment and quantification of PLMS.

History and physical examination remain the cornerstones for evaluating abnormal movements during sleep. Laboratory tests should always be considered subservient to history and physical examination. Furthermore, limitations of EEG, overnight PSG, and other laboratory tests must be taken into consideration. On the other hand, these tests can make critical contributions, and it is important to have a clear understanding of them. The following chapters discuss the different laboratory tests in detail.

10

Polysomnography

DAMIAN MCGOVERN AND BETH A. MALOW

POLYSOMNOGRAPHY (PSG) is defined as the recording of multiple physiologic variables during sleep. The technique is an important tool in the evaluation of patients with movements and complex behaviors during sleep in whom the history may be insufficient to provide a definitive diagnosis.

In sleep-related movement disorders, such as periodic limb movements of sleep (PLMS) or bruxism, PSG can characterize and quantify the events in question. In movement disorders associated with sleep dysfunction, such as Parkinson's disease, the PSG may reveal coexisting rapid eye movement (REM) sleep behavior disorder (RBD) or sleep apnea. In cases in which complex behaviors predominate, the PSG, combined with video and the electroencephalogram (EEG), allows behavioral analysis of the spell. Video-EEG polysomnography (VPSG), in which a video recording of the patient is combined with extended EEG coverage (12 or more channels) of the scalp, can be invaluable in differentiating among epileptic seizures, parasomnias, and other sleep disorders associated with movements and behaviors.[1] These entities include arousal disorders, RBD, rhythmic movement disorder, PLMS, dissociative disorders, and bruxism.[2] This chapter describes the methodology and indications for standard PSG and VPSG in the evaluation of patients with movement disorders or with complex behaviors during sleep. PSG evaluation of the patient with suspected epileptic seizures is discussed in Chapter 35.

METHODOLOGY

Technical Aspects of Polysomnography

The standard system for PSG recordings consists of a combination of alternating current (AC) and direct current (DC) amplifiers. The AC amplifiers record high-frequency signals, including the EEG, the electrooculogram (EOG), the electromyogram (EMG), and the electrocardiogram (ECG). The DC amplifiers record low-frequency signals such as oxyhemoglobin saturation. Airflow and respiratory effort can be monitored with either AC or DC amplifiers. The AC amplifiers have both low- and high-frequency filters, which allow isolation of the frequency bands of physiologic interest. The DC amplifiers lack a low-frequency filter. The digital specifications for routine sleep studies give the settings for sampling rates, low filter frequency, and high filter frequency. These impedances, sampling rates, and filter settings are defined in the *AASM Manual for the Scoring of Sleep and Associated Events*. The technologist carrying out a PSG study and the physician interpreting such a study must be skilled in the recognition of a variety of artifacts. Additional information regarding PSG technique, recording protocols, and artifact recognition is available in standard texts of sleep medicine.[3]

EEG electrodes and their placement are discussed in Chapter 35.

The EOG measures the potential difference between the cornea, which is positively charged, and the retina, which is negatively charged. For measurement of the EOG, electrodes are customarily applied at the outer canthus of the right eye, 1 cm above the horizontal, and at the outer canthus of the left eye, 1 cm below the horizontal (Fig. 10.1). Conjugate eye movements result in out-of-phase deflections. This electrode placement allows for recording of both horizontal and vertical eye movements. Typical filter settings for EOG channels, or combinations of electrodes, are a low-frequency filter of 0.3 Hz to enhance slow eye movements and a high-frequency filter of 35 Hz to diminish muscle artifact. Physiologic calibrations, which check the integrity and placement of EOG electrodes, should be performed before recording by having patients open and close their eyes; look to the left, right, up, and down; and blink.

The EMG measures activity from the mentalis and submentalis muscles (see Fig. 10.1). These electrodes aid in the scoring of REM sleep, the portion of the recording in which muscle tone is the lowest, and in the scoring of arousals from sleep, marked by an increase in EMG activity. In our laboratory, three chin EMG electrodes are applied, with one as a backup because chin electrodes are particularly likely to loosen during the recording. Additional EMG electrodes can be placed over the masseter muscle if bruxism is of concern (see Fig. 10.1). Typical filter settings for EMG channels are a low-frequency filter of 10 Hz to minimize slow-wave artifacts and a high-frequency filter of 100 Hz or greater to enhance myogenic activity. Physiologic calibrations include having patients grit their teeth, clench their jaws, and smile.[4]

Limb EMG recordings are especially important in patients with suspected PLMS and RBD. For leg movement recordings, electrodes are placed over the anterior tibialis muscles, approximately 2 to 3 cm apart. Because movements may occur in one leg only or switch from one leg to the other throughout the night, activity in both legs should be recorded. Calibration

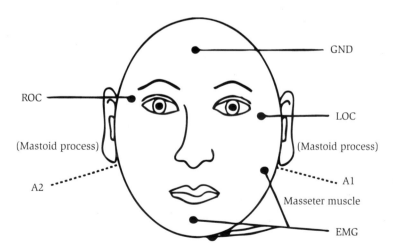

FIGURE 10.1 Schematic diagram shows placement of the electromyographic electrodes to record activity from the mental, submental, and masseter muscles. GND, ground (earth); LOC, left outer canthus; ROC, right outer canthus. (From Keenan SA: Polysomnographic technique: An overview. In Chokroverty S (ed): Sleep Disorders Medicine. Boston, Butterworth-Heinemann, 1999, p. 151.)

should be performed before recording by having patients slowly dorsiflex and plantarflex the great toe of each foot to approximately 30 degrees without resistance. When diagnoses such as PLMS or RBD are suspected, channels from each flexor and extensor compartment of the upper limb should be included to maximize the yield of the recording.[5] The minimum channels required for the diagnosis of parasomnia or sleep-related seizure disorder include sleep-scoring channels (EEG, EOG, chin EMG), EEG using an expanded bilateral montage, and EMG for body movements (anterior tibialis or extensor digitorum). Audiovisual recording and documented technologist observations during the period of study are also essential.[6]

Respiratory monitoring during sleep includes a variety of sensors for monitoring airflow and respiratory effort, as well as pulmonary gas exchange. Four signals used are the thermal sensor, the nasal pressure transducer, the respiratory inductance plethsmography, and the pulse oximeter.[7] These sensors range from the indirect, semiquantitative thermistor that is placed under the nose to the direct quantitative measurement of airflow obtained through a sealed face mask, such as occurs during the application of continuous positive airway pressure (CPAP).[8] Strain gauges and inductance plethysmography are indirect semiquantitative methods that sense changes in the thoracic and abdominal cross-sectional areas resulting from respiratory muscle contraction. They are easy to use and of relative comfort to the patient. In contrast, esophageal pressure monitoring provides a more reliable, but invasive, quantitative measure of respiratory effort. Pulmonary gas exchange is monitored with pulse oximetry and end-tidal carbon dioxide monitoring. Physiologic calibrations include inhaling, exhaling, and holding the breath.

EEG electrodes are applied to the surface of the skin just below the right clavicle and on the left side at the level of the seventh rib.

Impedances should be documented before recording, and adjustments should be made to EEG, EOG, ECG, or chin EMG electrodes with impedances greater than 5000 ohms.

DIGITAL ELECTROENCEPHALOGRAPHIC-POLYSOMNOGRAPHIC SYSTEMS

Computerized digital EEG-PSG systems are now widely available and have revolutionized the fields of EEG and PSG. Digital systems have advantages in both review and storage. These systems facilitate the review of large amounts of EEG-PSG data by displaying scoring and event information in a user-friendly fashion. The user can click on the stage or event of interest and bring up the corresponding EEG-PSG. The recording may be reviewed at a variety of display settings that correspond to different paper speeds of conventional recordings. For example, a PSG segment containing an abnormal movement may first be reviewed at the standard PSG paper speed (10 mm/second) (a minimum of 15 mm/second is now recommended and preferably 30 mm/second, with adequate sampling to identify brief paroxysmal discharges to determine the stage of sleep from which the event arises). It may then be reviewed at the standard EEG paper speed (30 mm/second) to review the pattern and evolution of the activity suspicious for an epileptic seizure. It may also be reviewed at a compressed speed (<10 mm/second) to aid in the review of respiratory parameters. Filters, sensitivities, and montages may be adjusted to assist in the visual analysis and help distinguish abnormalities from artifacts or normal variants.

Technical Aspects of Video-Electroencephalography-Polysomnography

VPSG combines video recording with an extended EEG montage, and PSG monitoring is useful for characterizing unusual behaviors and movements during sleep.[1] Events recorded with VPSG are reviewed to characterize (1) the motor and behavioral manifestations of the event and (2) the EEG-PSG features, including the stage of sleep preceding the event, the time of the event relative to sleep onset, and EEG and EMG patterns occurring during the event or between events. In patients with complex movements and behaviors during sleep, the information provided by VPSG can help distinguish movement disorders from parasomnias, psychiatric disorders, and epileptic seizures.

Video recordings are then synchronized with digital EEG-PSG recordings to allow review of the event in question. Time-locked video allows review of the event in real time or at slower speeds. Infrared cameras are useful for recording nighttime events. Movable cameras can be mounted in a patient's room and display close-ups or full-body views. Double cameras are useful to monitor the face and body simultaneously.

For review, the video signal can be combined with EEG-PSG on a single "split" screen so that the sleep-related movements and behaviors are time-linked to EEG-PSG changes. Alternatively, the EEG-PSG signal and video signal can be synchronously replayed on two monitors. The EEG-PSG also can be played back at a variety of speeds to display sleep features or EEG features as indicated.

The specific montage used depends on the number of channels available for EEG and the need to record additional PSG parameters. For example, in a patient in whom nocturnal seizures are the primary concern, most channels may be devoted to EEG. In a patient with spells suspicious for RBD but in whom nocturnal seizures are also a concern, a montage employing extensive EEG coverage and also additional limb leads may be employed. Table 10.1 lists sample recording montages.

Ambulatory Polysomnography

Although attended PSG performed in a sleep disorders laboratory is the accepted standard technique used for the diagnosis of sleep disorders, home PSG has been advocated as a means of increasing accessibility and minimizing costs. Systems are now available that provide at least 18 PSG channels and synchronized video recordings to facilitate correlation between EEG activity and clinical events. A major disadvantage of ambulatory monitoring relates to the fidelity of the recording in the absence of a technologist. If electrodes become detached, ground wires break, or conductive media become dry during the study, adjustments cannot be made. Furthermore, the patient is not under constant observation, and a technologist is not present. This limitation is most relevant to studies in which epileptic seizures are in question and is also essential in determining the nature of the involuntary movements in RBD and in disorders of partial arousal.

Practice parameters regarding the use of portable monitors (PMs) were recently published.[7, 9]

Using a categorization of sleep-monitoring procedures in which Type 1 is standard attended in-lab PSG, PMs are categorized into types 2–4. Type 2 is not used and Type 3 is a modified portable sleep apnea test referred to as a cardiorespiratory sleep study. These are

Table 10.1 Sample Electroencephalographic-Polysomnographic Montages

INDICATION	MONTAGE
Arousal disorder, possible nocturnal seizures (29 channels)	LEOG-A2, REOG-A1, chin EMG, C3-A2, C4-A1, LAT EMG, RAT EMG, Fp1-F7, F7-T3, T3-T5, T5-O1, Fp1-F3, F3-C3, C3-P3, P3-O1, Fp2-Fp8, F8-T4, T4-T6, T6-O2, Fp2-F4, F4-C4, C4-P4, P4-O2, Fz-Cz, Cz-Pz, nasal-oral airflow, thoracic effort, abdominal effort, ECG
RBD, possible nocturnal seizures (21 channels)	LEOG-A2, REOG-A1, chin EMG, C3-A2, C4-A1, LED EMG, RED EMG, LAT EMG, RAT EMG, Fp1-F7, F7-T3, T3-T5, T5-O1, Fp2-Fp8, F8-T4, T4-T6, T6-O2, nasal-oral airflow, thoracic effort, abdominal effort, ECG
RBD, possible nocturnal seizures (31 channels)	LEOG-A2, REOG-A1, chin EMG, C3-A2, C4-A1, LED EMG, RED EMG, LAT EMG, RAT EMG, Fp1-F7, F7-T3, T3-T5, T5-O1, Fp1-F3, F3-C3, C3-P3, P3-O1, Fp2-Fp8, F8-T4, T4-T6, T6-O2, Fp2-F4, F4-C4, C4-P4, P4-O2, Fz-Cz, Cz-Pz, nasal-oral airflow, thoracic effort, abdominal effort, ECG LEOG-A2, REOG-A1, chin EMG, C3-A2, C4-A1, O1-A2, O2-A1, LED EMG, LFD EMG, RED EMG
PLMS, extended limb coverage (19 channels)	RFD EMG, LAT EMG, LPT EMG, RAT EMG, RPT EMG, nasal-oral airflow, thoracic effort, abdominal effort, ECG

ECG, electrocardiogram; EMG, electromyogram; EOG, electrooculogram; L, left; LAT, left anterior tibialis; LED, left extensor digitorum; LFD, left flexor digitorum; LPT, left posterior tibialis; R, right; RAT, right anterior tibialis; RED, right extensor digitorum; RFD, right flexor digitorum; RPT, right posterior tibialis.

used in an attended setting and may rule in or rule out OSA when conducted on suitable patients and interpreted with manual scoring by trained personnel. Appropriate patients for this use should be free from significant comorbid conditions, and symptomatic patients with negative PM studies should undergo attended PSG to truly exclude OSA. Type 4 is the continuous single- or dual-bioparameter recording. Ambulatory overnight pulse oximetry is a Type 4 PM device. The utility of ambulatory oximetry varies depending on equipment, analysis methods, and patient population, and routine use is not recommended in specific situations.

INDICATIONS FOR POLYSOMNOGRAPHY AND VIDEO-ELECTROENCEPHALOGRAPHY-POLYSOMNOGRAPHY

Indications for VPSG include suspected sleep-related epileptic seizures, suspected non-REM arousal disorders, RBD, or suspected dissociative disorder.

Indications for PSG in the patient with complex movements and behaviors fall into three broad categories. First, PSG may quantify the event in question, such as in PLMS. Second, PSG may detect coexisting sleep disorders, such as RBD seen in association with narcolepsy. Finally, PSG can aid in diagnosis of the event in question. When the history does not allow the physician to diagnose nocturnal spells associated with complex movements and behaviors, recording the sleep-related event with PSG may allow definitive diagnosis. This section emphasizes the use of PSG and VPSG in the differential diagnosis of nocturnal spells. The reader is referred to other sections of the text dealing with specific disorders for information on diagnosis and quantification of these disorders with PSG. No standards or guidelines exist for when to choose specific monitoring techniques, and the reliability and validity of these have not been formally studied.[10,11]

With the exception of RBD, in which the diagnosis can be made even if an event is not recorded (see the following), the PSG and VPSG are generally reserved for patients with spells occurring at least several times a week. Generally it is useful to schedule a patient for two consecutive nights of study to maximize the yield of recording an event. The stage of sleep from which the spells emerge and the time of the spell, relative to sleep onset, provide useful diagnostic information. For example, arousal disorders arise from delta non-REM sleep usually in the first third of the sleep period (Chapter 28), whereas behaviors associated with RBD emerge out of REM sleep and may occur at intervals throughout the sleep period (Chapter 29). Epileptic seizures are more common during non-REM sleep, but they rarely occur during REM sleep (Chapter 35). Rhythmic movements associated with rhythmic movement disorder usually occur during sleep-wake transitions (Chapter 40). Psychiatric disorders that may mimic seizures or nocturnal movements are nocturnal dissociative disorder and panic disorder with nocturnal panic attacks. Posttraumatic stress disorder patients may have unusual transient behaviors upon awakening to dreams of trauma. In dissociative episodes, patients may appear to be asleep, but a key diagnostic point is that these events emerge from wakefulness. Nocturnal panic attacks occur from non-REM sleep, usually at the transition from stage 2 to stage 3.[12] Panic attacks also cause sudden awakenings without odd behaviors or involuntary movements. The indications for PSG and VPSG in the evaluation of specific types of nocturnal spells are discussed later. The indications for PSG and VPSG in the evaluation of suspected sleep-related epileptic seizures are discussed in Chapter 35.

The major disadvantage of VPSG in the evaluation of these disorders is the cost of the study. Additional technologist time is needed to place an extended EEG montage and to continuously observe patients throughout the study. Physicians must review each spell to assess behaviors and EEG patterns. At minimum, equipment must allow for review capabilities at EEG paper speed (30 mm/second) and preferably should also allow the interpreter to change montages, sensitivities, and filter settings to aid in review. These review capabilities are standard on most digital PSG equipment, although the additional channels and the ability to remontage require more space on storage media.

Suspected Arousal Disorder

Arousal disorders, which encompass confusional arousals, sleepwalking, and sleep terrors, are usually diagnosed by the clinical history (Chapter 28).[13] However, if there are clinical features that suggest seizures or RBD and spells are occurring at least several times a week, VPSG is indicated. Such features include behavioral characteristics that are atypical or stereotyped, multiple nightly episodes, onset in adulthood, or spells that do not respond to a trial of medications. The advantage of VPSG in the evaluation of suspected arousal disorders is the combination of video to characterize the spells, sleep scoring channels to determine the stage of sleep involved, and an extended EEG montage to exclude ictal EEG activity. The events characteristic of arousal disorders are less stereotyped than epileptic seizures and may be prolonged. Arousal disorders almost always emerge from stage N3 non-REM sleep, whereas seizures arise from all stages of non-REM sleep and less commonly from REM sleep. In contrast to the ictal EEG pattern characteristic of an epileptic seizure, which evolves in frequency and amplitude, the EEG pattern of an event characteristic of arousal disorder shows nonevolving high-voltage synchronous or asynchronous delta or theta activity, a drowsy pattern, or nonreactive alpha activity. However, differentiating seizures from arousal disorders on the basis of the EEG is not always straightforward, because the EEG may be normal in certain types of seizures or show only an arousal pattern. In addition, the most well-developed portion of the ictal EEG pattern may be rhythmic delta or theta without a clear evolution, or myogenic artifact may obscure the EEG.

Suspected REM Sleep Behavior Disorder

Although RBD may be suspected based on the history, definitive diagnosis requires either recording a behavioral event on a video recording or demonstrating abnormal muscle tone or excessive limb movements during REM sleep.[14] Specifically, a thorough history must be couple with an increased chin EMG or increased phasic muscle activity in the chin or limb leads to make a diagnosis. If a good history is not available, the event must be witnessed on PSG and at least one of the two EMG findings must be present for diagnosis. Because capturing a clinical event is not necessary for diagnosis, the yield of PSG is high, especially if two nights are recorded. An extended EEG montage can be used to exclude ictal EEG activity, and additional limb leads can be placed to evaluate for excessive limb movements. An example of a recording from a patient with RBD is shown in Figure 10.2. The clinical manifestations of RBD are discussed further in Chapter 29.

Suspected Dissociative Disorder

Dissociative episodes and other psychogenic spells occur during wakefulness, although patients may appear asleep and believe that they are asleep.[15] Because the manifestations of dissociative episodes may be quite bizarre, including thrashing, screaming, or bicycling movements, it is often impossible to determine whether these spells are seizures, parasomnias, or dissociative episodes by the history alone. The VPSG is useful in documenting the non-stereotyped nature of dissociative spells, the presence of waking background EEG preceding the onset of the spells and present during the spells, and the absence of ictal EEG activity. The major disadvantage of VPSG is the cost and time required for the extended lead placement and reading of this data.

Suspected Movement Disorders

Rhythmic movement disorder, PLMS, and bruxism occasionally mimic seizures, dissociative disorders, or other parasomnias. Rhythmic movement disorder, also known as head banging or body rocking, can occur during any sleep stage, although it is most commonly at the sleep-wake transition or in the lighter stages of sleep. It is manifested in a variety of ways, including recurrent banging of the head while the patient is prone or rocking of the body back and forth while on hands and knees (see Chapter 40). When rhythmic movement disorder resembles a dissociative disorder, VPSG may be useful in documenting that it arises from sleep or from wakefulness. The stereotyped nature of PLMS may suggest complex partial seizures. The PLMS have a characteristic appearance on PSG (see Chapter 49). Bruxism (see Chapter 41) may resemble the oral-lingual automatisms of sleep-related complex partial seizures. Bruxism has a characteristic pattern of myogenic artifact superimposed on the EEG background activity on the PSG, and the EEG does not evolve in bruxism.

In summary, PSG and VPSG can be extremely helpful diagnostic tools in evaluation of the patient with abnormal movements or behaviors during sleep. Digital PSG and VPSG have made a major impact on the field by facilitating review and storage of large amounts of physiologic data. Ambulatory PSG and VPSG continue to be refined and have the potential to allow for high-quality home recordings. PSG and VPSG are useful for diagnosis of abnormal

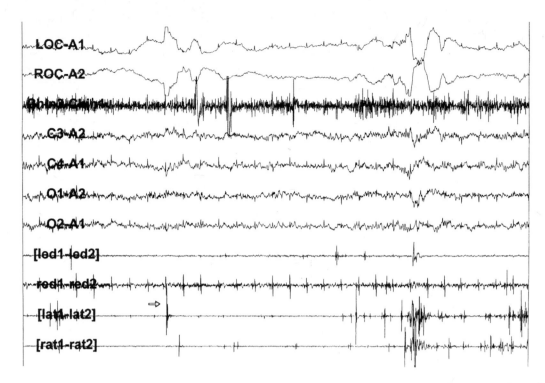

FIGURE 10.2 Use of additional limb leads to enhance the review of a patient with suspected rapid eye movement (REM) sleep behavior disorder. Note increased limb phasic activity (arrow) and persistent chin electromyographic (EMG) tone.

movements and behaviors in which the history is not definitive, quantification of movement disorders, and diagnosis of coexisting sleep disorders.

REFERENCES

1. Aldrich MS, Jahnke B. Diagnostic value of video-EEG polysomnography. *Neurology* 1991;41:1060–1066.
2. American Academy of Sleep Medicine. (2005) International Classification of Sleep Disorders. Diagnostic and Coding Manual, 2nd Edition. Westchester, IL:American Academy of Sleep Medicine.
3. Keenan S. Polysomnographic technique: an overview. In Chokroverty S, ed. *Sleep Disorders Medicine*. 2nd ed. Boston, MA: Butterworth-Heinemann; 1999:151.
4. *AASM Manual for the Scoring of Sleep and Associated Events*. Westchester, IL:American Academy of Sleep Medicine; 2007.
5. *American Sleep Disorders Association Task Force*. Recording and scoring leg movements. *Sleep* 1993;16:748–759.
6. American Academy of Sleep Medicine. Sleep-related breathing disorders in adults: recommendations for syndrome definition and measurement techniques in clinical research. The Report of an American Academy of Sleep Medicine Task Force. *Sleep* 1999;22:667–689.
7. Kushida CA, Littner MR, Morgenthaler T. Practice Parameters for the Indications for Polysomnography and Related Procedures: An Update for 2005. *Sleep* 2005;28(4):499–521.
8. A Technologist's Handbook for the AASM Manual for Understanding and Implementing the AASM Manual for the Scoring of Sleep. American Academy of Sleep Medicine, 2009.
9. Chesson AL, Jr., Berry RB, Pack A. Practice parameters for the use of portable monitoring devices in the investigation of suspected obstructive sleep apnea in adults. *Sleep* 2003;26(7):907–13.
10. Kryger MH, Roth T, Dement W. eds. *Principles and Practice of Sleep Medicine*. 5th ed. Philadelphia, PA: WB Saunders; 2011.

11. Fry J, DiPhillipo M, Curran K, et al. Full polysomnography in the home. *Sleep* 1998;21:635–642.

12. Mellman T, Uhde T. Electroencephalographic sleep in panic disorder. *Arch Gen Psychiatry* 1989;46:178–184.

13. Mahowald MW, Ettinger MG. Things that go bump in the night: the parasomnias revised. *J Clin Neurophysiol* 1990;7:119–143.

14. Mahowald M, Schenck C. REM Sleep Parasomnias. In Kryger M, Roth T, Dement W, eds. *Principles and Practice of Sleep Medicine*. 5th ed. Philadelphia, PA: WB Saunders; 2011:1083–1097.

15. Thacker K, Devinsky O, Perrine K, et al. Nonepileptic seizures during apparent sleep. *Ann Neurol* 1993;33:414–418.

11

Polysomnography

Scoring of Sleep Stages, Arousals, and Breathing

RODNEY A. RADTKE AND RAJDEEP SINGH

POLYSOMNOGRAPHY (PSG) is a commonly used test that evaluates a variety of sleep-related factors potentially impacting on a patient's daytime alertness, comorbid conditions, and long-term cardiovascular morbidity. The technical aspects involved in performing a PSG are discussed in Chapter 10. The clinical indications for overnight PSG are outlined in the next section, along with the indications for appropriate use of unattended home sleep studies. For most PSGs the main focus is on the assessment of sleep quality (as measured in total sleep time, sleep stages, and sleep disruption) along with the evaluation of accompanying respiratory events (as measured by hypopneas, apneas, oxygen desaturations, heart rate changes, and arousals). The focus of this chapter is the scoring of sleep stages, arousals from sleep, and respiratory events. Quantified assessments of movements during sleep are reviewed in Chapter 12.

INDICATIONS FOR POLYSOMNOGRAPHY

The American Academy of Sleep Medicine (AASM) has published practice parameters outlining the clinical indications for the use of PSG.[1,2] The main indication for PSG is the evaluation of sleep-related breathing disorders. The increasing awareness of sleep apnea and documentation of its effect on long-term cardiovascular health have led to a marked increase in PSG studies. While the classic obese hypersomnolent patient with sleep apnea is readily recognized, there are many less obvious candidates that also warrant PSG evaluation. Symptoms suggestive of possible sleep apnea include excessive daytime sleepiness, loud snoring, witnessed apneas, and unrefreshing sleep. Several medical conditions may also warrant consideration of sleep apnea given their frequent coexistence and the possibility that sleep apnea may be a major contributor to the presenting condition. These disorders include intractable hypertension, paroxysmal atrial fibrillation, intractable congestive heart failure, and stroke.

After documentation of the existence of significant sleep apnea, most patients then return for a repeat overnight PSG with the use of continuous positive airway pressure (CPAP). The primary goal during this study is to identify the ideal therapeutic pressure for CPAP that eliminates apneas, hypopneas, arousals, and snoring. The lowest effective pressure is usually chosen to assure effective treatment of the respiratory events but also to enhance tolerability and long-term compliance. Attention is focused on recording stage R sleep as well as supine sleep during the CPAP titration, as apneas and oxygen desaturations are usually more prominent during those recording situations. Patients that pursue other therapies for sleep apnea, such as upper airway surgery or an intra-oral appliance, are also recommended to return for a follow-up study to document the adequacy of that therapy and assure that additional therapeutic efforts are not required.

Even when sleep apnea is not suspected, a routine PSG is indicated for the evaluation of unexplained daytime sleepiness. The PSG is used to exclude the possibility of periodic limb movements of sleep (PLMS) or other cause of sleep disruption contributing to the patient's daytime dysfunction. A PSG is also done routinely the night preceding a multiple sleep latency test (MSLT). Besides excluding unsuspected sleep pathology, this PSG also documents total sleep time to assure adequate sleep prior to the MSLT. While patients with restless legs syndrome (RLS) often have nocturnal sleep complaints, PSGs are not routinely done in this setting. The diagnosis of RLS is made on a clinical basis and the restrained environment of the sleep lab can be very uncomfortable for the patient with symptomatic RLS. PSG may be appropriate if the RLS symptoms do not respond to therapy or if there is suspicion of a coexistent sleep apnea. Patients with a chief complaint of insomnia are not routinely evaluated with a PSG, as the diagnostic yield is low and rarely impacts on therapeutic approach. Both pharmacologic and behavioral approaches to treating insomnia are usually pursued before considering PSG evaluation.

Patients with unusual nocturnal behavior are also sometimes referred for PSG evaluation. Video recording is routinely done during a PSG, which allows assessment of patient behavior and its relationship to sleep stage or sleep-wake transition. Usually, the diagnosis of parasomnia or epileptic seizure can be reached on clinical evaluation alone. However, PSG may be warranted if there are unusual features or persistent diagnostic uncertainty surrounding the nocturnal behavior. Additional electroencephalographic (EEG) channels are recommended if nocturnal seizures are in the differential diagnosis as the limited EEG channels on a routine PSG are often inadequate to identify electrographic seizure activity or interictal epileptiform abnormalities.

INDICATIONS FOR AMBULATORY POLYSOMNOGRAPHIC RECORDING

In the past, ambulatory recording of sleep in the evaluation of sleep disorders had been used in a very limited fashion due to the inherent limitations of the technique and the lack of third-party reimbursement.[3] The Centers for Medicare and Medicaid Services (CMS) have recently approved coverage for home sleep tests (HSTs), which has led to the role of HSTs being reevaluated with respect to the diagnosis and treatment of sleep apnea. This reevaluation is understandable given the marked increase in laboratory PSG along with a desire to control health costs.[4] In-lab attended PSG (usually with 16 or more channels of physiologic recording) is the gold standard for the evaluation of sleep disorders and is classified as a type 1 study. An unattended home PSG with 7 or more channels, including the recording of EEG and respiratory assessment, is classified as a type 2 study. The main use of HSTs has been with the use of type 3 studies, which have 4–7 channels and focus only on the evaluation of respiratory parameters, but without recording of EEG. A type 3 HST does not evaluate sleep efficiency, sleep stages, or arousals. A type 4 study is a 1- or 2-channel overnight recording, with at least one of them being oximetry.[5]

When a home PSG is performed, the patient presents to the sleep lab or office during the day and is educated regarding use of the equipment and placement of electrodes and recording devices. After preparing for bed that night, the patient places the recording sensors and pushes a button indicating that he or she is retiring for the night. The button is pressed again upon awakening in the morning and a total recording time is determined. This objective measure of time in bed is supplemented by a brief sleep log from the patient outlining any sustained periods of wakefulness or other important information. This then allows an estimation of total sleep time. Usual parameters recorded in a type 3 study include nasal/oral airflow, respiratory effort, oxygen saturation, body position, snoring, and heart rate. The studies are scored utilizing automated scoring systems, but it is important to have the raw data reviewed by a technologist to assure that artifactual data are edited and not used as part of the assessment. An estimate of the patient's apnea/hypopnea index (AHI) and associated desaturation index is derived from the ambulatory recording.

Guidelines outlining the minimal technical standards for unattended home sleep studies have recently been published by the AASM.[5] HSTs should at a minimum record airflow, respiratory effort, and blood oxygenation. The same sensors used in the sleep laboratory should be used in carrying out the HSTs. Accurate data collection is paramount to successful use of the techniques, so the device should be used by technologists or physicians who have significant experience in sleep disorders and their evaluation. As noted earlier, review of the raw data is required to allow manual rescoring of the events or adjustment of the automated scoring algorithms.

The advantages of HSTs are obvious and include lower cost and greater patient accessibility. Patients who cannot access laboratory-based studies due to lab backlog or physical immobility can be evaluated with HST. Other patients with irregular or unusual sleep-wake cycles can also have an evaluation that does not have to fit into the usual lab schedule. The obvious disadvantages of HSTs include unreliable or lost data and the lack of any quantitative assessment of sleep stage or quality.

Portable or ambulatory sleep studies are not appropriate for all clinical settings. Both the AASM as well as the CMS guidelines support the use of HSTs as an alternative to in-lab PSGs in patients with a high probability of moderate to severe obstructive sleep apnea. However, both the CMS and AASM do not advocate the use of portable or ambulatory studies in many other clinical settings. HSTs are not indicated for patients with significant co-morbid illness such as chronic obstructive pulmonary disease, congestive heart failure, and neuromuscular disease. The coexistence of these disorders often leads to a greater degree of inaccuracy in evaluation of sleep-related breathing. Asymptomatic but high-risk individuals such as bariatric surgery patients or long-distance truck drivers have not been evaluated using HSTs, and as such its use as a screening tool in those clinical settings is not recommended.[4-7]

SCORING OF SLEEP STAGES

The publication of the Rechtschaffen and Kales sleep scoring atlas in 1968 represented a consensus agreement among sleep researchers of the time.[8] The goal was to standardize the scoring of sleep to assist in communication in sleep research studies. Thirty-second epochs (at a paper speed of 10 mm/sec) were proposed to assist in pattern recognition of sleep waveforms but also to limit the use of EEG paper. Limited four- or six-channel montages were proposed, as this was the limit of EEG or polygraph machines at that time. Similarly, the definition of the various sleep stages was somewhat arbitrary and not based on extensive research or experimental insight. Remarkably, this document remains the dominant force in sleep scoring for clinical sleep medicine today. With the recent publication of the American Academy of Sleep Medicine's Manual for the Scoring of Sleep and Associated Events, the standardization of sleep and event scoring has reached a new level of consensus.[9] The scoring of sleep in this recent document has only limited differences from that published in 1968.

With the recent AASM scoring manual, the nomenclature used for describing sleep stages has changed. The non–rapid eye movement (non-REM) sleep stages 1 and 2 have now been changed to stage N1 and N2, respectively. Non-REM stages 3 and 4 have now been combined and are labeled as stage N3. This change occurred both because of the poor reliability of differentiating stage 3 from stage 4 as well as the lack of documentation of any physiologic differences between those two stages. Stage REM is now labeled as stage R.

A sleep study is divided into 30 epochs and each is scored as stage W (or wakefulness), stage N1, stage N2, stage N3, or stage R. If more than one stage is identified in an epoch, the epoch is labeled as the stage that occupies the greatest portion of the epoch. Stage W represents the waking state ranging from full alertness through early drowsiness. Stage W is scored when more than 50% of the epoch demonstrates alpha frequency activity over the occipital region (Fig. 11.1). In the absence of alpha activity (which occurs in 10%–20% of normal individuals), Stage W is scored if eye blinks or irregular conjugate rapid eye movements are identified with accompanying evidence of chin muscle tone. The chin electromyogram (EMG) during stage W is quite variable but usually is higher than that seen during any sleep stage.

Stage N1 represents late drowsiness and light sleep. Stage N1 is identified by attenuation of alpha background with replacement by low-amplitude, mixed-frequency EEG activity. Once greater than 50% of an epoch is occupied by this pattern, the epoch is scored as stage N1 (Fig. 11.2). K complexes and sleep spindles are not seen during stage N1. If an individual does not generate alpha, stage N1 is scored when over 50% of the epoch demonstrates theta range slowing (4–7 Hz), vertex sharp waves, or slow eye movements. In individuals who do generate alpha, slow eye movements are frequently seen before the disappearance of alpha activity, so individuals who do not generate alpha activity may have N1 scored slightly earlier than those who do generate alpha activity. This small difference in defining sleep onset is of little concern in a PSG, but it may have some impact on the mean sleep latency determined during an MSLT

or maintenance of wakefulness test (MWT). Chin EMG is quite variable during stage N1, but it is usually lower than that seen in stage W.

The most easily defined and predominant sleep stage during an overnight PSG is stage N2. The scoring of stage N2 requires the appearance of either a sleep spindle (11–16 Hz sinusoidal activity lasting at least 0.5 seconds) or a K complex (Fig. 11.3). In sleep medicine, as opposed to traditional EEG nomenclature, a K complex is defined as a biphasic negative sharp wave that is maximum at the vertex and has a duration of at least 0.5 seconds. Delta activity (≤ 2 Hz, >75 microvolts) must occupy less than 20% of the epoch. Slow eye movements are sometimes seen during stage N2 but are usually absent. Axial EMG is variable but less than that seen in stage N1 or wakefulness. Stage N2 is scored from the first epoch of stage N2 until a clear epoch of stage W or another stage of sleep is identified.

Stage N3 is considered the deepest stage of sleep and is associated with increasing delta activity. Stage N3 is scored when greater than 20% of an epoch is delta activity (Fig. 11.4). In sleep medicine, delta activity is identified when EEG demonstrates waveforms in the range of 0.5–2 Hz that are at least 75 microvolts in amplitude (when recorded over the frontal or central regions). Sleep spindles are often identified in

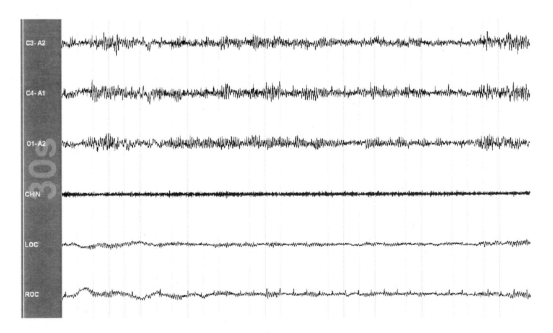

FIGURE 11.1 Thirty-second epoch of a limited polysomnographic montage that illustrates well-developed alpha activity consistent with stage W (wakefulness). Chin, submental electromyography; LOC, left outer canthus eye channel; ROC, right outer canthus eye channel.

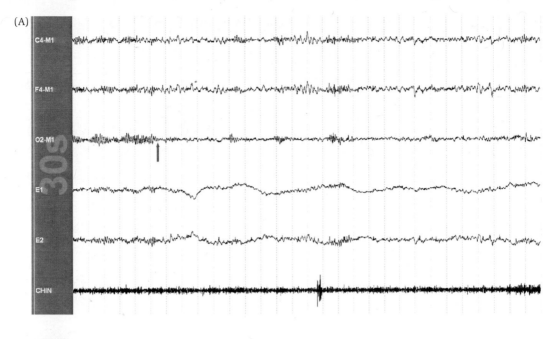

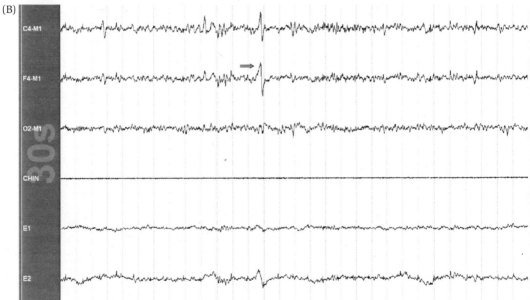

FIGURE 11.2 (*A*) Limited polysomnographic (PSG) montage that illustrates the dropout of alpha activity (arrow), which is replaced by low-amplitude theta activity accompanied by slow eye movements. This 30-second epoch is scored as stage N1. (*B*) Limited PSG montage, which demonstrates well-established stage N1 sleep with an absence of slow eye movements and a prominent vertex sharp wave (arrow). (30-second epoch)

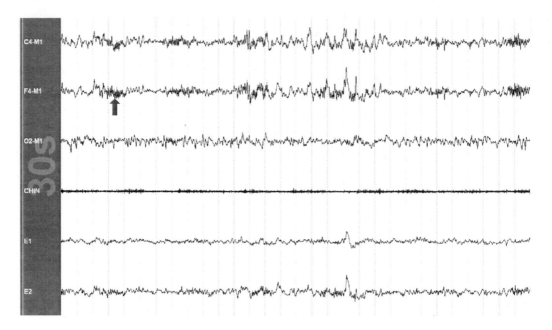

FIGURE 11.3   Limited polysomnographic montage illustrates sleep spindles (arrow) and broad vertex waves consistent with stage N2. (30-second epoch; chin, submental electromyography)

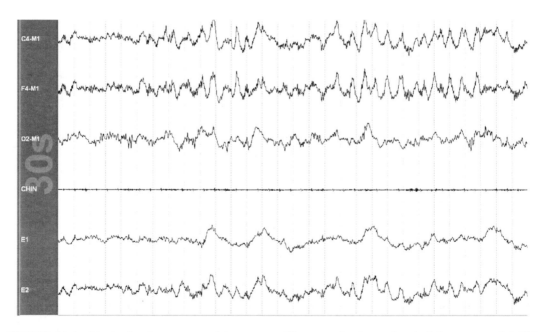

FIGURE 11.4   Limited polysomnographic montage illustrates high-amplitude delta activity (<2 Hz) occupying greater than 20% of the epoch and represents an example of stage N3. Delta frequency waveforms in two central channels are greater than 75 microvolts in amplitude. (30-second epoch; chin, submental electromyography)

stage N3 but are less well defined as compared to those seen in stage N2. Eye movements are rarely evident during stage N3 sleep. Axial EMG is usually lower in amplitude as compared to stage N2, but it remains higher than that subsequently seen in stage R sleep.

To score stage R, three components are required: the EEG must demonstrate low-amplitude, mixed-frequency activity that does not contain sleep spindles, K-complexes, or >20% delta activity; rapid eye movements must be present; and tonic EMG must be absent (or at least lower than at any other time during the study). Phasic bursts of EMG may occur, but tonic EMG should not be present. Sawtooth waves, which are 2–5 Hz vertex negative waves, are often seen especially just prior to phasic REM activity (Fig. 11.5).

Movement time (or stage M as described in Rechtschaffen and Kales[8]) is no longer scored. As noted in the new scoring manual, when major body movements occur and obscure greater than 50% of an epoch, the epoch is scored as stage W if alpha activity is present at any time in the epoch. If no alpha activity is identified, but an epoch of stage W precedes or follows the epoch with a major body movement, then the epoch is scored as stage W. If neither of these requirements can be met, then the movement is scored the same as the epoch that follows it.

SLEEP ARCHITECTURE

Each night's sleep has a predictable pattern of sleep stages that repeat themselves through several cycles of sleep. Sleep onset begins with a transition to N1 sleep followed quickly by stage N2. Stage N3 usually follows and is particularly sustained in this first sleep cycle in children and young adults. Sleep then briefly lightens to stage N2 and transitions briefly into stage R sleep for the first time, usually about 90 minutes after sleep onset. This completes the first sleep cycle, a pattern that repeats itself three to five times during the typical night's sleep. With each ensuing 90-minute sleep cycle there is a decreasing amount of stage N3 sleep and an increasing amount of stage R sleep. As such, the majority of stage N3 sleep occurs in the first half of the night, while the preponderance of stage R sleep is in the second half of the night. Predictable changes are noted in this sleep architecture with aging. Beginning in middle age, stage 3 sleep lessens and more wakefulness after sleep onset (WASO) is noted. The number of arousals and awakening continues

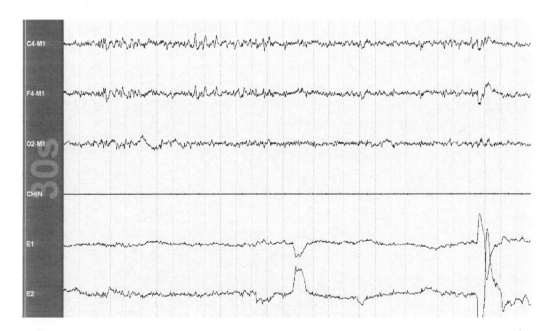

FIGURE 11.5 Limited PSG montage demonstrating stage R sleep with low-amplitude mixed-frequency electroencephalographic activity, absent axial electromyographic activity (chin channel represents submental electromyography) and rapid eye movements (out-of-phase activity in channels E1 and E2). (30-second epoch)

to increase with aging, becoming particularly notable in the elderly.[10,11]

SCORING OF AROUSALS

As discussed above, the original scoring guidelines of Rechtschaffen and Kales focused primarily on the scoring of the individual stages of sleep.[8] The R&K criteria did define the appearance of 30 seconds or more of waking background as representing an awakening. No other quantitative description of sleep disruption was addressed in the R&K manual. It was not until the publication of the position paper from the ASDA taskforce in 1992 that significant standardization of the scoring of arousals was introduced.[12] This consensus paper carefully defined rules for scoring an arousal from sleep. In the recent AASM scoring manual,[9] these rules were distilled to a single rule: Score arousal during sleep stages N1, N2, N3, or R if there is an abrupt shift of EEG frequency, including alpha, theta, and/or frequencies greater than 16 Hz (but not spindles) that lasts at least 3 seconds, with at least 10 seconds of stable sleep preceding the change. Scoring of arousals during stage R requires a concurrent increase in submental EMG lasting at least 1 second (Fig. 11.6).

The 3-second duration of EEG change is not based on any judgment of physiologic impact, but rather is an arbitrary value that was chosen by the taskforce due to improved interobsever reliability of arousal scoring (as compared to shorter duration events). The requirement for an accompanying EMG change in stage R is due to the appearance of faster EEG frequencies seen during normal sustained stage R sleep (Fig. 11.6c).

Given the subtle nature of the EEG events leading to an arousal, many authors refer to these events as microarousals. In any case, they are an important measure of sleep disruption. Despite the use of arousal scoring for over 20 years, comprehensive norms for arousals as a function of age have not been published. Bonnet and Arand[11] recently published carefully obtained normative data and identified a mean arousal index (AI, arousals per hour of sleep) for each decade of life. Between the ages of 21 and 30 years, the mean AI was 10.8 (+/−4.6), between 41 and 50 years the mean AI was 16.5 (+/−5.6), and between 61 and 70 years the mean AI was 21.9 (+/−6.8). No specific cutoff has been accepted clinically, but it is clear that arousals increase with age. Using the mean arousal index plus two standard deviations as the upper limits of normal, the normal for an arousal index would be approximately 21 at age 25 years, 28 at age 45 years, and 35 at age 65 years. These values are higher than the cutoffs that many sleep physicians use in assigning significance to the degree of sleep disruption.

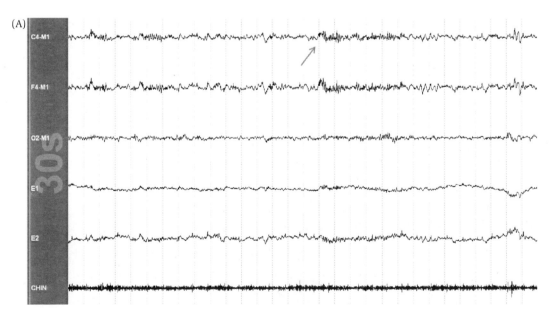

FIGURE 11.6　(Continued)

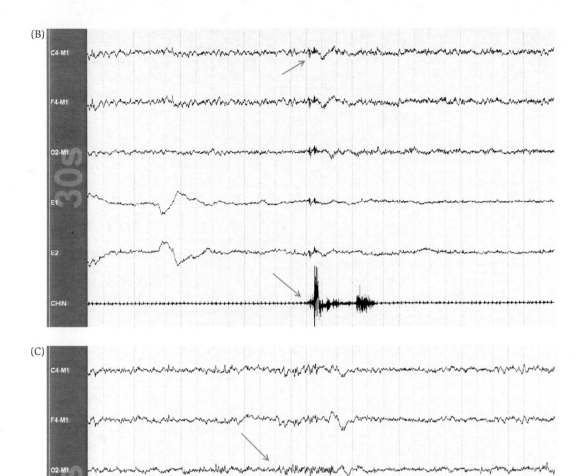

FIGURE 11.6 (*A*) Example of arousal from non-REM sleep with appearance of fast activity lasting greater than 3 seconds (arrow). No increase in electromyography (EMG) is required to score an arousal in stage N1, N2, or N3 sleep. (30-second epoch). (*B*) An arousal from stage R with appearance of >3 seconds of faster frequencies (top arrow) accompanied by the appearance of EMG in the axial (chin) EMG channel (bottom arrow). (30-second epoch). (*C*) Limited polysomnographic montage illustrating the appearance of fast activity (lasting greater than 3 seconds) in stage R sleep (arrow). The absence of any accompanying EMG activity (chin, submental EMG) precludes the scoring of an arousal. (30-second epoch)

SCORING OF ADULT RESPIRATORY EVENTS

With the initial recognition of apneic events during sleep,[13] the cessation of identified airflow for 10 seconds has been the standard definition of an apneic event. Subsequent recognition of the significance of partial airflow interruption (hypopneas) led to the quantification of both apneas and hypopneas. However, no consistent definition for what represented a hypopneic event was accepted and the technical and scoring standards for hypopneas varied widely. The recent AASM Scoring Manual defines both technical recording requirements as well as scoring rules[9] for apneas and hypopneas. This clear consensus statement has led to an improvement in the standardization of quantifying respiratory abnormalities during sleep.

Apneas are scored using the oronasal thermal sensor (thermistor or thermocouple), which has long been used to qualitatively assess airflow during a PSG recording. An apnea is scored when there is a >90% decrease in identified airflow by the thermal sensor lasting at least 10 seconds. Each apnea identified is then classified based on the accompanying respiratory effort. The ventilatory effort is measured using inductive plethysmography belts on the chest and abdomen. An apnea is labeled as obstructive if there is continued or increased respiratory effort throughout the entire period of absent airflow. The apnea is classified as central if the event has no associated inspiratory effort throughout the entire apneic period. The event is scored as a mixed apnea if there is initially an absence of inspiratory effort followed by resumption of inspiratory effort in the later portion of the event (Fig. 11.7). The duration of the absent respiratory effort required to score a mixed apnea is not defined, but it usually would be at least one complete breath cycle (4–6 seconds). It should be noted that there is no requirement for any accompanying oxygen desaturation or EEG arousal to score an apnea. While the inductive plethysmography belts represent the recommended technique in clinical sleep labs, the gold standard for identifying inspiratory effort remains esophageal manometry. The esophageal manometer can document negative intrathoracic pressure swings (that represent inspiratory efforts) when the inductive plethysmography belts are not able to identify any respiratory effort. As such, the plethysmography belts may overestimate the frequency of central apneas in some patients. Despite this superior sensitivity, esophageal manometry is not commonly used in clinical sleep labs due to its negative effect on sleep quality and patient comfort.

The sensor for detection of a hypopnea is the nasal air pressure transducer (NPT). The NPT is much more sensitive to the identification of a decrease in airflow and is appropriate to use for the identification of a hypopnea. It is a common occurrence during a PSG for a clear decrease in airflow to be identified in the NPT, with no evidence of change in the thermal sensor (Fig. 11.8). Previously, it was common to recognize cyclical arousal-associated loud snoring and oxygen desaturation that were not scorable using the less sensitive thermal sensors. This led to the recognition of the upper airway resistance syndrome (UARS).[23-26] UARS was diagnosed when the patient had a clinical syndrome consistent with obstructive sleep apnea but without scorable apneic or hypopneic events on PSG. With the use of NPT and the associated increased sensitivity to the scoring of hypopneas, it is uncommon to have a clinical suspicion of UARS using present PSG techniques. In fact, the NPT frequently is recognized to be overly sensitive in that it will demonstrate no airflow while the thermal sensor continues to demonstrate obvious airflow. As such, the NPT is not to be used for determination of apneic events, which are scored off of the thermal sensor recording.

Two separate rules for scoring hypopneas were presented in the AASM scoring manual. The "recommended" rule is that used by Medicare and was chosen in an attempt to be in concert with Medicare definitions and decisions regarding coverage of CPAP and other therapies. However, the "alternative" set of rules for scoring of hypopneas is actually more widely used and is more sensitive to the identification of hypopneas, particularly in individuals with healthy lungs where oxygen desaturations occur much less frequently.

The "recommended" rule for scoring a hypopnea requires the following:

1. NPT signal decreases by >30% for at least 10 seconds
2. There is an accompanying oxygen desaturation of 4% or more

The "alternative" rule for scoring a hypopnea requires the following:

1. NPT signal decreases by >50% for at least 10 seconds
2. There is an accompanying oxygen desaturation of at least 3% *or* the event is accompanied by an EEG arousal

Either scoring method is acceptable, but the rules used should be clearly defined in the PSG report. Most labs do not attempt to classify hypopneic events as obstructive or central due to the inaccuracy of assessing respiratory effort (using the standard inductive plethysmography belts) in the absence of complete airway obstruction.

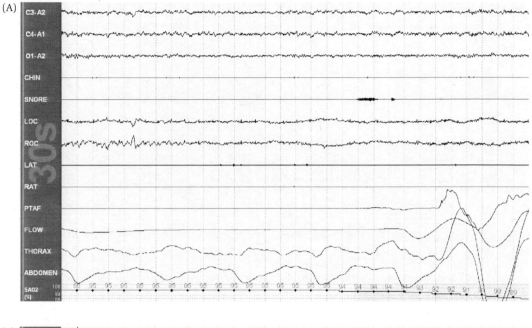

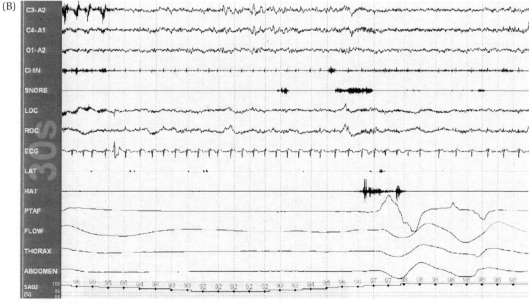

FIGURE 11.7   (Continued)

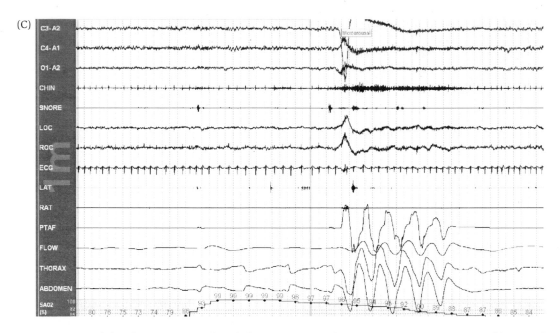

FIGURE 11.7 (*A*) Polysomnogram (PSG) demonstrating absence of airflow as measured by nasal pressure transducer (PTAF channel), oronasal thermocouple (flow channel) accompanied by evidence of continued ventilatory effort in the thoracic and abdominal channels (measured by respiratory inductive plethysmography belt). This is an example of an obstructive apnea. (30-second epoch). (*B*) PSG demonstrating no evidence of airflow as measured by nasal pressure transducer (PTAF channel), oronasal thermocouple (flow channel) accompanied by the absence of ventilatory effort in the thorax and abdominal channels (as measured by respiratory inductive plethysmography belts). This is an example of a central apnea. (30-second epoch). (*C*) PSG demonstrating an apneic event with no evidence of airflow is noted by the nasal pressure transducer (PTAF channel) or the oronasal thermocouple (flow channel) throughout the event identifying it as an apnea. During the first half of the apneic period, there is no evidence of ventilatory effort, but then increasing evidence of effort in the thorax and abdominal channel is seen leading up to the termination of the apneic event. This is an illustration of a mixed apnea, having central features at onset but then demonstrating obstructive features as the event progresses. Note the out-of-phase "paradoxical movement" of thorax and abdominal tracings often seen in obstructive apneic events (arrow). (60-second epoch)

An optional scoring rule outlines the scoring of respiratory effort-related arousals (RERAs). This may be particularly helpful in identifying potential clinically significant respiratory events if only the "recommended" rule for hypopnea identification is used. A RERA is scored if "there is a sequence of events lasting at least 10 seconds characterized by increasing respiratory effort or flattening of the nasal pressure waveform leading to an arousal from sleep when the sequence of breaths does not meet criteria for an apnea or hypopnea." Flattening of NPT waveform is thought to identify increased airway pressure, reflecting partial airway occlusion.

The total number of scored respiratory events identified in the study is then divided by the hours of sleep to yield an apnea-hypopnea index (AHI) that represents the number of respiratory events per hour of sleep. This value is most commonly used to categorize the severity of respiratory abnormality. The consensus statement from the American Academy of Sleep Medicine (AASM) classifies apnea severity as per the following criteria: AHI < 5: normal; AHI > 5 but < 15: mild apnea; AHI > 15 but < 30: moderate apnea; AHI > 30: severe apnea.[14] Many observers suggest this categorization of apnea severity may be too strict, particularly given the overlap with normative data noted in the literature. Several large studies have demonstrated that nonobese healthy middle-aged adults will have an AHI > 5 in 20% of individuals, and an AHI > 15 in approximately 6% of these same individuals. The AHI is also recognized to increase in age, even in individuals with no sleep complaint.[15–17]

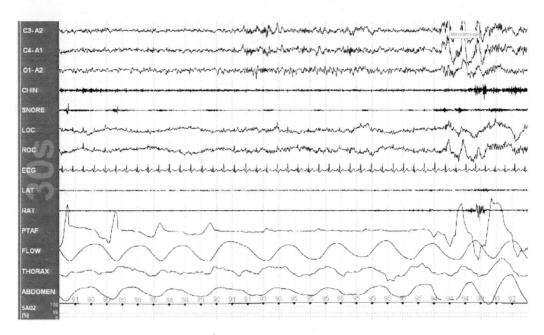

FIGURE 11.8 Polysomnogram demonstrating an example of a hypopnea lasting approximately 15 seconds. Note the absence of airflow in the nasal pressure transducer (PTAF channel) accompanied by continued flow as measured by the oronasal thermistor (flow channel). This illustrates how the nasal pressure transducer may overestimate the degree of flow limitation as compared to the oronasal thermistor. It also illustrates how the oronasal thermistor alone is inadequate to identify milder hypopneic events. Respiratory effort continues throughout the event. (30-second epoch)

SCORING OF PEDIATRIC RESPIRATORY EVENTS

Assessment of respiratory events in a pediatric population is technically similar to that recorded in adults. The major technical difference is that the scoring of respiratory events is supplemented by the recording of PCO_2. An elevated PCO_2 value is thought to reflect alveolar hypventilation and can be measured either by transcutaneous or end-tidal PCO_2 sensors.[9]

In pediatric sleep, an obstructive or mixed apnea is defined as lasting at least two breath cycles (as determined by the baseline breathing pattern). This is in contrast to the 10-second duration defined for apneas in an adult population. This two-breath value may be used up until 18 years of age, but many labs begin applying the adult rules after 13 years of age. The other rules for scoring obstructive and mixed apneas are the same as those used in the adult studies, as discussed earlier. Central apneas, however, have different scoring rules in pediatric patients. Two separate pediatric rules for

the scoring of central apneas are defined. Both require the absence of airflow along with the absence of any respiratory effort throughout the event. A central apnea is scored if the apnea lasts at least 20 seconds, or if the apnea lasts at least two breath cycles *and* is accompanied by an arousal, an awakening, or a 3% decline in oxygen saturation. The change in scoring central apneas in pediatric patients is based on the recognition that central apneas lasting less than 20 seconds occur in up to 30% of normal children.[18]

The scoring of hypopneas in children also uses the minimal duration of at least two breath cycles. The other required criteria for a hypopnea include a decrease in airflow by at least 50% (as measured by nasal pressure transducer) and an associated arousal, awakening, or 3% desaturation. These latter requirements are the same as the alternative adult hypopnea definition discussed earlier. As with adults, there is no attempt to categorize hypopneas as having obstrucitve, mixed, or central character unless esophageal manometry is used.

A respiratory event-related arousal (RERA) can be scored in a pediatric patient through the use of one of two rules, depending on whether a nasal pressure transducer or esophageal manometry is used during the study. Both rules require the event to last at least two breath cycles and have the accompanying demonstration of snoring, increased PCO_2, or visual evidence of increased work of breathing. With the use of a nasal pressure transducer, a RERA is scored if there is discernable fall in amplitude of the signal, which is also accompanied by a flattening of the nasal pressure transducer waveform. If an esophageal pressure transducer is used, a RERA is scored if there is progressive increase in inspiratory effort throughout the event. A RERA cannot be scored without an adequate signal from either the nasal pressure transducer or esophageal manometry.

Two other respiratory events may be scored in pediatric sleep studies. Sleep-related hypoventilation is scored if the measured PCO_2 (via transcutaneous or end-tidal CO_2 sensor) is above 50 mmHg for greater than 25% of the total sleep time. It should be recognized that the measurement of PCO_2 is technically challenging and false values are a common occurrence. Periodic breathing can also be scored in a pediatric patient. Periodic breathing requires at least three episodes of central apnea lasting at least 3 seconds and separated by less than 20 seconds of normal breathing.

SCORING OF CARDIAC EVENTS

Single channel ECG recordings have long been part of the routine recording of a PSG. However, prior to the AASM Scoring Manual[9] there had been no attempt to define or standardize the scoring or documentation of cardiac events during a PSG. The AASM Scoring Manual describes the use of a modified electrocardiogram lead II (recording electrodes placed on torso at approximately second rib to right of sternum and the sixth rib near the apex of the heart on the left chest). In morbidly obese patients excessive artifact is sometimes introduced by use of the left lower chest lead, and moving it to a position higher on the chest near the left shoulder many times eliminates the problem. The use of a single ECG lead limits any effort to identify cardiac ischemia or to define cardiac intervals. Identification of any of the arrhythmias discussed later is dependent on an adequate

tracing quality. It should be noted that the heart rate predictably slows during sleep, and as such the cutoff for identifying bradycardia and tachycardia has been lowered to 40 and 90 beats per minute, respectively. Brief periods of asystole up to 2 seconds are common during sleep in normals and cardiac pauses up to 3 seconds are not uncommonly noted in highly trained athletes. As a result of these observations, the AASM committee set the standard for determining asystole at 3 seconds.[19,20]

The following ECG scoring rules for adults were defined in the AASM scoring manual:

1. Score sinus tachycardia for sustained sinus heart rate >90 beats per minute
2. Score sinus bradycardia for sustained sinus heart rate <40 beats per minute
3. Score asystole for cardiac pauses >3 seconds
4. Score wide complex tachycardia for a rhythm of at least three consecutive beats at a rate greater than 100/min and a QRS duration of >120 milliseconds
5. Score narrow complex tachycardia for a rhythm of at least three consecutive beats at a rate >100/min and a QRS duration of <120 milliseconds
6. Score atrial fibrillation if there is an irregularly irregular ventricular rhythm associated with replacement of consistent P waves with variable rapid oscillations
7. Other significant arrhythmias (such as heart block) should be reported if quality of the single lead is sufficient for accurate identification.

COMPUTERIZED POLYSOMNOGRAPHY AND COMPUTER-ASSISTED SCORING

Despite the advent of digital recording of sleep studies and the associated software advances, visual scoring of sleep remains the standard for clinical PSG studies. Remarkably, the standardized scoring manual of Rechtschaffen and Kales remains the gold standard with only limited changes seen in the recently updated scoring manual.[8,9] When attempts are made at computerized scoring of sleep, they are patterned after these rules of visual sleep scoring. While the computerized analysis is extremely helpful in quantifying certain events (such as an oxygen desaturation), it remains inadequate for scoring sleep. This inadequacy is most evident in pathological studies where recurrent apneas, frequent arousals, and abundant movement artifacts limit the accuracy of computer analysis. Most commercially available sleep equipment does provide the potential for computerized analysis, but at the very least, sleep and event scoring needs to be reviewed and edited by a trained technologist.

The limitations of computerized analysis of sleep were discussed during the creation of the new scoring manual. The evidence reviewed suggested that "computer scoring and quantitative analysis is still in the formative stage of development" and has not been proven to be useful in clinical practice.[21] Computer analysis of sleep may still offer potential impact, but it is likely to be in the analysis of sleep in a way that does not try to mimic the arbitrary scoring in 30-second epochs.[22]

REFERENCES

1. Indications for PSG Task Force. Practice parameters for the indications for PSG and related procedures. *Sleep* 1997;20:406–22.
2. Kushida CA, Littner MR, Morgenthaler T, et al, Practice parameters for the indications for PSG and related procedures: an update for 2005. *Sleep* 2005;28:499–521.
3. Chesson AL, Jr., Berry RB, Pack A. Practice parameters for the use of portable monitoring devices in the investigation of suspected obstructive sleep apnea in adults. *Sleep* 2003;26:907.
4. Department of Health and Human Services, Center for Medicare and Medicaid Services. National Coverage Determination (NCD) for Continuous Positive Airway Pressure (CPAP) Therapy for Obstructive Sleep Apnea (240.4) Available at: http://www.cms.gov/medicare-coverage-database/details/ncd details.aspx?NCDId=226&ncdver=3&NCAId=204&NcaName=Continuous+Positive+Airway+Pressure+%28CPAP%29+Therapy+for+Obstructive+Sleep+Apnea+%28OSA%29&IsPopup=y&bc=AAAAAAAAIAAA& [accessed March 23, 2013].
5. Collop, NA, Anderson, WM, Boehlecke, B, et al. Clinical guidelines for the use of unattended portable monitors in the diagnosis of obstructive sleep apnea in adult patients. Portable Monitoring Task Force of the American Academy of Sleep Medicine. *J Clin Sleep Med* 2007;3:737–47.
6. Tonelli de Oliveira AC, Martinez D, Vasconcelos LF, et al. Diagnosis of obstructive sleep apnea syndrome and its outcomes with home portable monitoring. *Chest* 2009;135:330–6.
7. White DP, Gibb TJ, Wall JM, et al. Assessment of accuracy and analysis time of a novel device to monitor sleep and breathing in the home. *Sleep* 1995;18:115–26.
8. Rechtschaffen A, Kales A. A Manual of Standardized Terminology, Techniques and Scoring System for Sleep Stages of Human Subjects. Los Angeles, CA: Brain Information Service/Brain Research Institue, UCLA; 1968.
9. Ancoli-Israel S, Chesson A, and Quan SF for the American Academy of Sleep Medicine. The AASM Manual for the Scoring of Sleep and Associated Events: Rules, Terminology and Technical Specifications. Westchester, IL: American Academy of Sleep Medicine; 2007.
10. Williams RI, Karacan I, Hursch CJ. EEG of Human Sleep: Clinical Applications. New York: Wiley; 1974.
11. Bonnet MH, Arand DL. EEG arousal norms by age. *J Clin Sleep Med* 2007;3(3):271–4.
12. Bonnet M, Carley D, Carskadon M, et al. EEG arousals: scoring rules and examples: a preliminary report of the Sleep Disorders Atlas Task Force of the ASDA. *Sleep* 1992;15:173–184.
13. Gastaut H, Tassinari C, Duron B. Etude polygraphique des manifestations episodiques (hypniques et respiratoires) du syndrome de Pickwick. *Rev Neurol* 1965;112:568–79.
14. AASM Task Force. Sleep-related breathing disorders in adults: recommendations for syndrome definition and measurement techniques in clinical research. *Sleep* 1999;22(5):667–89.
15. Bixler EO, Vgontas AN, Ten Have T, et al. Effects of age on sleep apnea in men: prevalence and severity. *Am J Resp Crit Care Med* 1998;157:144–8.
16. Young T, Palta M, Dempsey J, et al. The occurrence of sleep disordered breathing among middle-ages adults. *N Engl J Med* 1993;328:1230–5.
17. Pavlova MK, Duffy JF, Shea SA. PSG respiratory abnormalities in aymptomatic individuals. *Sleep* 2008;31:241–8.
18. Marcus CL, Omlin KJ, Basinki DJ, et al. Normal PSG values for children and adolescents. *Am Rev Respir Dis* 1992;146:1235–9.
19. Brodsky M, Wu D, Denes P, et al. Arrhythmias documented by 24 hr ECG monitoring in

50 male medical students. *Am J Cardiol* 1977;39:390–395.

20. Viitasalo M, Kala R, Eisalo A. Ambulatory ECG recording in endurance atheletes. *Br Heart J* 1982;47:213–20.

21. Penzel T, Hirshkowitz M, Harsh J, et al. Digital analysis and technical specifications. *J Clin Sleep Med* 2007;3(2):109–20.

22. Schulz H. Rethinking sleep analysis: comment on the AASM Manual for Scoring Sleep and Associated Events. *J Clin Sleep Med* 2008;4:99–103.

23. Epstein MD, Chicoine SA, Hanumara RC. Detection of UARS using a nasal cannula/pressure transducer. *Chest* 2000;117:1073–7.

24. Exar E, Collop N. The Upper Airway Resistance Syndrome. *Chest* 1999;115:1127–39.

25. Guilleminault C, Stoohs R, Clerk A, et al A cause of daytime sleepiness: the upper airway resistance syndrome. *Chest* 1993;104:781–7.

26. Normal RG, Ahmed MM, Walsleben JA, et al. Detection of respiratory events during NPSG: nasal cannula/pressure sensor versus thermistor. *Sleep* 1997;20:1175–84.

12

Scoring of Sleep-Related Movements
Standard and Advanced Techniques

RAFFAELE FERRI, BIRGIT HÖGL, AND MARCO ZUCCONI

THE YEAR 2000 can be seen as a turnaround point for the analysis of polysomnographic (PSG) sleep recordings because, ideally, it can be considered as the approximate moment from which all PSG recordings have been stored digitally and paper has been definitely abandoned. The easy availability of data stored digitally has opened new frontiers for the automatic analysis of PSG signals. However, new unanswered questions have arisen, connected with the whole body of rules previously developed for the simple visual scoring of events on paper recordings, which can be considered as obsolete when a digital recording is available.

This chapter reflects the actual state of the art in the scoring of sleep-related movements, some of them with advanced techniques that take full advantage of the use of digital signals and computerized automatic analysis, and others that are still based on old criteria and rules developed for the visual analysis of events recorded on paper. Probably, in a few years, this gap will be filled by research, and

fully computerized techniques will be available for the detection and analysis of sleep-related movements.

LEG MOVEMENT ACTIVITY DURING SLEEP

Certainly, the most studied movements during sleep are those involving the lower limbs; they have been analyzed mostly by means of the recording of the surface electromyographic (EMG) activity of the tibialis anterior muscles, but, more recently, also the use of actigraphs has been introduced and validated. In this section we list several activities that can be recorded from the legs during sleep.

Periodic Leg Movements

The first "modern" PSG studies were performed in Bologna by the group led by Lugaresi, who described the details of periodic leg movements (PLMs) in patients with restless legs

• 161

syndrome (RLS) and characterized their appearance during wakefulness (PLMW), followed by their persistence during sleep (PLMS).[1,2] These observations constituted the evidence that RLS is not psychogenic.

Thus, the first method that was used for the measurement of PLMs was based on the EMG recording of the tibialis anterior muscles. However, it was only in 1982 that Coleman[3], after a visual-manual detection of LM on paper PSG studies of patients presenting with PLMS described this motor phenomenon in terms of duration, amplitude, periodicity, and symmetry, creating the basis of the scoring criteria accepted later by the American Sleep Disorders Association[4], which have been used for more than 20 years.

The current rules for scoring PLMs have been arranged after the development of some algorithms for the automatic detection of leg movements in PSG that have been made possible by the mathematical handling of parameters such as thresholds, intervals, and amplitude[5,6] and a detailed statistical analysis of additional parameters such as periodicity.[7] These rules were first introduced by a taskforce of the IRLSSG/WASM[8] and then substantially confirmed by the AASM[9,10]; the first, however, contain separate criteria for clinical or research purposes. We will list here briefly the rules currently used to score leg movements in PSG recordings.

Before the recording, a calibration should be carried out in order to obtain from the relaxed anterior tibialis muscles a nonrectified signal no greater than ±5 μV (or 10 μV peak to peak) for clinical purposes, and ±3 μV (or 6 μV peak to peak) for research; these values should be 5 and 3 μV, respectively, for rectified signals.

The onset of an event is identified when the EMG increases to ≥8 μV above the resting baseline and its offset is defined as the moment when the EMG decreases to <2 μV above the resting level and remains below that value for 0.5 seconds. An event may have one or more periods where the EMG drops below the offset criteria for less than 0.5 seconds. The duration of the event is defined as the time between its onset and offset as defined earlier and must be at least 0.5 seconds and no longer than 10 seconds (15 seconds are allowed for research purposes).

The interval between consecutive movements is measured from onset to onset. Events that are very short (<0.5 seconds) or very long (>10 seconds) do not affect the period duration measured from onset to onset of the candidate events. Figure 12.1 summarizes the detection parameters for leg movements.

The period length for two consecutive events to be considered as PLM must be at least 5 and no more than 90 seconds. A PLM sequence is then defined as a series of four or more leg movements separated from each other by at least 5 and no more than 90 seconds. These movements can occur in any stage of sleep or wake and the sequence of consecutive events continues across changes in the sleep-wake state. Thus, a PLM sequence starting in sleep can continue in waking and vice versa. An arousal occurring before or during a leg movement does not alter the assessment of that event.

Movements from the two legs can be combined, and bilateral movements are counted as one; movements that occur on the two legs are considered bilateral when they overlap or are separated (offset to onset) by less than 0.5 seconds. Bilateral movements can include two or more monolateral movements separated (offset to onset) by less than 0.5 seconds from each other.

A leg movement is considered associated with an arousal when there is less than 0.5 seconds between the end of one event and the onset of the other, regardless of which is first. Similarly, a leg movement is associated with the ending of an apnea/hypopnea event when they overlap or the offset of the earlier event precedes the onset of the other by less than 0.5 seconds, regardless

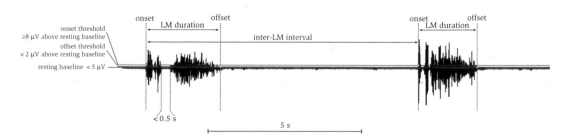

FIGURE 12.1   Detection parameters for leg movements (LM). (Adapted from Zucconi et al.[8])

of which is first; these leg movements are excluded from the computation of PLM-related parameters.

The following measures should always be computed and reported:

- PLMS index: Number of PLMS divided by the number of hours of sleep with leg movement recording (PLMS/hour)
- PLMS with arousals index. Number of PLMS associated with arousals divided by the number of hours of sleep with leg movement and arousal recording (PLMA/hour)
- PLMW index: Number of PLMW divided by the number of hours of wake with leg movement recording (PLMW/hour)

Additionally, it is recommended, whenever possible, to report PLMS index during non–rapid eye movement (non-REM) sleep only; PLMS index during REM sleep only; duration of PLMS and PLMW (separate PLMS duration for REM and non-REM sleep); and intermovement interval of PLMS and PLMW (separate PLMS interval for REM and non-REM sleep).

Optional parameters are PLMS by sleep stages (include duration and intermovement intervals) and isolated leg movements (leg movements separated by more than 90 seconds or movements in sequences formed by fewer than four PLMs).

Periodicity and Time Structure of Leg Movements during Sleep

Sleep PSGs of patients affected by RLS and PLMS and by other conditions usually also contain a significant amount of nonperiodic leg movements (LMs),[7,11–13] and LM activity during wakefulness in normal controls is essentially nonperiodic.[14] PLMS are usually embedded in a general oscillatory mechanism in which central, peripheral, and autonomic nervous system changes can be seen; however, other movements with shorter or longer intervals are also accompanied by such changes.[11,15] This points to the need to always consider these activities together for their combined effects on sleep neurophysiology.

Therefore, it seems more appropriate to use two additional indexes: Total LM index and Periodicity Index, the first indicating the total amount of LM activity recorded and the second indicating its degree of periodicity.[7] In particular, the Periodicity Index quantifies the proportion, over the total, of intermovement intervals with length $10 < i \leq 90$ seconds, which are preceded and followed by another interval with the same length (this is equivalent to a mini-series of four LMs all separated by intervals with length $10 < i \leq 90$ seconds). This index can vary between 0 (absence of periodicity, with none of the intervals having a length between 10 and 90 seconds) to 1 (complete periodicity, with all intervals having a length between 10 and 90 seconds).[7]

Both of these measures undergo significant age-related changes; thus, different normative reference values are needed for different age groups,[14,16] especially in children/adolescents and elderly people aged more than 75 years. These measures can also be applied to pediatric RLS[16]; a low degree of periodicity is expected at this age and the finding of a high degree of periodicity might prove to be a sign of severity of the syndrome, but this needs further research.

An additional essential feature to be considered is the time distribution of PLMS during the night, which shows in the majority of RLS patients a progressively decreasing course during the night.[16,17] Taken all together, these three parameters (total LM index, periodicity index, and time distribution) offer an important and sensitive help to support the diagnosis of RLS and have been found to differentiate LM activity of RLS from other clinical conditions previously reported to have PLMS, such as narcolepsy[18] and REM sleep behaviour disorder[19]; PLMS correlated to respiratory events are not counted.[8,9] Figure 12.2 shows the different features of PLMS found in different clinical conditions.

Actigraphy

Actigraphy has been used for decades to monitor sleep wake rhythms and movements during sleep. Basically two different types of use can be distinguished in actigraphy: longer time monitoring of rest-activity cycles, and shorter term monitoring of rest-activity rhythm combined with PLM measurements. Many current actigraphs have specific softwares to detect PLM. From the first attempts to analyze PLM with actigraphs[20] to today's systems, time resolution, storage capacity, and size have been much improved, and a great variety of additional channels added.

Several limitations have to be kept in mind when actigraphy is used:

1. The actigraph cannot distinguish between wakefulness and sleep.

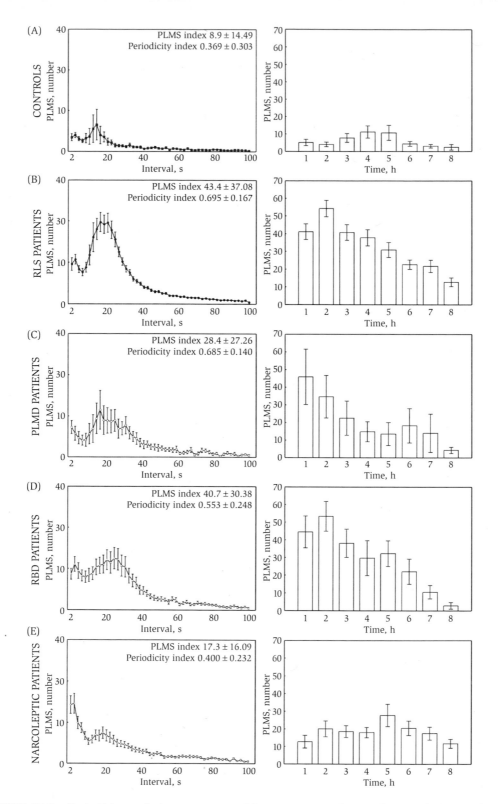

FIGURE 12.2   Periodicity and time structure of leg movements during sleep in different clinical conditions. (*A*) Normal controls (*n* = 35; age range, 25–80 years). (*B*) Restless legs syndrome (RLS) patients (*n* = 100; age range, 25–85 years; data from Ferri et al.[16]). (*C*) Periodic leg movement disorder (PLMD) patients (*n* = 12; age range, 30–67 years; data from Ferri et al.[21]). (*D*) REM sleep behavior disorder (RBD) patients (*n* = 20; age range, 61–80 years; data from Manconi et al.[19]). (*E*) Patients with narcolepsy/cataplexy (*n* = 40; age range, 18–61 years; data from Ferri et al.[18]).

2. A channel to record body position is important (otherwise other daytime activities, such as driving a car, working at the computer, or standing while observing something, can be falsely identified as PLM).

Several investigators have undertaken validation studies for actigraphy[22-24] compared to PSG, but in some of them only small time samples of PSG have been compared to actigraphy.[23] One study investigated two different actigraphs compared to PSG[22] and a very high correlation of PLM indices was found; the absolute values (e.g., PLM indices), however, differed significantly from PSG, according to the type of actigraph (both over- and underestimating PLM). In actimeters that allow for selecting specific settings, it was also shown that the filter settings have a significant impact on the PLM index.[22] This study showed that actigraphy can be used to detect PLM, but PLM measures obtained with actigraphy cannot be translated directly into PLM indices obtained from PSG. When choosing an actigraph, it is important to select a model that allows for understanding and modifying settings (for instance, duration of movement).

Actigraphs can be placed on the big toe, the dorsum of the foot, or the ankle.[25] They can measure movements in two or three movement axes, which are usually combined to one output. It has to be kept in mind that in conventional PSG, PLMs are measured as surface EMG activation of the tibialis anterior muscle, which can be present in the absence of visible movement. In contrast, actigraphy measures acceleration of the limb and can be positive also in the case of passive movement.

Actigraphy has been used successfully in large studies, even in subjects whose RLS status was not known[26]; it correlated better with genetic results than RLS status and this is probably due to the fact that actigraphy detects an objective phenotype, namely PLM. The stable detection of PLM, but with different absolute indices compared to PSG[22], also strengthens the argument that periodicity per se is more important than absolute indices.[7] In addition, actigraphy can be performed on several consecutive nights, and this is of paramount importance in light of the high intraindividual variability of PLM indices.[27]

Very recently, off-body video actigraphy systems have been proposed[28] and are under continuous improvement with the prospect of replacing on-body actigraphs to monitor movements during sleep. These systems seem to show some advantages and some disadvantages in comparison with other classical systems (EMG and actigraphy); the research in this field, however, is still at its very early stages and additional improvement and validation are needed. The old static charge-sensitive bed was also proposed as a method of measurement of activity.[29] It has been mostly used in Finland to evaluate sleep-related movements, respiration, and heart rate variability.[30,31]

OTHER LEG MOTOR ACTIVITIES DURING SLEEP

This section includes three very similar phenomena of small motor activations of the feet (and legs) occurring at sleep onset and correlated with arousals, usually in trains, with short-lasting bilateral alternating or unilateral (agonist/antagonist) activations. Sometimes the movements are so small that they can only be observed when the feet are filmed without a blanket. It remains to be determined how much these phenomena relate to PLM and/or RLS.

Alternating Leg Muscle Activation

The term *alternating leg muscle activation* (ALMA) during sleep indicates a quickly alternating pattern of anterior tibialis activation occurring at a frequency of approximately 1 to 2 Hz, lasting between 0.1 and 0.5 seconds, organized in sequences of alternating activations lasting up to 20–30 seconds. The phenomenon was reported to occur in all sleep stages but particularly during arousals.[33,33] It is not clear yet whether ALMA represents the PSG manifestation of a separate nosological entity or if it belongs to the wide spectrum of nocturnal motor activities of RLS. Figure 12.3 shows an example of an ALMA episode during sleep in the patient reported by Cosentino et al.[33]

Hypnagogic Foot Tremor

Hypnagogic foot tremor (HFT), first described by Broughton in 1988 and later by others,[34,35] is a clinical condition that has several similarities to ALMA; the patient complains of foot movements occurring at the transition between wake and sleep or during light sleep. PSG recordings show the presence of recurrent EMG potentials or foot movements typically at 1 to

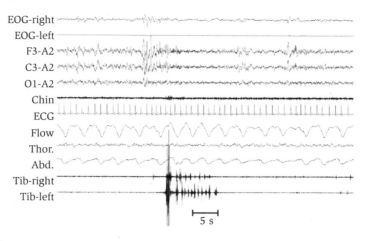

FIGURE 12.3   Alternating leg muscle activation during sleep and arousal event associated with an arousal during sleep stage 2. ECG, electroencephalogram; EOG, electro-oculogram.

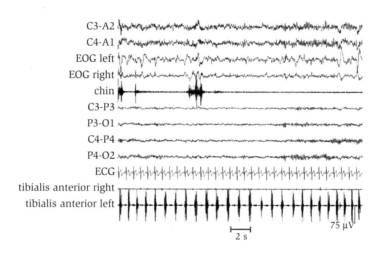

FIGURE 12.4   Polysomnographic recording of one patient with long runs of hypnagogic foot tremor involving the left side. ECG, electroencephalogram; EOG, electro-oculogram.

2 Hz (range 0.5–3 Hz) in one or both feet. The EMG bursts are longer than those of myoclonus (>250 ms), they last usually less than 1 second, and are organized in trains lasting 10 or more seconds.[9] Figure 12.4 shows the PSG recording of one patient with long runs of hypnagogic foot tremor involving the left side.

High-Frequency Leg Movements

The term *high-frequency leg movements* (HFLMs) was recently proposed for a similar phenomenon.[36] HFLM was defined as four or more discrete leg movements occurring at a frequency of 0.3–4 Hz, unilaterally, but sometimes with a bilateral pattern. Two thirds of the HFLM are observed during waking and approximately one third during sleep. However, the criteria to score this phenomenon have not been established yet, and additional studies and reports are needed to define their eventual relationship with RLS and their clinical relevance.

ALMA, Hypnagogic Foot Tremor, and High-Frequency Leg Movements: Are They Distinct Phenomena?

It is possible that ALMA,[32,33] HFT,[35] and HFLM[36] share many common features and might represent phenomena along the same spectrum? More research is needed to delineate better the differences, if any, among those phenomena and, finally, possibly to decide whether one name will be sufficient for all of them. In the opinion of the authors, HFLM[36] is the most neutral and precise term at the descriptive level; it accounts for the movements sometimes seen in video recordings. ALMA[32] is well known and recognized by sleep experts, and it has the advantage that a visible leg movement is not required because EMG muscle activation is enough, but it does not account for unilateral or simultaneous bilateral muscle activations. HFT[34,35] is a more problematic term because it is unlikely to be a tremor; moreover, the term *rhythmic foot movements*[35] is more descriptive but that this phenomenon fulfills the criteria for rhythmicity has not been demonstrated yet.

Table 12.1 reports a synopsis of the main EMG and clinical features of these three conditions, showing their many similarities and few differences.

EXCESSIVE FRAGMENTARY MYOCLONUS

Excessive fragmentary myoclonus (EFM) has been known for many years[37,38] and is characterized by small movements (or even no visible movements) of the fingers, toes, or corners of the mouth or small muscle twitches, resembling either physiologic hypnic myoclonus or fasciculations, that occur at the sleep-wake transition or during sleep. In PSG, recurrent and persistent, very brief (75 to 150 millisecond) EMG potentials in various muscles are recorded, occurring asynchronously and asymmetrically, in a sustained manner, without clustering. As an empirical quantitative criterion, it has been suggested that more than five potentials per minute should be sustained for at least 20 minutes of stage N2 or slow-wave sleep.[9] However, EFM can be quantified by means of the myoclonus index[39] that is defined as the number of 3-second mini-epochs containing at least one fragmentary myoclonus potential fulfilling the criteria, counted for each 30-second epoch and resulting in a number between 0 and 10. It should, however, be considered that fragmentary myoclonus is common and abundant in patients with sleep disorders who have been reported to show a mean fragmentary myoclonus index of 39.5 per hour of sleep; this index increases with age, is higher in men than in

women, and is correlated with the presence of sleep-related breathing disorders and respiratory variables. These data indicate that the definition of EFM needs a careful reconsideration based on statistically driven criteria.[40]

Figure 12.5 shows the PSG appearance of EFM at the transition between wakefulness and sleep and during sleep stage 2.

PROPRIOSPINAL MYOCLONUS (AT SLEEP ONSET)

Propriospinal myoclonus (PSM) is considered to be a rare motor disorder, first described in 1991.[41,42] PSM at sleep onset is characterized by generalized and symmetric jerks that arise during the transition between wakefulness and sleep, from axial muscles of the abdomen, thorax, or neck, and spread rostrally and caudally to the other myotomes by means of slow propriospinal polysynaptic pathways.[43] The jerks are typically facilitated by relaxed wakefulness or drowsiness and are inhibited by mental activation and sleep onset. PSM at sleep onset can be a cause of insomnia.[43,44]

PSM should be distinguished from PLMW, which have characteristics similar to PLMS but are generally longer in duration and less periodic; however, in PMS there is no urge to move, as the patient generally lies down calm and tries to get asleep without the need to get out of the bed. Nevertheless, it can cause insomnia because the patient is not able to reach a stable state of sleep for up to 2–3 hours, with the jerks appearing several times but not periodically. In general, different from RLS/PLMS, the jerks disappear during sleep. In some cases PLMS may appear if PSM is associated with RLS or PLMS.

No quantitative PSG features have been described and its description is basically qualitative.[9] Figure 12.6 shows the spreading of muscle activation, rostrally and caudally, starting from muscles at the 10th intercostal space in one patient with symptomatic propriospinal myoclonus.[45]

NECK MYOCLONUS (DURING SLEEP)

The term *neck myoclonus* (head jerks) has recently been proposed[46] to indicate the movement associated with a short stripe-shaped movement-induced artifact over the EEG leads during REM sleep (Fig. 12.7); it seems to be a

Table 12.1 Synopsis of the Electromyograph and Clinical Features of ALMA, HFT, and HFLM

	NAME (ABBREVIATION)	PREVALENCE (NO.)	BURST FREQUENCY	SINGLE BURST DURATION	BURST SERIES DURATION/ASPECT	OBSERVATIONS	COMORBIDITY, MEDICATIONS
Chervin *et al.* 2003	Alternating leg muscle activation during sleep and arousal (ALMA)	≈1.1% (16 out of ≈1500)	0.5–3 Hz (usually 1–2 Hz)	100–500 ms	1.4–22 s bilateral	Arise from all sleep stages including REM, in 12 patients around arousals and in 4 unrelated to arousals	Methylphenidate, pramipexole, benzodiazepines, antiepileptics
Wichniak *et al*, 2001	Rhythmic feet movements while falling asleep (RFM) Hypnagogic foot tremor (HFT)	7.1% (28 out of 375)	0.3–3 Hz (mostly 1–2 Hz)	510 ± 291 ms	10–15 s often >30 s, bilateral but asynchronous	High night-to-night variability, highest frequency in presleep wakefulness, S1 and S2, and during arousals	RBD, RLS, PLMS, narcolepsy, sleep walking, head banging, insomnia Dopaminergic, antidepressants, neuroleptics, antiepileptics
Yang and Winkelman 2010	High-frequency leg movements (HFLMs)	7.6% (37 out of 486)	1.6 ± 0.6 Hz (range 0.4–3.7 Hz)	100–700 ms	17.6 ± 1.1 s, 26.5 ± 5 sequences/ night usually unilateral, bilateral, alternating	Associated with cardiac acceleration, 2/3 arising from wakefulness and 1/3 from sleep	OSA 62%, PLMD 13.5%, OSA and PLMS 18.9% OR of having RLS 3.52

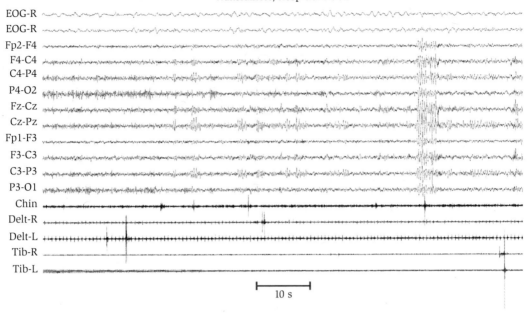

Wakefulness/sleep transition

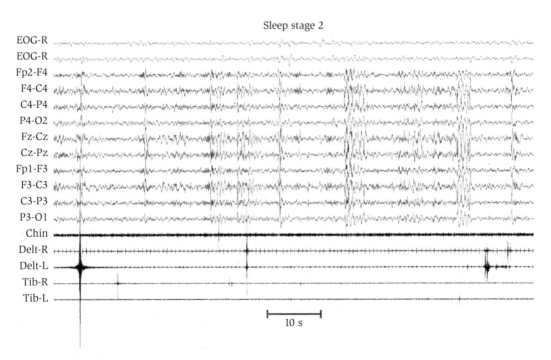

Sleep stage 2

FIGURE 12.5   Polysomnographic appearance of excessive fragmentary myoclonus at the transition between wakefulness and sleep (*top*) and during sleep stage 2 (*bottom*). EOG, electro-oculogram.

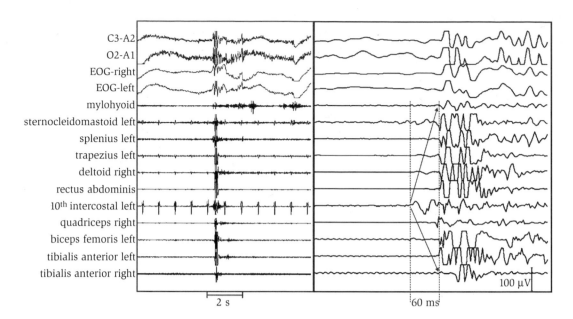

FIGURE 12.6   Rostral and caudal spreading of muscle activation, starting from the 10th inter-costals, in one patient with symptomatic propriospinal myoclonus (Manconi et al.[45]). EOG, electro-oculogram.

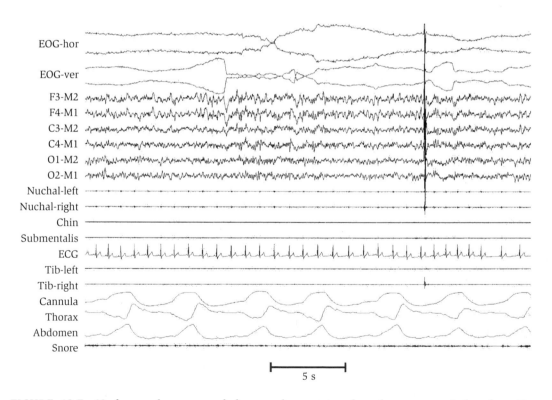

FIGURE 12.7   Neck myoclonus recorded as a short stripe-shaped movement-induced artifact over the electroencephalographic leads during REM sleep. ECG, electroencephalogram; EOG, electro-oculogram.

frequent finding in routine PSG, being present in >50% of patients, but with a low frequency during the night (1 ± 2.7 per hour of REM sleep) and an age-related decline, from younger to older patients. An elderly patient has also been reported with a similar phenomenon called faciomandibular myoclonus during REM sleep.[47] However, this patient had nocturnal awakenings following biting of the tongue and forceful jaw closings, which occurred in episodes of one to three contractions.

SLEEP BRUXISM

Sleep bruxism (SB) is defined as an oral activity characterized by grinding or clenching of the teeth during sleep, usually associated with sleep arousals, and different from the tooth grinding during wakefulness that may be present during the night or the day but related to wake activity.[48] The report of tooth grinding during the night by a bed partner, the observation of abnormal tooth wear, and the complaint of jaw muscle tenderness, fatigue, or pain are the clinical diagnostic features of SB. Headache, temporo-mandibular, and dental pain are also common consequences of clinically relevant SB. Besides the orofacial physical evaluation, use of psychoactive drugs, medication, or some neuropsychiatric conditions have to be considered when evaluating SB.[49]

From a sleep disorder point of view, PSG is indicated when SB is suspected in association with sleep disorders (OSA, REM sleep behavior disorder), epilepsy, or orofacial-mandibular disorders.

In routine clinical PSG, bruxism is represented by a typical EMG artifact recorded on the surface EEG leads, especially if referred to ear or mastoid electrodes. For the scoring of SB, the recommended chin EMG electrodes have been indicated to be sufficient,[9] but the clinical experiences of the group of Montreal suggest that additional masseter and/or temporal EMG should be recorded in accordance with discretion of the investigator or clinician.[50]

It should be considered that during normal sleep repetitive phasic jaw muscle contractions may occur 1–2 times per hour in most "healthy" subjects,[51] known as rhythmic masticatory muscle activity (RMMA). An episode of SB may consist of RMMA (at least three rhythmic phasic contractions at a frequency of 1 Hz, lasting between 0.25 and 2 seconds) and tonic (sustained contraction for more than 2 seconds) or mixed phasic-tonic masticatory muscle activities, associated with tooth grinding sound during sleep. Contractions shorter than 0.25 seconds are considered and scored as myoclonus that is present in a certain portion (around 10%) of patients with SB.[9,52] Each SB episode has to be separated by a period of at least 3 seconds of stable background EMG to be scored as a new SB episode. SB can be scored reliably by audio-video recording in combination with PSG, with a minimum of two audible tooth-grinding episodes per night, in the absence of epilepsy.

The diagnosis of SB requires the presence of at least four episodes of SB per hour of sleep or at least 25 individual masticatory muscle bursts per hour of sleep, accompanied by at least two audible episodes of tooth-grinding noise.[9,48] Figure 12.8 shows a PSG recording of a sequence of RMMA episodes in one subject with SB.

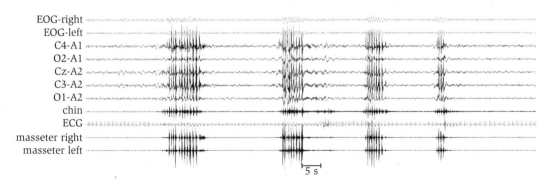

FIGURE 12.8   Polysomnographic recording of a sequence of rhythmic masticatory muscle activity episodes in one subject with sleep bruxism. ECG, electroencephalogram; EOG, electro-oculogram.

MUSCLE ACTIVITY OF REM SLEEP BEHAVIOR DISORDER

Electromyography

According to the *International Classification of Sleep Disorders*, second edition,[48] the diagnosis of REM sleep behavior disorder (RBD) can only be made in the presence of REM sleep without atonia in the PSG, with excessive tonic and/or phasic chin or extremity electromyographic (EMG) activation. Since the first descriptions of REM sleep without atonia and stage-1 REM in humans, different systems to analyze and possibly quantify EMG activity in RBD have been proposed. Lapierre und Montplaisir [53] were the first to publish a manual system to analyze submental EMG activity (tonic and phasic), and their system is still utilized without any or with only minor modifications by several investigators (for more details, see Chapter 29). In contrast to this system, which is based on chin EMG activity only, more recent studies also included extremity muscle analysis (mostly tibialis anterior EMG activity). A classification system on short- and long-lasting muscle activity was proposed,[54] while other authors focused on phasic muscle activity only introducing the Phasic EMG Metric or PEM.[55,56] The SINBAR group (Sleep Innsbruck Barcelona) performed a study to evaluate which is the most appropriate combination of EMG channels to investigate RBD. Out of 13 different body muscles investigated, a combination of EMG of the chin, one arm, and one leg muscle provided the highest yield of phasic EMG activity and was therefore recommended as appropriate montage for RBD detection.[57]

Cutoff values for phasic and tonic EMG activity during REM sleep have been provided for the chin activity.[58] A total correct classification of 81.9% was found for tonic chin EMG density ≥30% (i.e., the percentage of REM sleep epochs scored as tonic if chin EMG activity was present for >50% of the epoch duration, with activity defined as amplitude of chin EMG signal of at least twice that of the background or greater than 10 microvolts); moreover, a total correct classification of 83.8% was found for phasic chin EMG density ≥15% (percentage of 2-second REM sleep mini-epochs containing EMG events lasting 0.1 to 10 seconds, with an amplitude exceeding four times the amplitude of background EMG activity).

The SINBAR (Sleep Innsbruck Barcelona) group has recently provided extensive normative and cutoff values for EMG activity during REM sleep for RBD in 11 different body muscles obtained from 30 patients with RBD and 30 controls, who had been recruited from patients with effectively treated sleep breathing disorders. The study showed that recording of upper-extremity muscles, such as the biceps brachii or the flexor digitorum superficialis, was more sensitive and specific for RBD than the commonly recorded lower-extremity muscles, such as the tibial anterior muscle. This study also found that scoring of tonic, phasic, or any muscle activity in the mentalis muscle provided a good sensitivity and specificity for RBD. The authors therefore propose that simultaneous recording and quantitative analysis of any mentalis activity plus m. flexor digitorum superficialis recording in three second mini-epochs is appropriate for RBD and provided a 100% specificity for RBD, when activity was present in more than 31.9% microepochs. The authors also showed that analysis in 30-second epochs was feasible and provided reasonable sensitivity and specificity values.[59]

The issue of the quantitative EMG analysis in RBD is also addressed in Chapter 29.

Figure 12.9 shows an example of REM sleep without atonia (chin EMG) and PLMS (tibialis anterior EMG channels) in a PSG recording of one patient with RBD.

Automatic Analysis of the Chin Electromyographic Amplitude

Despite the crucial relevance of the increased chin EMG activity during REM sleep for the diagnosis of RBD, only a few systematic attempts have been carried out in order to analyze quantitatively submentalis muscle EMG activity during sleep, probably because of the use for decades of paper recordings in sleep research. Several methodological papers have appeared in the literature,[53,54,60] which have attempted to quantify submentalis muscle EMG activity in RBD patients by means of a visual approach, with the aim of counting the number of epochs without atonia (elevated background EMG activity) and the number of mini-epochs (2 to 3 seconds long) containing phasic EMG activity. In these studies, beside their simple and apparently quantitative parameters, no solid mathematical and quantitative definitions, in terms of amplitude and duration, have been provided for the elements taken into account: atonia, phasic, and tonic EMG activations.

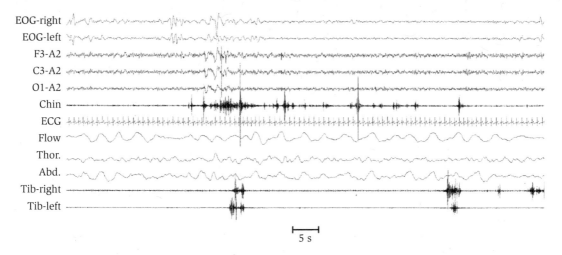

EOG-right
EOG-left
F3-A2
C3-A2
O1-A2
Chin
ECG
Flow
Thor.
Abd.
Tib-right
Tib-left

5 s

FIGURE 12.9   REM sleep without atonia (chin electromyography) and periodic leg movement during sleep (tibialis anterior electromyographic channels) in a polysomnographic recording of one patient with REM sleep behavior disorder. ECG, electroencephalogram; EOG, electro-oculogram.

In recent years, some algorithms have been proposed to quantify automatically the amplitude of the chin EMG during REM sleep, in order to provide a tool useful for the diagnosis of RBD.[61-64] Based on one of these algorithms, the REM sleep Atonia Index has been developed that can vary from 0, which means complete absence of EMG atonia, to 1 or stable EMG atonia in the epoch. This Index, which correlates closely with the results of the previous visual methods of quantification,[65] together with other measurements connected with the algorithm, was able to show differences between normal controls and patients. This index was also able to differentiate between nosologically different groups of RBD patients who might present a different type of REM sleep-related motor disturbance. So far, this index has been applied to a large number of subjects, including normal controls (young adults and elderly), idiopathic RBD patients, subjects with multiple system atrophy, narcoleptics,[65] patients with idiopathic hypersomnia, subjects with OSAS,[66] and patients with Parkinson's disease. This makes this index probably the best automated quantitative tool proposed so far for the detection of the main PSG marker of RBD.

Scoring of Video Recordings

Since time-synchronized video recording became widely available in PSG, several studies of RBD have incorporated video information, mainly to classify behaviors as simple or complex[67] or to subdivide them into different severity categories.[68] While the Sforza et al. system distinguishes between simple and complex events, Iranzo et al.'s approach distinguishes between mild, moderate, and severe RBD manifestations, based on the excursion amplitude of the limbs and volume of vocalizations.

Frauscher and coworkers performed detailed analyses of all, including the smallest movements and vocalizations in RBD, in order to describe clearly its motor and behavioral manifestations.[69,70]

Regarding video analyses in RBD, different approaches can be selected:

1. *Full analysis:* Studying the video in real time focusing on the eyes and different body parts for all REM sleep epochs was used mainly by the Innsbruck group, SINBAR,[69,70] and the Paris group.[71-73] This approach is very time consuming but necessary in research settings.

2. *Selective screening:* For clinical purposes, a more time-efficient video analysis is required. PSG recording simultaneous with video images can be studied epoch by epoch in 30-second epochs. This system is used in the Kassel classification system for RBD.[74] The SINBAR group has demonstrated that EMG activations or artifacts will point to video or vocal events with a high sensitivity but a low specificity.[57]

In summary, analysis of the video (in addition to analysis of PSG) is necessary in RBD. For clinical purposes, a time-efficient method to screen the video is acceptable.

RHYTHMIC MOVEMENT DISORDER

Rhythmic movement disorder (RMD) is characterized by recurrent episodes of stereotyped rhythmic body movements occurring predominantly during sleep or drowsiness before sleep, and it may involve the head, neck, trunk, or limbs in isolation or in combination. The occurrence of clinical consequences with interference with sleep because of body movements and significant impairment in daytime function or self-inflicted injuries are the required features for the diagnosis of the disorder. When the movements and behaviors are self-limited as frequently observed in healthy infants or young children, the term *rhythmic movements of sleep* (the benign form) is used to distinguish from the RMD[48]; however, no strict quantitative threshold has been indicated.

The duration of rhythmic movement episodes may be short (seconds) or long (several minutes) and may be present not only in sleep or during the transition from wakefulness to sleep but also during the wakefulness preceding sleep or after sleep onset, with a duration similar to those episodes occurring during sleep.

RMD is present in children, adolescents, and adults. The predominant pattern of movements involves the head (head banging or *jactatio capitis nocturna*, head rolling) but also the body (body rocking) or occasionally the legs (leg rolling or leg banging).

Although the clinical diagnosis is established on the basis of history and sometimes the video recording (home- and self-made), PSG simultaneous with video recording (video-PSG) showing the type and site of movements is useful when the diagnosis is doubtful or comorbid with other sleep disorders. The use of additional EEG and EMG leads, in particular, limbs leads, may help to distinguish RMD from other sleep-related repetitive movements such as PLMS, ALMA, or motor seizures.

Most of the rhythmic movements are related to sleep stages N1 and N2 and rarely SWS or REM sleep. Sometimes episodes have been reported in association with cyclic alternating patterns[75,76] and may follow or be associated with postapnea/hypopnea arousals. Single case reports described an epileptic etiology for RMD.[77]

The criteria for scoring RMD are essentially the features to define the PSG characteristics of the rhythmic movements[9] and include the following:

- Frequency of 0.5–2.0 Hz
- At least four single movements are required to form a rhythmic cluster
- The minimum amplitude of a single rhythmic movement is 2 times the background EMG activity

Finally, to achieve a correct diagnosis, the support of a synchronized video recording (video-PSG) is required.

CONCLUSIONS

The current rules for the measurement of sleep-related movements reflect some advanced computerized approach to the analysis of the EMG signals but also include, largely, criteria set up for the visual analysis of signals recorded on paper. Most of the rules involve the analysis of the EMG signal from the tibialis anterior, the submentalis, or other muscles that is a rapidly changing signal, containing a wide range of frequencies, extending from low- to very high-frequency bands (in biological terms). For this reason, setting up thresholds and measurements of its amplitude pose special problems that can be reliably solved only with strictly quantitative measures applied to digitally stored signals. On the contrary, all rules arranged for its visual measurement on paper can now be considered as almost obsolete and need to be updated, adapted, and refined for the digital era, allowing for an advanced, reliable, and fast analysis.

This does not mean that all old rules should be suddenly abandoned; instead, they should still be used consistently until new methods are validated and their relationship with the results obtained with the classical methods is analyzed in detail.

These concepts apply primarily to the analysis of the EMG signal and might be transferred also to the discussion of the results provided by actigraphy. On the contrary, the visual analysis of synchronized video-PSG recordings seems to be the current gold standard for the analysis of more complex patterns of movements or behaviors. The new computerized video image analysis techniques, however, seem to be promising, and it is hoped that they will be developed in the near future to provide fast and reliable tools for research and clinical applications.

Finally, at least for PLMs and submentalis muscle atonia, the new parameters derived from their automatic computerized analysis may play an important role in defining the criteria for some clinical conditions such as RLS and REM sleep behavior disorder.

REFERENCES

1. Lugaresi E, Coccagna G, Tassinari CA, et al. Rilievi poligrafici sui fenomeni motori nella sindrome delle gambe senza riposo. *Riv Neurol* 1965;35: 550–61.
2. Lugaresi E, Tate L, Coccagna G, et al. Particularités cliniques et polygraphiques du syndrome d'impatience des membres inferieurs. *Rev Neurol (Paris)* 1965;113: 545–55.
3. Coleman RM. Periodic movements in sleep (nocturnal myoclonus) and restless legs syndrome. In: Guilleminault C, ed. *Sleeping and Waking Disorders: Indications and Techniques.* Menlo Park, CA: Addison-Wesley; 1982:265–95.
4. American Sleep Disorders Association. Recording and scoring leg movements. The Atlas Task Force. *Sleep* 1993; 16:748–59.
5. Ferri R, Zucconi M, Manconi M, et al. Computer-assisted detection of nocturnal leg motor activity in patients with restless legs syndrome and periodic leg movements during sleep. *Sleep* 2005;28:998–1004.
6. Wetter TC, Dirlich G, Streit J, et al. An automatic method for scoring leg movements in polygraphic sleep recordings and its validity in comparison to visual scoring. *Sleep* 2004;27:324–8.
7. Ferri R, Zucconi M, Manconi M, et al. New approaches to the study of periodic leg movements during sleep in restless legs syndrome. *Sleep* 2006;29:759–69.
8. Zucconi M, Ferri R, Allen R, et al. The official World Association of Sleep Medicine (WASM) standards for recording and scoring periodic leg movements in sleep (PLMS) and wakefulness (PLMW) developed in collaboration with a task force from the International Restless Legs Syndrome Study Group (IRLSSG). *Sleep Med* 2006;7:175–83.
9. Iber C, Ancoli-Israel S, Chesson AL, et al. *The AASM manual for the scoring of sleep and associated events: rules, terminology, and technical specifications.* 1st ed. Westchester, IL: American Academy of Sleep Medicine; 2007.
10. Walters AS, Lavigne G, Hening W, et al. The scoring of movements in sleep. *J Clin Sleep Med* 2007;3:155–67.
11. Ferri R, Zucconi M, Rundo F, et al. Heart rate and spectral EEG changes accompanying periodic and non-periodic leg movements during sleep. *Clin Neurophysiol* 2007;118:438–48.
12. Ferri R, Zucconi M. Heart rate and spectral EEG changes accompanying periodic and isolated leg movements during sleep. *Sleep* 2008;31:16–17.
13. Manconi M, Ferri R, Zucconi M, et al. First night efficacy of pramipexole in restless legs syndrome and periodic leg movements. *Sleep Med* 2007;8:491–7.
14. Pennestrì M-H, Whittom S, Benoit A, et al. PLMS and PLMW in healthy subjects as a function of age: prevalence and interval distribution. *Sleep* 2006;29:1183–7.
15. Ferrillo F, Beelke M, Canovaro P, et al. Changes in cerebral and autonomic activity heralding periodic limb movements in sleep. *Sleep Med* 2004;5:407–12.
16. Ferri R, Manconi M, Lanuzza B, et al. Age-related changes in periodic leg movements during sleep in patients with restless legs syndrome. *Sleep Med* 2008;9:790–8.
17. Trenkwalder C, Hening WA, Walters AS, et al. Circadian rhythm of periodic limb movements and sensory symptoms of restless legs syndrome. *Mov Disord* 1999;14:102–10.
18. Ferri R, Zucconi M, Manconi M, et al. Different periodicity and time structure of leg movements during sleep in narcolepsy/cataplexy and restless legs syndrome. *Sleep* 2006;29:1587–94.
19. Manconi M, Ferri R, Zucconi M, et al. Time structure analysis of leg movements during sleep in REM sleep behavior disorder. *Sleep* 2007;30:1779–85.
20. Kazenwadel J, Pollmacher T, Trenkwalder C, et al. New actigraphic assessment method for periodic leg movements (PLM). *Sleep* 1995;18:689–97.
21. Ferri R, Gschliesser V, Frauscher B, et al. Periodic leg movements during sleep and periodic limb movement disorder in patients presenting with unexplained insomnia. *Clin Neurophysiol* 2009;120:257–63.
22. Gschliesser V, Frauscher B, Brandauer E, et al. PLM detection by actigraphy compared

to polysomnography: a validation and comparison of two actigraphs. *Sleep Med* 2009;10:306–11.

23. King MA, Jaffre MO, Morrish E, et al. The validation of a new actigraphy system for the measurement of periodic leg movements in sleep. *Sleep Med* 2005;6:507–13.

24. Sforza E, Johannes M, Claudio B. The PAM-RL ambulatory device for detection of periodic leg movements: a validation study. *Sleep Med* 2005;6:407–13.

25. Kemlink D, Pretl M, Sonka K, et al. A comparison of polysomnographic and actigraphic evaluation of periodic limb movements in sleep. *Neurol Res* 2008;30:234–8.

26. Stefansson H, Rye DB, Hicks A, et al. A genetic risk factor for periodic limb movements in sleep. *N Engl J Med* 2007;357:639–47.

27. Trotti LM, Bliwise DL, Greer SA, et al. Correlates of PLMs variability over multiple nights and impact upon RLS diagnosis. *Sleep Med* 2009;10:668–71.

28. Heinrich A, van Vugt H. A new video actigraphy method for non-contact analysis of body movement during sleep. *J Sleep Res* 2010;19(suppl 2):83–4.

29. Alihanka J, Vaahtoranta K. A static charge sensitive bed. A new method for recording body movements during sleep. *Electroencephalogr Clin Neurophysiol* 1979;46:731–4.

30. Anttalainen U, Polo O, Vahlberg T, et al. Reimbursed drugs in patients with sleep-disordered breathing: a static-charge-sensitive bed study. *Sleep Med* 2010;11:49–55.

31. Kirjavainen J, Ojala T, Huhtala V, et al. Heart rate variability in response to the sleep-related movements in infants with and without colic. *Early Hum Dev* 2004;79:17–30.

32. Chervin RD, Consens FB, Kutluay E. Alternating leg muscle activation during sleep and arousals: a new sleep-related motor phenomenon? *Mov Disord* 2003;18:551–9.

33. Cosentino FI, Iero I, Lanuzza B, et al. The neurophysiology of the alternating leg muscle activation (ALMA) during sleep: study of one patient before and after treatment with pramipexole. *Sleep Med* 2006;7:63–71.

34. Broughton R. Pathological fragmentary myoclonus, intensified hypnic jerks and hypnagogic foot tremor: three unusual sleep-related movement disorders. In: Koella WP, Obal F, Schultz H, Visser P, eds.

Sleep 86. Stuttgart, Germany: Gustav Fischer Verlag; 1988: 240–2.

35. Wichniak A, Tracik F, Geisler P, et al. Rhythmic feet movements while falling asleep. *Mov Disord* 2001;16:1164–70.

36. Yang C, Winkelman JW. Clinical and polysomnographic characteristics of high frequency leg movements. *J Clin Sleep Med* 2010;6:431–8.

37. Broughton R, Tolentino MA. Fragmentary pathological myoclonus in NREM sleep 1130. *Electroencephalogr Clin Neurophysiol* 1984;57:303–9.

38. Broughton R, Tolentino MA, Krelina M. Excessive fragmentary myoclonus in NREM sleep: a report of 38 cases 1068. *Electroencephalogr Clin Neurophysiol* 1985;61:123–33.

39. Lins O, Castonguay M, Dunham W, et al. Excessive fragmentary myoclonus: time of night and sleep stage distributions. *Can J Neurol Sci* 1993;20:142–6.

40. Frauscher B, Kunz A, Brandauer E, et al. Fragmentary myoclonus in sleep revisited: a polysomnographic study in 62 patients. *Sleep Med* 2011;12:410–15.

41. Brown P, Thompson PD, Rothwell JC, et al. Axial myoclonus of propriospinal origin. *Brain* 1991;114:197–214.

42. Chokroverty S. Propriospinal myoclonus. *Clin Neurosci* 1995;3:219–22.

43. Montagna P, Provini F, Vetrugno R. Propriospinal myoclonus at sleep onset. *Neurophysiol Clin* 2006;36:351–5.

44. Montagna P, Provini F, Plazzi G, et al. Propriospinal myoclonus upon relaxation and drowsiness: a cause of severe insomnia. *Mov Disord* 1997;12:66–72.

45. Manconi M, Sferrazza B, Iannaccone S, et al. Case of symptomatic propriospinal myoclonus evolving toward acute "myoclonic status." *Mov Disord* 2005;20:1646–50.

46. Frauscher B, Brandauer E, Gschliesser V, et al. A descriptive analysis of neck myoclonus during routine polysomnography. *Sleep* 2010;33:1091–6.

47. Wehrle R, Bartels A, Wetter TC. Facio-mandibular myoclonus specific during REM sleep. *Sleep Med* 2009;10:149–51.

48. American Academy of Sleep Medicine *International Classification of Sleep Disorders. Diagnostic and Coding Manual.* 2nd ed. Westchester, IL: American Academy of Sleep Medicine; 2005.

49. Huynh N. Sleep-related bruxism. In: Thorpy M, Plazzi G, eds. *The Parasomnias and Other*

Sleep-Related Movement Disorders. New York: Cambridge University Press; 2010:252–60.

50. Lavigne G, Manzini C, Huynh N. Sleep Bruxism. In: Kryger MH, Roth T, Dement WC, eds. *Principles and Practice of Sleep Medicine*. 5th ed. St. Louis, MO: Elsevier Saunders; 2011:1128–39.

51. Kato T, Thie NM, Montplaisir JY, et al. Bruxism and orofacial movements during sleep. *Dent Clin North Am* 2001;45:657–84.

52. Lavigne G, Manzini C, Kato T. Sleep Bruxism. In: Kryger MH, Roth T, Dement WC, eds. *Principles and Practice of Sleep Medicine*. Philadelphia, PA: Elsevier Saunders; 2005:946–59.

53. Lapierre O, Montplaisir J. Polysomnographic features of REM sleep behavior disorder: development of a scoring method. *Neurology* 1992;42:1371–4.

54. Eisensehr I, Ehrenberg BL, Noachtar S. Different sleep characteristics in restless legs syndrome and periodic limb movement disorder. *Sleep Med* 2003;4:147–52.

55. Bliwise DL, He L, Ansari FP, et al. Quantification of electromyographic activity during sleep: a phasic electromyographic metric. *J Clin Neurophysiol* 2006;23:59–67.

56. Bliwise DL, Rye DB. Elevated PEM (phasic electromyographic metric) rates identify rapid eye movement behavior disorder patients on nights without behavioral abnormalities. *Sleep* 2008;31: 853–7.

57. Frauscher B, Iranzo A, Hogl B, et al. Quantification of electromyographic activity during REM sleep in multiple muscles in REM sleep behavior disorder. *Sleep* 2008;31:724–31.

58. Montplaisir J, Gagnon JF, Fantini ML, et al. Polysomnographic diagnosis of idiopathic REM sleep behavior disorder. *Mov Disord* 2010;25:2044–51.

59. Frauscher B, Iranzo A, Gaig C, et al. Normative EMG values during REM sleep for the diagnosis of REM Sleep behavior disorder. *Sleep* 2012;35(6):835–47.

60. Consens FB, Chervin RD, Koeppe RA, et al. Validation of a polysomnographic score for REM sleep behavior disorder. *Sleep* 2005;28:993–7.

61. Burns JW, Consens FB, Little RJ, et al. EMG variance during polysomnography as an assessment for REM sleep behavior disorder. *Sleep* 2007;30:1771–8.

62. Ferri R, Manconi M, Plazzi G, et al. A quantitative statistical analysis of the submentalis muscle EMG amplitude during sleep in normal controls and patients with REM sleep behavior disorder. *J. Sleep Res* 2008;17:89–100.

63. Kempfner J, Sorensen G, Zoetmulder M, et al. REM behaviour disorder detection associated with neurodegenerative diseases. *Conf Proc IEEE Eng Med Biol Soc* 2010;2010:5093–6.

64. Mayer G, Kesper K, Ploch T, et al. Quantification of tonic and phasic muscle activity in REM sleep behavior disorder. *J Clin Neurophysiol* 2008;25:48–55.

65. Ferri R, Franceschini C, Zucconi M, et al. Searching for a marker of REM sleep behavior disorder: submentalis muscle EMG amplitude analysis during sleep in patients with narcolepsy/cataplexy. *Sleep* 2008;31:1409–17.

66. Ferri R, Rundo F, Manconi M, et al. Improved computation of the atonia index in normal controls and patients with REM sleep behavior disorder. *Sleep Med* 2010;11:947–9.

67. Sforza E, Zucconi M, Petronelli R, et al. REM sleep behavioral disorders. *Eur Neurol* 1988;28:295–300.

68. Iranzo A, Santamaria J, Rye DB, et al. Characteristics of idiopathic REM sleep behavior disorder and that associated with MSA and PD. *Neurology* 2005;65:247–52.

69. Frauscher B, Gschliesser V, Brandauer E, et al. Video analysis of motor events in REM sleep behavior disorder. *Mov Disord* 2007;22:1464–70.

70. Frauscher B, Gschliesser V, Brandauer E, et al. The relation between abnormal behaviors and REM sleep microstructure in patients with REM sleep behavior disorder. *Sleep Med* 2009;10:174–81.

71. De Cock V, Vidailhet M, Leu S, et al. Restoration of normal motor control in Parkinson's disease during REM sleep. *Brain* 2007;130:450–6.

72. Leclair-Visonneau L, Oudiette D, Gaymard B, et al. Do the eyes scan dream images during rapid eye movement sleep? Evidence from the rapid eye movement sleep behaviour disorder model. *Brain* 2010;133:1737–46.

73. Oudiette D, Leclair-Visonneau L, Arnulf I. Video-clinical corners. Snoring, penile erection and loss of reflexive consciousness during REM sleep behavior disorder. *Sleep Med* 2010;11:953–5.

74. Sixel-Doring F, Schweitzer M, Mollenhauer B, et al. Intraindividual variability of REM sleep

behavior disorder in Parkinson's disease: a comparative assessment using a new REM sleep behavior disorder severity scale (RBDSS) for clinical routine. *J Clin Sleep Med* 2011;7:75–80.

75. Manni R, Terzaghi M, Sartori I, et al. Rhythmic movement disorder and cyclic alternating pattern during sleep: a video-polysomnographic study in a 9-year-old boy. *Mov Disord* 2004;19:1186–90.

76. Terzano MG, Parrino L, Smerieri A, et al. Atlas, rules, and recording techniques for the scoring of cyclic alternating pattern (CAP) in human sleep. *Sleep Med* 2001;2:537–53.

77. Hoban T. Sleep-related rhythmic movements disorder. In: Thorpy M, Plazzi G, eds. *The Parasomnias and other Sleep-Related Movement Disorders*. New York: Cambridge University Press; 2010:270–7.

13

Cyclic Alternating Pattern in Sleep
Measurement and Clinical Significance

LIBORIO PARRINO, RAFFAELE FERRI, OLIVIERO BRUNI,
AND MARIO G. TERZANO

The average duration of syllables, the fundamental segmentation of speech in all languages, is approximately 250 milliseconds. Syllables cannot be stretched or sped up at will in spoken language beyond certain limits. Slowing down speech can be achieved only by introducing long pauses between syllables. This is the reason why it is difficult to understand the text of arias.

—Gyorgy Buzsaki, *Rhythms of the Brain*[1]

CYCLIC ALTERNATING pattern (CAP) is a well-defined marker of the physiologic cerebral activity occurring under conditions of reduced vigilance (sleep, coma), translating a state of arousal instability and involving muscle, behavioral, and autonomic functions.[1a]

During non–rapid eye movement (non-REM) sleep, CAP is organized in sequences. A CAP sequence is composed of a succession of CAP cycles. The CAP cycle is composed of a phase A and the following phase B. All CAP sequences (composed by a series of CAP cycles) begin with a phase A and end with a phase B. Each phase of CAP is 2–60 seconds in duration. This cutoff relies on the consideration that the great majority (about 90%) of A phases occurring during sleep are separated by an interval <60 seconds.

The absence of CAP for >60 seconds is scored as non-CAP. An isolated phase A (that is, preceded or followed by another phase A but separated by more than 60 seconds) is classified as non-CAP. The phase A that terminates a CAP sequence is counted as non-CAP.

The absence of CAP coincides with a condition of sustained physiologic stability and is defined as non-CAP.[2]

CAP and non-CAP can be consistently manipulated by sensorial inputs.

Applying separately the same arousing stimulus during the two electroencephalographic (EEG) components of CAP, phase B is the one that immediately assumes the morphology of the other component, whereas the inverse transformation never occurs when the stimulus is delivered during phase A. This stereotyped reactivity persists throughout the successive phases of CAP with lack of habituation. In contrast, when the same stimulus is presented during non-CAP, the EEG responses are generally brief, hypersynchronized (slow waves), and proceed toward progressive habituation.[3]

However, a robust or sustained stimulus delivered during non-CAP induces the immediate appearance of repetitive CAP cycles that display the same morphology and reactive behavior of spontaneous CAP sequences. The evoked CAP sequence may herald a lightening of sleep depth or continue as a damping oscillation before the complete recovery of non-CAP.

CAP sequences have no upper limits for duration and number of CAP cycles. In young adults, 2.5 minutes is the approximate mean duration of a CAP sequence, containing an average of six CAP cycles.[4]

At least two consecutive CAP cycles are required to define a CAP sequence (Fig. 13.1). Consequently, three or more consecutive A phases must be identified with each of the first two A phases followed by a phase B (interval <60 seconds) and the third phase A followed by a >60-second non-CAP interval.

General Rule

An A phase is scored within a CAP sequence only if it precedes and/or follows another phase A in the 2- to 60-second temporal range. CAP sequence onset must be preceded by non-CAP (a continuous non-REM sleep EEG pattern for >60 seconds), with the following three exceptions. There is no temporal limitation (1) before the first CAP sequence arising in non-REM sleep; (2) after a wake-to-sleep transition; or (3) after a REM to non-REM sleep transition.[2]

Stage Shifts

Within non-REM sleep, a CAP sequence is not interrupted by a sleep stage shift if CAP scoring requirements are satisfied. Consequently, because CAP sequences can extend across adjacent sleep stages, a CAP sequence can contain a variety of different phase A and phase B activities.[5]

Cyclic Alternating Pattern in REM Sleep

CAP sequences commonly precede the transition from non-REM to REM sleep and end just before REM sleep onset. REM sleep is characterized by the lack of EEG synchronization; thus, phase A features in REM sleep consist mainly of desynchronized patterns (fast low-amplitude rhythms), which are separated by a mean interval of 3–4 minutes.[5a] Consequently, under

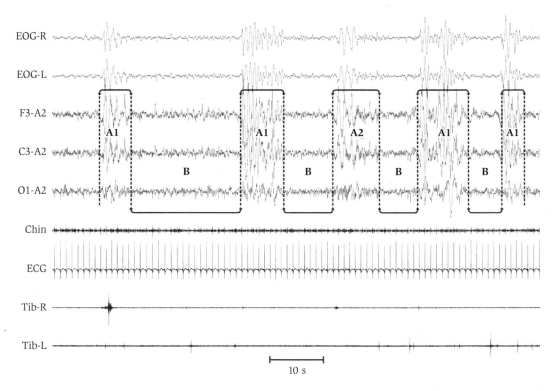

FIGURE 13.1 Example of a cyclic alternating pattern (CAP) sequence formed by four CAP cycles. ECG, electroencephalogram; EOG, electro-oculogram.

normal circumstances, CAP does not occur in REM sleep. However, pathologic conditions characterized by repetitive A phases recurring at intervals <60 seconds (for example, periodic REM-related sleep apnea events) can produce CAP sequences in REM sleep.

Recording Techniques and Montages

CAP is a global EEG phenomenon involving extensive cortical areas. Therefore, A phases should be visible on all or most EEG leads. Bipolar derivations such as Fp1-F3, F3-C3, C3-P3, P3-O1 or Fp2-F4, F4-C4, C4-P4, and P4-O2 guarantee a favorable detection of the phenomenon. A calibration of 50 mV/7 mm with a time constant of 0.1 seconds and a high-frequency filter in the 30 Hz range is recommended for the EEG channels. Monopolar EEG derivations (C3-A2 or C4-A1 and O1-A2 or O2-A1), eye movement channels, and submentalis electromyography (EMG), currently used for the conventional sleep staging and arousal scoring, are also essential for scoring CAP. For clinical studies, airflow and respiratory effort, cardiac rhythm, oxygen saturation, and leg movements should be included as part of standard polysomnographic technique.[6]

Amplitude Limits

Changes in EEG amplitude are crucial for scoring CAP. Phasic activities initiating a phase A must be a third higher than the background voltage (calculated during the 2 seconds before onset and 2 seconds after offset of a phase A). However, in some cases, a phase A can present ambiguous limits due to inconsistent voltage changes. Onset and termination of a phase A are established on the basis of an amplitude/frequency concordance in the majority of EEG leads. The monopolar derivation is mostly indicated when scoring is carried out on a single derivation. All EEG events that do not meet clearly the phase A characteristics cannot be scored as part of phase A.

Time Limits

The minimal duration of a phase A or a phase B is 2 seconds. If two consecutive A phases are separated by an interval <2 seconds, they are combined as a single phase A. If they are separated by a ≥2-second interval, they are scored as independent events.

THE A PHASES OF CYCLIC ALTERNATING PATTERN

Phase A activities can be classified into three subtypes. Subtype classification is based on the reciprocal proportion of high-voltage slow waves (EEG synchrony) and low-amplitude fast rhythms (EEG desynchrony) throughout the entire phase A duration. The three phase A subtypes are described next[7]:

- *Subtypes A1.*
- EEG synchrony (high-amplitude slow waves) is the predominant activity. If present, EEG desynchrony (low-amplitude fast waves) occupies <20% of the entire phase A duration. Subtype A1 specimens include delta bursts, K-complex sequences, vertex sharp transients, and polyphasic bursts with <20% of EEG desynchrony.
- *Subtypes A2.*
- The EEG activity is a mixture of slow and fast rhythms with 20%–50% of phase A occupied by EEG desynchrony. Subtype A2 specimens include polyphasic bursts with more than 20% but less than 50% of EEG desynchrony.
- *Subtypes A3.*
- The EEG activity is predominantly rapid low-voltage rhythms with >50% of phase A occupied by EEG desynchrony. Subtype A3 specimens include K-alpha, EEG arousals, and polyphasic bursts with >50% of EEG desynchrony. A movement artifact within a CAP sequence is also classified as subtype A3.[2]

CAP sequences include different phase A subtypes. The majority of arousals occurring in non-REM (87%) are inserted within the CAP sequences and basically coincide with a phase A2 or A3. In particular, 95% of subtypes A3 and 62% of subtypes A2 meet the AASM criteria for arousals.[8,9] The broad overlap between arousals and subtypes A2 and A3 is further supported by their similar evolution in relation to age and to their positive correlation with the amount of light non-REM sleep and negative correlation with the amount of deep non-REM sleep. However, some minor differences can be noticed resulting from the inclusion of slow waves in CAP events (see Fig. 13.2 for an example).

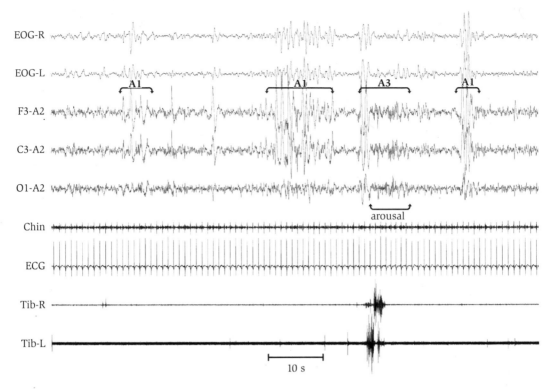

FIGURE 13.2   Example of the correspondence (and difference) between a cyclic alternating pattern (CAP) A3 phase and an arousal. Note that the criteria for the definition of the A3 phase of CAP include the slow waves immediately preceding the run of fast waves, while those for arousal do not. ECG, electroencephalogram; EOG, electro-oculogram.

RESPONSE OF COMPLEX NETWORKS TO STIMULI

Sleep is an excellent model of evolving brain state because it occurs without an outside influence. It evolves from within. Complex systems with a predictable "path" or trajectory in the state space are called deterministic. Sleep is such a detereministic evolving state. Each evolving sleep stage has its own characteristic oscillatory pattern. Oscillation is the inherent global behaviour of balanced systems, whose frequency is determined by some time constraints. Neurons in local or global regions of the cerebral cortex rapidly swing between excitable and less excitable (up and down) states. In the intact brain, properly timed exogenous influences (e.g., external sensory or body-movement-associated signals during sleep) can trigger upswing changes.

—Gyorgy Buzsaki, Rhythms of the Brain[1]

If the AASM arousal is a sign of transient sleep discontinuity, the finding of phasic EEG delta activities during enhancement of autonomic functions indicates the possibility of physiologic activation without sleep disruption. In effect, nonvisible sleep fragmentation induced by acoustic tones has been associated with increased daytime sleepiness, indicating that the processes of sleep consolidation may be impaired (in this case by sensorial stimulation) without evidence of sleep discontinuity.[10] Despite their EEG differences, slow EEG events (K-complexes and delta bursts) and AASM arousals (fast rhythms) may share functional properties, and therefore they may be included within the comprehensive term of *activating complexes.*

Such a variety of EEG manifestations relies on specific gates controlling the flow of internal and external inputs. The thalamic-basal forebrain gate is an ultimate step of resistance against arousing impulses. Initially the cortex tries to preserve sleep continuity with reinforcement of its gates that are indicated by the occurrence of K-complexes and delta bursts in the sleep EEG. However, when the thalamic gate cannot control the afferent inputs, a cortical change is seen translated by an alpha mixed or an alpha/beta frequency burst.[11] Anyway, the initial reaction of the cerebral cortex is a sleep-protective response as the majority of transient rapid activities are preceded by a slow high-amplitude EEG burst.[12] According to a recent review, mainly based on electrophysiologic recordings in animals, slow EEG events during non-REM sleep are an emergent property of cortico-thalamo-cortical networks. In particular, they originate from the dynamic interplay of three cardinal oscillators: the synaptically based cortical oscillator and two thalamic oscillators, that is, thalamocortical neurons and nucleus reticularis thalami. The functional implications of this dialogue provide permissive windows for cellular excitability and network plasticity during slow-wave sleep.[13]

CAP sequences reflect the balance between sleep-and wake-promoting systems. Accordingly, sleep instability in non-REM sleep elicits CAP sequences composed of sleep-like (K-complexes, delta waves) and wake-like (alpha and beta rhytms) bouts of EEG activity. In particular, subtypes A1 are a natural "delta injection" fueling deep stages and defending sleep against perturbations. On the contrary, CAP A2 and A3 responses drive the sleeper toward more superficial vigilance states. Therefore, CAP sequences represent a protective, short-term homeostatic mechanism of non-REM sleep in which the amount of slow-wave activity is buffered and sleep continuity preserved.[14] When delta power increases in sleep, after sleep deprivation, the CAP system reacts with a robust decrease of CAP rate.[15] Supplementation of sleep with slow waves after deprivation counteracts the production of CAP sequences probably because the sleep-promoting system is under saturation.

Power spectral analysis of CAP components shows that the different phase A subtypes in non-REM sleep are variants of a continuous two-fold process: an initial high-voltage slow-wave component, which predisposes the cerebral cortex to a greater readiness and opens the way to the more rapid activity, correlated with strong activating effects.[16–18] What distinguishes the single event is the buildup and reciprocal distribution of the EEG components. In the A1 phases of CAP, which host exclusively K-complexes and equivalent slow-wave

activities (vertex potentials and delta bursts), the starting delta power increase is maintained and prevails throughout the entire activation process. A balanced representation of slow and fast EEG frequency bands is the main characteristic of the A2 phases, while rapid EEG activities are the dominant feature of the A3 subtypes and of arousals. This does not mean that all activating complexes exert equivalent effects on sleep structure and on autonomic functions. A hierarchical activation from the slower EEG patterns (moderate autonomic activation without sleep disruption) to the faster EEG patterns (robust autonomic activation associated with visible sleep fragmentation) has been described in different studies.[14,19–22]

THE CONCEPT OF CORTICAL, SUBCORTICAL, AND AUTONOMIC AROUSAL

The conventional definition of arousal includes a cluster of physiologic manifestations expressed by an activation of electrocorticographic rhythms, an increase of blood pressure and muscle tone, and a variation of heart rate. During sleep, arousals provide an excitation drive to vital processes whenever respiratory and cardiovascular failure occurs. However, somatosensory and auditory stimulation during sleep may result in cardiac, respiratory, and somatic modifications apparently (visual analysis) without the EEG features of conventional arousals.[23] This observation implies that there is a range of partial arousal responses with EEG manifestations different from conventional arousals. The different arousal responses rely on the different combinations of the central and peripheral components, on the intensity scale of their manifestation, and on the morphological variations of the cortical reactions.

Different expressions of arousal can be identified:

1. *Behavioral arousal*: reported in the R&K manual[24] as movement arousal. Described as any increase in EMG activity that is accompanied by a change in any other EEG channel.

2. *Cortical arousal*: defined by the AASM committee[25] as EEG arousal, it is characterized by transient desynchronized EEG patterns interrupting sleep. It reflects a brief awakening of the cerebral cortex regardless of any concomitant participation of the autonomic system or behavioral components.

3. *Subcortical activation*: identified when autonomic activation is associated with a transient EEG pattern different from a conventional AASM arousal.[19,26,27]

Behavioral arousals and subcortical activations represent the two extremes of a gradual scale of cerebral activation. However, they are not separated by rigid boundaries. The temporal overlap between cortical, somatomotor, and autonomic events within the same arousal episode does not necessarily imply synchrony, and the order of activation of the single compartments can vary in the different physiologic or pathologic circumstances.

In arousal phenomena during sleep there is no mandatory chronological and etiologic subordination. The phenomenon takes place within interactive loops in which the cerebral cortex can be the starting or the ending point but anyway a source of control. The origin of arousal should be defined by the subsystem primarily activated or perturbed. The arousal can be generated directly by the brain under the impulse of the physiologic evolution of sleep, for example, the transition from non-REM to REM sleep, or in response to a sensorial perturbation, such as respiratory interruption, noisy environment, alteration of blood pressure or heart rate, or movements. In any case, it is the involvement of the brain that makes arousal a unitary phenomenon[28] in which activation is modulated through a hierarchy of phasic responses ranging from slow high-amplitude EEG patterns (CAP subtypes A1) to fast low-voltage (CAP subtypes A3).

CYCLIC ALTERNATING PATTERN AND BODY MOVEMENTS

Body movements can trigger or interrupt a CAP sequence. Body movements linked to one or more A phases in the temporal range of 2–60 seconds are included within the CAP sequence if the other scoring criteria are met. A previous study ascertained that 72% of all minor or major body movements occurring in non-REM appeared as inserted events, close (within 30 seconds) events, or far (> 30 seconds < 180 seconds) events. When a major dynamic event precedes a CAP sequence, the latter actively restores the steady-state conditions of non-CAP through its damped oscillations. When a major dynamic event appears as an inserted or following phenomenon, the CAP

sequence provides the excitatory background so as to overcome the sleep stage stability. In these cases, the major dynamic event can intervene as a stabilizing force in order to interrupt barren or threatening conditions of arousal instability. In other words, CAP sequence and major dynamic events interact within a consensual domain and represent reciprocal sources of adaptive strategies.

The activation of somatomotor epileptic seizures is only one of the functions of behavioral arousal within the CAP oscillation.[29-31] CAP can promote or release other motor activities ranging from physiologic body movements to periodic limb movements (PLMs), sleep bruxism, night terrors, and sleepwalking.[32]

The definition of clearcut boundaries between physiologic and pathologic movement patterns is in progress while promising indications are supplied by the accumulation of videopolysomnographic recordings of the motor events. It is known that the number and distribution of nocturnal movements is a personal trait, with a specific nightly profile for the accomplishment of motor episodes during sleep. Whether the outcome is a normal or a pathologic motor episode depends basically upon the nature of the putative underlying lesion, the susceptibility of the patient, and the location and extent of the neural circuits involved in the behavioral event.

Overall, the CAP A phase acts as an "amplifier" that may facilitate the occurrence of pathologic events, while the CAP B phase exerts a "filter" action.[7] The gating effects of phase A and phase B have been demonstrated in the last years in several sleep disturbances such as PLM,[33] sleep bruxism,[34] sleepwalking,[29,35] and sleep disordered breathing (Parrino et al., 2000).[6,30,36]

In movement disorders, the magnitude and temporal variations of cerebral activity and autonomic responses before and during the motor event support the hypothesis of a continuum in arousal reactivity present not only at visual analysis but also at the spectral level. Considering manual scoring, this continuum is translated by the progression of the arousal response from delta and K-complex bursts, to an EEG arousal and full awakening.[9,37] The same continuum can be detected by spectral analysis starting with an enhancement of delta activity and increase of heart and respiratory rates,[17,18,21,38,39] which may be followed by a transition to fast EEG activities. The hierarchy of the

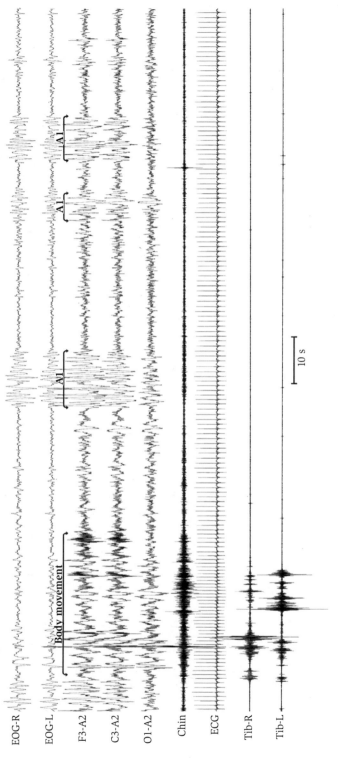

FIGURE 13.3 Example of a cyclic alternating pattern sequence triggered by a body movement. ECG, electroencephalogram; EOG, electro-oculogram.

arousal response is related to severity provided by emergency.

From a mechanistic point of view, postapnea arousals in sleep breathing disorders are the most evident example of automatic, purposeful, and ancestral periodic movement during sleep. In the upper airway resistance syndrome,[40,41] the esophageal pressure (Pes) reversal is associated with an increase in delta and thereafter in fast activities occurring 2 seconds before the Pes reversal and present even when EEG arousals do not occur. Similar results are observed in patients with sleep apnea syndrome in whom delta amplitude progressively rises throughout the apnea and continues to increase simultaneously with the appearance of alpha and fast activities just before the start of the hyperventilation period.[29]

CYCLIC ALTERNATING PATTERN AND PERIODIC LIMB MOVEMENTS

PLMs are a pattern of motor phenomena and EEG changes, both recurring at intervals of 20–40 seconds. Studies of biologic rhythms have identified several neurons and neural networks that generate rhythmic physiologic and behavioral events. Some of them are related to automatic physiologic patterns, and PLM is probably related to spinal flexor reflexes; it can involve one or both legs and occur also in spinal cord injury patients.[42,43] The periodicity of PLM parallels the recurrence of CAP cycles. Therefore, it is not surprising that the two PSG manifestations (PLM and CAP) are mutually connected. This does not imply that PLM is induced by CAP, but the latter represents a permissive framework that synchronizes rhytmicity. In patients with PLM, 92% of all jerks detected in non-REM sleep occurred in CAP with the great majority of limb movements (96%) were associated with a phase A (Fig. 13.4), especially subtypes A2 and A3 (95%). Ninety-four percent of the nocturnal jerks coupled with a phase A started jointly with the onset of the phase or when the latter had already begun. In particular, 67% of the myoclonic events occurred in the first 2.5 seconds of the A phase. PLM onset was heralded by a significant activation of delta activity power (the initial portion of the phase A2 or A3 subtype) starting approximately 3–4 seconds before the PLM onset ().[33,38,44]

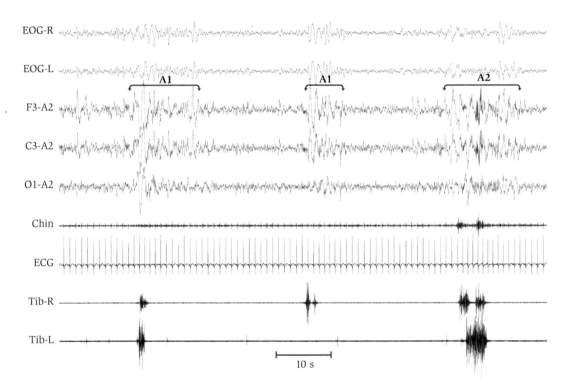

FIGURE 13.4 Example of the association between cyclic alternating pattern A phases and periodic leg movement events. ECG, electroencephalogram; EOG, electro-oculogram.

The appearance of the PLM coincides with the fast EEG frequencies of the phase A subtypes. CAP and PLM also appear to be related to the cyclic alternation of autonomic arousal and quiescence, as indicated by the increase in EKG-established heart rate that accompanies both the A phase and PLM.[21,45-48] In the sequence of events, cardiac and EEG changes take place before the onset of the motor phenomenon. The temporal relationship between delta activity, cardiac activation, and PLM onset suggests that these phenomena act as a preparatory condition, involving both central and autonomic nervous systems, exerting a permissive function on the activity of spinal motoneurons. According to Sforza et al.,[49] the rise of delta waves and heart rate could be considered as the first level of a transient activation from sleep. PLM, and the subsequent progressive activation of the faster EEG frequencies, should be considered as the second phase in the continuum of the arousal response associated with these movements.

The same stereotyped pattern of cerebral and autonomic variation has been described for EEG and heart rate changes associated with spontaneous arousals. These results support evidence of a central oscillatory mechanism regulating both EEG and autonomic functions. Irrespective of the arousal features, EEG and autonomic responses, consisting of a rise in heart rate and slow EEG frequencies, start before the arousal onset. In non-REM sleep, De Carli et al.[16] reported an increase in delta activity in the 3.5-second epoch preceding the arousal. There is converging evidence that a stereotyped pattern of cerebral and autonomic variations characterizes the microstructural fluctuations of the arousal level during non-REM sleep. Both in spontaneous arousals and in those related to motor phenomena, blood pressure variations or cardiac activations show a qualitatively common EEG spectral pattern, independent of the presence of a detectable arousing stimulus, its type or its strength.

Since all phenomena we have taken into consideration (CAP, PLM, spontaneous arousals, or arousals related to detectable stimuli) are always characterized by an initial increase in delta power and heart rate, followed by an inhibition and by a progressive activation of faster EEG frequencies, we agree with the hypothesis of a neural oscillatory network regulating the cyclic arousability of the sleeping brain.[50] In the hierarchy of the arousal response, the delta power and heart rate increase may be considered as the early sleep-maintaining response

of brain arousability to low-intensity stimuli, implicating the activation of thalamocortical networks.[51,52]

In PLM patients with myoclonic jerks occurring both in non-REM and in REM sleep, the pattern of EEG changes shows specific behaviors in the two states. While in non-REM sleep, the PLM is preceded by a rise in slow EEG activity and in heart rate, in REM sleep the changes in cerebral activity appear simultaneously with the PLM onset.[33] The sleep state-related EEG responses to PLM suggest that the mechanisms triggering PLM during REM sleep are different from those involved in non-REM sleep, the only sleep state during which the CAP phenomenon can be observed.

The relation between CAP and PLM varies also in different clinical conditions. A number of studies have clarified that the periodicity index exceeds 0.6 in restless legs syndrome (RLS) and PLM disorder, typically characterized by high CAP rate and a strong association between the A phases and myoclonic jerks, while it is under 0.5 in REM behavior disorder and narcolepsy associated with low amounts of sleep instability.[53] These findings reinforce the mutual interaction between central and peripheral mechanisms during non-REM sleep modulated by the permissive windows of CAP during non-REM sleep.

However, in RLS patients, a single dose of pramipexole drastically reduces PLM events during sleep but has no effect on the increased non-REM sleep instability measured by CAP analysis.[54] This suggests that dopaminergic treatment for RLS might be insufficient to correct the complete spectrum of sleep abnormalities of these patients. Exclusion of more central mechanisms can partially explain the subjective complaint of unrefreshed sleep reported by these patients in spite of the effective drug action on motor events.

CYCLIC ALTERNATING PATTERN AND PARASOMNIAS

Although the sleep architecture in disorders of arousal does not show significant differences from controls,[29,55,56] several studies have shown subtle alterations of non-REM sleep in adults, represented mostly by a high degree of arousal from SWS and by a peculiar EEG pattern defined as hypersynchronous delta (HSD) activity (Gadreau et al., 2000),[29,55-58] described as continuous high-voltage (>150 lV) delta waves occurring during SWS or immediately prior to an episode.[58]

HSD activity and sudden arousals from slow-wave sleep are features of non-REM sleep classically reported to occur in patients with non-REM parasomnias such as sleepwalking, night terrors, or confusional arousals. In most cases, several high-amplitude delta-frequency EEG waves occur immediately before the sudden arousal from SWS. Within the 10–12 seconds prior to the first EMG artifact associated with the complex behavior, there is a relative increase in the low delta power (0.75–2.0 Hz), compared to the previous background. This burst of high-amplitude repetitive and monomorphic slow delta waves visually correlates with the A1 subtypes of CAP.

Since high-amplitude waves are also part of the CAP, and hypersynchronous slow delta is part of the phase A1 and possibly A2 of the CAP,[35] different studies tried to evaluate CAP in sleepwalking and sleep terrors subjects, with conflicting results. Zucconi et al. (1995) found an increase of A1% and of CAP rate, and a decrease in phase B duration. Guilleminault et al.[57,59] also found an increase in CAP rate but also in A2 and A3 index, while A1 index was decreased.

A more recent study on 10 children with sleep terrors versus controls showed an increase of total CAP rate in SWS, of A1 index in SWS, and of the mean duration of A phases while B phases had a decreased duration, exclusively in SWS. The normalized CAP interval-distribution graphs showed significant differences in SWS with interval classes 10 seconds $\leq i < 35$ seconds higher in children with ST and interval classes above 50 seconds higher in normal controls. Therefore, this study clearly showed that children with ST presented faster alternations of the amplitude of slow EEG bursts during SWS (Fig. 13.5). This abnormally fast alternation of the EEG amplitude in SWS is linked to the frequent intrusion of CAP B phases interrupting the continuity of slow delta activity and could be considered as a neurophysiologic marker of sleep terrors and in general of disorders of arousals.[60,61]

Guilleminault,[59] when commenting the paper of Pilon et al.,[58] highlighted the importance of the CAP phase B, reporting that what is abnormal in sleepwalking is not the HSD per se, but the reappearance of the background activity (phase B) that interrupts the persistence of the slow delta and determines the bursting pattern of delta during SWS and, finally, questions why the delta burst (CAP A1) is abruptly interrupted.[59] It might be possible to hypothesize that the numerous recurrent arousals from SWS create a slow-wave activity (SWA) deficit within sleep, leading to a continued SWA reappearance due to an ultra-short intrasleep recovery process in SWS parasomnia. The coexistence of pressure for delta sleep and a high level of arousal intrusion in SWS might contribute to triggering SWS parasomnias, confirming the hypothesis of Broughton[62,63] that arousal disorders are precipitating factors for some sleep disturbances related to delta sleep, such as somnambulism and sleep terrors and also Espa et al.[55] concluded, in adults, that high SWS fragmentation might be responsible for the occurrence of sleepwalking or sleep terrors episodes.

Halasz et al.[64] found that in patients with sleepwalking/night terrors the number of slow type arousals increased and extended to every non-REM stage compared to normal subjects. Both Schenck et al.[65] and Gaudreau et al.[66] observed an increase of delta EEG hypersynchrony at the beginning of the sleepwalking event, suggesting a compensatory sleep defending action of slow activity against awakening. Guilleminault et al.[57] also hypothesize that the increase in relative low delta power just prior to the EMG increase may translate a feedback mechanism within a corticothalamic loop to maintain sleep and limit arousal.

This response may be responsible for the confused state seen as a consequence of these conflicting influences on the thalamus. In sleep bruxism, motor episodes show an impressive association with CAP cycles and a close temporal linkage with phase A. In contrast to other parasomnias, bruxism episodes often occur during subtypes A3[34].

Further support to the modulatory role of CAP to parasomnias has been provided by a PSG study carried out on a 9-year-old boy affected by a rhythmic movement disorder. Body banging and body rolling were found to be intimately linked to unstable non-REM sleep, as shown by their close association with the A phases of CAP.[67]

CENTRAL PATTERN GENERATORS AND THE UNIFYING ROLE OF AROUSAL

Virtually no nervous function exists without a time metric, be it the simplest motor or the most complex cognitive act. Bipedal walking is a periodic series of forward falls interrupted regularly by alternate extensions of each leg. It is almost as natural to us as breathing. This exercise is made

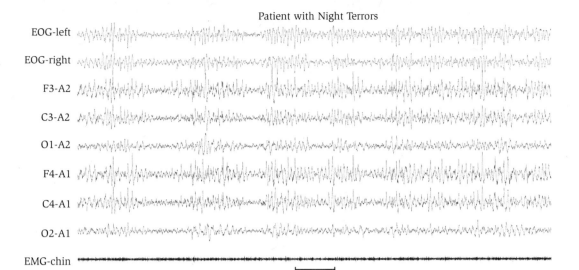

Patient with Night Terrors

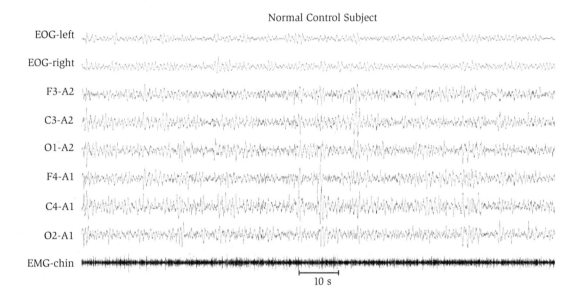

Normal Control Subject

FIGURE 13.5   Example of slow-wave sleep rich in short interruptions of the slow delta activity (B phases of cyclic alternating pattern) in a patient with sleep terrors, compared to the more continuous delta activity during the same sleep stage in a normal control. EMG, electromyogram; EOG, electro-oculogram.

possible by the predictive nature of the spinal cord oscillators. This general mechanism is the same in all animals, including eight-legged scorpions and centipedes. The notion that oscillators or "central pattern generators" are responsible for the coordination of motor patterns, such as breathing and walking, is a consolidated issue in neuroscience. Oscillators coordinate or "synchronize" various operations with and across

neuronal networks. Moreover, neuronal oscillators are involved in other brain-generated functions, including sleep. Sleep is the default state of the brain—default in the sense that it develops as a self-organized or spontaneaous state without an external supervisor.

Privileging a neuroethological interpretation,Tassinari and coworkers[68] have repeatedly assumed that the motor pattern of hyperkinetic automatisms observed in nocturnal frontal lobe epilepsy (NFLE) strongly resembles the ancient stereotyped behavior of reptiles or human neonates. Defensive postures, violent gestures, emotional behavior, and sudden arousals, which characterize most of the motor events in NFLE, recall archaic automatic motor sequences elicited not by direct epileptic activation, but triggered by the activation of ancient central pattern generators situated in subcortical structures. The release is due to an arousal activated by epileptic discharges during sleep.[69]

Oldani et al.,[70] Provini et al.,[71] and Zucconi et al.[72] described a continuum of motor phenomena from "minimal" to "major" seizure events in NFLE. The minor events were termed as fragments of the NFLE major episodes, although they often simulate normal behavior. The overlap between normal and pathologic events can be explored, matching the different motor patterns before and after effective treatment. In a patient with NFLE treated with carbamazepine, a number of global body movements evoked by an arousal and compatible with physiologic motor patterns replaced an equivalent number of arousal-induced major episodes recorder in the untreated baseline condition.[73] In a patient with NFLE with periodic leg movements, stereotactically implanted intracerebral multilead electrodes showed the presence of a left frontal lobe focus undetected on scalp EEG. During non-REM sleep, epileptic discharges always occurred in relation with an A phase, while PLMs occurred always within or immediately following an A phase.[74]

In a young subject, a given arousal event during non-REM sleep will evoke a nocturnal seizure if the cerebral frontal areas are activated by epileptic discharges, or a sleepwalking behavior if the frontal regions are depressed. Neuroimaging investigation has shown that the dorsolateral frontal cortex, which is responsible for high executive cognitive functions, appears functionally depressed during non-REM sleep.[75] Sustained functional depression, as occurs in conditions of sleep inertia, can cause a dissociation between sleep and wakefulness, which is the essential assumed mechanism behind "arousal disorders."[63]

Meletti et al.[76] described a case of teeth grinding as a constant and main manifestation of an epileptic seizure. The magnetic resonance imaging evidence of left-sided hippocampal sclerosis (confirmed by pathology) and the postsurgery seizure-free outcome supported evidence of the epileptic origin of this phenomenon in the patient. The clinical report indicated that a teeth-grinding event can be not only a parasomnia but also an epileptic-related motor event. Moreover, in the described patient, mesial temporal epileptic discharges led to the appearance not only of teeth grinding but also of rhythmic foot movements. The continuum from physiologic rhythmic mastication during sleep of a healthy subject to seizure-related bruxism, with intermediate values for sleep bruxism, suggests the activation of common central pattern generators involved in the regulation of masticatory rhythms in physiologic (sleep) or pathologic (seizure-related) conditions. In particular, these data suggest that brainstem central pattern generators for masticatory pattern can be set in motion by different conditions in order to generate rhythmic jaw muscle activities that share similar EMG and autonomic features.[77]

The trigger event can be an increased level of arousal, which can occur as a paraphysiologic manifestation, that is, sleep bruxism or chewing, or be induced by an epileptic discharge, as observed in the described patient.[78]

Taken together, these findings suggest that arousal during sleep is the common condition for the onset of motor patterns which are already written in the brain codes (central pattern generators) but that require a certain degree of activation (arousal) to become visibly apparent. In this case, arousal acts as a trigger releasing or facilitating an encoded "kinetic melody."[79]

In conclusion, arousal can appear either spontaneously or be elicited by internal or external stimuli. In non-REM sleep, where muscle tone is still operative, EEG synchrony reaches multiple levels of expression (from stage N1 to N3) and a variety of motor events can take place from seizures to parasomnias. Whether the outcome is a muscle jerk or a major epileptic attack will depend on a number of ongoing factors (sleep stage, delta power, motor chain, etc.) but all events will share the common trait of arousal-activated phenomena.

REFERENCES

1. Buzsaki G. *Rhythms of the Brain*. New York: Oxford University Press; 2006.
1a. Terzano MG, Mancia D, Salati MR, et al. The cyclic alternating pattern as a physiologic component of normal NREM sleep. *Sleep* 1985;8:137–45.
2. Terzano MG, Parrino L, Smerieri A, et al. Atlas, rules, and recording techniques for the

scoring of cyclic alternating pattern (CAP) in human sleep. *Sleep Med* 2001;2:537–53.

3. Terzano MG, Parrino L, Fioriti G, et al. JP. Modifications of sleep structure induced by increasing levels of acoustic perturbation in normal subjects. *Electroencephalogr Clin Neurophysiol* 1990;76:29–38.

4. Smerieri A, Parrino L, Agosti M, et al. Cyclic alternating pattern sequences and non-cyclic alternating pattern periods in human sleep. *Clin Neurophysiol* 2007;118:2305–13.

5. Terzano MG, Parrino L, Spaggiari MC, et al. Mutual cooperation between cyclic alternating pattern and major dynamic events of sleep. In: Barthouil P, ed. *Insomnie et Imidazopyridines.* Amsterdam, The Netherlands: Excerpta Medica; 1990:262–70.

5a. Schieber JP, Muzet A, Ferriere PJR. Les phases d'activation transitoire spontanées au cours du sommeil chez l'homme. *Arch Sci Physiol* 1971;25:443–65.

6. Terzano MG, Parrino L, Boselli M, et al. Polysomnographic analysis of arousal responses in obstructive sleep apnea syndrome by means of the cyclic alternating pattern (CAP). *J Clin Neurophysiol* 1996;13:145–55.

7. Terzano MG, Parrino L. Origin and significance of the cyclic alternating pattern (CAP). *Sleep Med Rev* 2000;4:101–23.

8. Parrino L, Smerieri A, Rossi M, et al. Relationship of slow and rapid EEG components of CAP to ASDA arousals in normal sleep. *Sleep* 2001;24:881–5.

9. Terzano MG, Parrino L, Rosa A, et al. CAP and arousals in the structural development of sleep: an integrative perspective. *Sleep Med* 2002;3:221–9.

10. Martin SE, Wraith PK, Deary IJ, et al. The effect of nonvisible sleep fragmentation on daytime function. *Am J Respir Crit Care Med* 1997;155:1596–601.

11. Hirshkowitz M. Arousals and anti-arousals. *Sleep Med* 2002;3:203–4.

12. Halasz P. Arousals without awakening. Dynamic aspect of sleep. *Physiol Behav* 1993;54:795–802.

13. Crunelli V, Hughes SW. The slow (<1 Hz) rhythm of non-REM sleep: a dialogue between three cardinal oscillators. *Nat Neurosci* 2010;13(1):9–17.

14. Halasz P. Hierarchy of micro-arousals and the microstructure of sleep. *Neurophysiol Clin* 1998;28:461–75.

15. De Gennaro L, Ferrara M, Spadini V, et al. The cyclic alternating pattern decreases as a consequence of total sleep deprivation and correlates with EEG arousals. *Neuropsychobiology* 2002;45(2):95–8.

16. De Carli F, Nobili L, Beelke M, et al. Quantitative analysis of sleep EEG microstructure in the time-frequency domain. *Brain Res Bull* 2004;63:399–405.

17. Ferri R, Rundo F, Bruni O, et al. Dynamics of the EEG slowwave synchronization during sleep. *Clin Neurophysiol* 2005;116:2783–95.

18. Ferri R, Bruni O, Miano S, et al. Topographic mapping of the spectral components of the cyclic alternating pattern (CAP). *Sleep Med* 2005;6:29–36.

19. Togo F, Cherniack NS, Natelson BH. Electroencephalogram characteristics of autonomic arousals during sleep in healthy men. *Clin Neurophysiol* 2006;117:2597–603.

20. Guilleminault C, Stoohs R. Arousal, increased respiratory efforts, blood pressure and obstructive sleep apnoea. *J Sleep Res* 1995;4:117–24.

21. Ferri R, Parrino L, Smerieri A, et al. Cyclic alternating pattern and spectral analysis of heart rate variability during normal sleep. *J Sleep Res* 2000;9:13–18.

22. Sforza E, Jouny C, Ibanez V. Cardiac activation during arousal in humans: further evidence for hierarchy in the arousal response. *Clin Neurophysiol* 2000;111:1611–19.

23. Thomas RJ. Arousals in sleep-disordered breathing: patterns and implications. *Sleep* 2003;26:1042–7.

24. Rechtschaffen A, Kales A. eds. *A Manual of Standardized Terminology, Techniques and Scoring System for Sleep Stages of Human Subjects. Brain Information Service/Brain Research Institute.* Los Angeles: University of California at Los Angeles; 1968.

25. American Sleep Disorders Association. EEG arousals: scoring rules and examples. *Sleep* 1992;15:173–84.

26. Rees K, Spence DP, Earis JE, et al. Arousal responses from apneic events during non-rapid eye movement sleep. *Am J Respir Crit Care Med* 1995;152:1016–21.

27. McNamara F, Lijowaska AS, Thach BT. Spontaneous arousal activity in infants during NREM and REM sleep. *J Physiol* 2002;538:263–9.

28. Parrino L, Halasz P, Tassinari CA, et al. CAP, epilepsy and motor events during sleep: the unifying role of arousal. *Sleep Med Rev* 2006;10:267–85.

29. Zucconi M, Oldani A, Ferini-Strambi L, et al. Arousal fluctuations in nonrapid eye movement parasomnias: the role of cyclic alternating pattern as a measure of sleep instability. *J Clin Neurophysiol* 1995;12:147–54.

30. Parrino L, Smerieri A, Boselli M, et al. Sleep reactivity during acute nasal CPAP in obstructive sleep apnea syndrome. *Neurology* 2000;54:1633–40.

31. Parrino L, Smerieri A, Spaggiari MC, et al. Cyclic alternating pattern (CAP) and epilepsy during sleep: how a physiological rhythm modulates a pathological event. *Clin Neurophysiol* 2000;111(Suppl. 2):S39–46.

32. Parrino L, Ferri R, Bruni O, et al. Cyclic alternating pattern (CAP): the marker of sleep instability. *Sleep Med Rev* 2012;16: 27–45

33. Parrino L, Boselli M, Buccino GP, et al. The cyclic alternating pattern plays a gate-control on periodic limb movements during non-rapid eye movement sleep. *J Clin Neurophysiol* 1996;13:314–23.

34. Macaluso GM, Guerra P, Di Giovanni G, et al. Sleep bruxism is a disorder related to periodic arousals during sleep. *J Dent Res* 1998;77:565–73.

35. Guilleminault C, Kirisoglu C, da Rosa AC, et al. Sleepwalking, a disorder of NREM sleep instability. *Sleep Med* 2006;7:163–70.

36. Parrino L, Thomas RJ, Smerieri A, Spaggiari MC, Del Felice A, Terzano MG. Reorganization of sleep patterns in severe OSAS under prolonged CPAP treatment. *Clin Neurophysiol* 2005;116:2228–39

37. Halasz P, Terzano MG, Parrino L, et al. The nature of arousal in sleep. *J Sleep Res* 2004;13:1–23.

38. Ferri R, Rundo F, Bruni O, et al. Small-world network organization of functional connectivity of EEG slow-wave activity during sleep. *Clin Neurophysiol* 2007;118:449–56.

39. Ferri R, Zucconi M, Rundo F, et al. Heart rate and spectral EEG changes accompanying periodic and non-periodic leg movements during sleep. *Clin Neurophysiol* 2007;118:438–48.

40. Poyares D, Guilleminault C, Rosa A, et al. Arousal, EEG spectral power and pulse transit time in UARS and mild OSAS subjects. *Clin Neurophysiol* 2002;113:1598–606.

41. Guilleminault C, Lopes MC, Hagen CC, et al. The cyclic alternating pattern demonstrates increased sleep instability and correlates with fatigue and sleepiness in adults with upper airway resistance syndrome. *Sleep* 2007;30:641–7.

42. Bara-Jimenez W, Aksu M, Graham B, et al. Periodic limb movements in sleep: state-dependent excitability of the spinal flexor reflex. *Neurology* 2000;54:1609–16.

43. Esteves AM, de Mello MT, Lancellotti CL, et al. Occurrence of limb movement during sleep in rats with spinal cord injury. *Brain Res* 2004;1017:32–8.

44. Ferrillo F, Beelke M, Canovaro P, et al. Changes in cerebral and autonomic activity heralding periodic limb movements in sleep. *Sleep Med* 2004;5:407–12.

45. Allena M, Campus C, Morrone E, et al. Periodic limb movements both in non-REM and REM sleep: relationships between cerebral and autonomic activities. *Clin Neurophysiol* 2009;120(7):1282–90

46. Winkelman JW. The evoked heart rate response to periodic leg movements of sleep. *Sleep* 1999;22:575–80.

47. Gosselin N, Lanfranchi P, Michaud M, et al. Age and gender effects on heart rate activation associated with periodic leg movements in patients with restless legs syndrome. *Clin Neurophysiol* 2003;114:2188–95.

48. Sforza E, Pichot V, Barthelemy JC, et al. Cardiovascular variability during periodic leg movements: a spectral analysis approach. *Clin Neurophysiol* 2005;116:1096–104

49. Sforza E, Juony C, Ibanez V. Time-dependent variation in cerebral and autonomic activity during periodic leg movements in sleep: implications for arousal mechanisms. *Clin Neurophysiol* 2002;113:883–91.

50. Steriade M, Nunez A, Amzica F. A novel slow (<1 Hz) oscillation of neocortical neurons in vivo: depolarizing and hyperpolarizing components. *J Neurosci* 1993;13:3252–65

51. Steriade M. The corticothalamic system in sleep. *Front Biosci* 2003;8:878–99.

52. Achermann P, Borbely AA. Low-frequency (<1 Hz) oscillations in the human sleep electroencephalogram. *Neuroscience* 1997;81:213–22.

53. Ferri R, Zucconi M, Manconi M, Plazzi G, Bruni O, Ferini-Strambi L.New approaches to the study of periodic leg movements during sleep in restless legs syndrome. Sleep. 2006 June;29(6):759–69.

54. Ferri R, Manconi M, Aricò D, et al. Acute dopamine-agonist treatment in restless legs syndrome: effects on sleep architecture and NREM sleep instability. *Sleep* 2010;33(6):793–800.

55. Espa F, Ondze B, Deglise P, et al. Sleep architecture, slow wave activity, and sleep spindles in adult patients with sleepwalking and sleep terrors. *Clin Neurophysiol* 2000;111:929–39.

56. Pressman MR. Hypersynchronous delta sleep EEG activity and sudden arousals from slow-wave sleep in adults without a history of parasomnias: clinical and forensic implications. *Sleep* 2004;27:706–10.

57. Guilleminault C, Lee JH, Chan A, et al. Non-REM-sleep instability in recurrent sleepwalking in pre-pubertal children. *Sleep Med* 2005;6:515–21.

58. Pilon M, Zadra A, Joncas S, et al. Hypersynchronous delta waves and somnambulism: brain topography and effect of sleep deprivation. *Sleep* 2006;29:77–84.

59. Guilleminault C. Hypersynchronous slow delta, cyclic alternating pattern and sleepwalking. *Sleep* 2006;29:14–15.

60. Bruni O, Ferri R, Novelli L, et al. NREM sleep instability in children with sleep terrors: the role of slow wave activity interruptions. *Clin Neurophysiol* 2008;119:985–92.

61. Bruni O, Novelli L, Miano S, et al. Cyclic alternating pattern: a window into pediatric sleep. *Sleep Med* 2010;11:628–36.

62. Broughton R, Billings R, Cartwright R, et al. Homicidal somnambulism: a case report. *Sleep* 1994;17(3):253–64.

63. Broughton RJ. Sleep disorders: disorders of arousal? Enuresis, somnambulism, and nightmares occur in confusional states of arousal, not in "dreaming sleep" *Science* 1968;159:1070–8.

64. Halasz P, Ujszaszi J, Gadoros J. Are microarousals preceded by electroencephalographic slow wave synchronization precursors of confusional awakenings? *Sleep* 1985;8:231–8.

65. Schenck CH, Pareja JA, Patterson AL, et al. Analysis of polysomnographic events surrounding 252 slow-wave sleep arousals in thirty-eight adults with injurious sleepwalking and sleep terrors. *J Clin Neurophysiol* 1998;15:159–66.

66. Gaudreau H, Joncas S, Zadra A, et al. Dynamics of slow-wave activity during the NREM sleep of sleepwalkers and control subjects. *Sleep* 2000;23:755–60.

67. Manni R, Terzaghi M, Sartori I, et al. Rhythmic movement disorder and cyclic alternating pattern during sleep: a video-polysomnographic study in a 9-year-old boy. *Mov Disord* 2004;19:1186–90.

68. Tassinari CA, Gardella E, Meletti S, et al. The neuroethological interpretation of motor behaviours in "nocturnal-hyperkinetic-frontal seizures": emergence of "innate" motor behaviours and role of central pattern generators. In: Beaumanoir A, Andermann F, Chauvel P, Mira L, Zifkin B, eds. *Frontal Seizures and Epilepsies in Children*. London: John Libbey Eurotext; 2003:43–8.

69. Tassinari CA, Rubboli G, Gardella E, et al. Central pattern generators for a common semiology in fronto-limbic seizures and in parasomnias. A neuroethologic approach. *Neurol Sci* 2005;26(Suppl 3):s225–32.

70. Oldani A, Zucconi M, Asselta R, et al. Autosomal dominant nocturnal frontal lobe epilepsy. A video-polysomnographic and genetic appraisal of 40 patients and delineation of the epileptic syndrome. *Brain* 1998;121:205–23.

71. Provini F, Plazzi G, Montagna P, et al. The wide clinical spectrum of nocturnal frontal lobe epilepsy. *Sleep Med Rev* 2000;4:375–86.

72. Zucconi M, Oldani A, Ferini-Strambi L, et al. Nocturnal paroxysmal arousals with motor behaviors during sleep: frontal lobe epilepsy or parasomnia? *J Clin Neurophysiol* 1997;14:513–22

73. Terzano MG, Monge-Strauss MF, Mikol F, et al. Cyclic alternating pattern as a provocative factor in nocturnal paroxysmal dystonia. *Epilepsia* 1997;38: 1015–25

74. Nobili L, Sartori I, Terzaghi M, et al. Relationship of epileptic discharges to arousal instability and periodic leg movements in a case of nocturnal frontal lobe epilepsy: a stereo-EEG study. *Sleep* 2006;29(5):701–4.

75. Braun AR, Balkin TJ, Wesenten NJ, et al. Regional cerebral blood flow throughout the sleep–wake cycle. An H2(15)O PET study. *Brain* 1997;120:1173–97.

76. Meletti S, Cantalupo G, Volpi L, et al. Rhythmic teeth grinding induced by temporal lobe seizures. *Neurology* 2004;62:2306–9.

77. Lavigne G, Kato T, Kolta A, et al. Neurobiological mechanisms involved in sleep bruxism. *Crit Rev Oral Biol Med* 2003;14:30–46.

78. Halasz P, Ujszaszi J. Chewing automatisms in sleep connected with micro-arousals: an indicator of propensity to confusional awakening? In: Koella WP, Obal H, Schulz H, Visser P, eds. *Sleep 86*. Stuttgart, Germany: Gustav Fischer Verlag; 1998:235–9.

79. Luria AR. *The Working Brain*. London: Penguin; 1973.

14

Assessment of Daytime Sleepiness

ANITA VALANJU SHELGIKAR AND RONALD D. CHERVIN

EXCESSIVE DAYTIME sleepiness (EDS) is among the most important consequences of disrupted or insufficient nocturnal sleep. Some neurological disorders can also cause EDS directly, without commensurate disruption of nocturnal sleep. Defined as difficulty with maintenance of alert wakefulness, sleepiness is considered excessive when it occurs in inappropriate circumstances.[1] The complaint of EDS is among those most commonly encountered by sleep medicine specialists and also arises often in the practices of primary clinicians and neurologists. Movement disorders that can disrupt nocturnal sleep and cause EDS are covered in detail in subsequent chapters. This chapter describes approaches to the assessment of EDS more generally. Careful assessment of EDS can generate important diagnostic clues, help define the impact of a disorder, and provide a measure of treatment response.

The clinical history is the most important tool in the assessment of EDS. The physical examination plays only a minor role, in part because the stimulating environment of the examination room often eliminates physical signs that might otherwise be informative. Formal tests of sleepiness are useful when the history is unclear, EDS is an essential diagnostic consideration, treatment decisions are affected by the extent of sleepiness, or a more reliable longitudinal measure of sleepiness is desired. Such tests can be subjective or objective: Both types can follow standard, validated methods, but the former rely on a patient's self-assessment, whereas the latter are usually based on neurophysiologic measures. Tests do not obviate the need for a thorough history, and interpretations must be made in the context of other clinical information that has been obtained.

HISTORY

Direct questions about EDS are often a useful starting point, and chronic EDS is the reason that many patients seek a clinician's help. However, for some individuals sleepiness has been present so long that the condition may not be considered abnormal. Patients' innate ability to perceive sleepiness or willingness to admit it may also vary widely.

An essential component of the sleep history is determination of the sleep schedule, which may vary from weekdays and weekends. The patient's bedtime, latency to sleep, wake time, and final rise time from bed should be ascertained. The frequency, duration, and etiology of nocturnal awakenings should also be discussed. Endorsement of daytime sleepiness warrants further questioning to elucidate symptoms of sleep disorders commonly associated with daytime sleepiness, such as obstructive sleep apnea, narcolepsy, or behaviorally induced insufficient sleep syndrome. A thorough medical and psychiatric history, including medication use, should be obtained to determine other factors that may exacerbate daytime sleepiness. The patient's need for daytime naps and propensity to doze unintentionally should also be discussed in detail.

One of the ways to refine the reliability and comparability of historical information is to ask questions about the types of situations in which sleepiness is likely to be a problem. Such questions also allow better assessment of both the severity and functional impact of EDS. A report of dozing during a 1-hour morning commute by train does not suggest a degree of sleepiness as unusual as sleepiness that might allow a patient to doze off during a personal meeting with an employer. Questions about sleepiness while driving are particularly important because automobile accidents, injuries, and deaths represent some of the most severe potential consequences of EDS.[2] Sleepiness also can affect quality of life due to impaired ability to enjoy hobbies, free time, and social events. Work productivity and job performance can also decline due to daytime sleepiness. Complaints associated with sleepiness may include poor concentration, impaired memory, irritability, and emotional lability; these, in turn, can adversely affect an individual's interpersonal relationships.

Whenever possible, the history also should be obtained from the patient's family and bed partner. The bed partner's reports are often invaluable aids in diagnosis of a nocturnal sleep disorder. The bed partner's or other family members' descriptions about the patient's daytime behavior may differ considerably from the history given by the patient; the additional information may help to illustrate the effect that EDS has on the patient's overall function. Signs of sleepiness may be much more apparent to family members than to the patient: What may be vaguely recalled as occasional pleasant naps after dinner by the patient may be described by a spouse as a more worrisome inability to participate in family affairs. Some evidence suggests that men in particular, as compared with women, fail to recognize or admit EDS documented with objective testing. In one study of 190 male and female sleep apneics, the odds ratios for female gender and reports of frequent sleepiness, fatigue, tiredness, and lack of energy were respectively 2.1, 2.8, 3.4, and 4.1 (all $p < .05$), and results showed little change after controlling for multiple sleep latency test (MSLT) results, apnea severity, and age.[3]

Traditional teaching suggests that although complaints of sleepiness are likely to represent a sleep disorder, symptoms such as fatigue, tiredness, and lack of energy suggest other medical problems, for example, thyroid dysfunction or depression. However, patients with obstructive sleep apnea syndrome usually prefer terms other than *sleepiness*—in particular, *fatigue*, *tiredness*, and *lack of energy*—to describe their major problem[3] or to describe treatment benefits that are most important to them.[4] Further research is needed to better define how patients use these terms and how to quantify these other symptoms, so that they can be better identified and followed. Clinicians should realize that some overlap exists and investigations of EDS should also include questions about related symptoms.

PHYSICAL EXAMINATION

Although the absence of physical signs of sleepiness contributes little to an evaluation for a complaint of EDS, positive findings can help confirm a severe problem. Some patients fall asleep while waiting for the clinician or even while the clinician is present. Occasional patients can be observed to yawn excessively, remain unusually still, have difficulty keeping their eyes open, blink less often than might be expected, or lose concentration easily. Often a subjectively sleepy facial appearance is present but only recognized in retrospect after diagnosis and treatment have rendered the patient considerably more refreshed. Dark, "baggy" circles under the eyes, as a sign of sleepiness, are a popular notion but have received scant medical study.

A general physical exam should be performed to assess for systemic abnormalities, such as cardiac arrhythmia or signs of hypothyroidism, which may contribute to sleepiness or fatigue. Thorough examination of the nasal and oral airways is particularly important in the clinical assessment for sleep-disordered breathing. A neurological examination should also be performed and may be particularly helpful in rare circumstances. For example, tumors in the region of the third ventricle or myotonic dystrophy can cause EDS; weakness precipitated by laughter and accompanied by loss of previously demonstrated reflexes can confirm cataplexy.

TESTING
Subjective Tests

The Stanford Sleepiness Scale and Karolinska Sleepiness Scale provide well-validated, standardized ways to quickly assess instantaneous sleepiness. They each ask the patient to select, from among several descriptions of sleepiness levels, the one level that best describes his or her current state.[5–8]

A more long-term assessment is provided by the Epworth Sleepiness Scale (ESS) (Fig. 14.1), now the most commonly used subjective standardized assessment for adult EDS. This instrument asks the respondent to rate, on a Likert scale of 0, 1, 2, or 3, the likelihood of dozing during eight different sedentary situations. The popularity of this instrument stems, in part, from face validity, initial reports of criterion validity, good reliability, and cost savings in comparison to objective testing. Some studies have utilized the ESS as a measure of treatment response to continuous positive airway pressure (CPAP) in patients with obstructive sleep apnea.[9,10] However, studies that established

Epworth Sleepiness Scale

Name: _____ Today's date: _____

Your age (Yrs): _____ Your sex (Male = M, Female = F): _____

How likely are you to doze off or fall asleep in the following situations, in contrast to feeling just tired?

This refers to your usual way of life in recent times.

Even if you haven't done some of these things recently try to work out how they would have affected you.

Use the following scale to choose the **most appropriate number** for each situation:

> 0 = would **never** doze
> 1 = **slight chance** of dozing
> 2 = **moderate chance** of dozing
> 3 = **high chance** of dozing

It is important that you answer each question as best you can.

Situation	Chance of Dozing (0–3)
Sitting and reading _____	____
Watching TV _____	____
Sitting, inactive in a public place (e.g. a theatre or a meeting) _____	____
As a passenger in a car for an hour without a break _____	____
Lying down to rest in the afternoon when circumstances permit _____	____
Sitting and talking to someone _____	____
Sitting quietly after a lunch without alcohol _____	____
In a car, while stopped for a few minutes in the traffic _____	____

THANK YOU FOR YOUR COOPERATION
© M.W. Johns 1990–97

FIGURE 14.1 The Epworth Sleepiness Scale. (From Johns MW. A new method for measuring daytime sleepiness: the Epworth sleepiness scale. Sleep 1991;14:540–5.)

validity of the instrument reported only weak to moderate associations between ESS scores and objective assessments of sleepiness.[7,8] Some more recent reports have failed to identify any statistically significant associations between ESS results and objective measures of sleepiness or nocturnal sleep pathology.[11-13] The ESS was developed as a tool to distinguish individuals with excessive daytime sleepiness from alert individuals,[14] and some data support its use in the assessment of treatment response.[15] These issues are discussed in more detail later, but in short, the ESS may not serve well as a substitute for objective neurophysiologic measures, although it can provide a standardized measure that facilitates comparisons of self-assessed sleepiness between different persons, time points, or treatment conditions.

Whereas the questionnaire instruments discussed earlier seek to measure sleepiness, the Functional Outcomes of Sleep Questionnaire (FOSQ) provides some assessment of the impact EDS may have on a patient's health-related quality of life.[16] Generic quality-of-life measures, such as the Short Form-36 (SF-36) and the Nottingham Health Profile,[17-19] also reflect the effects of sleep disorders, but the FOSQ offers a validated measure more specific for EDS.

The Medical Outcomes Study-Sleep Scale (MOS-Sleep) is a self-administered tool that assesses the responder's sleep over the prior 4 weeks.[20] The MOS-Sleep is a 12-item scale, though information can be summarized across nine items as well. This scale is divided into six sections: "sleep disturbance," "snoring," "sleep awakening short of breath or with headache," "sleep adequacy," "somnolence," and "quantity of sleep/optimal sleep."[20] The MOS-Sleep was initially developed and tested in a sample of 3445 individuals with chronic illness[20]; reliability and validity for this tool have been reported in the general population and in patients with neuropathic pain,[21] and in patients with overactive bladder.[22]

Subjective measures of sleepiness and its impact in children have not been extensively developed or tested. The Sleep Disturbance Scale for Children is a parental questionnaire that contains several items about excessive somnolence, and results appear to distinguish children with sleep disorders from controls.[23] A four-item sleepiness subscale from another parental questionnaire, the Pediatric Sleep Questionnaire, similarly appears to distinguish children with obstructive sleep-disordered breathing from controls.[24] This is the only subjective pediatric sleepiness scale that has been validated against objective Multiple Sleep Latency Tests.[25] However, the Epworth Sleepiness Scale has also been modified for use in children.[26] The Pediatric Daytime Sleepiness Scale (PDSS) has been developed to assess EDS in middle school-aged children.[27]

Nocturnal Polysomnography

Nocturnal polysomnography, described in detail as a diagnostic tool in another chapter, also provides some objective information about a patient's sleepiness. Findings that suggest EDS include short sleep latencies, increased sleep efficiency, and increased slow-wave sleep. However, sleep disorders that cause EDS may also obscure sleep architectural clues. Perhaps for that reason, a study of 147 patients suspected on clinical grounds to have EDS found that the only valid and statistically significant polysomnographic correlate of MSLT results was nocturnal sleep latency (Spearman $rho = .45, p < .0001$).[28] In some individuals with obstructive sleep apnea, even this correlate may be inaccurate, because respiratory events may begin within the first seconds of sleep onset and cause enough wake time to delay scoring of the first 30-second epoch of sleep. A study of 42 Parkinson's disease patients and 30 healthy controls showed that PD patients as a group had lower sleep efficiency, greater amount of Stage 2 sleep, and a lower percentage of REM sleep compared to controls.[29] These findings were seen in Parkinson's disease patients with and without EDS, which suggests that daytime sleepiness in Parkinson's disease is multifactorial and not only attributable to changes in sleep architecture. Nocturnal polysomnographic evidence of excessive sleepiness is more reliable when the underlying cause is insufficient sleep, an environmental problem at home, or some other disorder that is not an intrinsic dyssomnia. Polysomnography generally is not considered reliable enough as a measure of EDS to be used alone as an objective test for that condition. Nocturnal polysomnography can definitively evaluate for sleep-disordered breathing, which, depending upon the clinical history, may contribute to the patient's daytime sleepiness.

Multiple Sleep Latency Test

In clinical practice, the MSLT is an imperfect but essentially gold-standard objective test for

EDS.[30] The test requires a patient to try to fall sleep at several intervals spaced throughout the day, and the main result is the mean sleep latency (MSL) as determined by polysomnography. The MSLT was developed in the 1970s by researchers at Stanford,[31] who described it as a test of physiologic sleep tendency.[32] Experimental sleep deprivation paradigms were used to validate the MSLT. Utility in the diagnosis of narcolepsy was quickly established,[33] and clinicians soon discovered that patients with hypersomnolence resulting from several different sleep disorders could be distinguished from normal subjects by the results of the MSLT.[34] Advantages of the MSLT over other objective tests of sleepiness include its measurement of an important functional consequence of sleepiness (falling asleep) and its assessment of daytime sleepiness at several different circadian time points instead of just one.[35]

Technical guidelines for recording MSLTs require that a referential electroencephalogram (EEG) is recorded from central (C3-A2, C4-A1) and occipital (O1-A2, O2,-A1) leads.[30] Two electrodes near the outer canthus of each eye provide an electrooculogram (EOG). Mental or submental surface electromyogram (EMG) and echocardiogram (EKG) are also recorded. Equipment to record airflow, chest and abdominal excursion, and respiratory sounds is not required to distinguish wakefulness from sleep, though these added measures can sometimes help clarify the point of sleep onset. The additional leads may also reveal, on occasion, that the MSL is confounded by the arousing effects of a primary sleep disorder, such as obstructive sleep apnea.

Recommendations for the MSLT protocol, detailed in Figure 14.2, include maintenance of a 2-week sleep diary prior to testing, complete discontinuation of antidepressant and stimulant medication for a minimum of 2 weeks, and performance of a nocturnal polysomnogram with at least 6 hours of recorded sleep prior to administration of the first nap trial. The recommended MSLT protocol (Fig. 14.2) includes five nap attempts spaced throughout the day, usually at 2-hour intervals.[30] The environment should be quiet, dark, comfortable, and conducive to sleep. The patient is instructed to lie quietly, close the eyes, and try to sleep. Sleep onset is defined as the first 30-second epoch during which at least 15 seconds of sleep is recorded.[30] The nap attempt is terminated after 20 minutes if no sleep has occurred. If sleep does occur, the patient is allowed to remain in bed at least 15 minutes from that point forward to observe whether rapid eye movement (REM) sleep is obtained. The sleep latencies recorded at each nap attempt, and 20 minutes if no sleep occurred, are averaged across the five nap attempts to generate the MSL. Another result that is important in some cases is the number of naps during which REM sleep occurs: two or more sleep-onset REM periods (SOREMPs) support a diagnosis of narcolepsy in the appropriate clinical context.

Although many clinicians view the MSL as a continuous variable that reflects sleepiness, interpretation of what constitutes normal or abnormal results is not yet based on adequate data with which to link specific MSLT results with significant health-related outcomes. Instead, published clinical observational data have led to consensus recommendations that an MSL below 5 minutes reflects abnormal sleepiness, whereas an MSL above 10 minutes is a normal result. Many recognize a diagnostic "gray zone" between 8 and 10 minutes.[34,36] These limits have arisen from sleep-deprivation paradigms and clinical experience rather than from well-designed, prospective, and outcome-based clinical research among patients and controls. Prior to the 2005 publication of *Practice Parameters for Clinical Use of the MSLT*,[30] some sleep laboratories used four-nap trials while others used five-nap trials during the MSLT. Normative data differ depending upon the testing protocol utilized. A summary of pooled control mean sleep latency values obtained during MSLT across all age groups showed that the MSL over four naps is 10.4 minutes +/– 4.3 minutes, whereas the MSL over five naps is 11.6 minutes +/– 5.2 minutes.[30] In addition, results of the MSLT vary with age. Normal children have MSLs that average between 15 and 20 minutes, whereas adults between 21 and 35 years of age average 10 minutes, 30- to 49-year-old adults average 11 to 12 minutes, and 50- to 59-year-old adults average 9 minutes.[37,38]

Despite its intuitive appeal and frequent use as a gold standard, many factors may conspire to reduce the accuracy of the MSLT as a measure of sleepiness. Levels of anxiety or discomfort among patients who undergo an MSLT can vary widely and may obscure short sleep latencies in some cases.[39] The current MSLT recommendations include a number of precautions that may facilitate test uniformity and sensitivity to EDS; these include that the testing environment should be dark and quiet, a sleep

Box 1
Recommendations for the MSLT Protocol
(Adapted from Carskadon and colleagues, Guidelines for the multiple sleep latency test (MSLT): a standard measure of sleepiness [9].
Modified by collective expert opinion using Rand/UCLA Appropriateness Method)

1. The MSLT consists of five nap opportunities performed at two hour intervals. The initial nap opportunity begins 1.5 to 3 hours after termination of the nocturnal recording. A shorter four-nap test may be performed but this test is not reliable for the diagnosis of narcolepsy unless at least two sleep onset REM periods have occurred.

2. The MSLT must be performed immediately following polysomnography recorded during the individual's major sleep period. The use of MSLT to support a diagnosis of narcolepsy is suspect if TST on the prior night sleep is less than 6 hours. The test should not be performed after a split-night sleep study (combination of diagnostic and therapeutic studies in a single night).

3. Sleep logs may be obtained for 1 week prior to the MSLT to assess sleep-wake schedules.

4. Standardization of test conditions is critical for obtaining valid results. Sleep rooms should be dark and quiet during testing. Room temperature should be set based on the patient's comfort level.

5. Stimulants, stimulant-like medications, and REM suppressing medications should ideally be stopped 2 weeks before MSLT. Use of the patient's other usual medications (e.g., antihypertensives, insulin, etc.) should be thoughtfully planned by the sleep clinician before MSLT testing so that undesired influences by the stimulating or sedating properties of the medications are minimized. Drug screening may be indicated to ensure that sleepiness on the MSLT is not pharmacologically induced. Drug screening is usually performed on the morning of the MSLT but its timing and the circumstances of the testing may be modified by the clinician. Smoking should be stopped at least 30 minutes prior to each nap opportunity. Vigorous physical activity should be avoided during the day and any stimulating activities by the patient should end at least 15 minutes prior to each nap opportunity. The patient must abstain from any caffeinated beverages and avoid unusual exposures to bright sunlight. A light breakfast is recommended at least 1 hour prior to the first trial, and a light lunch is recommended immediately after the termination of the second noon trial.

6. Sleep technologists who perform MSLTs should be experienced in conducting the test.

7. The conventional recording montage for the MSLT includes central EEG (C3-A2, C4-A1) and occipital (O1-A2, O2-A1) derivations, left and right eye electrooculograms (EOGs), mental/submental electromyogram (EMG), and electrocardiogram (EKG).

8. Prior to each nap opportunity, the patient should be asked if they need to go to the bathroom or need other adjustments for comfort. Standard instructions for bio-calibrations (i.e., patient calibrations) prior to each nap include: (1) lie quietly with your eyes open for 30 seconds, (2) close both eyes for 30 seconds, (3) without moving your head, look to the right, then left, then right, then left, right and then left, (4) blink eyes slowly for 5 times, and (5) clench or grit your teeth tightly together.

9. With each nap opportunity the subject should be instructed as follows: "Please lie quietly, assume a comfortable position, keep your eyes closed and try to fall asleep." The same instructions should be given prior to every test. Immediately after these instructions are given, bedroom lights are turned off, signaling the start of the test. Between naps, the patient should be out of bed and prevented from sleeping. This generally requires continuous observation by a laboratory staff member.

10. Sleep onset for the clinical MSLT is determined by the time from lights out to the first epoch of any stage of sleep, including stage 1 sleep. Sleep onset is defined as the first epoch of greater than 15 sec of cumulative sleep in a 30-sec epoch. The absence of sleep on a nap opportunity is recorded as a sleep latency of 20 minutes. This latency is included in the calculation of mean sleep latency (MSL). In order to assess for the occurrence of REM sleep, in the clinical MSLT the test continues for 15 minutes from after the first epoch of sleep. The duration of 15 minutes is determined by "clock time", and is not determined by a sleep time of 15 minutes. REM latency is taken as the time of the first epoch of sleep to the beginning of the first epoch of REM sleep regardless of the intervening stages of sleep or wakefulness.

11. A nap session is terminated after 20 minutes if sleep does not occur.

12. The MSLT report should include the start and end times of each nap or nap opportunity, latency from lights out to the first epoch of sleep, mean sleep latency (arithmetic mean of all naps or nap opportunities), and number of sleep-onset REM periods (defined as greater than 15 sec of REM sleep in a 30-sec epoch).

13. Events that represent deviation from standard protocol or conditions should be documented by the sleep technologist for review by the interpreting sleep clinician.

FIGURE 14.2 Recommendations for the multiple sleep latency test (MSLT) protocol. (From Littner MR, et. al. Standards of Practice Committee of the American Academy of Sleep Medicine. Practice parameters for clinical use of the multiple sleep latency test and the maintenance of wakefulness test. Sleep 2005;28(1):113–121.)

technologist experienced with MSLT should conduct the test, and the patient's comfort needs should be addressed prior to each nap opportunity.[30] In clinical practice, MSLT interpretation should include consideration of sleep duration on the previous night, current medications, recently discontinued medications, caffeine consumption, use of nicotine or illicit drugs, medical or psychological conditions, recent sleep schedules and schedule variability, and other factors specific to each patient.

Test-retest reliability of the MSLT is good among healthy individuals with consistent sleep-wake schedules,[40] but it may be significantly lower among patients with insomnia.[41] In addition to biologic variation from day to day, interrater differences can add to test-retest differences, although one study of 21 patients with EDS showed good levels of agreement between three different readers.[42] A larger study of 200 sleep center patients, including individuals with and without sleep disorders, showed high interrater and intrarater reliability for both sleep latency and REM onset scores.[43] A study of 44 subjects randomly selected from an ongoing narcolepsy family study showed excellent intra- and interrater reliability among three readers for five-nap MSLT performed in this study population.[44]

Variants of the Multiple Sleep Latency Test

In part because an inability to stay awake may be more relevant to important outcomes than an ability to fall asleep quickly, the maintenance of wakefulness test (MWT) is preferred over the MSLT by some clinicians. The recording montage and spaced nap attempts of the MWT are identical to those of the MSLT, but the patient is instructed to try to remain awake, rather than sleep, during the nap opportunities. The currently recommended protocol includes four, 40-minute nap trials,[30] but 20- or 40-minute nap trials have been used in the past. Sleep onset is identified as the first 30-second epoch to include at least 15 seconds of sleep. Nap trials are ended at 40 minutes if no sleep occurs or after unequivocal sleep, which is defined as three consecutive epochs of stage I sleep or one epoch of any other stage of sleep.[30] Published normative data are not extensive for the MWT, but comparisons between data from 64 normal adults[45] in one study and patients with obstructive sleep apnea[46] or narcolepsy[47] in other studies suggest good discriminant ability.

In one clinical series of 258 patients, mean sleep latencies on MSLT and MWT trials interdigitated into the same testing day showed a correlation of only .41.[48] The large differences between these results could reflect underlying discrepancies between abilities to stay awake and fall asleep, but poor accuracy and reliability of the tests could also account for the findings. Limited data exist to link MWT or MSLT results to future health-related outcomes of importance. One study failed to find an association between MSLT results and motor vehicle accidents.[49] However, a more recent study of 618 subjects found that those who were excessively sleepy, defined as a mean sleep latency of <5 minutes on MSLT, had a significantly greater risk of motor vehicle collision than alert individuals as documented in accident records over a 10-year period that included the time of MSLT administration.[50] Another study reported that results of the MWT correlated better than those of the MSLT with daytime function.[51] The MWT may be more sensitive than the MSLT to treatment effects among EDS patients with sleep disorders.[52] Implementation of the recommended test protocol and scoring criteria may partially attenuate the lack of standardization that influenced older MWT studies. However, relative disadvantages of the MWT in routine practice include inapplicability to the diagnosis of narcolepsy and unfamiliarity among clinicians. Both the MWT and MSLT lack large, multicenter, prospectively collected data on the extent to which "real-world" outcomes can be predicted.

Additional modifications of the MSLT have been suggested or tested but none have been widely adopted. One group proposed the addition of a simple cognitive task to the MSLT nap trials; the task is also sensitive to sleep deprivation, but the main advantage is distraction from other sources of mental excitement or anxiety.[39] Another group proposed to use the sleep architecture of naps, rather than just sleep latency, in a formula that would generate an overall polygraphic score of sleepiness.[53] One study found that mean wake efficiency (100 − percentage of time asleep during nap attempt), in comparison to MSL, provided a result that was better correlated with measures of sleep apnea severity.[54] In contrast, another report found that calculation of MSL based only on successful nap attempts, or only among patients able to fall asleep on each nap attempt, failed to improve correlations between the MSL and measures of apnea severity.[28] Finally, in the proposed Oxford Sleep Resistance Test, sleep onset during four 40-minute nap trials was defined by a participant's failure to respond to a recurring light signal rather than by more complicated and expensive polysomnographic means; results were similar to those of MWTs among 10 participants tested with both protocols.[55] Punjabi et al.[56] described the use of the technique of survival analysis to determine independents of apnea-hypopnea frequency, nocturnal hypoxemia, and sleep fragmentation on daytime sleepiness in patients with sleep-disordered breathing. Each of the 741 patients included in the study had a baseline polysomnogram followed by MSLT; the variable of interest was the median time to sleep onset during the MSLT. Multivariate analyses were done with the stepwise addition of covariates to the proportional hazards regression model to determine the independent effect of each risk factor studied (age, sex, body mass index, apnoea/hypopnoea index [AHI], oxyhemoglobin desaturation, amount of time in sleep stages 1 and 2, time in slow-wave sleep, and total sleep time). AHI, nocturnal hypoxemia, and sleep fragmentation were found to be individual determinants of hypersomnolence in patients with sleep-disordered breathing.[56] While this survival analysis technique may not be applicable to individual patients, it may be useful for research studies of cohorts of patients.

OTHER OBJECTIVE TESTS OF SLEEPINESS

Besides the MSLT and its variants, other electrophysiologic measures are sensitive to sleepiness, although none are used commonly as a measure of EDS in clinical practice. Comparisons of pupillometric recordings in pathologically sleepy patients and controls, during wakefulness in dark environments, have suggested that miosis and increased fluctuation of pupil diameter (hippus) are associated with sleepiness.[57,58] Sleep-deprived normal subjects can show similar changes,[59] but pupillary oscillations may provide better discrimination than miosis between control participants and sleep apneics or narcoleptics.[60,61] Pupillometry may be reliable when following responses in a given individual over time, but comparisons between individuals may be less reliable.[62] Pupillometry is not a simple technique, has not been widely adopted, and requires further development before it can serve more routinely in clinical practice as an accurate measure of sleepiness.[60,63]

Quantitative EEG (qEEG), which evaluates the ratio of slow (delta and theta) frequencies to fast (alpha and beta) frequencies,[64] may provide an objective measure of sleepiness that reflects treatment response. One study of 14 subjects with moderate to severe obstructive sleep apnea performed qEEG before and after 6 months of CPAP therapy and found significant improvement in qEEG slowing after CPAP, along with statistically significant increase in the mean sleep latency on MSLT.[65] However, the

posttreatment MSLT results remained significantly lower than those of 10 control subjects. Changes in sleep architecture and qEEG have been described in a number of neurogenerative diseases.[66] Quantitative EEG may evolve to be a useful tool for assessment of sleepiness and treatment response in this patient population.

The bispectral index (BIS), which measures cortical integration as an indicator of consciousness, is used as an assessment of the depth of sedation and anesthesia.[67] The BIS values range from 0 to 100 depending upon whether low and high EEG frequencies are in phase; the higher the index, the higher the level of consciousness. A BIS of 40 to 55 usually occurs during general anesthesia.[67] There may be a role for use of the BIS as a marker of depth of sleep. A study of five subjects compared changes in the BIS with stages of sleep as determined by conventional EEG and found that light sleep, slow-wave sleep, and REM sleep occurred at BIS values of 75–90, 20–70, and 75–92, respectively.[68] However, another study of 10 patients found a wide range of BIS values during each sleep stage, with considerable overlap between stages.[69]

Brainstem auditory evoked responses (BAERs) may show delays and sometimes topographic abnormalities in patients with severe obstructive sleep apnea, idiopathic hypersomnolence, and narcolepsy, although reports are not all consistent.[70-72] Reports of evoked response abnormalities in several different disorders associated with hypersomnolence support a potential relationship between BAERs and sleepiness. However, correlations between BAER P300 latencies and MSLT results ($r = .12$) or MWT results ($r = .15$) are too weak to confirm clinical utility of the evoked responses as measures of sleepiness.[73] Some sleep apneics without clear objective evidence of sleepiness still have prolonged BAERs,[74] and BAERs may[70] or may not[75] improve after treatment of sleep apnea. Some studies have also reported abnormal visual evoked responses in patients with sleep apnea,[71,74] but again these abnormalities have not resolved after treatment that improved sleep-related breathing and MSLT results.[75]

Although rarely part of routine clinical evaluations, several cognitive and performance tests can show important functional deficits in people with an underlying sleep disorder or insufficient sleep quantity. In general, long tedious tasks tend to be most sensitive to sleepiness, but participants' motivation also affects scores. Functional imaging studies have shown changes in brain activity and cerebral metabolism in sleep-deprived individuals. For example, a positron emission tomography study of 17 normal subjects before and after 24-hour sleep deprivation showed decreases in regional and global cerebral metabolism.[76] These changes after sleep deprivation also correlated with an increase in the Stanford Sleepiness Scale score and decrease in performance on a Serial Addition/Subtraction test. Conversely, reversal of sleep deprivation, either by treatment of an identified sleep disorder or by an increase in total sleep time, may improve performance on cognitive and performance testing. Previous data suggest that sustained attention and vigilance, measured by instruments such as Steer Clear[77] or the Psychomotor Vigilance Test,[78] may improve with CPAP as compared with placebo. Mental flexibility measured by Trail-Making B results may also improve.[79] A large, randomized controlled trial is needed to substantiate these preliminary data and confirm that cognitive tests may well provide measures of functionally important outcomes in patients with EDS.

Ancillary Studies

On occasion, other tests relevant to a differential diagnosis for EDS but not actually measuring sleepiness are important. For example, a diagnosis may emerge from magnetic resonance imaging in a patient with EDS along with other central neurologic deficits, or from thyroid function tests in a patient with EDS, fatigue, weight gain, and lower-extremity edema. A urine or serum drug screen can be considered if EDS may be secondary to illicit drug use or inappropriate use of prescription medication.

INTEGRATION OF INFORMATION FROM DIFFERENT SOURCES

The differential diagnosis for EDS is extensive, and arriving at a final diagnosis often requires more than collection of results from various assessments at the bedside, home, medical facility, or sleep laboratory. Sound clinical judgment is essential as available information is weighed and combined into an overall assessment of EDS severity and likely causes. Although rules to cover every possible set of circumstances are not available, the following considerations are likely to be useful.

Historical complaints of sleepiness, tiredness, fatigue, or lack of energy should not assume less importance when tests fail to provide more standardized or objective corroboration of those complaints. In particular, the results of the ESS should not be used to minimize a patient's complaint, which may vary substantially with an ESS score.[80] Use of the ESS as a standardized sleepiness measure grew quickly since its introduction in 1991[11,14] as reflected by its translation into multiple languages, such as French, Norwegian, and Portuguese.[81-83] However, investigators who attempted to validate the ESS against the MSLT or MWT reported somewhat discrepant enthusiasm for the ESS as a clinical tool. Those authors who found a small but statistically significant association with the objective tests generally supported use of the ESS—perhaps even as a measure that assesses sleepiness in a wider variety of situations than that tested by the MSLT[84]—whereas those authors who could find no statistically significant associations with objective results suggested that the ESS should not be considered a replacement for objective testing.[11,13]

Other potential sources of ESS validity data were studies that compared its results with measures of sleep apnea severity. One author initially reported a correlation of $r = .55$ ($p < .001$) between ESS scores and rates of apneas and hypopneas per hour of sleep (AHI).[14] In a subsequent and larger study by the same author, the correlation was $r = .44$ ($p < .001$).[85] A recent comparison of home polysomnography and ESS results from 1824 community-dwelling older adults showed that participants with an AHI less than 5 had an average ESS score of 7.2, whereas those with an AHI greater than or equal to 30 averaged 9.3; the percentage of participants with an ESS score greater than or equal to 11 was 21% in the first group and 35% in the second.[86] Studies such as these confirmed statistically significant relationships between ESS results and apnea severity, but the magnitudes of these associations were weak. Other studies failed to find any statistically significant associations between ESS results and measures of apnea severity.[11,28]

Associations of small magnitude between ESS scores and expected correlates suggest that the clinical usefulness of the ESS alone, as a measure of EDS, is somewhat limited. Whether the ESS is a worthwhile addition to a clinician's less standardized interview has not been tested and may depend to some extent on how well the instrument improves prediction of important health-related outcomes. Two studies reported an association between EDS and motor vehicle accidents, at least retrospectively,[87,88] but another failed to find any such relationship.[89] The ESS may also be useful to the extent that it reflects improvement with treatment for sleep disorders. One study of 50 sleep apnea patients found that 2 months of treatment was associated with a reduction in mean ESS scores from 16.4 to 7.0.[90] Another study randomized 107 male sleep apneics to receive CPAP or subtherapeutic CPAP for 1 month and found that the ESS, among other measures, improved substantially in the first group (from a median score of 15.7 to 7.0) but much less among controls (from 15.0 to 13.0).[91] Another study of 283 narcoleptics showed that the median ESS score decreased from approximately 18 to 12 after 9 weeks of treatment with modafinil at 400 mg per day; this study was randomized and placebo controlled, improvements in ESS scores were highly significant ($p < .001$), and the decrement in ESS scores paralleled simultaneous improvement in MSLT and MWT scores.[47]

If the ESS should not replace a patient's complaints as a prime consideration in the clinical assessment of EDS, neither should objective tests, especially when they fail to confirm a patient's complaint. In clinical series, patients' reports of the extent to which they have a problem with sleepiness may show little or no relationship to MSLT results.[11,28,80] Furthermore, like the ESS scores, MSLT results may show surprisingly weak or absent correlations with measures of nocturnal sleep quality or pathology.[11,28,92]

The MSLT was developed in part because of early observations by sleep clinicians that a patient with a sleep disorder can be falling asleep in the examination room while denying EDS,[70] and, therefore, no test should be expected to match complaints precisely. However, the accuracy of the MSLT can be affected by patient anxiety, direct effects of sleep disorders on sleep onset, biologic night-to-night variation, and interrater variability. In clinical practice, a normal MSLT should not be used alone to exclude the possibility of significant EDS in a patient who complains of this problem. In contrast, a short MSL on a properly performed MSLT is a strong indication that excessive physiologic sleep tendency is likely to be present, regardless of whether the patient has expressed awareness of the problem. Generally physicians believe that such a result is an important finding, although literature yields conflicting results about the predictive value of short MSLs on important outcomes, such as driving accidents.[49,50] However, the most recent study of 10-year crash data, as verified by the Department of Motor Vehicles, in patients who underwent MSLT provides some prospective data that objectively documented excessive sleepiness is predictive of increased risk of motor vehicle crashes (Fig. 14.3).[50] This association is augmented in single-occupant

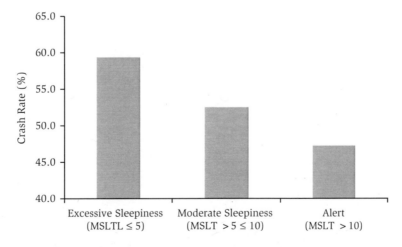

FIGURE 14.3   Crash prevalence in each multiple sleep latency test (MSLT)–based sleepiness group for the primary study endpoint—police-verified motor vehicle crashes during the 10-year study assessment period. Cochran-Armitage trend test, $p < .05$. (From Drake C; Roehrs T; Breslau N; Johnson E; Jefferson C; Scofield H; Roth T. The 10-year risk of verified motor vehicle crashes in relation to physiologic sleepiness. Sleep 2010;33(6):745–752.)

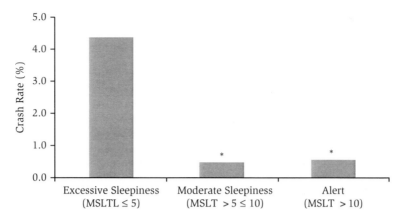

FIGURE 14.4 Crash prevalence in each multiple sleep latency test (MSLT)–defined sleepiness group for single occupant motor vehicle crashes during the 10-year study assessment period. Cochran-Armitage trend test, $p < .05$; *post hoc $\chi 2$, $p < .05$; severe injury accidents were those that "prevent normal activities and require hospitalization." (From Drake C; Roehrs T; Breslau N; Johnson E; Jefferson C; Scofield H; Roth T. The 10-year risk of verified motor vehicle crashes in relation to physiologic sleepiness. Sleep 2010;33(6):745–752.)

motor vehicle crashes documented during the study period (Fig. 14.4).[50] The MWT may be used to gauge response to treatment;[30] the result should not be interpreted in isolation but should instead be considered in the overall clinical context. While a trend in MWT results may be informative, the degree of change that represents a significant treatment response remains unclear.[30]

The clinician must often integrate other information with that obtained from tests of sleepiness. Experience in sleep laboratories suggests that nocturnal polysomnographic measures of sleep continuity, efficiency, architecture, and pathology sometimes show little association with assessments of sleepiness, subjective or objective. For example, clinicians should not be surprised by a patient who has more than 60 apneas or hypopneas per hour of sleep but an MSL of 16 minutes, or by another patient who has 6 such respiratory events per hour of sleep and an MSL of 2 minutes. In each case, treatment may well result in important improvements in the chief complaint and quality of life.

A PRACTICAL CLINICAL APPROACH

The clinical evaluation of EDS should be constructed based on the needs of each patient and the experience of the clinician. The evaluation must include a clinical history. To further measure, clarify, or document EDS, the most useful test is usually an MSLT. An MSLT is especially helpful when the history of EDS is ambiguous and treatment for sleep-related abnormalities, identified by history or polysomnography, is motivated by a more definitive assessment of daytime consequences. For example, very mild obstructive sleep apnea is highly prevalent but is not proven to affect cardiovascular health or longevity, and the decision to treat any particular patient may rest on evidence of significant EDS.

The ESS, which requires a tiny fraction of the time and cost of an MSLT, may also be useful for office-based longitudinal assessments of a patient's progress at frequent intervals. Results of the ESS and any other measures should be integrated and interpreted with knowledge of their strengths and weaknesses, typical relations or lack thereof to other measures, and likely implications given the clinical setting. Use of strict cutoffs between normal and abnormal values on the ESS, the MSLT, and other polysomnographic tests should be avoided because results from people with sleep disorders and without sleep disorders often overlap and the relationship of test results to important health-related outcomes remains unclear. The use of cognitive or performance tested can be considered on a case-by-case basis, when thought most pertinent to an individual's complaints. A thorough clinical history, with appropriate consideration of subjective or objective test results in some cases, is likely to provide the most accurate impression of the severity of EDS and its likely causes.

REFERENCES

1. American Academy of Sleep Medicine. *The International Classification of Sleep Disorders: Diagnostic and Coding Manual.* 2nd ed. Westchester, IL: American Academy of Sleep Medicine; 2005.
2. Lyznicki JM, Doege TC, Davis RM, et al. Sleepiness, driving, and motor vehicle crashes. Council on Scientific Affairs, American Medical Association. *JAMA* 1998;279:1908–13.
3. Chervin RD. Sleepiness, fatigue, tiredness, and lack of energy in obstructive sleep apnea. *Chest* 2000;118:372–9.
4. Chotinaiwattarakul W, O'Brien LM, Fan L, et al. Fatigue, tiredness, and lack of energy improve with treatment for OSA. *J Clin Sleep Med* 2009;5:222–7.
5. Hoddes E, Dement W, Zarcone V. The development and use of the Stanford Sleepiness Scale (SSS). *Psychophysiology* 1972;9:150.
6. Hoddes E, Zarcone V, Smythe H, et al. Quantification of sleepiness: a new approach. *Psychophysiology* 1973;10:431–6.
7. Herscovitch J, Broughton R. Sensitivity of the stanford sleepiness scale to the effects of cumulative partial sleep deprivation and recovery oversleeping. *Sleep* 1981;4:83–91.
8. Akerstedt T, Gillberg M. Subjective and objective sleepiness in the active individual. *Int J Neurosci* 1990;52:29–37.
9. Ballester E, Badia JR, Hernandez L, et al. Evidence of the effectiveness of continuous positive airway pressure in the treatment of sleep apnea/hypopnea syndrome. *Am J Respir Crit Care Med* 1999;159:495–501.
10. Engleman HM, Kingshott RN, Wraith PK, et al. Randomized placebo-controlled crossover trial of continuous positive airway pressure for mild sleep Apnea/Hypopnea syndrome. *Am J Respir Crit Care Med* 1999;159:461–7.
11. Chervin RD, Aldrich MS. The Epworth Sleepiness Scale may not reflect objective measures of sleepiness or sleep apnea. *Neurology* 1999;52:125–31.
12. Furuta H, Kaneda R, Kosaka K, et al. Epworth Sleepiness Scale and sleep studies in patients with obstructive sleep apnea syndrome. *Psychiatry Clin Neurosci* 1999;53:301–2.
13. Benbadis SR, Mascha E, Perry MC, et al. Association between the Epworth sleepiness scale and the multiple sleep latency test in a clinical population. *Ann Intern Med* 1999;130:289–92.
14. Johns MW. A new method for measuring daytime sleepiness: the Epworth sleepiness scale. *Sleep* 1991;14:540–5.
15. Miletin MS, Hanly PJ. Measurement properties of the Epworth sleepiness scale. *Sleep Med* 2003;4:195–9.
16. Weaver TE, Laizner AM, Evans LK, et al. An instrument to measure functional status outcomes for disorders of excessive sleepiness. *Sleep* 1997;20:835–43.
17. Fornas C, Ballester E, Arteta E, et al. Measurement of general health status in obstructive sleep apnea hypopnea patients. *Sleep* 1995;18:876–9.
18. Gall R, Isaac L, Kryger M. Quality of life in mild obstructive sleep apnea. *Sleep* 1993;16:S59–61.
19. Jenkinson C, Stradling J, Petersen S. Comparison of three measures of quality of life outcome in the evaluation of continuous positive airways pressure therapy for sleep apnoea. *J Sleep Res* 1997;6:199–204.
20. Hays RD, Stewart AL. Sleep measures. In: Stewart AL, Ware JE, eds. *Measuring Functioning and Well-Being: The Medical Outcomes Study Approach.* Durham, NC: Duke University Press; 1992:xxiii, 449.
21. Hays RD, Martin SA, Sesti AM, et al. Psychometric properties of the Medical Outcomes Study Sleep measure. *Sleep Med* 2005;6:41–4.
22. Lau DT, Morlock RJ, Hill CD. Psychometric evaluation of the medical outcomes study-sleep scale in persons with overactive bladder. *Clin Ther* 2006;28:2119–32.
23. Bruni O, Ottaviano S, Guidetti V, et al. The Sleep Disturbance Scale for Children (SDSC). Construction and validation of an instrument to evaluate sleep disturbances in childhood and adolescence. *J Sleep Res* 1996;5:251–61.
24. Chervin RD, Hedger K, Dillon JE, et al. Pediatric sleep questionnaire (PSQ): validity and reliability of scales for sleep-disordered breathing, snoring, sleepiness, and behavioral problems. *Sleep Med* 2000;1:21–32.
25. Chervin RD, Weatherly RA, Garetz SL, et al. Pediatric sleep questionnaire: prediction of sleep apnea and outcomes. *Arch Otolaryngol Head Neck Surg* 2007;133:216–22.

26. Melendres MC, Lutz JM, Rubin ED, et al. Daytime sleepiness and hyperactivity in children with suspected sleep-disordered breathing. *Pediatrics* 2004;114:768–75.

27. Drake C, Nickel C, Burduvali E, et al. The pediatric daytime sleepiness scale (PDSS): sleep habits and school outcomes in middle-school children. *Sleep* 2003;26:455–8.

28. Chervin RD, Kraemer HC, Guilleminault C. Correlates of sleep latency on the multiple sleep latency test in a clinical population. *Electroencephalogr Clin Neurophysiol* 1995;95:147–53.

29. Shpirer I, Miniovitz A, Klein C, et al. Excessive daytime sleepiness in patients with Parkinson's disease: a polysomnography study. *Mov Disord* 2006;21:1432–8.

30. Littner MR, Kushida C, Wise M, et al. Practice parameters for clinical use of the multiple sleep latency test and the maintenance of wakefulness test. *Sleep* 2005;28:113–21.

31. Carskadon M, Dement W. Sleep tendency: an objective measure of sleep loss. *Sleep Res* 1977;6:200.

32. Carskadon MA, Dement WC. The multiple sleep latency test: what does it measure? *Sleep* 1982;5(Suppl 2):S67–72.

33. Richardson GS, Carskadon MA, Flagg W, et al. Excessive daytime sleepiness in man: multiple sleep latency measurement in narcoleptic and control subjects. *Electroencephalogr Clin Neurophysiol* 1978;45:621–7.

34. van den Hoed J, Kraemer H, Guilleminault C, et al. Disorders of excessive daytime somnolence: polygraphic and clinical data for 100 patients. *Sleep* 1981;4:23–37.

35. American Sleep Disorders Association. The clinical use of the multiple sleep latency test. *Sleep* 1992;15:268.

36. Carskadon MA, Dement WC, Mitler MM, et al. Guidelines for the multiple sleep latency test (MSLT): a standard measure of sleepiness. *Sleep* 1986;9:519–24.

37. Levine B, Roehrs T, Zorick F, et al. Daytime sleepiness in young adults. *Sleep* 1988;11:39–46.

38. Roehrs T, Zorick F, McLenaghan A, et al. Sleep and MLST norms for middle aged adults. *Sleep Res* 1984;13.

39. Naitoh P, Kelly T. Modification of the multiple sleep latency test. In: Ogilvie RD, Harsh JR, eds. *Sleep Onset: Normal and Abnormal Processes*. Washington, DC: American Psychological Association; 1994:xxviii, 397.

40. Zwyghuizen-Doorenbos A, Roehrs T, Schaefer M, et al. Test-retest reliability of the MSLT. *Sleep* 1988;11:562–5.

41. Roehrs T, Roth T. Multiple Sleep Latency Test: technical aspects and normal values. *J Clin Neurophysiol* 1992;9:63–7.

42. Benbadis SR, Qu Y, Perry MC, et al. Interrater reliability of the multiple sleep latency test. *Electroencephalogr Clin Neurophysiol* 1995;95:302–4.

43. Drake CL, Rice MF, Roehrs TA, et al. Scoring reliability of the multiple sleep latency test in a clinical population. *Sleep* 2000;23:911–13.

44. Chen L, Ho CK, Lam VK, et al. Interrater and intrarater reliability in multiple sleep latency test. *J Clin Neurophysiol* 2008;25:218–21.

45. Doghramji K, Mitler MM, Sangal RB, et al. A normative study of the maintenance of wakefulness test (MWT). *Electroencephalogr Clin Neurophysiol* 1997;103:554–62.

46. Poceta JS, Timms RM, Jeong DU, et al. Maintenance of wakefulness test in obstructive sleep apnea syndrome. *Chest* 1992;101:893–7.

47. US Modafinil in Narcolepsy Multicenter Study Group. Randomized trial of modafinil for the treatment of pathological somnolence in narcolepsy. US Modafinil in Narcolepsy Multicenter Study Group. *Ann Neurol* 1998;43:88–97.

48. Sangal RB, Thomas L, Mitler MM. Maintenance of wakefulness test and multiple sleep latency test. Measurement of different abilities in patients with sleep disorders. *Chest* 1992;101:898–902.

49. Aldrich MS. Automobile accidents in patients with sleep disorders. *Sleep* 1989;12:487–94.

50. Drake C, Roehrs T, Breslau N, et al. The 10-year risk of verified motor vehicle crashes in relation to physiologic sleepiness. *Sleep* 2010;33:745–52.

51. Kingshott RN, Engleman HM, Deary IJ, et al. Does arousal frequency predict daytime function? *Eur Respir J* 1998;12:1264–70.

52. Sangal RB, Thomas L, Mitler MM. Disorders of excessive sleepiness. Treatment improves ability to stay awake but does not reduce sleepiness. *Chest* 1992;102:699–703.

53. Roth B, Nevsimalova S, Sonka K, et al. An alternative to the multiple sleep latency test for determining sleepiness in narcolepsy and hypersomnia: polygraphic score of sleepiness. *Sleep* 1986;9:243–5.

54. Pollak CP. How should the multiple sleep latency test be analyzed? *Sleep* 1997; 20:34–9.

55. Bennett LS, Stradling JR, Davies RJ. A behavioural test to assess daytime sleepiness in obstructive sleep apnoea. *J Sleep Res* 1997;6:142–5.

56. Punjabi NM, O'Hearn D J, Neubauer DN, et al. Modeling hypersomnolence in sleep-disordered breathing. A novel approach using survival analysis. *Am J Respir Crit Care Med* 1999;159:1703–9.

57. Yoss RE, Moyer NJ, Ogle KN. The pupillogram and narcolepsy. A method to measure decreased levels of wakefulness. *Neurology* 1969;19:921–8.

58. Yoss RE, Moyer NJ, Hollenhorst RW. Pupil size and spontaneous pupillary waves associated with alertness, drowsiness, and sleep. *Neurology* 1970;20:545–54.

59. Wilhelm B, Wilhelm H, Ludtke H, et al. Pupillographic assessment of sleepiness in sleep-deprived healthy subjects. *Sleep* 1998;21:258–65.

60. Newman J, Broughton R. Pupillometric assessment of excessive daytime sleepiness in narcolepsy-cataplexy. *Sleep* 1991;14:121–9.

61. Wilhelm H, Ludtke H, Wilhelm B. Pupillographic sleepiness testing in hypersomniacs and normals. *Graefes Arch Clin Exp Ophthalmol* 1998;236:725–9.

62. Mathis J, Hess CW. Sleepiness and vigilance tests. *Swiss Med Wkly* 2009;139:214–19.

63. O'Neill WD, Oroujeh AM, Keegan AP, et al. Neurological pupillary noise in narcolepsy. *J Sleep Res* 1996;5:265–71.

64. Morisson F, Lavigne G, Petit D, et al. Spectral analysis of wakefulness and REM sleep EEG in patients with sleep apnoea syndrome. *Eur Respir J* 1998;11:1135–40.

65. Morisson F, Decary A, Petit D, et al. Daytime sleepiness and EEG spectral analysis in apneic patients before and after treatment with continuous positive airway pressure. *Chest* 2001;119:45–52.

66. Petit D, Gagnon JF, Fantini ML, et al. Sleep and quantitative EEG in neurodegenerative disorders. *J Psychosom Res* 2004;56:487–96.

67. Vernon JM, Lang E, Sebel PS, et al. Prediction of movement using bispectral electroencephalographic analysis during propofol/alfentanil or isoflurane/alfentanil anesthesia. *Anesth Analg* 1995;80:780–5.

68. Sleigh JW, Andrzejowski J, Steyn-Ross A, et al. The bispectral index: a measure of depth of sleep? *Anesth Analg* 1999;88:659–61.

69. Nieuwenhuijs D, Coleman EL, Douglas NJ, et al. Bispectral index values and spectral edge frequency at different stages of physiologic sleep. *Anesth Analg* 2002;94:125–9.

70. Walsleben JA, Squires NK, Rothenberger VL. Auditory event-related potentials and brain dysfunction in sleep apnea. *Electroencephalogr Clin Neurophysiol* 1989;74:297–311.

71. Sangal RB, Sangal JM. P300 latency: abnormal in sleep apnea with somnolence and idiopathic hypersomnia, but normal in narcolepsy. *Clin Electroencephalogr* 1995;26:146–53.

72. Sangal RB, Sangal JM, Belisle C. Longer auditory and visual P300 latencies in patients with narcolepsy. *Clin Electroencephalogr* 1999;30:28–32.

73. Sangal RB, Sangal JM. Measurement of P300 and sleep characteristics in patients with hypersomnia: do P300 latencies, P300 amplitudes, and multiple sleep latency and maintenance of wakefulness tests measure different factors? *Clin Electroencephalogr* 1997;28:179–84.

74. Sangal RB, Sangal JM. Obstructive sleep apnea and abnormal P300 latency topography. *Clin Electroencephalogr* 1997;28:16–25.

75. Sangal RB, Sangal JM. Abnormal visual P300 latency in obstructive sleep apnea does not change acutely upon treatment with CPAP. *Sleep* 1997;20:702–4.

76. Thomas M, Sing H, Belenky G, et al. Neural basis of alertness and cognitive performance impairments during sleepiness. I. Effects of 24 h of sleep deprivation on waking human regional brain activity. *J Sleep Res* 2000;9:335–52.

77. Findley L, Unverzagt M, Guchu R, Fabrizio M, Buckner J, Suratt P. Vigilance and automobile accidents in patients with sleep apnea or narcolepsy. *Chest* 1995;108:619–24.

78. Kribbs NB, Pack AI, Kline LR, et al. Effects of one night without nasal CPAP treatment on sleep and sleepiness in patients with obstructive sleep apnea. *Am Rev Respir Dis* 1993;147:1162–8.

79. Engleman HM, Martin SE, Deary IJ, et al. Effect of continuous positive airway pressure treatment on daytime function in sleep apnoea/hypopnoea syndrome. *Lancet* 1994;343:572–5.

80. Chervin RD, Aldrich MS, Pickett R, et al. Comparison of the results of the Epworth Sleepiness Scale and the Multiple Sleep Latency Test. *J Psychosom Res* 1997;42:145–55.

81. Kaminska M, Jobin V, Mayer P, et al. The Epworth Sleepiness Scale: self-administration

versus administration by the physician, and validation of a French version. *Can Respir J* 2010;17:e27–34.

82. Beiske KK, Kjelsberg FN, Ruud EA, et al. Reliability and validity of a Norwegian version of the Epworth sleepiness scale. *Sleep Breath* 2009;13:65–72.

83. Bertolazi AN, Fagondes SC, Hoff LS, et al. Portuguese-language version of the Epworth sleepiness scale: validation for use in Brazil. *J Bras Pneumol* 2009;35:877–83.

84. Johns MW. Sleepiness in different situations measured by the Epworth Sleepiness Scale. *Sleep* 1994;17:703–10.

85. Johns MW. Daytime sleepiness, snoring, and obstructive sleep apnea. The Epworth Sleepiness Scale. *Chest* 1993;103:30–6.

86. Gottlieb DJ, Whitney CW, Bonekat WH, et al. Relation of sleepiness to respiratory disturbance index: the Sleep Heart Health Study. *Am J Respir Crit Care Med* 1999;159:502–7.

87. Maycock G. Sleepiness and driving: the experience of UK car drivers. *J Sleep Res* 1996;5:229–37.

88. Noda A, Yagi T, Yokota M, et al. Daytime sleepiness and automobile accidents in patients with obstructive sleep apnea syndrome. *Psychiatry Clin Neurosci* 1998;52:221–2.

89. Barbe F, Pericas J, Munoz A, et al. Automobile accidents in patients with sleep apnea syndrome. An epidemiological and mechanistic study. *Am J Respir Crit Care Med* 1998;158:18–22.

90. Hardinge FM, Pitson DJ, Stradling JR. Use of the Epworth Sleepiness Scale to demonstrate response to treatment with nasal continuous positive airways pressure in patients with obstructive sleep apnoea. *Respir Med* 1995;89:617–20.

91. Jenkinson C, Davies RJ, Mullins R, et al. Comparison of therapeutic and subtherapeutic nasal continuous positive airway pressure for obstructive sleep apnoea: a randomised prospective parallel trial. *Lancet* 1999;353:2100–5.

92. Chervin RD, Aldrich MS. Characteristics of apneas and hypopneas during sleep and relation to excessive daytime sleepiness. *Sleep* 1998;21:799–806.

15

Ambulatory Activity Monitoring

RICHARD P. ALLEN

IT HAS now been over 30 years since Colburn and colleagues introduced piezoelectric sensors to the measurement of physical activity.[1,2] They cleverly recognized the power of this type of very small sensor to reliably detect small accelerations with minimal power demands. They produced the first self-contained, battery-operated monitor of human physical activity. It was designed to be worn on the wrist and to continuously record all arm accelerations for small units of time over several days. This ingenious development was followed shortly thereafter by a careful engineering analysis by Redmond and Hegge,[3] who demonstrated that this sensor could capture the full range of human physiological movements. The initial monitors had limited dynamic range, single axis of movement detection, and inadequate time resolution for adequately describing significant human movements. Subsequent advances in technology provided a three-dimensional sensor, much enhanced memory, and faster sampling rates, permitting better description of human motor activity. There remains, however, a rather limited attention to the basic measurement concepts for most ambulatory activity monitors in all its potential uses for assessing human activity. Many investigators or clinicians using these devices appear to understand neither how these measurements are obtained nor what is being measured. Thus, there are references to "activity counts" referring to some period of time with activity levels that are then correlated with some physical characteristic such as exercise levels. These studies generally fail to clearly define an "activity count." This approach treats the activity meter as some sort of black box producing some sort of counts of activity, but there is often no actual recognition of the physical dimensions being measured.

The application of the activity monitor to sleep medicine has a very spotty history. Most of the effort has been the sort of blind "black box" approach of simply looking for the level of inactivity suggesting sleep. The goal has been to develop an easily used meter that inexpensively records the sleep patterns over several days for evaluation of possible sleep problems. This sadly asks both too much and too little of activity measurements for sleep medicine. The rather sad history of using ambulatory activity monitoring for sleep was noted in the first edition of this book and has changed little in the ensuring 8 years. On one hand, the considerable amount of work focused on activity recording for assessing sleep length, primarily for insomnia studies, has been overall rather disappointing. On the other hand, the very promising approaches to measuring actual movements during sleep have remained rather inchoate with only limited although promising development mostly for assessing periodic leg movements in sleep (PLMS).

This chapter reviews first some of the areas of potential development for ambulatory activity monitoring that appear promising and then looks very briefly at the issue of sleep-wake state determination by activity measurement. The promise of better assessments of movements related to sleep medicine was noted in the first edition, but aside from work on PLMS there has been little further development. The claims about sleep-wake determination and the efforts to use activity monitoring for insomnia have increased with some actual practice guidelines developed,[4] but as noted these remain inherently limited by the physics of activity monitoring. These guidelines unfortunately fail to adequately assess the basic physics and limitations of activity monitoring as detailed in this chapter. No amount of effort can overcome these significant limitations. So the good news is the increased use of activity monitoring for PLMS assessment in sleep; the sad news is the failure to develop this much further for PLMS or to explore possible other areas with significant movements in sleep. The following provides a brief introduction to the areas of significance for ambulatory activity monitoring for movement disorders related to sleep.

CIRCADIAN RHYTHM DETERMINATIONS

The rest-activity cycle provides a reasonable surrogate measure for intrinsic circadian cycle that so dominates much of human biology, including the balance between sleep and waking. It has multiple problems requiring adjustments for divergent events disrupting the normal daily cycle. But various tools have been developed

to adjust for this. The cosinor and similar analytic methods provide descriptions of phase and amplitude based on wrist activity recordings over several days.[5–8] These wrist activity recordings have been found to provide a reasonable assessment of sleep phase compared to dim-light melatonin onset.[5] This can be improved by adding other simply recorded information, including skin temperature and ambient light in the critical blue spectral band.[9] One of the problems with the activity measures of circadian phase is the rather large amount of time with little or no activity. This complicates the mathematics of most measurements and remains poorly handled in some circadian phase models. Thus, body temperature continues to decrease during the sleep period, while the floor effects of activity measures fail to show this progressive change. The mathematics of the analyses partly adjust for the truncated data. The floor effect of activity measurements may be reduced some by increasing more the dynamic and frequency range of the activity meters, but this will always remain a problem for activity assessment of circadian phase. Thus, as noted earlier, recordings of multiple physiological signals as well as activity are likely to be required to produce circadian phase assessment considered satisfactory for use with sleep disorder patients.

PERIODIC LIMB MOVEMENTS

One area of sleep medicine where activity monitoring has become fully accepted is that of measuring actual movement events during sleep, particularly for leg movements during sleep. Here the monitor is placed at the site of the movement, usually the ankle or foot, and the recording is established to detect events of clinical significance. Validation is provided by agreement with full physiological electromyogram (EMG) recordings of the muscles involved in the movements (mostly anterior tibialis for the PLMS).

Ambulatory leg activity monitors have several major advantages for recording PLMS. First, they are inexpensive and easily accessible for the patient. This removes these major limitations to evaluating these movements. Second, they can record for several nights. PLMS have marked night-to-night variability.[10] One well-done study noted that it took about 5 nights of recording to provide a reasonably stable measure of the PLMS/hour of sleep for one individual.[11] They have some limitations.

Sleep-disordered breathing can produce episodic arousals with leg movements that confound any assessment of the leg movements in sleep. But for most subjects this is a minor problem. The activity monitor records both wake and sleep movements, but it has now been recognized that both of these are significant for assessment of movement disorders in sleep, including restless legs syndrome (Willis-Ekbom disease) and also periodic limb movement disorder.

Thus, at this point the assessment of leg movements in sleep is probably best done by excluding possible sleep-disordered breathing by history or examination and then obtaining an ambulatory activity monitoring for five or more nights. The accuracy of these monitors is very good with outputs that closely follow the amplitude of the EMG activation as shown for one monitor now available from Phllips-Respironics (PAM-RL) in Figure 15.1. Data from the PAM-RL in the laboratory setting with well-calibrated meters show an excellent agreement with the nocturnal PSG. The number of leg movements form the PAM-RL correlated very well (r = .997) with independent measurement of PLM from the EMG recordings and the average error for rates per hour of less than 1.0.[12] The monitors when used off the shelf in a standard clinical setting also have very good

agreement with results from the PSG and are considered validated for this use.[13] The PAM-RL also has the advantage for at-home use that it records separately the PLM rates when the legs are stretched out from when they are upright (subject sitting or standing). The PLM/hour can be measured for the sleep position excluding times sitting up or out of bed, which can be significant for restless legs syndrome (RLS) patients.

The leg activity can also be reliably measured using activity meters during the suggested immobilization test (SIT) developed by Jacques Montplaisir[14] for evaluating the severity of the RLS. In that test the subject sits up in bed for 1 hour awake with legs stretched out. Observation can be used to ensure the eyes remain open, indicating the patient remains awake. The patient is asked to record every 5 or 10 minutes the degree of sensory discomfort in the legs. The leg activity is recorded continuously during the test. For this test there is no problem of sleep-disordered breathing or other sleep-arousing events altering the basic rate of PLM. The leg activity monitor, therefore, provides an adequate assessment of the leg movements without needing the standard EMG recordings. There is, however, a problem with the standard "off-the-shelf" detection criteria for these monitors. These criteria were developed and validated for nocturnal leg

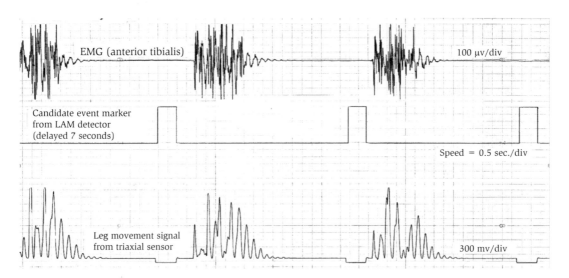

FIGURE 15.1 Simultaneous leg movement recordings from EMG and the PAM-RL activity monitor (Phillips Respironics) from an RLS patient. Note the close agreement of the envelope for the EMG and the activity monitor record of acceleration. The EMG is not calibrated to a physical unit, but the activity meter is calibrated to give the acceleration in g units. The Signal here is the RMS of the acceleration from the 3 orthogonal axes.

movements that tend to be both stereotyped and reasonably large. The SIT, however, produces leg movements during prolonged waking that are modulated by the wake state when the patient is attempting to relax and stay still. This produces a very wide range of movements, including many very small movements not usually seen during sleep. The PAM-RL has been validated only for detection of PLMS during sleep in RLS patients[13] and has not been validated for the SIT. The differences in the leg movements during the waking SIT compared to sleep suffice to likely require adjustment of the criteria for detecting the events. The criteria to detect the small movements during a SIT may need to be visually adjusted so that the offset ending a movement is slightly above the noise level for that monitor at that test time. Hopefully further studies will be done to determine the appropriate settings for accurate detection of leg movements during the SIT. At this point visual adjustment of detection criteria and scoring of the SIT ambulatory leg activity data are recommended.

As with all movement analyses, the engineering details of the monitor need to match the physical movements expected. Ideally the monitor will actually provide the average force measurements over the sample time in some units of force (e.g., g force). The sampling rate needs to be at least twice the minimum frequency of the desired movements, and the storage of information needs to be at least twice as often as the minimum detection duration. For PLM the minimum detection time is 0.5 seconds, with a desired resolution of 0.1 seconds. The activity is therefore ideally stored at 10 to 20 Hz and must be recorded for at least every 0.1 seconds. The sampling for small EMG changes needs to be at about 20 to 40 Hz to capture the 10 to 20 Hz small rapid movements. The data need to be recorded for at least 5 nights with some marker for time in and out of bed. A leg position detector on the monitor would be ideal, but button presses or logs giving the times for these events also suffice. The leg position monitor can indicate when the leg is vertical or horizontal and thereby give the ideal separation of leg movements by body position. It is strongly recommended that this be included in any assessment of PLM. The PAM-RL leg activity meter sold by Phillips Respironics currently provides a measure of leg position and separates the PLM into those occurring with legs vertical or horizontal.

PARASOMNIAS WITH MOVEMENTS DURING SLEEP

The major parasomnias involve abnormal or at least unusual movements during sleep. Documenting the time and nature of these movements can be helpful. This of course can be done with video polysomnogram. The parasomnia events, however, often do not occur every night. Sleep walking and REM behavior disorder (RBD), in particular, may occur only once a week or month. Both have characteristic features that can be detected on a single-night polysomnogram even when the behaviors are not present, but these can sometimes be difficult to detect. The loss of REM atonia in RBD can be fairly dramatic and thus the usual polysomnogram is the standard for RBD diagnosis. The increased synchronized delta activity usually associated with sleepwalking or sleep terrors is, however, neither particularly unique nor always present for these conditions. The differential between these events and seizures while not usually difficult can be a problem, especially since the nocturnal seizures often have no daytime EEG abnormalities. The standard diagnosis by history of these movement events in sleep would be aided by several nights of activity monitoring. The requirements for this, unfortunately, have not been well developed. It is unclear where the ambulatory motion detector should be placed—leg, wrist, or maybe the head. The range of normal motor events during sleep in a setting outside of the sleep laboratory remains poorly documented.

The motor activity during sleep might also be a potential trigger for alarms. This could be used to reduce the risks inherent in episodes of sleepwalking or other sleep-related movements out of bed. It might be able to support arousal to abort an event or timing of arousals prior to the usual times of events to prevent the events. These potential benefits from ambulatory activity monitoring of movement events in sleep have, however, received little attention.

TREMORS, TICS, AND DYSKINESIAS IN SLEEP

Although both tremors and tics generally decrease or cease in sleep, they sometimes persist and may even be more expressed or better observed in drowsy resting or lighter stages of sleep. Some episodes of unusual foot and leg myoclonic or rapid rhythmic activity have also been reported in sleep. The clinical significance of any of these events remains unclear, in part because of the lack of adequate documentation or study of these events. Standard wrist and leg monitors generally do not provide the frequency data needed to categorize the movements or permit separating normal from abnormal movements.

One example of a promising approach is a monitor marketed by IM Systems, Inc (Baltimore, MD). This produces a fast Fourier transform of the data from consecutive small time units over several hours. It can be used to record from the leg, wrist, or head. The level of analyses from this meter should be able to differentiate tremors, tics, and dyskinesias. Figure 15.2 shows the graphic data output from this monitor. Despite the promise of this technology, it has unfortunately been little used.

SLEEP-WAKE DETERMINATIONS

It intuitively seems the rest-activity patterns provide a good surrogate measure for sleep-wake states. Sleep-wake states are defined by the brain state assessed directly by scalp EEG recordings. Sleep certainly occurs with decreased activity. Increased motor activity generally both prevents and disrupts sleep, but the contrary is not the case. Decreased activity occurs in many conditions that are not sleep. Moreover, we now appreciate that sleep is not a passive process, but rather an active one with many episodes of motor activity during sleep. Thus, activity both fails to be very sensitive for sleep, and it certainly is not specific. This becomes particularly problematic for patients with a sleep disorder, who are likely to either increase movement during sleep or be unable to sleep.

There have been multiple claims that various activity measurements at the wrist provide a reasonable measure of sleep times for subjects who have normal sleep patterns without any sleep disorder. These claims, unfortunately, mostly involve incorrect statistical considerations. Normal healthy sleepers have sleep efficiencies usually greater than 90%, that is, 90% of the time in bed they are asleep. A meter that simply reports all the recording time as sleep will then have a 90% accurate detection of sleep (correlation of about .95) and it will be very hard with any adjustment to do much better given the small amount of time awake during the night. The important measure that should be calculated is the accuracy of detecting the wake periods during the night. These data are rarely analyzed for accuracy of detecting wake during the night. Similarly the situation is reversed during the normal waking day. Sleep periods or naps are rare and the meters' accuracy of detecting these is also not generally reported. Thus, the critical measurements assessing the accuracy of these meters are rarely even considered.

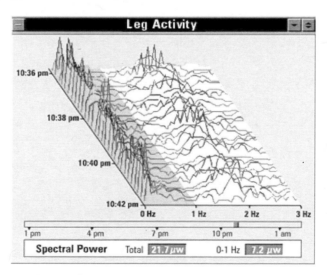

FIGURE 15.2   An example of an ambulatory monitoring showing FFT power spectrum by frequency continuously recorded over time. This is from IM System's Digitrac. (Reproduced with permission from IM Systems Inc., Baltimore, MD).

The situation is even more complicated by the use of gross overall sleep measures rather than epoch-by-epoch evaluation of the EEG compared to the activity meter determination of the sleep-wake state. At this point the degree of accuracy for the wrist activity monitoring of sleep has to be considered not much better than a written sleep log. One study including older as well as younger subjects reported the critical measures of the accuracy of predicting sleep and wake states over the 24-hour day. Multiple criteria were used to evaluate the activity compared to physiological data. The best accuracy from the activity meter looking only at usual sleep periods was 82% compared with 78% accuracy from sleep-wake logs maintained by the subjects.[15] The use of the best analytic program produced only a 77% prediction of sleep-wake state over the 24-hour day. Moreover, the accuracy for predicting the sleep state during the times the patient was out of bed was 0%. This technique simply does not work well for assessing sleep-wake states, except where the measurement is rather trivial

Given all the clear limitations of using activity to discriminate between sleep and waking, it should hardly come as a surprise to discover failure in populations known to have more activity in sleep, including both younger and older adults. These meters in particular fail to accurately report the sleep of adolescents[16] and children.[17] Thus, activity meters if they have any role for sleep-wake detection are limited to healthy young adults without a significant sleep disorder. *The sleep specialist should always remain aware that activity monitors measure activity, not sleep, and low activity should never be confused with the sleep state.*

SUMMARY

Ambulatory activity monitoring holds considerable promise for evaluating movement disorders related to sleep, but unfortunately this promise has been largely unfulfilled. The efforts spent on using activity as a surrogate for sleep-wake state have largely ignored the obvious limitation of this approach. Activity is not very sensitive for sleep, and it is certainly not specific. It essentially cannot work alone, although it might be useful with other measures or in very special populations. It might, for example, be useful in assessing agitated patients who are only inactive when asleep such as happens to some after a closed head injury.

Hopefully future development of ambulatory activity monitoring will focus less on sleep and more on movement detection and characterization. Detailed movement analyses hold considerable promise for movement disorders of sleep yet to be explored.

REFERENCES

1. Colburn TR, Smith BM, Guarini JJ, et al. An ambulatory activity monitor with solid state memory. *Biomed Sci Instrum* 1976;12:117–22.
2. Colburn TR, Smith BM, Guarini JJ, et al. An ambulatory activity monitor with solid state memory. *ISA Trans* 1976;15(2):149–54.
3. Redmond DP, Hegge FW. Observations on the design and specification of a wrist-worn activity monitor. *Behav Res Meth Instr Comp* 1985;17(6):639–69.
4. Morgenthaler T, Alessi C, Friedman L, et al. Practice parameters for the use of actigraphy in the assessment of sleep and sleep disorders: an update for 2007. *Sleep* 2007;30(4):519–29.
5. Lockley SW, Skene DJ, Arendt J. Comparison between subjective and actigraphic measurement of sleep and sleep rhythms. *J Sleep Res* 1999;8(3):175–83.
6. Teicher MH. Actigraphy and motion analysis: new tools for psychiatry. *Harv Rev Psychiatry* 1995;3(1):18–35.
7. Brown A, Smolensky M, D'Alonzo G, et al. Circadian rhythm in human activity objectively quantified by actigraphy. *Prog Clin Biol Res* 1990;341A:77–83.
8. Brown AC, Smolensky MH, D'Alonzo GE, et al. Actigraphy: a means of assessing circadian patterns in human activity. *Chronobiol Int* 1990;7(2):125–33.
9. Kolodyazhniy V, Spati J, Frey S, et al. Estimation of human circadian phase via a multi-channel ambulatory monitoring system and a multiple regression model. *J Biol Rhythms* 2011;26(1):55–67.
10. Sforza E, Haba-Rubio J. Night-to-night variability in periodic leg movements in patients with restless legs syndrome. *Sleep Med* 2005;6(3):259–67.
11. Trotti LM, Bliwise DL, Greer SA, et al. Correlates of PLMs variability over multiple nights and impact upon RLS diagnosis. *Sleep Med* 2009;10:668–71.
12. Gorny SW, Allen RP, Krausman DT, et al. Evaluation of the PAM-RL system for the

detection of periodic leg movements during sleep in the lab and home environments. *Sleep* 1998;21(Suppl):183.

13. Sforza E, Johannes M, Claudio B. The PAM-RL ambulatory device for detection of periodic leg movements: a validation study. *Sleep Med* 2005;6(5):407–13.

14. Montplaisir J, Boucher S, Nicolas A, et al. Immobilization tests and periodic leg movements in sleep for the diagnosis of restless leg syndrome. *Mov Disord* 1998;13(2):324–9.

15. Pollak CP, Tryon WW, Nagaraja H, et al. How accurately does wrist actigraphy identify the states of sleep and wakefulness? *Sleep* 2001;24(8):957–65.

16. Short MA, Gradisar M, Lack LC, et al. The discrepancy between actigraphic and sleep diary measures of sleep in adolescents. *Sleep Med* 2012;13(4):378–84.

17. Meltzer LJ, Walsh CM, Traylor J, et al. Direct comparison of two new actigraphs and polysomnography in children and adolescents. *Sleep* 2012;35(1):159–66.

16

Clinical Neurophysiology of Movement Disorders

MARK HALLETT AND SUDHANSU CHOKROVERTY

MOVEMENT DISORDERS certainly occur during the night, but have received much less attention than those that occur during the day. Some disorders occur during both night and day; these are more easily studied than those disorders that occur only during the night. In disorders that look superficially similar, it is critical to make the right diagnosis because therapies might differ. Clinical neurophysiologic methods can be helpful in extending the physical examination. One reason is that small differences in timing, easily measured with simple techniques, can be impossible to tell by eye. For example, what is the burst duration of electromyography (EMG) underlying an involuntary movement? What is the latency of a muscle jerk after a stimulus?

Movement disorders can be classified as involuntary movement disorders, voluntary movement disorders, and disorders of tone. Involuntary movement disorders are often called the hyperkinesias; there are many different kinds and many occur during sleep (see Table 22.1 in Chapter 22).

Voluntary movement disorders, such as bradykinesia, are also called hypokinesias but also include problems such as clumsiness. Tone disorders are most commonly spasticity and rigidity. It is only the involuntary movement disorders that are an issue in relation to sleep.

This chapter focuses on the clinical neurophysiologic testing that helps make the diagnosis of an involuntary movement disorder. More complete accounts are published elsewhere.[1,2] Sleep-related changes in diurnal movement disorders are discussed in Chapter 39.

ELECTROMYOGRAPHY

Involuntary movements can be characterized by the body part affected, the frequency of the movements, the relationship of the timing of the movement in the different body parts, the triggers for the movements, and the duration of each movement. It is the latter feature that is most easily studied with EMG methods. Because mechanical events take so long compared with the electrical events that control them, observations of the mechanical events are often ambiguous. In addition, EMG can determine the relationship between the activity in antagonist muscle pairs and the relative timing of different body parts, which are other difficult observations to make clinically.

EMG data can be measured with surface, needle, or wire electrodes.[1,3] The advantages of surface electrodes are that they are not painful and they record from a relatively large volume of muscle. Because they integrate over many muscle fibers, there is some correlation between the amplitude of the EMG and force. The advantage of needle electrodes is that they are more selective, sometimes a necessity when recording from small or deep muscles. However, traditional needle electrodes are stiff, and it is best to use them when recording from muscles during movements that are close to isometric. Otherwise needles are very painful. Pairs of fine-wire electrodes have the advantage of selectivity similar to that of needle electrodes, but they are flexible, permitting free movement with only minimal pain. It is important to avoid movement artifact, which can contaminate the EMG signal in all these circumstances. Wire movement should be limited. Low-frequency content of the EMG signal can be restricted with filtering, and, because movement artifact is mostly less than 10 Hz, such filtering preserves most of the EMG signal. Impedance of surface electrodes should be reduced.

There are three EMG patterns that may underlie involuntary movements.[1,3-5] One pattern, which can be called "tonic," resembles slow voluntary (tonic) movements and is characterized by continuous or almost continuous EMG activity lasting for the duration of the movement, from 200 to 1000 msec or longer. Activity can be solely in the agonist muscle, or there can be some cocontraction of the antagonist muscle with the agonist. Another pattern, which can be called "ballistic," resembles voluntary ballistic movements with a triphasic pattern; there is a burst of activity in the agonist muscle lasting 50 to 100 msec, a burst of activity in the antagonist muscle lasting 50 to 100 msec, and then return of activity in the agonist, often in the form of another burst. The third pattern, which can be called "reflex," resembles the burst occurring in many reflexes, including H reflexes and stretch reflexes. The EMG burst duration is 10 to 40 msec, and EMG activity in the antagonist muscle is virtually

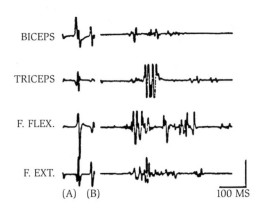

FIGURE 16.1 Comparison of (A) "reflex" and (B) "ballistic" electromyogram appearance underlying different types of myoclonus. (A) From a patient with reticular reflex myoclonus. (B) From a patient with ballistic movement overflow myoclonus. Vertical calibration is 1 mV for A and 0.5 mV for B. (From Chadwick D, Hallett M, Harris R, et al. Clinical, biochemical, and physiological features distinguishing myoclonus responsive to 5-hydroxytryptophan, tryptophan with a monoamine oxidase inhibitor, and clonazepam. Brain 100:455, 1977.)

always synchronous. Categorizing the EMG pattern is a first valuable step in making a physiologic diagnosis (Fig. 16.1).

MYOCLONUS

Myoclonus is characterized by quick muscle jerks, either irregular or rhythmic.[1,4,5] Because there are many types of myoclonus and no common etiologic, physiologic, or therapeutic features bind them together, it is critical to make a more explicit diagnosis. Myoclonus can be focal, involving only a few adjacent muscles; generalized, involving many or most of the muscles in the body; or multifocal, involving many muscles but in different jerks. Myoclonus can be spontaneous, activated, or accentuated by voluntary movement (action myoclonus), and activated or accentuated by sensory stimulation (reflex myoclonus). Rhythmic (segmental) myoclonus has the appearance of a rest tremor but is typically unaffected by action, stimulation, or even sleep. In this disorder, a segment of the spinal cord (spinal myoclonus) or brainstem (palatal myoclonus) produces persistent rhythmic repetitive discharges usually unaffected by sleep. A number of contiguous muscles produce synchronous contractions at a rate of 1 to 3 Hz. Because of the slow speed of the movements, palatal myoclonus is now often called palatal tremor (see following).

By defining epileptic myoclonus as myoclonus that is a fragment of epilepsy, it is possible to divide irregular myoclonus into epileptic and nonepileptic myoclonus.[1,4,5] The physiologic characteristics of epileptic myoclonus are (1) EMG burst length of 10 to 50 msec, (2) synchronous antagonist activity, and (3) an electroencephalographic (EEG) correlate (the technique of EMG-EEG correlation is described in the following). The EMG shows a reflex pattern. Nonepileptic myoclonus shows (1) EMG burst lengths of 50 to 300 msec, (2) synchronous or asynchronous antagonist activity, and (3) no EEG correlate. The EMG patterns are either ballistic or tonic.

Examples of epileptic myoclonus are cortical reflex myoclonus, reticular reflex myoclonus, and primary generalized epileptic myoclonus; these are discussed later. Examples of nonepileptic myoclonus include dystonic myoclonus; essential myoclonus, such as ballistic movement overflow myoclonus; exaggerated startle; and physiologic phenomena, such as hypnic jerks. Frequent myoclonus may have the appearance of tremor. In the case of action myoclonus, this may be confusing clinically, but EMG analysis is definitive.

For sorting out the different types of myoclonus, it can be useful to look for EEG events at the time of a movement.[1] Events in the ongoing EEG can be correlated with EMG events, but it is more informative to average the EEG with respect to the EMG.[3] Just as sensory-evoked cerebral potentials are time locked to the stimulus, these movement-related EEG potentials must be time-locked to a phase of the EMG, such as its onset. A great deal of attention is devoted to that part of the potential preceding movement onset because it may relate to generation of the movement; the part of the potential after movement onset includes feedback from the movement itself. The movement potential can be analyzed for the presence of consistent positive and negative waves, and the topography and time relationship of these to the movement can be determined.

Stimulation may produce involuntary movements, like reflex myoclonus, and evoke responses in the EEG. The waves in the evoked response that precede the provoked movement can be analyzed for their relationship to the movement. If the timing and topography of an event in the movement potential before a spontaneous involuntary movement are similar to the timing and topography of an event in the evoked response before the provoked movement, a similarity of the physiologic mechanism can be suggested.

With reflex myoclonus, a late response may appear in a relaxed muscle after stretch, mixed nerve stimulation, or cutaneous nerve stimulation. This response, which is not normally present, may also be seen in muscles outside of the region of the nerve stimulated or even throughout the body. This additional response, sometimes called a C-reflex, is a myoclonic movement produced by the stimulation.[1,5,6] Such responses are manifestations of hyperexcitability of the nervous system and typically reflect exaggerations of a normal reflex.

EPILEPTIC MYOCLONUS

The use of the aforementioned techniques can distinguish the three types of epileptic myoclonus described earlier.[1,5–7] Cortical reflex myoclonus is a fragment of focal or partial epilepsy. Each myoclonic jerk involves only a few adjacent muscles, but larger jerks with involvement of more muscles can be seen. The disorder is commonly multifocal and accentuated by action and sensory stimulation. The genesis of cortical reflex myoclonus is thought to be hyperexcitability of sensorimotor cortex, with each jerk representing the discharge of a small region activated by a paroxysmal depolarization shift. The EEG recognizes the discharge as a focal negative event preceding spontaneous and reflexively induced myoclonic jerks. The event with reflex jerks is a giant P1-N2 component of the somatosensory evoked potential.

Reticular reflex myoclonus is a fragment of a type of generalized epilepsy. These jerks are usually generalized with proximal more than distal, and flexor more than extensor, predominance. Voluntary action and sensory stimulation increase the jerking. The genesis of the myoclonus is thought to be hyperexcitability of a portion of the caudal brainstem reticular formation. A spike can be seen in the EEG often associated with the myoclonic jerk; but because it follows the first EMG manifestation and is not time locked to the jerk, it does not seem responsible for the jerk. The first activated muscles are those innervated by the 11th cranial nerve; this strongly suggests the brainstem origin. The somatosensory evoked potential is not enlarged, but there can be a C-reflex.

Primary generalized epileptic myoclonus is a fragment of primary generalized epilepsy. The most common clinical manifestation is a small, focal jerk that often involves only the fingers and has sometimes been called minipolymyoclonus. Generalized body jerks can also be seen. This type of myoclonus is thought to arise from the firing of a hyperexcitable cortex driven synchronously by ascending subcortical impulses. The EEG correlate is a slow, bilateral, frontocentrally predominant negativity similar to the wave of a primary generalized paroxysm. In this circumstance there is neither an enlarged somatosensory evoked response nor a C-reflex.

NONEPILEPTIC MYOCLONUS
Essential Myoclonus

The term *essential myoclonus* be used for those patients whose sole neurologic abnormality is myoclonus and specifically do not have seizures, dementia, or ataxia. The EEG and other laboratory investigations should be normal. Familial cases, as well as sporadic cases, are seen. The most common features of the familial cases are autosomal dominant inheritance with variable severity, equal involvement of males and females, onset in the first or second decade of life, and benign course compatible with normal life span. Essential myoclonus can be generalized or multifocal. The myoclonus is variable in amplitude, and, in some cases, the jerks are so small that the disability can be minimal. Jerks can be present at rest and may be improved or worsened by action. Reflex myoclonus has not been described in this group.

In some families with essential myoclonus, some involved patients also have essential tremor, and some family members have essential tremor without myoclonus. Some of these patients also may exhibit dystonia. The essential tremor, myoclonus, and dystonia may all be sensitive to alcohol in these patients.[8] It is likely that in these families the disorder is myoclonus dystonia, a known genetic condition.

The Startle Reflex

The startle reflex is a rapid, generalized motor response to a sudden, surprise stimulus.[9-12] The most extensively studied human startle response is that which occurs to loud noises (See Chapter 17). It is an oligosynaptic reflex mediated in the brainstem. The startle response is distinctive on EMG testing with surface electrodes (Fig. 16.2). The pattern is bilaterally symmetric with an invariable blink; other craniocervical muscles almost always are activated, but recruitment in the limbs is variable. The

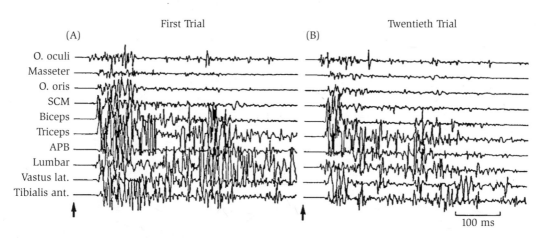

FIGURE 16.2 Multichannel surface electromyographic recordings of startle responses in a 13-year-old girl with hereditary hyperekplexia. (*A*) An initial 103-dB acoustic stimulus given at the arrow is followed by a generalized electromyographic startle response. Note the early activation of the orbicularis oculi followed by the sternocleidomastoid (SCM). (*B*) The twentieth startle response after repetitive acoustic stimuli given every 1 minute shows little habituation. (From Matsumoto J, Fuhr P, Nigro M, Hallett M: Physiological abnormalities in hereditary hyperekplexia. Ann Neurol 32:41, 1992.)

onset latency of EMG activity is 30 to 40 msec in orbicularis oculi, 55 to 85 msec in masseter and sternocleidomastoid, 85 to 100 msec in biceps brachii, 100 to 125 msec in hamstrings and quadriceps, and 130 to 140 msec in tibialis anterior. There is synchronous activation of antagonist muscles with an EMG burst duration of 50 to 400 msec. Habituation generally occurs after four or five stimuli. Increased startle responses are recognized by being excessive or being evoked by stimuli that are not effective in most people. This is most easily identified by loss of habituation. Increased startle reflexes are characteristic of a variety of disorders, called the hyperekplexias, including hereditary hyperekplexia due to abnormal glycine neurotransmission. Increased startle is also seen in posttraumatic stress syndrome.

Spinal Myoclonus

In spinal myoclonus a segment of the spinal cord produces spontaneous, persistent rhythmic repetitive discharges usually unaffected by sleep. A number of contiguous muscles produce synchronous contractions at a rate of 0.5 to 3 Hz, and this seems to be due to heightened spinal excitability.[13] Involved regions can be one limb, one limb and adjacent trunk, or both legs. Lesions of the spinal cord giving rise to focal movements include infection, degenerative disease, tumor, cervical myelopathy, and demyelinating disease, and it may follow spinal anesthesia or the introduction of contrast media into the cerebrospinal fluid.

Propriospinal Myoclonus

Propriospinal myoclonus is a special type of spinal myoclonus.[14,15] It is clinically characterized by axial jerks that are nonrhythmic and that lead to symmetric flexion of neck, trunk, hips, and knees. Jerks can be spontaneous or stimulus induced. Propriospinal myoclonus has been described as appearing mainly during drowsiness and being a possible forerunner of periodic limb movements in sleep. Recently, it has also been recognized that at least some cases of propriospinal myoclonus are psychogenic.

Asterixis

Asterixis is characterized by a brief lapse in tonic innervation.[1,16] It appears as an involuntary jerk superimposed on a postural or intentional movement. Careful observation often reveals that the jerk is in the direction of gravity, but this can be difficult because the lapse is often followed by a quick, compensatory, antigravity movement to restore limb position. The jerks may show rapid flexion-extension movements of the wrists and fingers. The involuntary movement is usually irregular, but when asterixis comes rapidly there may be the appearance of tremor. EMG analysis shows characteristic synchronous pauses in antagonist muscles. Asterixis is also called negative myoclonus.[16] When there is an EEG correlate, the physiology is likely similar to epileptic myoclonus as described previously.

Sleep-Related Movements

There are several types of movements seen at sleep onset or during sleep (see also Chapter 22): some are physiologic, whereas others are pathologic (abnormal). Physiologic types include physiologic fragmentary myoclonus and hypnic jerks. Pathologic movements that occur during sleep include non–rapid eye movement (non-REM) parasomnias, rapid eye movement (REM) parasomnias, sleep-related movement disorders, isolated sleep-related motor symptoms, abnormal movements comorbid with obstructive sleep apnea syndrome (OSAS), and daytime involuntary movements persisting in sleep.

SLEEP-RELATED MYOCLONUS

There are a variety of types of myoclonus that occur during drowsiness and sleep, and these are described in detail in subsequent chapters. Physiologic hypnic fragmentary myoclonus is characterized by small multifocal jerks maximal in hands and face.[17,18] Polymyographic study shows random transient phasic bursts of motor units discharging asynchronously or in clusters seen in stage N1 and REM sleep, decreasing progressively in sleep stages N2 and N3.

Pathologic types of myoclonus include excessive fragmentary myoclonus (EFM) in both REM and non-REM sleep (see also Chapter 22).[19,20] The EMG pattern consists of brief (duration up to 250 msec) bursts occurring randomly on both sides of the body accompanied by brief muscle jerks that are not associated with any specific EEG changes. Quantitative measurement requires at least five EMG bursts per minute and their presence during at least 20 minutes of non-REM sleep during polysomnogram

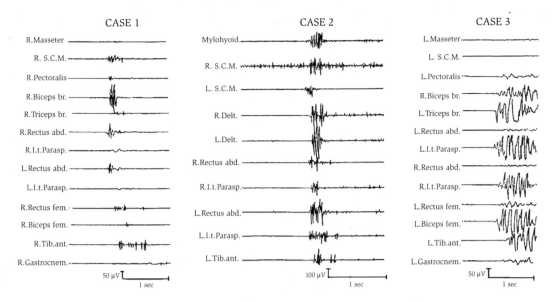

CASE 1

R.Masseter
R. S.C.M.
R.Pectoralis
R.Biceps br.
R.Triceps br.
R.Rectus abd.
R.I.t.Parasp.
L.Rectus abd.
L.I.t.Parasp.
R.Rectus fem.
R.Biceps fem.
R.Tib.ant.
R.Gastrocnem.

50 μV
1 sec

CASE 2

Mylohyoid
R. S.C.M.
L. S.C.M.
R.Delt.
L.Delt.
R.Rectus abd.
R.I.t.Parasp.
L.Rectus abd.
L.I.t.Parasp.
L.Tib.ant.

100 μV
1 sec

CASE 3

L.Masseter
L. S.C.M.
L.Pectoralis
R.Biceps br.
L.Triceps br.
L.Rectus abd.
L.I.t.Parasp.
R.Rectus abd.
R.I.t.Parasp.
L.Rectus fem.
L.Biceps fem.
L.Tib.ant.
L.Gastrocnem.

50 μV
1 sec

FIGURE 16.3 Wire electrode polygraphic recordings in three patients with propriospinal myoclonus when drowsy. SCM, sternocleidomastoid; t.l.parasp, thoracolumbar paraspinal muscles. (From Montagna P, Provini F, Plazzi G, et al. Propriospinal myoclonus upon relaxation and drowsiness: a cause of severe insomnia. Mov Disord 12:66, 1997.)

recording.[21] Myoclonus associated with epilepsy, intention myoclonus associated with semivolitional movements, and segmental myoclonus also occur in sleep but are not primarily nocturnal.

As noted earlier, propriospinal myoclonus may be present at sleep onset, induced by drowsiness and relaxation.[22] The myoclonus is identified with electrodiagnostic studies that show the myoclonus starting in the midthoracic region and propagating slowly, about 5 m/second, both rostrally and caudally (Fig. 16.3).

HYPNIC JERKS

Hypnic jerks are physiologic phenomena characterized by sudden transient nonstereotyped (unlike the stereotyped jerks of myoclonic seizures), purposeless jerks of the limbs and trunk experienced by up to 70% of the adult population at the moment of sleep onset sometime in their life. Polymyographic recordings most commonly show bilaterally synchronous, patterned, and symmetrical EMG bursts with a duration in the myoclonic range (up to about 250 msec). The jerks most likely originate in the subcortical region without any cortical prepotential on back-averaging (EMG-EEG correlate).

SLEEP-RELATED MOVEMENT DISORDERS

The ICSD-2[21] introduced a new category of sleep-related movement disorders in its latest classification encompassing restless legs syndrome (now renamed as Willis-Ekbom disease), periodic limb movement disorder, sleep-related leg cramps, sleep-related bruxism, and sleep-related rhythmic movement disorder. These along with those included in the ICSD-2 under "isolated sleep-related motor symptoms" (e.g., hypnagogic foot tremor, alternating leg muscle activation, hypnic jerks, propriospinal myoclonus) have been described in various sections of this book.

PERIODIC LIMB MOVEMENTS IN SLEEP

Periodic limb movements in sleep (PLMS) occurs in virtually all groups of patients referred to a sleep disorders laboratory, and the clinical correlation is not always clear. Although originally classified as nocturnal myoclonus, the movement is typically too long in duration to fit this category. Patients with the restless legs syndrome often have PLMS.[20,21] Certainly, PLMS can be asymptomatic for the patient, although, as with all types of nocturnal movements, the disorder may cause distress to the patient's spouse. On some rare occasions, however, PLMS can induce sleep fragmentation and excessive daytime sleepiness, when it is called periodic limb movement disorder (PLMD).[21] The etiology of PLMS seems to be increased excitability of the flexor reflex mechanism of the spinal cord.[23]

TICS

Tics are quick, involuntary, repetitive movements that occur at irregular intervals.[1] The unique feature of a tic is that it is not completely involuntary. Most patients describe a psychic tension that builds up inside them and can be relieved by the tic movement. Hence, the tics can be voluntarily suppressed for some period at the expense of increasing psychic tension; patients "let the tic happen" (or perhaps even "make the tic") to relieve the tension. Tic movements, which can be simple or complex, look like quick, voluntary movements both clinically and electromyographically. EMG bursts vary from 50 to 200 msec in duration and may have a ballistic or tonic pattern.

Both motor and verbal tics may persist during non-REM and REM sleep.[24] The tics have a similar appearance to those during wakefulness. This indicates that the generating mechanism for the tics does not require volition, an ambiguity when patients are awake. In addition, the generator is not fully suppressed by sleep. The tics may cause arousals and disturb sleep.[25]

CHOREA, DYSKINESIA, AND BALLISM

The most appropriate adjective to describe chorea is "random."[1] Random muscles throughout the body are affected at random times and make movements of random duration. Movements can be brief, such as myoclonus, or long, such as dystonia. Usually they are totally beyond voluntary control, but in some mild cases the movements can be temporarily suppressed. EMG patterns are reflex, ballistic, and tonic. Dyskinesia describes choreic movements seen in selected circumstances, such as a late consequence of neuroleptic drugs or with levodopa toxicity. Ballism describes wild, large-amplitude choreic movements; these usually involve one side of the body and are then called hemiballismus. Choreic movements may persist in stage N1 but with decreased intensity. Ballistic movements progressively diminish in intensity and frequency from stages N1 to N3 and REM sleep.[20,26,27]

DYSTONIA AND ATHETOSIS

The involuntary movements of dystonia and athetosis are similar, and the use of one term rather than the other seems more a matter of situation and semantics than physiology.[1] The movements are typically slow but can be quick and may be "sustained for a second or longer at the height of the involuntary contraction." Dystonia is often used to describe proximal "twisting" movements; athetosis is often used to describe distal "flowing" movements. Dystonic and athetotic movements are often characterized by cocontraction of antagonist muscles.[28] Although normal voluntary movement is often characterized by reciprocal inhibition, there may be some cocontraction. The cocontraction of dystonia and athetosis is excessive, with the appearance of increased tension at the joint. Some dystonic and athetotic movements are fully involuntary, arising at rest independent of will. Other movements arise as excessive, unwanted concomitants to voluntary movements. This phenomenon is called overflow, with the implication that the motor control command is sent to too many muscles with too much intensity. EMG studies can document these phenomena. The shortest EMG bursts seen even with dystonic myoclonus are in the range of 100 to 300 msec.

The physiology of dystonia has been studied in detail and generally can be characterized by loss of inhibition at all levels of the neuraxis.[28-30] Some clinical neurophysiologic tests are often abnormal in patients with dystonia, but none have specificity. Hence, such studies can be employed to see if a consistent abnormality is present. Three tests are worthy of mention in this regard.

Reciprocal inhibition can be assessed at the spinal cord level. It is evaluated in the upper extremity by studying the effect of stimulating the radial nerve at various times before producing an H-reflex with median nerve stimulation (Fig. 16.4). The radial nerve afferents come from muscles that are antagonist to median nerve muscles. Via various pathways, the radial afferent traffic can inhibit motoneuron pools of median nerve muscles. Reciprocal inhibition is reduced in patients with dystonia, including those with generalized dystonia, writer's cramp, spasmodic torticollis, and blepharospasm.[31-35]

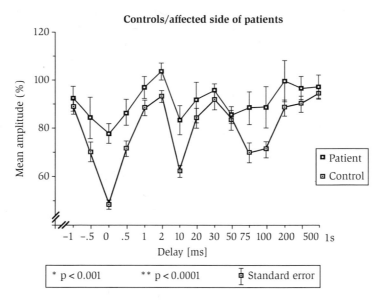

Controls/affected side of patients

FIGURE 16.4 Reciprocal inhibition study of the affected hands of patients with focal hand dystonia compared with a group of normal control subjects. (From Panizza ME, Hallett M, Nilsson J: Reciprocal inhibition in patients with hand cramps. Neurology 39:85, 1989.)

The blink reflex can be used to assess inhibition at the level of the brainstem. Abnormalities of blink reflex recovery were first identified for blepharospasm[36] and have also been demonstrated in generalized dystonia, spasmodic torticollis, and spasmodic dysphonia.[37] In the last two conditions, abnormalities can be found even without clinical involvement of the eyelids. Inhibition can also be shown to be deficient at the level of the motor cortex using a method with transcranial magnetic stimulation (TMS)[38] that evaluates intracortical inhibition with the "double-pulse paradigm." Motor evoked potentials are inhibited when conditioned by a prior subthreshold TMS stimulus to the same position at intervals of 1 to 5 msec. Inhibition was less in both hemispheres of patients with focal hand dystonia showing that the test is sufficiently sensitive to detect subclinical abnormality.

Dystonic movements decrease markedly from stage N1 to stage N2 and are absent in N3 and REM sleep.[20]

TREMOR

Physiology varies in different forms of human tremor.[39,40] Tremors may come from mechanical oscillations, mechanical-reflex oscillations (EMG activity is entrained with a mechanical oscillation), normal central oscillators, and pathologic central oscillators.[41] Any physical object has mechanical properties that obey the laws of physics, and this certainly includes a joint with its associated muscles. Any perturbation of a mechanical system causes it to oscillate at its resonant frequency. Muscles are connected to the central nervous system via reflex loops. These loops operate over related fixed time intervals and may oscillate at frequencies inversely proportional to the loop delay. In certain circumstances, when the frequencies of the mechanical and reflex oscillations are similar, the two frequencies can be mutually entrained to a single frequency. Such a mutually entrained oscillation may behave just like a mechanical system and is referred to as a mechanical-reflex. Central oscillators differ, at least theoretically, from central nodes of reflexes by their independence of peripheral input. Central oscillators might arise from the properties of individual neurons, from the properties of neuronal networks, or a combination of the two.

Tremor can be examined with accelerometry. The output of an accelerometer is a time-varying analog signal proportional to instantaneous acceleration. Accelerometers in common use measure movement only in one axis so that they must be oriented carefully in the direction of movement. Also available are triaxial accelerometers that measure movement in three orthogonal axes and permit the accurate, three-dimensional description of movement. Gyroscopes measure rotations rather than linear movements and can be used instead of, or together with, accelerometers.

An excellent method for determining the physiology consists of combined accelerometry and EMG using spectral analysis and study of the tremor with and without weighting of the body part.[39-41] Because mechanical or mechanical-reflex tremors reduce frequency with increasing inertia, it is possible to separate such tremors using weighting from those coming from a central oscillator. In a pure mechanical tremor, such as a physiologic tremor, there is a tremor peak in the acceleration trace, but the EMG is relatively the same over different frequencies. With weighting, the tremor peak shifts down and the EMG remains nondescript. In a mechanical-reflex tremor, seen when a physiologic tremor is enhanced, the EMG now participates at a similar frequency as the accelerometry record. With weighting in this condition, the peaks for both the accelerometer and the EMG shift down similarly. These two situations can be compared with the result when there is a central oscillator. For example, some normal subjects have a contribution to their physiologic tremor from an 8- to 12-Hz central oscillator.[39,40] In this circumstance without weighting, the EMG shows an 8- to 12-Hz peak, and the accelerometer record may be the same or different depending on the mechanical characteristics. With weight, the accelerometer record shows two peaks, one shifting downward, the mechanical peak, and the other staying at 8 to 12Hz. A component of tremor with a constant frequency with weighting presumably comes from a central oscillator.

Tremor can be divided into those at rest and those seen with action. Rest is only relative; some slight tonic postural maintenance is often required. Action tremors must be subdivided into those seen just with postural maintenance (postural or static tremor) and those requiring goal-directed movement (intentional or kinetic tremor). A third division of action tremors is those seen only with specific types of kinetic movement, such as handwriting.

PARKINSONIAN TREMOR AT REST

The most frequent tremor at rest is that seen with Parkinson's disease or other parkinsonian states, such as that produced by neuroleptics.[1,39,40,42] The tremor is usually seen in the context of other basal ganglia symptoms but on rare occasions can be the sole clinical finding. It is present at rest and disappears with action, but it may resume with a static posture, particularly late in the disease, and can be called re-emergent tremor. The frequency is 3 to 5 Hz. EMG studies show antagonist muscles to be active alternately (Fig. 16.5A). The tremor frequency is not altered by weighting and, hence, has its origin in a central oscillator, but its location is not known. Rest tremor tends to persist in drowsiness; it is occasionally seen in stage N1 sleep and rarely in stage N3 but is absent in REM sleep. It can, however, reappear on arousals and during transition to stage N1 and N2.[20]

EXAGGERATED PHYSIOLOGIC TREMOR

Physiologic tremor is a normal postural action tremor. In certain circumstances, such as anxiety, fatigue, thyrotoxicosis, and excessive use of caffeine, the tremor can be increased in magnitude and may be symptomatic. The frequency usually is in a range from 5 to 12 Hz, varying in part because of the weight of the tremulous body part. The EMG in mild cases may look just like a normal interference pattern without well-defined bursting. In more severe cases, bursting may appear; it is usually synchronous in antagonist muscles. The accelerometric and EMG spectral peaks are the same and shift together with weighting. There may also be a component from an 8- to 12-Hz central oscillator also seen in this condition.[1,39,40,42]

ESSENTIAL TREMOR

Essential tremor is a common neurologic disorder that often runs as an autosomal-dominant trait in families.[1] It may appear in childhood or late life and runs a slowly progressive course. Typically it is a postural tremor; in some patients there is some increase in tremor with intention (kinetic movement), and in others the tremor occurs primarily with goal-directed movement (intentional essential tremor). Rarely it appears to persist with rest. In most circumstances it is seen as the sole neurologic abnormality; there is no known pathology and the pathophysiology is not clear. The frequency ranges from 5 to 8 Hz and there is often an associated component of physiologic tremor (8–13 Hz). EMG studies commonly

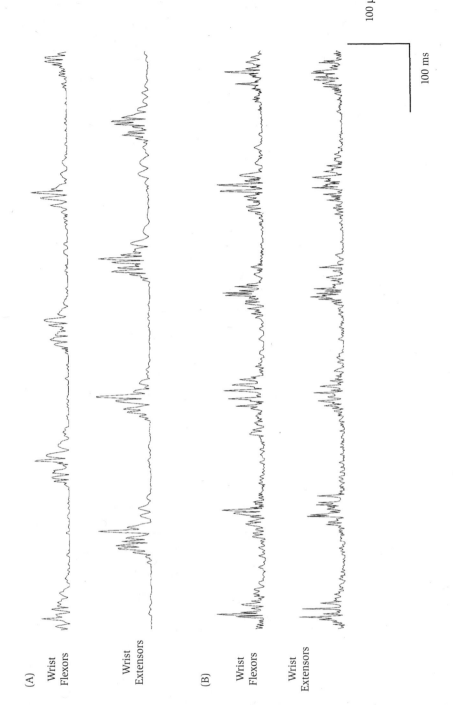

FIGURE 16.5   Electromyographic recordings of tremor. (A) The typical rest tremor of Parkinson's disease with alternating activity in antagonist muscles. (B) The commonest pattern in essential tremor with synchronous activity in antagonist muscles. Electromyogram is rectified. (Courtesy of Dr. Holly Shill.)

show synchronous activity in antagonist muscles (Fig. 16.5B), but alternating activity is also possible. Sometimes it is clinically difficult to separate exaggerated physiologic tremor and essential tremor. Using accelerometry and EMG, there is a constant frequency with weighting, which is clearly different from that seen with exaggerated physiologic tremor.[39,40] This observation indicates that essential tremor originates from a generator in the central nervous system. The cerebellum and cerebellar circuits seem involved,[43] and one commonly considered candidate is the inferior olivary nucleus.[44]

CEREBELLAR TREMOR

Tremor with cerebellar lesions can be postural, as well as the more well-known kinetic tremor.[1,42,45] Typically it has a frequency of 2.5 to 4 Hz, affects proximal muscles more than distal muscles, waxes and wanes, and has a tendency to increase progressively in amplitude with prolonged posture. It persists or worsens with goal-directed movement and is associated with dysmetria. EMG studies show bursts of activity lasting 125 to 250 msec and alternation of activity in antagonist muscles. The responsible lesion appears to be in the superior cerebellar peduncle. The most common etiology in general neurologic practice is multiple sclerosis, but there may be other causes, such as strokes, tumors, or head trauma.

Kinetic tremor without postural tremor is usually ascribed to cerebellar dysfunction and is often called cerebellar intention tremor. It certainly can be seen also together with a postural tremor. The lesions can be in the cerebellum or cerebellar pathways. Kinetic tremor is characterized by rhythmic oscillations about the target of movement; EMG studies show alternating activity in antagonist muscles. It should be differentiated from sequential irregular, inaccurate movements toward the target, which have been named serial dysmetria.[1,42,45]

OTHER TREMORS

Wilson's disease can present with tremor as its sole manifestation, although other movement disorders and psychiatric disturbances are often present as well. The tremor is an action tremor present with posture and kinetic movement. Physiologic analysis shows alternating activity in antagonist muscles at 3 to 5 Hz.[45]

Neuropathic Tremor

This may be seen in the setting of congenital or acquired peripheral neuropathies.[1] The pathophysiology is obscure. The tremor seen with hereditary sensorimotor neuropathy type 1 may simply be essential tremor that is coinherited. Physiologically, the frequency is in the range of 6 to 8 Hz, and EMG studies show a mixture of synchronous and alternating activity in antagonist muscles. It is likely that in many circumstances, particularly in IGM (sometimes IgG) paraproteinemic demyelinating neuropathy, slowing of nerve conduction in the peripheral loop will give rise to delays that create instability.[46]

Palatal tremor, also known as palatal myoclonus, is characterized by rhythmic movements of the palate at approximately 3 Hz. There are two separate disorders: essential palatal tremor (EPT), which manifests an ear click, and symptomatic palatal tremor (SPT), which is associated with cerebellar disturbances.[1,47] The palatal movements are due to activation of the tensor veli palatini muscle in EPT and of the levator veli palatini muscle in SPT. In SPT, the palatal movements may be accompanied by synchronous movements of adjacent muscles such as the external ocular muscles, tongue, larynx, face, neck, diaphragm, or even limb muscles. SPT is associated with hypertrophy of the inferior olive and many authorities consider it to arise there, but the generator for EPT likely differs. SPT continues during sleep but may become irregular, whereas EPT typically ceases.

Psychogenic Tremor

This is commonly encountered by movement disorder specialists and neurologists in general. Its physiology is largely unknown, but the movement despite being involuntary has characteristics of voluntary movement. It is often highly variable in nature and may disappear with distraction. It may be present in rest, posture, and kinetic action. Clinical neurophysiologic assessment may include (1) measurement of frequency and amplitude; (2) measurement in two body parts simultaneously; (3) entrainment testing; and (4) monitoring tremor while asking the patient to make a sudden rapid movement of another body part.[48]

Accelerometry is the best method to record frequency and amplitude, although EMG can also be used. Characteristically psychogenic tremor is highly variable in frequency and amplitude and can be seen synchronous between two limbs. The most useful clinical test that can be measured accurately and quantified physiologically is the entrainment test in which the patient is asked to voluntarily tap at various frequencies, preferably with a body part unaffected or least affected by the tremor. The tremor is entrained if it takes up the frequency of the voluntary tapping measurement. Measurement will show the same frequency in all body parts in psychogenic tremor, whereas in organic tremors there is often a slightly different frequency in different body parts. The other test that may be useful is the ballistic movement test in which the patient is asked to make a sudden rapid movement of another body part. In psychogenic disorder the tremor may transiently stop in contrast to that in parkinsonian or essential tremor (there may be false positives or false negatives).

Stiffness

Stiffness is generally not a specific complaint at night, but often it is helpful in the differential diagnosis to find out whether the stiffness continues during the night. In disorders such as Parkinson's disease and dystonia, the stiffness and involuntary movements typically melt away when the patient is asleep unless contractures have developed. Stiff-person syndrome is a disorder characterized by continuous muscle contraction giving rise to severe stiffness, most severe axially.[49,50] Patients have difficulty moving and make voluntary movements slowly. Sensory stimulation often induces a worsening of the spasms.[51] The disorder is often associated with circulating antibodies to glutamic acid decarboxylase, and the resultant deficiency of gamma-aminobutyric acid may play a role in its pathophysiology. EMG demonstrates continuous activity of motor units in a normal pattern but that cannot be silenced even with contraction of the antagonist muscle.[52] The stiffness does disappear, however, with sleep.

The syndrome of neuromyotonia, on the other hand, is a condition of muscle stiffness that does not disappear with sleep. This disorder, also called Isaacs syndrome or continuous muscle fiber activity, is due to activity arising in the peripheral nerve. There may be a variety of etiologies, but a common link appears to be an abnormality of potassium channels in the nerve membrane.[53] With EMG, there is continuous muscle activity with myokymia and neuromyotonic discharges.

CONCLUSION

It is important for sleep specialists, other physicians practicing sleep medicine, and movement disorder specialists to have a basic knowledge about various movements that are frequently seen during sleep. Clinically there is often diagnostic confusion, particularly between various parasomnias and nocturnal seizures. An optimal history and physical examination followed by a set of clinical neurophysiologic tests often clarify a seemingly complex movement disorder encountered at sleep onset or during sleep. This chapter briefly addressed some of these common movements and their neurophysiologic tests, which should help in making a correct diagnosis and designing appropriate treatment.

AUTHORS' NOTE

Many portions of the text are similar to previous chapters written by the senior author.[1,4,6]

REFERENCES

1. Hallett M. Electrophysiologic evaluation of movement disorders. In: Aminoff MJ, ed. *Electrodiagnosis in Clinical Neurology*. 5th ed. Philadelphia, PA: Elsevier, Churchill Livingstone; 2005:389–405.
2. Hallett M. Electrodiagnosis in movement disorders. In: Levin KH, Lüders HO, eds. *Comprehensive Clinical Neurophysiology*. Philadelphia, PA: WB Saunders; 2000:281.
3. Hallett M, Berardelli A, Delwaide P, et al. Central EMG and tests of motor control. Report of an IFCN Committee. *Electroencephalogr Clin Neurophysiol* 1994;90:404.
4. Hallett M, Marsden CD, Fain S. Myoclonus. In: Vinken PJ, Bruyn GW, Klawans HL, eds. *Handbook of Clinical Neurology*. Vol 5. Amsterdam, The Netherlands; Elsevier Science; 1987:609.
5. Hallett M. Myoclonus and myoclonic syndromes. In: Engel JJ, Pedley TA, eds. *Epilepsy: A Comprehensive Textbook*. Vol. 3. Philadelphia, PA: Lippincott Williams & Wilkins;20082765–70.
6. Toro C, Hallett M. Pathophysiology of myoclonic disorders. In: Watts RL, Standaert D, Obeso J, eds. *Movement Disorders*. 3rd ed. New York: McGraw Hill Medical; 2012:761–79.
7. Chokroverty S. An approach to a patient with disorders of voluntary movements.

In: Chorkoverty S, ed. *Movement Disorders.* PMA Publishing; 1990:1–43.

8. Quinn NP. Essential myoclonus and myoclonic dystonia. *Mov Disord* 1996;11:119.

9. Brown P, Rothwell JC, Thompson PD, et al. The hyperekplexias and their relationship to the normal startle reflex. *Brain* 1991;114:1903.

10. Matsumoto J, Fuhr P, Nigro M, et al. Physiological abnormalities in hereditary hyperekplexia. *Ann Neurol* 1992;32:41.

11. Matsumoto J, Hallett M. Startle syndromes. In: Marsden CD, Fahn S, eds. *Movement Disorders 3.* Oxford, England: Butterworth-Heinemann; 1994:418.

12. Chokroverty S, Walczak T, Hening W. Human startle reflex: technique and criteria. *Electroencephalogr Clin Neurophysiol* 1992;85(4):236–42.

13. Di Lazzaro V, Restuccia D, Nardone R, et al. Changes in spinal cord excitability in a patient with rhythmic segmental myoclonus. *J Neurol Neurosurg Psychiatry* 1996;61:641.

14. Chokroverty S, Walters A, Zimmerman T, et al. Propriospinal myoclonus: a neurophysiologic analysis. *Neurology* 1992;42:1591.

15. Brown P, Thompson PD, Rothwell JC, et al. Axial myoclonus of propriospinal origin. *Brain* 1991;114:197.

16. Shibasaki H. Pathophysiology of negative myoclonus and asterixis. In: Fahn S, Hallett M, Lüders HO, Marsden CD, eds. *Negative Motor Phenomena. Advances in Neurology.* Vol. 67. Philadelphia, PA: Lippincott-Raven; 1995:199.

17. Dagnino N, Loeb C, Massazza G, et al. Hypnic physiological myoclonias in man: an EEG-EMG study in normals and neurological patients. *Eur Neurol* 1969;2:47.

18. Montagna P, Liguori R, Zucconi M, et al. Physiological hypnic myoclonus. *Electroencephalogr Clin Neurophysiol* 1988;70:172.

19. Broughton R, Tolentino MA, Krelina M. Excessive fragmentary myoclonus in NREM sleep: a report of 38 cases. *Electroencephalogr Clin Neurophysiol* 1985;61:123.

20. Lysenko L, Hanna P, Chokroverty S. Sleep disruption from movement disorders. In: Barkoukis TJ, Matheson JK, Ferber R, Doghramji K, eds. *Therapy in Sleep Medicine.* Philadelphia, PA: Elsevier/Saunders; 2012:345–60.

21. American Academy of Sleep Medicine. *International Classification of Sleep Disorders. Diagnostic and Coding Manual.* 2nd ed. Westchester, IL: American Academy of Sleep Medicine; 2005.

22. Montagna P, Provini F, Plazzi G, et al. Propriospinal myoclonus upon relaxation and drowsiness: a cause of severe insomnia. *Mov Disord* 1997;12:66.

23. Bara-Jimenez W, Aksu M, Graham B, et al. Periodic limb movements in sleep: state-dependent excitability of the spinal flexor reflex. *Neurology* 2000;54:1609.

24. Glaze DG, Frost JD, Jankovic J. Sleep in Gilles de la Tourette's syndrome: disorder of arousal. *Neurology* 1983;33:586.

25. Drake ME, Jr., Hietter SA, Bogner JE, et al. Cassette EEG sleep recordings in Gilles de la Tourette syndrome. *Clin Electroencephalogr* 1992;23:142.

26. Mano T, Shiozawa Z, Sobue I. Extrapyramidal involuntary movements during sleep. *Electroencephalogr Clin Neurophysiol Suppl* 1982;35:431–42.

27. Dyken ME, Rodnitzky RL. Periodic, aperiodic and rhythmic motor disorders of sleep. *Neurology* 1992;42:68–74.

28. Hallett M. Physiology of dystonia. In: Fahn S, Marsden CD, DeLong M, eds. *Dystonia 3. Advances in Neurology.* Vol. 78. Philadelphia, PA: Lippincott-Raven; 1998:11.

29. Berardelli A, Rothwell JC, Hallett M, et al. The pathophysiology of primary dystonia. *Brain* 1998;121:1195.

30. Hallett M. The neurophysiology of dystonia. *Arch Neurol* 1998;55:601.

31. Nakashima K, Rothwell JC, Day BL, et al. Reciprocal inhibition in writer's and other occupational cramps and hemiparesis due to stroke. *Brain* 1989;112:681.

32. Panizza ME, Hallett M, Nilsson J. Reciprocal inhibition in patients with hand cramps. *Neurology* 1989;39:85.

33. Panizza M, Lelli S, Nilsson J, et al. H-reflex recovery curve and reciprocal inhibition of H-reflex in different kinds of dystonia. *Neurology* 1990;40:824.

34. Chen RS, Tsai CH, Lu CS. Reciprocal inhibition in writer's cramp. *Mov Disord* 1995;10:556.

35. Deuschl G, Seifert G, Heinen F, et al. Reciprocal inhibition of forearm flexor muscles in spasmodic torticollis. *J Neurol Sci* 1992;113:85.

36. Berardelli A, Rothwell JC, Day BL, et al. Pathophysiology of blepharospasm and

oromandibular dystonia. *Brain* 1985; 108:593.

37. Cohen LG, Ludlow CL, Warden M, et al. Blink reflex excitability recovery curves in patients with spasmodic dysphonia. *Neurology* 1989;39:572.

38. Ridding MC, Sheean G, Rothwell JC, et al. Changes in the balance between motor cortical excitation and inhibition in focal, task specific dystonia. *J Neurol Neurosurg Psychiatry* 1995;59:493.

39. Elble RJ, Koller WC. *Tremor.* Baltimore, MD: Johns Hopkins University Press; 1990.

40. Elble RJ. The pathophysiology of tremor. In: Watts RL, Koller WC, eds. *Movement Disorders. Neurologic Principles and Practice.* New York: McGraw-Hill; 1997:405.

41. Hallett M. Overview of human tremor physiology. *Mov Disord* 1998;13(Suppl 3):43.

42. Hallett M. Classification and treatment of tremor. JAMA 266:1115, 1991.

43. Jenkins IH, Bain PG, Colebatch JG, et al. A positron emission tomography study of essential tremor: evidence for overactivity of cerebellar connections. *Ann Neurol* 1993;34:82.

44. Hallett M, Dubinsky RM. Glucose metabolism in the brain of patients with essential tremor. *J Neurol Sci* 1993;114:45.

45. Hallett M. Differential diagnosis of tremor. In: Vinken PJ, Bruyn GW, Klawans HL, eds. *Handbook of Clinical Neurology: Extrapyramidal Disorders.* Vol 5. Amsterdam, The Netherlands: Elsevier Science; 1987:583.

46. Bain PG, Britton TC, Jenkins LH, et al. Tremor associated with benign IgM paraproteinaemic neuropathy. *Brain* 1996;119:789.

47. Deuschl G, Toro C, Valls-Solé J, et al. Symptomatic and essential palatal tremor. 1. Clinical, physiological, and MRI analysis. *Brain* 1994;117:775.

48. Hallett M. Physiology of psychogenic movement disorders. *J Clin Neurosci* 2010;17:959–65.

49. Brown P, Marsden CD. The stiff man and stiff man plus syndromes. *J Neurol* 1999;246:648.

50. Levy LM, Dalakas MC, Floeter MK. The stiff-person syndrome: An autoimmune disorder affecting neurotransmission of gammaaminobutyric acid. *Ann Intern Med* 1999;131:522.

51. Matsumoto JY, Caviness JN, McEvoy KM. The acoustic startle reflex in stiff-man syndrome. *Neurology* 1994;44:1952.

52. Toro C, Jacobowitz DM, Hallett M. Stiffman syndrome. *Semin Neurol* 1994;14:154.

53. Hart IK. Acquired neuromyotonia: a new autoantibody-mediated neuronal potassium channelopathy. *Am J Med Sci* 2000;319:209.

17

Clinical Neurophysiology of Acoustic Startle

JOSEP VALLS-SOLÉ

A STIMULUS of any kind that is presented unexpectedly and with sufficient intensity may trigger a motor response in all living creatures equipped with appropriate afferent and efferent circuits. Such a generalized motor reaction is known as the startle reaction. Literally, a startle is defined as a sudden involuntary movement of the body triggered by a stimulus causing surprise or alarm. The motor reaction to a startling stimulus is usually a reflex involuntary reaction intended to protect our body from the potential danger related to the stimulus. It is common to all animals but manifests in different ways in different species. For instance, it is difficult to freely watch animal behavior since they show an apparently inevitable reaction to the visual and auditory signals of our presence. Such signals act as a warning stimulus for the alertness system and prepare the animal's motor apparatus for escaping from such eventual threat. Small reptiles freeze or curl when touched as a reaction of protection, since they are unlikely to escape. In animals and human beings, the initial protecting reaction is followed by the so-called orienting reaction, which sets the body in a fight-or-flight condition. Probably, human beings are not different from animals in regard to the physiological mechanisms underlying the startle and orienting reactions. One difference is that our reactions are contextually modulated in accordance with the motor set and behavior. We may learn that the auditory stimulus does not actually evoke any danger and, with some training, we may not even bother about the presence of such a stimulus. Humans have certainly more control than animals on reflex responses, but abnormalities of such a control system may lead to diseases characterized by either reduced or enhanced reactivity. Among the disorders with enhanced startle responses, the best known is likely hyperekplexia,[1] whereas among those leading to reduced startle, the best known ones are probably those that present with parkinsonism.

The circuit conveying the startle reaction should be a phylogenetically very old nervous tract with widespread connections to motoneurons. The system fitting with these requirements is the reticular formation and the lateral ponto-medullary reticulospinal tract. This is a descending motor tract that originates in the nuclei gigantocellularis and reticularis pontis caudalis, projecting directly to alpha motoneurons, mainly those of proximal and axial muscles. The medial part of the reticulospinal tract terminates in interneurons of the lamina VII and lamina VIII of the spinal cord and innervates mainly antigravity muscles. The extent to which this subcortical motor system contributes to voluntary movement is difficult to know, but it probably contributes largely to movement preparation in anticipatory postural adjustments or automatic movements.

This chapter is dealing with the physiology of startle reaction in humans, the abnormalities in the control of motor responses, and the relationship between voluntary movement and startle reactions. A control system should be involved in many aspects of the startle reaction and its relationship with voluntary movements. One of these control mechanisms is the so-called prepulse inhibition, a concept that is defined as any attention-drawing sensory signal that, while being processed, prevents reaction to a subsequent suprathreshold stimulus that would otherwise be followed by a response. This applies to the domain of the startle reaction, where prepulse inhibition can be obtained with stimuli of the same or different sensory modality as the one producing the startle reaction. The inhibitory effect is probably a consequence of the attentional displacement required to process the information brought about by the prepulse.[2] It is likely that abnormalities in the control of the startle reaction are related to functional disturbances of prepulse inhibition.

PHYSIOLOGICAL MECHANISMS OF THE NORMAL HUMAN STARTLE REACTION

Startle Response Circuits

Usually, the startle reaction is examined experimentally using auditory stimuli, although other sensory modalities are also capable of inducing the response. In humans, visual,[3] somatosensory,[4] or vestibular stimuli[5] have been also used. The circuits of the auditory startle reaction have been delineated after research

in animals.[6-9] The circuits of the startle reaction were localized at the brainstem.[10] These authors found that the response was preserved in decerebrated animals and obtained to direct stimulation of the nucleus reticularis pontis caudalis (nRPC), but not of the nucleus reticularis gigantocellularis.[6] The circuit proposed by Davis et al.[6] involved the cochlear nucleus, the nucleus of the lateral lemniscus, the nRPC, and the motoneurones of the brainstem and the spinal cord, activated through the medial reticulospinal tract. Later, Lingenhöhl and Friauf[7] described direct afferent inputs from the cochlear nucleus to the nRPC, and Lee et al.[11] demonstrated that the nucleus of the lateral lemniscus was not necessary for elicitation of the reflex response. At present, the auditory startle reaction is considered to be conveyed through a very simple circuit,[8-10,12] with activation of the reticulospinal and reticulobulbar neurons after direct synaptic activation from the cochlear nucleus to the nRPC.

The nRPC neurons are not modality specific[13] and, hence, they respond to sensory afferents other than the auditory ones. The nRPC receives continuous inputs from many sources. One of the sources relevant for the startle circuit is the pedunculopontine nucleus (PPn), which cholinergic neurons are strongly influenced by the output from the basal ganglia (Fig. 17.1). This brings up an explanation for the presence of abnormalities in the startle reaction in diseases caused by dysfunction of the basal ganglia. The inputs arriving at the nRPC from the PPn are inhibitory[14] and tune down transiently

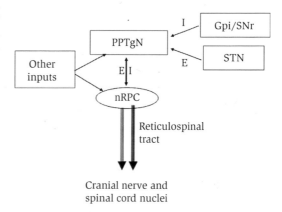

FIGURE 17.1 Schematic representation of the relationship between the basal ganglia, the pedunculopontine nucleus, and the nucleus reticularis pontis caudalis for the generation of the startle reaction.

the sensitivity of the nRPC to high-intensity stimuli. Other, uncontrolled influences set the membrane potential of PPn cholinergic neurons to various levels, differing from one moment to another, with the consequence of varying the size of the startle reaction. Probably, the interaction of many inputs in the PPn is the crucial factor for an appropriate control of the startle reactions.

An alternative pathway, comprising neurons of inferior colliculus and midbrain reticular formation, has been suggested by Hori et al.[15] to account for the peculiarities of the response recorded from the orbicularis oculi muscle (OOc) to sound stimuli, known as the auditory blink reflex.

Prepulse Inhibition Circuits

The best known mechanism of control over the startle reaction is prepulse inhibition.[2] The functional anatomy of prepulse inhibition is not completely known, although there is evidence from various sources that the PPn may be involved.[14,16,17] The PPn is the main structure within the first level of higher order hierarchical circuits governing the primary startle circuit. In rats, PPn lesions increase baseline auditory startle reaction amplitude and abolish prepulse inhibition without affecting long-term habituation.[18,19] The effect is likely mediated by cholinergic projections, since direct injections of the acetylcholine antagonist scopolamine into the nRPC in rats increase the basal startle reaction amplitude.[20] Aging goes with loss of cholinergic neurons of the PPn.[21] This could account for the observation reported by Kofler et al.[22] of an age-related increase in the size of the startle response. The PPn receives basal ganglia inputs (Fig. 17.1) mainly from the substantia nigra pars reticulata and the globus pallidus.[23] This startle modulation circuit is further regulated by higher brain circuitry via the pontine tegmentum, which involves limbic cortical inputs to the ventral striatum, striatal connections with the pallidum, and pallidal inputs to the pontine tegmentum.[24]

Prepulse inhibition is effective not only on the startle reaction but also on the blink reflex elicited by electrical stimulation of the supraorbital nerve.[25–27] Recently, Costa et al.[28] studied the effects of low-intensity electrical stimuli, applied through the electrodes inserted for therapeutic purposes in the subthalamic nucleus of Parkinson's disease patients, on the blink reflex

induced by supraorbital nerve stimulation. The inhibitory effect was significant already at very short intervals (5 ms) and lasted for less than 100 ms, suggesting that the structures responsible for prepulse inhibition were probably at a very short distance from the stimulation site. Connections between the internal pallidum and the PPn, adjacent to the subthalamic nucleus, were the most likely candidates for the effect.

Recording Human Startle and Orienting Reactions

Typically, a loud auditory stimulus gives rise to an early brief and generalized muscle contraction, the (short-latency) startle reaction, and a later more elaborated activity, resulting from the central integration of sensory information carried by the stimulus, known as the orienting reaction. While the short-latency startle reaction serves a basic protective function, the orienting reaction is the partial expression of a behavioral change in preparation for defense or attack. Figure 17.2 shows an example of the startle and orienting reactions in a healthy subject.

SHORT-LATENCY STARTLE REACTION

The most prominent features of the short-latency startle reaction are forceful closure of the eyes; raising of bent arms over the head; and flexion of the neck, trunk, elbows, hips, and knees.[29] The response can be recorded with surface electromyography (EMG) electrodes, to show the progression of the latency of the response in face, trunk, and limb muscles in relation to the distance from the startle generator at the medulla.[32] The shortest latencies are about 50 ms for the orbicularis oculi muscle, which is probably the consequence of a special circuit impinging on orbicularis oculi motoneurons.[15,31] The next muscle showing a response and the one considered the most representative for the generalized startle response in human being is the sternocleidomastoid muscle, at a latency variable between 60 and 100 ms. The EMG responses of the intrinsic hand and foot muscles are particularly delayed, if obtained, with respect to the responses of other muscles of the same limb.

The response of the orbicularis oculi to auditory stimuli is known also as the auditory blink reflex. Some recordings show two

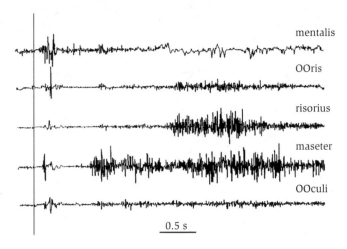

FIGURE 17.2 The two components of the startle reaction to an auditory stimulus of 130 dB in a naïve healthy subject (S, startle reflex; O, orienting reaction). The sound was obtained by discharging the coil of a magnetic stimulator at 100% of the stimulator output intensity on top of a metallic platform at about 1 m distance from the subject. Activity was recorded from facial muscles. Note the early brief component and the late and much longer component corresponding, in this case, to a nodding and a comment on the surprisingly loud stimulus.

responses, identified as the auditory blink reflex and the component of the auditory startle in the orbicularis oculi. There are physiological differences between the auditory blink reflex and the auditory startle reaction. The auditory blink reflex is induced more frequently, is more consistent, and is less prone to habituation with repeated presentation of the stimuli than the auditory startle reaction. However, even if the circuits are indeed different, Koch et al.[13] demonstrated in the rat that the facial and extremity muscle responses are mediated by the same neurons located in the nRPC. Bisdorff et al.[5] proposed that the peculiarities of the auditory blink reflex are due to a differentially patterned organization of the orbicularis oculi response to startling stimuli in comparison to other muscles, regardless of whether the circuit is a different one. The response would be organized according to the type and strength of sensory inputs and the degree of muscle preparation to react. A similar reasoning was put forward by Matsumoto et al.[33] in their explanation of the results obtained in patients with hyperekplexia (see later). If these hypotheses are correct, the different behavior of the auditory blink reflex could be due to tonic facilitation of the OOc,[34] which would need to react faster and more consistently than other muscles to protect the eyes from potentially dangerous stimuli.

THE ORIENTING REACTION

Apart from the early, involuntary, fast reaction, subjects submitted to an unexpected loud sound present with later components (the orienting reaction) have received relatively less attention in neurophysiology than the short-latency components. The orienting reaction is a poorly defined behavioral response that probably results from a combination of curiosity, fear, annoyance, and so on.[35] An orienting response consists of a shift of attention and perception, autonomic changes and postural adjustments, and orientation toward the stimulus, as shown in EMG. The orienting response shows variable, complex behaviors, possibly due to psychological factors. It includes a motor reaction consisting of maneuvers involving the whole body in preparation for defense or attack,[36] but these are largely dependent on the experimental setup. In most subjects, the orienting reaction is limited to relatively slow movements of the head or the upper limbs, laughter, or guttural vocal expressions. This is so when using headphones for sound presentation. However, if the source of the stimulus is located in the space nearby, some subjects may exhibit complex reactions such as fast rising from the chair and heading for the door before any attempt to look for a reasonable explanation for the noise. The orienting reaction also entails changes in the galvanic skin resistance, transient increase in blood pressure, and acceleration of heartbeat frequency.[37-39]

OTHER PHYSIOLOGICAL EFFECTS OF A LOUD UNEXPECTED AUDITORY STIMULUS

Apart from the elicitation of the auditory startle reaction, the auditory stimulus causes also changes in the excitability of structures along the motor pathway. Furubayashi et al.[40] were the first to report the effects of an auditory stimulus of high intensity on motor cortex excitability. These authors showed that auditory stimuli of an intensity louder than 80 dB induced transient inhibition of the motor evoked potentials elicited by transcranial magnetic stimulation (TMS) over the motor area but no effect on those elicited by transcranial electrical stimuli. Such findings were confirmed later by Fisher et al.,[41] who examined the effects after habituation of the auditory startle reaction, to avoid interference with the response to TMS. Kühn et al.[42] demonstrated nicely that the effect takes place at a cortical level, because inhibition was only seen in motor evoked potentials to TMS but not on the motor responses obtained with focal stimulation using electrodes inserted in the subthalamic nucleus for deep brain stimulation in patients with Parkinson's disease. Delwaide et al.[43] recorded time-locked facilitation of the soleus H reflex after a startling auditory stimulus, suggesting that activity in the descending reticulospinal tract caused a transient enhancement of alpha motoneuronal excitability. The effect of a startling auditory stimulus on heart rate was reported by Valls-Solé et al.,[44] suggesting that this effect would help assessing the autonomic component of the startle reaction.

The speeding up of a voluntary movement by a startling stimulus, an effect known as StartReact,[45,47,48] will be the subject of a specific selection later. However, the physiological mechanisms underlying this observation are briefly described here. In short, the application of a startling stimulus unexpectedly at the same time as the imperative signal in simple reaction time task experiments causes a significant shortening of reaction time to values typical of the startle reaction. One possible explanation for that finding is that, in simple reaction time tasks, subcortical motor circuits are extremely ready for movement execution and, therefore, reflex activation of a subcortical motor center with enough widespread effect may be able to trigger the prepared response.[45,49] Another possibility is that the addition of a high-intensity stimulus to the imperative signal causes a larger amount of sensory input, facilitating sensorimotor processing as in the intersensory facilitation.[50] Finally, a startling stimulus causes an enhancement of arousal that is likely related to the generation of a galvanic skin response and the enhancement of heart rate. The consequences of such an increased arousal are many. The increased attention and alertness may lead to a faster processing of sensory stimuli and a faster reaction to the presentation of a sensory cue.[51]

HUMAN STARTLE RESPONSES TO SOMATOSENSORY STIMULI

As mentioned earlier, auditory stimuli are not the only ones giving rise to the startle reaction. Other than that, visual,[3] somatosensory,[4] and vestibular stimuli[5] have been used. Using electrical stimuli of unexpectedly high intensity, Alvarez-Blanco et al.[52] reported differences in the composition of the response in relation to whether the stimulus was applied to the median nerve or to the posterior tibial nerve. With the former, responses were prominent and of shortest latency in the orbicularis oculi, while with the later, the shortest latency response was that of the sternocleidomastoid. The authors speculated that the composition of the afferent volley and the pathways followed by that volley in its way to the startle center are different for arm and leg in humans.

The response of the orbicularis oculi to somatosensory stimuli is known as the somatosensory blink reflex[53] and may be the one actually accounting for the shortest latency of the orbicularis oculi response. An abnormal somatosensory blink reflex has been reported in patients with various neurological disorders.[53] Remarkably, focal brainstem lesions may affect the somatosensory blink reflex (to median nerve stimulation) but not the auditory blink reflex or the trigeminally induced blink reflex,[54] suggesting the specificity of the afferent arm of brainstem circuits impinging on the reticular formation.

Somatosensory startle and somatosensory blink reflexes are prone to habituation, which occurs faster than with the auditory stimuli. Also, they respond dramatically to the presentation of a prepulse, which often inhibits the whole response. This was found to be in contrast with the withdrawal reflex, a response that is unavoidably accompanying the somatosensory startle reaction to median nerve or posterior tibial nerve electrical stimuli. In their characterization of the somatosensory startle, Alvarez-Blanco et al.[52] found that the only remaining response to the test stimuli after a prepulse was the one elicited in the same limb as part of the withdrawal reaction. These results could help in distinguishing between withdrawal and somatosensory startle reactions.

Factors Influencing the Magnitude of the Startle Reaction

AROUSAL

The startle reaction is a defensive and protective reflex and, therefore, it would be expected that the size of the startle reaction relates to the level of assumed danger from a stimulus. Animals show an increased startle when a potentially startling stimulus is paired with an electrical stimulus to their paw, and the enhancement remains for a certain time even when the electrical stimulus is not anymore present. Therefore, the animal has been conditioned by the aversive stimulus. The same has been seen to occur in humans exposed to aversive pictures.[55,56] Startle potentiation is obtained while viewing highly unpleasant pictures (threat and mutilation), while a significant decrease in the size of the startle is obtained while viewing pleasant pictures (erotica and romance). The circuit proposed to account for such fear-mediated potentiation of the startle reflex involves the projections from the central nucleus of the amygdala to the reticular formation.[57]

Slightly arousing, nonthreatening pictures increase the subject's attention and evoke an overt orienting reaction toward that specific sensory input. This may initially lead to a slight decrease of the startle reaction, together with a decrease in heart rate, which in healthy subjects change dramatically when the aversive situation becomes more negative or a threat is detected toward a defensive reaction, implying heightened startle reflex and sympathetically mediated acceleration of the heart rate. Phobic subjects have a different behavior, lacking the first phase of increased attention. Possibly in relation to that, they increase their arousal-related startle levels more than healthy subjects.[58,59] Arousal-potentiated startle reactions may be underlying clinical findings in patients with posttraumatic stress disorders.[60,61]

Startle modification by stress and arousal has its counterpart in the effects of such conditions on prepulse inhibition. This is regulated by fear-anticipation, emotion, attention, and other behavioral conditions through top-down circuits.[62,63] Enhanced attention should go with increased prepulse inhibition and consequently diminished startle. The opposite is true in certain disorders such as schizophrenia and attention-deficit-hyperactivity disorder in which prepulse inhibition is diminished and subjects may not be able to avoid disruption of sensory processing by concomitant sensory stimuli.[63]

HABITUATION

The startle reaction is the product of a multisynaptic activity and, as many other polysynaptic reflexes, it habituates relatively fast. In normal subjects in a quiet environment, the third stimulus in a sequence may not elicit responses other than a burst in the orbicularis oculi.[64] As previously mentioned, habituation rate to subsequent stimuli is significantly different for the orbicularis oculi response and for the responses of other muscles, which indicates again the distinctive behavior of the orbicularis oculi responses. Habituation of the auditory startle reaction is thought to result from synaptic depression of the pontine reticular formation.[65] A relationship between long-term habituation of the startle reaction and nonassociative learning has been pointed out by Timmann et al.[66] Guidelines for the study of the startle response have been issued that take into account many of the variables influencing the size of the response.[67]

Habituation is an inconvenient feature for clinical studies on the assessment of the characteristics of the startle reaction. After the first response, the auditory startle reaction may be completely absent in muscles other than the OOc in some normal individuals. Various strategies have been used to diminish habituation: Brown et al.[31,32] used long interstimuli intervals, Kofler et al.[22,68] used auditory stimuli of varying characteristics, and Valldeoriola et al.[69] used attention focusing to an impending imperative sensor signal for voluntary reaction.[64]

PREPULSE INHIBITION

Undoubtedly, the most important aspect to consider in the modulation of the startle reaction is whether the stimulus is preceded by another sensory input, or prepulse. A prepulse is any low-intensity stimulus, unable to cause a recordable response by itself, that induces changes in the response to a subsequent suprathreshold stimulus. Inhibition of the startle reaction by a prepulse can be obtained with stimuli of the same or different sensory modality as the one producing the startle reaction (Fig. 17.3). Prepulse inhibition has been long ago described by various authors using different concepts such as reflex modification,[70,71] stimulus anticipation,[25] and sensorimotor modulation.[19,72] Prepulse inhibition neither depends on learning nor on previous experiences with a similar type of stimuli. The inhibitory effect is probably a consequence of the attentional displacement required to process the information brought about by the prepulse.[2,73]

Most of prepulse inhibition studies have been carried out in the field of psychophysiology and behavior, using the response of the OOc as the only probe for the startle reaction.[2,74–76] The issue is important if we consider that the auditory blink reflex may actually reflect activity in a circuit different from that of the startle reaction.[15,31] However, even if the circuits for the auditory blink reflex and the auditory startle reaction are indeed different, this does not seem to affect prepulse inhibition since the amount of inhibition was the same for the auditory blink reflex and the auditory startle reaction with somatosensory or auditory prepulses.[46]

Healthy subjects are probably able to integrate at the subcortical level impulses generated by the environmental conditions of daily life, such as visual, acoustic, or somatosensory impulses. These environmental impulses may adopt the role of prepulse stimuli and cause inhibition of undesired motor reactions, which would otherwise interfere with sensory processing of relevant inputs. Hoffman and Fleshler[77] reported significant startle reaction reduction in rats located in an environment of pulsed auditory stimuli in comparison to rats submitted to continuous noise. Consistent with these findings, the startle reaction was found to be larger in humans when common environmental noises were masked by background noise.[64]

Prepulse inhibition occurs also with the blink reflex elicited by electrical stimuli to the supraorbital nerve. This allows observing an effect of the prepulse that is not obvious with other stimuli: prepulse facilitation. This occurs in the R1 component of the blink reflex at a relatively short interstimulus interval between the prepulse and the supraorbital nerve stimulus. With auditory or somatosensory prepulses, facilitation of the R1 component occurs at intervals between 40 and 100 ms, while inhibition of the R2 and R2c responses occurs at intervals of 70 ms or longer.[25–27,46,75] The dissociation of the prepulse effects on the R1 and R2 components of the blink reflex suggests that prepulse inhibition takes place at a presynaptic level.

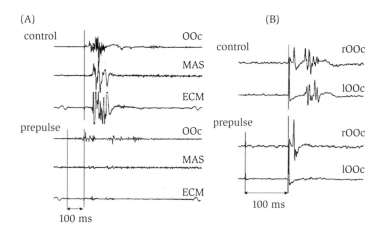

FIGURE 17.3 Prepulse effects (A) on the startle reaction and (B) on the blink reflex. The top traces are baseline recordings to a startling auditory stimulus (A) and to a supraorbital nerve electrical stimulus (B). The bottom traces are test trials in which the same stimuli were applied 100 ms after a somatosensory prepulse, a weak electrical stimulus to the digital nerves of the third finger. Note the absence of the responses in both cases (except for the R1 of the blink reflex) when the prepulse is applied.

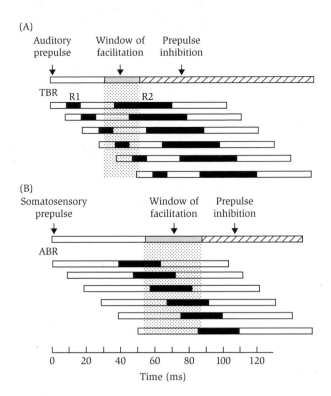

(A)

Auditory prepulse · Window of facilitation · Prepulse inhibition

TBR · R1 · R2

(B)

Somatosensory prepulse · Window of facilitation · Prepulse inhibition

ABR

0   20   40   60   80   100   120

Time (ms)

FIGURE 17.4 Schematic representation of the effects of an auditory prepulse on the blink reflex to a supraorbital nerve stimulus (*A*) and that of a somatosensory stimulus on the orbicularis oculi response to an auditory stimulus (*B*), based on data from Valls-Solé et al.[46] The input generated by the prepulse stimulus carries a window of facilitation followed by a long-lasting inhibition. The timing is slightly different for each prepulse modality and, therefore, the facilitatory effects may or may not be seen depending on the interstimulus interval. ABR, auditory blink reflex; TBR, trigeminally induced blink reflex.

A facilitatory effect of prepulse takes place also on the R2 component with a time frame that depends on the combination of stimuli (Boelhouwer et al. 1991).[46] This is likely resulting from the short-latency facilitatory effect of any sensory input reaching the brainstem. Figure 17.4 shows a schematic representation of the effects of an auditory prepulse on the blink reflex to trigeminal inputs and of a somatosensory prepulse on the auditory blink reflex.

OTHER FACTORS

Corticospinal projections exert inhibitory effects on the auditory startle reflex. This is probably the explanation for larger startle responses in children with cerebral palsy and in patients with either hemiplegia caused by cerebral infarction[78] or paraplegia after spinal cord injury.[79] The size of the startle reaction is a probe for the subject's emotional state.[74] These emotional influences are strong enough to have made the auditory startle reflex an important method in the investigation of affective systems.

Magnitude and latency of the startle reaction vary between individuals. Maintaining stimulus intensity and frequency of presentation stable, authors have examined the effect of some physiological factors. Several authors have reported experiments done in animals (rats or mice). In a study of the effects of the circadian rhythm, Chabot and Taylor[80] showed that the auditory startle reaction was significantly increased at night. The effect of environmental noise was shown by Hoffman and Fleshler,[77] who reported larger startle responses in environments with steady noise levels in comparison to those with punctiform noise inputs. The size of the response is also increased with high illumination levels.[81] Paylor and Crawley[82] have been able to modify genetically the size of the auditory startle reflex by means of inducing more or less prepulse inhibition. In humans, Kofler et al.[22,68] reported the influence of gender and age on the auditory startle reaction. Women had higher probability and larger responses than men, while older subjects had larger responses than younger subjects in leg muscles. Interestingly, age-related differences were not observed in facial or neck muscles. The excitability of the startle circuits is also modulated by mood, attention, fear, and other emotional states.[74,83–85] Lang and Davis[86] pointed out the parallelism between the size of the startle reaction and the degree of emotional arousal derived from the stimulus and the engagement of the whole body in preparation for reaction to it. The pattern of the auditory startle reaction is modified according to posture[32] and laterality.[87] Brown et al.[32] found that the responses of leg muscles were of shorter latency and twice as frequent when standing than when sitting. Kofler et al.[87] found larger responses in the sternocleidomastoid contralateral, and in the biceps brachii ipsilateral, to hand dominance. All these observations reflect the importance of this basic motor system in all human motor actions.

CLINICALLY RELEVANT ABNORMALITIES IN THE STARTLE REACTION

The division between normal and abnormal startle reaction is difficult to establish. Some healthy persons can display intense startle reactions to unexpected stimuli even if they are of low intensity, whereas others would have a minimum reaction to the same or greater stimulus intensity. However, abnormalities in regard to the size of the startle reaction have been described for reduced as well as for exaggerated responses. In case of abnormal response reduction, the examiner has to take into account the fast habituation of the startle response with repetition of stimuli. In the case of exaggerated reactions, the examiner has to take into account how easy it is to add voluntary muscle contraction on top of the involuntary reaction.

Abnormal Reduction of the Startle Reaction

Vidailhet et al.[88] showed for the first time the abnormal decrease of the startle reaction in patients with parkinsonism. These authors reported a delay in the latency of the startle reaction in idiopathic Parkinson's disease and a marked reduction or even absence of the response in progressive supranuclear palsy. This was replicated by Valldeoriola et al.,[69] who, instead of using just unexpected auditory stimuli, prone to fast habituation, delivered the loud auditory stimuli together with the imperative signal in the context of a reaction time task. In this condition, habituation is significantly reduced.[64] Apart from the absence of the startle reaction, Valldeoriola et al.[69] showed that patients with progressive supranuclear palsy were unable to speed up their reaction, while this was not the case in patients with other degenerative disorders presenting with parkinsonism.

In patients with multiple system atrophy, the startle reaction was found normal in facial and cervical muscles by Valldeoriola et al. (1997).[89] Later on, however, Kofler et al.[90,91] reported a higher response probability, shortening of the initial latency, and increase in response magnitude with respect to normal controls when the cranial and limb muscle responses were analyzed together. Opposite to patients with multisystem atrophy, those with dementia with Lewy bodies had a reduction in response probability, latency delay, and decrease in duration of the responses recorded in limb muscles with respect to control subjects.[90] Two more details are worth pointing out from the works of Kofler and coworkers on patients with parkinsonism. One is the fact that three patients with multisystem atrophy had absent startle reaction, which indicates that the dysfunction of the startle circuit is not uniform in these patients and that absence of the startle reaction is not an exclusive feature of patients with progressive supranuclear palsy. Possibly, a particularly large increase in oligodendroglial cytoplasmatic inclusions in the areas of the reticular formation where the startle reaction is generated could have accounted for the absent response in these patients. The other detail is the existence of subtle differences in the characteristics of the startle response between patients with the parkinsonian (strio-nigral) type and those with the cerebellar variant of multisystem atrophy. Whereas those with strio-nigral degeneration had higher response probability and shorter latency, those with cerebellar degeneration presented with reduced habituation. The inhibitory effect of cerebellar inputs on the motor tract might contribute to these differences. [91]

Abnormal Enhancement of the Startle Reaction

Syndromes with exaggerated startle reaction are known by the general term of *hyperekplexia*,[92,93] although this term should better be preserved for the hereditary rather than for any condition presenting with enhanced startle. Although there are criteria published to define the abnormality of the startle reaction,[65] there are no objective methods for a positive diagnosis of idiopathic or primary hyperekplexia, since signs of structural damage or typical functional alterations have not been observed.[94] A typical feature of primary hyperekplexia is that patients complain of involuntary motor reactions interfering with their work or social activities. A good interview with the patient can already detect differences between abnormally exaggerated startle reaction and exaggerated voluntary reactions. Electrophysiological examination shows also some differences in the response pattern.[95] However, before determining that the exaggerated startle reaction is primary, there should be a thorough investigation for a possible cause.

IDENTIFIABLE CAUSES FOR AN EXAGGERATED STARTLE REACTION

Exaggerated startle reaction can be due to residual anoxic cerebral injuries, malformations, traumatisms, or metabolic diseases. In some patients, startle is accompanied by seizures (startle epilepsy). Also, an exaggeration of the startle reaction has been described in patients with the stiff-person syndrome, occurring predominantly in axial and lower-limb muscles.[96] Stell et al.[97] described an abnormal decrease of habituation in two out of eight patients with Gilles de la Tourette's syndrome. Exaggerated startle has been reported also in patients with restless legs syndrome[98] and in patients with postraumatic stress disorder.[60]

Diffuse cerebral damage leads usually to exaggerated startle reaction. The exception is the infarct in the auditory area at the temporal lobe.[84] Voordecker et al.[78] and Jankelowitz and Colebatch[99] reported that a startling stimulus caused responses of shorter latency in patients with stroke than in control subjects. They demonstrated also that vestibulospinal responses were not enhanced and, therefore, the enhancement of activity in the reticulospinal tract must be due to a particular influence of the lesion on the reticular formation but not on the vestibular nuclei. Brainstem and spinal lesions also induce exaggerated startle reflexes.[99–102] A pontine lesion was suggested to be responsible for secondary hyperekplexia in a patient reported by Kimber and Thompson.[103] One consequence of central nervous system lesions is a change in the neural representation of the body, associated with alterations in the location of cortical representation sites and in cortical excitability.[104] This could lead to plastic changes that could have the consequence of startle response enhancement. An indirect piece of evidence for such a pathophysiological mechanism is the finding of a positive correlation between the size of the startle response and the duration of the disorder in patients with spinal cord injury.[102]

A series of stimulus-induced reactions should also be considered when delivering a startling stimulus. It can induce seizures in patients with epilepsy ("startle-induced epilepsy"). In progressive myoclonus epilepsy, the presence of myoclonus makes it more difficult to observe the startle reaction. Reticular and propriospinal myoclonus resemble exaggerated startle. A difference between stimulus-induced myoclonus and exaggerated startle exists in the sensory stimulus provoking the response. Hyperekplexia is clinically characterized by stimulus sensitivity to the mantle area and the presence of tonic spasms. By contrast, stimulus sensitivity is usually over the limbs in reticular myoclonus and abdominal in propriospinal myoclonus, with spontaneous jerks occurring between induced jerks.[32] In the differential diagnosis of hyperekplexia, there should be considered the stiff-person syndrome in which there is also stiffness induced by an unexpected stimulus.[33] In the stiff-person syndrome, there is a defect in GABA-mediated inhibition, rather than in the glycine-mediated inhibition as in hyperekplexia. In paroxysmal kinesigenic choreoathetosis, abnormal movements are initiated by an unexpected stimulus, but the movements are chorea or dystonia rather than a startle reflex. Patients with cataplexy show a loss of muscle tone with unexpected stimuli rather than an increase in tone as in the major form of hyperekplexia. In tic disorders, a normal startle reflex can induce a tic. The phenomenology and pathophysiology of stimulus-induced disorders is diverse. To discriminate between hyperekplexia, neuropsychiatric startle syndromes, and other stimulus-induced disorders, a detailed history, video registration, and electrophysiological testing are needed.

HYPEREKPLEXIA AND EXAGGERATED STARTLE WITH NO EVIDENCE FOR A CAUSE

The best known among the conditions presenting with exaggerated startle is hyperekplexia, which can be familiar or sporadic and consists of involuntary motor reactions that sometimes cause falls to the ground, induced by unexpected stimuli. There are two forms of the syndrome, the major and the minor form.[93,105,106] For the diagnosis of the major form, three features are required: generalized stiffness at birth, excessive startling to unexpected stimuli, and a generalized stiffness after a startle reflex that lasts a few seconds.[92] The minor form of hyperkplexia can be sporadic and the term is used too broadly to include any patient with exaggerated startle. Specific diagnostic cues for the minor form of hyperkplexia are lacking and, therefore, every effort has to be made to rule out disorders that can lead to exaggerated startle reactions before assuming that the syndrome is genetically mediated.

Excessive startle reflex can be a symptomatic condition in which there is damage to the brainstem, such as neurochemical abnormalities in the nuclei of the reticular formation. In the major form of hyperekplexia, a mutation in the α1 subunit of the glycine receptor gene, GLRA1, has been identified in most pedigrees, indicating that this defect can be regarded as the defining element of autosomal dominant major hyperekplexia. Actually, it is in the brainstem reticular formation where the largest concentration of glycine receptors is found in humans. The major form of hereditary hyperekplexia can be revealed in newborns as a generalized stiffness ("stiff-baby syndrome"). In adults, stiffness reveals in the legs while walking with a wide base. No other clinical signs may be found in many patients with hyperekplexia. If anything, tendon reflexes may be slightly increased. A somatosensory stimulus is able also to lead to an exaggerated reaction. This is observed in the head-retraction sign in which patients with hyperekplexia perform an involuntary backward jerk when a tap is delivered to the base of the nose. Latency of such response is in the order of 20 ms in the trapezius. Additionally, patients with hyperekplexia might have periodic limb movements in sleep and hypnagogic myoclonus. Sudden infant death may occur if stiffness is very severe. Standard tests of serum, urine, cerebrospinal fluid, neuroimaging, and electroencephalography reveal no abnormalities. TMS revealed no abnormalities regarding stimulus response curves, cortical inhibition, and facilitation.

As expected, the actual startle reaction is larger in patients with hyperekplexia than in healthy subjects. Conduction along the sensory central nervous system pathways is normal. Latency of the startle reflex is abnormally short in the major form. Habituation to repeated stimuli may be normal.[106] The minor can be seen in members of families with genetically proven hyperekplexia but, in this case, the startle reflex has a longer latency than in the major form. One hypothesis is that the minor form might represent a learned behavioral response in patients who are in contact with family members exhibiting organic startle attacks. Although the exact nature of the minor form of hyperekplexia is far from understood, the prolonged latencies and other features can be taken as an indication of a psychogenic or psychiatric origin of the exaggerated startle reflex.[95,107]

An interesting group of disorders akin to the minor form of hyperekplexia are those occurring in certain communities as part of rituals or specific behaviors. This is the case of the Latah in Indonesia and Malaysia, the "Jumping Frenchmen of Maine," the Myriachit in Siberia, and other rare entities. All these various forms of culture-specific syndromes involve nonhabituating hyperstartling reactions, evoked by loud noises or by being poked forcefully in the side. After a startle reflex, various other responses might be seen, including "forced obedience," echolalia, and echopraxia. Unfortunately, there are no detailed physiological studies documenting the nature of the startle reflexes in these culture-specific, startle-matching syndromes. The cause of the jumping disorder seems to be situational because of the type of response, the peculiar circumstances of onset, and clinical development.[108] It is to note that, as already stated, arousal increases significantly the size of the startle response in healthy persons and more so in patients with anxiety, fear, or other kinds of emotional disturbances or psychiatric conditions.[74]

Abnormal Prepulse Inhibition

Prepulse inhibition is a very robust phenomenon in healthy subjects and in many disease conditions. However, it was soon discovered that it was abnormally reduced in patients with schizophrenia.[109] These patients have impaired inhibition of intrusive or irrelevant stimuli, which can lead to attention deficit and abnormal information processing.[110] These alterations underlie the difficulties of schizophrenics in selecting relevant information from the continuous arrival of sensory inputs. The investigation of prepulse inhibition in schizophrenia and related conditions has led to a large number of reports and continues yielding interesting views and opinions.[111] Similar abnormalities have been reported in patients with panic disorder, in whom the defective inhibition could reflect a more generalized cognitive impairment.[112] A defective prepulse inhibition leads usually to enhancement of the startle reaction or lack of habituation with repeated stimulation. This is the case in most psychiatric disorders, in which both abnormalities have been correlated with the gray matter volume measured in the dorsolateral prefrontal, middle frontal, and the orbital/medial prefrontal cortices.[113]

Prepulse inhibition has been examined relatively scarcely in patients with Parkinson's disease. Nakashima et al.[114] found that auditory prepulse of the blink reflex was significantly reduced with respect to the values obtained in normal controls. In a comparative study of Parkinson's disease and Huntington's disease, Valls-Solé et al.[115] confirmed these findings and observed that the proportion of patients with abnormal somatosensory prepulse inhibition was considerably smaller than the one with abnormal auditory prepulse inhibition. This probably indicates subtle differences between stimuli of different sensory modality. Patients with progressive supranuclear palsy also show a significant decrease of both auditory and somatosensory prepulse inhibition, revealing again the marked dysfunction of brainstem circuits in these patients. The phenomenon of prepulse inhibition in patients with multisystem atrophy has still not been properly examined, although preliminary data indicate dysfunction of the inhibitory effect of somatosensory prepulses, at least in patients with parkinsonian-type multisystem atrophy.[116]

Other groups of patients with abnormal reduction of prepulse inhibition are those exhibiting hyperactivity such as in Huntington's disease[76,115] and dystonia.[117] It is interesting to note that prepulse inhibition is similarly abnormal in two diseases that have been considered the prototypical opposite regarding the dysfunction of the basal ganglia (Huntington's disease and Parkinson's disease). Therefore, it could be that structures outside the basal ganglia circuit that are dysfunctional in the two diseases are responsible for the defective prepulse inhibition or that either excessive or defective output leads to the same type of dysfunction in both diseases.

Patients with dystonia can transiently alleviate their symptoms using relatively subtle sensory stimuli ("geste antagonistique"). The patients with blepharospasm use tricks such as touching the forehead or holding the upper eyelid with a piece of tape. Gómez-Wong et al.[119] thought that the degree to which a "geste antagonistique" was effective in patients with blepharospasm could be related to whether PPI was effectively decreasing reflex responses in the OOc. Therefore, they studied prepulse inhibition in dystonic patients separated in two groups according to whether they benefited from the "geste antagonistiques." The results showed that prepulse inhibition was significantly more preserved in patients who experienced benefit in comparison to those who did not.

THE STARTLE REACTION IN THE CONTEXT OF VOLUNTARY MOVEMENTS: THE STARTREACT EFFECT

The startle reaction is the fastest generalized motor reaction of humans and animals. Thus, it would be convenient to use the startle reaction pathways for the execution of voluntary movements requiring great speed. However, to do so with efficacy, the central nervous system must have developed the appropriate mechanisms of control, as is the case with other subcortical motor reactions such as the cutaneo-muscular or stretch reflexes.

The execution of a voluntary motor act requires activation of cerebral neuronal circuits. Voluntary commands may be generated in loops involving the basal ganglia and the premotor and supplementary motor areas. However, if rapid movement execution is needed, subjects usually prepare their motor system in such a way that it is ready for releasing the energy in the form of muscle contraction at the appropriate moment. The mechanisms involved in motor preparation are not known, but they certainly involve a buildup of excitability in subcortical structures in accordance with the program to be executed. In such a situation, an unexpected and abrupt sensory input may trigger the motor response by direct activation of the prepared subcortical structures, a phenomenon termed "StartReact".[45,48,49,118]

The reaction time task paradigm is a useful tool for investigation of the temporal characteristics of sensory information processing and its integration in motor circuits in humans. The paradigm in which the voluntary reaction is faster is the simple reaction time task, in which subjects are able to prepare sufficiently in advance their motor programs because they know exactly what to do. Latencies as short as 150 ms are common in simple reaction time tasks to visual stimuli. However, when subjects prepared for execution of a voluntary movement receive an unexpected startling stimulus, their reaction becomes significantly faster, with latencies of 70 to 80 ms.[45,48,49,118,119] In these conditions, the movement executed is the one that had been prepared. For instance, the simplest motor program of performing a ballistic wrist movement is executed much faster but otherwise unchanged, and saccadic eye movements reach the target faster but with the same precision,[120] in the presence of the startling stimulus in comparison to a control condition. Figure 17.5 illustrates these observations. The StartReact effect could theoretically be due to various possibilities. One is that the increase in energy of the sensory input may accelerate sensorimotor coupling and all synaptic processes necessary for task execution. This is exemplified by intersensory facilitation,[50,121] a process by which the reaction to a given sensory cue is advanced when another cue of a different sensory modality is applied simultaneously. Another possibility is that the startling stimulus activates the whole set of neural structures needed for execution of the task at a subcortical level, bypassing cortical sensorimotor integration processes.[45,48,122] Probably both mechanisms

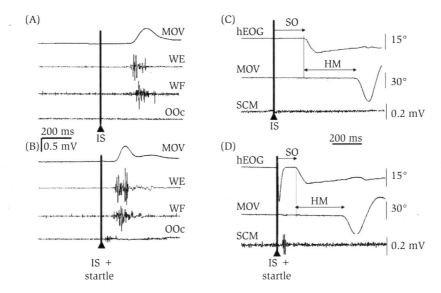

FIGURE 17.5   Two examples of the StartReact effect. The graphs in *A* and *B* show the recordings from a wrist extension simple reaction time task paradigm, with accelerometric signal (ACC), surface electromyographic signals from the wrist extensors (WE) and wrist flexors (WF), as well as from the orbicularis oculi (OOc) muscles. In *A*, the subject responded to a visual imperative signal (IS), while in *B*, the IS was accompanied by a loud auditory startling stimulus (IS + startle). The graphs in *C* and *D* show the recordings from a horizontal saccadic movement recorded with electrooculography (hEOG), which was to be followed by a choice wrist movement (HM) toward flexion or extension depending on the cue that could be seen only after the saccade. We also recorded from the sternocleidomastoid muscle (SCM) to monitor for startle-related activity. In *C*, subjects were asked to start the saccadic movement at the presentation of a visual imperative signal (IS), while in *D* the IS was accompanied by a startling auditory stimulus (IS + startle). Note the significant shortening of reaction time with preservation of the pattern of EMG activity in *B*, and the shortening of the saccadic movement with preservation of HM in *D*.

contribute in part to the StartReact effect. The increase of energy with the addition of a startling stimulus is substantial, and it may account for some effect. However, the largest amount of simple reaction time shortening reported so far with intersensory facilitation is around 50 ms, and the absolute value for the StartReact effect is usually larger. A third possibility is that arousal is increased in the presence of a startling stimulus, leading to the use of more resources in the performance.[123] Whatever the case, one important conclusion stands out from the first observations of the effect: that the reticulospinal tract may contribute significantly to the execution of prepared voluntary movements. Otherwise, one would expect that collision between the voluntary commands and the involuntary descending volley generated by the startling stimulus would modify the motor program. For this not to be the case, the motor program must have been represented and ready to be launched in the subcortical motor structures activated by the startling stimulus.

The StartReact effect is convincingly present in simple reaction time tasks. It is also present with some reservations in choice reaction time tasks. While Carlsen et al.[48] reported lack of effect of the startling stimulus on choice reaction time tasks when error trials were eliminated from the analysis, Valls-Solé[124] found that there was a significant StartReact effect even if subjects reacted with the wrong hand in a percentage of cases. The latter means that there is some degree of subcortical preparation in choice reaction time task paradigms that possibly goes along with a general pre-movement increase of arousal and could lead to the characteristic precipitation error that we might have seen in a number of situations in which there are time constraints for a reaction (i.e., the goal-keeper trying to stop a penalty shot may be throwing himself toward the wrong side of the goal line even before the ball has begun to move). The StartReact effect has been reported when performing relatively complex movements in a number of articles published recently by different research groups: Tresilian and Plooy[125] reported it with interceptive actions in a short time window; Nijhuis et al.[126] reported it with head rotation, pointing out that the effect is independent on stimulus direction. Reynolds and Day[127] reported it with foot movements to a visual target, where the startling stimulus accelerated the already fast visuomotor processing, and MacKinnon et al.[128] showed the speeding

up of stepping to visual targets. The StartReact effect is also present during the first period of the sit-to-stand maneuver[129] or the initiation of gait,[131] but it does not interfere with its execution if the startling stimulus is delivered during execution of the maneuver. Queralt et al.[130] showed also that stepping over an obstacle was done faster and more effectively when a loud auditory sound was presented together with the obstacle.

There is another consequence of the application of auditory stimuli during movement preparation: the startle reaction becomes larger and shows less habituation than if the same high-intensity stimulus is applied with no previous instruction of preparation.[64,118,132]

Measuring the Excitability of the Startle Circuit before Voluntary Reaction

The observation that the startle reaction is larger in the StartReact phenomenon than in resting conditions indicates that there is enhanced excitability in subcortical motor structures at the time of presentation of the imperative signal. It is known that corticospinal tract excitability increases in the premotor time of a simple reaction time task experiment.[133,134] However, such cortical changes may not reflect adequately changes occurring in subcortical centers. In view of that, Kumru and Valls-Solé[135] analyzed changes in the size of the auditory startle reaction recorded in cranial and cervical muscles as a measure of the excitability of subcortical motor structures during the premotor time in simple reaction time task paradigms. High-intensity auditory stimuli were applied at various intervals preceding the onset of EMG activity in a simple reaction time task. As expected, the startling stimulus induced a larger auditory startle reaction in sternocleidomastoid muscle (SCM) during motor preparation than at rest. However, in contrast to the progressive increase in excitability found with cortical stimulation,[133,134] the size of the auditory startle reaction did not increase or otherwise change during the 100 ms preceding onset of voluntary movement. Therefore, the excitability enhancement of subcortical motor structures seems not to depend on the proximity of task execution. Rather, this may be a situation in which higher centers should exert some form of control on hyperexcitable subcortical motor structures. Release of such inhibition could lead to task execution. An argument in favor of such a possibility is the finding of decreased intracortical inhibition that has been reported just preceding the increase in cortical excitability before movement onset.[136,137] However, the modulation of cortico-cortical inhibition does not seem to be related to the type of contraction. We hypothesized that the amount of inhibition (and, hence, the amount of release before reaching the appropriate level of excitability in the corticospinal tract) would be different in simple and choice reaction time tasks because of the different requirements of the two tasks before execution. Theoretically, the amount of inhibitory control of muscle activity should be larger in choice than in simple reaction time tasks. However, this was not the case; the decrease in short-interval intracortical inhibition was not significantly different in simple versus choice reaction time tasks.[138] Another form of inhibitory control, prepulse inhibition, was also not likely participating in the control of task execution in the StartReact phenomenon.[139] We examined whether the inhibitory effect of a prepulse was present when given in the context of a reaction time task paradigm. Subjects engaged in a simple reaction time task received, together with the "go" signal in test trials, either a startling stimulus alone or the combination of a startling stimulus preceded by a prepulse 100 ms earlier. The results showed that prepulses were effectively inhibiting the startle response (i.e., the responses of the OOc and the SCM were significantly reduced in trials with a prepulse), but they did not modify the StartReact effect (i.e., the reaction time shortening induced by the auditory stimulus was similar in trials with and without prepulse).

If there is an increase in excitability in subcortical motor pathways at the time of the imperative signal, we may hypothesize that it is also present some time before. This was tested by applying the startling auditory stimulus at various time intervals preceding the presentation of the imperative signal.[124] Subjects executed the prepared reaction to presentation of the startling stimulus for a mean of about −400 ms before imperative signal presentation in simple reaction time tasks and −100 ms for complex reaction time tasks. These results together with those reported by Kumru and Valls-Solé[135] suggest that the excitability of subcortical motor tracts begins to increase some time after forewarning and builds up to a plateau that remains more or less stable until task execution.

When a response to a startling stimulus is detected in the SCM, reaction time becomes significantly shorter than when no SCM response is elicited, regardless of the intensity of the stimulus.[141] In the same line, Kumru et al.[140] showed that, compared to rest, the size of the SCM component of the auditory startle reaction was larger in forced-choice reaction time and smaller in Go/noGo paradigms. Again, the size of the EMG burst in the SCM was significantly and inversely correlated with the percentage reaction time shortening induced by the startle in the two conditions. The authors concluded that the excitability of the subcortical motor pathways is relatively enhanced when subjects know that they will move either way, while it is less so when the task includes a "not-to-move" option. The substantial difference between the two tasks should be related to the amount of inhibitory activity used to stop the intention to move. Such correlation was not found in the OOc response,[140,142] pointing again to a different behavior of the OOc and the SCM in startle-related responses.

Subjective Perception of Movement and the StartReact Effect

The subjective perception of one's own movement has received little attention. Libet et al.[143] studied the conscious perception of movement in various psychological states related to voluntary actions. The paradigm consists of the graphical representation of a clock face with 60 marks, and a needle gives a whole turn of the circumference in precisely 2560 ms. Subjects are requested to press a button and describe the position of the needle at the moment in which they believe they have performed the action. The comparison of the real position of the needle and its subjective appraisal gives a measure of the subjective error.

Sanegre et al.[123] examined whether perception of the action varied when movement execution was shortened in the StartReact phenomenon. As expected, the simultaneous application of a high-intensity auditory stimulus with the imperative signal accelerated both movement onset and task execution, but it did not substantially modify the subjective perception of the movement. Furthermore, subjects estimated the time of imperative signal presentation with no significant differences with respect to the condition without startling stimulus. These results indicate that, in certain conditions, subjective appraisal of reaction time can be dissociated from task execution, a concept consistent with previous investigations.[144,145] Subjective appraisal of reaction time is probably generated by processes during motor preparation and has been related to the appearance of the lateralized premotor readiness potential, recorded as a differential potential between motor areas of both sides.[146,147] The results mentioned earlier indicate that the StartReact effect takes place at a level different from the one where perception of movement is generated.

CONCLUSIONS

The startle reaction is an involuntary reflex reaction under some form of voluntary control. We all have experienced a startle reflex and most of us have learned how to control the involuntary reaction either by letting it happen or by inhibiting it when it is inappropriate. Nevertheless, our control of such reaction is not complete. There is always the possibility that unexpected stimuli make us have an unwanted twitch. The startle circuit is an important part of our motor behavior. Apart from the neurological disorders that lead to hyper- or hyporeactivity of the startle circuit, there is evidence for the contribution of startle pathways to the execution of fast reactions. The startle reaction is generated at a relatively high hierarchic level in the motor system, leading to activation of a sufficient number of muscles for a motor response to be effective in movement execution. Fast voluntary movements may be prepared, taking into account the startle circuits. The motor programs underlying such fast movements may contain an inhibitory component to prevent execution once they are fully prepared. There is, therefore, a very critical balance between movement preparation and inhibition of movement execution that sometimes may lead to movement precipitation and errors. We think that the control of excitability of subcortical motor structures is a very important aspect of motor preparation for an incoming task. Prepulse inhibition is likely the most important mechanism of control of the startle reaction but does not seem to participate in the StartReact effect. Abnormalities in either the startle reaction or the prepulse inhibitory circuits can lead to an expression of abnormally exaggerated or reduced reaction. The circuits of the startle reaction and prepulse inhibition offer an interesting field for neurophysiological studies in healthy subjects and in patients with neurological disorders.

Very limited scientific studies on the clinical application of startle reflex are available in movement disorders, and almost none are available in sleep-related movements. Abnormal reduction of startle reflex has been noted in progressive supranuclear palsy, Parkinson's disease, diffuse Lewy body disease with dementia, and some patients with multiple-system atrophy. In contrast, an abnormal enhancement of startle reaction has been described in the hyperekplexia syndrome, posttraumatic stress disorder, restless legs syndrome, and stiff-person syndrome.

REFERENCES

1. Bakker MJ, van Dijk JG, van den Maagdenberg AM, et al. Startle syndromes. *Lancet Neurol* 2006;5:513–24.
2. Graham FK. The more or less startling effects of weak prestimulation. *Psychophysiology* 1975; 12:238–48.
3. McManis MH, Bradley MM, Berg WK, et al. Emotional reactions in children: verbal, physiological, and behavioral responses to affective pictures. *Psychophysiology* 2001;8:222–31.
4. Gokin AP, Karpukhina MV. Reticular structures in the cat brain involved in startle to somatic stimuli of various modalities. *Neurophysiology* 1985;17:278–86.
5. Bisdorff AR, Bronstein AM, Gresty MA. Responses in neck and facial muscles to sudden free fall and a startling auditory stimulus. *Electroenceph Clin Neurophysiol* 1994;93:409–16.
6. Davis M, Gendelman DS, Tischler MD, et al. A primary acoustic startle circuit: lesion and stimulation studies. *J Neurosci* 1982;2:791–805.
7. Lingenhöhl K, Friauf E. Giant neurons in the rat reticular formation: a sensorimotor interface in the elementary acoustic startle circuit? *J Neurosci* 1994;14:1176–94.
8. Yeomans JS, Frankland PW. The acoustic startle reflex: neurons and connections. *Brain Res Rev* 1996;21:301–14.
9. Koch M. The neurobiology of startle. *Progr Neurobiol* 1999;59:107–28.
10. Davis M, Gendelman PM. Plasticity of the acoustic startle response in the acutely decerebrate rat. *J Comp Physiol Psychol* 1977;91:549–63.
11. Lee Y, López DE, Meloni EJ, et al. A primary acoustic startle pathway: obligatory role of cochlear root neurons and the nucleus

reticularis pontis caudalis. *J Neurosci* 1996;16:3775–89.

12. Nodal FR, López DE. Direct input from cochlear root neurons to pontine reticulospinal neurons in albino rat. *J Comp Neurol* 2003;460:80–93.

13. Wu MF, Suzuki SS, Siegel JM. Anatomical distribution and response patterns of reticular neurons active in relation to acoustic startle. *Brain Res* 1988;457:399–406.

14. Koch M, Kungel M, Herbert H. Cholinergic neurons in the pedunculopontine tegmental nucleus are involved in the mediation of prepulse inhibition of the acoustic startle response in the rat. *Exp Brain Res* 1993;97:71–82.

15. Hori A, Yasuhara A, Naito H, et al. Blink reflex elicited by auditory stimulation in the rabbit. *J Neurol Sci* 1986;76:49–59.

16. Inglis WL, Winn P. The pedunculo-pontine tegmental nucleus: where the striatum meets the reticular formation. *Prog Neurobiol* 1995;47:1–29.

17. Reese NB, Garcia-Rill E, Skinner RD. The pedunculopontine nucleus—auditory input, arousal and pathophysiology. *Prog Neurobiol* 1995;47:105–33.

18. Kodsi MH, Swerdlow NR. Regulation of prepulse inhibition by ventral pallidal projections. *Brain Res Bull* 1997;43:219–28.

19. Swerdlow NR, Geyer MA. Prepulse inhibition of acoustic startle in rats after lesions of the pedunculopontine tegmental nucleus. *Behav Neurosci* 1993;107:104–17.

20. Fendt M, Koch M. Cholinergic modulation of the acoustic startle response in the caudal pontine reticular nucleus of the rat. *Eur J Pharmacol* 1999;370:101–7.

21. Ransmayr G, Faucheux B, Nowakowski C, et al. Age-related changes of neuronal counts in the human pedunculopontine nucleus. *Neurosci Lett* 2000;288:195–8.

22. Kofler M, Muller J, Reggiani L, et al. Influence of age on auditory startle responses in humans. *Neurosci Lett* 2001;307:65–8.

23. Parent A, Hazrati LN. Functional anatomy of the basal ganglia. II. The place of subthalamic nucleus and external pallidum in basal ganglia circuitry. *Brain Res Brain Res Rev* 1995;20:128–54.

24. Swerdlow NR, Braff DL, Geyer MA. Animal models of deficient sensorimotor gating: what we know, what we think we know, and what we hope to know soon. *Behav Pharmacol* 2000;11:185–204.

25. Ison JR, Sanes JN, Foss JA, et al. Facilitation and inhibition of the human startle blink reflexes by stimulus anticipation. *Behav Neurosci* 1990;104: 418–29.

26. Rossi A, Scarpini C. Gating of trigemino-facial reflex from low-threshold trigeminal and extratrigeminal cutaneous fibres in humans. *J Neurol Neurosurg Psychiatry* 1992;55:774–80.

27. Valls-Solé J, Cammarota A, Alvarez R, et al. Orbicularis oculi responses to stimulation of nerve afferents from upper and lower limbs in normal humans. *Brain Res* 1994;650:313–16.

28. Costa J, Valls-Solé J, Valldeoriola F, et al. Single subthalamic nucleus deep brain stimuli inhibit the blink reflex in Parkinson's disease patients. *Brain* 2006;129:1758–67.

29. Landis C, Hunt WA. *The Startle Pattern*. New York: Farrar, Strauss and Giroux; 1939.

30. Wilkins DE, Hallett M, Wess MM. Audiogenic startle reflex of man and its relationship to startle syndromes. *Brain* 1986;109:561–73.

31. Brown P, Rothwell JC, Thompson PD, et al. New observations on the normal auditory startle reflex in man. *Brain* 1991;11:1891–902.

32. Brown P, Day BL, Rothwell JC, et al. The effect of posture on the normal and pathological auditory startle reflex. *J Neurol Neurosurg Psychiatry* 1991;54:892–7.

33. Matsumoto JY, Caviness JN, McEvoy KM. The acoustic startle reflex in stiff-man syndrome. *Neurology* 1994;44:1952–5.

34. Jenny AB, Saper CB. Organization of the facial nucleus and the corticofacial projection in the monkey: a reconsideration of the upper motor neuron facial palsy. *Neurology* 1987;37:930–9.

35. Gogan P. The startle and orienting reactions in man. A study of their characteristics and habituation. *Brain Research* 1970;18:117–35.

36. Turpin G. Effects of stimulus intensity on autonomic responding: the problem of differentiating orienting and defense reflexes. *Psychophysiology* 1986;23:1–14.

37. Gautier CH, Cook EW. Relationship between startle and cardiovascular reactivity *Psychophysiology* 1997;34:87–96.

38. Dimberg U. Facial electromyographic reactions and autonomic activity to auditory stimuli. *Biol Psychol* 1990;31:137–47.

39. Holand S, Girard A, Laude D, et al. Effects of an auditory startle stimulus on blood pressure and heart rate in humans. *J Hypertens* 1999;17:1893–7.

40. Furubayashi T, Ugawa Y, Terao Y, et al. The human hand motor area is transiently

suppressed by an unexpected acoustic stimulus. *Clin Neurophysiol* 2000;111:78–83.

41. Fisher RJ, Sharott A, Kühn AA, et al. Effects of combined cortical and acoustic stimuli on muscle activity. *Exp Brain Res* 2004;157:1–9

42. Kühn AA, Sharott A, Trottenberg T, et al. Motor cortex inhibition induced by acoustic stimulation. *Exp Brain Res* 2004;158:120–4.

43. Delwaide PJ, Schepens B. Auditory startle (audio-spinal) reaction in normal man: EMG responses and H reflex changes in antagonistic lower limb muscles. *Electroenceph Clin Neurophysiol* 1995;97:416–23.

44. Valls-Solé J, Veciana M, León L, et al. Effects of a startle on heart rate in patients with multiple system atrophy. *Mov Disord* 2002;17:546–9.

45. Valls-Solé J, Rothwell JC, Goulart F, et al. Patterned ballistic movements triggered by a startle in healthy humans. *J Physiol* 1999;516:931–8.

46. Valls-Solé J, Valldeoriola F, Molinuevo JL, et al. Prepulse modulation of the startle reaction and the blink reflex in normal human subjects. *Exp Brain Res* 1999;129:49–56.

47. Valls-Solé J, Kumru H, Kofler M. Interaction between startle and voluntary reactions in humans. *Exp Brain Res* 2008;187:497–507.

48. Carlsen AN, Chua R, Inglis JT, et al. Can prepared responses be stored subcortically? *Exp Brain Res* 2004;159:301–9.

49. Carlsen AN, Chua R, Inglis JT, et al. Prepared movements are elicited early by startle. *J Mot Behav* 2004;36:253–64.

50. Nickerson RS. Intersensory facilitation of reaction time: energy summation or preparation enhancement? *Psychol Rev* 1973;80:489–509.

51. Anzak A, Tan H, Pogosyan A, et al. Doing better than your best: loud auditory stimulation yields improvements in maximal voluntary force. *Exp Brain Res* 2011;208:237–43.

52. Alvarez-Blanco S, Leon L, Valls-Solé J. The startle reaction to somatosensory inputs: different response pattern to stimuli of upper and lower limbs. *Exp Brain Res* 2009;195:285–92.

53. Miwa H, Nohara C, Hotta M, et al. Somatosensory-evoked blink response: investigation of the physiological mechanisms. *Brain* 1998;121:281–91.

54. León L, Casanova-Molla J, Lauria G, et al. The somatosensory blink reflex in upper and lower brainstem lesions. *Muscle Nerve* 2011;43:196–202.

55. Davis M. Neural systems involved in fear-potentiated startle. *Ann NY Acad Sci* 1989;563:165–83.

56. Lang PJ, Bradley MM, Cuthbert BN. Emotion, motivation, and anxiety: brain mechanisms and psychophysiology. *Biol Psychiatry* 1998;44:1248–63

57. Hitchcock JM, Sananes CB, Davis M. Sensitization of the startle reflex by foot-shock: blockade by lesions of the central nucleus of the amygdala or its efferent pathway to the brainstem. *Behav Neurosci* 1989;103:509–18.

58. Grillon C. Models and mechanisms of anxiety: evidence from startle studies. *Psychopharmacology* 2008;199:421–37.

59. Bakker MJ, Tijssen MA, van der Meer JN, et al. Increased whole-body auditory startle reflex and autonomic reactivity in children with anxiety disorders. *J Psychiatry Neurosci* 2009;34:314–22.

60. Siegelaar SE, Olff M, Bour LJ, et al. The auditory startle response in post-traumatic stress disorder. *Exp Brain Res* 2006;174:1–6.

61. McTeague LM, Lang PJ, Laplante MC, et al. Aversive imagery in posttraumatic stress disorder: trauma recurrence, comorbidity, and physiological reactivity. *Biol Psychiatry* 2010;67:346–56.

62. Grillon C, Davis M. Effects of stress and shock anticipation on prepulse inhibition of the startle reflex. *Psychophysiology* 1997;34:511–17.

63. Li L, Du Y, Li N, et al. Top-down modulation of prepulse inhibition of the startle reflex in humans and rats. *Neurosci Biobehav Rev* 2009;33:1157–67.

64. Valls-Solé J, Valldeoriola F, Tolosa E, et al. Habituation of the auditory startle reaction is reduced during preparation for execution of a motor task in normal human subjects. *Brain Res* 1997;751:155–9.

65. Chokroverty S, Walczak T, Hening W. Human startle reflex: technique and criteria for abnormal response. *Electroenceph Clin Neurophysiol* 1992;85:236–42.

66. Timmann D, Musso C, Kolb FP, et al. Involvement of the human cerebellum during habituation of the acoustic startle response: a PET study. *J Neurol Neurosurg Psychiatry* 1998;65:771–3.

67. Blumenthal TD, Cuthbert BN, Filion DL, et al. Committee report: guidelines for human startle eyeblink electromyographic studies. *Psychophysiology* 2005;42:1–15

68. Kofler M, Muller J, Reggiani L, et al. Influence of gender on auditory startle responses. *Brain Res* 2001;921:206–10

69. Valldeoriola F, Valls-Solé J, Tolosa E, et al. Effects of a startling acoustic stimulus on reaction time in different parkinsonian syndromes. *Neurology* 1998;51:1315–20.

70. Hoffman HS, Ison JR. Reflex modification in the domain of startle: I. Some empirical findings and their implications for how the nervous system processes sensory input. *Psychol Rev* 1980;87:175–89.

71. Ison JR, Hoffman HS. Reflex modification in the domain of startle. II. The anomalous history of a robust and ubiquitous phenomenon. *Psychol Bull* 1983;94:3–17

72. Boulu P, Willer JC, Cambier J. Analyse électrophysiologique du réflexe de clignement chez l'homme: interaction des afferences sensitives segmentaires et intersegmentaires, des afferences auditives et visuelles. *Rev Neurol* 1981;137:523–33.

73. Blumenthal TD, Gescheider GA. Modification of the acoustic startle reflex by a tactile prepulse: the effects of stimulus onset asynchrony and prepulse intensity. *Psychophysiology* 1987; 24: 320–7.

74. Lang PJ, Bradley MM, Cuthbert BN. Emotion, attention and the startle reflex. *Psychol Rev* 1990;97:377–95.

75. Boelhouwer AJW, Teurlings RJMA, Brunia CHM. The effect of an acoustic warning stimulus upon the electrically elicited blink reflex in humans. *Psychophysiology* 1991;28:133–9.

76. Swerdlow NR, Paulsen J, Braff DL, et al. Impaired prepulse inhibition of acoustic and tactile startle response in patients with Huntington's disease. *J Neurol Neurosurg Psychiatry* 1995;58:192–200.

77. Hoffman HS, Fleshler M. Startle reaction: modification by background acoustic stimulation. *Science* 1963;141:928–30.

78. Voordecker P, Mavroudakis N, Blecic S, et al. Audiogenic startle reflex in acute hemiplegia. *Neurology* 1997;49:470–3

79. Kumru H, Vidal J, Kofler M, et al. Alterations in excitatory and inhibitory brainstem interneuronal circuits after severe spinal cord injury. *J Neurotrauma* 2010;27:721–8

80. Chabot CC, Taylor DH. Circadian modulation of the rat acoustic startle response. *Behav Neurosci* 1992;106:846–52.

81. Walker DL, Davis M. Anxiogenic effects of high illumination levels assessed with the acoustic startle response in rats. *Biol Psychiatry* 1997;42:461–71.

82. Paylor R, Crawley JN. Inbred strain differences in prepulse inhibition of the mouse startle response. *Psychopharmacology* 1997;132:169–80.

83. Ho KJ, Kileny P, Paccioretti D, et al. Neurologic, audiologic, and electrophysiologic sequelae of bitemporal lobe lesions. *Arch Neurol* 1987;44:982–7

84. Liegeois-Chauvel C, Morin C, Musolino A, et al. Evidence for contribution of the auditory cortex to audiospinal facilitation in man. *Brain* 1989;112:375–91.

85. Grillon C, Ameli R, Wood SW, et al. Fear-potentiated startle in humans: effects of anticipatory anxiety on the acoustic blink reflex. *Psychophysiology* 1991;28:588–95.

86. Lang PJ, Davis M. Emotion, motivation, and the brain: reflex foundations in animal and human research. *Prog Brain Res* 2006;156:3–29.

87. Kofler M, Müller J, Rinnerthaler-Weichbold M, et al. Laterality of auditory startle responses in humans. *Clin Neurophysiol* 2008;119:309–14.

88. Vidailhet M, Rothwell JC, Thompson PD, et al. The auditory startle response in the Steele-Richardson-Olszewski syndrome and Parkinson's disease. *Brain* 1992;115:1181–92.

89. Valldeoriola F, Valls-Solé J, Tolosa E, Nobbe FA, Muñoz JE, Martí J. The acoustic startle response is normal in patients with multiple system atrophy. *Mov Disord*. 1997 Sep;12(5):697–700.

90. Kofler M, Müller J, Wenning GK, et al. The auditory startle reaction in parkinsonian disorders. *Mov Disord* 2001;16:62–71.

91. Kofler M, Müller J, Seppi K, et al. Exaggerated auditory startle responses in multiple system atrophy: a comparative study of Parkinson and cerebellar subtypes. *Clin Neurophysiol* 2003;114:541–7.

92. Andermann F, Keene DL, Andermann E, et al. Startle disease or hyperekplexia: further delineation of the syndrome. *Brain* 1980;103:985–97.

93. Tijssen MA, Vergouwe MN, van Dijk JG, et al. Major and minor form of hereditary hyperekplexia. *Mov Disord* 2002;17:826–30.

94. Tijssen MA, Brown P, MacManus D, et al. Magnetic resonance spectroscopy of cerebral cortex is normal in hereditary hyperekplexia due to mutations in the GLRA1 gene. *Mov Disord* 2003;18:1538–41.

95. Thompson PD, Colebatch JG, Brown P, et al. Voluntary stimulus sensitive jerks and jumps mimicking myoclonus or pathological startle syndromes. *Mov Disord* 1992;7:257–62.

96. Matsumoto J, Fuhr P, Nigro M, et al. Physiologicalabnormalities in hereditary hyperekplexia. *Ann Neurol* 1992;32:41–50.

97. Stell R, Thickbroom GW, Mastaglia FL. The audiogenic startle response in Tourette's syndrome. *Mov Disord* 1995;10:723–30.

98. Frauscher B, Löscher W, Högl B, et al. Auditory startle reaction is disinhibited in idiopathic restless legs syndrome. *Sleep* 2007;30:489–93.

99. Jankelowitz SK, Colebatch JG. The acoustic startle refl ex in ischemic stroke. *Neurology* 2004;62:114–16.

100. Watson SR, Colebatch JG. Focal pathological startle following pontine infarction. *Mov Disord* 2002;17:212–18.

101. Della Marca G, Restuccia D, Mariotti P, et al. Pathologic startle following brainstem lesion. *Neurology* 2007;68:437.

102. Kumru H, Vidal J, Kofler M, et al. Exaggerated auditory startle responses in patients with spinal cord injury. *J Neurol* 2008;255:703–9.

103. Kimber TE, Thompson PD. Symptomatic hyperekplexia occurring as a result of pontine infarction. *Mov Disord* 1997;12:814–16

104. Lotze M, Laubis-Herrmann U, Topka H. Combination of TMS and fMRI reveals a specific pattern of reorganization in M1 in patients after complete spinal cord injury. *Restor Neurol Neurosci* 2006;24:97–107.

105. Tijssen MA, Padberg GW, van Dijk JG. The startle pattern in the minor form of hyperekplexia. *Arch Neurol* 1996;53:608–13.

106. Tijssen MA, Voorkamp LM, Padberg GW, et al. Startle responses in hereditary hyperekplexia. *Arch Neurol* 1997;54:388–93.

107. Brown P, Thompson PD. Electrophysiological aids to the diagnosis of psychogenic jerks, spasms, and tremor. *Mov Disord* 2001;16:595–9

108. Saint-Hilaire MH, Saint-Hilaire JM, Granger L. Jumping Frenchmen of Maine. *Neurology* 1986;36:1269–71.

109. Geyer MA, Swerdlow NR, Mansbach RS, et al. Startle response models of sensorimotor gating and habituation deficits in schizophrenia. *Brain Res Bull*1990;25:485–98.

110. Braff DL, Geyer MA. Sensorimotor gating and schizophrenia. *Arch Gen Psychiatry* 1990;47:181–8.

111. Braff DL. Prepulse inhibition of the startle reflex: a window on the brain in schizophrenia. *Curr Top Behav Neurosci* 2010;4:349–71.

112. Ludewig S, Geyer MA, Ramseier M, Vollenweider FX, Rechsteiner E, Cattapan-Ludewig K. Information-processing deficits and cognitive dysfunction in panic disorder. *J Psychiatry Neurosci.* 2005 Jan;30(1):37–43.

113. Kumari V, Fannon D, Geyer MA, et al. Cortical grey matter volume and sensorimotor gating in schizophrenia. *Cortex* 2008;44:1206–14.

114. Nakashima K, Shimoyama R, Yokoyama Y, et al. Auditory effects on the electrically elicited blink reflex in patients with Parkinson's disease. *Electroencephalogr Clin Neurophysiol* 1993;89:108–12.

115. Valls-Solé J, Muñoz JE, Valldeoriola F. Abnormalities of prepulse inhibition do not depend on blink reflex excitability. A study in Parkinson's disease and Huntington's disease. *Clinical Neurophysiology* 2004;115:1527–36.

116. Mascia MM, Valls-Solé J, Marti MJ, et al. Sensorimotor integration in patients with Parkinsonian type multisystem atrophy. *J Neurol* 2005;252:473–81.

117. Gómez-Wong E, Martí MJ, Tolosa E, et al. Sensory modulation of the blink reflex in patients with blepharospasm. *Arch Neurol* 1998;55:1233–7.

118. Valls-Solé J, Solé A, Valldeoriola F, et al. Reaction time and acoustic startle in normal human subjects. *Neurosci Lett* 1995;195:97–100.

119. Siegmund GP, Inglis JT, Sanderson DJ. Startle response of human neck muscles sculpted by readiness to perform ballistic head movements. *J Physiol* 2001;535:289–300.

120. Castellote JM, Kumru H, Queralt A, et al. A startle speeds up the execution of externally guided saccades. *Exp Brain Res* 2007;177:129–36.

121. Gielen SC, Schmidt RA, Van den Heuvel PJ. On the nature of intersensory facilitation of reaction time. *Percept Psychophys* 1983;34:161–8.

122. Sanegre MT, Castellote JM, Haggard P, et al. The effects of a startle on awareness of action. *Exp Brain Res* 2004;155:527–31.

123. Schmidt L, Cléry-Melin ML, Lafargue G, et al. Get aroused and be stronger: emotional facilitation of physical effort in the human brain. *J Neurosci* 2009;29:9450–7.

124. Valls-Solé J. Contribution of subcortical motor pathways to the execution of ballistic movements. *Suppl Clin Neurophysiol* 2004;57:554–62.

125. Tresilian JR, Plooy AM. Effects of acoustic startle stimuli on interceptive action. *Neuroscience* 2006;142:579–94.

126. Nijhuis LB, Janssen L, Bloem BR, et al. Choice reaction times for human head rotations are shortened by startling acoustic stimuli, irrespective of stimulus direction. *J Physiol* 2007;584:97–109.

127. Reynolds RF, Day BL. Fast visuomotor processing made faster by sound. *J Physiol* 2007;583:1107–15.

128. MacKinnon CD, Bissig D, Chiusano J, et al. Preparation of anticipatory postural adjustments prior to stepping. *J Neurophysiol* 2007;97:4368–79.

129. Queralt A, Valls-Solé J, Castellote JM. The effects of a startle on the sit-to-stand manoeuvre. *Exp Brain Res* 2008;185:603–9.

130. Queralt A, Weerdesteyn V, van Duijnhoven HJ, et al. The effects of an auditory startle on obstacle avoidance during walking. *J Physiol* 2008; 586:4453–63.

131. Queralt A, Valls-Solé J, Castellote JM. Speeding up gait initiation and gait-pattern with a startling stimulus. *Gait Posture* 2010;31:185–90.

132. Carlsen AN, Chua R, Inglis JT, et al. Startle response is dishabituated during a reaction time task. *Exp Brain Res* 2003;152:510–18.

133. Starr A, Caramia M, Zarola F, et al. Enhancement of motor cortical excitability in humans by non-invasive electrical stimulation appears prior to voluntary movement. *Electroencephalogr Clin Neurophysiol* 1988;70:26–32.

134. Pascual-Leone A, Valls-Solé J, Wassermann EM, et al. Effects of focal transcranial magnetic stimulation on simple reaction time to acoustic, visual and somatosensory stimuli. *Brain* 1992;115:1045–59.

135. Kumru H, Valls-Solé J. Excitability of the pathways mediating the startle reaction before execution of a voluntary movement. *Exp Brain Res* 2006;169:427–32.

136. Reynolds C, Ashby P. Inhibition in the human motor cortex is reduced just before a voluntary contraction. *Neurology* 1999;53:730–5.

137. Floeter MK, Rothwell JC. Releasing the brakes before pressing the gas pedal. *Neurology* 1999;53:664–5.

138. Soto O, Valls-Solé J, Kumru H. Paired-pulse transcranial magnetic stimulation during preparation for simple and choice reaction time tasks. *J Neurophysiol* 2010;104:1392–400.

139. Valls-Solé J, Kofler M, Kumru H, et al. Startle-induced reaction time shortening is not modified by prepulse inhibition. *Exp Brain Res* 2005;165:541–8.

140. Kumru H, Urra X, Compta Y, et al. Excitability of subcortical motor circuits in Go/noGo and forced choice reaction time tasks. *Neurosci Lett* 2006;406:66–70.

141. Carlsen AN, Dakin CJ, Chua R, et al. Startle produces early response latencies that are distinct from stimulus intensity effects. *Exp Brain Res* 2007;176:199–205.

142. Lipp OV, Kaplan DM, Purkis HM. Reaction time facilitation by acoustic task-irrelevant stimuli is not related to startle. *Neurosci Lett* 2006;409:124–7.

143. Libet B, Gleason CA, Wright EW, et al. Time of conscious intention to act in relation to onset of cerebral activity (readiness-potential). *Brain* 1983;106:623–42.

144. McCloskey DI, Colebatch JG, Potter EK, et al. Judgments about onset of rapid voluntary movements in man. *J Neurophysiol* 1983;49:851–63.

145. Haggard P, Magno E. Localising awareness of action with transcranial magnetic stimulation. *Exp Brain Res* 1999;127:102–7.

146. Eimer M. The lateralized readiness potential as an on-line measure of selective response activation. *Behav Res Methods Instrum Comput* 1998;30:146–56.

147. Haggard P, Eimer M. On the relation between brain potentials and the awareness of voluntary movements. *Exp Brain Res* 1999;126:128–33.

18

Electroencephalography in Relation to Abnormal Movements during Sleep

JOANNA FONG AND NANCY FOLDVARY-SCHAEFER

THE WORD *epilepsy* is derived from the Greek word *epilambanein*, meaning "to seize." The oldest reference to epilepsy is found on Babylonian cuneiform tablets called "Sakkiku" meaning "all diseases," dating back to the middle of the first millennium BC.[1] Two of the tablets described epilepsy as "the falling disease." The Babylonians believed epilepsy to be the work of ghosts and demons that could possess one temporarily. Over the ages, epilepsy remained a poorly understood, stigmatized disorder.

In the 19th century, John Hughlings Jackson revolutionized understanding of the pathophysiology of epilepsy, theorizing that seizures were the result of electrical activity in the brain.[2] By observing his wife's seizures, Jackson recognized that abnormal electrical discharges originating from one region of the brain could spread to another, producing variable clinical manifestations depending on the area(s) of cortex activated. He detailed the clinical features of focal motor seizures arising from activation of primary motor cortex, known as the "Jacksonian march" or "Jacksonian epilepsy."

With the advancement in clinical medicine and diagnostic technologies, epilepsy is now recognized as a brain disorder characterized by an enduring predisposition to generate epileptic seizures and by the neurobiologic, cognitive, psychological, and social consequences of the condition.[3] An epileptic seizure is a transient occurrence of signs and/or symptoms due to abnormal excessive or synchronous neuronal activity in the brain.

In contrast to the rich history of clinical epilepsy, the history of the electroencephalogram (EEG) began less than a century ago. Hans Berger discovered EEG in 1929 and it has remained the key diagnostic tool for epilepsy. Basic concepts of EEG remain the same, despite the evolution of technology from paper to digital recordings. EEG procedures are categorized by the length and location of the recording (routine EEG, sleep-deprived EEG, polysomnography [PSG] with video EEG [VEEG], ambulatory home EEG, long-term VEEG), as well as the type of electrode placement (scalp, semi-invasive, invasive). The indication of each procedure and choice of electrode placement vary by the clinical question and the degree of precision required in localizing the epileptic focus.

The relationship between sleep and epilepsy has been recognized since the time of Hippocrates. In 1885, Gowers was the first to observe the diurnal pattern of seizures.[4] Due to the predisposition of some epileptic disorders to arise from sleep, seizures may be mistaken for other abnormal movements in sleep, including parasomnias and sleep-related movement disorders.

In this chapter, we will address EEG in relation to abnormal movements in sleep through a review of (1) technical aspects of EEG; (2) procedure types and indications; (3) sleep and sleep deprivation as activation maneuvers; (4) noninvasive EEG and its limitations; and (5) invasive EEG and its limitations. Cases of sleep-related abnormal movements will be used to illustrate important EEG findings and ways to tailor EEG to address specific clinical questions.

TECHNICAL ASPECTS OF ELECTROENCEPHALO-GRAPHY

Basic Concepts of Electroencephalography

EEG potentials are a reflection of the intrinsic electrophysiological properties of the central nervous system, particularly the six neocortical layers with neurons arranged perpendicular to the cortical surface. The EEG is generated by inhibitory and excitatory postsynaptic potentials of neurons and reflects summation of these potentials generated by the underlying cortex. With neuronal depolarization, a tangential net negativity is seen on the cortical surface with a relative positivity in the deeper neocortical layers, forming a "dipole" (Fig. 18.1). Generators that are deep-seated or dipoles that are horizontal to the cortical surface may not produce recognizable EEG potentials when recording from scalp electrodes. A cortical surface area of at least 10 cm² with synchronous activation is required to generate an interictal epileptiform discharge (IED) on scalp EEG.[5]

Electrical potentials recorded by scalp electrodes are processed through a series of differential amplifiers and filters before being displayed

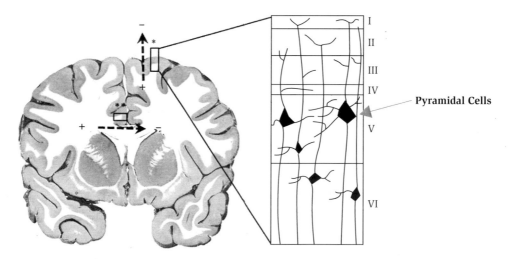

FIGURE 18.1 Schematic illustrating the generation of electrical potentials on a coronal brain section. Six neocortical layers with pyramidal cells arranged perpendicular to the cortical surface, dentritic trees located in more superficial neocortical layers, and cell bodies in the deeper neocortical layers are shown to the right. A tangential potential generated by cortex near the convexity (*) produces a dipole with a net negativity on the cortical surface and a net positivity in the deep neocortical layers. In contrast, a potential generated in the interhemispheric region (**) produces a horizontal dipole that is not appreciable on the scalp electroencephalogram.

as the EEG. Differential amplifiers have a dual input, G1 and G2, and are constructed to amplify only the potential difference between the two inputs. Signals from G1 and G2 are compared to augment the relative voltage differences between the two signals. The amplifier rejects signals common to both inputs. This process is called "common mode rejection." The common mode rejection allows for better detection of abnormal activity by eliminating unwanted shared background noise. The digital EEG signal can be filtered for display. The settings for the low-frequency (or high-pass) filter and high-frequency (or low-pass) filter are 0.2–1 Hz and 15–70 Hz, respectively. The low-frequency filter attenuates unwanted slow EEG activity such as sweat artifact, whereas low-pass filter attenuates unwanted fast EEG activity such as muscle artifact. A notch filter is used to remove artifact caused by electrical power lines (60 Hz in the United States).

Polarity and Localization Rules

A basic understanding of polarity is required to correctly localize electrical signals on the EEG. The direction of the waveform deflection depends on which of the two inputs (G1 or G2) is relatively more active. Upward deflection signifies either a relative negativity at G1 or a relative positivity at G2. Similarly, a downward deflection is a result of either a relative positivity at G1 or a relative negativity at G2.[6] On a bipolar montage (see later), the localization of an IED is determined by identifying the phase reversal, where two adjacent channels show deflections in opposite directions. An inward or negative phase reversal (deflections point toward each other) on a bipolar montage identifies the electrode of maximum negativity, and therefore, the area from which the discharge arises. The majority of potentials seen on noninvasive (scalp) EEG are surface negative. Positive potentials are more common in depth and electrocorticographic recordings; in patients with skull defects, head trauma, and malformations of cortical development; and in cases where the generator produces a horizontally oriented dipole.

Electrodes and Placement

The 10–20 System of the International Federation of Societies for EEG and Clinical Neurophysiology is the method of electrode placement used in EEG (Fig. 18.2). The system is based on measurements of 10% and 20% of the distance between standard cranial landmarks. Each electrode site is identified by a letter and a number. The letter represents the underlying region of the brain, and the number indicates a specific position in that region. Odd numbers indicate the left hemisphere; even numbers indicate the right hemisphere. Each recording channel represents the difference in electrical potential between a pair of electrodes. Several pairs of electrodes are combined to form a montage. Additional rows of electrodes in between the coronal and sagittal rows of the 10–20 System may be placed for more precise localization of epileptiform activity. Known as the 10/10 System, this method of electrode

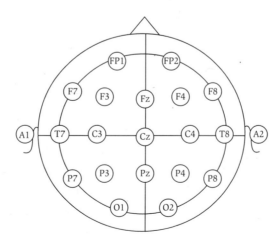

FIGURE 18.2   10–20 International Electrode System is the method of electrode placement used in conventional electroencephalography. The nasion is at the top of the illustration.

placement is used primarily during long-term VEEG.[7] Additional, closely spaced scalp electrode placement increases the detection of EEG abnormalities, notably, epileptiform activity, by enhancing spatial resolution.[8] Depending on the type and purpose of the study, electrode density can be reduced or expanded to optimize the yield of the recording.

Sphenoidal electrodes are commonly used to increase the yield of scalp EEG in the presurgical assessment of patients with drug-resistant epilepsy suspected to arise from the temporal lobe or connected structures.[9] Sphenoidal electrodes are semi-invasive electrodes placed through the cheek at the mandibular recess with the tip of the electrode ideally laying inferior to the foramen ovale. The utility of sphenoidal electrodes is controversial.[10,11] Overall, evidence has shown that sphenoidal electrodes are superior to laterally placed scalp electrodes in the detection of mesial temporal IEDs and seizures. However, several studies reported no significant difference in IED detection using sphenoidal and mandibular notch or anterior temporal scalp electrodes.[12]

EEG electrodes are made of metals, including silver-silver chloride, silver, gold-plated silver, platinum, stainless steel, and tin.[13] Silver-silver chloride and gold are preferred for their minimal electrode potential drift and long-time constant properties. Plastic-covered metal electrodes are inferior to metal electrodes but available for EEG recording during magnetic resonance imaging (MRI). EEG electrodes are cup-shaped discs secured onto the scalp with an adhesive. Collodion has long been recognized as the most reliable adhesive for electrode placement, especially during long-term VEEG. In other settings such as in PSG, electrode adhesive cream may be preferred due to ease of application, odorless nature, shorter recording duration, and reduced likelihood of movement-related artifact. Electrolyte gel is used to fill the disc cups to allow for optimal contact between the skin and electrode. The scalp must be adequately prepared by removing dead skin and oily residue that can produce unacceptable electrode impedance and degradation of signal quality.

Montages

EEG electrodes are connected in a variety of configurations called montages. Montages may be either referential, in which one of the electrodes in each pair is connected to a common electrode, or bipolar, in which there is no common electrode.

Bipolar montages are usually arranged in a chain with a common electrode in adjacent derivations. The EEG is typically viewed on an anterior-posterior (AP) bipolar montage, although any configuration of electrodes may be used. The AP bipolar montage, also known as a "double-banana," connects electrodes from anterior to posterior, creating a parasagittal and a temporal chain of electrodes over each cerebral hemisphere. This configuration allows for comparison of adjacent electrode pairs in a sequential fashion and highlights hemispheric asymmetries. A transverse montage is another type of bipolar montage in which adjacent electrodes are connected in a coronal fashion from left to right, highlighting the midline and anterior-to-posterior differences. A transverse or coronal montage is most commonly used to identify IEDs or seizures arising from midline or interhemispheric structures, such as in epilepsy arising from the supplementary sensorimotor area (SSMA).

In contrast, referential montages compare differences in electrical activity between each recording electrode and a common reference electrode(s), such as the auricular electrode placements, A1 and A2, in the 10–20 system of electrode placement. Referential montages are often used to confirm hemispheric asymmetries suspected on a bipolar montage and assist in the localization of epileptiform abnormalities. In this regard, it is critical to select a reference electrode that is least involved in the region of interest. For example, the use of an ear or mastoid reference is not advised when mapping the distribution of a temporal lobe discharge. In this case, the referential electrode is likely to be within the field of the electrical abnormality and will be "active," contaminating the montage with unnecessary artifact. An average reference in which the outputs of all of the amplifiers are summed and averaged, or a midline position, such as CZ or PZ, would be preferred in this situation.

PROCEDURE TYPES AND INDICATIONS

A Routine Electroencephalogram

The routine EEG is performed in an outpatient laboratory during the day. It is typically a 15–20 minute recording, but it can be lengthened particularly for purposes of recording sleep. Activation maneuvers, including hyperventilation (HV) and intermittent photic stimulation (IPS), are performed during the routine EEG to increase the yield of abnormalities. The technique of HV consists of deep breathing at a rate of 20 per minute for 2 to 4 minutes that produces a drop in plasma carbon dioxide and cerebral vasoconstriction. IPS utilizes a strobe light with 1.5 million candlepower and a flash duration of 10 seconds to present flashing lights at variable rates during an EEG. Several effects may be produced, the most important of which is the photoconvulsive or photoparoxysmal response, characterized by generalized or posteriorly dominant spike or polyspike and wave complexes that convey a predisposition for epileptic seizures when accompanied by certain electrographic features. Both techniques are effective in eliciting IEDs in individuals with idiopathic generalized epilepsy and rarely yield significant abnormalities in patients with focal epilepsy. Therefore, while generally the first procedure performed, the routine EEG is usually normal in patients being evaluated for abnormal movements in sleep. Arguably, the most effective way to enhance the yield of a routine EEG for investigation of abnormal sleep-related behaviors is to record sleep. This is generally done by recording a prolonged EEG during the daytime after a night of sleep deprivation, partial or total, depending on the laboratory protocol. See later for a more detailed discussion.

Video-Electroencephalography-Polysomnography

Video-EEG-PSG (VPSG) combines PSG and VEEG to evaluate patients with abnormal sleep-related motor activity. This technique has several advantages over routine PSG, including the ability to analyze behavior, correlate behavior with neurophysiologic parameters, and detect epileptiform activity. High-quality video recording is a necessary component of VPSG, as unambiguous epileptic semiology such as tonic-clonic motor activity, automatisms, and versive head movements provide important clues to seizure localization. Minor motor manifestations characteristic of some focal epilepsies, including brief bilateral or focal tonic posturing and myoclonus, are more difficult to characterize using the clinical history alone. Negative motor activity, including behavior arrest, staring, and

subtle loss of postural tone, may not be recognized even by experienced observers without video recordings and patient interaction. The sleep technologist must have the skills to assess and manage patients with abnormal sleep-related movements. Technologists should be trained to identify behaviors that are likely to be epileptic in nature and interact with the patient to determine level of consciousness. The degree of unresponsiveness, recollection of dream content, and presence of lateralizing signs, including postictal language deficits and Todd's paralysis, during and immediately following nocturnal events, provide important clues to the diagnosis and localization of epileptic disorders. In addition, sleep technologists should be educated on patient safety in the setting of generalized motor seizures and management of postictal violent or aggressive behavior and be able to recognize potentially injurious situations, including prolonged seizures and complications such as respiratory distress and aspiration.

The indications of VPSG include the evaluation of sleep-related movements, particularly those that are violent or otherwise potentially injurious to the patient or others, sleep behaviors suggestive of parasomnia that are unusual or atypical, situations with forensic considerations, presumed parasomnia or sleep-related seizures not responsive to conventional therapy, and behaviors suspected to be seizures when the initial clinical evaluation and routine EEG are inconclusive.[14-16] The differential diagnosis of abnormal motor behavior in sleep includes epileptic seizures, non-REM arousal disorders, REM behavior disorder, rhythmic movement disorder, and psychiatric disorders such as panic or dissociative disorder. The accuracy of differentiating seizures from other motor behaviors in sleep increases with the number of EEG electrodes incorporated in the VPSG montage.[17] In a study comparing 8- and 18-channel EEG recordings, seizure identification and localization were significantly greater using the expanded montage.

Seizures arising from the temporal or parieto-occipital regions are more likely to be correctly identified and localized than those arising from the frontal lobe. This is particularly important for the evaluation of sleep-related movements since frontal lobe seizures are most apt to be confused with other types of nocturnal events.

Ambulatory Electroencephalography

Ambulatory EEG is performed in the home, typically in patients with infrequent events or who are unwilling or unable to undergo long-term VEEG. The procedure is initiated in the outpatient EEG laboratory, where scalp electrodes are placed and connected to the portable EEG recorder. An event button is pushed by the patient or an observer to mark the timing of a clinical event. Ambulatory EEG is generally limited to 24 to 48 hours, largely due to challenges of maintaining good-quality recordings as electrode integrity is readily compromised by patient movement. The absence of a skilled observer and video recording reduces the diagnostic yield of this procedure, though the cost is substantially less than long-term VEEG.

Long-Term Video Electroencephalography

Long-term VEEG monitoring is performed in an inpatient setting, typically in a specialized unit dedicated to the care of patients with epilepsy. This procedure is indicated for the diagnosis of epileptic paroxysmal electrographic and/or behavioral abnormalities, classification of clinical seizure type(s) in patients with documented epilepsy, characterization (lateralization, localization, distribution) of EEG abnormalities associated with seizure disorders, quantification of the number or frequency of seizures and/or IEDs and their relationship to naturally occurring events or cycles, and quantitative documentation of the EEG response to a therapeutic intervention or modification.[14] This type of EEG evaluation aids in the diagnosis of patients with normal or inconclusive outpatient EEG recordings and is most often performed in patients with frequent spells in whom epilepsy is strongly suspected.

Long-term VEEG identifies interictal and ictal abnormalities, correlates clinical behavior and electrographic findings, and assists in the recognition of disabling or potentially injurious effects of ictal and postictal behaviors, such as seizure-induced cardiac arrhythmias. The length of the evaluations is usually in the range of 3 to 7 days depending on its purpose. Antiepileptic drugs are typically reduced or tapered in order to precipitate seizures. As in the case of VPSG, technical and nursing staff should be adequately trained to recognize epileptic and nonepileptic behaviors, and to interact with patients to increase the value of the recording and maintain patient safety. Recordings are generally reviewed every 24 hours to identify IEDs and seizures and assess the need for additional monitoring. Commercial EEG monitoring systems provide a variety of analysis tools allowing for spike detection, mapping, and extensive re-montaging to increase the yield of the recording and localize abnormalities.

SLEEP AND SLEEP DEPRIVATION AS ACTIVATION MANEUVERS

Effects of Sleep on the Electroencephalogram

Sleep is a potent activator of IEDs and seizures in patients with epilepsy.[18,19] The activating effect of sleep on the EEG was first illustrated by Gibbs and Gibbs in 1947, who reported IEDs on the wake EEG in 36% of 500 epilepsy cases compared with 82% on the sleep EEG.[20] A more detailed analysis performed decades later found that compared to wakefulness, the rate of IEDs is increased in non-REM sleep and decreased in REM sleep.[21] Additionally, the distribution of IEDs was found to be more restricted in REM compared to non-REM sleep and wakefulness, suggesting that localization of the primary epileptogenic focus may be more reliable in REM sleep than any other stage. Similarly, nocturnal seizures more often arise from non-REM sleep, especially stages N1 and N2, and rarely during REM sleep.[22]

The activating property of non-REM sleep is purportedly due to the state-dependent neurophysiologic characteristics of neuronal synchronization.[23,24] Non-REM sleep represents a state of EEG synchronization and relative preservation of antigravity (tonic) muscle tone. Synchronous oscillations of cortical neurons that generate sleep spindles, K complexes, and tonic background slow waves during non-REM sleep promote seizure propagation. The preservation of tonic muscle tone during non-REM sleep permits the expression of clinical ictal manifestations. In contrast, REM sleep is a state of EEG desynchronization and loss of tonic muscle tone. This EEG desynchronization impedes seizure propagation during REM sleep and wakefulness. Similarly, the absence of tonic muscle tone during REM sleep blocks the clinical expression of seizures.

Effects of Sleep Deprivation on the Electroencephalogram

The occurrence of seizures following sleep deprivation was noted by Hippocrates in the fifth century BC. In 1962, Janz described this phenomenon in relation to different types of epileptic disorders, most notably in military populations.[24a] In soldiers returning from Vietnam in the 1970s, the risk of a seizure after 24 to 36 hours of total sleep deprivation was 1 in 10,000; after 48 hours of sleep loss, 1 in 2500.[25] Lesser amounts of sleep loss can also trigger seizures in vulnerable populations. In a study involving 14 patients with temporal lobe epilepsy (TLE) with nearly 5000 nights of sleep, the probability of having a seizure was significantly higher after a night of modest sleep loss compared to a night of normal sleep.[26]

Similarly, concurrent EEG studies of healthy subjects and patients referred for diagnostic evaluation of suspected epilepsy demonstrate an increase in IEDs after sleep deprivation.[27,28] Sleep deprivation has been shown to activate IEDs beyond the effects of sleep alone. In one series, the percentage of EEGs demonstrating IEDs during wakefulness, sleep, and sleep deprivation states was 25%, 50%, and 80%, respectively.[29] A sleep EEG performed in subjects who had an initial routine EEG confirmed findings in 54% and provided additional information that led to a more accurate diagnosis in 20% of subjects.[30] In a prospective study involving 2000 patients, a significantly greater yield of IEDs occurred after total sleep deprivation as compared to a second routine EEG (22.6% vs. 9.5%).[31]

NONINVASIVE ELECTRO-ENCEPHALOGRAPHY

Noninvasive EEG is routinely used as an initial tool in the evaluation of patients with abnormal movements during sleep and/or suspected epilepsy. EEG provides for the detection of IEDs and localization of an epileptic focus not possible using PSG due to the limited number of electrode placements in routine sleep testing. EEG interpretation requires knowledge of the clinical and electrographic manifestations of seizures and nonepileptic sleep-related movements. Epileptic seizures are classified as focal or generalized based on their clinical and electrographic features. Epilepsy syndromes are constellations of specific signs and symptoms that can be used to predict the natural history of a disorder.

Electroencephalographic Manifestations of Epilepsy

Sharp waves and spikes are the two most common paroxysmal discharges seen in the EEG of people with epilepsy. Sharp waves (70–200 milliseconds) and spikes (20–70 milliseconds) are differentiated only by duration. Other types of IEDs include spike or sharp waves complex (single spike or sharp wave followed by a slow wave), polyspikes (successive of three or more spikes with a frequency of more than 10 Hz) that can be followed by a slow wave (polyspike and wave), and paroxysmal fast activity (high-frequency oscillations in the beta- and gamma-frequency band).[32,33] These waveforms have four fundamental features, including an electrical field that extends beyond one electrode, a sharply contoured component, mostly electro-negativity on the cerebral surface, and disruption of the background activity.[34] Unlike IEDs, ictal EEG patterns typically consist of repetitive, rhythmical activity with a clear onset and offset that evolve in space, amplitude, and/or frequency.

Generalized Seizures and Epilepsies

Generalized epileptic seizures are those conceptualized as originating at some point within, and rapidly engaging, bilaterally distributed networks. Such bilateral networks can include cortical and subcortical structures, but they do not necessarily include the entire cortex.[35] While classically defined as lacking localizing features, it is now accepted that some generalized seizures appear asymmetric both clinically and electrographically. However, most generalized epilepsies are characterized by IEDs having a generalized, bi-anterior maximal distribution (F3/F4 or FP1/FP2) with progressive amplitude decay posteriorly. These discharges are typically detected when recording from frontal and central electrode placements. During generalized seizures, the EEG typically shows diffuse rhythmic activity or repetitive epileptic discharges, reflecting initial involvement of both cerebral hemispheres.

Focal Seizures and Epilepsies

Focal epileptic seizures are those conceptualized as originating within networks limited to one hemisphere. They may be discretely localized or more widely distributed. Focal seizures may originate in subcortical structures.[35] The electrographic manifestations of focal epilepsy depend upon a variety of factors, including the size and location of the ictal generator, location and number of recording electrodes, and the attenuating characteristics of the skull and other intervening tissues.[36] In many cases, the EEG shows IEDs from the region harboring the epileptogenic lesion. This is particularly true in TLE where a unilateral focal preponderance of IEDs predicts the area of seizure origin with a probability of more than 95%.[37] Similarly, regional ictal EEG patterns are more common in TLE (90%), specifically those arising from the mesial temporal structures (93%), compared to epilepsies arising from outside the temporal lobe (50%), in particular from the mesial frontal lobe (24%).[38]

The EEG may be normal in patients with epileptogenic lesions arising from deep or midline regions or show generalized epileptiform activity due to rapid propagation to the contralateral hemisphere. The involvement of basal and mesial cortical areas not directly accessible to scalp EEG, rapid spreading of electric activity within and outside these areas, and tangential orientation of the spike source are responsible for the lower yield of scalp EEG in these cases.[39] Lateralized, generalized, or non-lateralized ictal EEG patterns are characteristic of some extratemporal focal epilepsies.[38] This is critically important in the evaluation of abnormal movements during sleep as some of the sleep-related epilepsies arise from deep structures that are not apparent on noninvasive EEG even with the finest of recording techniques. Most focal seizures are characterized by rhythmic activity that evolves in frequency, distribution (field), and/or amplitude.[40] Repetitive spikes or sharp waves and sudden attenuation of activity over one region or cerebral hemisphere are also observed. Seizures characterized by excessive motor activity may be obscured by muscle artifact, rendering the EEG uninterpretable. This is most commonly observed in patients with frontal lobe epilepsy (FLE) in whom parasomnias or psychogenic seizures may be erroneously diagnosed due to the apparent lack of an EEG correlate. The EEG may be normal even during a seizure if the event is brief and the epileptogenic focus is distant from the recording electrodes, another feature of FLE. Similarly, EEG changes may not be apparent when a seizure remains confined to a limited area. The absence of epileptic abnormalities does not definitively exclude the diagnosis of epilepsy.

LIMITATIONS OF NONINVASIVE ELECTRO-ENCEPHALOGRAPHY

EEG relies on scalp electrodes to record coherent electrical discharges from the underlying brain, resulting from synchronously activated populations of neurons.[41,42] One fundamental limitation is that sources must originate from cortical areas of at least 10 cm^2 to enable detection from the scalp.[5,43,44] Furthermore, scalp electrodes are relatively insensitive to activity arising within sulci that comprise nearly 70% of the cortical surface.[45] Other deep structures are too distant for reliable detection, such as mesial and basal cortices. Lastly, electrical propagation through multiple nonneural layers (cerebrospinal fluid, dura, skull, and scalp) produces a "smearing effect," reducing source localization.[46,47] High-frequency EEG patterns are often observed during the evolution of seizures. These fast frequencies are dampened more than lower frequencies on noninvasive EEG recordings. Overall, the ictal noninvasive EEG is not adequately localized in one quarter to one third of cases, varying by the location, size, and pathological substrate of the generator.[38,48]

INVASIVE ELECTRO-ENCEPHALOGRAPHY

Invasive (intracranial) EEG using subdural or depth electrodes is applied to patients with drug-resistant focal epilepsy when noninvasive EEG and neuroimaging fail to provide an adequate estimation of the epileptic focus and resective surgery is being considered. The role of invasive EEG in the surgical management of epilepsy can be best appreciated by an introduction to the five epileptogenic zones used in localization of focal epilepsy.[49]

The Five Epileptogenic Zones

Despite the emergence of new antiepileptic medications (AEDs), as many as one third of patients have drug-resistant epilepsy. The International League Against Epilepsy recently established a task force to find a consensus in the definition of drug-resistant epilepsy. The proposed definition is failure of adequate trials of two tolerated, appropriately chosen AEDs to achieve sustained seizure freedom.[50] Surgery for drug-resistant epilepsy aims to produce a seizure-free state, which is best done through complete removal of the epileptogenic zone. The epileptogenic zone is the conceptual area necessary for generating seizure activity that, when removed, eliminates seizures. Since the epileptogenic zone is a theoretical concept, there are no diagnostic techniques that measure and delineate it directly. With current technology, the epileptogenic zone cannot be visualized directly. However, it can be estimated by a combination of five other cortical zones that are defined in the presurgical evaluation[49]:

- The *symptomatogenic zone* is responsible for the initial symptoms of an aura or a seizure; thus, it can be defined using history and video recordings of seizures.
- The *functional deficit zone* corresponds to interictal neurological or neuropsychological deficits that may be detected through the neurological examination, neuropsychological testing, or functional imaging.
- The *irritative zone* generates IEDs; it is estimated through the interictal EEG.
- The *ictal onset zone* creates the initial seizure discharges; it can be approximated through ictal EEG recordings and ictal single photon emission computed tomography (SPECT).
- An *epileptogenic lesion* is a structural imaging abnormality that is responsible for the generation of seizures; it may be visualized by MRI.

The long-term effects and comorbidities associated with drug-resistant epilepsy have significant impact, including medication side effects, behavioral and psychiatric effects such as major depression, and quality of life issues such as employment, education, driving, and social stigmata.[51-53] In addition, the risk of sudden unexplained death, the most common cause of mortality in people with epilepsy, is 0.35 per 1000 person-years, 24-fold higher in epilepsy compared to the general population.[54]

Indications for Invasive Electroencephalography

Invasive EEG is indicated in a variety of settings where the findings from the clinical history and examination, noninvasive EEG, and structural and functional imaging fail to provide adequate

localization of the epileptogenic zone. These include the following:

- MRI-negative (non-lesional) focal epilepsy
- Discordant findings on noninvasive EEG and imaging studies
- Suspected pathology extending beyond the structurally visible lesion
- Multiple structural lesions (e.g., tuberous sclerosis or other dual pathologies)
- Poorly localized noninvasive EEG (e.g., diffuse interictal spikes, nonlocalizing ictal patterns)
- Epileptogenic zone is in close proximity to functionally eloquent cortex

The implantation strategy is driven by the surgical hypothesis and the risk-benefit ratio of the proposed procedure. Since the risk of complications increases with the number of electrodes implanted, the more focused the hypothesis, the more likely it can be adequately and safely tested.[55] Subdural electrodes are platinum or stainless-steel contacts imbedded in sheets of plastic that can be cut in a variety of arrays. Subdural electrodes allow for a better signal to noise ratio than noninvasive EEG electrodes since they record directly from the cortical surface. They are also less sensitive to the orientation of the dipole generated by neuronal activity. When the suspected epileptogenic zone involves deep-seated or interhemispheric structures, depth electrodes can be placed freehandedly or stereotactically (SEEG). Depth electrodes consist of arrays of contacts along the length of the wire. Subdural and depth electrodes can be combined to optimally cover networks of interest. Invasive EEG electrodes are implanted in the operating room under general anesthesia. Co-registration of invasive electrodes and brain anatomy is carried out using conventional skull radiographs, computerized tomography, or MRI to confirm electrode placement. Electrical stimulation is typically performed after interictal activity and spontaneous seizures are recorded in order to map eloquent cortex, areas that subserve language and sensorimotor function.

LIMITATIONS OF INVASIVE ELECTROENCEPHALOGRAPHY

While invasive EEG records directly from brain tissue, it samples only the region in or near the recording electrodes. Unlike noninvasive EEG, invasive EEG can record only from the specific targets chosen by the working hypothesis of the epileptogenic zone. Therefore, if the ictal onset zone is not part of the targets sampled, findings from the invasive EEG evaluation may be misleading, leading to an unsuccessful surgical resection or eliminating a potential candidate from surgical consideration. The risk of complications increases with the number of implanted electrodes (more than 60), longer recording duration (more than 10 days), older age, and left-sided grid implantation.[55] Complications occur in approximately one quarter of cases, the majority not associated with permanent injury. These include infection, transient neurologic deficits, hemorrhage, increased intracranial pressure, and infarction.

CASE ILLUSTRATIONS
Case 1

B.S. is a 25-year-old obese female who presented with unexplained bruising for several months. She had woken up with bruises on her extremities about once weekly, and on one occasion, discovered she had urinated in bed with the nightstand lamp knocked to the floor. She had enuresis and sleepwalking that remitted spontaneously at 8 years of age and underwent tonsillectomy for snoring. On further questioning, she reported two witnessed episodes during wakefulness in which she experienced a sudden sense of fear and anxiety. One of these was followed by staring and repetitive chewing movements described by a friend, for which she had no awareness. A routine PSG was performed prior to presentation that was unremarkable, as was a routine awake EEG. A prolonged, sleep-deprived EEG was recommended (Figs 18.3 and 18.4).

Discussion

Based on the history, the differential diagnosis of unexplained bruising includes non-REM arousal disorder, nocturnal seizures, sleep apnea, and sleep-related movement disorders. However, the daytime episodes make epilepsy the most probable diagnosis. The lack of abnormal findings on PSG and routine awake EEG does not exclude this diagnosis, since the EEG montage in routine PSG is limited and a routine awake EEG recording may be normal in cases of epilepsy. The sleep-deprived EEG (Fig. 18.3)

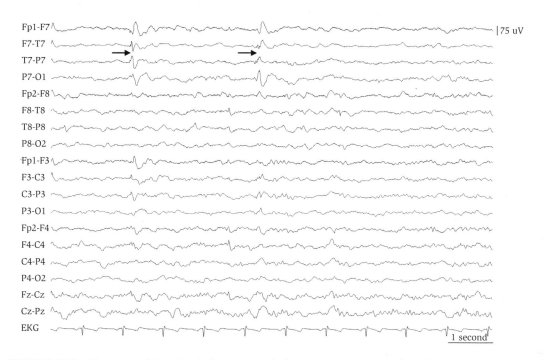

FIGURE 18.3 Ten-second interictal electroencephalogram tracing after sleep deprivation, showing left temporal sharp waves displayed on an 18-channel anterior-posterior (AP) bipolar montage. A negative phase reversal is best seen at the T7 (mid-temporal) electrode (arrows). EKG, electrocardiogram.

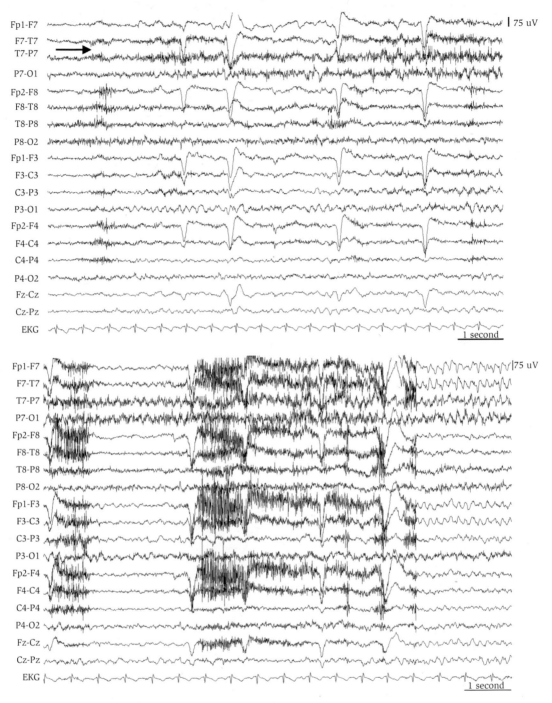

FIGURE 18.4   (Continued)

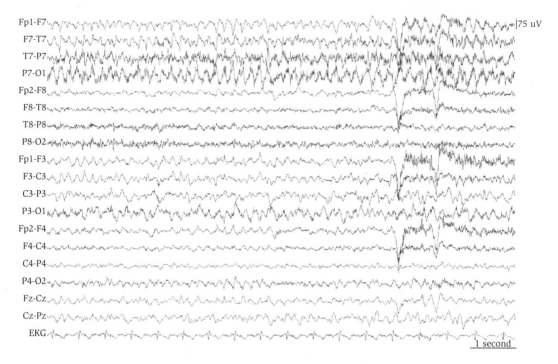

FIGURE 18.4 Three consecutive 10-second epochs showing a seizure arising from the left temporal region on an 18-channel anterior-posterior (AP) bipolar montage performed after sleep deprivation. Seizure onset is characterized by a change in background frequencies that is initially arrhythmic, later evolving to rhythmic 5-to-8 Hz activity in the left temporal region with propagation to the left parasagittal region. This was associated with an arrest of activity with intermittent eye blinking. The patient did not recall the event after the procedure. EKG, electrocardiogram.

revealed repetitive left temporal sharp waves. Somewhat surprising was the recording of a spontaneous focal seizure (Fig. 18.4) arising from the left temporal region.

Temporal lobe epilepsy is the most common focal epilepsy in adolescents and adults. A variety of clinical features may be used to distinguish TLE from other forms of focal epilepsy.[56] Seizures of temporal origin typically begin with an aura of a rising epigastric sensation, fear, déjà vu (an illusion of familiarity), or depersonalization (a feeling of lack of reality of one's sense of self). Common ictal manifestations include behavioral arrest with staring and oroaliminary (lip smacking, chewing, or licking) or limb automatisms. The etiologies of TLE include hippocampal sclerosis, malformations of cortical development, trauma, and vascular or neoplastic lesions. An estimated 9% of patients in one TLE series had seizures restricted to sleep.[57] Temporal nocturnal seizures arise most commonly from no-REM

sleep, especially N2 sleep.[58] Similarly, IEDs are more common in non-REM sleep than REM sleep, peaking in N2 (95%) and N3 (98%) followed by N1 (53%) and REM sleep (12.5%).[19,21,29]

Case 2

M.M. is an 8-year-old male with sleepwalking since 4 years of age who presented with abnormal motor activity in sleep for the past 2 months. The episodes were described as right facial twitching spreading to the right arm and leg and associated with drooling and grunting sounds. Birth, development, neurological examination, and brain MRI were normal. A PSG with 18-channel EEG was performed. The patient snored, though there was no evidence for periodic limb movements or sleep-disordered breathing. Epileptiform discharges were recorded, but no abnormal movements were seen (Fig. 18.5A-B).

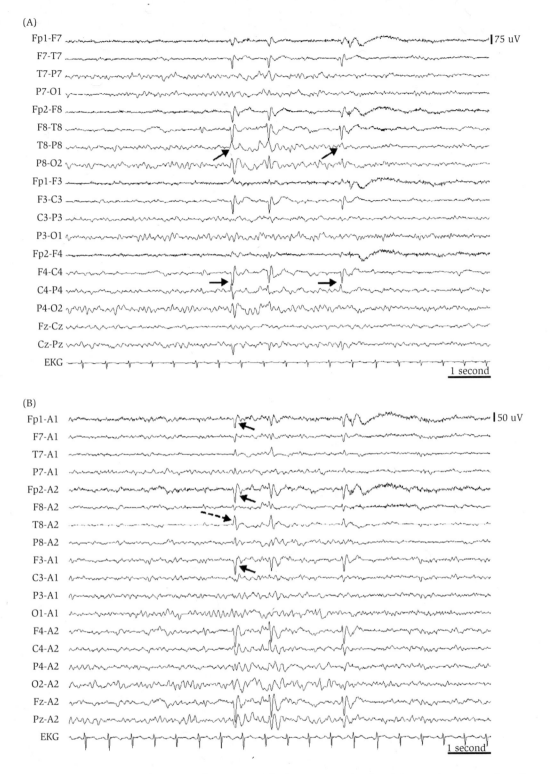

FIGURE 18.5 Ten-second interictal tracing with sharp waves in the right centrotemporal region displayed on (A) an 18-channel anterior-posterior (AP) bipolar and (B) A1/A2 referential montage. The morphology and distribution of the discharges are characteristic of benign focal epileptiform discharges. Note the negative phase reversal at C4 and T8 with conduction to the left hemisphere on the bipolar montage (A, arrows) and the dipole (relative negativity at T8 [dashed arrow] and C4 and positivity at F3 and the frontopolar electrodes [solid arrows]) on the referential tracing (B). EKG, electrocardiogram.

Discussion

The clinical history is suggestive of benign focal epilepsy of childhood (BFEC). This syndrome accounts for 15%–25% of childhood epilepsy and features seizures arising from rolandic area in close proximity to motor cortex.[59] Patients with BFEC have characteristic unilateral focal sensorimotor seizures typically involving the face and arm that frequently evolve into generalized tonic clonic seizures (GTCs). Seizures restricted to sleep are observed in 51%–80% of cases.[60,61] The EEG is characterized by benign focal epileptiform discharges (BFEDs), commonly localized to the centrotemporal region with a stereotyped morphology consisting of a small positivity followed by a prominent negativity and a subsequent negative slow wave of lower amplitude than the sharp wave. BFEDs can be unilateral or bilateral; the latter is more typical in sleep. Discharges are typically markedly activated in non-REM sleep. On a referential montage, the stereotyped dipole field has a negative polarity in the centrotemporal region and positive polarity anteriorly in the frontal region (Fig. 18.5). This is due to the orientation of the generator that is tangential to the cortical surface in the lower rolandic region. Patients with BFEC have good prognosis with spontaneous remission typically in the second decade of life.

Case 3

D.R. is a 33-year-old female with a history of night terrors who presented with new onset of nocturnal awakenings associated with bizarre movements of her limbs and trunk with variable degrees of impaired consciousness. During these episodes, the right arm was notably stiff and flexed. Episodes lasted less than 1 minute. She had no daytime complaints other than fatigue on days followed nights of activity. Routine awake and sleep-deprived EEGs were normal. An all-night EEG recorded several typical spells (Fig. 18.6).

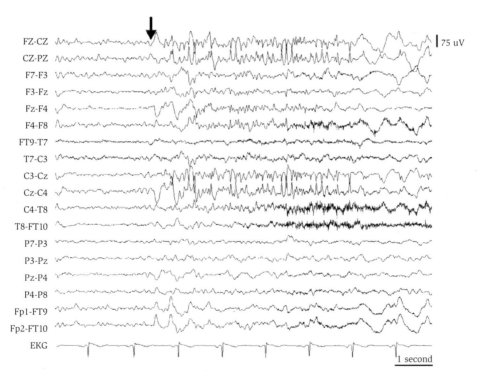

FIGURE 18.6   Ten-second ictal electroencephalogram (EEG) tracing on a transverse bipolar montage of one of several recorded seizures. Seizure onset (arrow) is characterized by repetitive fast spiking in the vertex (Fz, Cz) region, later evolved into delta activity in the frontocentral regions bilaterally. In this seizure, the patient had an arousal from sleep, elevated her head off the bed, and appeared confused with dystonic posturing of the right arm. The ictal EEG was compromised by excessive movement artifact in more typical seizures involving larger body movements and vocalization. EKG, electrocardiogram.

Discussion

The seizure semiology and prolonged sleep EEG findings are suggestive of epilepsy arising from or activation of the SSMA, located in the mesial aspect of the superior frontal gyrus (Brodmann's area 6). Seizures are brief (10–40 seconds), with abrupt tonic or dystonic posturing of the extremities or truck or violent, thrashing movements. In its classic form known as the "fencing posture," extremity posturing is asymmetric with shoulder abduction, flexion of one elbow, and extension of the other with the head turned as though looking toward the flexed arm.[62] The legs are also involved with abduction of the hips and flexion or extension of the knees. Sensory symptoms consisting of a feeling of pulling, heaviness, or a sensation that a limb is about to move can precede the tonic component.[62,63] Seizures arising from the SSMA have a tendency to occur predominantly or exclusively in sleep [63] as described in 65% of 330 recorded SSMA seizures in a large series.[64]

Due to its deep, interhemispheric location, the noninvasive EEG is often normal or devoid of convincing epileptiform features in cases of SSMA epilepsy. If present, IEDs and seizures appear localized to the vertex region and are best appreciated during non-REM sleep using a transverse montage incorporating midline electrode placements. Seizures are commonly obscured by artifact due to the prominent motor features of SSMA seizures.

Case 4

J.K. is a 29-year-old male was in his usual state of health until 3 months prior to presentation when he developed abnormal behaviors in sleep. The nocturnal episodes were described as brief, violent movements occurring in clusters during sleep nearly every night. His wife noticed that the patient's eyes were open and he appeared to be awake. Immediately after episodes, he was able to recall vaguely what had transpired. He was diagnosed with epilepsy and started on carbamazepine. The frequency of episodes decreased dramatically for 1 year. Seizures then recurred and failed to respond to trials of multiple AEDs. He underwent long-term VEEG as part of a presurgical evaluation during which five typical seizures were recorded. Seizures consisted of sudden tonic posturing of the upper extremities, vocalization, and facial distortion lasting 10 to 20 seconds with

preserved awareness. One seizure evolved to right version followed by a GTC. The interictal EEG was unremarkable. The ictal EEG was uninterpretable due to excessive movement artifact (Fig. 18.7A). A high-resolution MRI revealed a hyperintensity on fluid attenuated inversion recovery (FLAIR) imaging extending from the ependymal surface of the superior margin of the left frontal horn to the overlying cortex of the ventral aspect of the left superior frontal sulcus with thickened cortex suggestive of a malformation of cortical development (Fig. 18.7B). A positron emission tomography scan showed hypometabolism in the superior left frontal pole corresponding to MRI lesion. A functional MRI suggested left hemisphere language dominance. Invasive EEG was performed to localize the epileptogenic zone, delineate the posterior extent of resection, and map eloquent cortex (Fig. 18.7C). Interictal discharges and ictal onset in 27 recorded seizures were localized to the depth electrode in the MRI lesion (Fig. 18.7C-D). Electrical stimulation found no speech or motor function in the area of EEG abnormalities. A left superior frontal premotor resection was performed. The pathology revealed marked architectural disorganization and neuronal cytomegaly consistent with a malformation of cortical development. The patient has been seizure-free for 3 years.

Discussion

The clinical history, seizure semiology, and noninvasive EEG are suggestive of FLE. Sleep activates frontal seizures much more often than temporal seizures, and secondary generalization is less common in seizures of frontal origin.[58] Patients with seizures arising predominately or exclusively from sleep are classified as nocturnal frontal lobe epilepsy (NFLE). NFLE is a heterogeneous disorder.[65] Asymmetric tonic posturing, dystonic, dyskinetic, and hypermotor activity, as well as agitated wandering, are observed. Most attacks are brief and repetitive, with sudden onset and offset and accompanied by marked autonomic activation. Seizures can appear violent due to involvement of large, proximal body movements of high amplitude and velocity. Consciousness is often preserved. Due to the bizarre motor manifestations in sleep and normal noninvasive EEG, NFLE may be misdiagnosed as a parasomnia. A personal or family history of non-REM arousal disorder is common in patients with NFLE.[66]

Consequently, a shared pathophysiology involving the cholinergic pathway in the ascending arousal system has been proposed. The familial form, known as autosomal dominant nocturnal frontal lobe epilepsy (ADNFLE), constitutes as many as 25% of cases. Linkage studies localized genes for ADNFLE to chromosomes 20q13 and 15q24 with mutations in the transmembrane region of the neuronal nicotinic acetylcholine receptor (nAChR) alpha4-subunit (CHRNA4), beta2-subunit (CHRNB2), and alpha2-subunit (CHRNA2). The nAChRs are ion channels distributed widely on neuronal and glial membranes in cortical and subcortical regions of the brain that regulate the release of acetylcholine, gamma-hydroxybutyric acid, and glutamate

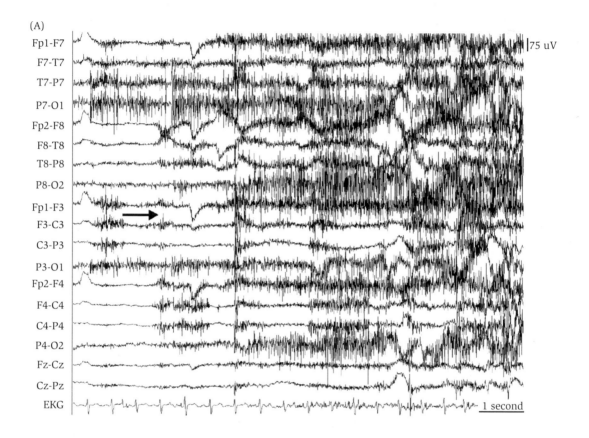

(A)

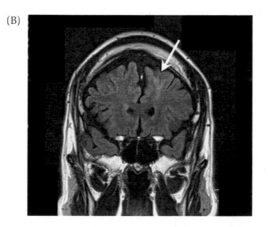

(B)

FIGURE 18.7   (Continued)

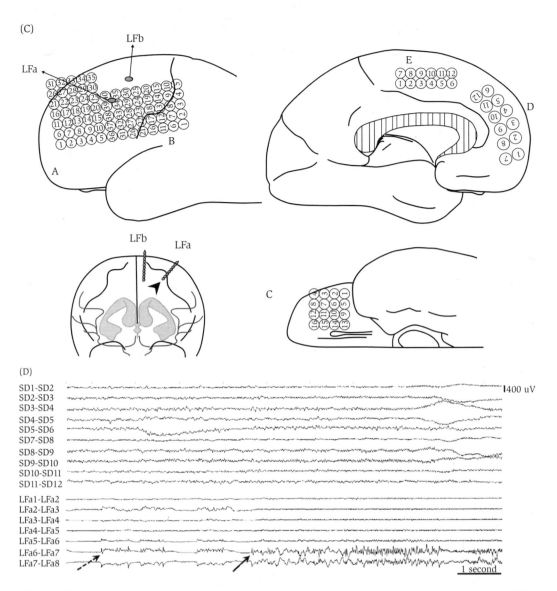

FIGURE 18.7   (*A*) Shown is a 10-second epoch of the noninvasive ictal electroencephalogram (EEG) displayed on an 18-channel anterior-posterior (AP) bipolar montage. EEG seizure onset (arrow) was obscured by artifact due to the hypermotor features of the seizure. (*B*) Coronal fluid attenuated inversion recovery (FLAIR) magnetic resonance imaging (MRI) revealed an area of hyperintensity extending from the ependymal surface of the superior margin of the left frontal horn to the overlying cortex of the ventral aspect of the left superior frontal sulcus with thickened cortex suggestive of a malformation of cortical development (arrow). (*C*) Schematic map of the invasive EEG implantation using subdural and depth electrodes. Frequent runs of interictal discharges were localized to a depth contact (LFa 7–8; arrowhead) in the lesion in the superior frontal gyrus. (*D*) Invasive ictal EEG tracing, including the depth electrode in the MRI lesion and the anterior interhemispheric subdural grid. EEG seizure onset was preceded by baseline interictal spiking in LFa 7–8 (dashed arrow). Seizure onset (solid arrow) was characterized by an abrupt cessation of interictal spiking and an evolution of fast frequencies involving electrode recording from the superior frontal gyrus around the MRI lesion, which later spread to the remaining frontal lobe. EKG, electrocardiogram.

and have a modulatory effect on arousals at the cortical and thalamic levels. Receptor mutations are thought to cause changes in neuronal excitability, preferentially affecting the mesial prefrontal area and regulating microarousals, thereby destabilizing sleep.[67]

Case 5

G.R. is a 38-year-old male who presented to the sleep clinic with his wife with abnormal behaviors in sleep and snoring for over 10 years. Episodes were sporadic, typically occurring once or twice per month, and increased in the setting of stress, sleep deprivation, and alcohol consumption. His wife described that he would wake up within 1 hour of going to sleep and wander around the bedroom without recollection. If not coaxed back to bed, he might walk into other rooms or around the outside of their house. He had sustained minor bruising on many occasions, but he had fallen down

a flight of stairs several weeks prior to presentation, sustaining an ankle fracture. He had no recollection of these events and denied negative dream content.

A VPSG with 18 channel EEG was performed. There was no evidence of sleep apnea or periodic limb movements, although snoring was recorded. Limited REM and N3 sleep was recorded, though muscle tone was not augmented in REM and no abnormal behaviors or EEG abnormalities were recorded. Due to persistent disruptive nocturnal behaviors despite alcohol cessation and attempts to avoid sleep deprivation and manage stress, long-term VEEG was performed. On the fourth night of the evaluation after two nights of partial sleep deprivation, a typical, though milder, episode was recorded, characterized by arousal with nonspecific limb movements and repeated attempts to get out of bed and disconnect the EEG (Fig. 18.8). The evaluation failed to reveal any evidence of epilepsy.

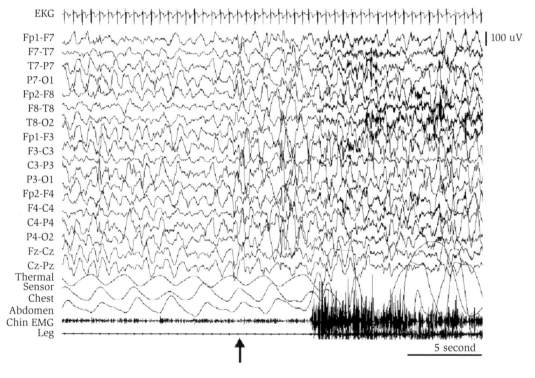

FIGURE 18.8   Shown is an arousal from N3 sleep displayed on a video polysomnogram montage and 30-second epoch length. The electroencephalographic arousal (arrow) heralds the onset of the clinical arousal. Generalized hypersynchronous delta activity is observed, supporting the diagnosis of an arousal disorder having features of both a confusional arousal and somnambulism. EKG, electrocardiogram; EMG, electromyogram.

Discussion

This case illustrates the spectrum of complex behaviors seen in disorders of arousal. Most episodes of sleepwalking and confusional arousals occur in the first third of the sleep period when N3 sleep predominates. EEG changes associated with arousal disorders usually consist of hypersynchronous delta waves with superimposed faster frequencies not evolving appreciably and generalized in distribution.[68] The differentiation of seizures and parasomnias can be challenging, due to the overlapping features of NFLE and disorders of arousal, shared precipitating factors, and limitations of noninvasive EEG to detect seizures arising from deep or midline structures. In this case, the single-night VPSG study failed to clarify the diagnosis, and attempts to treat the presumed diagnosis of a disorder of arousal were unsuccessful. Given this and the injurious nature of episodes, long-term VEEG was performe,d which provided confirmatory support for the diagnosis.

REFERENCES

1. Wilson JV, Reynolds EH. Translation and analysis of a cuneiform text forming part of a Babylonian treatise on epilepsy. *Med Hist* 1990;34:185–98.
2. Hogan RE, Kaiboriboon K. The dreamy state: John Hughlings-Jackson's ideas of epilepsy and consciousness. *Am J Psychiatry* 2003;160:1740–7.
3. Fisher RS, van Emde BW, Blume W, et al. Epileptic seizures and epilepsy: definitions proposed by the International League Against Epilepsy (ILAE) and the International Bureau for Epilepsy (IBE). *Epilepsia* 2005;46:470–2.
4. Gowers WR. General characteristics of epileptic fit. In: Gowers WR, ed. *Epilepsy and other chronic convulsive disease: their causes, symptoms, and treatment*. New York: Williams Wood; 1885:29.
5. Tao JX, Ray A, Hawes-Ebersole S, et al. Intracranial EEG substrates of scalp EEG interictal spikes. *Epilepsia* 2005;46:669–76.
6. Niedermeyer E. The EEG signal: polarity and field determination. In: Niedermeyer E, Lopes da Silva F, eds. *Electroencephalography: basic principles, clinical applications, and related fields*. Baltimore, MD: Urban & Schwarzenberg; 1987:79–83.
7. American Electroencephalographic Society. Guideline thirteen: guidelines for standard electrode position nomenclature. *J Clin Neurophysiol* 1994;11:111–3.
8. Morris HH, III, Lüders H, Lesser RP, et al. The value of closely spaced scalp electrodes in the localization of epileptiform foci: a study of 26 patients with complex partial seizures. *Electroencephalogr Clin Neurophysiol* 1986;63:107–11.
9. Jasper HH. Second international congress symposia. *Electroencephalogr Clin Neurophysiol* 1940;1:789–90.
10. Blume WT. The necessity for sphenoidal electrodes in the presurgical evaluation of temporal lobe epilepsy. *J Clin Neurophysiol* 2003;20: 305–10.
11. Sperling MR, Guina L. The necessity for sphenoidal electrodes in the presurgical evaluation of temporal lobe epilepsy. *J Clin Neurophysiol* 2003;20:299–304.
12. Fernández Torre JL, Alarcón G, Binnie CD, et al. Comparision of sphenoidal, foramen ovale and anterior temporal placements for detecting interictal epileptiform discharges in presurgical assessment for temporal lobe epilepsy. *Clin Neurophysiol* 1999;110:895–904.
13. Tallgran P, Vanhatalo S, Kaila K, et al. Evaluation of commercially available electrodes and gels for recording of slow EEG potentials. *Clin Neurophysiol* 2005;116:799–806.
14. American Clinical Neurophysiology Society. Guideline twelve: guidelines for long-term monitoring for epilepsy. *Am J Electroneurodiagnostic Technol* 2008;48:265–86.
15. Aldrich MS, Jahnke B. Diagnostic value of video-EEG polysomnography. *Neurology* 1991;41:1060–6.
16. Kushida CA, Littner MR, Morgenthaler T, et al. Practice parameters for the indications for polysomnography and related procedures: an update for 2005. *Sleep* 2005;28:406–22.
17. Foldvary-Schaefer N, De Ocampo J, Mascha E, et al. Accuracy of seizure detection using abbreviated EEG during polysomnogram. *J Clin Neurophysiol* 2006;23:68–71.
18. Ajmone Marsan C, Ziven LS. Factors related to the occurrence of typical paroxysmal abnormalities in the EEG records of epileptic patients. *Epilepsia* 1970;11: 361–81.
19. Rossi GF, Colicchio G, Pola P. Interictal epileptic activity during sleep: a stereo-EEG study in patients with partial epilepsy. *Electroencephalogr Clin Neurophysiol* 1984;58:97–106.

20. Gibbs EL, Gibbs FA. Diagnostic and localizing value of electroencephalographic studies in sleep. *Res Pbl Assoc Res Nerv Ment Dis* 1947;26:366–76.

21. Sammaritano M, Gigli G, Gotman J. Interictal spiking during wakefulness and sleep and the localization of foci in temporal lobe epilepsy *Neurology* 1991;4:290–7.

22. Herman ST, Walczak TS, Bazil CW. Distribution of partial seizures during the sleep-wake cycle: difference by seizure onset site. *Neurology* 2001;56:1453–9.

23. Steriade M, Conteras D, Amzica F. Synchronized sleep oscillations and their paroxysmal developments. *Grends Neurosci* 1994;17:199–208.

24. Shouse MN, Farber RR, Staba RJ. Physiological basis: how NREM sleep components can promote and RE sleep components can suppress seizure discharge propagation. *Clin Neurophysiol* 2000;111:S9–18.

24a. Janz D. The grand-mal epilepsies and the sleeping-waking cycle. *Epilepsia* 1962;3:69–109.

25. Gunderson C, Dunne PB, Feyer TL. Sleep deprivation seizures. *Neurology* 1973;23:678–86.

26. Rajna P, Veres J. Correlations between night sleep duration and seizure frequency in temporal lobe epilepsy. *Epilepsia* 1993;34:574–9.

27. Rodin EA, Luby ED, Gottlieb JS. The electroencephalograms during prolonged experimental sleep deprivation. *Electroencephalogr Clin Neurophysiol* 1962;14:544–51.

28. Pratt KL, Mattson RH, Weikers NJ, et al. EEG activation of epileptics following sleep deprivation: a prospective study of 114 cases. *Electroencephalogr Clin Neurophysiol* 1968;24:11–15.

29. Rowan AJ, Veldhuisen JF, Nagelkerke NJD. Comparative evaluation of sleep deprivation and sedated sleep EEGs as a diagnostic aid in epilepsy. *Electroencephalogr Clin Neurophysiol* 1982;54:357–64.

30. Roger J, Rey M, Bureau M, et al. Apport de l'EEG du sommeil en epileptogie: Bilan d'une etude portent sur une annee [Contribution of sleep EEG to epileptology: evaluation of a year-long study]. *Rev Electroencephalogr Neurophysiol Clin* 1986;16:249–55.

31. Ropakiotis SC, Gatzonis SD, Triantafyllou N, et al. The usefulness of sleep and sleep deprivation as activating methods in electroencephalographic recording: contribution to a long-standing discussion. *Seizure* 2000;9:580–4.

32. Lüders HO, Noachtar S. *Atlas and Classification of Electroencephalography*. Philadelphia, PA: WB Saunders; 2001:26–61.

33. Westmoreland BF. Epileptiform electroencephalographic patterns. *Mayo Clin Proc* 1996;71:501–11.

34. Stern JM, Engel J. *An Atlas of EEG patterns*. Pennsylvania, PA: Lippincott Williams & Wilkins; 2005:161–3.

35. Berg AT, Berkovic SF, Brodie MJ, et al. Revised terminology and concepts for organization of seizures and epilepsies: report of the ILAE commission on classification and terminology, 2005–2009. *Epilepsia* 2010;51: 676–85.

36. Jaykar P, Duchowny M, Resnick TJ. Localization of seizure foci: pitfalls and caveats. *J Clin Neurophysiol* 1991;8:414–31.

37. Holmes MD, Dodrill CB, Wilensky AJ, et al. Unilateral focal preponderance of interictal epileptiform discharges as a predictor of seizure origin. *Arch Neurol* 1996;53:228–32.

38. Foldvary N, Klem G, Hammel J, et al. The localizing value of ictal EEG in focal epilepsy. *Neurology* 2001;57:2022–8.

39. Stuve O, Dodrill CB, Holmes MD, et al. The absence of interictal spikes with documented seizures suggests extratemporal epilepsy. *Epilepsia* 2001;42:778–81.

40. Sharbrough FW. Scalp-recorded ictal patterns in focal epilepsy. *J Clin Neurophysiol* 1993;10:262–7.

41. Creutzfeldt OD, Watanabe S, Lux HD. Relations between EEG phenomena and potentials of single cortical cells. II. Spontaneous and convulsoid activity. *Electroencephalogr Clin Neurophysiol* 1966;20:19–37.

42. Elul R. The genesis of the EEG. *Int Rev Neurobiol* 1971;15:227–72.

43. Copper R, Winter AL, Crow HJ, et al. Comparison of subcortical, cortical and scalp activity using chronically indwelling electrodes in man. *Electroencephalogr Clin Neurophysiol* 1965;18:217–28.

44. Lutzenberger W, Elbert T, Rockstroh B, A brief tutorial on the implication of volume conduction for the interpretation of the EEG. *J Psychophysiol* 1987;1:81–9.

45. Carpenter MB. *Core Text of Neuroanatomy*. Baltimore, MD: Lippincott, Williams and Wilkins; 1991.

46. Neshige R, Luders H, Shibasaki H. Recording of movement-related potentials from scalp and cortex in man. *Brain* 1988;111: 719–36.

47. Nunez PL. *Electrical Fields of the Brain: The Neurophysics of EEG*. New York: Oxford University Press; 1981.

48. Spencer SS, Guimaraes P, Shewmon A. Intracranial electrodes. In: Engel J, Jr., Pedley TA, eds. *Epilepsy: A Comprehensive Textbook*. New York: Lippincott–Raven; 1998:1719–48.

49. Lüders HO, Najm I, Nair D, et al. The epileptogenic zone: general principles. *Epileptic Disord* 2008;10:191.

50. Kwan P, Arzimanoglou A, Berg AT, et al. Definition of drug resistant epilepsy: consensus proposal by the ad hoc task force of the ILAE commission on therapeutic strategies. *Epilepsia* 2010;51:1069–77.

51. Gilliam FG, Kuzniecky R, Meador K. Patient-oriented outcome assessment after temporal lobectomy for refractory epilepsy. *Neurology* 1999;53:687–94.

52. Hermann BP, Seidenberg M, Dow C, et al. Cogntive prognosis in chronic temporal lobe epilepsy. *Ann Neurol* 2000;60:80–7.

53. Schuele SU, Lüders HO. Intractable epilepsy: management and therapeutic alternatives. *Lancet Neurol* 2008;7:514–24.

54. Ficker DM, So EL, Shen WK, et al. Population-based study of the incidence of sudden unexplained death in epilepsy. *Neurology* 1998;51:1270–4.

55. Hamer HM, Morris HH, Mascha EJ, et al. Complications of invasive video-EEG monitoring with subdural grid electrodes. *Neurology* 2002;58:97–103.

56. Unnwongse K, Wehner T, Foldvary-Schaefer N. Selecting patients for epilepsy surgery. *Curr Neurol Neurosci Rep* 2010;10:299–307.

57. Billiard M. Epilepsies and the sleep-wake cycle. In: Sterman MB, Shouse MN, Passouant P, eds. *Sleep and Epilepsy*. New York: Academic Press; 1982:269–86.

58. Crespel A, Baldy-Moulinier M, Coubes P. The relationship between sleep and epilepsy in frontal and temporal lobe epilepsies: practical and physiologic considerations. *Epilepsia* 1998;39:150–7.

59. Lerman P, Kivity S. Benign focal epilepsy in childhood. *Arch Neurol* 1974;15:229–34.

60. Beaussart M. Benign epilepsy of children with rolandic (centro-temporal) paroxysmal foci-a clinical entity. Study of 221 cases. *Epilepsia* 1972;13:527.

61. Gregory DL, Wong PK. Topographical analysis of the centrotemporal discharges in benign rolandic epilepsy in childhood. *Epilepsia* 1984;25:705–11.

62. Penfield W, Jasper H. *Epilepsy and the Functional Anatomy of the Human Brain*. Boston, MA: Little Brown; 1954.

63. Morris H III, Dinner D, Luders HO, et al. Supplementary motor seizures: clinical and electroencephalographic findings. *Neurology* 1988;38:1075–82.

64. Anand I, Dinner DS. Relation of supplementary motor area epilepsy and sleep. *Epilepsia* 1997;8:48.

65. Oldani A, Zucconi M, Asselta R, et al. Autosomal dominant nocturnal frontal lobe epilepsy: a video-polysomnographic and genetic appraisal of 40 patients and delineation of the epileptic syndrome. *Brain* 1998;121:205–23.

66. Bisulli F, Vignatelli L, Naldi I, et al. Increased frequency of arousal parasomnias in families with nocturnal frontal lobe epilepsy: a common mechanism? *Epilepsia* 2010;51:1852–60.

67. Marini C, Guerrini R. The role of the nicotinic acetylcholine receptors in sleep-related epilepsy. Biochem Pharmacol 2007;74:1308–14.

68. Schenck CH, Pareja JA, Patterson AL, et al. Analysis of polysomnographic events surrounding 252 slow-wave sleep arousals in thirty-eight adults with injurious sleepwalking and sleep terrors. *JCNP* 1998;15:159–66.

19

Sleep and Movement Disorders
Neuroimaging Aspects

THIEN THANH DANG-VU, MARTIN DESSEILLES, PIETRO-LUCA
RATTI, PHILIPPE PEIGNEUX, AND PIERRE MAQUET

BRAIN IMAGING techniques, such as positron emission tomography (PET) or functional magnetic resonance imaging (fMRI), have characterized the specific distribution of cerebral activity for each stage of sleep in healthy subjects (for review, see Maquet,[1] Dang-Vu et al.[2]). Functional neuroimaging studies have demonstrated regional increases and decreases of brain activity in areas responsible for the generation of rapid eye movement (REM) sleep and some important characteristics of dreams.[3] During non-REM sleep, as compared to wakefulness, they have evidenced mostly decreases of brain responses, in various associative cortical areas and subcortical structures.[1] Beyond sleep stages, recent fMRI studies have also described the neural responses associated with brain oscillations of sleep.[4] In particular, they have shown increased brain responses associated with spindles and slow waves of non-REM sleep, demonstrating that non-REM sleep is not merely a passive state of brain deactivation.[5,6] Altogether these data have refined our understanding of the mechanisms and functions of normal human sleep.

An increasing number of neuroimaging studies dedicated to the disorders of sleep have been published in the last decade (for review, see Dang-Vu et al.,[2] Desseilles et al.[7]), bringing an important contribution to the pathophysiology of sleep disorders. For instance, in the case of narcolepsy-cataplexy, brain imaging studies have shown structural and functional abnormalities in the hypothalamus and multiple associative cortical areas, in agreement with a loss of hypocretinergic neurons in this disease.[8]

In this chapter, we will focus on neuroimaging studies of sleep-related movement disorders. We will consider specific sleep disorders such as restless legs syndrome (RLS), often associated with periodic limb movements during sleep (PLMS), and parasomnias taking place either during non-REM sleep (such as sleepwalking) or REM sleep (REM sleep behavior disorder [RBD]). Several neurological disorders associated with specific sleep disturbances, such fatal familial insomnia (FFI), and specific epileptic syndromes occurring during sleep, such as nocturnal frontal lobe epilepsy (NFLE), benign epilepsy with centro-temporal lobe spikes (BECTS), Landau-Kleffner syndrome (LKS), and the syndrome of continuous spike-and-wave discharges during slow-wave sleep (CSWS), will also be discussed.

We will review the brain imaging studies published to date in each of these disorders. Various modalities have been used and will be considered successively. These include neuroanatomical studies using magnetic resonance imaging (MRI) to analyze changes in gray matter with voxel-based morphometry (VBM), white matter changes with diffusion tensor imaging (DTI), or neuronal integrity with proton magnetic resonance spectroscopy (^{1}H-MRS). Functional studies were carried out with single photon emission computed tomography (SPECT), PET, and fMRI to assess brain responses throughout the sleep-wake cycle (mostly during wakefulness) or in association with symptomatic events. Finally, SPECT and PET were also coupled with specific ligands to measure local neurotransmitter function, such as for dopamine (DA).

It should be noted that acquiring brain imaging data in patients with movement disorders constitutes in many instances a technical challenge. The presence of movements during acquisition produces artifacts both on structural and functional sequences. Techniques such as SPECT, however, allow scan acquisition to be performed well after the radio-labeled compound has been injected during the episode of interest, therefore minimizing the interference of movements on the imaging procedure.

RESTLESS LEGS SYNDROME AND PERIODIC LIMB MOVEMENTS

Restless Legs Syndrome

Restless legs syndrome (RLS) is a sensorimotor disorder characterized by a nearly irresistible urge to move the lower limbs (less frequently the upper limbs), usually associated with a discomfort sensation deep inside the limbs, which is exacerbated by rest or inactivity, especially when lying or sitting at evening or night.[9,10] Around 94% of patients report sleep-onset insomnia or nocturnal awakenings due to RLS-related symptoms, which is corroborated by patterns of disrupted sleep at polysomnography.[11] RLS can present as an isolated phenomenon (i.e., *idiopathic* forms) or

being *secondary* to other medical conditions.[9,10] Among these latter forms, the one associated with iron deficiency anemia is by far the most common. Multiple interacting mechanisms seem to underlie this disease, including various cortical and subcortical brain structures, the spinal cord, the peripheral nervous system, and multiple biochemical pathways and neurotransmitter systems. Nevertheless, the exact pathophysiological "puzzle" of RLS has not been solved so far.[12] Important clues on RLS pathophysiology have arisen from clinical experience and point to a role for iron metabolism and dopaminergic system.[13,14] Neuroimaging studies of RLS have investigated the changes in brain anatomy and function associated with this condition.

STRUCTURAL NEUROIMAGING

Structural brain imaging studies of RLS are summarized in Table 19.1.

VBM and DTI Studies. Structural abnormalities in RLS were studied with MRI, using a VBM approach. A first study comparing 51 RLS patients to 51 controls evidenced a gray matter increase in the dorsal thalamus bilaterally, in a region compatible with the pulvinar nuclei.[15] Another VBM study, conducted on a larger sample of 63 patients (and 40 controls), found decreases of gray matter in primary sensorimotor cortices.[16] Interestingly, gray matter values in these cortical areas were also negatively correlated with RLS severity and disease duration.[16] The same group also investigated differences in white matter in 45 RLS patients (compared to 30 controls), using MRI with DTI sequences.[17] In line with their previous study, they found white matter alterations in the vicinity of sensorimotor cortices and in thalamic structures. These findings of sensorimotor thalamocortical pathways alterations in RLS seem to be in line with the patients' description of their symptoms. Whether these changes reflect neural mechanisms underlying the disease or secondary changes induced by chronic afferent input still needs to be elucidated. Additionally, patients in these three studies were medicated, mostly with dopaminergic agents, which might have affected the results. In favor of this last interpretation, three other VBM studies conducted on unmedicated patients showed no significant change between RLS and controls,[18-20] with the exception of a slight gray matter increase in the hippocampus and orbitofrontal gyrus.[18] The

Table 19.1 Structural Neuroimaging of Restless Legs Syndrome

STUDY	IMAGING	NO. PAT. // CTRL.	MEDICATION*	RESULTS
Etgen et al.[15]	MRI / VBM	51 // 51	Yes	GM increase in dorsal thalamus
Unrath et al. [16]	MRI / VBM	63 // 40	Yes	GM decreases in primary sensorimotor cortices
Unrath et al. [17]	MRI / DTI	45 // 30	Yes	WM changes near sensorimotor and thalamic areas
Hornyak et al. [18]	MRI / VBM	14 // 14	No	Slight GM increase in hippocampus and orbitofrontal gyrus
Celle et al. [19]	MRI / VBM	17 // 54	No	No difference
Comley et al.[20]	MRI / VBM	16 // 16	No	No difference
Allen et al. [24]	MRI / R2	5 // 5	Yes	Decrease of iron concentration in SN
Earley et al. [25]	MRI / R2	41 // 39	No	Decrease of iron concentration in SN, for early-onset RLS
Godau et al. [26]	MRI / R2 & TCS	6 // 19	No	Decrease of iron concentration in SN, thalamus, and caudate
Schmidauer et al. [29]	TCS	20 // 20	Yes	Decrease of iron concentration in SN
Godau et al. [28]	TCS	49 // 49	Yes	Decrease of iron concentration in SN

*Medication at the time of imaging (mostly dopaminergic agents).

DTI, diffusion tensor imaging; GM, gray matter; MRI, magnetic resonance imaging; RLS, restless legs syndrome; SN, substantia nigra; TCS, transcranial ultrasound; VBM, voxel-based morphometry; WM, white matter.

number of patients was, however, much lower in these these studies (ranging from 15 to 17), which could have contributed to a lack of significant difference between RLS and controls.

Iron Studies. Iron metabolism has been suggested to play a crucial role in RLS pathophysiology. Indeed, RLS association with iron deficiency is well known. Moreover, iron is closely associated to the DA system since it is an important cofactor for tyrosine hydroxylase, the rate-limiting enzyme in DA synthesis.[21] Furthermore, a decrease of ferritin level in cerebrospinal fluid has been found in RLS,[22] while neuropathologic studies have shown a reduction of H-ferritin (ferritin heavy chain) and iron staining in the substantia nigra (SN) of these patients.[23] MRI studies have brought additional evidence for a central iron deficiency in RLS. In a study of five idiopathic RLS patients compared to five controls, Allen and colleagues have shown a decrease of iron concentration in SN, as reflected by R2' measurements on MRI sequences.[24] Iron decrease correlated with RLS severity from clinical scales. Another study from the same group confirmed this finding on a higher sample of patients ($n = 41$) and additionally showed that the decreased iron concentration in SN was restricted to early-onset RLS patients (<45 years; $n = 22$).[25] An MRI study from a different group using similar measurements in a small sample of six RLS patients showed decreased iron concentrations in other brain areas such as thalamus and caudate, suggesting that central iron deficiency might be multiregional rather than limited to SN only.[26] Iron brain concentration can also be assessed by transcranial ultrasound (TCS), since echogenicity of SN is associated with local iron content.[27] Three studies using this technique have consistently shown a hypoechogenicity of SN in RLS patients, further supporting the evidence for a reduction of iron concentration in this area.[26,28,29]

FUNCTIONAL NEUROIMAGING

fMRI Studies. Few studies have attempted to describe the neural mechanisms underlying RLS using functional brain imaging with fMRI. In an early fMRI study, seven idiopathic RLS patients were scanned during periods of sensory leg discomfort. During these symptomatic periods, there was a bilateral activation of the cerebellum and a contralateral activation of the thalamus.[30] Recently a preliminary study used fMRI with simultaneous leg electromyography (EMG) to assess the brain responses associated with tonic EMG at rest in seven RLS patients.[31] Indeed, tonic EMG was found inversely correlated with subjective sensory leg discomfort, thereby providing an objective reflection of RLS symptoms. This study showed that tonic EMG was positively correlated with

fMRI response in sensorimotor cortical areas, cingulate gyrus, precuneus and occipital cortex, and negatively correlated in the cerebellum.[31] Altogether these preliminary results suggest an involvement of thalamocortical sensorimotor pathways, in agreement with several VBM studies cited earlier, as well as additional structures (including cerebellum) in the pathophysiology of RLS.

SPECT and PET Ligand Studies. Most functional neuroimaging studies of RLS have used SPECT or PET in association with various radio-labeled compounds to assess neurotransmission abnormalities (Table 19.2). Two systems were of particular interest: DA and opiate systems. Indeed, dopaminergic agents and opioids constitute the main therapeutic options in RLS patients.[32] SPECT and PET studies have explored both presynaptic DA transporter (DAT) and postsynaptic D2-receptor binding, mainly in the striatum. Striatal DAT reflects the density of DA neurons in SN. SPECT studies using [123]I-2betacarbomethoxy-3beta-(4-iodophenyl)tropane(^{123}I-β-CIT)[33,34] or ^{123}I-N-(3-iodopropen-2-yl)-2β-carbomethoxy-3β-(4-chlorophenyl)tropane (^{123}I-IPT) [35,36] failed to demonstrate any difference in DAT between RLS and controls. In contrast with SPECT data, PET studies using ^{18}F-dopa [37,38] or ^{11}C-methylphenidate [39] found decreased presynaptic DA function in the striatum of RLS compared to controls. This discrepancy might be due to distinct pharmacokinetic properties of the different SPECT and PET compounds. In the recent PET study with ^{11}C-methylphenidate from Earley and coworkers, RLS patients were scanned either in the morning ($n = 20$) or in the evening ($n = 16$), which allowed the researchers to assess the diurnal differences in DAT.[39] No significant difference was observed between patients scanned in the morning and those scanned in the evening, which suggests that DAT is not modulated by time of day. Furthermore, there was no significant correlation between DAT binding and RLS symptom severity. Results for postsynaptic D2-receptor binding were also quite divergent. ^{123}I-iodobenzamide (^{123}I-IBZM) SPECT found no change[35,40,41] or a mild decrease[33] of striatal D2-receptor binding in RLS patients compared to controls. PET using ^{11}C-raclopride showed either a decreased[37] or an increased [42] D2-receptor binding in the striatum. Differences between these two studies might be related to the inclusion of RLS patients

Table 19.2 SPECT- and PET-Ligand Studies in Restless Legs Syndrome

STUDY	IMAGING	TARGET	NO. PAT. // CTRL.	MEDICATION*	RESULTS
Michaud et al.[33]	SPECT 123I-β-CIT & 123I-IBZM	DAT & D2	10 // 10	No	No change in DAT, decrease in D2
Mrowka et al. [34]	SPECT 123I-β-CIT	DAT	6 // 7	Yes	No change
Eisensehr et al.[35]	SPECT 123I-IPT & 123I-IBZM	DAT & D2	14 // 10	No	No change
Linke et al. [36]	SPECT 123I-IPT	DAT	14 // 23	No	No change
Turjanski et al. [37]	PET 18F-dopa and 11C-raclopride	DAT & D2	13 // 14	Yes	Decrease in DAT and D2
Ruottinen et al. [38]	PET 18F-dopa	DAT	9 // 27	No	Decrease in DAT
Earley et al. [39]	PET 11C-methylphenidate	DAT	36 // 34	No	Decrease in DAT
Tribl et al. [40]	SPECT 123I-IBZM	D2	14 // 9	No	No change
Tribl et al. [41]	SPECT 123I-IBZM	D2	14 // 10	No	No change
Cervenka et al. [42]	PET 11C-raclopride & 11C-FLB457	D2	16 // 16	No	Increase in D2
von Spiczak et al. [44]	PET 11C-diprenorphine	Opioid receptor	15 // 12	No	No change

*Medication at the time of imaging (mostly dopaminergic agents).

D2, dopaminergic D2-receptor binding; DAT, dopamine transporter binding; PET, positron emission tomography; SPECT, single photon emission computed tomography.

who had been exposed to DA drugs in the first study, while patients in the second study were naïve to DA drugs. Indeed, chronic D2 receptor stimulation by drug treatment has been shown to induce receptor downregulation, thereby resulting in lower radioligand binding.[43] In the study of Cervenka and colleagues, RLS patients ($n = 16$) were also scanned with PET using 11C-FLB457, which allowed the researchers to measure D2-receptor binding in extrastriatal structures.[42] Increased binding potential in RLS patients was found not only in the striatum but also in the thalamus, insula, and anterior cingulate cortex. Since increased receptor levels can be caused by receptor upregulation

in response to depletion of endogenous DA, this study is consistent with a hypoactive DA neurotransmission in RLS. The areas showing changes in D2 receptor binding are part of the medial nociceptive system, which regulates the affective component of pain. Therefore, these results are in agreement with the view of RLS as a disorder of somatosensory processing. Finally, since scans were performed both in the morning and evening, the authors were able to evaluate the diurnal changes in D2 receptor binding. Interestingly, they found no significant change between evening and morning scans.[42] In addition, there was no significant correlation between D2 receptor binding and RLS symptom ratings. Therefore, both presynaptic [39] and postsynaptic [42] studies suggest that diurnal variations in RLS symptoms (being prominent in the evening and night) as well as symptom severity cannot be explained by parallel changes in DA neurotransmission. As regards the opiate system, only one study has compared RLS and controls using PET with ^{11}C-diprenorphine (a nonselective opioid receptor radioligand).[44] Although some correlations were found between ligand binding and RLS severity or pain scores in multiple brain areas, no significant difference in opioid receptor binding was found between patients and controls. This result is in agreement with the available data suggesting that the efficacy of opioids in the treatment of RLS may not be related to specific deficiencies of the endogenous opioid system but rather mediated by DA.[45]

Periodic Limb Movements

Periodic limb movements (PLMs) are stereotyped repetitive movements occurring at rest, which typically involve extension of the big toe, often in combination with partial flexion of the ankle, knee, and sometimes hip. They can occur during sleep (PLMS) or during wakefulness (PLMW) and both PLMS and PLMW can coexist in the same subject.[10] RLS frequently associates with the presence of PLMS or PLMW, but PLMS and PLMW are themselves nonspecific, occurring in other sleep disorders (narcolepsy, sleep apnea, etc.) and in healthy individuals.[46] Because of the frequent association of RLS and PLMS/PLMW, most neuroimaging studies have considered these conditions together. Only a few have attempted to consider PLMs in a more specific way.

In their fMRI study cited earlier, Bucher and colleagues not only scanned RLS patients during periods of sensory leg discomfort but also scanned them in a combined leg discomfort and PLMW condition.[30] While leg discomfort alone induced brain responses in the thalamus and cerebellum, combined sensory symptoms and PLMW were associated with an additional activation in the red nuclei and brainstem (12 patients). When these patients were instructed to voluntarily imitate PLMW, there was no activation of the brainstem but instead an activation of the motor cortex and globus pallidus. These results suggested a subcortical origin for PLM, involving red nucleus and other brainstem structures.

Dopaminergic neurotransmission has also been investigated in association with PLM. One study has assessed striatal presynaptic DA transmission in 11 patients with Parkinson's disease (PD) using SPECT with ^{123}I-β-CIT.[47] As expected, they found a robust reduction in striatal binding values in PD compared to healthy controls. Importantly, these patients were also recorded with polysomnography, which allowed measuring the number of PLMs during their sleep. A negative correlation was found between the number of PLMs and striatal binding values, suggesting that a presynaptic DA deficiency might be involved in the generation of PLMs in PD. At the postsynaptic level, Staedt and colleagues conducted a few studies assessing D2-receptor binding in the striatum of patients with PLMS, using SPECT using ^{123}I-IBZM.[48-50] They found a lower D2-receptor occupancy in PLMS patients.[48,49] This pattern can be corrected by DA replacement therapy, which also leads to an improvement in sleep quality.[50]

Summary

Neuroimaging findings in RLS and PLMs can be summarized as follows:

1. RLS is associated with alterations in *thalamus*, *sensorimotor* cortical areas, and *cerebellum*, as evidenced by functional and some structural brain imaging studies.
2. Functional studies suggest a *subcortical* origin for PLMs, encompassing structures located in the brainstem.
3. MRI and ultrasound studies are consistent with a central *iron* deficiency in RLS patients, located in SN and possibly other subcortical structures.
4. A hypoactivity of DA neurotransmission can be found in the striatum at both pre- and postsynaptic levels in patients with RLS and PLMs.

If RLS and PLMs still appear as complex conditions involving various brain areas and mechanisms, neuroimaging studies seem to demonstrate a deficiency in the DA system, in association with a depletion of iron concentration in SN, which ultimately affects brain structures responsible for sensorimotor control. Future studies are needed to confirm these findings and extend them to unexplored aspects of RLS and PLM pathophysiology, such as brain activity patterns during sleep itself (e.g., for PLMS).

PARASOMNIAS

Parasomnias are defined as undesirable physical events and experiences occurring during entry into sleep, within sleep, or during arousals from sleep. They are classified according to the sleep stage from which they arise and therefore divided into two main categories: REM and non-REM sleep-related parasomnias.[10]

Non-REM Parasomnias

Non-REM parasomnias are also referred to as *arousal parasomnias*, to indicate that they come out at state transitions from non-REM sleep—and especially from slow-wave sleep (SWS)—to wakefulness. They include different subtypes: sleepwalking, confusional arousals, and sleep terrors. Common features are automatic behaviors and the lack of full awareness or memory of the behavioral events themselves.[10] Their pathogenesis is hypothesized to rely on a state dissociation, in which non-REM sleep and wakefulness overlap or occur simultaneously[51]: cortical locomotor centers likely exhibit an activity that is dissociated from the neural state of non-REM sleep.[52]

The only neuroimaging study to date in non-REM parasomnias is a single-case ^{99m}Tc-ethylcysteinate dimer (^{99m}Tc-ECD) SPECT study of a 16-year-old patient with frequent sleepwalking episodes.[53] In this patient, SPECT was acquired in two conditions, each during a separate nighttime recording: during undisturbed SWS and 24 seconds after the onset of a sleepwalking episode arising from SWS. Compared to quiet SWS, sleepwalking was associated with an increased perfusion in the posterior cingulate cortex and in the cerebellum (vermis). Data from awake normal volunteers were also used as a control condition, and a decrease of perfusion was observed in frontoparietal associative cortices during sleepwalking as compared to normal wakefulness. Posterior cingulate cortex, cerebellum, and frontoparietal associative cortices are usually found deactivated during SWS compared to wakefulness in normal volunteers.[1] The brain perfusion patterns found during sleepwalking are therefore in agreement with the hypothesis of a dissociated state, in which certain areas display activities typical of SWS (frontoparietal cortices), while other structures (cerebellum, posterior cingulate) maintain activities similar to wakefulness. In addition, the deactivation of frontoparietal associative areas might also explain the lack of insight and the amnesia typical of sleepwalking episodes.[53] This finding needs to be confirmed on larger samples. It should also be noted that, given the brief duration of sleepwalking episodes, it is difficult to precisely isolate the brain activity patterns of the episode from those of the wakefulness period that follows (in the present study, the injection was done 24 seconds after the onset of the episode, and the electroencephalogram [EEG] at that time showed fast activities resembling wakefulness). Finally, there was no comparison with the patient's own wakefulness and with SWS in normal subjects; inclusion of these conditions is needed to confirm the specificity of the results to the sleepwalking state.

REM Sleep Behavior Disorder

Among REM parasomnias, REM sleep behavior disorder (RBD) is characterized by excessive sustained or phasic muscle activity during REM sleep (REM sleep without atonia), typically associated with unpleasant dreams and dream enactment behaviors.[10] RBD can present as an isolated phenomenon (*idiopathic* or *cryptogenic RBD*) or in association with neurological or general medical conditions (*secondary RBD*). The secondary forms usually occur within the context of some neurodegenerative diseases or narcolepsy,[54] or they can also represent an "incidental" phenomenon within the context of various brain lesions (vascular, demyelinating, tumor, inflammatory, postsurgical, toxic, etc.).[55] Neuroimaging studies, and anatomical MRI in particular, play a pivotal role in the diagnosis of these forms of RBD. Growing evidence in the literature indicates that idiopathic RBD actually represents an early stage of a neurodegenerative process involving the central nervous system.[56–58] The long-term risk for patients with RBD to develop a neurodegenerative disease (especially synucleinopathies: PD, dementia with Lewy bodies, progressive supranuclear palsy, and multiple-system atrophy) has been estimated at around 17.7% at 5 years and 52.4% at 12 years.[59] RBD physiopathology has been explored in relationship with various models of REM sleep regulation in animals. In one of these models, REM sleep regulatory circuits hinge on the so-called *REM-on* and *REM-off* areas, which mainly contain GABA-ergic neurons located in the pontine tegmentum.[60,61] Among REM-on areas, the sublaterodorsal nucleus (SLD) sends projections to interneurons in the brainstem and spinal cord, which finally exert an inhibitory action on motoneurons, leading to muscle tone suppression during REM sleep. In RBD, lesions to the SLD would be responsible for a disinhibition of motoneurons, resulting in excessive muscle activity during REM sleep.[60,61] This model is corroborated by several human case reports and case series describing RBD occurrence following focal lesions at brainstem level, independently of their origin: ischemic,[62-64] hemorrhagic,[65] neoplastic,[58,66,] demyelinating,[67-69] and inflammatory.[70] In all these observations, lesions involved the pons, usually (when specified) in the medial and tegmental region.

STRUCTURAL NEUROIMAGING

Structural brain imaging studies of RBD are summarized in Table 19.3.

VBM and DTI Studies. Besides these case reports of standard anatomical neuroimaging procedures cited earlier, it was not until very recently that quantification of morphological changes was assessed in RBD patients, for both gray (VBM) and white (DTI) matter. In a first report, Ellmore and colleagues studied five patients with RBD (and without Parkinson disease), five patients with PD at an early stage (and with subclinical or clinical RBD), and seven healthy controls.[71] All subjects underwent MRI, and their data were processed for VBM. The main outcome measures were volumes of caudate and putamen nuclei. There was no significant difference for caudate volume across groups. RBD patients had reduced putaminal volume compared to controls but also, surprisingly, compared to patients with early PD. While these results might be related to changes in DA neurotransmission in RBD and PD (see later), this study is limited by the small sample size. Microstructural changes in the white matter were assessed in an MRI study with DTI scans in 12 patients with idiopathic RBD compared to 12 healthy control subjects.[72] Changes were located in multiple brain areas such as the internal capsule, the left superior temporal lobe, the right occipital lobe, and the fornix. Alterations were also found in the pons, in agreement with animal and human data suggesting a role for pontine lesions in RBD pathophysiology. Finally, changes were observed in the olfactory region and in the SN, in line with the concept of RBD as an early stage of neurodegenerative diseases, especially for PD. Very recently, Scherfler

and collaborators conducted a large multimodal MRI study combining both DTI and VBM in 26 patients with idiopathic RBD compared to 14 healthy controls.[73] DTI identified significant changes in the tegmentum of the midbrain and rostral pons, in line with the results of the previous study. VBM detected gray matter increases in the hippocampus bilaterally in RBD patients compared to controls. While the significance of this last finding remains unclear, it is interesting to note that increased hippocampal perfusion has been observed with SPECT in RBD [74] and PD patients[75] (see later).

Spectroscopy. A single case study of a 69-year-old idiopathic RBD patient scanned with ^{1}H-MRS found increased choline/creatine ratio in the brainstem,[76] when compared to values from a previously published group of healthy young subjects.[77]

The specificity of this finding to RBD is quite uncertain, since it could be confounded by other factors such as age (reference values were taken from subjects aged 21–32 years). Indeed, this result was not confirmed by two subsequent larger ^{1}H-MRS studies. Iranzo and colleagues found no differences of metabolic ratios in the midbrain and pontine tegmentum between 15 idiopathic RBD patients and 15 age- and sex-matched healthy controls.[78] A more recent study compared 12 PD patients with RBD to 12 PD patients without RBD and assessed ^{1}H-MRS metabolic ratios in the pons.[79] No significant difference was found between groups. In summary, in contrast to other structural (see earlier) or functional methods (see later), ^{1}H-MRS does not detect consistent alterations in pontine structures of RBD patients.

Transcranial Ultrasound. Increased echogenicity of SN has been associated with PD, and it is thought to reflect the stage of degeneration of this structure.[80] Given that RBD often precedes the onset of a synucleinopathy, several studies have used TCS to assess echogenicity of SN in RBD patients, in order to evaluate whether SN hyperechogenicity (defined as a size of echogenic SN above 0.20 cm^2) could also be consistently found in RBD as it is in PD. A preliminary report investigated five patients with idiopathic RBD and found hyperechogenic SN in two of them.[81] No control subject was recruited. In a subsequent study, Iwanami and colleagues recruited 34 idiopathic RBD patients, 17 PD patients with a history of RBD and 21 control

Table 19.3 Structural Neuroimaging of REM Sleep Behavior Disorder

STUDY	IMAGING	N PAT. // CTRL.	MEDICATION*	RESULTS
Ellmore et al. (2010)[71]	MRI / VBM	5 // 7	No	GM decrease in putamen
Unger et al. (2010)[72]	MRI / DTI	12 // 12	No	WM changes in pons, midbrain, olfactory region, internal capsule, temporo-occipital, fornix
Scherfler et al. (2011)[73]	MRI / VBM & DTI	26 // 14	No	WM changes in pons, midbrain; GM increase in hippocampus
Miyamoto et al. (2000)[76]	MRI / 1H-MRS	1 // 0**	No	Cho/Cr increase in brainstem
Iranzo et al. (2002)[78]	MRI / 1H-MRS	15 // 15	No	No difference in brainstem
Hanoglu et al. (2006)[79]	MRI / 1H-MRS	12 // 12***	Yes****	No difference in brainstem
Unger et al. (2008)[81]	TCS	5 // 0	No	SN hyperechogenicity in 2 pat.
Iwanami et al. (2010)[82]	TCS	34 // 21	No	SN hyperechogenicity in 42% of pat. (9.5% of ctrl.)
Stockner et al. (2009)[83]	TCS	55 // 165	No	SN hyperechogenicity in 37% of pat. (11% of ctrl.)
Iranzo et al. (2010)[84]	TCS	39 // 149	No	SN hyperechogenicity in 36% of pat. (11% of ctrl.)

MRI = magnetic resonance imaging; VBM = voxel-based morphometry; DTI = diffusion tensor imaging; 1H-MRS = proton magnetic resonance spectroscopy; Cho/Cr = choline / creatine ratio; TCS = transcranial ultrasound; GM = grey matter; WM = white matter; SN = substantia nigra.

*Medication at the time of imaging (sleep-modifying or dopaminergic medication).

**Values were compared to a database of controls from another study (Ref. 77).

***In this particular study, patients and controls had Parkinson's disease (with and without REM sleep behavior disorder, respectively).

****Participants were treated with levodopa, but levodopa dosage was matched between groups.

subjects.[82] While 9.5% of the control group showed SN hyperechogenicity, this pattern was found in 42.1% of the idiopathic RBD group, and at an even higher proportion of 52.6% of the PD group. This finding suggested a continuum of SN degenerative changes from RBD to PD.

Another group conducted a study on a larger sample of 55 idiopathic RBD patients and 165 controls and confirmed the higher proportion of SN hyperechogenicity in RBD (37.3%) compared to controls (10.7%).[83] The same group conducted a follow-up study on idiopathic RBD patients and found that 30% of these patients developed a neurodegenerative disorder (PD, dementia with Lewy bodies or multiple-system atrophy) within 2.5 years.[84] Among those who developed a neurodegenerative disease, 62.5% had SN hyperechogenicity at baseline. This result suggests that TCS could be useful to identify RBD patients at increased risk for the development of full-blown neurodegenerative disorders (see later).

FUNCTIONAL NEUROIMAGING

Regional Brain Activity Patterns. Distribution of brain perfusion in RBD patients was assessed in several studies using SPECT. A first study compared 20 male idiopathic RBD patients to seven healthy elderly men with N-isopropyl-p-^{123}I-iodoamphetamine (^{123}I-IMP) SPECT.[85] Decreased perfusion was found in the superior frontal gyrus and the pons of RBD patients. SPECT scans were performed at night in both groups, but it is not clear in which state of vigilance the subjects were during scan acquisition. Hypoperfusion in the frontal lobe was confirmed in a ^{99m}Tc-ECD SPECT study, along with additional hypoperfusion in temporo-parietal cortices.[74] In this study, which included eight idiopathic RBD patients and nine control subjects scanned during wakefulness, the pons did not display decreased but increased perfusion in RBD patients, a pattern that was also found in the putamen and the right hippocampus. Since hyperperfusion of putamen and right hippocampus is likewise found in the early stages of PD,[75] this pattern is in agreement with the hypothesis of RBD as an early stage of a neurodegenerative disorder. The same group then conducted a larger and independent study on 20 idiopathic RBD patients and 20 controls during wakefulness using the same ^{99m}Tc-ECD SPECT technique.[86] They found that RBD patients displayed decreased perfusion in frontal and medial parietal (precuneus) areas, and increased perfusion in the pons, putamen, and hippocampus bilaterally, which is mostly consistent with their previous results. Interestingly, a recent follow-up study investigated the clinical evolution of these patients over an average period of 3 years, and examined the differences in brain perfusion at baseline (with ^{99m}Tc-ECD SPECT) between those who would later convert to PD or dementia with Lewy bodies and those who would remain clinically stable.[87] Out of 20 RBD patients, 10 converted and displayed increased perfusion in the hippocampus at baseline compared to the 10 remaining patients who did not convert (Fig. 19.1), but also compared to healthy controls matched for age and sex. Furthermore, this study also found an association in RBD patients between hippocampal hyperperfusion and worse clinical scores for motor function and color vision, both associated with neurodegenerative evolution.[87–89] Altogether, these results demonstrate that increased perfusion in the hippocampus constitutes a consistent biomarker for clinical evolution towards neurodegenerative diseases in RBD patients. Another group used ^{123}I-IMP SPECT to study brain perfusion in 24 idiopathic RBD patients and 18 controls.[90] Unlike previous reports, this study did not find any significant difference between groups in the brainstem and frontal areas. However, hypoperfusions were found for the RBD group in the precuneus, cerebellum, and uncus. Discrepancies with previous studies might be related to differences in the acquisition technique (^{123}I-IMP), study population (mostly male patients), or vigilance state/time at which the study was performed (not specified). Two studies assessed brain glucose metabolism with ^{18}F-fluorodeoxyglucose (^{18}F-FDG) PET in subjects with dream-enactment behavior suggestive of RBD.[91,92] In contrast with the SPECT studies presented earlier, no polysomnographic recording was conducted to confirm a diagnosis of RBD and subjects were selected following questionnaires and interview only, which limits the interpretation of the findings. Decreases of brain glucose metabolism were found in subjects with dream-enactment behavior in multiple cortical areas (occipital, frontal, parietal, temporal, cingulate), and results were discussed in comparison with similar patterns found in patients with neurodegenerative diseases such as dementia with Lewy bodies. Finally, a recent ^{99m}Tc-ECD SPECT study reported the brain perfusion patterns associated with an episode of RBD in a single patient with multiple-system atrophy.[93] Perfusion in the supplementary motor area was increased during the episode as compared to wakefulness. This pattern was not found when comparing REM sleep and wakefulness in two healthy controls. It was concluded that the supplementary motor area might play a role in the generation of dream-enactment behavior in RBD. However, there was no SPECT acquisition during the patient's REM sleep per se (outside the episode) in this study. Future studies including REM

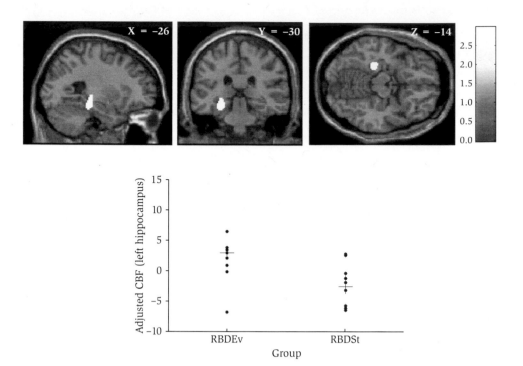

FIGURE 19.1 Hippocampal perfusion predicts clinical evolution in REM sleep behavior disorder (RBD). (Upper panels) Brain perfusion increases at baseline in RBD patients who would convert to neurodegenerative disease (RBDEv), compared to those who would not (RBDSt), were located in the hippocampus. The panels show the peak hyperperfusion, centered on the left hippocampus, and represented on sagittal, coronal and transverse sections (from left to right panels) ($P^{corr} < 0.05$). The level of section is indicated on the top of each panel (x, y, and z coordinates, in mm). The color scale indicates the range of t values for this contrast.

(Lower panel) Plot of the adjusted regional cerebral blood flow values (arbitrary units) in the left hippocampus (x=−30mm, y=−30mm, z=−14mm), showing the distinct distribution in RBDEv and RBDSt patients. Each circle represents one subject. Horizontal bars represent mean values.

This figure shows results from a ^{99m}Tc-ECD SPECT study. (Reproduced from Dang-Vu et al.,[87] with permission.) (See color insert.)

sleep assessments and more patients are needed to confirm the specificity of this finding.

SPECT and PET Ligand Studies. Given the frequent association between RBD and conditions associated with a DA dysfunction (such as PD, dementia with Lewy bodies, multiple-system atrophy), several neuroimaging studies have targeted the nigrostriatal DA system in RBD patients (Table 19.4). At the presynaptic level, two SPECT studies with ^{123}I-IPT conducted by the same group demonstrated a decrease of DAT in the striatum of idiopathic RBD patients compared to controls.[94,95] In a first study, DAT in 5 RBD patients was found lower than in 7 controls, but higher than in 14 early-stage PD.[94] In a subsequent report, 8 RBD

patients were compared to 8 subjects with "subclinical" RBD (i.e., with loss of muscular atonia during REM sleep in polysomnography, but no behavioral episodes), 11 controls, and 8 early-stage PD.[95] There was a decrease of DAT from controls to subclinical RBD, from subclinical RBD to manifest RBD, and then from RBD to PD. Altogether these results suggest a continuum of striatal presynaptic DA dysfunction in patients with subclinical RBD, clinical RBD, and PD. This finding was confirmed by a PET study using ^{11}C-dihydrotetrabenazine (^{11}C-DTBZ) to probe the density of striatal DA terminals in 6 idiopathic RBD patients compared to 19 controls.[96] Decreases in striatal binding were found in the striatum, especially in the posterior putamen, in agreement with a presynaptic

Table 19.4 SPECT- and PET-Ligand Studies in REM Sleep Behavior Disorder

STUDY	IMAGING	TARGET	NO. PAT. // CTRL.	MEDICATION*	RESULTS
Eisensehr et al. [92]	SPECT 123I-IPT & 123I-IBZM	DAT & D2	5 // 7	No	Decrease in DAT, no change in D2
Eisensehr et al. [93]	SPECT 123I-IPT & 123I-IBZM	DAT & D2	8 // 11	No	Decrease in DAT, no change in D2
Albin et al. [94]	PET 11C-DTBZ	DAT	6 // 19	Yes	Decrease in DAT
Gilman et al. [95]	PET 11C-DTBZ	DAT	13** // 15	No	Decrease in DAT, neg. correl. with REM atonia loss
Stiasny-Kolster et al. [96]	SPECT 123I-FP-CIT	DAT	11 // 10	Yes	Decrease in DAT in 2 patients
Unger et al. [81]	SPECT 123I-FP-CIT	DAT	5 // 0	No	Decrease in DAT in 2 patients
Kim et al. [97]	SPECT 123I-FP-CIT	DAT	14 // 12	No	Decrease in DAT
Iranzo et al. [84]	SPECT 123I-FP-CIT	DAT	43 // 18	No	Decrease in DAT in 40% of patients
Iranzo et al (link to iranzo 2011)	SPECT 123I-FP-CIT	DAT	20 // 20	No	Decrease in DAT over time
Miyamoto et al. [98]	PET 11C-CFT	DAT	1 // 6	No	Decrease in DAT

* Medication at the time of imaging (sleep-modifying or dopaminergic medication).

** In this particular study, patients had multiple-system atrophy and a history of RBD.

D2, dopaminergic D2-receptor binding; DAT, dopamine transporter binding; PET, positron emission tomography; SPECT, single photon emission computed tomography.

DA impairment in RBD. Interestingly, another PET study using ^{11}C-DTBZ was conducted in 13 patients with probable multiple-system atrophy compared to 15 control subjects.[97] Not only was striatal binding decreased in the patients' group, but binding was also negatively correlated with the severity of REM atonia loss. This finding suggests that presynaptic DA deficit might contribute to the frequent occurrence of RBD in patients with multiple-system atrophy. Four studies assessed presynaptic DAT in RBD patients using SPECT with ^{123}I-2βcarbomethoxy-3β-(4-iodophenyl)-N-(3-fluoropropyl)-nortropane (^{123}I-FP-CIT). Two reports found decreases of striatal DAT only in a minor proportion of RBD patients: 2 out of 11[98] and 2 out of 5 patients,[81] respectively. A third study reported group comparisons between 14 idiopathic RBD patients,

14 early-stage PD patients, and 12 controls.[99] RBD patients showed a lower binding in the striatum, in particular in the putamen, compared to controls but higher when compared to PD. This result is in line with the ^{123}I-IPT SPECT studies from Eisensehr and colleagues,[94,95] and with the concept of a continuum in striatal DA impairment from RBD to PD. In a fourth, recent and longitudinal study, 43 idiopathic RBD and 18 controls were assessed for striatal DAT.[84] Reduced binding was found in 40% of RBD patients. The same study included a clinical follow-up showing the appearance of a neurodegenerative disorder (PD, dementia with Lewy bodies or multiple-system atrophy) in 8 of these patients within 2.5 years after neuroimaging. Importantly, 6 of these 8 RBD patients who would develop a neurodegenerative disease had a reduced striatal DAT at baseline. This study also associated TCS to measure echogenicity of SN (see earlier), and the combination of ^{123}I-FP-CIT SPECT and TCS allowed the detection of anomalies at baseline in all 8 RBD patients who would convert to a full-blown neurodegenerative disorder. These results suggest that ^{123}I-FP-CIT SPECT in association with TCS might constitute methods of interest in the identification of RBD patients at higher risk for the development of synucleinopathies.

A case report described the changes over time of nigrostriatal presynaptic DA function in RBD. PET using ^{11}C-carbomethoxy flurophenyl tropane (^{11}C-CFT) was acquired twice in a 73-year-old man: 1 year and 3.5 years after RBD onset, respectively.[100] While only a slight binding decrease was noted in the posterior putamen after 1 year (compared to controls), the decrease was more pronounced in the striatum after 3.5 years, with an estimate of a 4%–6% decrease per year. The progressive decrease in striatal DAT was confirmed by a prospective ^{123}I-FP-CIT SPECT study conducted in 20 idiopathic RBD patients.[101] In this study, patients were evaluated for presynaptic DA function at baseline, after 1.5 years, and again after 3 years, showing a progressive decline in striatal DAT over time.

Finally, concerning postsynaptic DA function, the two studies from Eisensehr and colleagues also included acquisitions with ^{123}I-IBZM SPECT, targeting striatal postsynaptic D2 receptor density.[94,95] No significant change was observed between RBD and other groups (controls, PD), demonstrating that postsynaptic DA function is not affected in RBD patients.

Summary

Neuroimaging findings in sleepwalking and RBD can be summarized as follows:

1. *Sleepwalking* appears as a *dissociated state*, with mixed functional brain patterns of SWS and wakefulness.
2. Structural and functional studies have demonstrated alterations in the *pons* of *RBD* patients, supporting the involvement of pontine nuclei in RBD pathophysiology.
3. Structural and functional studies suggest degenerative changes of the *SN* and presynaptic dysfunction of *DA* nigro-striatal pathways in *RBD*, which are in agreement with the hypothesis that RBD actually represents an early stage of a *neurodegenerative* disease, in particular a synucleinopathy (PD, dementia with Lewy bodies and multiple-system atrophy).
4. Neuroimaging provides objective *biomarkers* of RBD evolution towards neurodegenerative disorders, in particular with TCS, striatal DAT and hippocampal perfusion patterns.

While an increasing number of neuroimaging studies are devoted to RBD, only one study with a single patient is available in sleepwalking. Additional studies are needed to confirm and extend this study, especially as regards the role of SWS alterations in the pathophysiology of somnambulism. Neuroimaging studies have brought important support to theories suggesting a role for pontine structures and DA dysfunction in RBD. Future studies are needed to further explore the relationship between RBD and neurodegenerative diseases, and especially the evolution from RBD to full-blown neurodegenerative disorders. They should also address the role of structures such as the hippocampus in RBD, along with cognitive aspects of the disease. Finally, the investigation of brain activity patterns during behavioral episodes as well as during sleep itself should be further documented in the next neuroimaging studies of RBD.

FATAL FAMILIAL INSOMNIA

Fatal familial insomnia (FFI) is a hereditary autosomal dominant disease caused by prion-protein gene (PRNP) mutation. It is linked to a mutation of PRNP at codon 178, and to the presence of a methionine codon at position 129. Clinical features include insomnia, autonomic hyperactivity, and motor abnormalities.[102,103]

This disease is invariably lethal, hence its name.[102] The disrupted sleep profile presents a loss of sleep spindles and SWS, and enacted dreams during REM sleep.[103]

A prominent hypometabolism was observed in the anterior part of the thalamus in four patients investigated with ^{18}F-FDG PET during wakefulness.[104] Two of those patients exhibited symptoms restricted to insomnia and dysautonomia: in one subject, hypometabolism was exclusively located in the thalamus; in the other one, hypometabolism was also found in frontal, anterior cingulate, and temporal polar areas in addition to the thalamus. In the two remaining patients, who had a more complex clinical presentation, hypometabolism was more widespread and involved many cortical areas, the basal ganglia, the cerebellum, and the thalamus. This widespread pattern was found significantly aggravated as the disease progressed in one patient reexamined several months later. However, whether widespread hypometabolism is indicative of the more advanced stages of the disease or indicates a different variant of this disorder (disseminated vs. thalamic) still remains to be confirmed.

The same group then studied seven FFI patients with ^{18}F-FDG PET, to examine regional cerebral glucose utilization in FFI and its relation with neuropathology.[105] A severe decrease of glucose utilization in the thalamus and a milder decrease in the cingulate cortex were detected in all FFI patients. Six of these patients also displayed a hypometabolism of the basal and lateral frontal cortex, the caudate nucleus, and the middle and inferior temporal cortex. Further comparison between homozygous (n = 4) or heterozygous (n = 3) patients at codon 129 showed that the hypometabolism was more widespread in the heterozygous group, which had longer symptom duration at the time of study. A comparison with neuropathologic data showed that areas with neuronal loss were among those that were shown hypometabolic in the PET study. However, hypometabolism extended beyond areas demonstrated by neuropathologic data, and it significantly correlated with the amount of prion protein across brain areas. Altogether these data indicate that hypometabolism of the thalamus and cingulate cortex is a common feature of FFI, while the involvement of other brain regions may depend on various factors, such as symptom duration.[105] Interestingly, thalamic hypometabolism was also found in a case of genetically confirmed FFI with atypical clinical presentation (ataxia, dementia, and dysautonomic signs, no obvious insomnia per se).[106]

Recently, an ^{18}F-FDG PET study assessed the changes in brain metabolism in carriers of the mutation involved in FFI before the actual onset of the symptoms. In one of these subjects, selective thalamic hypometabolism was detected 13 months before disease onset, suggesting that thalamic metabolic changes constitute an early, even preclinical, marker of FFI[107] (Fig. 19.2).

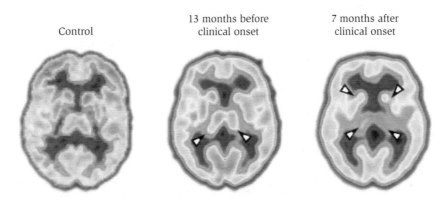

Control 13 months before clinical onset 7 months after clinical onset

FIGURE 19.2 Brain glucose metabolism in fatal familial insomnia (FFI). Decrease of glucose metabolism in the thalamus has been consistently shown in FFI. Thalamic hypometabolism is manifest in this patient with symptomatic FFI, along with metabolic decrease in the basal ganglia (*right*), as compared to controls (*left*). A milder decrease of glucose metabolism in the thalamus was already detected in that FFI patient more than 1 year before the onset of symptoms (*middle*). This figure shows results from an ^{18}F-FDG PET study. (Reproduced from Cortelli et al.,[104] with permission.) (*See* color insert.)

This observation is highly important since the thalamus plays a key role in sleep regulation, especially in the generation of brain oscillations of sleep such as spindles.[108] Indeed, spectral analysis in the frequency band of spindles showed a reduction of spindle activity 13 months before disease onset in that patient who also exhibited a reduced thalamic metabolism at the same time.[107]

Only one imaging study investigated the changes of neurotransmission in FFI. Serotonin transporters of two FFI patients were examined with ^{123}I-β-CIT SPECT as compared to age-expected control values.[109] This study showed a reduced availability of serotonin transporters of 57% and 73%, respectively, in a diencephalic region of the two FFI patients. Although this finding suggests an involvement of the serotonergic neurotransmission, its eventual causative role in FFI pathophysiology still remains to be established.[109]

NOCTURNAL EPILEPSY
Nocturnal Frontal Lobe Epilepsy

Nocturnal frontal lobe epilepsy (NFLE) is a peculiar form of epilepsy with seizures arising from foci within the frontal lobe and occurring almost exclusively during sleep. Three main phenotypes can be identified within the clinical spectrum of NFLE seizures: paroxysmal arousals (PAs), defined as brief (<20 seconds) and recurrent arousals associated with a stereotypical motor activity; nocturnal paroxysmal dystonia (NPD), constituted by recurrent and longer (<2 minutes) motor attacks with dystonic or hyperkinetic features; and episodic nocturnal wanderings (ENWs), which are agitated and stereotyped behaviors resembling somnambulism.[110] Differential diagnosis might be difficult, especially with parasomnias, since epileptic activity is often not visible on standard scalp EEG recordings.[111] Vetrugno and colleagues reported a case study of one patient with a history of PA, NPD, and ENW.[112] In this patient, ^{99m}Tc-ECD SPECT was acquired twice: during an episode of PA (ictal), and during sleep (interictal) at a 1-week interval. Comparing ictal and interictal scans showed that PA was associated with increased perfusion in the cerebellum and anterior cingulate gyrus. Ictal scans in this patient were also compared with scans of 20 age-matched healthy volunteers during wake: compared to controls, the episode was still associated with hyperperfusion

of cerebellum and anterior cingulate gyrus but also with a decreased perfusion of frontal and temporal associative areas. The authors interpreted this finding as reflecting a dissociative state, with the activity of anterior cingulate and cerebellum responsible for a state of behavioral arousal, and the decreased perfusion in associative frontal-temporal areas accounting for an impaired awareness during the episodes.[112] The consistency and specificity of this result still need to be confirmed. In particular, these patterns are strikingly similar to those found during a sleepwalking episode [53] and could thus be related to nonspecific central patterns common to parasomnias and seizures arising from sleep.[113] Another patient was likewise studied with ^{99m}Tc-ECD SPECT during an episode of NPD.[114] In agreement with the study on PA, this report described an increased perfusion in the anterior cingulate cortex during ictal compared with interictal scans.

NFLE can also be inherited as an autosomal dominant trait. In this case, it is termed autosomal dominant nocturnal frontal lobe epilepsy (ADNFLE). ADNFLE is associated with different mutations in the genes encoding two subunits (α4 and β2) of the neural nicotinic acetylcholine receptor (nAChR). This condition has been associated with abnormal brain activity during the interictal period (awake state) in a study using PET with ^{18}F-FDG, that is, decreased glucose uptake over the left middle and superior frontal gyri and the left central regions, including anterior parietal lobe.[115] These patterns were described in 6 members of a same Korean family compared to 14 control subjects, and they were consistent with the EEG features showing epileptiform activity over frontocentral areas. Previously another study had shown in one ADNFLE patient a left frontal hypometabolism on interictal ^{18}F-FDG PET, which was congruent with left frontopolar onset on EEG but also a focal hyperperfusion in the same area on ictal ^{99m}Tc-hexamethylpropyleneamineoxime (^{99m}TcH-MPAO) SPECT.[116] In a more recent ^{18}F-FDG PET study, Picard and colleagues likewise found a frontal hypometabolism (right orbitofrontal cortex) during the interictal period (awake state) in 5 ADNFLE patients compared to 30 controls.[117] In the same study, these authors were also able to report the regional density of nAChRs using PET with ^{18}F-A-85380, a radiotracer with a high affinity for α4β2 receptors. Comparing eight patients and seven controls, they found that ADNFLE was associated with a lower nAChR density in the right dorsolateral prefontal cortex—in agreement with the frontal origin of this epilepsy—and with a higher density in the mesencephalon and cerebellum (Fig. 19.3). The exact significance of these localized increases in nAChR density remains unclear, but they seem to indicate an overactivated brainstem ascending cholinergic system.[117]

Benign Epilepsy of Childhood with Centrotemporal Spikes

Benign epilepsy of childhood with centrotemporal spikes (BECTS) or benign rolandic epilepsy is an idiopathic localization-related epilepsy of childhood with no recognized underlying cause other than a possible hereditary predisposition. Seizures are typically nocturnal and confined to sleep and are accompanied by abnormal motor movement, including the face, the leg, or the full body. Structural imaging studies (CT scans and MRI) have shown that brain lesions can be found in approximately 15% of patients with BECTS (e.g., enlargement of ventricles or hippocampal atrophy).[118] This association seems to be coincidental, since the presence of such lesions did not affect the prognosis of the disease. More recently, a study using anatomical MRI has confirmed the high prevalence of abnormal findings in BECTS: more than 40% of patients had lesions such as hippocampal atrophy, malformation of cortical development, or Chiari malformation.[119] These lesions were still of unclear clinical significance. Functional imaging remains to be systematically studied in patients with BECTS.

Landau-Kleffner Syndrome and Syndrome of Continuous Spike-and-Wave Discharges during Slow-Wave Sleep

The Landau-Kleffner syndrome (LKS) and the syndrome of continuous spike-and-wave discharges during SWS (CSWS) have been originally described and are still considered separately. LKS is characterized by acquired aphasia and paroxysmal sleep-activated EEG predominating over the temporal or parietal-occipital regions.[120] Paroxysmal events are spike-and-wave discharges that are activated by SWS. Secondary symptoms include psychomotor or behavioral disturbances. LKS has a favorable outcome for seizure control.[121] CSWS is characterized by continuous spike-and wave discharges during SWS, usually combined with global intellectual deterioration and epileptic seizures.[122] These two syndromes share many features in common, including early onset during childhood, deterioration of cognitive function (previously acquired normally), seizure type, EEG pattern, and pharmacological reactivity. They have also in common the regression of neuropsychological symptoms, EEG abnormalities, and seizures before the end of adolescence. Structural lesions evaluated by CT scan or MRI are usually absent or nonspecific.[121–124]

In both conditions, initial functional neuroimaging studies using PET[121,125–128] and SPECT[127,129–135] described metabolic abnormalities that predominantly involved the temporal lobes. Focal or regional areas of decreased and increased metabolism were reported. A normal distribution of cerebrospinal fluid was reported in one isolated case.[136] These early results were difficult to interpret in terms of pathogenesis.

In a restrospective analysis of ^{18}F-FDG PET data during sleep and wakefulness in a population of patients with CSWS, regional increases and decreases in cerebral glucose metabolism were again observed.[137] The metabolic patterns were found to be variable from one patient to another and grossly related to the neuropsychological deterioration. Moreover, metabolic patterns in individual patients were reported to change over time. Four basic metabolic characteristics were drawn up from this study. First, patients with CSWS have a higher rate of metabolism in the cortical mantle than in the thalamic nuclei. This metabolic pattern is characteristic of an immature brain. Second, they show focal or regional metabolic abnormalities of the cortex, suggesting a focal origin of the spike-and-wave discharges. Third, they have metabolic disturbances predominantly involving associative cortices, compatible with a deterioration of cognitive functions. Fourth, glucose metabolism in thalamic nuclei remains symmetrical despite significant cortical asymmetries, suggesting that corticothalamic neurons either do not participate in the generation of spike-and-wave discharges or are being inhibited by pathological mechanisms.

More recently, voxel-based analyses of cerebral glucose metabolism were performed in a group of 18 children with CSWS.[138] Each patient was compared with a control group and the influence of age, epileptic activity, and corticosteroid treatment on metabolic

2-[^{18}F]-F-A-85380   [^{18}F]-FDG

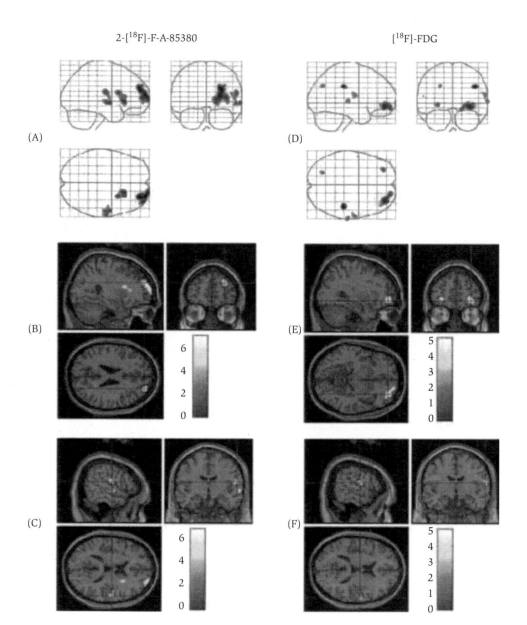

FIGURE 19.3   Brain glucose metabolism and nicotinic acetycholine receptor density in autosomal dominant nocturnal frontal lobe epilepsy. The right panels (*D–F*) illustrate the decrease of glucose metabolism in the right prefrontal region (*E*) and right opercular cortex (*F*), in ADNFLE as compared to controls, during the interictal period (^{18}F-FDG PET study). Given that ADNFLE is associated with mutations in the genes encoding subunits α4 and β2 of nAChR, the brain regional density of nAChR has also been investigated. As shown in the left panels (*A–C*), ADNFLE is associated with a lower nAChR density in the right prefontal region (*B*) and right opercular cortex (*C*), as compared to controls (^{18}F-A-85380 PET study). Note the similarity between glucose metabolism and nAChR distributions, both of which being in agreement with the frontal origin of ADNFLE. (Reproduced from Picard et al.,[114] with permission.) (*See* color insert.)

abnormalities was assessed. Cerebral metabolic patterns were heterogeneous across patients with CSWS. Age and intensity of interictal spiking did not significantly differ in patients showing focal hypermetabolism compared with the other ones. Treatment with corticosteroids corrected focal hypermetabolism. Altered parietofrontal connectivity observed in patients with hypermetabolism was interpreted as a phenomenon of remote inhibition of the frontal lobes induced by highly epileptogenic and hypermetabolic posterior cortex.

Altogether these studies suggest that CSWS is produced by an alteration in the maturation of one or more associative cortices, potentially leading to disturbed neuronal wiring. An imbalance of inhibitory and excitatory drives would lead to a deterioration of associated higher cerebral functions and would create conditions favorable for the generation of neuronal discharges. Epileptic discharges would be triggered during SWS because of the physiological reinforced synchronization of neuronal firing characteristic of SWS.[139]

CONCLUSION

Neuroimaging has brought an important contribution to sleep medicine, and especially to the topic of movements disorders in sleep. The development of techniques and methods of analysis has allowed an increasing number of complex neuroimaging studies to emerge. The systematic study of anatomical changes in both gray and white matter has allowed, for instance, the detection of subtle structural changes in key structures for RBD pathogenesis.[73] Recent ligand studies were able to confirm the existence of striatal DA dysfunction in RLS.[39] The identification of brain regions involved in the generation of paroxysmal episodes in nocturnal epilepsy was made possible by brain metabolism studies.[112,117] Future studies will further explore the patterns of brain function predictive of clinical evolution, as well as the neuroimaging longitudinal changes in the course of disease progression. This is illustrated, for example, by the relationship between neuroimaging data at baseline and clinical progression of RBD toward neurodegenerative disorders.[84,87] Beyond the understanding of pathophysiology, neuroimaging techniques also constitute promising tools for the diagnostic and prognostic evaluation of sleep-related movement disorders.

ACKNOWLEDGMENTS

TD is supported by the Canadian Institutes of Health Research and the Belgian College of Neuropsychopharmacology and Biological Psychiatry.

REFERENCES

1. Maquet P (2000) Functional neuroimaging of normal human sleep by positron emission tomography. J Sleep Res 9:207–31.
2. Dang-Vu TT, Desseilles M, Petit D, Mazza S, Montplaisir J, Maquet P (2007) Neuroimaging in sleep medicine. Sleep medicine 8:349–72.
3. Dang-Vu TT, Desseilles M, Albouy G, Darsaud A, Gais S, Rauchs G, Schabus M, Sterpenich V, Vandewalle G, Schwartz S, Maquet P (2005) Dreaming: A Neuroimaging View. Swiss Archives of Neurology and Psychiatry 156:415–25.
4. Dang-Vu TT, Schabus M, Desseilles M, Sterpenich V, Bonjean M, Maquet P (2010) Functional neuroimaging insights into the physiology of human sleep. Sleep 33:15891603.
5. Schabus M, Dang-Vu TT, Albouy G, Balteau E, Boly M, Carrier J, Darsaud A, Degueldre C, Desseilles M, Gais S, Phillips C, Rauchs G, Schnakers C, Sterpenich V, Vandewalle G, Luxen A, Maquet P (2007) Hemodynamic cerebral correlates of sleep spindles during human non-rapid eye movement sleep. Proc Natl Acad Sci U S A 104:1316413169.
6. Dang-Vu TT, Schabus M, Desseilles M, Albouy G, Boly M, Darsaud A, Gais S, Rauchs G, Sterpenich V, Vandewalle G, Carrier J, Moonen G, Balteau E, Degueldre C, Luxen A, Phillips C, Maquet P (2008) Spontaneous neural activity during human slow wave sleep. Proc Natl Acad Sci U S A 105:15160–5.
7. Desseilles M, Dang-Vu T, Schabus M, Sterpenich V, Maquet P, Schwartz S (2008) Neuroimaging insights into the pathophysiology of sleep disorders. Sleep 31:777–94.
8. Dang-Vu TT, Desseilles M, Schwartz S, Maquet P (2009) Neuroimaging of narcolepsy. CNS Neurol Disord Drug Targets 8:254–63.
9. Allen RP, Picchietti D, Hening WA, Trenkwalder C, Walters AS, Montplaisi J (2003) Restless legs syndrome: diagnostic criteria, special considerations, and epidemiology. A report from the restless legs syndrome diagnosis and epidemiology workshop at the National Institutes of Health. Sleep medicine 4:101–19.

10. AASM (2005) International classification of sleep disorders, 2nd ed.: Diagnostic and coding manual. Westchester, IL: American Academy of Sleep Medicine.

11. Montplaisir J, Boucher S, Poirier G, Lavigne G, Lapierre O, Lesperance P (1997) Clinical, poly-somnographic, and genetic characteristics of restless legs syndrome: a study of 133 patients diagnosed with new standard criteria. Mov Disord 12:61–5.

12. Scalise A (2009) Patho-physiology of restless legs syndrome: a very tedious puzzle! Sleep medicine 10:1073–4.

13. Garcia-Borreguero D, Stillman P, Benes H, Buschmann H, Chaudhuri KR, Gonzalez Rodriguez VM, Hogl B, Kohnen R, Monti GC, Stiasny-Kolster K, Trenkwalder C, Williams AM, Zucconi M (2011) Algorithms for the diagnosis and treatment of restless legs syndrome in primary care. BMC Neurol 11:28.

14. Montplaisir J, Allen RP, Walters AS, Ferini-Strambi L (2011) Chapter 90. Restless Legs Syndrome and Periodic Limb Movements during Sleep. In: Principles and Practice of Sleep Medicine 5th ed(Kryger, M. H. et al., eds), pp 1026–37 St. Louis, Missouri, U. S. A.: Elsevier Saunders.

15. Etgen T, Draganski B, Ilg C, Schroder M, Geisler P, Hajak G, Eisensehr I, Sander D, May A (2005) Bilateral thalamic gray matter changes in patients with restless legs syndrome. Neuroimage 24:1242–7.

16. Unrath A, Juengling FD, Schork M, Kassubek J (2007) Cortical grey matter alterations in idiopathic restless legs syndrome: An optimized voxel-based morphometry study. Mov Disord 22:1751–6.

17. Unrath A, Muller HP, Ludolph AC, Riecker A, Kassubek J (2008) Cerebral white matter alterations in idiopathic restless legs syndrome, as measured by diffusion tensor imaging. Mov Disord 23:1250–5.

18. Hornyak M, Ahrendts JC, Spiegelhalder K, Riemann D, Voderholzer U, Feige B, van Elst LT (2007) Voxel-based morphometry in unmedicated patients with restless legs syndrome. Sleep medicine 9:22–6.

19. Celle S, Roche F, Peyron R, Faillenot I, Laurent B, Pichot V, Barthelemy JC, Sforza E (2010) Lack of specific gray matter alterations in restless legs syndrome in elderly subjects. Journal of neurology 257:344–8.

20. Comley RA, Cervenka S, Palhagen SE, Panagiotidis G, Matthews JC, Lai RY, Halldin C, Farde L, Nichols TE, Whitcher BJ (2012) A Comparison of Gray Matter Density in Restless Legs Syndrome Patients and Matched Controls Using Voxel-Based Morphometry. J Neuroimaging 22(1):28–32.

21. Allen R (2004) Dopamine and iron in the pathophysiology of restless legs syndrome (RLS). Sleep medicine 5:385–91.

22. Earley CJ, Connors JR, Allen RP (1999) RLS patients have abnormally reduced CSF ferritin compared to normal controls. Neurology 52:A111-A112.

23. Connor JR, Boyer PJ, Menzies SL, Dellinger B, Allen RP, Ondo WG, Earley CJ (2003) Neuropathological examination suggests impaired brain iron acquisition in restless legs syndrome. Neurology 61:304–9.

24. Allen RP, Barker PB, Wehrl F, Song HK, Earley CJ (2001) MRI measurement of brain iron in patients with restless legs syndrome. Neurology 56:263–5.

25. Earley CJ, P BB, Horska A, Allen RP (2006) MRI-determined regional brain iron concentrations in early-and late-onset restless legs syndrome. Sleep medicine 7:458–61.

26. Godau J, Klose U, Di Santo A, Schweitzer K, Berg D (2008) Multiregional brain iron deficiency in restless legs syndrome. Mov Disord 23:1184–7.

27. Berg D, Roggendorf W, Schroder U, Klein R, Tatschner T, Benz P, Tucha O, Preier M, Lange KW, Reiners K, Gerlach M, Becker G (2002) Echogenicity of the substantia nigra: association with increased iron content and marker for susceptibility to nigrostriatal injury. Arch Neurol 59:999–1005.

28. Schmidauer C, Sojer M, Seppi K, Stockner H, Hogl B, Biedermann B, Brandauer E, Peralta CM, Wenning GK, Poewe W (2005) Transcranial ultrasound shows nigral hypoechogenicity in restless legs syndrome. Ann Neurol 58:630–4.

29. Godau J, Schweitzer KJ, Liepelt I, Gerloff C, Berg D (2007) Substantia nigra hypoechogenicity: definition and findings in restless legs syndrome. Mov Disord 22:187–92.

30. Bucher SF, Seelos KC, Oertel WH, Reiser M, Trenkwalder C (1997) Cerebral generators involved in the pathogenesis of the restless legs syndrome. Ann Neurol 41:639–45.

31. Spiegelhalder K, Feige B, Paul D, Riemann D, van Elst LT, Seifritz E, Hennig J, Hornyak M (2008) Cerebral correlates of muscle tone fluctuations in restless legs syndrome: a pilot study with combined functional magnetic resonance imaging and anterior tibial

muscle electromyography. Sleep medicine 9:177–83.

32. Trenkwalder C, Hening WA, Montagna P, Oertel WH, Allen RP, Walters AS, Costa J, Stiasny-Kolster K, Sampaio C (2008) Treatment of restless legs syndrome: an evidence-based review and implications for clinical practice. Mov Disord 23:22672302.

33. Michaud M, Soucy JP, Chabli A, Lavigne G, Montplaisir J (2002) SPECT imaging of striatal pre-and postsynaptic dopaminergic status in restless legs syndrome with periodic leg movements in sleep. J Neurol 249:164–70.

34. Mrowka M, Jobges M, Berding G, Schimke N, Shing M, Odin P (2005) Computerized movement analysis and beta-CIT-SPECT in patients with restless legs syndrome. Journal of neural transmission 112:693–701.

35. Eisensehr I, Wetter TC, Linke R, Noachtar S, von Lindeiner H, Gildehaus FJ, Trenkwalder C, Tatsch K (2001) Normal IPT and IBZM SPECT in drug-naive and levodopa-treated idiopathic restless legs syndrome. Neurology 57:1307–9.

36. Linke R, Eisensehr I, Wetter TC, Gildehaus FJ, Popperl G, Trenkwalder C, Noachtar S, Tatsch K (2004) Presynaptic dopaminergic function in patients with restless legs syndrome: are there common features with early Parkinson's disease? Mov Disord 19:1158–62.

37. Turjanski N, Lees AJ, Brooks DJ (1999) Striatal dopaminergic function in restless legs syndrome: 18F-dopa and 11C-raclopride PET studies. Neurology 52:932–7.

38. Ruottinen HM, Partinen M, Hublin C, Bergman J, Haaparanta M, Solin O, Rinne JO (2000) An FDOPA PET study in patients with periodic limb movement disorder and restless legs syndrome. Neurology 54:502–4.

39. Earley CJ, Kuwabara H, Wong DF, Gamaldo C, Salas R, Brasic J, Ravert HT, Dannals RF, Allen RP (2011) The dopamine transporter is decreased in the striatum of subjects with restless legs syndrome. Sleep 34:341–7.

40. Tribl GG, Asenbaum S, Klosch G, Mayer K, Bonelli RM, Auff E, Zeitlhofer J, Happe S (2002) Normal IPT and IBZM SPECT in drug naive and levodopa-treated idiopathic restless legs syndrome. Neurology 59:649–50.

41. Tribl GG, Asenbaum S, Happe S, Bonelli RM, Zeitlhofer J, Auff E (2004) Normal striatal D2 receptor binding in idiopathic restless legs syndrome with periodic leg movements in sleep. Nucl Med Commun 25:55–60.

42. Cervenka S, Palhagen SE, Comley RA, Panagiotidis G, Cselenyi Z, Matthews JC, Lai RY, Halldin C, Farde L (2006) Support for dopaminergic hypoactivity in restless legs syndrome: a PET study on D2-receptor binding. Brain: a journal of neurology 129:2017–28.

43. Stanwood GD, Lucki I, McGonigle P (2000) Differential regulation of dopamine D2 and D3 receptors by chronic drug treatments. J Pharmacol Exp Ther 295:1232–40.

44. von Spiczak S, Whone AL, Hammers A, Asselin MC, Turkheimer F, Tings T, Happe S, Paulus W, Trenkwalder C, Brooks DJ (2005) The role of opioids in restless legs syndrome: an [11C]diprenorphine PET study. Brain: a journal of neurology 128:906

45. Barriere G, Cazalets JR, Bioulac B, Tison F, Ghorayeb I (2005) The restless legs syndrome. Prog Neurobiol 77:139–65.

46. Pennestri MH, Whittom S, Adam B, Petit D, Carrier J, Montplaisir J (2006) PLMS and PLMW in healthy subjects as a function of age: prevalence and interval distribution. Sleep 29:1183–7.

47. Happe S, Pirker W, Klosch G, Sauter C, Zeitlhofer J (2003) Periodic leg movements in patients with Parkinson's disease are associated with reduced striatal dopamine transporter binding. Journal of neurology 250:83–6.

48. Staedt J, Stoppe G, Kogler A, Munz D, Riemann H, Emrich D, Ruther E (1993) Dopamine D2 receptor alteration in patients with periodic movements in sleep (nocturnal myoclonus). J Neural Transm Gen Sect 93:71–4.

49. Staedt J, Stoppe G, Kogler A, Riemann H, Hajak G, Munz DL, Emrich D, Ruther E (1995) Nocturnal myoclonus syndrome (periodic movements in sleep) related to central dopamine D2-receptor alteration. Eur Arch Psychiatry Clin Neurosci 245:8–10.

50. Staedt J, Stoppe G, Kogler A, Riemann H, Hajak G, Munz DL, Emrich D, Ruther E (1995) Single photon emission tomography (SPET) imaging of dopamine D2 receptors in the course of dopamine replacement therapy in patients with nocturnal myoclonus syndrome (NMS). J Neural Transm Gen Sect 99:187–93.

51. Zadra A, Pilon M, Joncas S, Rompre S, Montplaisir J (2004) Analysis of postarousal EEG activity during somnambulistic episodes. J Sleep Res 13:279–84.

52. Terzaghi M, Sartori I, Tassi L, Didato G, Rustioni V, LoRusso G, Manni R, Nobili L

(2009) Evidence of dissociated arousal states during NREM parasomnia from an intracerebral neurophysiological study. Sleep 32:409–12.

53. Bassetti C, Vella S, Donati F, Wielepp P, Weder B (2000) SPECT during sleepwalking. Lancet 356:484–5.

54. Boeve BF (2010) REM sleep behavior disorder: Updated review of the core features, the REM sleep behavior disorder-neurodegenerative disease association, evolving concepts, controversies, and future directions. Ann N Y Acad Sci 1184:15–54.

55. Iranzo A, Ratti PL, Casanova-Molla J, Serradell M, Vilaseca I, Santamaria J (2009) Excessive muscle activity increases over time in idiopathic REM sleep behavior disorder. Sleep 32:1149–53.

56. Schenck CH, Mahowald MW (2002) REM sleep behavior disorder: clinical, developmental, and neuroscience perspectives 16 years after its formal identification in SLEEP. Sleep 25:120–38.

57. Iranzo A, Molinuevo JL, Santamaria J, Serradell M, Marti MJ, Valldeoriola F, Tolosa E (2006) Rapid-eye-movement sleep behaviour disorder as an early marker for a neurodegenerative disorder: a descriptive study. Lancet Neurol 5:572–7.

58. Iranzo A, Aparicio J (2009) A lesson from anatomy: focal brain lesions causing REM sleep behavior disorder. Sleep medicine 10:9–12.

59. Gagnon JF, Postuma RB, Montplaisir JY (2009) [Neurodegenerative disorder in idiopathic REM sleep behaviour disorder]. Med Sci (Paris) 25:782–3.

60. Lu J, Sherman D, Devor M, Saper CB (2006) A putative flip-flop switch for control of REM sleep. Nature 441:589–94.

61. Boeve BF, Silber MH, Saper CB, Ferman TJ, Dickson DW, Parisi JE, Benarroch EE, Ahlskog JE, Smith GE, Caselli RC, Tippman-Peikert M, Olson EJ, Lin SC, Young T, Wszolek Z, Schenck CH, Mahowald MW, Castillo PR, Del Tredici K, Braak H (2007) Pathophysiology of REM sleep behaviour disorder and relevance to neurodegenerative disease. Brain 130:2770–88.

62. Culebras A, Moore JT (1989) Magnetic resonance findings in REM sleep behavior disorder. Neurology 39:1519–23.

63. Kimura K, Tachibana N, Kohyama J, Otsuka Y, Fukazawa S, Waki R (2000) A discrete pontine ischemic lesion could cause REM sleep behavior disorder. Neurology 55:894–5.

64. Xi Z, Luning W (2009) REM sleep behavior disorder in a patient with pontine stroke. Sleep medicine 10(1):143–6.

65. Provini F, Vetrugno R, Pastorelli F, Lombardi C, Plazzi G, Marliani AF, Lugaresi E, Montagna P (2004) Status dissociatus after surgery for tegmental ponto-mesencephalic cavernoma: a state-dependent disorder of motor control during sleep. Mov Disord 19:719–23.

66. Zambelis T, Paparrigopoulos T, Soldatos CR (2002) REM sleep behaviour disorder associated with a neurinoma of the left pontocerebellar angle. J Neurol Neurosurg Psychiatry 72:821–2.

67. Plazzi G, Montagna P (2002) Remitting REM sleep behavior disorder as the initial sign of multiple sclerosis. Sleep medicine 3:437–9.

68. Tippmann-Peikert M, Boeve BF, Keegan BM (2006) REM sleep behavior disorder initiated by acute brainstem multiple sclerosis. Neurology 66:1277–9.

69. Gomez-Choco MJ, Iranzo A, Blanco Y, Graus F, Santamaria J, Saiz A (2007) Prevalence of restless legs syndrome and REM sleep behavior disorder in multiple sclerosis. Mult Scler 13:805–8.

70. Limousin N, Dehais C, Gout O, Heran F, Oudiette D, Arnulf I (2009) A brainstem inflammatory lesion causing REM sleep behavior disorder and sleepwalking (parasomnia overlap disorder). Sleep medicine 10:1059–62.

71. Ellmore TM, Hood AJ, Castriotta RJ, Stimming EF, Bick RJ, Schiess MC (2010) Reduced volume of the putamen in REM sleep behavior disorder patients. Parkinsonism Relat Disord 16:645–9.

72. Unger MM, Belke M, Menzler K, Heverhagen JT, Keil B, Stiasny-Kolster K, Rosenow F, Diederich NJ, Mayer G, Moller JC, Oertel WH, Knake S (2010) Diffusion tensor imaging in idiopathic REM sleep behavior disorder reveals microstructural changes in the brainstem, substantia nigra, olfactory region, and other brain regions. Sleep 33:767–73.

73. Scherfler C, Frauscher B, Schocke M, Iranzo A, Gschliesser V, Seppi K, Santamaria J, Tolosa E, Hogl B, Poewe W (2011) White and gray matter abnormalities in idiopathic rapid eye movement sleep behavior disorder: a

diffusion-tensor imaging and voxel-based morphometry study. Ann Neurol 69:400–7.

74. Mazza S, Soucy JP, Gravel P, Michaud M, Postuma R, Massicotte-Marquez J, Decary A, Montplaisir J (2006) Assessing whole brain perfusion changes in patients with REM sleep behavior disorder. Neurology 67:1618–22.

75. Imon Y, Matsuda H, Ogawa M, Kogure D, Sunohara N (1999) SPECT image analysis using statistical parametric mapping in patients with Parkinson's disease. Journal of nuclear medicine: official publication, Society of Nuclear Medicine 40:1583–9.

76. Miyamoto M, Miyamoto T, Kubo J, Yokota N, Hirata K, Sato T (2000) Brainstem function in rapid eye movement sleep behavior disorder: the evaluation of brainstem function by proton MR spectroscopy (1H-MRS). Psychiatry and clinical neurosciences 54:350–1.

77. Michaelis T, Merboldt KD, Bruhn H, Hanicke W, Frahm J (1993) Absolute concentrations of metabolites in the adult human brain in vivo: quantification of localized proton MR spectra. Radiology 187:219–27.

78. Iranzo A, Santamaria J, Pujol J, Moreno A, Deus J, Tolosa E (2002) Brainstem proton magnetic resonance spectroscopy in idiopathic REM sleep behavior disorder. Sleep 25:867–70.

79. Hanoglu L, Ozer F, Meral H, Dincer A (2006) Brainstem 1H-MR spectroscopy in patients with Parkinson's disease with REM sleep behavior disorder and IPD patients without dream enactment behavior. Clin Neurol Neurosurg 108:129–34.

80. Becker G, Seufert J, Bogdahn U, Reichmann H, Reiners K (1995) Degeneration of substantia nigra in chronic Parkinson's disease visualized by transcranial color-coded real-time sonography. Neurology 45:182–4.

81. Unger MM, Moller JC, Stiasny-Kolster K, Mankel K, Berg D, Walter U, Hoeffken H, Mayer G, Oertel WH (2008) Assessment of idiopathic rapid-eye-movement sleep behavior disorder by transcranial sonography, olfactory function test, and FP-CIT-SPECT. Mov Disord 23:596–9.

82. Iwanami M, Miyamoto T, Miyamoto M, Hirata K, Takada E (2010) Relevance of substantia nigra hyperechogenicity and reduced odor identification in idiopathic REM sleep behavior disorder. Sleep medicine 11:361–5.

83. Stockner H, Iranzo A, Seppi K, Serradell M, Gschliesser V, Sojer M, Valldeoriola F, Molinuevo JL, Frauscher B, Schmidauer C, Santamaria J, Hogl B, Tolosa E, Poewe W (2009) Midbrain hyperechogenicity in idiopathic REM sleep behavior disorder. Mov Disord 24:1906–9.

84. Iranzo A, Lomena F, Stockner H, Valldeoriola F, Vilaseca I, Salamero M, Molinuevo JL, Serradell M, Duch J, Pavia J, Gallego J, Seppi K, Hogl B, Tolosa E, Poewe W, Santamaria J (2010) Decreased striatal dopamine transporter uptake and substantia nigra hyperechogenicity as risk markers of synucleinopathy in patients with idiopathic rapid-eye-movement sleep behaviour disorder: a prospective study [corrected]. Lancet Neurol 9:1070–7.

85. Shirakawa S, Takeuchi N, Uchimura N, Ohyama T, Maeda H, Abe T, Ishibashi M, Ohshima Y, Ohshima H (2002) Study of image findings in rapid eye movement sleep behavioural disorder. Psychiatry Clin Neurosci 56:291–2.

86. Vendette M, Gagnon JF, Soucy JP, Gosselin N, Postuma RB, Tuineag M, Godin I, Montplaisir J (2011) Brain perfusion and markers of neurodegeneration in rapid eye movement sleep behavior disorder. Mov Disord 26:1717–24.

87. Dang Vu, T. T., Gagnon, J. F., Vendette, M., Soucy, J. P., Postuma, R., & Montplaisir, J. (2012). Hippocampal perfusion predicts impending neurodegeneration in REM sleep behavior disorder. Neurology, 79(24):2302–6.

88. Postuma, R. B., Gagnon, J. F., Vendette, M., Desjardins, C., & Montplaisir, J. Y. (2011). Olfaction and color vision identify impending neurodegeneration in rapid eye movement sleep behavior disorder. Annals of neurology, 69(5), 811–818, doi:10.1002/ana.22282.

89. Postuma, R. B., Lang, A. E., Gagnon, J. F., Pelletier, A., & Montplaisir, J. Y. (2012). How does parkinsonism start? Prodromal parkinsonism motor changes in idiopathic REM sleep behaviour disorder. Brain : a journal of neurology, 135(Pt 6), 1860–1870, doi:10.1093/brain/aws093.

90. Hanyu H, Inoue Y, Sakurai H, Kanetaka H, Nakamura M, Miyamoto T, Sasai T, Iwamoto T (2011) Regional cerebral blood flow changes in patients with idiopathic REM sleep behavior disorder. Eur J Neurol 18(5):784–8.

91. Caselli RJ, Chen K, Bandy D, Smilovici O, Boeve BF, Osborne D, Alexander GE,

Parish JM, Krahn LE, Reiman EM (2006) A preliminary fluorodeoxyglucose positron emission tomography study in healthy adults reporting dream-enactment behavior. Sleep 29:927–33.

92. Fujishiro H, Iseki E, Murayama N, Yamamoto R, Higashi S, Kasanuki K, Suzuki M, Arai H, Sato K (2010) Diffuse occipital hypometabolism on [18 F]-FDG PET scans in patients with idiopathic REM sleep behavior disorder: prodromal dementia with Lewy bodies? Psychogeriatrics 10:144–52.

93. Dauvilliers Y, Boudousq V, Lopez R, Gabelle A, Cochen De Cock V, Bayard S, Peigneux P (2011) Increased perfusion in supplementary motor area during a REM sleep behaviour episode. Sleep medicine 12:531–2.

94. Eisensehr I, Linke R, Noachtar S, Schwarz J, Gildehaus FJ, Tatsch K (2000) Reduced striatal dopamine transporters in idiopathic rapid eye movement sleep behaviour disorder. Comparison with Parkinson's disease and controls. Brain 123 (Pt 6):1155–60.

95. Eisensehr I, Linke R, Tatsch K, Kharraz B, Gildehaus JF, Wetter CT, Trenkwalder C, Schwarz J, Noachtar S (2003) Increased muscle activity during rapid eye movement sleep correlates with decrease of striatal presynaptic dopamine transporters. IPT and IBZM SPECT imaging in subclinical and clinically manifest idiopathic REM sleep behavior disorder, Parkinson's disease, and controls. Sleep 26:507–12.

96. Albin RL, Koeppe RA, Chervin RD, Consens FB, Wernette K, Frey KA, Aldrich MS (2000) Decreased striatal dopaminergic innervation in REM sleep behavior disorder. Neurology 55:1410–12.

97. Gilman S, Koeppe RA, Chervin RD, Consens FB, Little R, An H, Junck L, Heumann M (2003) REM sleep behavior disorder is related to striatal monoaminergic deficit in MSA. Neurology 61:29–34.

98. Stiasny-Kolster K, Doerr Y, Moller JC, Hoffken H, Behr TM, Oertel WH, Mayer G (2005) Combination of "idiopathic" REM sleep behaviour disorder and olfactory dysfunction as possible indicator for alpha-synucleinopathy demonstrated by dopamine transporter FP-CIT-SPECT. Brain 128:126–37.

99. Kim YK, Yoon IY, Kim JM, Jeong SH, Kim KW, Shin YK, Kim BS, Kim SE (2010) The implication of nigrostriatal dopaminergic degeneration in the pathogenesis of REM sleep behavior disorder. Eur J Neurol 17:487–92.

100. Miyamoto T, Orimo S, Miyamoto M, Hirata K, Adachi T, Hattori R, Suzuki M, Ishii K (2010) Follow-up PET studies in case of idiopathic REM sleep behavior disorder. Sleep medicine 11:100–1.

101. Iranzo, A., Valldeoriola, F., Lomena, F., Molinuevo, J. L., Serradell, M., Salamero, M., et al. (2011). Serial dopamine transporter imaging of nigrostriatal function in patients with idiopathic rapid-eye-movement sleep behaviour disorder: a prospective study. Lancet Neurology, 10(9), 797–805. doi:10.1016/S1474-4422(11)70152-1.

102. Lugaresi E, Medori R, Montagna P, Baruzzi A, Cortelli P, Lugaresi A, Tinuper P, Zucconi M, Gambetti P (1986) Fatal familial insomnia and dysautonomia with selective degeneration of thalamic nuclei. N Engl J Med 315:997–1003.

103. Montagna P, Gambetti P, Cortelli P, Lugaresi E (2003) Familial and sporadic fatal insomnia. Lancet Neurol 2:167–76.

104. Perani D, Cortelli P, Lucignani G, Montagna P, Tinuper P, Gallassi R, Gambetti P, Lenzi GL, Lugaresi E, Fazio F (1993) [18F]FDG PET in fatal familial insomnia: the functional effects of thalamic lesions. Neurology 43:2565–9.

105. Cortelli P, Perani D, Parchi P, Grassi F, Montagna P, De Martin M, Castellani R, Tinuper P, Gambetti P, Lugaresi E, Fazio F (1997) Cerebral metabolism in fatal familial insomnia: relation to duration, neuropathology, and distribution of protease-resistant prion protein. Neurology 49:126–33.

106. Bar KJ, Hager F, Nenadic I, Opfermann T, Brodhun M, Tauber RF, Patt S, Schulz-Schaeffer W, Gottschild D, Sauer H (2002) Serial positron emission tomographic findings in an atypical presentation of fatal familial insomnia. Arch Neurol 59:1815–18.

107. Cortelli P, Perani D, Montagna P, Gallassi R, Tinuper P, Provini F, Avoni P, Ferrillo F, Anchisi D, Moresco RM, Fazio F, Parchi P, Baruzzi A, Lugaresi E, Gambetti P (2006) Pre-symptomatic diagnosis in fatal familial insomnia: serial neurophysiological and 18FDG-PET studies. Brain 129:668–75.

108. Steriade M, McCormick DA, Sejnowski TJ (1993b) Thalamocortical oscillations in the sleeping and aroused brain. Science 262:679–85.

109. Kloppel S, Pirker W, Brucke T, Kovacs GG, Almer G (2002) Beta-CIT SPECT demonstrates reduced availability of serotonin transporters in patients with Fatal Familial Insomnia. J Neural Transm 109:1105–10.

110. Provini F, Plazzi G, Tinuper P, Vandi S, Lugaresi E, Montagna P (1999) Nocturnal frontal lobe epilepsy. A clinical and polygraphic overview of 100 consecutive cases. Brain: a journal of neurology 122 (Pt 6):1017–31.

111. Tinuper P, Provini F, Bisulli F, Vignatelli L, Plazzi G, Vetrugno R, Montagna P, Lugaresi E (2007) Movement disorders in sleep: guidelines for differentiating epileptic from non-epileptic motor phenomena arising from sleep. Sleep medicine reviews 11:255–67.

112. Vetrugno R, Mascalchi M, Vella A, Della Nave R, Provini F, Plazzi G, Volterrani D, Bertelli P, Vattimo A, Lugaresi E, Montagna P (2005) Paroxysmal arousal in epilepsy associated with cingulate hyperperfusion. Neurology 64:356–8.

113. Tassinari CA, Rubboli G, Gardella E, Cantalupo G, Calandra-Buonaura G, Vedovello M, Alessandria M, Gandini G, Cinotti S, Zamponi N, Meletti S (2005) Central pattern generators for a common semiology in fronto-limbic seizures and in parasomnias. A neuroethologic approach. Neurol Sci 26 Suppl 3:s225–32.

114. Schindler K, Gast H, Bassetti C, Wiest R, Fritschi J, Meyer K, Kollar M, Wissmeyer M, Lovblad K, Weder B, Donati F (2001) Hyperperfusion of anterior cingulate gyrus in a case of paroxysmal nocturnal dystonia. Neurology 57:917–20.

115. Cho YW, Motamedi GK, Laufenberg I, Sohn SI, Lim JG, Lee H, Yi SD, Lee JH, Kim DK, Reba R, Gaillard WD, Theodore WH, Lesser RP, Steinlein OK (2003) A Korean kindred with autosomal dominant nocturnal frontal lobe epilepsy and mental retardation. Arch Neurol 60:1625–32.

116. Hayman M, Scheffer IE, Chinvarun Y, Berlangieri SU, Berkovic SF (1997) Autosomal dominant nocturnal frontal lobe epilepsy: demonstration of focal frontal onset and intrafamilial variation. Neurology 49:969–75.

117. Picard F, Bruel D, Servent D, Saba W, Fruchart-Gaillard C, Schollhorn-Peyronneau MA, Roumenov D, Brodtkorb E, Zuberi S, Gambardella A, Steinborn B, Hufnagel A, Valette H, Bottlaender M (2006) Alteration of the in vivo nicotinic receptor density in ADNFLE patients: a PET study. Brain: a journal of neurology 129:2047–60.

118. Gelisse P, Corda D, Raybaud C, Dravet C, Bureau M, Genton P (2003) Abnormal neuroimaging in patients with benign epilepsy with centrotemporal spikes. Epilepsia 44:372–8.

119. Sarkis R, Wyllie E, Burgess RC, Loddenkemper T (2010) Neuroimaging findings in children with benign focal epileptiform discharges. Epilepsy research 90:91–8.

120. Hirsch E, Valenti MP, Rudolf G, Seegmuller C, de Saint Martin A, Maquet P, Wioland N, Metz-Lutz MN, Marescaux C, Arzimanoglou A (2006) Landau-Kleffner syndrome is not an eponymic badge of ignorance. Epilepsy research 70 Suppl 1:S239–47.

121. Pearl PL, Carrazana EJ, Holmes GL (2001) The Landau-Kleffner Syndrome. Epilepsy Curr 1:39–45.

122. Smith MC, Hoeppner TJ (2003) Epileptic encephalopathy of late childhood: Landau-Kleffner syndrome and the syndrome of continuous spikes and waves during slow-wave sleep. J Clin Neurophysiol 20:462–72.

123. Hirsch E, Marescaux C, Maquet P, Metz-Lutz MN, Kiesmann M, Salmon E, Franck G, Kurtz D (1990) Landau-Kleffner syndrome: a clinical and EEG study of five cases. Epilepsia 31:756–67.

124. Marescaux C, Hirsch E, Finck S, Maquet P, Schlumberger E, Sellal F, Metz-Lutz MN, Alembik Y, Salmon E, Franck G (1990) Landau-Kleffner syndrome: a pharmacologic study of five cases. Epilepsia 31: 768–77.

125. Cole AJ, Andermann F, Taylor L, Olivier A, Rasmussen T, Robitaille Y, Spire JP (1988) The Landau-Kleffner syndrome of acquired epileptic aphasia: unusual clinical outcome, surgical experience, and absence of encephalitis. Neurology 38:31–8.

126. Maquet P, Hirsch E, Dive D, Salmon E, Marescaux C, Franck G (1990) Cerebral glucose utilization during sleep in Landau-Kleffner syndrome: a PET study. Epilepsia 31:778–83.

127. Rintahaka PJ, Chugani HT, Sankar R (1995) Landau-Kleffner syndrome with continuous

spikes and waves during slow-wave sleep. J Child Neurol 10:127–33.

128. da Silva EA, Chugani DC, Muzik O, Chugani HT (1997) Landau-Kleffner syndrome: metabolic abnormalities in temporal lobe are a common feature. J Child Neurol 12:489–95.

129. O'Tuama LA, Urion DK, Janicek MJ, Treves ST, Bjornson B, Moriarty JM (1992) Regional cerebral perfusion in Landau-Kleffner syndrome and related childhood aphasias. J Nucl Med 33:1758–65.

130. Mouridsen SE, Videbaek C, Sogaard H, Andersen AR (1993) Regional cerebral blood-flow measured by HMPAO and SPECT in a 5-year-old boy with Landau-Kleffner syndrome. Neuropediatrics 24:47–50.

131. Park YD, Hoffman JM, Radtke RA, DeLong GR (1994) Focal cerebral metabolic abnormality in a patient with continuous spike waves during slow-wave sleep. J Child Neurol 9:139–43.

132. Guerreiro MM, Camargo EE, Kato M, Menezes Netto JR, Silva EA, Scotoni AE, Silveira DC, Guerreiro CA (1996) Brain single photon emission computed tomography imaging in Landau-Kleffner syndrome. Epilepsia 37:60–7.

133. Harbord MG, Singh R, Morony S (1999) SPECT abnormalities in Landau-Kleffner syndrome. J Clin Neurosci 6:9–16.

134. Sayit E, Dirik E, Durak H, Uzuner N, Anal O, Cevik NT (1999) Landau-Kleffner syndrome: relation of clinical, EEG and Tc-99m-HMPAO brain SPECT findings and improvement in EEG after treatment. Ann Nucl Med 13:415–18.

135. Raybarman C (2002) Landau-Kleffner syndrome: a case report. Neurol India 50:212–13.

136. Hu SX, Wu XR, Lin C, Hao SY (1989) Landau-Kleffner syndrome with unilateral EEG abnormalities—two cases from Beijing, China. Brain Dev 11:420–2.

137. Maquet P, Hirsch E, Metz-Lutz MN, Motte J, Dive D, Marescaux C, Franck G (1995) Regional cerebral glucose metabolism in children with deterioration of one or more cognitive functions and continuous spike-and-wave discharges during sleep. Brain: a journal of neurology 118 (Pt 6):1497–520.

138. De Tiege X, Goldman S, Laureys S, Verheulpen D, Chiron C, Wetzburger C, Paquier P, Chaigne D, Poznanski N, Jambaque I, Hirsch E, Dulac O, Van Bogaert P (2004) Regional cerebral glucose metabolism in epilepsies with continuous spikes and waves during sleep. Neurology 63:853–7.

139. Steriade M, Contreras D, Curro Dossi R, Nunez A (1993a) The slow (< 1 Hz) oscillation in reticular thalamic and thalamocortical neurons: scenario of sleep rhythm generation in interacting thalamic and neocortical networks. J Neurosci 13:3284–99.

20

Autonomic Evaluation in Sleep-Related Movement Disorders

PAOLA A. LANFRANCHI, MARIE-HELENE PENNESTRI,
RONALD B. POSTUMA, AND JACQUES Y. MONTPLAISIR

THE AUTONOMIC nervous system (ANS) is a highly integrated system, with centers located in the spinal cord, brainstem, hypothalamus, and the limbic cortex. This network is broadly divided into two anatomically distinct efferent operating components, the sympathetic system (SNS) and the parasympathetic system (PNS). Both the SNS and PNS consist of a two-neuron chain, divided into pre- and postganglionic parts. Acetylcholine is released by all the preganglionic neurons, and postganglionic parasympathetic neurons, while postganglionic sympathetic neurons release norepinephrine. The exception is the release of acetylcholine by sympathetic stimulation of sweat glands.

The preganglionic neurons of the SNS are located in the lateral horn of the gray matter spanning from levels T1 to L1 of the spinal cord, termed the intermediolateral cell column. The myelinated axons of the preganglionic neurons synapse with the paravertebral ganglia located lateral to the spinal cord in a collection known as the truncus sympathicus. The axons of the postganglionic neurons travel to target organs.

The PNS consists of two parts: the cranial portion in the brainstem (cranial nerves III, VII, IX, and X) and the sacral portion in the spinal cord at levels S2 to S4 in the intermediolateral cell column. Distinctive from the SNS, the parasympathetic postganglionic neurons form ganglia located near the target organ. Depending upon the target organ, sympathetic and parasympathetic stimulation can elicit either excitatory or inhibitory effects.

The cardiovascular autonomic nervous system is a highly integrated network that controls visceral functions. On a short timescale (seconds to hours) it adjusts the circulation in keeping with behavior, the environment, and emotions. In the longer term, this neural circulatory regulation appears to be coupled with the circadian rhythm, the wake-sleep cycle, and some ultradian rhythms, including non-REM-REM sleep processes, as well as hormones implicated in long-term blood pressure (BP) regulation.

The primary role of the cardiovascular autonomic nervous system is to ensure an adequate cardiac output to the vital organs through continuous and rapid adjustments of heart rate (HR), arterial BP, and redistribution of blood flow. Neural control of the circulation operates via parasympathetic neurons to the heart, and sympathetic neuronal efferents to the heart, blood vessels, kidneys, and adrenal medulla.

Autonomic impulses to the vasculature and heart originate from the vasomotor center in the brainstem, located bilaterally in the reticular substance of the medulla and pons.

The vasomotor center is in turn modulated by higher nervous system regions in the pons, mesencephalon, and diencephalon, including the hypothalamus and many portions of the cerebral cortex.

Finally, neurons from the reticular formation of the common brainstem system (CBS) are implicated in the regulation and coordination of several systems such as cardiovascular, respiratory, vigilance, and motor systems. The CBS, which receives somatosensory, visceral, and higher brain structure afferences, is modulated by the baroreceptor activation and excited by the chemoreceptor activation, and it influences peripheral somatic and autonomic response and synchronizes them with higher brain structures.

ASSESSMENT OF AUTONOMIC FUNCTION IN CLINICAL AND RESEARCH SETTINGS: COMMON TECHNIQUES AND THEIR PHYSIOLOGICAL SIGNIFICANCE

Techniques to evaluate autonomic function are numerous, but only a limited number are considered well established and suitable for routine clinical application.[1,2] Table 20.1 describes standardized recommended testing commonly used in the assessment of autonomic function either in a clinical or research setting and the type of sleep-related movement disorders in which they have been employed. A more detailed description is herein provided on tests or techniques employed in the autonomic assessment of sleep-related movement disorders.

The most established, reliable, and easy to perform are tests based on HR and BP responses to endogenous or exogenous challenges, for instance, in response to respiratory changes, postural changes, or mental or physical stress.

Spectral analysis techniques are also widely used in research in the quantification of spontaneous oscillatory components of HR and BP variability and their variation in relationship with different states, such as, for instance, supine and standing, mental stress, and sleep stages.

Parasympathetic Tests

Three simple tests evaluate cardiovagal function. They have high sensitivity, are valuable, and are safe.

CYCLIC DEEP BREATHING

In this test both afferent and efferent pathways are vagally mediated and blunted by anticholinergic agents. The effect is maximal with 6 breaths per minute (1 cycle every 10 seconds). The simplest measure considers the average of Expiration- Inspiration difference (E-I) or Expiration- Inspiration ratio (E/I) between the highest and the lowest HR or R-R interval within each breathing cycle. E-I HR responses <10 bpm are usually considered abnormal.[3] However, HR changes during deep breathing vary considerably with age, with highest values in young individuals (median E-I = 30 bpm) and lowest after the age of 70 (median E-I = 12 bpm).[4] Other more complex analytic techniques partially adjust for confounding factors, such as resting HR and HR drift during the test.

VALSALVA RATIO

The Valsalva maneuver is a complex test of both cardiovagal and sympathetic reflex response to a transient decrease in venous return to the heart.[1] Traditionally it is used to assess HR responses: the ratio between the maximal HR to minimal HR is regarded as an index of cardiovagal control. Normative values are well established (normal values ≥ 1.21)[3] and slightly decline with age.[4] Currently, the use of beat-to-beat noninvasive BP monitoring across the maneuver also provides a measure of the integrity of sympathetic vasoconstrictor activity.[5]

HEART RATE RESPONSE TO STANDING

Transition from the sitting to the standing position forces the cardiovascular system to adapt to gravity and the subsequent hemodynamic downward shift, translating in lowering of systolic BP (SBP). Consequently, standing initiates a coordinated sequence of reflexes to maintain BP and therefore cerebral perfusion. Response to orthostatic stress can be assessed by active standing or passive head-up tilt.

Responses to standing have been reviewed by several authors.[1] The short-term circulatory responses to active standing have been subdivided into two phases: an initial phase (first 30 seconds) and an early steady-state response (after 1–2 minutes standing); prolonged standing is defined as at least 5 minutes upright. In healthy subjects the initial response to active standing is an abrupt increase in heart rate (occurring at around 15 seconds) followed by a bradycardia (around 30 seconds). The magnitude of this HR change decreases with age. The ratio between the longest RR interval (occurring around the 30th heart beat after standing) and the shortest RR interval (occurring around the 15th heart beat) is regarded as an index of cardiovagal function (normal values ≥ 1.04).[3]

Assessment of Sympathetic Activity

Sympathetic activity is critical for thermoregulation (through vasomotor and sudomotor innervation) and arterial BP control. A number of techniques have been developed throughout the years to evaluate sympathetic activity in humans.[6] Some can be presently regarded as unreliable or almost obsolete, while others represent the most valuable tools so far available to assess adrenergic drive to the heart and peripheral circulation. Sympathetic outflow is functionally heterogeneous and does not discharge massively, but rather it produces a patterned control on specific organs. Thus, in normal conditions, there is not a generalized sympathetic tone, but there is coordinated activity of a specific subset of sympathetic neurons. The expression of patterned autonomic responses reflects the activity of spatially segregated and functionally related sympathetic preganglionic neurons located in T-1 to L-2 segments of the intermedio-lateral cell column.

Cardiovascular adrenergic activation has been inferred in the past from the evaluation of the pressor and tachycardic responses to standardized stressful stimuli, such as in response to standing, or other stressors such as the cold pressor test, isometric exercise, and mental stress. As a limitation to be considered, an "abnormal" pressor response to stress maneuvers may be secondary to abnormalities in vessel wall composition

and structure (for example, in hypertension, arteriolar or arterial hypertrophy), which may amplify the vasoconstrictor effects of a given stimulus, rather than being due primarily to augmented adrenergic nerve firing.

BLOOD PRESSURE RESPONSE TO ORTHOSTATIC POSITION

BP response to standing, either active standing or head-up tilt, is an established test to assess adrenergic function and is an essential part of any evaluation in patients suspected of adrenergic failure. Orthostatic hypotension during active standing is defined as a persistent decrease in SBP of more than 20 mmHg or DBP of 5 mmHg within 3 minutes of change from the supine into standing position.[2]

The response to passive standing (head-up tilt) is especially helpful in the assessment of the dynamic of postural failure and syncope, but it is also widely used in research to assess spectral analysis of HR and BP variability in response to sustained orthostatic stimulus.

TESTS OF SUDOMOTOR FUNCTION

Thermal homeostasis is a complex process that relies on both sweating and vasomotor control for heat elimination or heat production and conservation. Several tests have been used for years in the assessment of peripheral polyneuropathies (Table 20.1).[1] The sympathetic skin response is the most widely used test and is usually measured at the palm and sole in response to a variety of arousal stimuli, including electric shock, cough, startle, deep breathing, and mental stress, to name a few. This response relies on a highly complex multisynaptic reflex with sudomotor activity as final arm. The precise mechanisms are not well defined, but they probably implicate different central generators likely located in orbitofrontal cortex, posterior hypothalamus, and brainstem.

MICRONEUROGRAPHIC RECORDING OF SYMPATHETIC NERVE ACTIVITY

Microneurography provides direct information on regional postganglionic sympathetic vasomotor and sudomotor activity to muscle and skin. Muscle sympathetic nerve activity (MSNA), usually measured at the peroneal nerve, induces vasoconstriction and is modulated by the baroreflex.[7] MSNA also increases in

Table 20.1 Selected Tests of Autonomic Function

TEST OF AUTONOMIC FUNCTIONS	SLEEP MOTOR DISORDERS
HR and HRV	
HR variability to cyclic deep breathing	RBD, RLS, narcolepsy, bruxism
HR response to the Valsalva maneuver (Valsalva ratio)	RBD, RLS, narcolepsy, bruxism
HR response to standing (30:15 ratio)	RBD, RLS, narcolepsy, bruxism
Spectral analysis of HR variability (frequency domain)	
At rest	RBD, RLS, narcolepsy, bruxism
During sleep	RBD, RLS, narcolepsy, bruxism
Response to tilt	Narcolepsy
BP	
BP response to the Valsalva maneuver (Phases IV and late phase II)	—
BP response to orthostatic stress	
Active standing	Narcolepsy, bruxism
Passive standing (head-up tilt)	RBD, RLS, narcolepsy
Sustained handgrip test	Narcolepsy
Others	
Plasma catecholamine levels (supine/standing)	Bruxism
Microneurography (muscle sympathetic nerve activity)	Narcolepsy (during cataplexy)
Mental stress tests	—
Cold pressure test	Narcolepsy
Spectral analysis of BP variability	—
Cardiac fluorodopamine PET scanning	—
Cardiac[123] MIBG SPECT scanning	RBD
Sympathetic skin response (SSR)	RLS, narcolepsy (during cataplexy)
Quantitative sudomotor axon reflex test (QSART)	—
Thermoregulatory sweat test (TST)	—

BP, blood pressure; HR, heart rate; HRV, heart rate variability; RBD, REM behavior disorder; RLS, restless legs syndrome; PET, positron emission tomography; SPECT, single-photon emission computed tomography.

response to hypoxic and hypercapnic chemoreceptor stimulation.[8] Skin sympathetic nerve activity (SSNA) reflects thermoregulatory output related to sudomotor and vasomotor activity and is affected by emotional stimuli but not by the baroreflex.

While microneurography provides a direct measure of peripheral sympathetic drive, it is invasive and technically demanding for both operator and patient. MSNA decreases during sleep as compared to wakefulness, and is higher during REM sleep as compared to non-REM sleep.[9]

CARDIAC NEUROIMAGING

Imaging methodologies of several types, involving both single-photon emission computed tomography (SPECT) and positron emission tomography (PET) have been applied to visualize the sympathetic innervations of human organs,[10-12] primarily the heart. Many autonomic tracers are available that mimic endogenous neurotransmitters and transporters and variably allow the assessment of presynaptic and postsynaptic sympathetic integrity of autonomic innervation.[123] MIBG SPECT imaging is the most widely used method to assess cardiac sympathetic function. [123]-MIBG is an analogue of norepinephrine with the same mechanisms of uptake, storage, and release, and it is retained at sympathetic endings. Decreased or absent [123]-MIBG accumulation can occur in the presence of denervation of postganglionic cardiac nerve, in diabetes, in cardiac disorders, and central nervous system disorders. [^{11}C]-hydroxyephedrine (HED) and 6-[^{18}F]fluorodopamine are the most widely used PET tracers.[12] [^{11}C]-hydroxyephedrine is used for cardiac neuronal imaging and allows the assessment of regional presynaptic sympathetic integrity of the heart, whereas 6-[^{18}F] fluorodopamine allows the assessment of both cardiac and extracardiac sympathetic innervation (mainly thyroid gland and kidneys).

Sympathetic denervation can be readily demonstrated with these imaging techniques in patients with pure autonomic failure, in subjects with heart transplantation, in subjects with Parkinson disease and REM behavior disorders.

SYSTEMIC CATECHOLAMINES

Measurements of plasma and urinary catecholamines (epinephrine and norepinephrine) provide an estimate of global sympathetic activity. The rate of overflow of noradrenaline is determined not only by the rate of noradrenaline release (and hence sympathetic nerve firing and sympathetic nerve density) but also by the activity of the competing disposition mechanisms of uptake, metabolism, and diffusional flow to the circulation. However, blood norepinephrine reflects only a small percentage (8%–10%) of neurotransmitter release during sympathetic activation. Moreover, the relatively rapid clearance of catecholamine from the bloodstream may limit the ability to detect transient changes in sympathetic activity. The measure of urinary excretion of catecholamine and their metabolites is a simpler approach to provide an estimate of the cumulative catecholamine secretion over time and has been used widely in the clinical and sleep research settings. Systemic epinephrine and norepinephrine physiologically decrease with nocturnal sleep,[13,14] but they may persist high in the presence of insomnia and sleep deprivation.[15,16] Urinary catecholamine has been assessed in sleep bruxism.[17]

Spectral Analysis of Heart Rate and Blood Pressure Variabilities

Spectral analysis of RR and BP variability is the most extensively used tool to assess cardiovascular autonomic regulation. It provides an estimate on the variance of RR and BP variabilities as a function of frequency. In the short period, that is, in a frequency range between 0 and 0.5 Hz, RR and BP manifest oscillations that appear to be under the influence of intrinsic autonomic rhythms and of respiratory inputs.[18] Indeed, RR and BP variability appear to be organized in three major components, the high-frequency (HF) (>0.15 Hz) respiratory band, the low-frequency band (LF) (around 0.1 Hz), and the very low-frequency band (VLF) (0.003–0.039 Hz). The HF components of RR variability primarily reflect the respiration-driven modulation of sinus rhythm, evident as sinus arrhythmia, and have been used as an index of tonic vagal drive. Nonneural mechanical mechanisms, linked to respiratory fluctuations in cardiac transmural pressure, atrial stretch, and venous return, are also determinants of HF power and may become especially important after cardiac denervation such as heart transplantation.[19] The LF rhythm, which appears to have a widespread neural genesis,[20] is believed to reflect in part the sympathetic modulation of the heart,[21] as well as the baroreflex responsiveness to the beat-to beat variations in arterial BP,[22] but it can also be modulated by low-frequency or irregular breathing patterns. The LF/HF ratio is used to provide an index of the sympathovagal balance on the sinus node,[23] providing measurements are obtained in strictly controlled conditions. Finally, the VLF has been hypothesized to reflect thermoregulation and the renin-angiotensin system.[24] Regarding BP variability, LF components in systolic BP variability are considered an index of efferent sympathetic vascular modulation, whereas the HF components reflect mechanical effects of respiration on BP changes.[21]

Although sensitivity and specificity of the powers expressed in these LF and HF components in the spectra are not always optimal in quantifying the sympathetic and parasympathetic tone, given that other mechanisms may be implicated in these fluctuations, the informative content that they provide remains high when they are coupled with information from other biological systems (including the sleep-wake cycle, sleep stages, steady sympathetic challenge) and when assessing the integrity of autonomic modulation in various study population. For example, spectral analysis of RR variability has consistently revealed that, in normal subjects, different rhythms dominate in non-REM and REM sleep: a shift toward HF components of R-R variability characterizes non-REM sleep, while the cardiovascular excitation and instability of REM sleep are reflected by a significant increase of the LF components.[25,26] This response has been shown to be absent in patients with REM behavior disorder[27] (Fig. 20.1).

More advanced algorithms of signal processing can be used to assess dynamic changes in autonomic cardiovascular control during transient events[28] and help define the temporal relationship between dynamic changes occurring in different systems, such as for instance encephalogram (EEG), electrocardiogram, and BP.[29–30] The most commonly used algorithms include Short Time Fourier Transform, Wigner-Ville distribution, Time Variant Autoregressive Models, Wavelets, and Wavelet-Packets.[28] These algorithms have been applied to assess the temporal relationship between autonomic, cortical, and motor response of periodic leg movements during sleep (PLMS).[30]

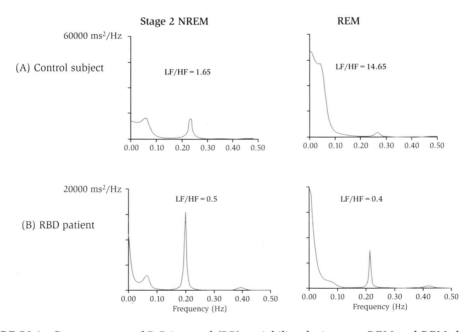

FIGURE 20.1 Power spectra of R-R interval (RR) variability during non-REM and REM sleep in a control subject (*A*) and in a patient with REM behavior disorder (RBD, *B*). Note the increase in LF power and hence LF/HF ratio from stage 2 non-REM to REM in the control, but note how strikingly similar are the LF/HF ratios between non-REM and REM sleep in the RBD patient.

ASSESSMENT OF AUTONOMIC FUNCTION IN SLEEP-RELATED MOTOR DISORDERS

Autonomic Responses Associated with Periodic Leg Movements

Periodic leg movements (PLMs) are described as a repetitive rhythmic extension of the big toe and dorsiflexion of the ankle, with occasional flexion at the knee and hip. PLMs can occur during wakefulness as well as during sleep (PLMS). PLMS recur frequently in several sleep disorders (such as restless legs syndrome,[31,32] narcolepsy,[32-34] REM sleep behavior disorder,[34-35] and sleep apnea[34,36,37]) and in patients with congestive heart failure[38] but are also a frequent finding in healthy, asymptomatic subjects especially with advancing age.[39]

The analyses of beat-to-beat changes in HR and BP changes associated with PLMS and their temporal relationship with EEG events have provided new insights into the physiological mechanisms of PLMS. Several studies showed that PLMS are associated with HR increase (tachycardia) followed by a HR decrease (bradycardia) and subsequent return to baseline level.[35,40,41] This is a sensitive measure, considering that these HR changes are present in 99% of PLMS[40] and are present in patients with PLMS such as RLS,[40,42] PLMD,[41] RBD,[35] narcolepsy,[43] and children with PLMS.[44] More recently, two studies using beat-to-beat noninvasive BP recording reported that PLMS are also associated with significant BP increments (~ 20 mmHg in systolic BP and ~ 10 mmHg in diastolic BP).[45,46] HR and BP changes are present regardless of whether the PLMS are associated with arousals. However, the magnitude of the cardiovascular response is greater when PLMS are associated with cortical arousals.[40,41,45,46] In addition, the amplitude of cardiovascular responses of PLMS is greater during sleep than that associated with spontaneous or simulated PLMS during wake.[41,45,47] These observations suggest that the intensity of cardiovascular response observed with PLMS is related to the degree of central brain activation (brainstem to cortical activation) which accompanies PLMS and much less to the somatomotor response (i.e., not a classical sensory-motor reflex).

Studies assessing the temporal relationship between the leg motor event and autonomic and cortical activation consistently reported that changes in HR and EEG activity precede by several seconds the leg movement.[40,45,48] Specifically, HR and EEG delta waves rise first, followed by motor activity and eventually progressive activation, of faster EEG frequencies (i.e., in the alpha, beta, and sigma frequencies). A recent study assessing the dynamic time course of RR variability changes and EEG changes in association with PLMS confirmed the LF components of RR variability to be the first physiological change to occur, followed by EEG changes in delta frequencies, and thereafter the leg movement with or without faster EEG frequencies.[30] These data corroborate an original hypothesis suggesting the presence of an integrative hierarchy of the arousal response primarily involving the autonomic responses with sympatho-excitation, then progressing toward EEG synchronization (represented by bursts of delta waves) and finally EEG desynchronization (arousal) and eventually awakening.[40] In this view, leg movements are part of the same periodic activation process that is responsible for cardiovascular and EEG changes during sleep.[48]

The measure of HR changes associated with PLMS could also represent a model providing information on the integrity of cardiovascular autonomic modulation in different physiological and clinical conditions (Fig. 20.2). For instance, ageing is one of the factors known to blunt cardiac response to sympathetic stimuli.[49] Accordingly, in a study investigating age-related HR response to PLMS in three groups of RLS patients (young, middle-aged, and elderly), the magnitude of the tachycardia and the bradycardia associated with PLMS was blunted in older patients compared to younger subjects.[42] The same type of analysis has shown that the PLMS-related HR response is attenuated in some specific sleep disorders such as REM behavior disorders[38] and narcolepsy,[43] conditions associated with autonomic dysfunction,[27,50-52] as discussed later.

Restless Legs Syndrome

Restless legs syndrome (RLS) is a neurologic condition characterized by an urge to move, usually associated with paresthesia/dysesthesia, which occurs or worsens at rest, especially in the evening or night, interfering with sleep onset and causing frequent awakenings. Epidemiological studies suggest the presence of a link between RLS and risk for cardiovascular diseases.[53-56] However, the precise interaction between this condition and cardiovascular disease and the explanation of the pathophysiological mechanisms involved remain to be elucidated. Approximately 80% of subjects with restless legs syndrome (RLS) have

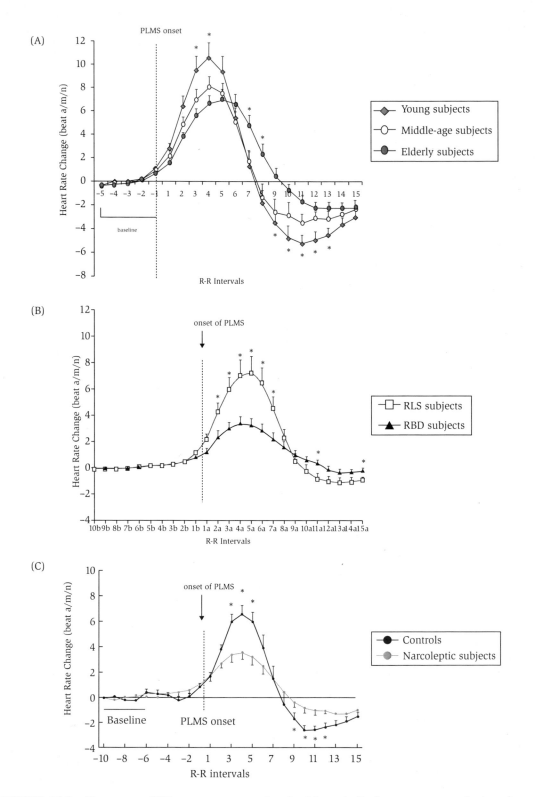

FIGURE 20.2   Heart rate (HR) responses associated with periodic leg movements during sleep (PLMS). (*A*) HR responses in young, middle-aged, and elderly subjects with restless legs syndrome. (Reprinted and modified from Gosselin et al.,[39] with permission of the publisher.) (*B*) HR responses in subjects with REM behavior disorders compared to subjects with restless legs syndrome (RLS). (Reprinted from Fantini et al.,[32] with permission of the publisher.) (*C*) HR responses in subjects with narcolepsy and controls. (Reprinted from Dauvilliers et al.,[30] with permission of the publisher.)

repetitive PLMS.[31] The cardiovascular response to PLMS described earlier has been documented in RLS and invoked as a potential contributing factor of increased risk. Other components of RLS physiopathology, for instance, insomnia and sleep deprivation or other unknown factors, could be invoked to have a harmful effect on the cardiovascular system via an increased sympathetic drive. However, to date, only a few studies have explored the autonomic function independent of PLMS in RLS patients.

A recent study assessing HR responses to deep breathing and Valsalva maneuver, BP response to active standing, and skin sympathetic response to electric shocks found comparable responses between 27 RLS subjects and 26 controls.[57] A different study using spectral analysis of HR variability assessed in RLS with PLMS showed an increase in RR variability power in the low frequencies (0,04–0,15 Hz) and very low frequencies (<0,04 Hz), that is, in the frequency range of PLMS occurrence.[44,58] However, no differences were seen between RLS patients and controls when spectral analysis of HR variability was performed in segments without PLMS.[59] Preliminary data from our laboratory found no differences in day-to-night BP measures between RLS patients, controls with PLMS, and controls without PLMS.[60] However, altered nocturnal BP appeared associated with poor sleep in all subjects.

Although limited, all these studies are consistent with a preserved autonomic function in RLS. In a recent cohort of 73 RLS and 34 controls, it was found that RLS exhibit higher urinary excretion of cortisol, which correlated, although weakly, with indices of sleep fragmentation.[61] Increased cortisol has been featured in subjects with insomnia with polysomnographic indices of poor sleep and correlated with indices of adrenergic hyperactivity.[62] Therefore, autonomic abnormalities might exist in RLS subjects as an effect of insomnia and its neuroendocrine and autonomic derangement. The investigation of insomnia and sleep impairment as mediators of the link between RLS and cardiovascular diseases via an increase in sympathetic influences could represent an avenue for research.

REM Sleep Behavior Disorder

Autonomic dysfunction is a common manifestation of neurodegenerative diseases, especially diseases characterized by deposition of α-synuclein (so-called synucleinopathies); these include Parkinson's disease (PD), multiple-system atrophy, and Lewy body dementia (LBD). Synucleinopathies are associated with a broad degeneration of nuclei involved in autonomic function.[63] Staging systems of PD have suggested that these abnormalities are present very early in the disease process, often before development of hallmark manifestations of motor and cognitive dysfunction. Of special interest, there is broad-based degeneration of peripheral autonomic ganglia and the dorsal nucleus of the vagus in incidental Lewy body disease, a potential "preclinical" stage of synucleinopathy.[64] Given that idiopathic RBD is known to occur before development of defined synucleinopathies,[65-67] a working hypothesis of several investigators in the past few years has been that autonomic abnormalities may be present in RBD and may even help predict those who will develop neurodegenerative disease.

MARKERS OF AUTONOMIC DYSFUNCTION IN REM BEHAVIOR DISORDER

The hypothesis that subjects with idiopathic REM behavior disorder (RBD) have autonomic dysfunction was previously proposed by Mahowald and Schenck, who noted a lack of HR changes in association with the vigorous REM sleep behaviors shown by these patients.[68] This hypothesis was supported by two studies reporting an attenuation of the HR response to motor activity during non-REM and REM sleep in RBD subjects compared to both controls[54] and subjects with restless legs syndrome.[35] The normal autonomic activation seen during transitions from non-REM to REM sleep has also been shown to be attenuated in RBD subjects.[27] As additional demonstration of adrenergic failure, BP response to standing appears also to be more frequently altered in these patients compared to controls, with approximately 60% demonstrating a SBP drop ≥10 mm Hg and 33% with a drop ≥20 mm Hg.[69,70]

In a larger population of RBD patients we found a reduced RR variability also during wakefulness.[71,72] Spectral analysis revealed that this is present at all frequencies (VLF, LF, and HF), suggesting that there is a broad autonomic dysfunction affecting both sympathetic and parasympathetic systems.

Finally, [123]MIBG scintigraphy has also been shown to be significantly altered in RBD subjects. The initial report of abnormal MIBG scintigraphy in RBD was in 2006 by Miyamoto et al., who noted reduced cardiac MIBG scintigraphy, indicating sympathetic denervation in 100% of RBD patients studied (presumably this would indicate that none of those patients were in preclinical stages of MSA).[73] This has subsequently been confirmed by other investigators.[74,75] Scintigraphy abnormalities are more severe in RBD than in early-stage Parkinson disease (scintigraphy is also worse in LBD than PD),[74] suggesting a close relationship between RBD and autonomic dysfunction, potentially independent of the presence of PD.

All of these findings point to a broad and reproducible degeneration of autonomic cardiac innervation in RBD, consistent with its association with synuclein-mediated neurodegeneration.

In addition, data from our laboratory indicate that patients with idiopathic RBD also have a higher prevalence of constipation, urinary dysfunction, and erectile dysfunction compared to controls,[70] indicating broad autonomic denervation may occur outside the heart in this condition.

DOES AUTONOMIC DYSFUNCTION PREDICT OUTCOME IN REM BEHAVIOR DISORDER?

Given that models of synucleinopathy progression suggest that autonomic dysfunction may be present at an early stage of the disease, it is logical that autonomic abnormalities may be able to predict those who eventually develop a defined neurodegenerative disorder. For most markers, these studies have not been performed. One study recently described baseline cardiac autonomic dysfunction in 21 patients with RBD who eventually converted to defined disease, compared to 21 who did not. Surprisingly, despite clear differences between RBD patients and controls, there was absolutely no evidence that those who eventually developed disease had worse cardiac denervation on the baseline examination 7 years before[71] (Fig. 20.3). This could be consistent with a causative role of autonomic dysfunction in the symptoms of

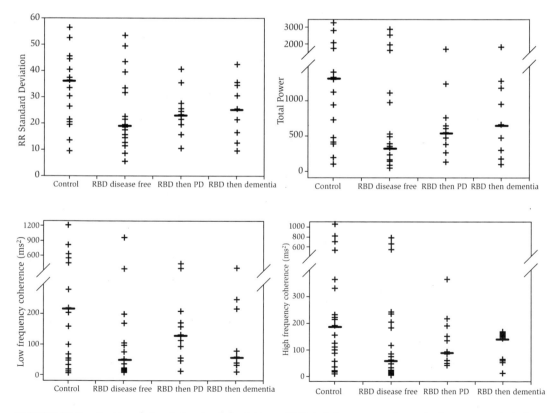

FIGURE 20.3 Scatterplots of standard deviation of RR, total power, and spectral components in low and high frequency in control subjects and in patients with REM behavior disorders (RBD) according to disease outcome (RBD disease free, patients who developed Parkinson disease [PD], and patients who developed dementia). (Reprinted from Postuma et al.,[65] with permission of the publisher.)

RBD, a counterintuitive concept which is supported by observations that autonomic dysfunction related to Guillain-Barre syndrome (a peripheral nervous system disorder can cause RBD). Alternatively, the absence of predictive ability could suggest that autonomic dysfunction is in fact the "perfect" marker, occurring in all patients in idiopathic RBD and at floor by the time a patient presents with RBD. So far, other than case reports describing MIBG abnormalities in RBD patients who eventually developed disease,[75] there have been no systematic studies assessing whether other markers of neurodegeneration can predict outcome. Therefore, the role of autonomic markers as predictors of disease remains uncertain.

Narcolepsy

Narcolepsy with cataplexy is a clinical condition characterized by excessive daytime sleepiness, cataplexy and disturbed nocturnal sleep. Narcolepsy is associated with the loss of hypocretin-producing cells of the lateral and posterior hypothalamus and markedly reduced level of hypocretin-1 in the cerebrospinal fluid. Significant neuroanatomical and neurophysiological data indicate that hypocretin plays a significant role in the regulation of the autonomic nervous system.[76]

Autonomic complaints (fainting spells, low body temperature, erectile dysfunction, gastric complaints, dry mouth, and others) have been described but do not appear to be common among unmedicated narcoleptic patients.[76] A number of studies have also been undertaken to assess subclinical signs of autonomic dysfunction in this condition. To date, the data available are not consistent and rather puzzling. The response to deep breathing and Valsalva maneuver was reported to be altered in narcoleptic subjects by some authors[77] and normal by others.[78] Early studies found HR and BP responses to active standing to be preserved.[78] A more recent study investigating the response to head-up tilt (passive standing) confirmed that HR and BP response to tilt were similar between controls and narcoleptics.[79] However, at baseline narcoleptic subjects had higher HR, and by using the more sensitive techniques of spectral analysis narcoleptics appeared to have enhanced sympathetic influences at rest (higher LF/HF ratio) with an attenuation of the response to tilt.[79] Finally, when examining HRV associated with wake-sleep cycle, Ferini-Strambi et al. noted a higher ratio of low to high frequency (as presumable index of sympathetic dominance) in narcoleptics compared to controls during presleep wakefulness, but the sympathovagal balance was comparable between the two groups across non-REM and REM sleep.[52] On the other hand, when assessing HR response to PLMS, this appeared significantly attenuated in narcoleptic subjects.[43] In conclusion, some studies, but not all, seem to indicate that sympathetic activation is higher at rest but attenuated in response to sympathetic stimuli.

CATAPLEXY

Cataplexy is a transient loss of muscle tone with preserved consciousness, triggered by intense emotion. Autonomic changes have been reported to occur in association with cataplexy. Investigations using continuous monitoring of cardiovascular variables before, during, and after attacks of cataplexy found that a cardio-acceleration can occur few seconds before the cataplectic attack, followed by a significant deceleration and subsequent steady bradycardia throughout the entire attack.[80] One study found an increase in MSNA activity to occur simultaneously with the bradycardia, indicating sympathetic and cardiovagal activation, during the attack (Fig. 20.4).[81] The observed simultaneous activation of peripheral sympathetic drive and cardiovagal inhibitory drive in association with cataplexy is similar to what is seen in other reflexes such as the diving reflex and the so-called startle-defense orienting reflex.[81] According to some authors, these findings corroborate the hypothesis that cataplexy may not only be a tonic REM state into wake as traditionally thought[82] but also a freezing-like perturbation of the orienting response, which includes somatic and autonomic responses, linked to a downstream dysfunction of brainstem reflex mechanisms.[81,83-85]

Sleep Bruxism

Sleep bruxism (SB) is defined by grinding or clenching of the teeth and a rhythmic masticatory muscle activity (RMMA) mainly occurring during non-REM sleep.

Subjects with SB are generally good sleepers with normal overall sleep macrostructure when compared to controls. Studies suggest that RMMA and tooth grinding may be secondary to sleep-increased arousal. The vast proportion

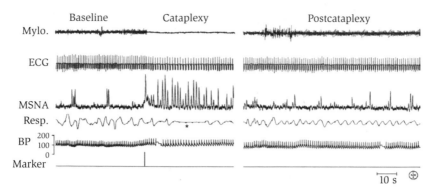

FIGURE 20.4 Continuous recording of mylohyoideus muscle (mylo), one electrocardiaphic lead (ECG), muscle sympathetic nerve activity (MSNA), respiration, and blood pressure (BP) in association with a cataplectic episode (marker indicates cataplexy onset). A marked increase in muscle sympathetic nerve activity (MSNA) and in blood pressure (BP) simultaneous with a slowing of heart rate (HR) appears in concomitance with muscle atonia. MSNA, BP, and HR returned to baseline after the episode when the muscle tone reappeared (asterisk). (Reprinted from Donadio et al.,[78] with permission of the publisher.)

of SB have been shown to be associated with microarousal[86] and to occur in phase A of the cyclic alternating pattern (CAP).[87] Indices of enhanced autonomic activation have been found during daytime in children as well as in adults[88] with sleep bruxism.[17] For instance, in a large sample of 6- to 8-year-old children, bruxism was linked to heightened nocturnal urinary excretion of epinephrine and dopamine.[17] Other authors found sleep bruxism subjects to have enhanced BP response to standing[89] and greater LF power and LF/HF ratio of heart rate variability in resting condition while awake.[88] Whether increased sympathetic drive may stem from an underlying autonomic dysregulation or is a physiological correlate of enhanced psychological stress in these subjects is not known.

More recent studies examined cardiac autonomic modulation during sleep as well as in association with RMMA/sleep bruxism episodes. HR has been shown to precede cortical activation and RMMA episodes.[86,87] One study comparing spectral components of HR variability in subsequent 3-minute segments across the night found no differences in these measures between the two groups across sleep stages but found that LF/HF started to increase approximately 8 minutes before RMMA occurrence.[90] From the same authors, the use of time-frequency analysis showed that LF/HF increased further during the minute preceding the RMMA episode.[90] In this same study

clonidine, a potent sympathetic-inhibitory agent, appeared to reduce LF/HF across the night, suppress the adrenergic drive preceding RMMA episodes, and significantly reduce the incidence of RMMA/sleep bruxism episodes. Therefore, these findings suggest that by modulating the sequence of cardiac autonomic changes preceding sleep bruxism, it may be possible to prevent the occurrence of these episodes during sleep, supporting a potential role of sympathetic influences in the genesis of this sleep-related motor disorder.

CONCLUSION

The autonomic nervous system is intimately linked to central neural state changes, including physiological and disordered sleep. Although limited, available studies indicate clearly that sleep-related movement disorders and autonomic function are closely linked. Current data also pinpoint the importance of broadening polysomnography and daytime assessment of sleep-related movement disorders to autonomic evaluation to help in understanding their physiopathology and clinical implications.

REFERENCES

1. Weimer LH. Autonomic testing: common techniques and clinical applications. *Neurologist* 2010;16(4):215–22.

2. Assessment: clinical autonomic testing report of the Therapeutics and Technology Assessment Subcommittee of the American Academy of Neurology. *Neurology* 1996;46(3):873–80.

3. Ewing DJ, Martyn CN, Young RJ, Clarke BF. The value of cardiovascular autonomic function tests: 10 years experience in diabetes. *Diabetes Care* 1985; 8(5):491–8.

4. Low PA, Denq JC, Opfer-Gehrking TL et al. Effect of age and gender on sudomotor and cardiovagal function and blood pressure response to tilt in normal subjects. *Muscle Nerve* 1997;20(12):1561–8.5. Benarroch EE, Opfer-Gehrking TL, Low PA. Use of the photoplethysmographic technique to analyze the Valsalva maneuver in normal man. *Muscle Nerve* 1991;14(12):1165–72.

6. Grassi G, Esler M. How to assess sympathetic activity in humans. *J Hypertens* 1999;17(6):719–34.

7. Vallbo AB, Hagbarth KE, Torebjork HE, et al. Somatosensory, proprioceptive, and sympathetic activity in human peripheral nerves. *Physiol Rev* 1979;59(4):919–57.

8. Somers VK, Dyken ME, Mark AL, et al. Parasympathetic hyperresponsiveness and bradyarrhythmias during apnoea in hypertension. *Clin Auton Res* 1992;2(3):171–6.

9. Somers VK, Dyken ME, Mark AL, Abboud FM. Sympathetic-nerve activity during sleep in normal subjects. *N Engl J Med* 1993; 328(5):303–7.

10. Yamashina S, Yamazaki J. Neuronal imaging using SPECT. *Eur J Nucl Med Mol Imaging* 2007;34(Suppl 1):S62–73.

11. Goldstein DS, Chang PC, Eisenhofer G, et al. Positron emission tomographic imaging of cardiac sympathetic innervation and function. *Circulation* 1990;81(5):1606–21.

12. Lautamaki R, Tipre D, Bengel FM. Cardiac sympathetic neuronal imaging using PET. *Eur J Nucl Med Mol Imaging* 2007;3 (4 Suppl 1):S74–85.

13. Linsell CR, Lightman SL, Mullen PE, et al. Circadian rhythms of epinephrine and norepinephrine in man. *J Clin Endocrinol Metab* 1985;60(6):1210–15.

14. Dodt C, Breckling U, Derad I, et al. Plasma epinephrine and norepinephrine concentrations of healthy humans associated with nighttime sleep and morning arousal. *Hypertension* 1997;30(1 Pt 1):71–6.

15. Irwin M, Thompson J, Miller C, et al. Effects of sleep and sleep deprivation on catecholamine and interleukin-2 levels in humans: clinical implications. *J Clin Endocrinol Metab* 1999;84(6):1979–85.

16. Irwin M, Clark C, Kennedy B, et al. Nocturnal catecholamines and immune function in insomniacs, depressed patients, and control subjects. *Brain Behav Immun* 2003;17(5):365–72.

17. Vanderas AP, Menenakou M, Kouimtzis T, et al. Urinary catecholamine levels and bruxism in children. *J Oral Rehabil* 1999;26(2):103–10.

18. Heart rate variability: standards of measurement, physiological interpretation and clinical use. Task Force of the European Society of Cardiology and the North American Society of Pacing and Electrophysiology. *Circulation* 1996;93:1043–65.

19. Bernardi L, Salvucci F, Suardi R, et al. Evidence for an intrinsic mechanism regulating heart rate variability in the transplanted and the intact heart during submaximal dynamic exercise? *Cardiovasc Res* 1990;24(12):969–81.

20. Montano N, Porta A, Malliani A. Evidence for central organization of cardiovascular rhythms. *Ann NY Acad Sci* 2001;940:299–306.

21. Pagani M, Lombardi F, Guzzetti S, et al. Power spectral analysis of heart rate and arterial pressure variabilities as a marker of sympatho-vagal interaction in man and conscious dog. *Circ Res* 1986;59(2):178–93.

22. Sleight P, La Rovere MT, Mortara A, et al. Physiology and pathophysiology of heart rate and blood pressure variability in humans: is power spectral analysis largely an index of baroreflex gain? *Clin Sci (Lond)* 1995;88(1):103–9.

23. Malliani A, Pagani M, Lombardi F, et al. Cardiovascular neural regulation explored in the frequency domain. *Circulation* 1991;84(2):482–92.

24. Akselrod S, Gordon D, Ubel FA, et al. Power spectrum analysis of heart rate fluctuation: a quantitative probe of beat-to-beat cardiovascular control. *Science* 1981;213(4504):220–2.

25. Bonnet MH, Arand DL. Heart rate variability: sleep stage, time of night, and arousal influences. *Electroencephalogr Clin Neurophysiol* 1997;102(5):390–6.

26. Van de Borne P, Nguyen H, et al. Effects of wake and sleep stages on the 24-h autonomic control of blood pressure and heart rate in recumbent men. *Am J Physiol* 1994;266(2 Pt 2):H548–54.

27. Lanfranchi PA, Fradette L, Gagnon JF, et al. Cardiac autonomic regulation during sleep in idiopathic REM sleep behavior disorder. *Sleep* 2007;30(8):1019–25.

28. Cerutti S, Bianchi AM, Mainardi LT. Advanced spectral methods for detecting dynamic behaviour. *Auton Neurosci* 2001;90(1–2):3–12.

29. Blasi A, Jo J, Valladares E, et al. Cardiovascular variability after arousal from sleep: time-varying spectral analysis. *J Appl Physiol* 2003;95(4):1394–404.

30. Guggisberg AG, Hess CW, Mathis J. The significance of the sympathetic nervous system in the pathophysiology of periodic leg movements in sleep. *Sleep* 2007;30(6):755–66.

31. Montplaisir J, Boucher S, Poirier G, et al. Clinical, polysomnographic, and genetic characteristics of restless legs syndrome: a study of 133 patients diagnosed with new standard criteria. *Mov Disord* 1997;12(1):61–5.

32. Montplaisir J, Michaud M, Denesle R, et al. Periodic leg movements are not more prevalent in insomnia or hypersomnia but are specifically associated with sleep disorders involving a dopaminergic impairment. *Sleep Med* 2000;1(2):163–7.

33. Dauvilliers Y, Pennestri MH, Petit D, et al. Periodic leg movements during sleep and wakefulness in narcolepsy. *J Sleep Res* 2007;16(3):333–9.

34. Coleman RM, Pollak CP, Weitzman ED. Periodic movements in sleep (nocturnal myoclonus): relation to sleep disorders. *Ann Neurol* 1980;8(4):416–21.

35. Fantini ML, Michaud M, Gosselin N, et al. Periodic leg movements in REM sleep behavior disorder and related autonomic and EEG activation. *Neurology* 2002;59(12):1889–94.

36. Carelli G, Krieger J, Calvi-Gries F, et al. Periodic limb movements and obstructive sleep apneas before and after continuous positive airway pressure treatment. *J Sleep Res* 1999;8(3):211–16.

37. Fry JM, DiPhillipo MA, Pressman MR. Periodic leg movements in sleep following treatment of obstructive sleep apnea with nasal continuous positive airway pressure. *Chest* 1989;96(1):89–91.

38. Javaheri S. Sleep disorders in systolic heart failure: a prospective study of 100 male patients. The final report. *Int J Cardiol* 2006;106(1):21–8.

39. Pennestri MH, Whittom S, Adam B, et al. PLMS and PLMW in healthy subjects as a function of age: prevalence and interval distribution. *Sleep* 2006;29(9):1183–7.

40. Sforza E, Nicolas A, Lavigne G, et al. EEG and cardiac activation during periodic leg movements in sleep: support for a hierarchy of arousal responses. *Neurology* 1999;52(4):786–91.

41. Winkelman JW. The evoked heart rate response to periodic leg movements of sleep. *Sleep* 1999;22(5):575–80.

42. Gosselin N, Lanfranchi P, Michaud M, et al. Age and gender effects on heart rate activation associated with periodic leg movements in patients with restless legs syndrome. *Clin Neurophysiol* 2003;114(11):2188–95.

43. Dauvilliers Y, Pennestri MH, Whittom S, et al. Autonomic response to periodic leg movements during sleep in narcolepsy-cataplexy. *Sleep* 2011;34(2):219–23.

44. Walter LM, Foster AM, Patterson RR, et al. Cardiovascular variability during periodic leg movements in sleep in children. *Sleep* 2009;32(8):1093–9.

45. Pennestri MH, Montplaisir J, Colombo R, et al. Nocturnal blood pressure changes in patients with restless legs syndrome. *Neurology* 2007;68(15):1213–18.

46. Siddiqui F, Strus J, Ming X, et al. Rise of blood pressure with periodic limb movements in sleep and wakefulness. *Clin Neurophysiol* 2007;118(9):1923–30.

47. Lavoie S, de Bilbao F, Haba-Rubio J, et al. Influence of sleep stage and wakefulness on spectral EEG activity and heart rate variations around periodic leg movements. *Clin Neurophysiol* 2004;115(10):2236–46.

48. Ferrillo F, Beelke M, Canovaro P, et al. Changes in cerebral and autonomic activity heralding periodic limb movements in sleep. *Sleep Med* 2004;5(4):407–12.

49. Lakatta EG. Cardiovascular regulatory mechanisms in advanced age. *Physiol Rev* 1993;73(2):413–67.

50. Fronczek R, Overeem S, Reijntjes R, et al. Increased heart rate variability but normal resting metabolic rate in hypocretin/orexin-deficient human narcolepsy. *J Clin Sleep Med* 2008;4(3):248–54.

51. Ferini-Strambi L, Oldani A, Zucconi M, et al. Cardiac autonomic activity during wakefulness and sleep in REM sleep behavior disorder. *Sleep* 1996;19(5):367–9.

52. Ferini-Strambi L, Spera A, Oldani A, et al. Autonomic function in narcolepsy: power

spectrum analysis of heart rate variability. *J Neurol* 1997;244(4):252–5.

53. Ohayon MM, Roth T. Prevalence of restless legs syndrome and periodic limb movement disorder in the general population. *J Psychosom Res* 2002;53(1):547–54.

54. Winkelman JW, Finn L, Young T. Prevalence and correlates of restless legs syndrome symptoms in the Wisconsin Sleep Cohort. *Sleep Med* 2006;7(7):545–52.

55. Winkelman JW, Shahar E, Sharief I, et al. Association of restless legs syndrome and cardiovascular disease in the Sleep Heart Health Study. *Neurology* 2008;70(1):35–42.

56. Ulfberg J, Nystrom B, Carter N, et al. Prevalence of restless legs syndrome among men aged 18 to 64 years: an association with somatic disease and neuropsychiatric symptoms. *Mov Disord* 2001;16(6):1159–63.

57. Isak B, Agan K, Ergun A, et al. Where is the core of the volcano? The undetermined origin of primary restless legs syndrome. *Int J Neurosci* 2011;121(3):130–6.

58. Sforza E, Pichot V, Barthelemy JC, et al. Cardiovascular variability during periodic leg movements: a spectral analysis approach. *Clin Neurophysiol* 2005;116(5):1096–104.

59. Manconi M, Ferri R, Zucconi M, et al. Effects of acute dopamine-agonist treatment in restless legs syndrome on heart rate variability during sleep. *Sleep Med* 2011;12(1):47–55.

60. Pennestri MH, Lanfranchi PA, Amyot R, et al. Nocturnal blood pressure dipping in restless legs syndrome. *Sleep* 2010;33:A257.

61. Schilling C, Schredl M, Strobl P, et al. Restless legs syndrome: evidence for nocturnal hypothalamic-pituitary-adrenal system activation. *Mov Disord* 2010;25(8):1047–52.

62. Vgontzas AN, Bixler EO, Lin HM, et al. Chronic insomnia is associated with nyctohemeral activation of the hypothalamic-pituitary-adrenal axis: clinical implications. *J Clin Endocrinol Metab* 2001;86(8):3787–94.

63. Beach TG, Adler CH, Sue LI, et al. Multi-organ distribution of phosphorylated alpha-synuclein histopathology in subjects with Lewy body disorders. *Acta Neuropathol* 2010;119(6):689–702.

64. Braak H, Del Tredici K. Invited article: nervous system pathology in sporadic Parkinson disease. *Neurology* 2008;70(20):1916–25.

65. Postuma RB, Gagnon JF, Vendette M, et al. Quantifying the risk of neurodegenerative

disease in idiopathic REM sleep behavior disorder. *Neurology* 2009;72(15):1296–300.

66. Iranzo A, Molinuevo JL, Santamaria J, et al. Rapid-eye-movement sleep behaviour disorder as an early marker for a neurodegenerative disorder: a descriptive study. *Lancet Neurol* 2006;5(7):572–7.

67. Schenck CH, Bundlie SR, Mahowald MW. Delayed emergence of a parkinsonian disorder in 38% of 29 older men initially diagnosed with idiopathic rapid eye movement sleep behaviour disorder. *Neurology* 1996;46(2):388–93.

68. Mahowald MW, Schenck CH. REM sleep behaviour disorder. In: Kriger MDW, Roth T, eds. *Principle and Practice of Sleep Medicine.* Philadelphia, PA: WB Saunders; 1989:389–401.

69. Postuma RB, Lang AE, Massicotte-Marquez J, et al. Potential early markers of Parkinson disease in idiopathic REM sleep behavior disorder. *Neurology* 2006;66(6):845–51.

70. Postuma RB, Gagnon JF, Vendette M, et al. Markers of neurodegeneration in idiopathic rapid eye movement sleep behaviour disorder and Parkinson's disease. *Brain* 2009;132(Pt 12):298–307.

71. Postuma RB, Lanfranchi PA, Blais H, et al. Cardiac autonomic dysfunction in idiopathic REM sleep behavior disorder. *Mov Disord* 2010;25(14):2304–10.

72. Valappil RA, Black JE, Broderick MJ, et al. Exploring the electrocardiogram as a potential tool to screen for premotor Parkinson's disease. *Mov Disord* 2010;25(14):2296–303.

73. Miyamoto T, Miyamoto M, Inoue Y, et al. Reduced cardiac 123I-MIBG scintigraphy in idiopathic REM sleep behavior disorder. *Neurology* 2006;67(12):2236–8.

74. Kashihara K, Imamura T, Shinya T. Cardiac 123I-MIBG uptake is reduced more markedly in patients with REM sleep behavior disorder than in those with early stage Parkinson's disease. *Parkinsonism Relat Disord* 2010;16(4):252–5.

75. Oguri T, Tachibana N, Mitake S, et al. Decrease in myocardial 123I-MIBG radioactivity in REM sleep behavior disorder: two patients with different clinical progression. *Sleep Med* 2008;9(5):583–5.

76. Plazzi G, Moghadam KK, Maggi LS, et al. Autonomic disturbances in narcolepsy. *Sleep Med Rev* 2011;15(3):187–96.

77. Sachs C, Kaijser L. Autonomic regulation of cardiopulmonary functions in sleep

apnea syndrome and narcolepsy. *Sleep* 1982;5(3):227–38.

78. Hublin C, Matikainen E, Partinen M. Autonomic nervous system function in narcolepsy. *J Sleep Res* 1994;3(3):131–7.

79. Grimaldi D, Pierangeli G, Barletta G, et al. Spectral analysis of heart rate variability reveals an enhanced sympathetic activity in narcolepsy with cataplexy. *Clin Neurophysiol* 2010;121(7):1142–7.

80. Vetrugno R, D'Angelo R, Moghadam KK, et al. Behavioural and neurophysiological correlates of human cataplexy: a video-polygraphic study. *Clin Neurophysiol* 2010;121(2):153–62.

81. Donadio V, Plazzi G, Vandi S, et al. Sympathetic and cardiovascular activity during cataplexy in narcolepsy. *J Sleep Res* 2008;17(4):458–63.

82. American Academy of Sleep Medicine. *International Classification of Sleep Disorders. Diagnostic and Coding Manual.* 2nd ed. Westchester, IL: American Academy of Sleep Medicine; 2005.

83. Rubboli G, d'Orsi G, Zaniboni A, et al. A video-polygraphic analysis of the cataplectic attack. *Clin Neurophysiol* 2000;111(Suppl 2):S120–8.

84. Lammers GJ, Overeem S, Tijssen MA, et al. Effects of startle and laughter in cataplectic subjects: a neurophysiological study between attacks. *Clin Neurophysiol* 2000;111(7):1276–81.

85. Overeem S, Lammers GJ, van Dijk JG. Cataplexy: "tonic immobility" rather than "REM-sleep atonia"? *Sleep Med* 2002;3(6):471–7.

86. Kato T, Rompre P, Montplaisir JY, et al. Sleep bruxism: an oromotor activity secondary to micro-arousal. *J Dent Res* 2001;80(10):1940–4.

87. Macaluso GM, Guerra P, Di Giovanni G, et al. Sleep bruxism is a disorder related to periodic arousals during sleep. *J Dent Res* 1998;77(4):565–73.

88. Marthol H, Reich S, Jacke J, et al. Enhanced sympathetic cardiac modulation in bruxism patients. *Clin Auton Res* 2006;16(4):276–80.

89. Sjoholm TT, Piha SJ, Lehtinen I. Cardiovascular autonomic control is disturbed in nocturnal teethgrinders. *Clin Physiol* 1995;15(4):349–54.

90. Huynh N, Kato T, Rompre PH, et al. Sleep bruxism is associated to micro-arousals and an increase in cardiac sympathetic activity. *J Sleep Res* 2006;15(3):339–46.

PART FOUR

Clinical Science

A

General Introductory Section

21

An Introduction

CHRISTIAN GUILLEMINAULT

SLEEP IS a period of rest and relaxation. Therefore, it must involve a suppression of much of the normal waking motor activity. Even in the approach to sleep, the motor system becomes quiescent. Humans, along with many mammals, have a presleep behavior that is defined by a multiplicity of features. In it, a comfortable body position is sought, limbs are positioned to avoid discomfort and strain, eyelids droop, and a decrease in peripheral sensory stimulation is experienced. These form part of the phenomenon of sleep onset. These are, in turn, associated with changes in the pattern of neuronal firings that can lead subsequently to the development of non–rapid eye movement (non-REM) and rapid eye movement (REM) sleep. This phenomenon of sleep onset is associated with a decreased activity of the hypocretin neurons located in the postero-lateral hypothalamus, projecting to many places in the brain through five different bundles[1] that impinge on dopaminergic, cholinergic, and histaminergic neurons involved in maintenance of wakefulness and an increased activity of neurons in the ventrolateral preoptic area in the anterior hypothalamus with many GABA-ergic neurons with inhibitory activity on structures involved in maintenance of non-REM sleep. As sleep becomes established, a notable decrease in muscle tone also occurs in the postural muscles, particularly in the neck, trunk, and proximal leg muscles. When later REM sleep is reached, the muscles are then characterized by maximal hypotonia or atonia. This requires, during REM sleep, the activation of the medullary reticular neurons that generate an active spinal inhibition of the alpha motor neurons, as well as a reduction in excitation. Different neurotransmitters have been identified in promoting this active inhibition. Although this is the normal progression, varying influences may alter the typical depressed motor state of sleep. For instance, sleep may occur in mammals even without the mediation of presleep relaxing behaviors. However, this may require particular pathologic conditions or special circumstances.

Villablanca and Salinas-Zeballos[2] performed a complete ablation of the thalamus in cats creating an "athalamic" cat model that still presented the abrupt appearance of non-REM sleep, but without the preparatory behavior of curling and limb retraction that is normally seen. The cat will sleep in bizarre postures of very limited comfort, as if it had been abruptly frozen in place at sleep onset.

Following a long period of sleep deprivation, humans also succumb to sleep while in the most uncomfortable and even painful positions. In such cases, posture collapses in association with an abrupt reduction of the tonic neuronal firing seen during wakefulness. Non-REM and REM sleep, thus, are physiologically defined by the reduction or inhibition of muscular activity, such that movements are clearly reduced during normal sleep.

However, reduction is not abolition. Movements can occur and may display a temporal pattern. Takahashi, Guillemnault, and Dement in 1974[3] studied the occurrence of gross body movements during sleep and found a periodicity to large movements of about 20 minutes. In addition, sleep history can be an important influence on motor activity during the sleep stages. The abrupt muscle jerks that reoccur during REM sleep, and are part of the phasic events of REM sleep, increase in frequency and in amplitude after REM sleep deprivation, as does REM density. Even under ordinary circumstances, muscle tone is continuously varying during sleep.

POSITIVE AND NEGATIVE MOTOR PHENOMENA

Abnormal motor activity during wake is often subdivided into negative and positive motor phenomena.[4] To observe a negative motor phenomenon, a background activation of the muscle tone is necessary. As a result, most motor phenomena during sleep are positive motor phenomena. There are many neural structures that contribute to the development or modulation of such phenomena. The positive motor phenomenon in waking is typically induced by an activation that starts in the cerebral cortex and propagates down to the spinal cord via the pyramidal tract. However, subcortical structures can also elicit positive phenomena by acting on the brainstem reticular formation, sending excitation down to the spinal cord via the reticulospinal system. Excitatory influences[4] over the

spinal motor apparatus originate from different brainstem reticular nuclei but particularly from the gigantocellular medial reticular zone[5] of the lower pons and upper medulla (in experimental studies of the cat, the spinal motor apparatus originates from the nucleus reticularis pontis caudalis and the nucleus reticularis gigantocellularis). These structures receive input from widely distributed brain centers, including the cerebral cortex (from areas 6 and 4), the superior colliculus (deeper layers), the pedunculopontine tegmental nucleus, the deep nuclei (fastigial) of the cerebellum, the limbic system, the hypothalamus, and the amygdala. Similarly, the spinal motor neuron pool can be excited by the locus coeruleus subcoeruleus alpha, and midline cell groups while reciprocally exciting those sites. Finally, spinal cord autonomic neurons can participate in a positive motor response, and similar effects can occur with stimulation of other autonomic centers such as the limbic system, the hypothalamus, and the amygdala. The circuitry that modulates tone and motor activity is diverse, and many neurotransmitter systems are involved at different points of these circuits. Certain neurotransmitters such as serotonin (5HT) have been shown to have an excitatory effect on the spinal motor neurons, whereas cholinergic, noradrenergic, and dopaminergic compounds have been shown to be present at synapses within the excitatory pathways.

Neurologic lesions have an impact on the structures and pathways involved in excitatory motor activity, and freeing the spinal motor neurons from the active sleep-related inhibition induces an abnormal motor activity, a positive motor phenomenon, during sleep. The severity and evolution of any disease process influence positive and negative motor activity.

NEGATIVE MOTOR PHENOMENA AND NEUROLOGIC DISORDERS

During the period of sleep onset, physiologic negative myoclonus,[6] defined as transient jerky involuntary movements resulting from an abrupt interruption of electromyographic (EMG) activity of very short duration, may occur, causing a sudden loss of postural muscle tone, and it may be speculated to be responsible for the physiologic hypnic jerk. Other negative phenomena disturbing sleep may include negative myoclonus,[6] REM muscle atonia, sleep paralysis, and cataplexy. Negative myoclonus may be observed in epileptic negative myoclonus[7] and posthypoxic myoclonus (Lance-Adams syndrome), which also displays positive myoclonus and asterixis, a form of subcortical negative myoclonus. Epileptic negative myoclonus and atonic or astatic seizures result from a sudden loss of postural muscle tone. Electromyogram shows periods of electrical silence (negative phenomenon) that may be preceded by positive jerks. The interruption of tonic muscle activity is time locked to an electroencephalographic spike or sharp wave.[6] Magnetic stimulation study has revealed evidence of pure inhibitory motor areas. Epileptic negative myoclonus is thought to result from an activation of cortical inhibitory areas.[7] Toro, Hallett, and Rothwell[8] postulated an alternative hypothesis that the same abnormal cortical event may be responsible for both the positive and negative phenomena and, therefore, both may coexist.

Their expression depends on many factors, including the pathways of spread, the time course, sleep-wake cycles, posture, and fatigue. Cataplexy is the most studied negative motor phenomenon.[9] It mimics what is observed during the normal occurrence of REM sleep, which is associated with an abrupt decrease in the motor tone of volitional muscles.[10] It is induced by emotional response to abrupt, mostly humorous events. Anomalous hypothalamic responses in the hypothalamus have been reported in narcoleptic-cataplectic patients. Also cataplectic-related neurons have been reported in the amygdala, with abnormal activity of these neurons that normally receive input from hypothalamic hypocretin neurons, during humor processing in humans.[11-14] It is an abrupt, reversible inhibition of volitional muscle tone associated with inhibition of mono- and polysynaptic motor reflexes.[10] It is an event of short duration, varying from a few seconds to a few minutes, and may be associated with complete fall. When present, it is pathognomic of the narcolepsy syndrome. The complete disappearance of the postero-lateral hypocretin neurons has been shown in histologic material of cataplectic-narcoleptic patients, and abnormally low or complete absence of measurable hypocretin level in the cerebrospinal fluid is noted.[15,16] An autoimmune disorder is strongly suspected in the development of narcolepsy-cataplexy syndrome with genetic involvement of both Human-Leucocyte-Antigen (HLA) DQ beta1-0602[17] and a specific T-cell receptor haplotype. The trigger of the autoimmune reaction is unknown at this date. Direct lesions of the postero-lateral hypothalamus will also lead to isolated cataplexy. Infectious, vascular, and tumoral lesions have been identified.[18] Craniopharyngioma appears to be the most common process leading to secondary cataplexy. Rarely, lesions on the pathway controlling the active inhibition of muscle tone during wakefulness and non-REM sleep from the locus coeruleus and adjacent region with either relay in the medulla or directly descending without relay to the spinal cord and impinging on a spinal cord motor interneuron may be involved. It has been documented in brainstem glioma; these cases, however, are rare because the brainstem lesions most commonly will eliminate the descending pathways responsible for the inhibition and will lead to a positive motor phenomenon.

POSITIVE MOTOR PHENOMENA AND NEUROLOGIC DISEASES

The positive motor phenomena are usually much better known to sleep specialists, and often they are associated with obvious neurologic lesions. Patients with Parkinson's disease, for example, have major sleep dysfunction that has a clear impact on their lives. The sleep disorder may be related to the disappearance of the normal REM sleep-related muscle atonia that accompanies the development of the typical features of REM sleep behavior disorder.[19] Patients with parkinsonism, particularly those with multiple-system atrophy, may have the same loss of REM sleep atonia and abnormal behavior. REM behavior disorder (RBD) may precede appearance of other symptoms of Parkinson syndrome by many (up to 30) years difference. In this case, simultaneous disappearance of good olfaction is a key symptom. Idiopathic RBD may exist despite the fact that autopsy material has shown presence of Lewy body disease[20, 21] in neurons involved in maintenance of REM sleep atonia without extension to substantia nigra sufficiently to induce clinical manifestations. Synucleinopathy is the most common pathological association with RBD, but many other disease entities, particularly neurodegenerative and brainstem disorders ranging from Korsakoff's syndrome and brainstem glioblastoma to Leigh disease or olivopontocerebellar degeneration,[22] may present with abnormal movements during REM sleep and REM sleep behavior disorder. Direct lesions of brainstem pathways involved in the control of the active inhibition of muscle tone during REM sleep will lead to RBD. These lesions may be traumatic, vascular, inflammatory, or tumoral. A special case is the narcolepsy syndrome. Abnormal control of muscle tone is related to the disappearance of the hypocretin neurons and the absence of state control: narcoleptic-cataplectic patients are unable to maintain the state of alertness (wakefulness, non-REM and REM sleep) in which they are and will abruptly switch from one state to another or will have reappearance of a component of one state in another such as abrupt reappearance of wakefulness muscle tone while in REM sleep. The use of some drugs may also lead to the elimination of REM sleep muscle atonia. This occurs with antidepressant drugs and certain antihypertensive and many illicit drugs. This is related to the interaction between neurotransmitters identified as involved in the normal occurrence of muscle atonia of REM sleep and the pharmacological agents. Certain metabolic conditions may also lead to abnormal motor activity during REM sleep.

As mentioned earlier, Parkinson syndrome and multiple-system atrophy patients may present with RBD; but the most common cause of sleep disturbance in Parkinson's patients is related to the abnormal control of rigidity during sleep and poor therapeutic control at night. Patients often present a rebound of rigidity during the night because of a lack of appropriate drug coverage during total nocturnal sleep time.

Undoubtedly, late daytime intake of dopamine precursors and agonists may lead to an increased alertness near bedtime, and one may face the problem of a "drug-induced insomnia." However, sleep disturbance resulting from rebound rigidity associated with poor nocturnal drug coverage is a much more common problem than the dopamine-related insomnia.

Positive motor phenomena may occur in hyperekplexia.[8,23,24] Hereditary and symptomatic hyperekplexia is a pathologic exaggeration of the normal startle reflex.[8,23-25] It is greatly exaggerated in amplitude and in body distribution and shows impaired habituation. The hereditary form is inherited as an autosomal dominant trait caused by mutations of the alpha 1 subunit of the inhibitory glycine receptor. The condition presents with three abnormal motor responses: tonic spasms, pathologic startle response, and episodes of sustained jerking either spontaneously or in response to unexpected stimuli. Episodes of repetitive, violent myoclonic jerks while falling asleep and during non-REM sleep are common early features. Symptomatic hyperekplexia is seen in neurologic syndromes that have an impact on the medial bulbo-pontine reticular formation. The neurologic lesions include static encephalopathies (static perinatal encephalopathies without tonic spasm, postanoxic encephalopathy, posttraumatic encephalopathy), brainstem encephalopathies (viral encephalomyelitis, sarcoidosis, encephalomyelitis with rigidity, multiple sclerosis, paraneoplastic encephalitis), and structural lesions (brainstem hemorrhage or infarct, cerebral abscess, Arnold-Chiari malformation). At sleep onset, patients with familial or symptomatic hyperekplexia may present long episodes of sustained jerking that reoccur during stage I and sometimes stage II non-REM sleep. This activity may involve repetitive flexion of the limbs, particularly of the legs. Some diseases, like Tourette's syndrome,[26] hexosaminidase A deficiency, and static perinatal encephalopathy with epileptic tonic spasm or startle epilepsy[27] may also cause disruption of sleep through motor activities.

The epilepsies during sleep that are most commonly associated with sleep onset, sleep offset (that is to say with state changes), and non-REM sleep rather than REM sleep are another example of a positive motor phenomenon leading to a significant disturbance of sleep. A mesiofrontal focus may lead to the development of a complex behavior in sleep usually during non-REM sleep.[28,29] The abnormal motor activity may begin in any non-REM sleep stage and at any time during the night and usually mimics the features of a non-REM dyssomnia. Clinically, it may present during sleep as a night terror that occurs with limb movements, as a somnambulistic episode, or even as an abnormal sexual behavior such as repetitive masturbation. To differentiate nocturnal seizure from parasomnia, one must be willing to perform a nocturnal sleep video-electroencephalographic recording for several successive days if necessary. One must also remember that 99% of abnormal nocturnal behaviors reported in the literature have been found to have a nonepileptic origin.[30]

Many positive motor phenomena and abnormal movements abate during sleep. However, it is important to emphasize that neurologic lesion or pharmacologic treatment may eliminate the normal active motor inhibition that occurs during REM sleep. Alzheimer's disease and vascular encephalopathy may be associated with positive motor phenomena. The abnormal behavior and abnormal movements may be part of a sundowning syndrome.[31] Systematic recordings have shown that patients are most often awake for several minutes before engaging in disruptive motor activity. Darkness and sleep inertia worsen their confusion and disorientation, providing an impetus to their abnormal behavior.

Restless legs syndrome is not a sleep-related disorder per se: it occurs during wakefulness and inhibits at the onset of sleep, but it is associated during sleep with periodic leg or limb movements.[32] Periodic limb movement is a well-described phenomenon: the movements are involuntary, repetitive, stereotypic, short-lasting, segmental movements of the lower and sometime upper extremities. When the movements of lower extremities are visually observed, the movements consist of dorsiflexion of the big toe with fanning of the small toes sometimes accompanied by a flexion of the ankles, knees, and sometime thighs, closely related to a "Babinski maneuver."[33] The scoring of periodic leg movements (PLMs) is based on the amplitude of anterior tibialis EMG discharges.

Similar movements have been simultaneously observed in the upper limbs but to a much lesser frequency than in the lower limbs.[34] When seen during nasal continuous positive airway pressure titration, they may occur in association with simultaneous burst monitored in abdominal expiratory muscles. The EMG bursts monitored with the movements reoccur with a clear periodicity with EMG muscle activity of short duration (seconds), initially monitored in the tibial anterialis muscles of both legs. The pathophysiology behind these short EMG bursts is still unknown. These positive motor phenomena are seen in some but not all patients with restless legs syndrome (RLS) but also in association with other neurological syndromes such as lesions of the spinal cord, radiculopathies, motor neuron disease, and stiff-person syndrome. They have been recorded with chronic uremia, where they are particularly violent,

with cardiac failure, with abnormal breathing during sleep, and during nasal continuous positive-airway-pressure titration. In association with RLS, they have been shown to follow the circadian distribution similar to the one shown in RLS; that is, they are present mostly during the first two sleep cycles at the beginning of sleep and are absent in the early morning hours. The occurrence of PLMs in so many different syndromes suggests that they may be related to a nonspecific response to many different biological disturbances involving the motor system.

CONCLUSION

Many neurologic insults are associated with a negative or positive motor phenomenon during sleep. Depending on the type of insult, the active inhibitory motor activity that occurs during REM sleep is abolished or an abnormal increase (a positive phenomenon) or abnormal decrease (a negative phenomenon) in muscle tone occurs, which leads to the presence of an abnormal movement disorder during sleep. Abnormal motor activity may also lead to abnormal behaviors. When seen during the confusional arousal that occurs in tandem with the abnormal motor activity in sleep, it carries a risk of violence to others or to self. It is important to recognize the presence of abnormal motor phenomena during sleep because they lead to sleep disruption and sleep fragmentation, which always have an impact on daytime motor function and rehabilitation efforts. The abnormal motor behavior may be ignored by the sleeping patient for a long time, but it will nonetheless diminish quality of life and may be expressed only by nonspecific complaints such as daytime tiredness, sleepiness, or by sleep fragmentation.

REFERENCES

1. Peyron C, Tighe DK, van Den Pol AN, et al. Neurons containing hypocretin (orexin) project to multiple neuronal systems. *J Neurosci* 1998;18:9996–10015.
2. Villablanca J, Salinas-Zeballos ME. Sleepwakefulness EEG and behavioral studies on chronic cats without the thalamus: the athalamic cat. *Arch Ibal Biol* 1972;110:383.
3. Takahashi S, Guillemnault C, Dement WC. A study of body movements in pseudo insomniacs. *Sleep Res* 1974;3:146.

4. Fahn S, Hallett M, Luders HO, et al. eds. *Negative Motor Phenomena. Advances in Neurology*. Vol 67. Philadelphia, PA: Lippincott Williams & Wilkins; 1995.

5. Vertes RP. Brain-stem giganto cellular nervous: patterns of activity during behavior and sleep in the freely moving rat. *J Neurophysiol* 1979;42:214.

6. Obeso JA, Artieda J, Burleigh A. Clinical aspects of negative myoclonus. In: Fahn S, Hallett M, Luders HO, Marsden CD, eds. *Negative Motor Phenomena. Advances in Neurology*. Vol 67. Philadelphia, PA: Lippincott Williams & Wilkins.

7. Tassinari C, Rubboli G, Parmeggiani L, et al. Epileptic negative myoclonus. In: Fahn S, Hallett M, Luders HO, Marsden CD, eds. *Negative Motor Phenomena. Advances in Neurology*. Vol 67. Philadelphia, PA: Lippincott Williams & Wilkins; 1995:181.

8. Toro C, Hallett M, Rothwell JC. Physiology of negative myoclonus. In: Fahn S, Hallett M, Luders HO, Marsden CD, eds. *Negative Motor Phenomena. Advances in Neurology*. Vol 67. Philadelphia, PA: Lippincott Williams & Wilkins;1995:211.

9. Guilleminault C. Cataplexy. In: Guilleminault C, Dement WC, Passouant P, eds. *Narcolepsy*. New-York: Spectrum; 1976:125–43.

10. Guilleminault C, Wilson R, Dement WC. A study on cataplexy. *Arch Neurol* 1974;31:255–61.

11. Gulyani S, Wu MF, Nienhuis R, et al. Cataplexy-related neurons in the amygdala of the narcoleptic dog. *Neuroscience* 2002;112:355–65.

12. Poryazova R, Schnepf B, Werth E, et al. Evidence for metabolic hypothalamo-amygdala dysfunction in narcolepsy. *Sleep* 2009;32:607–13.

13. Khatami R, Birkmann S, Basseti CL. Amygdala dysfunction in narcolepsy-cataplexy. *J Sleep Res* 2007;16:226–9.

14. Reiss AL, Hoeft F, Tenforde AS, et al. Anomalous hypothalamic responses to humor in cataplexy. *PLoS One* 2008;3:e2225.

15. Peyron C, Faraco J, Rogers WW, et al. A mutation in a case of early onset narcolepsy and a generalized absence of hypocretin peptides in human narcoleptic brain. *Nat Med* 2000;6:991–7.

16. Nishino S, Ripley B, Overeem S, et al. Hypocretin (orexin) deficiency in human narcoleptics *Lancet* 2000;355:39–40.

17. Mignot E, Lin X, Arrigoni J, et al. DQBeta1-0602 and DQA1-0102 (DQ!) are better markers than DR2 for narcolepsy in Caucasian and black Americans. *Sleep* 1994;17:S60–7.

18. Arii j, Kambayashi T, Tanabe Y, et al A hypersomnolent girl with decrease CSF hypocretin levels after removal of a hypothalamic tumor. *Neurology* 2001;56:1775–6.

19. Schenck CH, Mahowalg MW. REM sleep behavior disorder: clinical, developmental and neuroscience perspective 16 years after its formal identification in sleep. *Sleep* 2002;25:125–30.

20. Uchiyama M, Isse K, Tanaka K, et al. Incidental Lewy body disease in a patient with REM sleep behavior disorder *Neurology* 1995;45:709–17.

21. Boeve BF, Silber MH, Parisi JE, et al. Synucleinopathy pathology often underlies REM sleep behavior disorder and dementia, or Parkinson. *Neurology*. 2003;61:40–5.

22. Quera Salva MA, Guilleminault, C. Olivo-ponto-cerebellar degeneration, abnormal sleep, and REM sleep without atonia. *Neurology* 1986;36:576–7.

23. Brown P. Physiology of startle phenomena. In: Fahn S, Hallett M, Luders HO, Marsden CD, eds. *Negative Motor Phenomena. Advances in Neurology*. Vol 67. Philadelphia, PA: Lippincott Williams & Wilkins; 1995:125–43.

24. Brown P, Thompson PD, Rothwell JC, et al. The hyperekplexias and their relationship to the normal startle reflex. *Brain* 1991;114:1903.

25. Suhren O, Brwyn GW, Tuynman JA. Hyperexplexia: a hereditary startle syndrome. *J Neurol Sci* 1966;3:577.

26. Kurlan R. ed. *Handbook of Tourette's Syndrome and Related Tic and Behavioral Disorders*. New York: Dekker; 1993.

27. Cirignotta R, Lugaresi E. Partial epilepsy with "negative myoclonus" *Epilepsia* 1991;32:54.

28. Pedley TA, Guilleminault C. Episodic nocturnal wanderings responsive to anticonvulsant drug therapy. *Ann Neurol* 1977;2:30–5.

29. Guilleminault C, Leger D, Philip P, et al. Nocturnal wandering and violence: review of a sleep clinic population. *J Forensic Sci* 1998;43:158.

30. Manelis J, Bental E, Loeber JN, Dreifus FE. eds *Advances in Epileptology. XVIIth Epilepsy International Symposium*. New York: Raven Press; 1989:295.

31. Bliwise DL. What is sundowning? *J Am Geriatr Soc* 1994;42:1009–11.

32. Walter AS, Restless leg and periodic limb movements in sleep. In: Guilleminault C, ed. *Clinical Neurophysiology of Sleep Disorders-Handbook of Clinical Neurophysiology*. Vol.6. New York: Elsevier; 2005:273–80.

33. Smith RC. Relationship of periodic movements in sleep (nocturnal myoclonus) and the Babinski sign. *Sleep* 1985;8:239–43.

34. Chabli A, Michaud M, Montplaisir J. Periodic arm movements in patients with the restless leg syndrome. *Eur.Neurol* 2000;44:133–8.

22

An Approach to a Patient with Movement Disorders during Sleep and Classification

SUDHANSU CHOKROVERTY, RICHARD P. ALLEN,
AND ARTHUR S. WALTERS

AN APPROACH to a patient complaining of abnormal movements and behavior during sleep must begin with a clear understanding of the nature and prevalence of such abnormal movements and a rational system of classification of normal and abnormal movements occurring during sleep. The epidemiology of abnormal movements and behavior during sleep is still incompletely understood. There are many anecdotal reports and some limited studies of prevalence of abnormal behavior and movements or physiologic events occurring during different sleep stages and at sleep-wake transition. Most of the parasomnias, which are defined as abnormal movements and behavior intruding into sleep but not necessarily disrupting sleep architecture, occur during childhood and disappear by adulthood or adolescence. There are some limited studies to show a prevalence of 2%–5% of sleepwalking in the adult, general population, but this ranges from 5% to 30% in childhood. There is no gender preference, and it is virtually never reported in older adults except in occasional patients with sleep apnea. The prevalence of sleep terror in children varies from 1% to 6.5% and that of confusional arousal in the general population is around 4.2%. Only a few surveys are available for sleep-wake transition disorders. Sleep talking is frequent in younger age groups, in which 3% report frequent sleep talking and 21.3% report infrequent sleep talking. The prevalence of nocturnal leg cramps is not well known but appears to be frequent in older subjects and those with severe daytime sleepiness. Rapid eye movement behavior disorder (RBD) is a modern phenomenon and very little is known about its prevalence, but Ohayon estimated it at 0.5% in the general population. Nightmares, which are other rapid eye movement (REM) sleep parasomnias, have been reported to occur at least once a week in approximately 5% of the adult population.[1]

Paroxysmal involuntary movements, postures, and behavior often labeled by the patient or caregiver as "shakes, jerks, and screams" occurring during sleep at night are always challenging to clinicians and are difficult to diagnose. All these paroxysmal dyskinesias and behaviors encompass a number of different entities forming a heterogeneous collection of phenomena. Some of these diurnal and nocturnal movement disorders are especially triggered by sleep or occur preferentially during sleep, whereas others are overlapping (i.e., those movements seen during the daytime may persist during sleep at night).

The problem of diagnosis and differential diagnosis of such abnormal movements and behaviors can be exemplified by the following case scenario:

> *John is a 10-year-old boy who was brought to the family physician by his parents for peculiar "spells" at night. During sleep at night John has thrashing movements; he sits up in bed looking confused, and sometimes he screams. The parents also noted that on some occasions John has slow twisting movements of the arms and legs, and he may get out of bed and attempt to walk. Except for occasional transient generalized jerking movements, particularly in response to noise, John does not have any diurnal movements.*

What does John have?

Is it a motor parasomnia[9]
Is it a nocturnal seizure?
Is it nocturnal paroxysmal dystonia (NPD)?
Is it a psychogenic seizure?
Is it a diurnal movement disorder persisting in sleep?

In the following sections we try to address this dilemma by outlining a rational classification, brief description of some entities causing diagnostic difficulties, and approach to such patients.

CLASSIFICATION OF MOVEMENT DISORDERS DURING SLEEP

Based on behavioral manifestations of motor activities, movement disorders during sleep can be classified into physiologic (normal) and pathologic (abnormal) types (Table 22.1). Physiologic motor activity during sleep includes postural shifts, body and limb movements,

physiologic fragmentary myoclonus consisting of phasic muscle bursts seen typically in REM sleep, hypnic jerks, hypnagogic foot tremor, and rhythmic leg movements.

Abnormal movements that occur during sleep consist of motor parasomnias, sleep-related movement disorders, isolated sleep-related motor symptoms (apparently named variants), nocturnal seizures (traditionally not classified with movement disorders), miscellaneous nocturnal motor activities, and diurnal involuntary movements persisting during sleep.

Clinical characteristics of some common movement disorders during sleep are described in the following sections. The reader is referred to chapters throughout this volume for more detailed discussion.

Motor parasomnias are abnormal movements intruding into sleep without generally disturbing sleep architecture and may be classified into three categories[2-4]: non-REM sleep parasomnias, REM sleep parasomnias, and other motor parasomnias without any stage preference (see Table 22.1). Several parasomnias occurring in non-REM and REM sleep may be mistaken for seizures, particularly complex partial seizures. Somnambulism, night terror, confusional arousals, somniloquy, bruxism, head banging, RBD, nightmares, and dissociated disorders are some of the parasomnias that may be mistaken for seizures. RBD and nightmares are associated with REM sleep. Characteristic clinical features combined with electroencephalography (EEG) and polysomnographic (PSG) recordings are essential to differentiate these conditions.[5,6]

Somnambulism (Sleepwalking)

Somnambulism occurs most commonly in children between 5 and 12 years of age (Table 22.2). Sometimes it persists in adulthood or rarely begins in adults. Sleepwalking begins with abrupt motor activity arising out of slow-wave sleep during the first third of sleep but occasionally arises out of other non-REM stages of sleep. Episodes generally last less than 10 minutes. There is a high frequency of positive family histories in sleepwalking patients. Injuries and violent actions have been reported during sleepwalking episodes, but generally individuals can negotiate their way around the room. Sleep deprivation, fatigue, sedatives, and concurrent illness may act as precipitating factors.

Table 22.1 Classification of Motor Activities during Sleep

I. *Physiologic (Normal) Motor Activity during Sleep and at Sleep Onset*
  A. Postural shifts, body and limb movements during sleep
  B. Physiologic fragmentary myoclonus
  C. Hypnic jerks
  D. Hypnagogic foot tremor
  E. Rhythmic leg movements

II. *Pathologic (Abnormal) Motor Activity during Sleep*
  A. *Motor Parasomnias*
    1. *Non–Rapid Eye Movement (non-REM) Sleep Parasomnias*
      a. Confusional arousals
      b. Sleep walking
      c. Sleep terror
    2. *Rapid Eye Movement (REM) Sleep Parasomnias*
      a. REM sleep behavior disorder
      b. Nightmare disorder
      c. Recurrent isolates sleep paralysis
    3. *Other Motor Parasomnias*
      a. Sleep-related eating disorder
      b. Sleep-related groaning (catathrenia)
      c. Sleep-related dissociative disorders
  B. *Sleep-Related Movement Disorders*
    a. Restless Legs Syndriome (RLS)
    b. Periodic Limb Movements in Sleep (PLMS)
    c. Sleep related leg cramps
    d. Sleep related bruxism
    e. Sleep related rhythmic movement disorder
  C. *Isolated Sleep-Related Motor Symptoms (Apparently Normal Variants)*
    1. Sleep talking
    2. Hypnic jerks (sleep starts), including intensified hypnic jerks
    3. Benign sleep myoclonus of infancy
    4. Hypnagogic foot tremor
    5. Alternating leg muscle activation
    6. Propriospinal myoclonus at sleep onset
    7. Excessive fragmentary myoclonus
  D. *Nocturnal Seizures*
    1. True nocturnal seizures
      a. Tonic seizure
      b. Benign rolandic seizure
      c. Nocturnal frontal lobe epilepsy (NFLE)
        • Nocturnal paroxysmal dystonia
        • Paroxysmal arousals and awakenings
        • Episodic nocturnal wanderings
      d. Autosomal dominant nocturnal frontal lobe epilepsy (ADNFLE)
      e. Nocturnal temporal lobe epilepsy
      f. Continuous spike waves during sleep wave sleep (CSWS) or electrical status epilepticus in sleep (ESRS)
    2. Nocturnal and diurnal seizures
      a. Juvenile myoclonic epilepsy
      b. Generalized tonic-clonic seizures on awakening
      c. Infantile spasms (West syndrome)
      d. Generalized tonic-clonic seizures
      e. Partial complex seizures

Table 22.1 Continued

   f. Frontal lobe seizures
   g. Epilepsia partialis continua
E. *Miscellaneous Nocturnal Motor Hyperactivity*
   1. Drug-induced nocturnal dyskinesias
   2. Nocturnal jerks and shakes in obstructive sleep apnea syndrome
   3. Nocturnal panic attacks
   4. Posttraumatic stress disorder
   5. Agrypnia excitata, including fatal familial insomnia, Morvan's fibrillary chorea, and delirium tremens
   6. Hyperekplexia or exaggerated startle syndrome
   7. Rhythmic leg movements on termination of apneas-hypopneas
   8. High-frequency leg movements (rhythmic leg movements) during sleep and wakefulness
   9. Neck myoclonus (head jerks) during REM sleep
   10. Faciomandibular myoclonus during REM sleep
F. *Involuntary Movement Disorders*
   1. Usually persisting during sleep
      a. Symptomatic palatal myoclonus/palatal tremor
   2. Frequently persisting during sleep
      a. Spinal myoclonus
      b. Tics in Tourette's syndrome
      c. Hemifacial spasms
      d. Hyperekplexia
   3. Sometimes persisting during sleep
      a. Tremor
      b. Chorea
      c. Dystonia
      d. Hemiballismus

Pavor Nocturnus (Sleep Terrors)

Peak onset of sleep terrors is between 5 and 7 years of age, but sometimes they may persist into adulthood (see Table 22.3). The episodes also occur during slow-wave sleep. As with sleepwalking, there is a high frequency of familiar cases in sleep terror. The spell begins with an abrupt set of intense autonomic and motor symptoms, including a loud, piercing scream. Patients appear confused and fearful. Many patients also have a history of sleepwalking episodes. Precipitating factors are similar to those described with sleepwalking.

Confusional Arousals

Confusional arousal episodes occur mostly before the age of 5 years. As in sleepwalking and sleep terrors, these episodes arise out of slow-wave sleep (but may also occur out of stage N2) with confusion (Table 22.4). Patients may have some automatic and inappropriate behavior, but most spells are benign. Multiple

Table 22.2 Features of Somnambulism (Sleepwalking)

- Onset: common between ages 5 and 12 years
- High frequency of a positive family history
- Abrupt onset of motor activity arising out of slow-wave sleep during the first third of night
- Duration: less than 10 minutes
- Injuries and violent activity reported occasionally
- Precipitating factors: sleep deprivation, fatigue, concurrent illness, sedatives
- Treatment: precautions, benzodiazepines, imipramine

Table 22.3 Sleep Terror (Pavor Nocturnus)

1. Onset: peak occurs between ages 5 and 7 years
2. High frequency of familial cases
3. Abrupt arousal from slow-wave sleep during the first third of night with loud, piercing scream
4. Intense autonomic and motor components
5. Many patients also sleepwalk
6. Precipitating factors: stress, sleep deprivation, fever
7. Treatment: psychotherapy, benzodiazepines, tricyclics

episodes of confusional arousal in the same night are not uncommon. Confusional arousals may be considered part of a spectrum of sleep-walking and sleep terrors.

Rhythmic Movement Disorder

Rhythmic movement disorder is noted mostly before 18 months of age and is occasionally associated with mental retardation. It is a sleep-wake transition disorder occurring immediately before sleep during relaxed wakefulness and may continue into light sleep with these characteristic movements: head banging, head rolling, body rolling, and body rocking. These are stereotyped repetitive movements of large muscles at a rate of 0.5–2 Hz that last for a few minutes at a time but sometimes last up to 30 minutes or longer. Rhythmic movement disorder is a benign condition, and the patient outgrows the episodes.

Nocturnal Leg Cramps

Nocturnal leg cramps are intensely painful sensations accompanied by muscle tightness that occur during sleep. The spasms generally last for a few seconds but sometimes persist for several minutes. Cramps during sleep are in general associated with awakening. Many normal people experience nocturnal leg cramps; the cause remains unknown. Local massage or movement of the limbs usually relieves the cramps.

Somniloquy (Sleep Talking)

Somniloquy is a benign phenomenon that consists of speech or sounds uttered by people during sleep without awareness of behavior. Sleep talking becomes a problem when it occurs frequently and is loud enough to disturb the sleep of others. There is a report of a dialogue between two sleepers, neither of whom recalls it on awakening. Sleep talking most commonly occurs in non-REM stages N1 and N2 and REM sleep; rarely it occurs in slow-wave sleep. Sleep talking is a common disorder in the general population and most commonly occurs between 3 and 10 years of age and sometimes in adults. Stress and sleep deprivation may be triggering factors. Sometimes there is a family history of sleep talking.

Propriospinal Myoclonus at the Transition from Wakefulness to Drowsiness

This is a recently described special type of spinal myoclonus originating from a myoclonic generator usually in the midthoracic region with propagation up and down the spinal cord along the propriospinal pathways at a very

Table 22.4 Pertinent Features of Confusional Arousals

- Onset: peak onset before 5 years
- Abrupt onset out of slow wave sleep in the first third of the night but may also occur out of stage N2
- Appears confused with vacant look and may have automatic and inappropriate behavior lasting for a few seconds or minutes
- Multiple confusional episodes in the same night are not uncommon
- May be part of a spectrum of sleep walking and sleep terror; all three may occur in the same individual

slow speed. Montagna, Provini, Plazzi, et al.[7] described three patients with propriospinal myoclonus in the period between wakefulness and the moment of sleep onset, the state termed the *predormitum* by Critchley.[8] The myoclonic jerks involve predominately the axial muscles. The patients complain of insomnia or difficulty falling asleep. The differential diagnosis includes intensified hypnic jerks and periodic limb movements during sleep (PLMS). The hypnic jerks occur as soon as the patient falls asleep, in contrast to this particular type of propriospinal myoclonus that disappears as the patient goes into stage N1 or N2 sleep. PLMS occur mostly during non-REM sleep and not in the stage of the predormitum, except in some RLS patients. The mechanism in propriospinal myoclonus is thought to be supraspinal disinhibition of the spinal generator, and this particular propriospinal myoclonus is classified in the ICSD-2[3] under the category of isolated sleep-related motor symptoms (apparently normal variants).

Nightmares

Nightmares (also known as dream anxiety attacks) are fearful, vivid, and often frightening dreams that occur during REM sleep that are mostly visual but sometimes auditory. Nightmares may accompany sleep talking and body movements and most commonly occur during the middle to late part of sleep at night. Nightmares are mostly a normal phenomenon. About 50% of children, perhaps even more, have nightmares beginning at age 3 to 5 years. Frequencies of nightmares continuously decrease as children grow older, and older adults have few or no nightmares. Frightening and recurring nightmares (e.g., one or more nightmares per week) are not common and occur in less than 1% of individuals.

Nightmares can also occur as side effects of certain medications such as antiparkinsonian drugs (e.g., pergolide, levodopa); anticholinergics; and antihypertensive drugs, particularly beta-blockers. Nightmares commonly occur after sudden withdrawal of REM-suppressant drugs (e.g., tricyclic antidepressants, selective serotonin reuptake inhibitors). Benzodiazepines (e.g., diazepam or clonazepam) often suppress nightmares, but withdrawal from these drugs may precipitate nightmares. Nightmares have also been reported after alcohol ingestion or sudden withdrawal from barbiturates. Nightmares may sometimes be the initial manifestation of schizophreniform psychosis along with severe sleep disturbance. Many people with a certain personality type have nightmares throughout life. Nightmares generally do not require treatment except reassurance. In patients with recurring and fearful nightmares, however, combined behavioral or psychotherapy and REM-suppressant medications may be helpful.

Rapid Eye Movement Behavior Disorder

RBD is an important REM sleep parasomnia commonly seen in older adults (Table 22.5). A characteristic feature of RBD is intermittent loss of REM-related muscle hypotonia or atonia and the appearance of various abnormal motor activities during sleep. The patient experiences violent dream-enacting behavior during REM sleep, often causing self-injury or injury to the bed partner. The condition may be either idiopathic or more commonly occurs after a neurologic illness, particularly neurodegenerative diseases (e.g., Parkinson's

---

Table 22.5 Pertinent Features of Rapid Eye Movement Behavior Disorder

- Onset: middle-aged or older adult men
- Presents with violent dream-enacting behavior during sleep, causing injury to self or bed partner
- Often misdiagnosed as psychiatric disorder or nocturnal seizure (partial complex seizure)
- Etiology: 40% idiopathic, 60% causal association with neurodegenerative or other structural central nervous system lesion or related to alcohol or drugs (sedatives, hypnotics, tricyclics, anticholinergics)
- Polysomnography: REM sleep without muscle atonia or with excessive transient muscle bursts
- Experimental model: bilateral perilocus coeruleus lesions
- Treatment: 90% respond to clonazepam

---

disease, multisystem atrophy, diffuse Lewy body disease, and other structural lesions of the brainstem). RBD is sometimes associated with withdrawal of REM suppressant medications, barbiturates, and alcohol, or ingestion of drugs (e.g., sedative-hypnotics, tricyclic antidepressants, and anticholinergics). The most prominent finding in a PSG recording is REM sleep without muscle atonia and excessive transient phasic muscle bursts. Multiple muscle electromyograms (EMGs) from the upper and lower extremities should be obtained during the PSG recording in addition to the traditional chin and tibialis anterior muscle EMG because absence of muscle atonia may not be seen in all muscles. In experiments, similar behavior was produced by bilateral perilocus coeruleus lesions in cats many years before discovery of human RBD.

Bruxism (Tooth Grinding)

Bruxism occurs most commonly between the ages of 10 and 20 years. It is also commonly noted in children with mental retardation or cerebral palsy. Bruxism is noted most commonly during stages N1 and N2 and REM sleep. The episode is characterized by stereotypical tooth grinding and often precipitated by anxiety, stress, and dental disease. Occasionally, familial cases have been described.

Benign Sleep Myoclonus of Infancy

Benign sleep myoclonus of infancy occurs during the first few weeks of life and is generally seen in non-REM sleep, but it is sometimes seen during REM sleep. Episodes often occur in clusters involving arms, legs, and sometimes the trunk. The movements consist of jerky flexion, extension, abduction, and adduction. The condition is benign, needs no treatment, and generally subsides within several months.

NOCTURNAL SEIZURES

Seizures have been shown to occur predominately during sleep (nocturnal seizures), predominately in the daytime (diurnal seizures), or both during sleep at night and daytime (diffuse epilepsy).[9] The incidence of sleep epilepsy shows a wide variation, but the most likely figure is approximately 10%. Because of inconsistencies and contradictions in the classification of seizures based on biorhythmicity, modern epileptologists use the International Classification of Epilepsy, which divides seizures into primarily generalized seizures and partial seizures with or without secondary generalization.

True nocturnal seizures may include tonic seizures, benign focal epilepsy of childhood with rolandic spikes, juvenile myoclonic epilepsy, electrical status epilepticus during sleep or continuous spike and waves during sleep, and some varieties of frontal lobe seizures, particularly nocturnal paroxysmal dystonia (NPD) and autosomal dominant frontal lobe seizures. There is a special type of nocturnal temporal lobe seizure. Many patients with generalize tonic-clonic and partial complex seizures also have predominantly nocturnal seizures. Nocturnal seizures may be mistaken for motor and behavioral parasomnias or other movement disorders persisting during sleep or reactivating during stage transitions or on awakenings during the middle of the night.

Primary Generalized Tonic-Clonic (Grand Mal Seizures)

These may occur only during sleep, only during daytime, or may be randomly distributed. The nocturnal seizures occur almost exclusively in non-REM sleep and are frequently seen 1 to 2 hours after sleep onset and again at 5:00 am to 6:00 am. The interictal discharges on EEG increase in non-REM and disappear in REM sleep.

Juvenile Myoclonic Seizures

The onset of myoclonic epilepsy of Janz is usually between 13 and 19 years and is manifested by massive bilateral synchronous myoclonic jerks. The seizures are noted to increase shortly after awakening in the morning and occasionally on awakening in the middle of the night. A typical EEG shows polyspikes and spike and wave discharges synchronously and symmetrically. The interictal discharges are predominant at sleep onset and then on awakening but are virtually nonexistent during the rest of the sleep cycle.

Tonic Seizures

Tonic seizures are characteristic of Lennox-Gastaut syndrome; other types, however, such as myoclonic, generalized tonic-clonic, atonic, and atypical absences are also seen. Tonic seizures are typically activated by sleep and are much more frequent during non-REM sleep than during wakefulness and are never seen during REM sleep. A typical interictal EEG finding is slow spike and waves intermixed with trains of fast spikes during sleep.

Benign Focal Epilepsy of Childhood

This is a childhood seizure disorder seen mostly during drowsiness and non-REM sleep and is characterized by focal clonic facial twitchings, often preceded by perioral numbness. Many patients may have secondary generalized tonic-clonic seizures. The characteristic EEG finding consists of centrotemporal or rolandic spikes or sharp waves. These discharges are present in all stages of sleep. The seizures generally stop by the age of 15 to 20 years without any neurologic sequelae.

Partial Complex Seizure

Some patients with partial complex seizure may have predominantly sleep epilepsy, which mostly presents as focal seizures with or without secondary generalization. The interictal EEG discharges increase during non-REM and diminish during REM sleep. During non-REM sleep, the discharges spread ipsilaterally and contralaterally from the primary focus, whereas during REM sleep discharges tend to remain focal without propagation. It is often difficult to differentiate partial complex seizures of temporal origin from partial complex seizures of extratemporal (frontal) focus. A special subset of temporal lobe epilepsy patients has been described recently to have exclusively nocturnal seizure.[10]

Nocturnal Paroxysmal Dystonia and Frontal Lobe Seizures

It was Lugaresi and his group who brought this entity to the forefront of the medical community.[11-14] The spells occur during non-REM sleep and are characterized by dystonic, choreoathetoid, or ballismic movements during non-REM sleep almost every night (Table 22.6) in a stereotypical fashion. Ictal and interictal EEGs are generally normal. The patients respond to carbamazepine satisfactorily. Currently, it is believed that short-duration NPD attacks represent a form of frontal lobe seizures that are evoked specifically during sleep at night.[15] Three other entities—paroxysmal arousals, paroxysmal awakenings, and episodic nocturnal wanderings—share a common feature with NPD: abnormal paroxysmal motor activities during sleep and favorable response to anticonvulsants. All these entities most likely represent partial seizures arising from discharging foci in the deeper regions of the frontal cortex without any concomitant scalp EEG evidence of epileptiform activities.

Frontal lobe seizures may be nocturnal in addition to diurnal or may sometimes be exclusively nocturnal in nature (Table 22.7).[16-18] The onset is relatively sudden with sudden termination with short postictal confusion and scant recall of the events. The spells often occur in clusters. A special autosomal dominant nocturnal frontal lobe epilepsy has recently been described in several families, and this is often misdiagnosed as parasomnias.[19] Frontal lobe seizures are often difficult to differentiate from psychogenic nonepileptic seizure (NES).

Table 22.6 Salient Features of Nocturnal Frontal Lobe Epilepsy

- Onset: infancy to fifth decade of life
- Usually sporadic, rarely familial
- Sudden onset from non–rapid eye movement sleep
- Short lasting (15 seconds to <2 minutes)
- Semiology: ballismic, choreoathetotic, or dystonic movements, tonic, clonic, bipedal, bimanual, bicycling
- Stereotyped movements (Note: most other sleep-related movements including parasomnias are non-stereotypical movements
- Often occurs in clusters
- Short postictal confusion
- Mistaken for nonepileptic seizures
- Electroencephalogram (EEG): generally normal (both ictal and interictal EEG)
- Treatment: carbamazepine effective in most of the patients

Table 22.7 Features of Frontal Lobe Seizures

- Age of onset: infancy to middle age
- Sporadic, occasionally familial (dominant)
- Both diurnal and nocturnal spells, sometimes exclusively nocturnal
- Sudden onset in non–rapid eye movement sleep with sudden termination
- Duration: mostly less than 1 minute, sometimes 1–2 minutes with short postictal confusion
- Often occurs in clusters
- Semiology: tonic, clonic, bipedal, bimanual, and bicycling movements; motor and sexual automatisms; contralateral dystonic posturing or arm abduction with or without eye deviation
- Ictal electroencephalogram (EEG) may be normal; interictal EEG may show spikes; sometimes depth recording is needed

Psychogenic Nonepileptic Seizures (Pseudoseizures)

It is important to diagnose and differentiate nonepileptic seizures (NES) from true seizures because of the difference in the management.[20,21] NES is not common during sleep but rarely can occur on awakening from sleep at night and be mistaken for true nocturnal seizures (Table 22.8). These spells are emotionally triggered. The spells superficially resemble epilepsy but are bizarre and atypical. An important feature is out-of-phase clonic movements contrasting with in-phase clonic movements in true seizures. Onset is often gradual with gradual termination in contrast to sudden paroxysmal onset and sudden termination of true epileptic seizure. Postictally, there is no confusion in NES, in contrast to the postictal confusion in true seizures. The ictal and interictal EEGs in NES are normal and show no postictal slowing.

INVOLUNTARY DAYTIME MOVEMENT DISORDERS

These involuntary movements are traditionally seen by the movement disorder specialists and general neurologists. Many of these diurnal movement disorders persist during sleep, particularly during stage N1 sleep and stage shifts and on awakening in the middle of the night. These movements, therefore, must be considered in the differential diagnosis of abnormal motor activities during sleep at night. Certain diurnal involuntary movements frequently persist during sleep (e.g., spinal and propriospinal myoclonus, tics in Tourette's syndrome, hemifacial spasms, and hyperekplexia or exaggerated startle syndrome, palatal myoclonus or palatal tremor), whereas others are sometimes seen infrequently during sleep, such as tremor, chorea, dystonia, and hemiballismus (see Table 22.1).

INVOLUNTARY MOVEMENTS ALWAYS PERSISTING IN SLEEP

Palatal Myoclonus (Palatal Tremor) [See also Chapter 57]

There has been controversy in the terminology since the initial description of palatal myoclonus more than 100 years ago.[22,23] The term adopted by the movement disorder specialists

Table 22.8 Psychogenic Nonepileptic Seizure

- Can be mistaken for true nocturnal seizure
- Gradual onset with gradual termination
- No postictal confusion
- Out-of-phase clonic movements
- Forward pelvic thrust
- Repetitive stereotyped bizarre movements
- To-and-fro head movements without eye deviation
- Duration: longer than several minutes
- Ictal and interictal electroencephalogram: normal
- May also have true seizures (15%–20% in some monitoring units)

recently is the palatal tremor, which describes involuntary rhythmic movements of the soft palate and pharynx at a rate of 1.5 to 3.0 Hz. These movements are sometimes associated with rhythmic ocular, buccal, lingual, laryngeal, and diaphragmatic movements and occasionally also movements of the upper limbs. With rare exceptions, palatal tremor persists throughout the day and night for the remaining life span of the patient. Two types have been described: a primary or essential palatal myoclonus or tremor and a secondary or symptomatic type, resulting from brainstem infarction, tumors, trauma, demyelinating disease, degenerative disorders, encephalitis, or encephalopathy. The characteristic complaint of the patient in the essential type is a clicking noise in the ears as a result of rhythmic contraction of the tensor veli palatini muscle. This type may disappear during sleep. In the secondary variety, the palatal movement is thought to be due to activation of the levator veli palatini muscle, and the patient presents with a variety of brainstem findings. Palatal tremor results from an involvement of the Guillain-Mollaret triangle, which is formed by the cerebellar dentate nucleus and its outflow tract in the superior cerebellar peduncle crossing over to the contralateral side in the vicinity of the red nucleus and descending down along the central tegmental tract to the inferior olivary nucleus with a final connection from the inferior olivary nucleus back to the contralateral dentate nucleus. The lesions are generally found in the dentate nucleus or its outflow tract and in the central tegmental tract. In the rare case of unilateral palatal tremor, the lesions are noted in the contralateral central tegmental tract or inferior olivary nucleus or in the ipsilateral dentate nucleus or its outflow tract. A characteristic pathologic finding is olivary hypertrophy. Palatal tremor is mostly refractory to treatment. There are occasional reports of response to anticholinergics or botulinum toxin injections, baclofen, valproic acid, lamotrigine, tetrabenazine, and carbamazepine.[24-28]

INVOLUNTARY MOVEMENTS FREQUENTLY PERSISTING IN SLEEP

Spinal Myoclonus

Spinal myoclonus, like palatal myoclonus, is a segmental myoclonus.[29] Spinal myoclonus generally presents with rhythmic myoclonic movements of one limb, trunk, or both legs, resulting from discharges from a myoclonic generator in one or more contiguous segments of the spinal cord affecting the muscles supplied by the corresponding segments. Frequently, spinal myoclonus persists during sleep. Sometimes the myoclonus can be arrhythmic and stimulus sensitive. In most cases, an etiologic agent is recognized, for example, spinal cord tumor or trauma, cervical spondylotic myelopathy, herpes zoster infection, myelitis, demyelinating myelopathy, anesthetic agents, intrathecal medication, or arteriovenous malformation. A special type of spinal myoclonus, called propriospinal myoclonus, has recently been described.[30,31] The myoclonic generator is usually in the midthoracic region, and the myoclonic movements of the trunk and the limbs result from activation of the slowly conducting propriospinal systems. Spinal myoclonus frequently responds to clonazepam.

Tics in Tourette's Syndrome

Tics in Tourette's syndrome persist during all stages of sleep as documented by overnight PSG, accelerometric, and video monitoring studies. In 11 of 12 Tourette's patients studied by Glaze, Frost, and Jankovic et al.,[32] tics and rare vocalization were noted in all stages of sleep. Tourette's patients also have repeated awakenings and have been shown to have an increased incidence of somnambulism and night terrors.

Hemifacial Spasm

Hemifacial spasm consists of intermittent contraction of one side of the face that can be repetitive and jerk-like or sustained. It is believed to arise from irritation of the facial nerve or the muscles.

Hemifacial spasms persist during the lighter stages of sleep but progressively decrease as the patients drift from wakefulness into the deepening stages of sleep. Both central and peripheral (ephaptic transmission between adjacent nerve fibers without synapses) factors are responsible for hemifacial spasm.

Involuntary Movements Sometimes Persisting during Sleep

Many of the involuntary movements (e.g., parkinsonian tremor, dystonic spasms, chorea, tics, hemiballismus, and hyperekplexia) are shown to reappear during awakenings from sleep or during stage N1 and rarely during stage N2 sleep, and these are absent during slow-wave sleep. Physiologic motor activities such as postural shifts and body and limb movements in normal individuals are also seen under similar circumstances during sleep at night, suggesting similar modulation by sleep of normal physiologic and disordered movements. Fish, Sawyers, Allen, et al.[33] have clearly documented these findings in Parkinson's disease, Huntington's chorea, torsion dystonia, and Tourette's syndrome following a careful PSG study using multiple muscle EMGs, split-screen video monitoring, and accelerometric study.

Drug-Induced Nocturnal Dyskinesias

In some patients on medications, drug-induced nocturnal dyskinesias must be considered in the differential diagnosis of abnormal motor activities during sleep at night. Many patients with moderately to severely affected Parkinson's disease on levodopa treatment have myoclonic movements during sleep at night. These movements should be differentiated from PLMS by the history of Parkinson's disease and levodopa treatment, a lack of periodicity in these drug-induced dyskinesias, and reduction or disappearance of these movements on reducing the dose of the medication or changing to another therapeutic agent. PLMS have also been noted in patients on tricyclic antidepressants or lithium treatment. An additional cause of drug-induced nocturnal dyskinesia is secondary or symptomatic RLS, which has been described in those taking neuroleptics, lithium, calcium channel antagonists (e.g., nifedipine), or selective serotonin reuptake inhibitors and in withdrawal from sedatives or narcotics.

Nocturnal Jerks and Body Movements in Obstructive Sleep Apnea Syndrome

Patients with obstructive sleep apnea syndrome (OSAS) may have flailing and jerking movements of the body and limbs repeatedly throughout the night associated with repeated apneas or hypopneas and hypoxemias.[33a] These movements need to be differentiated from other motor abnormalities during sleep at night by paying close attention to the history and overnight PSG study. Sometimes respiratory-related leg movements during resumption of breathing following apnea or hypopnea may occur in a periodic fashion resembling PLMS, but in some OSAS patients true PLMS are unmasked after continuous positive airway pressure titration. OSAS patients may also have increased prevalence of sleep walking[34] and confusional arousals, which are occasionally associated with sleep violence and sexsomnia.

Excessive Fragmentary Myoclonus

Excessive fragmentary myoclonus (EFM) may represent intensified physiologic fragmentary myoclonus and may be seen during all stages of non-REM sleep and stage R, and it is noted to accompany a variety of primary sleep disorders.[3] Further evidence is needed to prove that EFM has any biological consequence.

Hyperekplexia or Exaggerated Startle Syndrome

In this condition, nocturnal leg jerking has been described. These myoclonic jerks occur in response to stimulus (e.g., startle) during wakefulness in the daytime and during sleep.[35]

Restless Legs Syndrome

Restless legs syndrome (RLS) is characterized by intense disagreeable feelings in the legs with an urge to move the legs to get relief[36] (Table 22.9). The symptoms appear mostly or exclusively when the patient is at rest, as when sitting for a sustained period or lying down in bed, particularly in the evening and nightfall.[37,38] The symptoms occur at sleep onset and may also occur on awakenings in the middle of the night. Idiopathic RLS is often a lifelong condition. Its pathophysiologic cause is not well worked out, although dopamine and iron abnormalities have been implicated. A major genetic contribution is suggested by the high percent of patients with affected first-degree relatives (often more than 50% in some studies), with many pedigrees suggesting a dominant inheritance. Secondary RLS may be associated with a variety of suggested causes.

Periodic Limb Movements in Sleep

PLMS is characterized by periodically recurring movements, particularly dorsiflexion of the ankles and sometimes flexion of the knees

Table 22.9 Clinical Criteria for Restless Legs Syndrome (RLS)

Essential criteria for diagnosis of RLS:
1. An urge to move the legs, usually accompanied or caused by uncomfortable or unpleasant sensations in the legs
2. The urge to move, or unpleasant sensations that begin or worsen during periods of rest or inactivity such as lying or sitting
3. The urge to move, or unpleasant sensations that are partially or totally relieved by movement, such as walking or stretching, at least as long as the movement continues
4. The urge to move, or unpleasant sensations that are worse in the evening or night than during the day, or that occur only in the evening or night

Supportive criteria for the diagnosis of RLS:
1. Response to dopaminergic therapy
2. Positive family history
3. Periodic limb movements (during wakefulness or sleep)

Associated features of RLS:
1. Progressive clinical course
2. Physical examination normal in patients with primary RLS, unless other disorders are present; in secondary RLS, signs of the causal condition may be present
3. Sleep disturbance, especially problems with initiating and maintaining sleep (insomnia), often leading to reduced total sleep time and daytime fatigue and sleepiness

and hips occurring periodically at an average interval of 20 to 40 seconds (range of 5 to 90 seconds) during non-REM sleep[36] (Table 22.10). PLMS is noted in at least 80% of cases of RLS, and RLS is noted in approximately 30% of cases of PLMS. PLMS may occur in normal individuals, particularly in subjects older than 65 years in whom there is an incidence of approximately 30%. There are a variety of other causes of PLMS.

Fatal Familial Insomnia

Fatal familial insomnia (FFI) is a rare autosomal dominant prion disease.[39] Clinical manifestations of this disorder include impaired control of the sleep-wake cycle (e.g., circadian dysrhythmia, autonomic and neuroendocrine dysfunction), in addition to somatic neurologic, cognitive, and behavioral manifestations. From the onset of illness, profound sleep disturbances (particularly severe insomnia) are noted. Ataxia, corticospinal deficit, myoclonus, and tremor are characteristic neurologic deficits that occur in FFI. The condition runs a rapidly progressive course. PSG study shows an almost total absence of sleep pattern; only short periods of REM sleep exist, lasting for a few seconds or minutes but without the normal muscle atonia. These brief REM periods may be associated with dream-enacting behavior that manifests as complex movements and gestures (resembles RBD). Characteristic neuropathologic findings consist of severe atrophy of the thalamus (especially anterior ventral and dorsomedial thalamic nuclei) associated with variable involvement of the inferior olive, striatum, and cerebellum.

Table 22.10 Diagnostic Criteria for Periodic Limb Movements in Sleep

- Repetitive, often stereotyped movements mostly during non–rapid eye movement sleep
- Usually noted in the legs, consisting of extension of the great toe, dorsiflexion of the ankle, and flexion of the knee and hip; sometimes seen in the arms
- Periodic or quasiperiodic at an average interval of 20–40 seconds (range, 5–90 seconds) with a duration of 0.5–10.0 seconds and as part of at least four consecutive movements
- Occurs at any age but prevalence increases with age
- May occur as an isolated condition or may be associated with a large number of other medical, neurologic, or sleep disorders and medications
- Seen in at least 80% of patients with restless legs syndrome

Sleep-Related Panic Attacks

Panic attacks commonly occur during daytime, but up to 30% of these patients may also have nocturnal panic attacks during sleep, and rarely isolated panic attacks in sleep[40] have been described. Sleep panic attacks are characterized by extreme anxiety, and the patients wake up during transition from non-REM stage N2 to N3. Other features besides extreme anxiety include palpitation, choking, shortness of breath, sweating, shakes in the form of trembling, dizziness, and extreme fear of dying. Up to 70% of patients with panic disorder have sleep complaints such as insomnia and fear of going to bed or falling asleep. The nocturnal panic attacks should be differentiated from sleep terrors, nocturnal seizures, and nightmares.

Dissociative Disorders

Status dissociatus is characterized by a complete breakdown of state boundaries and can be considered an extreme form of RBD.[41,42] During the attacks, the patient has complex motor and behavioral manifestations characterized by jerks, shakes, and screams. PSG study shows features of wakefulness, non-REM, and REM sleep, making it impossible to score wakefulness, REM, or non-REM sleep. For example, there may be a mixture of sleep spindles, REMs, alpha intrusions, and absence of REM muscle atonia. The condition may be precipitated by withdrawal from prolonged alcohol abuse and has also been noted occasionally in patients with narcolepsy, after open heart surgery, and in olivopontocerebellar atrophy. FFI almost invariably manifests features of status dissociatus.

There is a condition known as psychogenic dissociative state,[42,43] which is characterized by complex and often injurious behavior noted occasionally during apparent sleep at night. PSG study, however, shows an EEG wakeful pattern during the abnormal behavior. Patients frequently give a history of physical or sexual abuse as a child.

Posttraumatic Stress Disorder

Posttraumatic stress disorder (PTSD) is characterized by preoccupation with and the reenactment of severely traumatic or life- threatening past events such as war experience, torture, or other situations involving physical or sexual abuse.[44] Symptoms include flashbacks and anxiety-prone dreams. During the reenactment of the past traumatic events, patients may sometimes strike out violently, hide under the bed, or run out of the bed. Patients with PTSD experience chronic insomnia caused by states of hyperarousal. These patients may also have increased PLMS and other body movements during sleep. PSG findings in PTSD include decreased total sleep time, reduced slow-wave and REM sleep, increased number of awakenings, and impaired sleep efficiency. Frequent nightmares that may occur during non-REM and REM sleep are hallmarks of PTSD. REM sleep findings in PTSD are contradictory. Some experts consider PTSD a disorder of the REM sleep mechanism and associate it with RBD.

APPROACH TO A PATIENT WITH MOVEMENT DISORDERS DURING SLEEP

The first step in assessing a patient presenting with abnormal movements and behavior during sleep is obtaining a history, which should include directed inquiries on detailed sleep history and sleeping habits; history of current or previous medical, neurologic, and psychiatric illnesses; and history of drug and alcohol consumption, as well as family history.[45] Laboratory tests must be confirmatory and subservient to the clinical history and physical examination (see Table 22.11).

Sleep History

Sleep histories must encompass the entire 24-hour span, not just symptoms occurring at sleep onset or during sleep at night. Particular

Table 22.11 Clinical Approach to a Patient with Abnormal Movements and Behavior during Sleep

- History
  - Sleep history
  - Sleep questionnaire
  - Sleep log or diary
  - Drug and alcohol history
  - Psychiatric history
  - General medical history
  - Neurologic history
  - History of previous illnesses
  - Family history
- Physical examination

attention must be paid to the frequency, type, and time of onset of the complex or abnormal behavior and the pattern of behavior. The history must also address nocturnal behavior and forensic implications. Time of onset of symptoms, including complex movements and abnormal behavior, is important in making a clinical diagnosis in a patient presenting with abnormal motor activity and behavior during sleep. Arousal disorders (e.g., sleepwalking, sleep terrors, confusional arousals), RBD, and disorders occurring at sleep onset or at sleep-wake transition all present at a particular time during the night or during certain stages of sleep. Symptoms occurring in the early evening while the patient is lying in bed or at sleep onset (e.g., paresthesias and uncontrollable limb movements) may suggest RLS. Repeated awakenings throughout the night, snoring, and cessation of breathing during sleep at night may suggest a diagnosis of OSAS. Similarly, symptoms of exhaustion and sleepiness on awakening first thing in the morning may suggest fragmented sleep or OSAS. Daytime fatigue and excessive somnolence in the late morning and afternoon are additional symptoms pointing to a diagnosis of OSAS. Excessive sleepiness in the daytime, "sleep attacks," and an irresistible desire for brief episodes of sleep followed by a feeling of being refreshed are characteristic symptoms of narcolepsy. Abnormal movements and behavior occurring during the first third of the night followed by partial or complete amnesia next morning may suggest arousal disorders. The occurrence of complex motor behavior with or without injuries to the self or the bed partners during the middle and late part of the night is characteristic of RBD. Symptoms occurring during sleep-wake transition or at sleep onset may suggest a diagnosis of rhythmic movement disorder, sleep talking, or propriospinal myoclonus at the transitional stage. Leg jerks throughout the night, often occurring in a periodic or quasiperiodic fashion, may suggest PLMS. Inquiries should be made about the possible daytime involuntary movements, which might persist during sleep or reemerge during stage shifts. A history of daytime seizures may help in establishing a diagnosis of possible nocturnal seizures in a patient with appropriate history.

Understanding patient problems requires consideration of psychological, social, medical, and biologic factors and how they interact. The physician should inquire about the patient's functional status and mood during the day and should also analyze the onset, frequency, duration, and severity of the complex behavior and movements. The progression, evaluation, and fluctuation over time and any triggering factors that might have initiated the movements should be considered in the history. An analysis of these factors may differentiate transient disorder from persistent ones.

An interview with the patient's bed partner and caregiver (or, in the case of a child, a parent) is important for diagnosing abnormal movements (e.g., PLMS or other body movements), abnormal behavior (e.g., parasomnias, nocturnal seizures), and breathing disorders during sleep. The bed partner may also be able to answer questions about the patient's sleeping habits, history of drug use, psychosocial problems (e.g., stress at home, work, or school), and changes in his or her sleep habits. Home videotaping by the bed partners or other observers may also be helpful.

Sleep history must also include any confounding medical or psychiatric conditions and medication history, including alcohol or illicit drugs.

The physician should pay particular attention to the pattern of behavior as each movement disorder occurring during sleep at night may present with a set of complex motor acts and behavior. Patients with RBD may present with complex motor acts and are often violent and injurious to themselves and their bed partner. Patients with arousal disorders (sleepwalking, sleep terror, confusional arousals) present with characteristic movements and behavior as described in the previous section. Patients with frontal lobe seizures, including NPD, may present with choreoathetotic and other complex stereotypical movements. Patients with partial complex seizures of temporal or extratemporal origin or other types of nocturnal seizures present with characteristic clinical manifestations, which may be diagnostic of a particular entity. Patients presenting with abnormal movements accompanied by tongue biting or nocturnal enuresis are highly suggestive of nocturnal seizures. Sudden onset followed by sudden termination and postictal confusion favors a seizure disorder, whereas gradual onset and gradual termination, and occurrence of bizarre movements and behavior during wakeful stage in the middle of the night without any accompanying postictal confusion strongly suggest NES.

Sleep Questionnaire

Patients may fill out a sleep questionnaire containing a list of pertinent questions relating to sleep complaints (e.g., sleep hygiene; sleep patterns; medical, psychiatric, and neurologic disorders; drug and alcohol use). This can reduce professional interview time.

Sleep Log or Sleep Diary

A sleep log or diary kept over a 2-week period is also a valuable indicator of sleep hygiene. Such a log should document bedtime, arising time, and daytime nap information; amount of time needed to go to sleep; number of nighttime awakenings; total sleep time; and feelings on arousal (e.g., whether the patient is refreshed or drowsy). Other information in the sleep log should include patient's mood and naps taken during the daytime and, in women, the relation of abnormal movements and behavior to their menstrual cycles.

The Drug and Alcohol History

The physician should inquire about drugs that may induce or exacerbate the symptoms of RBD (e.g., selective serotonin reuptake inhibitors, tricyclic antidepressants). The physician should also elicit from history any causal relationship between medications and abnormal behavior and movements. Certain medications may trigger arousal disorders (e.g., lithium, zolpidem, triazolam, and other central nervous system depressants). Withdrawal of REM suppressant medications may trigger REM parasomnias (e.g., RBD, nightmares). Alcohol or barbiturate withdrawal may also precipitate RBD.

Psychiatric History

Attention should be paid to signs of possible psychiatric or psychophysiologic disorder (e.g., depression, anxiety, psychosis, obsession, life stress, personality traits). If the abnormal movements and behavior are secondary to a psychiatric illness, treating it eliminates the sleep disturbance in most cases. If sleep complaint persists after such treatment, an additional cause or a primary sleep disorder should be suspected. Psychiatric history is also very important in patients suspected of psychogenic dissociative disorders and PTSD.

Medical and Neurologic History

It is very important to go into the details of neurologic history as certain abnormal movements and behavior during sleep at night may be the manifestations of an underlying neurologic disorder, or the abnormal movements and behavior may sometimes precede neurodegenerative disorder. For example, complex movements and behavior of RBD may be the forerunner of a neurodegenerative disease or may accompany many neurodegenerative diseases. Many daytime movement disorders may persist during sleep or reemerge during stage shifts, and, therefore, it is important to inquire about the neurologic or other medical disorders.

History of Past Illness

The patient history should contain information about past medical, psychiatric, or neurologic disorders that may be responsible for the patient's complaint of abnormal movements and behavior during sleep at night.

Family History

Family history is important because approximately one third of patients with narcolepsy and about 40% of patients with RLS have a family history of sleep disorder. OSAS, with or without obesity, has also been described as affecting other family members. Prevalence of sleepwalking and sleep terrors in other family members is high. Many neurologic disorders, including FFI, have family histories.

Physical Examination

A careful physical examination is important and may uncover various medical disorders such as respiratory, cardiovascular, endocrine, or neurologic disorders that might be responsible for the abnormal behavior and movements during sleep at night. Physical examination in OSAS may uncover upper-airway anatomic abnormalities. Physical examination may also reveal systemic hypertension, often associated with sleep apnea. A total physical examination, including detailed neurologic examination, should direct attention to any underlying structural cause, including evidence of neurodegenerative disease, for the abnormal movements or may uncover the presence of characteristics typical of diurnal movement disorders.

Clinical Scales to Assess Subjective Measurement of Sleepiness

A variety of scales have been developed to assess subjective degree of sleepiness.[45] Some patients presenting with abnormal movements and behavior may complain of excessive daytime sleepiness. The following features suggest the presence of excessive sleepiness: falling asleep in inappropriate places and under inappropriate circumstances (e.g., the patient dozes while sitting down, watching television, reading, watching movies, sitting in classes or conferences, listening to a lecture, or, in severe cases, talking on the telephone or in person face to face or while eating or engaged in other activities, even driving); dozing off during routine tasks such as driving; poor attention span and difficulty coping at work and school; involvement in accidents at work; nonrefreshing sleep; and frequent napping throughout the day.

The Stanford Sleepiness Scale (see Chapter 14) is a 7-point scale used to measure subjective sleepiness; however, it may not be reliable in patients with persistent sleepiness. Another scale used to assess sleepiness is the Visual Analog Scale of alertness and well-being, in which subjects indicate their feelings and alertness at an arbitrary point on a line. This scale has been used successfully in treating circadian rhythm disorders. The Epworth Sleepiness Scale evaluates general levels of sleepiness in each. The patients rate eight situations on a scale of 0 to 3, with 3 indicating a situation in which chances of dozing off are highest. The maximum score is 24 and a score of 10 suggests the presence of excessive sleepiness (see Chapter 14). This scale has been weakly correlated with multiple sleep latency test (MSLT) scores. There are other scales and questionnaires to assess sleep-related movements, for example, the validated RBD questionnaire and two sleep scales.

LABORATORY ASSESSMENT

Laboratory assessment should be considered an extension of the history and physical examination. Laboratory tests should include diagnostic workup for primary conditions that may be responsible for abnormal movements and behavior during sleep at night as well as workup for the sleep disturbance caused by abnormal movements and behavior (Table 22.12). Laboratory tests for patients with parasomnias, nocturnal seizures, or other abnormal

Table 22.12 Laboratory Asseement for Abnormal Movement and Behavior during Sleep

- Diagnostic workup for the primary condition causing secondary sleep disturbance
- Laboratory tests for the diagnosis of sleep disorder
- Overnight polysomnographic study
- Multiple sleep latency test
- Maintenance of Wakefulness Test
- Actigraphy
- Video-polysomnography
- Neuroimaging study in cases of suspected neurologic illness causing sleep disorders
- Pulmonary function tests in cases of suspected bronchopulmonary diseases causing sleep apnea

movements and behavior during sleep at night include overnight PSG recording, particularly video PSG, MSLTs, actigraphy, long-term video-EEG monitoring, and EEG, including 24-hour EEG.[9,45]

Polysomnographic and Video-Polysomnographic Recording

PSG study is not routinely indicated in uncomplicated and typical parasomnias. PSG is, however, indicated for patients who experience unusual or atypical parasomnias or for those whose behaviors are violent or otherwise potentially injurious to themselves or others. Video-PSG recordings should be performed to correlate behavior with PSG recordings (see Chapter 10). Video PSG may also be indicated in situations with forensic considerations. Because certain parasomnias may mimic seizure disorders, PSG or video-PSG is essential when a seizure disorder is suspected.[46] To document nocturnal epilepsy, video-PSG using multiple channels of EEG and multiple montages is required. If sleep epilepsy is suspected, EEG analysis should be performed using the standard EEG speed of 30 mm per second to identify epileptiform discharges.

For patients with suspected RBD, multiple muscle EMGs from all four limbs and orofacial region are essential—there is often dissociation in the activities between upper limb, lower limb, and cranially innervated muscles in these patients. Hence, if multiple muscle EMGs are not included in the recording, REM sleep without atonia or transient muscle bursts may be missed in some cases.

In diurnal movement disorders persisting during sleep, special neurophysiologic studies to record tremor and characterize myoclonus may be needed combining EEG and EMG recordings (see Chapter 16 for details).

Indications for PSG and video-PSG in patients suspected of abnormal movements and behavior may be listed as follows[9]: to differentiate between epileptic and nonepileptic nocturnal events (e.g., parasomnias, seizures, and pseudoseizures); to clarify the classification of patients with known sleep epilepsy; to diagnose continuous spike waves during slow-wave sleep; to diagnose benign epilepsy of childhood with rolandic spikes; to lateralize and localize the main focus, which may be important before surgical treatment for seizure is contemplated; to unmask the primary focus in a patient with secondary bilateral synchrony during REM sleep, which can suppress generalized discharges; to diagnose tonic seizures in patients with Lennox-Gastaut syndrome; to diagnose sleep apnea or other primary sleep disorders, which may be mistaken for epilepsy or other abnormal movements during sleep; for investigation of patients who present with excessive daytime sleepiness, which cannot be explained by the seizures, the abnormal movements, or the anticonvulsant medication; and to document sleep disturbances and sleep architecture in epileptics so that these disturbances may be treated to prevent chronic sleep deprivation, which may have deleterious effects on epilepsy.

Utility of Sleep in the Diagnosis of Epilepsy

Utility of sleep in the diagnosis of epilepsy is well established. Table 22.13 lists recordings that may be recommended for patients with suspected nocturnal seizures. An EEG is the single most important diagnostic test in patients with suspected epilepsy.[47] The EEG study must routinely include activation procedures such as sleep, hyperventilation, and photic stimulation. In suspected partial complex seizures, special basal temporal electrodes (e.g., T1, T2, or sphenoidal electrodes) should be used. Certain EEG waveforms are correlated with a high percentage of patients with clinical seizures and are considered potentially epileptogenic (e.g., spikes, sharp waves, spike and wave, or sharp and slow-wave complexes;

Table 22.13 Laboratory Recordings for Patients with Suspected Nocturnal Seizures

- Standard daytime sleep-wake electroencephalographic recording
- Prolonged daytime electroencephalographic recording after sleep deprivation
- Twenty-four hour ambulatory electroencephalographic recording
- Long-term video-electroencephalographic monitoring
- Intracranial recording in selected cases

an evolving pattern of focal, rhythmic theta or delta waves, especially in neonatal seizures; and temporal intermittent rhythmic delta activity). It should be noted that a single normal EEG does not exclude a diagnosis of epilepsy. Epilepsy is a paroxysmal event and, therefore, during a short EEG recording, paroxysmal discharges are not necessarily seen. Therefore, the chance of getting positive interictal EEG findings improves if several EEGs can be obtained. The initial EEG recording may show normal results in 50% of patients with true epilepsy. Even after three or four EEG recordings, 8% to 10% of patients with seizures may show only normal EEG findings. The yield after three to four EEG recordings obtained after activation procedures does not increase significantly. Increasing the duration of recording to several hours or days, however, increases the chance of obtaining a positive EEG result. The other reason for obtaining a normal EEG recording in a patient with true epilepsy is that the epileptic foci may be located in a deep location (e.g., orbitofrontal and medial interhemispheric region). Surface electrodes may not pick up these discharges in a deep location. Furthermore, the epileptiform discharges may have been attenuated considerably or may have changed morphologically by the time the discharges are seen at the surface.

Twenty-Four-Hour Ambulatory Electroencephalogram Recording

Ambulatory EEG recording permits 24-hour continuous recording in the patient's normal day- to-day environment. This type of recording is very valuable in documenting interictal epileptiform discharges in presence of normal routine EEGs. However, the presence of movements and muscle artifacts and lack of video documentation of the behavior are distinct disadvantages of ambulatory recording.

Long-Term Video-Electroencephalographic Recording

Documentation of ictal epileptiform discharges coupled with characteristic behavioral pattern in a long-term video-EEG monitoring unit provides unambiguous evidence of the presence of true seizure.

Intracranial Recordings

If the result of the EEG, including long-term monitoring and neuroimaging, is discordant in localizing the focus, the patient should then be referred to a specialized epilepsy center for intracranial recordings.

Multiple Sleep Latency Tests

MSLT is important for objectively documenting excessive sleepiness and sleep onset rapid eye movements (SOREMs). A mean sleep latency of less than 8 minutes, which is consistent with pathologic sleepiness, in conjunction with SOREMs in two or more of the four to five recordings during MSLT, strongly suggests narcolepsy. Maintenance of Wakefulness Test (MWT) is a variant of the MSLT that measures the patient's ability to stay awake. This test is important for monitoring effective stimulant treatment in narcolepsy or positive pressure therapy in OSAS, but it is not as good as MSLT for measuring daytime sleepiness.

Actigraphy

Actigraphy is a technique of motion detection that records activities during sleep and waking (see Chapter 15). It complements a sleep diary or sleep log data. The actigraphic instrument is a small device, slightly larger than a wristwatch, worn generally on the wrist but also on the ankle for 1 to 2 weeks. It is a cost-effective method for assessing a sleep-wake pattern. Actigraph is very useful in the diagnosis of circadian rhythm sleep disorders, sleep-state misperception, and other types of insomnias, as well as in detecting and quantifying PLMS. Its role in evaluating varieties of movements during sleep at night has been evolving. It appears to be a promising technique for assessment of

patients with abnormal movements during sleep at night.

Other Laboratory Tests

Neuroimaging study (computed tomography [CT] and magnetic resonance imaging [MRI]) of the brain is essential when a neurologic illness is suspected of causing abnormal movements and behavior during sleep or a structural neurologic disease is responsible for such abnormal movements. All adults with new-onset seizures and children without any characteristic epilepsy syndrome should have MRI performed to identify any structural brain disorders. MRI is more sensitive than CT and, therefore, the preferred procedure. Positron emission tomography (PET) and single-photon emission computed tomography (SPECT) may detect areas of cerebral hypometabolism or relative reduction of blood flow in patients with partial seizures during interictal period. During ictal episodes, these studies demonstrate focal hypermetabolism and hyperperfusion. PET and SPECT scans are not performed routinely in patients presenting with abnormal movements and behavior but are mostly research tools. In RBD special sophisticated MRI procedures (not available in every center) such as diffusion tensor imaging showing anisotrophy or diffusibility to detect brainstem microstructural alterations, and voxel based morphometry may be useful.[48,49]

SUMMARY AND CONCLUSION

In this chapter we have outlined an approach to a patient with abnormal motor activity during sleep and a rational practical classification, which we hope should help the practicing sleep and movement disorder specialists in the diagnosis and differential diagnosis of abnormal motor activity during sleep. Such an approach should begin with a careful clinical analysis of the patient's symptoms and behavior not only during sleep at night but also during the entire 24-hour day-night cycle. The analysis should include a history of past illnesses, including neurologic, general medical, and psychiatric disorders, as well as the patient's history of drug and alcohol intake and the patient's family history of transmitted disorders. The historical analysis should be followed by physical examination that pays particular attention to the nervous system. Based on the history and physical examination, a presumptive diagnosis and possible differential diagnosis should be formulated. The physician can then determine appropriate laboratory tests based on the history and physical examination. In many patients with abnormal motor activity during sleep, the diagnosis can be made clinically without the additional expense and inconvenience of the laboratory tests. Laboratory investigations, however, must be performed in uncertain or difficult cases, those with a history of violence to self or others or of unusual movements evading clear categorization, and in those suspected of nocturnal seizures. Laboratory tests are also needed for medicolegal purposes or for assessing severity and establishing prognosis. Movement disorders during sleep constitute a group of the most challenging sleep disorders. If we rise to this challenge, however, we will find that most of these disorders are amenable to treatment. Many patients with movement disorders during sleep remain undiagnosed or misdiagnosed for years and are subjected to inappropriate treatment (e.g., treating intensified hypnic jerks with antiepileptic medications for a mistaken diagnosis of myoclonic seizures or inappropriately treating a true nocturnal seizure as an arousal disorder). We must gather all our resources to heal and comfort the unfortunate victims of nocturnal movement disorders and to do no further harm.

REFERENCES

1. Ohayon M. Epidemiology of parasomnias. In: Thorpy MJ, Plazzi G, eds. *The Parasomnias and Other Sleep Related Movement Disorders.* Cambridge, England: Cambridge University Press; 2010:7.
2. Broughton R. Behavioral parasomnias. In: Chokroverty S, ed. *Sleep Disorders Medicine: Basic Science, Technical Considerations and Clinical Aspects.* Boston, MA: Butterworth-Heinemann; 1999:635.
3. American Academy of Sleep Medicine. *International Classification of Sleep Disorders. Diagnostic and Coding Manual.* 2nd ed. Westchester, IL: American Academy of Sleep Medicine; 2005.
4. Lysenko L, Hanna P, Chokroverty S. Sleep disruption from movement disorders. In: Barkoukis TJ, Matheson JK, Farber R, Doghramji K, eds. *Therapy in Sleep Medicine.* Philadephia: Elsevier/Saunders; 2012:345–60.
5. Chokroverty S. *Clinical Companion to Sleep Disorders Medicine.* 2nd ed. Boston, MA: Butterworth-Heinemann; 2000:107.
6. Chokroverty S. Approach to the patient with sleep complaints. In: Chokroverty S, ed. *Sleep Disorders Medicine: Basic Science, Technical Considerations and Clinical Aspects.* Philadelphia, PA: Saunders/Elsevier; 2009:255.
7. Montagna P, Provini F, Plazzi G, et al. Propriospinal myoclonus upon relaxation and drowsiness: a cause of severe insomnia. *Mov Disord* 1997;12:66.
8. Critchley M. The pre-dormitum. *Rev Neurol (Paris)* 1955;93:101.
9. Chokroverty S, Montagna P: Sleep and epilepsy. In Chokroverty S ed. *Sleep Disorders Medicine: Basic Science, Technical Considerations and Clinical Aspects.* Philadelphia, PA: Saunders/Elsevier, 2009:499.
10. Bernasconi A, Andermann F, Cendes F, et al. Nocturnal temporal lobe epilepsy. *Neurology* 1998;50:1772.
11. Lugaresi E, Cirignotta F. Hypnogenic paroxysmal dystonia: epileptic seizure or a new syndrome? *Sleep* 1981;4:129.
12. Lugaresi E, Cirignotta F, Montagna P. Nocturnal paroxysmal dystonia. *J Neurol Neurosurg Psychiatry* 1986;49:375.
13. Tinuper P, Cerullo A, Cirignotta F, et al. Nocturnal paroxysmal dystonia with short-lasting attacks: three cases with evidence of an epileptic frontal lobe origin of seizures. *Epileptia* 1990;31:549.
14. Montagna P. Nocturnal paroxysmal dystonia and nocturnal wandering. *Neurology* 1992;42(Suppl 17):61.
15. Meierkord H, Fish DR, Smith SJM, et al. Is nocturnal paroxysmal dystonia a form of frontal lobe epilepsy? *Mov Dis* 1992;7:38.
16. Bancaud J, Talairach J. Clinical semiology of frontal lobe seizures. In: Chauvel P, Delgado Escueta A, Halgren E, Bancaus H, eds. *Frontal Lobe Seizures and Epilepsies. Advances in Neurology.* Vol 57. New York: Raven Press; 1992:
17. Williamson PD, Spencer DD, Spencer SS, et al. Complex partial seizures of frontal lobe origin. *Ann Neurol* 1985;18:497.
18. Wada JA. Nocturnal frontal lobe seizure. *Epilepsia* 1988;29:209.
19. Scheffer IE, Bhatia KP, Lopes-Candes I, et al. Autosomal dominant nocturnal frontal lobe epilepsy: a distinctive clinical disorder. *Brain* 1995;118:61.

20. Gulick TA, Spinks IP, King DW. Pseudoseizures: ictal phenomena. *Neurol* 1982;32:24.

21. Gates JR, Ramani V, Whalen S, et al. Ictal characteristics of pseudoseizures. *Arch Neurol* 1985;42:1183.

22. Lapresle J. Palatal myoclonus. In: Fahn S, Marsden CD, Van Woert MH eds. *Myoclonus*. New York: Raven Press; 1986:265.

23. Deuscl G, Mischke G, Schenck E, et al. Symptomatic and essential rhythmic palatal myoclonus. *Brain* 1990;113:1645.

24. Jabbari B, Scherokman B, Gunderson CH, et al. Treatment of movement disorders with trihexyphenidyl. *Mov Disord* 1989;4:202.

25. Cho JW, Chu K, Jeon BS. Case of essential palatal tremor. Atypical features and remarkable benefit from botulinum toxin injection. *Mov Disord* 2001;16:779.

26. Deuschel G, Lohle E, Heinen F, et al. Ear click in palatal tremor: its original treatment with botulinum toxin. *Neurology* 1991;41:1677.

27. Nasr A, Brown N. Palatal myoclonus responding to lamotrigine. *Seizure* 2002;11:136.

28. Fahn S, Jankovic J. Hallett M. *Principles and Practice of Movement Disorders*. Philadelphia, PA: Churchill-Livingstone/Elsevier/Saunders 2011: 451.

29. Brown P. Spinal myoclonus. In: Marsden CD, Fahn S, eds. *Movement Disorders 3*. Oxford, England: Butterworth-Heinemann; 1994:458.

30. Brown P, Thompson PD, Rothwell JC, et al. Axial myoclonus of propriospinal origin. *Brain* 1991;114:197.

31. Chokroverty S, Walters A, Zimmerman T, et al. Propriospinal myoclonus: a neurophysiologic analysis. *Neurology* 1992;42:1591.

32. Glaze DG, Frost JD, Jr., Jankovic J. Sleep in Gilles de la Tourette syndrome: disorders of arousal. *Neurology* 1983;33:586.

33. Fish DR, Sawyers D, Allen PJ, et al. The effect of sleep on the dyskinetic movements of Parkinson's disease, Gilles de la Tourette syndrome, Huntington's disease, and torsion dystonia. *Arch Neurol* 1991;48:210.

33a. Lysenko L, Bhat S, Patel D, Salim S, Chokroverty S. Complex sleep behavior in a patient with obstructive sleep apnea and nocturnal hypoglycemia: A diagnostic dilemma. *Sleep Med* 2012; 1321–3.

34. Guilleminault C, Kirisoglu C, Bao G, et al. Adult chronic sleep walking and its treatment based on polysomnography. *Brain* 2005;128(Pt 5):1062–9.

35. Shiang R, Ryan SG, Zhu YZ, et al. Mutations in the alpha 1 subunit of the inhibitory glycine receptor cause the dominant neurologic disorder, hyperekplexia. *Nat Genet* 1993;5:351.

36. Hening WA, Allen R, Walters AS, et al. Motor functions and dysfunctions of sleep. In: Chokroverty S, ed. *Sleep Disorders Medicine: Basic Science, Technical Considerations and Clinical Aspects*. Philadelphia, PA: Saunders/Elsevier; 2009: 397.

37. Walters AS. Group organizer and correspondent: the International Restless Legs Syndrome Study Group. Toward a better definition of the restless legs syndrome. *Move Dis* 1995;10:634.

38. Allen R, Picchietti D, Hening W, et al. Restless legs syndrome: Diagnostic criteria, special considerations and epidemiology. A report from the Restless Legs Syndrome Diagnosis and Epidemiology Workshop at the National Institute of Health. *Sleep Med* 2003;4:101.

39. Medori R, Tritscher J, Leblanc AA, et al. Fatal familial insomnia, a prion disease with a mutation at codon 178 of the prion protein gene. *N Engl J Med* 1992;326:444.

40. Rosenfeld DS, Furman Y. Pure sleep panic: two case reports and a review of the literature. *Sleep* 1994;17:462.

41. Mahowald MW, Schenck CH. Status dissociatus: a perspective on states of being. *Sleep* 1991;14:69.

42. Schenck CH, Milner D, Huwitz TD, et al. Dissociative disorders presenting as somnambulism: polysomnographic, video and clinical documentation (8 cases). *Dissociation* 1989;2:194.

43. Kluft RP. Dissociative disorders. In: Talbott JA, Hales RE, Yudofsky SC eds. *Textbook of Psychiatry*. Washington, DC: American Psychiatric Press; 1988:557.

44. Pillar G, Malhotra A, Lavie P. Post-traumatic stress disorder and sleep-what a nightmare. *Sleep Med Rev* 2000;4:183.

45. Chokroverty S. Approach to the patient with sleep complaints. In: Chokroverty S ed. *Sleep Disorders Medicine: Basic Science, Technical Considerations and Clinical Aspects*. Philadelphia, PA: Saunders/Elsevier; 2009:255–274.

46. Aldrich MS, Jahnke B: Diagnostic value of video-EEG polysomnography. *Neurology* 1991;41:1060.

47. Chokroverty S. Role of electroencephalography in epilepsy. In: Chokroverty S ed. *Management of Epilepsy*. Boston, MA: Butterworth-Heinemann; 1996:67.

48. Scherfler C, Frauscher B, Schocke M, et al. White and gray matter abnormalities in idiopathic rapid eye movement sleep behavior disorder: A diffusion tensor imaging and voxel-based morphometric study. *Ann Neurol* 2011;69:400–7.

49. Unger MM, Belke M, Menzler K, et al. Diffusion tensor imaging in idiopathic REM sleep behavior disorder reveals microstructrual changes in the brainstem, substantia nigra, olfactory region, and other brain regions. *Sleep* 2010;33:767–73.

23

Epidemiology of Sleep-Related Movement Disorders

MAURICE M. OHAYON

THE 2005 edition of the *International Classification of Sleep Disorders* (*ICSD*) includes a chapter on sleep-related movement disorders. It comprises eight diagnoses: restless legs syndrome (RLS), periodic limb movement disorder (PLMD), sleep-related leg cramps, sleep-related bruxism, sleep-related rhythmic movement disorder (seen only in infants and children), and sleep-related movement disorder unspecified, due to a medical condition or due to drug or substance. These disorders involve characteristic, stereotyped movements that often disturb sleep.

In other parasomnias, which involve body movements and lead to sleep disruption such as sleepwalking or REM sleep behavior disorder, the movements are more complex and appear as purposeful and goal-directed behaviors. At the other extreme is sleep paralysis, which is characterized by the impossibility of movement for seconds or minutes upon sleep onset or upon awakening.

Apart from RLS, the epidemiology of these sleep movement disorders has been seldom studied in the general population or even in clinical settings.

RESTLESS LEGS SYNDROME

RLS is a sleep disorder affecting a significant portion of the general population. It is characterized by disagreeable leg sensations of an urge to move the legs occurring often at sleep onset. Patients with RLS typically complain of itching, creeping, tingling in their legs, usually between the ankle and the knee. These unpleasant sensations occur when the individual is at rest and are more pronounced in the evening or at night. The unpleasant sensations are relieved temporarily with leg movements.

Since 2000, nearly 50 epidemiological studies on RLS (see also Chapter 43) in community samples have been published.[1] Thirty-five of these studies were using the 1995 or 2003 criteria proposed by the International Restless Legs Syndrome Study Group (IRLSSG).

The estimates for prevalence of RLS depends on how it is assessed. Studies that assessed RLS with a single question generally reported higher rates of RLS, ranging from 9.4% to 15% in adults samples (18–20 years and older) and up to 23% when older samples were used (participants 40 years and older).

Studies that assessed RLS using the 1995 or 2003 four minimal IRLSSG criteria[2] without differential diagnoses have reported lower prevalences. Tables 23.1 and 23.2 summarize the findings of 14 European and North America studies by gender and age groups. Rates considerably vary between studies, especially when smaller samples were used. Overall, women are twice more likely than men to have RLS. This is observed for all age groups. In both genders, RLS prevalence increases until about 45 years old and remains unchanged until 75 years old and slightly decreases after that age.

Some epidemiological studies have provided additional information regarding the frequency and severity of the symptoms. According to these studies, between 50% and 60% of the participants who met minimal IRLSSG criteria had symptoms at least one time per week.[3–11]

Table 23.1 Prevalence of Restless Legs Syndrome Using International Restless Legs Syndrome Study Group Criteria by Age Groups among Men

FIRST AUTHOR, REFERENCE	N	AGE GROUPS						
		18–27	28–37	38–47	48–57	58–67	65–74	≥75
		%	%	%	%	%	%	%
Tasdemir[44]	1007	1.0	0.0	3.0	1.8	6.3	1.8	—
Benediktsdottir[21]								
Iceland	369	—	—	11.0	20.0	6.0	10.0	—
Sweden	288	—	—	10.0	7.0	12.0	5.0	—
Happe[7]	614	—	3.9	3.9	8.5	8.5	8.5	—
Hadjigeorgiou[45]	1419	1.0	1.9	2.2	3.3	2.0	3.2	3.0
Tison[4]	4762	3.9	5.0	6.2	8.0	7.5	6.7	4.0
Allen[3]	7388	0.8	1.0	0.9	2.0	1.8	2.5	2.0
Högl[46]	335	—	—	—	7.8	6.6	6.4	2.8
Rijsman[47]	687	—	—	—	4.0	5.1	7.9	8.4
Berger[48]	2018	3.0	3.5	5.0	7.5	13.2	11.0	—
Sevim[49]	1591	1.9	1.8	2.0	3.4	3.9	4.6	—
Ulfberg[15]	2608	1.2	4.0	6.2	8.0	10.5	—	—
Rothdach[50]	196	—	—	—	—	—	7.3	3.7
Total	23,282	1.9	2.6	3.7	5.2	5.9	5.2	3.1

Some prevalences are estimates derived from graphic presentation of data. Age groups are approximation and might differ between studies. Total prevalences are adjusted for the sample sizes.

Table 23.2 Prevalence of Restless Legs Syndrome Using International Restless Legs Syndrome Study Group Criteria by Age Groups among Women

FIRST AUTHOR, REFERENCE	N	AGE GROUPS 18–27 %	28–37 %	38–47 %	48–57 %	58–67 %	65–74 %	≥75 %
Tasdemir[43]	1104	1.8	4.0	8.0	7.0	9.8	7.9	—
Benediktsdottir[21]								
Iceland	400	—	—	24.0	24.0	28.0	21.0	—
Sweden	313	—	—	12.0	17.0	6.0	20.0	—
Wesström[19]	3516	—	11.0	11.7	18.1	20.9	—	—
Happe[7]	698	—	8.6	8.6	11.1	11.1	11.1	—
Hadjigeorgiou[44]	1614	1.4	3.8	4.0	6.7	7.8	8.5	4.3
Tison[4]	5501	6.0	9.0	10.0	13.0	15.0	12.0	12.0
Allen[3]	8003	1.2	2.1	3.6	5.0	6.0	6.2	2.4
Hogl[45]	366	—	—	—	13.9	16.3	12.6	13.5
Rijsman[46]	730	—	—	—	3.0	6.7	7.1	8.7
Berger[47]	2089	4.9	10.5	10.5	19.4	18.0	17.5	—
Sevim[48]	1643	3.1	3.9	4.3	4.4	4.0	4.6	—
Rothdach[49]	173	—	—	—	—	—	13.7	13.0
Total	26,150	3.1	6.2	7.6	10.4	11.7	9.6	6.4

Some prevalences are estimates derived from graphic presentation of data. Age groups are approximation and might differ between studies. Total prevalences are adjusted for the sample sizes.

Therefore, setting the frequency of leg symptoms to at least one time per week decreased the prevalence by about 40%, and setting the frequency to at least two times per week decreased prevalence by about 50%. Daily or near-daily occurrence of RLS symptoms occurred in about 20% of individuals with minimal IRLSSG criteria.

However, using only minimal IRLSSG criteria without differential diagnosis may lead to a high number of false-positive RLS individuals. This is well illustrated in epidemiological studies conducted in primary care settings with the advantage that the physicians could confirm the diagnosis and eliminate cases where RLS symptoms could be attributed to other diseases. Three studies have applied differential diagnosis process. In one study,[12] prevalence dropped from 7.4% (four minimal IRLSSG criteria) to 2.8%; in another[13] from 9.0% to 4.6%; and in the last[14] from 7.6% to 4.4%.

Associated Factors with Restless Legs Syndrome

Sleep disturbances are a common complaint among individuals with RLS. Depending on the age of the samples, the proportion of RLS individuals who reported having difficulty initiating sleep (DIS) varied from 27.9% to 69.2% and difficulty in maintaining sleep varied from 24% to 50.5%. Nonrestorative sleep was seldom studied but appeared to be at least twice more frequent in RLS individuals.[15,16]

Excessive sleepiness, measured with the Epworth Sleepiness Scale (ESS), had mixed results in community samples: three studies found that RLS participants had higher ESS scores, and three other studies did not find such an association. On the other hand, when excessive sleepiness was assessed with subjective questions on somnolence, all studies found that RLS individuals were two to three times more likely to report excessive sleepiness than non-RLS participants: between 32% and 42% of RLS individuals complained of excessive sleepiness.[15,17-21]

Several medical conditions have been less consistently associated with RLS, including cardiovascular diseases, hypertension, diabetes, obesity, and pain. The effects of medications on RLS symptoms have not been investigated in epidemiological studies.

PERIODIC LIMB MOVEMENT DISORDER

This disorder, originally called nocturnal myoclonus by Symonds,[22] is characterized by periodic episodes of repetitive and highly stereotyped limb movements occurring during sleep and by clinical sleep disturbance that cannot be explained by another primary sleep disorder. It occurs most frequently in the lower extremities. The diagnosis relies essentially on polysomnography results and is a diagnosis of exclusion: it is given only in the absence of other sleep, medical, or neurological disorders that could explain the repetitive limb movements.

On the other hand, periodic limb movement during sleep (PLMS) refers to the leg movements (dorsiflexion of the ankle, of the toes, and partial flexion of the knee and sometimes the hip) recorded during sleep regardless of the cause.

It is therefore very difficult to assess PLMS and PLMD in community samples or even in clinical settings because of the extensive efforts it requires to confirm the diagnosis.

Older studies reported a PLMS prevalence of 5%–11% in small populations.[23,24] One large epidemiological study[25] evaluating the simultaneous presence of PLMS and sleep complaints (PLMD) reported a 3.9% prevalence in 18,980 subjects from the European general population aged 15–100 years. This telephone interview survey used the *ICSD* criteria. The study identified several factors associated with PLMD, such as female gender, caffeine intake, stress, and the presence of mental disorders.

SLEEP-RELATED LEG CRAMPS

Sleep-related leg cramps are caused by sudden and intense painful involuntary contractions of muscles or muscle groups usually in the lower limbs (calf, thighs, or feet). Cramps may last a few seconds or several minutes and usually remit spontaneously.

Prevalence data on sleep-related leg cramps are nearly nonexistent. The pathology is mostly considered benign and has therefore raised little interest on the epidemiological level. It is estimated that nearly everybody will experience nocturnal leg cramps at least once but without consequences. One survey conducted with 515 war veterans, aged 60.4 years on average, reported that 56% experienced nocturnal leg cramps, 24% of them experienced them on a daily basis and 26% between 1 and 4 times per week.[26] Leg cramps were assessed with a single question: "Have you had trouble with cramps in your calves or feet at night?" Another small study investigated 218 patients taken from a general practice register.[27] In that study, women were aged on average 73 years and men were aged 66 years. A total of 37% of the sample responded reporting "rest" cramps occurring at night in 93% of cases. The cramps occurred at least three times per week in 40% of cases. Another study with 350 elderly outpatients[28] reported a prevalence of 50%.

One study has assessed nocturnal leg cramps in 2527 healthy children aged between 3 and 18 years. The overall prevalence was 7.3%, but episodes were most infrequent: once or several times a year; only 4.3% of them had cramps on a weekly basis.[29] No nocturnal leg cramps were reported before the age of 8 years.

Sleep-related leg cramps have been understudied in the general population. It is estimated they are mostly idiopathic, but little is known about associated medical conditions and psychiatric disorders.

SLEEP PARALYSIS

Sleep paralysis is one of the main symptoms associated with narcolepsy, but it can also occur individually (i.e., isolated sleep paralysis). Téllez-Lòpez et al.[30] found that 11.3% of their general population sample had sleep paralysis episodes at least sometimes.

An epidemiological study[31] performed with 8085 subjects between 15 and 99 years of age found that 6.2% had at least one episode of sleep paralysis in their lifetime, 0.8% experienced severe sleep paralysis (at least one episode per week), and 1.4% moderate sleep paralysis (at least one episode per month).

Overall, it is estimated that about 7.6% of the general population will experience at least one episode of sleep paralysis in their lifetime. Studies conducted with psychiatric patients reported lifetime prevalence around 32%.

In more narrowly defined populations, Goode[32] and Everett[33] observed rates of 4.7% and 15.4%, respectively, for self-reported sleep paralysis in medical students, and Bell et al.[34] noted a prevalence of 41% in Black Americans. In a study of adults living on the northeast coast of Newfoundland, Ness[35] reported a rate of 62% for "old hag" attacks, as sleep paralysis is popularly known in that part of Canada. The overall prevalence of lifetime sleep paralysis in students is around 28%.

REM-SLEEP BEHAVIOR DISORDER

REM-sleep behavior disorders were first described in the late 1970s by Japanese researchers and labeled as such by Schenck et al.[36] This sleep disorder is characterized by a loss of generalized skeletal muscle REM-related atonia and the presence of physical dream enactment. The individual has no consciousness of acting out a dream but is generally able to recount the dream upon awakening. This syndrome often results in behavior dangerous to oneself or others.[36-38] Their initial sample[36] included four men and one woman, all aged 60 years or over. Four of them had neurological disorders. Most of these cases had excessive slow-wave sleep for their age. This is not however, a sine qua non condition. Indeed, Tachibana et al. (1990)[39] reported seven cases of REM sleep behavior disorder without neurological or psychiatric disorder, who had a normal quantity of slow-wave sleep.

In all studies, this disorder is observed almost exclusively in men.

According to Schenck and Mahowald,[40] prodromal symptoms of REM sleep behavior disorder appeared 10 to 40 years before the full manifestation of the disorder in 25% of the studied cases. This prodrome is characterized by sleep talking, yelling, or limb jerking during sleep.

The mechanism underlying this disorder is not yet fully understood. Polysomnographic recordings of individuals with REM sleep behavior disorder showed a reduction of the tonic phenomena of REM sleep and the activation of the phasic phenomena. Destruction of the brainstem regions responsible for the REM sleep atonia had been hypothesized as responsible for such phenomena.

Prevalence of REM sleep behavior disorder in the general population is little documented. Ohayon et al.[41] estimated it to 0.5% in the general population using minimal criteria proposed by the International Classification of Sleep Disorder. However, as many as 2% of the general population reported experiencing violent behaviors during sleep with a male predominance.[41] In a more recent study, violent behaviors during sleep were found in 1.6% of the population[42] with a predominance among younger participants. Injuries to self or others were reported in 31.4% of the cases. These violent behaviors were not specific to REM sleep behavior disorder and were found in several parasomnias (sleepwalking, sleep terrors, nightmares, hypnagogic and hypnopompic hallucinations). A strong family link was also observed: the odds of having a family member also displaying violent behaviors during sleep were nine times higher among participants reporting this type of behavior compared to nonviolent participants.

CONCLUSIONS

Our knowledge about prevalence and incidence of most sleep-related movement disorders, with the exception of RLS, is still limited compared to other sleep disorders such as insomnia or obstructive sleep apnea syndrome. Most of the available data are based on the main symptoms of the disorders and not the diagnoses.

RLS is common in the general population, but a full appreciation of its severity and impact on daily life remains unclear. The overwhelming majority of prevalence rates reported in epidemiological studies of RLS are based solely on the presence of one symptom or a constellation of symptoms (four minimal criteria proposed by the IRLSSG group) that might occur only infrequently, regardless of the severity of the symptoms. While this may be defensible from an epidemiological point of view, for the physician it raises the question of "When does one need to treat these people?" As the International RLS Study Group has pointed out, the minimal criteria were not intended to confirm the presence of RLS but to indicate the possibility of the syndrome. Minimal RLS criteria without applying frequency and severity yield a false-positive rate of around 50%. Another consequence of using cases with infrequent RLS in general population-based studies is that it can mask the presence of some risk factors. This is probably one of the reasons why there are so many conflicting results when it comes to identifying medical conditions associated with RLS.

PLMD was rarely studied in community settings because the diagnosis is based on polysomnographic measures that are costly to realize outside sleep clinic studies. However, the association of PLMS with other sleep disorders and specific diseases has shown its high frequency in several diseases such as congestive heart failure, hypertension, Parkinson's disease, and obstructive sleep apnea syndrome.[43]

Similarly, sleep-related leg cramps seem frequent in the general population, especially among elderly people, but the data are clearly insufficient. Information regarding associated medical conditions and impacts on quality of life is undocumented.

Parasomnias involving more complex body movements have also been sparsely investigated.

REFERENCES

1. Ohayon MM, O'Hara R, Vitiello MV. Epidemiology of restless legs syndrome: a synthesis of the literature. *Sleep Med Rev* July 25, 2011. [Epub ahead of print]
2. Allen RP, Picchietti D, Hening WA, et al. Restless Legs Syndrome Diagnosis and Epidemiology workshop at the National Institutes of Health; International Restless Legs Syndrome Study Group. Restless legs syndrome: diagnostic criteria, special considerations, and epidemiology. A report from the restless legs syndrome diagnosis and epidemiology workshop at the National Institutes of Health. *Sleep Med* 2003;4:101–19.
3. Allen RP, Walters AS, Montplaisir J, et al. Restless legs syndrome prevalence and impact: REST general population study. *Arch Intern Med* 2005;165:1286–92.
4. Tison F, Crochard A, Léger D, et al. Epidemiology of restless legs syndrome in French adults: a nationwide survey: the INSTANT Study. *Neurology* 2005;65:239–46.
5. Cho YW, Shin WC, Yun CH, et al. Epidemiology of restless legs syndrome in Korean adults. *Sleep* 2008;31:219–23.
6. Lee HB, Hening WA, Allen RP, et al. Restless legs syndrome is associated with DSM-IV major depressive disorder and panic disorder in the community. *J Neuropsychiatry Clin Neurosci* 2008;20:101–5.
7. Happe S, Vennemann M, Evers S, et al. Treatment wish of individuals with known and unknown restless legs syndrome in the community. *J Neurol* 2008;255:1365–71.
8. Winkelman JW, Shahar E, Sharief I, et al. Association of restless legs syndrome and cardiovascular disease in the Sleep Heart Health Study. *Neurology* 2008;70:35–42.
9. Gao X, Schwarzschild MA, Wang H, et al. Obesity and restless legs syndrome in men and women. *Neurology* 2009;72:1255–61.
10. Erer S, Karli N, Zarifoglu M, et al. The prevalence and clinical features of restless legs syndrome: a door to door population study in Orhangazi, Bursa in Turkey. *Neurol India* 2009;57:729–33.
11. Yilmaz K, Kilincaslan A, Aydin N, et al. Prevalence and correlates of restless legs syndrome in adolescents. *Dev Med Child Neurol* 2011;53:40–7.
12. O'Keeffe ST, Egan D, Myers A, et al. The frequency and impact of restless legs syndrome in primary care. *Ir Med J* 2007;100:539–42.
13. Baos Vicente V, Grandas Pérez F, Kulisevsky Bojarski J, et al. El síndrome de piernas inquietas: detección, diagnóstico, consecuencias sobre la salud y utilización de recursos sanitarios. *Rev Clin Esp* 2009;209:371–81.
14. Allen RP, Stillman P, Myers AJ. Physician-diagnosed restless legs syndrome in a large sample of primary medical care patients in Western Europe: prevalence and characteristics. *Sleep Med* 2010;11:31–7.
15. Ulfberg J, Nyström B, Carter N, et al. Prevalence of restless legs syndrome among men aged 18 to 64 years: an association with somatic disease and neuropsychiatric symptoms. *Mov Disord* 2001;16:1159–63.

16. Ulfberg J, Nyström B, Carter N, et al. Restless legs syndrome among working-aged women. *Eur Neurol.* 2001;46:17–19.
17. Bjorvatn B, Leissner L, Ulfberg J, et al. Prevalence, severity and risk factors of restless legs syndrome in the general adult population in two Scandinavian countries. *Sleep Med* 2005;6:307–12.
18. Ulfberg J, Bjorvatn B, Leissner L, et al. Comorbidity in restless legs syndrome among a sample of Swedish adults. *Sleep Med* 2007;8:768–72.
19. Wesstrom J, Nilsson S, Sundstrom-Poromaa I, et al. Restless legs syndrome among women: prevalence, co-morbidity and possible relationship to menopause. *Climacteric* 2008;11:422–8.
20. Juuti AK, Läärä E, Rajala U, et al. Prevalence and associated factors of restless legs in a 57-year-old urban population in northern Finland. *Acta Neurol Scand* 2010;122:63–9.
21. Benediktsdottir B, Janson C, Lindberg E, et al. Prevalence of restless legs syndrome among adults in Iceland and Sweden: lung function, comorbidity, ferritin, biomarkers and quality of life. *Sleep Med* 2010;11:1043–8.
22. Symonds CP. Nocturnal myoclonus. *J Neurol Neurosurg Psychiatry* 1953; 16:166–71.
23. Kales A, Wilson T, Kales JD, et al. Measurements of all-night sleep in normal elderly persons: effects of aging. *J Am Geriatr Soc* 1967;15:405–14.
24. Bixler EO, Kales A, Vela-Bueno A, et al. Nocturnal myoclonus and nocturnal myoclonic activity in the normal population. *Res Commun Chem Pathol Pharmacol* 1982;36:129–40.
25. Ohayon MM, Roth T. Prevalence of restless legs syndrome and periodic limb movement disorder in the general population. *J Psychosom Res* 2002;53:547–54.
26. Oboler SK, Prochazka AV, Meyer TJ. Leg symptoms in outpatient veterans. *West J Med* 1991;155:256–9.
27. Naylor JR, Young JB. A general population survey of rest cramps. *Age Ageing* 1994;23:418–20.
28. Abdulla AJ, Jones PW, Pearce VR. Leg cramps in the elderly: prevalence, drug and disease associations. *Int J Clin Pract* 1999;53:494–6.
29. Leung AK, Wong BE, Chan PY, et al. Nocturnal leg cramps in children: incidence and clinical characteristics. *J Natl Med Assoc* 1999;91:329–32.
30. Téllez-Lòpez A, Sánchez EG, Torres FG, et al. Hábitos y trastornos del dormir en residentes del área metropolitana de Monterrey. *Salud Mental* 1995; 18:14–22.
31. Ohayon MM, Zulley J, Guilleminault C, et al. Prevalence and pathological associations of sleep paralysis in the general population. *Neurology* 1999;52:1194–200.
32. Goode GB. Sleep paralysis. *Arch Neurology* 1962; 2:228–34.
33. Everett HC. Sleep paralysis in medical students. *J Nerv Ment Dis* 1963;3:283–7.
34. Bell CC, Shakoor B, Thompson B, et al. Prevalence of isolated sleep paralysis in black subjects. *J Natl Med Assoc* 1984; 76:501–8.
35. Ness RC. The Old Hag phenomenon as sleep paralysis: a biocultural interpretation. *Cult Med Psychiatry* 1978;2:15–39.
36. Schenck CH, Bundlie SR, Ettinger MG, et al. Chronic behavioral disorders of human REM sleep: a new category of parasomnia. *Sleep* 1986; 9:293–308.
37. Schenck CH, Bundlie SR, Patterson AL, et al. Rapid eye movement sleep behavior disorder. A treatable parasomnia affecting older adults. *JAMA* 1987;257:1786–9.
38. Schenck CH, Hurwitz TD, Mahowald MW. REM sleep behavior disorder: an update on a series of 96 patients and a review of the world literature. *J Sleep Res* 1993; 2:224–31.
39. Tachibana N, Sugita Y, Terashima K, et al. Polysomnographic characteristics of healthy elderly subjects with somnambulism-like behaviors. Biol Psychiat1991; 30:4–14.
40. Schenck CH, Mahowald MW. Injurious sleep behavior disorders (parasomnias) affecting patients on intensive care units. *Intensive Care Med* 1991; 17:219–24.
41. Ohayon MM, Caulet M, Priest RG. Violent behaviour during sleep. *J Clin Psychiatry* 1997; 58:369–78.
42. Ohayon MM, Schenck CH. Violent behavior during sleep: prevalence, comorbidity and consequences. *Sleep Med* 2010;11:941–6.
43. Hornyak M, Feige B, Riemann D, et al. Periodic leg movements in sleep and periodic limb movement disorder: prevalence, clinical significance and treatment. *Sleep Med Rev* 2006;10:169–77.
44. Taşdemir M, Erdoğan H, Börü UT, et al. Epidemiology of restless legs syndrome in Turkish adults on the western Black Sea coast

of Turkey: a door-to-door study in a rural area. *Sleep Med* 2010;11:82–6.

45. Hadjigeorgiou GM, Stefanidis I, Dardiotis E, et al. Low RLS prevalence and awareness in central Greece: an epidemiological survey. *Eur J Neurol* 2007;14:1275–80.

46. Högl B, Kiechl S, Willeit J, et al. Restless legs syndrome: a community-based study of prevalence, severity, and risk factors. *Neurology* 2005;64:1920–4.

47. Rijsman R, Neven AK, Graffelman W, et al. Epidemiology of restless legs in The Netherlands. *Eur J Neurol* 2004;11:607–11.

48. Berger K, Luedemann J, Trenkwalder C, et al. Sex and the risk of restless legs syndrome in the general population. *Arch Intern Med* 2004;164:196–202.

49. Sevim S, Dogu O, Camdeviren H, et al. Unexpectedly low prevalence and unusual characteristics of RLS in Mersin, Turkey. *Neurology* 2003;61:1562–9.

50. Rothdach AJ, Trenkwalder C, Haberstock J, et al. Prevalence and risk factors of RLS in an elderly population: the MEMO study. Memory and morbidity in Augsburg elderly. *Neurology* 2000;54:1064–8.

51. American Academy of Sleep Medicine. The International Classification of Sleep Disorders- Second Edition: Diagnostic and Coding Manual. Rochester Minnesota: American Academy of Sleep Medicine, 2005.

52. Shimizu T, Jnami Y, Sugita Y, et al. REM sleep without muscle atonia (stage 1-REM) and its relation to delirious behavior during sleep in patients with degenerative diseases involving the brain stem. *Jpn J Psychiatr Neurol* 1990; 44:681–92.

24

General Sleep Difficulties in Patients with Movement Disorders

ANTONIO CULEBRAS

THERE IS an intimate relationship between neurological alterations commonly included under the label of "movement disorders" and sleep. In general, movement disorders that are apparent during wakefulness diminish in amplitude during sleep with some exceptions, such as recurrence of parkinsonian tremors during rapid eye movement (REM) sleep, periodic limb movements, and persistence of palatal myoclonus secondary to brainstem stroke. Persistent movement disorders may delay, prevent, or reduce the quality and continuity of sleep. The restless legs syndrome (RLS) is emblematic of the movement disorders that disturb sleep. Its presence may delay for hours the initiation of sleep and when sleep occurs, its restoring quality may be reduced by the emergence of periodic leg (limb) movements during sleep (PLMS), a common companion of RLS. Recent reports (vide infra) have challenged, however, this seemingly intuitive pathogenetic mechanism and suggest a divorce between RLS and insomnia. Parkinsonian tremors that recur during

REM sleep interrupt its maintenance. On the other hand, sound sleep has a beneficial effect on many of the manifestations of Parkinson's disease (PD), and some patients may not need to take medication until mid-morning. Medications that are administered to patients for the alleviation of daytime movement disorders, in particular antiparkinsonian medications, may induce inappropriate sleep, cause excessive somnolence, inhibit normal sleep, and precipitate behavioral or motoric side effects that interrupt sleep.

Hypnic jerks or sleep starts are normal companions in the transition to sleep; yet when excessive, they may delay the onset of sleep and concern patients. Other more unusual disorders like rhythmic movement disorders, propriospinal myoclonus at sleep onset, excessive fragmentary myoclonus, and hypnagogic foot tremor may alter the initiation or the continuity of sleep depending on the time of their occurrence. In general, movement disorders affect mostly the initiation of sleep and disturb its continuity if recurring during periods of wakefulness. Thus, movement disorders have the potential to alter the three pillars of good quality sleep—duration, continuity, and depth—and sleep modifies the occurrence and severity of movement disorders.

Specialists in sleep disorders and in movement disorders should be well acquainted with the sleep-wake manifestations of patients with movement disorders and the numerous interactions between one and the other before and after treatment. This chapter presents an overview of the general pathologic manifestations of sleep presented by patients with movement disorders.

PREVALENCE

Surveys of patients with PD have indicated that sleep-wake alterations are common. In an early study,[1] 74% of 100 respondents with PD noted sleep complaints that were unrelated to patient age and duration of disease but increased in prevalence with longer periods of levodopa therapy. Insomnia was generally followed by daytime somnolence, although patients also complained of altered dreams, nocturnal vocalizations, and myoclonus. Based on a strong relationship between sleep alterations and levodopa-induced psychiatric symptoms, the authors felt that antiparkinsonian medication was principally responsible for sleep alterations. In another study,[2] the authors observed that 93% of 220 patients with PD complained of sleep abnormalities at night or on waking, including inability to turn over or get out of bed, along with frequent urination or urinary incontinence disrupting sleep. Only 6% were taking antiparkinsonian medication at night, suggesting that sleep alterations are inherently common in patients with PD.

PLMS are present in 5% or more of the population 30 to 49 years of age and in 30% or more of the population 50 years of age or older.[3] The tendency for PLMS to occur spontaneously at higher frequency with advancing age has also been demonstrated for PLMS associated with restless legs syndrome.[4] In children there is considerable individual night-to-night random variability of PLMS,[5] but some studies report that up to 11.9% of 5- to 7-year-old children have a periodic limb movement index higher than 5.[6] PLMS are increased in RLS (80% or more), and in patients with narcolepsy, unexplained insomnia, and sleep apnea. PLMS have also been described in association with neurological disorders such as multiple-system atrophy, dopa-responsive dystonia, and PD (in about 32% of patients),[7] especially when associated with camptocormia.[8] It has also been associated with Huntington disease, corticobasal degeneration, Tourette syndrome, stiff-person syndrome, Isaacs syndrome, motor neuron disease, post-polio syndrome, hyperekplexia (startle disease), various myelopathies, stroke, and peripheral neuropathy.

MANIFESTATIONS

Cardinal symptoms of sleep alteration are excessive sleepiness or protracted sleeplessness. Excessive sleepiness is characterized by a tendency to fall asleep and an uncomfortable feeling of struggle when the sleepiness is inopportune. Excessive and inappropriate sleepiness, if persistent, may lead to social disruption and decreased job productivity, as well as accidents in situations in which full alertness is critical for survival, such as when driving or operating heavy machinery and equipment. Sleeplessness, or insomnia, is the inability to initiate or maintain sleep sufficient to satisfy the requirements of full daytime vigilance. Patients with insomnia may develop secondary excessive daytime sleepiness as a principal manifestation of their alteration.

Parasomnias are undesirable motor behaviors or sensory phenomena occurring during entry to sleep, within sleep, or during awakenings. Parasomnias are characterized by a peculiar event that is motor, sensory, or dream-like in nature that disrupts the continuity of sleep and often but not obligatorily leads to complaints of insomnia or of excessive sleepiness.

Circadian dysrhythmias are characterized by a mismatch of the desired sleep time with the timing of the circadian rhythm of sleep and wake propensity. Misalignments of individual sleep-wake timings with the 24-hour social environment lead to chronic sleep disturbance.

Physicians need to learn when it is appropriate to refer a patient with a sleep-wake problem to the sleep center and to correlate the diagnostic interpretation of the sleep alteration with the overall condition of the patient. Medication tolerance, interaction with other products, and loss of efficacy are common occurrences. Movement disorders affecting the ability to initiate or maintain sleep or diminishing the quality of nocturnal sleep should be considered for study with polysomnography. Movement disorder specialists should be acquainted with the cardinal manifestations of sleep-wake disorders and their clinical evaluation, treatment options, and follow-up.

EXCESSIVE SLEEPINESS

Sleepiness is the unavoidable consequence of the unsatisfied need of periodic sleep, the result of an intrinsic phenomenon, or the effect of medication. Sleepy individuals may fall asleep inadvertently, other times inappropriately, and more rarely abruptly. They take naps, either planned or unscheduled, and remain asleep for variable periods of time. The term *hypersomnia* should be reserved for situations in which excessive amounts of sleep predominate in the 24-hour period. A common accompaniment of sleepiness is the struggle to stay awake when falling asleep is inopportune. Individuals experience the uncomfortable sensation of a losing battle to remain aware and connected with the environment. Fluctuations in the level of alertness occur in response to a variable intent to stay awake. In this transitional period, attention wanes, learning declines, and memory fails to record accurately data from the moment. Reaction time is prolonged and the individual may fail to react promptly and accurately to unexpected occurrences. Physical activity helps maintain alertness, but relaxed environments with background noise such as waiting rooms, lecture halls, and theaters facilitate the tendency to enter sleep. Watching TV, reading the newspaper, and driving a vehicle are common precipitating factors.

As sleepiness persists, some individuals may reach a state of automatic behavior in which reaction time is decreased, memory is weak and defective, perceptions become distorted, and lapses of attention occur. Mental ability is compromised, and unexpected variations may increase the incidence of errors and the risk of accident. During such instances, individuals may drive a car for many miles, take the wrong turn, trespass properties, wander around, and even commit criminal acts. Automatic behavior is common in patients with narcolepsy, advanced sleep apnea syndrome, and severe sleep deprivation.

Sleepiness in patients with PD is pervasive, multifactorial, and commonly associated with medication effect. Levodopa, amantadine, dopamine agonists, and anticholinergic agents have the potential to induce excessive daytime somnolence. Selegiline has not been associated with sleepiness. Levodopa induces somnolence 30 minutes following its administration by mouth. Some patients report less somnolence with standard carbidopa/levodopa preparations than with sustained-release forms.

Sudden irresistible attacks of sleep have been described in patients with PD taking pramipexole or ropinirole.[9] These episodes were the cause of accidents when occurring while driving. Of eight patients reported in the original study, five experienced no warning before falling asleep. Sleep attacks ceased when the drugs were stopped. Somnolence is common in patients receiving pramipexole at doses of 1.5 mg/day or more. Manifestations of somnolence have appeared as long as 1 year after initiation of treatment. Drug interactions, in particular those that increase pramipexole plasma levels (such as cimetidine), may worsen the condition. Dose reduction reduces the tendency to fall asleep, but ordinarily patients developing significant daytime sleepiness should be switched to another antiparkinsonian medication. Patients should be advised not to drive a motor vehicle until they have tested their ability to function on a daily basis under the influence of the medication. Other sedating drugs or alcohol may potentiate the sedative effect of pramipexole.

Excessive daytime sleepiness may also be the consequence of sleep of poor quality, commonly a function of fragmentation and discontinuity of sleep caused by awakenings and arousals. Awakenings are defined in the polysomnogram as alerting episodes of more than 30 seconds duration; they are recorded in memory if lasting more than 3 minutes. Awakenings may occur for a variety of internal or external reasons, from idiopathic to an urge to urinate or in response to a loud noise. Arousals are brief, alerting responses lasting less than 30 seconds. They are not recorded in memory and, thus, individuals are unaware of their occurrence. Arousals are recorded in the polysomnogram as brief (1 to 3 seconds) bursts of cortical activity interrupting the continuity of the ongoing stage of sleep. Arousals typically occur at the termination of sleep apnea episodes and in relation to episodes of periodic leg movements. Awakenings may occur dozens of times and arousals hundreds of times in the course of the night, altering the continuity of sleep and its homeostatic value. In consequence, patients with advanced sleep apnea syndrome or with severe periodic limb movement disorder (PLMD) and many arousals typically exhibit excessive daytime sleepiness.

Sleepiness, like many other sleep-wake parameters, shows a circadian pattern. Sleepiness manifested by shorter latencies to sleep is more marked with body temperature reductions. Bedtime normally coincides with the initiation of the body temperature downturn and an increase in sleepiness. As the nocturnal period progresses, body temperature continues to decline and sleepiness becomes increasingly marked, as noted when patients are awakened and allowed to fall asleep again.[10] A modest midday body temperature reduction is also associated with mild sleepiness in most people. Patients with intrinsic forms of excessive sleepiness are sleepy as a result of central nervous system dysfunction. In narcolepsy, sleepiness is persistent and may appear in attacks over which the patient has little control. Short naps satisfy temporarily, although partially, the pressure to fall asleep, unlike idiopathic hypersomnia in which sleepiness is chronic and never satisfied by sleep. Pathologic sleepiness differs from excessive sleepiness secondary to sleep deprivation or nocturnal fragmentation in that it cannot be eliminated to the patient's satisfaction by sleep, regardless of how prolonged it is. Sleepiness and napping in the morning, following a night in bed allegedly asleep, are strong markers of a sleep-wake pathologic condition.

Excessive sleepiness may have profound social consequences. In a survey conducted in New York State, 24.7% of drivers admitted having fallen asleep at the wheel sometime in their life.[11] The rate of traffic accidents increases considerably between 1am and 7 am when, ironically, road traffic is most scarce but vigilance is at its lowest. Job-related accidents are more common during the night shift when alertness is low. Twenty percent of shift workers have fallen asleep on the job as shown by continuous electroencephalographic ambulatory recordings performed at night.[12] Excessive sleepiness may also interfere with the learning process in children and may lead to family pathologic conditions in adults.

Sleepiness in patients with narcolepsy has been associated with low production of hypocretin by lateral and posterior hypothalamic nerve cells. Loss of the physiologic hypocretin excitatory influence on histaminergic, dopaminergic, and cholinergic systems may

reduce thalamocortical arousal and underlie manifestations typically associated with narcolepsy. In a study of the histopathology of the hypothalamus in patients with narcolepsy, hypocretin-producing cells were reduced by 85% to 95%.[13] Most cases of narcolepsy with cataplexy are associated with the loss of approximately 50,000 to 100,000 hypothalamic neurons containing hypocretin. Studies of hypocretin content in cerebrospinal fluid (CSF) in humans have shown that hypocretin was undetectable in CSF in 7 of 9 patients with narcolepsy.[14] It has been determined that hypocretin 110 pg/mL in CSF is the cutoff value to diagnose narcolepsy.[15] Patients with idiopathic hypersomnia, sleep apnea, restless legs syndrome, or insomnia have normal hypocretin levels. Sleepiness has been associated with hypothalamic lesions in resection of craniopharyngioma, resection of an astrocytoma, irradiation of the pituitary gland in acromegaly, in multiple sclerosis, in myotonic dystrophy, and in traumatic brain injury. These observations suggest that symptomatic narcolepsy may be caused by damage to the hypocretin system. In PD excessive daytime sleepiness is more frequent in patients with dementia than in patients without dementia. Lumbar CSF hypocretin-1 levels are normal and unrelated to severity of sleepiness or the cognitive status.[16] Lumbar CSF does not accurately reflect the hypocretin cell loss known to occur in the hypothalamus of advanced PD. Mechanisms other than hypocretin cell dysfunction may be responsible for excessive daytime sleepiness in patients with PD.

Assessment and measurement of excessive sleepiness can be done in various ways. Sleepiness that interferes with job performance, social and family activities, or scholastic achievement is a marker of severity that needs management. Sleepiness that is associated by the patient with occupational or automobile accidents should always be considered serious, requiring urgent attention and immediate counseling pending full workup.

Excessive sleepiness can be documented with the Stanford Sleepiness Scale, which is a subjective rating scale of sleepiness.[17] Patients rate their daytime state of alertness every 2 hours using various levels of vigilance: full, high but not at peak, decreased, cannot stay awake, and asleep. The Epworth Sleepiness Scale[18] identifies sleep propensity by asking how likely the patient would be to fall asleep in everyday situations such as watching TV, reading, talking to others, as a passenger in a vehicle, or sitting in a car waiting for a traffic light to turn.

The objective measurement of sleepiness has been standardized with the multiple sleep latency test (MSLT).[19] Following nocturnal polysomnographic recording in the sleep laboratory, patients are asked to return to bed at 2-hour intervals during daytime hours starting at 8 am. Four or five segments of sleep are recorded, each segment lasting 20 minutes or less. The objective is to identify the average time it takes to engage stage I of sleep, defined by a reduction of 50% or more in alpha activity over 50% or more of the epoch. An average sleep latency of 8 minutes or less indicates excessive sleepiness, whereas a score between 8 and 10 minutes is suggestive but not indicative of excessive sleepiness. The MSLT has the advantage of detecting episodes of daytime REM sleep in patients with narcolepsy, allowing confirmation of this diagnosis when there are two or more REM sleep episodes with a latency of 15 minutes or less. The Maintenance of Wakefulness Test (MWT) is intended to measure the ability to stay awake in a quiet, controlled, laboratory environment. The average sleep latency for four segments indicates the ability to stay awake. Most clinicians will consider an average latency of 10 minutes or less an indication of excessive sleepiness.

INSOMNIA

Insomnia refers to the inability to initiate or to maintain sleep. Insomnia is not a disease but a symptom of the failure to engage timely, satisfying sleep. Insomnia becomes a disorder when daytime alertness is compromised.[20] The inability to initiate and the difficulty to maintain sleep are often associated in the same person, disturbing the quantity and quality of nocturnal sleep. The patient unable to fall asleep is commonly troubled by anxiety or develops a state of increasing anguish as precious time elapses. The anticipation of a difficult entry into sleep increases the tension. Other patients may have no difficulty falling asleep but wake up 1 or 2 hours later and then are either unable to continue sleeping or enter a state in which sleep comes and goes at brief intervals, finally driving the patient out of bed. Insomnia may take various clinical forms and have multiple causes. Transient insomnia, also known as adjustment or acute insomnia, is a common complaint secondary to a defined stressor. Once the problem is removed, the

insomnia tends to disappear. If the difficulty with sleep persists beyond 3 months, the clinician should suspect occult underlying factors and conditioned mechanisms responsible for sleeplessness. A peculiar form of insomnia is characterized by relatively sound sleep during the first part of the night followed by inability to continue asleep. Early morning awakenings when persistent are generally a manifestation of depression. In sleep-state misperception, timing of sleep seems to have been lost and patients complain of subjective insomnia when in reality they sleep sufficiently during the night. Patients with RLS may have difficulty initiating sleep as a result of the leg discomfort. Sleep quality may be frequently compromised when associated periodic limb movements with arousals appear during the night. However, sleep loss may be independent of PLMS in patients with RLS. A recent report suggests that patients with RLS may be afflicted with a hyperarousal disorder that in preliminary studies has been correlated with increased glutamate signal in the thalamus,[21] a finding that requires further verification.

Nocturnal restlessness is a common accompaniment of insomnia in patients with PD. These patients may exhibit an elevated nocturnal activity level along with an increased proportion of time with movement indicating a disturbed sleep.[22] Inability to turn in bed or recurrence of tremors in REM sleep may alter the continuity of sleep in patients with PD. REM sleep behavior disorder and other forms of parasomnia interrupt sleep and disturb both patient and bedmate. Some forms of insomnia may be the consequence of medication effect, whereas others remain unexplained.

Extreme insomnia leading to death, or fatal familial insomnia, has been described in patients with degeneration of the dorsomedial nucleus of the thalamus caused by a prion agent. REM sleep behavior disorder with agitation, dementia, dysautonomia, and end-stage stupor are principal manifestations.

The differential diagnosis of insomnia must be made with circadian rhythm abnormalities that mimic the condition. Sleep-phase delays are more common in young patients. In this condition the occurrence of sleep is retarded beyond conventional hours of the night, resembling insomnia. In sleep-phase advance, a disorder almost exclusively found in older individuals, the early consumption of sleep may awaken the patient at an early morning hour giving the appearance of an early morning awakening. Finally, the clinician must keep in mind that there are patients who fail to sleep well and sufficiently because of external factors such as environmental noises, temperature elevations, or traffic that continuously interrupts sleep. Somatic complaints may also cause insomnia, the paramount example being chronic pain that prevents the entry into sleep or arouses the individual.

Individuals who complain of insomnia are also distressed by the anticipation of inability to function properly during waking hours. These subjects report tiredness, irritability, loss of motivation, poor memory, decreased concentration, and vague physical manifestations. Muscle aches are common, particularly during morning hours. Despite sleepiness, patients are unable or unwilling to take naps because they are worried about the effect of daytime slumber on nocturnal sleep. Preoccupation about the ensuing night struggle to fall asleep heightens the tension surrounding the entire process and contributes importantly to sleeplessness, closing a vicious circle that loops anxiety and insomnia.

Polysomnographic evaluation of patients with movement disorders and insomnia may reveal various patterns of insomnia. In some patients the study merely confirms prolongation of the latency to sleep and fragmentation of sleep architecture. In others the study documents early morning awakenings. Polysomnography is justified when a movement disorder affecting sleep requires investigation. An extended electroencephalogram and electromyogram montage along with video-monitoring are recommended to capture abnormal motor events. In patients with suspected REM sleep behavior disorder, video recording may capture nocturnal enactment of dreams and the tracing may record REM sleep without atonia that confirms the diagnosis. PLMS are recorded in either leg as brief 0.5-second duration episodes of electromyographic activation occurring at intervals of 5 to 90 seconds. There is good justification to proceed with expensive testing when the sleep apnea syndrome is suspected as a factor underlying sleeplessness.

Bruxism, or tooth grinding during sleep, is a very common movement alteration that can be recorded in polysomnography as recurrent phasic activation of masseter muscles, sometimes associated with arousals. Bruxism is an uncommon cause of insomnia.

CIRCADIAN DYSRHYTHMIA

Older patients with advanced PD commonly exhibit some form of reversal or alteration of the circadian rhythm. This is manifested by fragmentation of nocturnal sleep and frequent napping during daytime hours. PD patients share in late age the troubles with circadian rhythmicity that are so common in older adults. In addition, dopamine-dependent functions influenced by medication effect may change patterns of motor behavior throughout the day that in turn affect the circadian rhythm. The sedative and hypnotic effect of dopaminergic agents may increase napping time during daytime hours, altering the circadian balance. The advanced sleep phase disorder is common in patients with PD, particularly if a period of immobility coincides with evening hours.

Actigraphy is a valuable method for recording sleep-wake behaviors. The actigraph is a device worn on the wrist that detects motion for periods lasting several weeks. The information can be downloaded and expressed as a graph showing periods of motor activity and inactivity, presumably sleep, in each 24-hour period. Circadian rhythm alterations and their response to therapy can thus be identified with relative ease.

SNORING AND APNEA

Snoring is the act of breathing during sleep with a rough hoarse noise. Pathologic or obnoxious snoring that is persistent and loud disturbs the sleep of others. Commonly, the bedmate describes irregular breathing and respiratory pauses that are as disturbing as the noise. Snoring occurs with the turbulent passage of air through a narrow oropharynx, causing vibration of soft tissues. During sleep the pharyngeal dilator muscles that maintain tautness of the pharyngeal wall during inspiration tend to relax, narrowing the space behind the tongue. Many anatomic factors can contribute to narrowing the oropharyngeal space. These include large tonsils, accumulation of adipose tissue in the soft palate, large tongue, large uvula, and redundant engorged soft palate tissues. Weakness and incoordination of pharyngeal dilator muscles in patients with neuromuscular disorders, including PD, may result in loud snoring.

The stenosis that creates increasing air turbulence and snoring may eventually reach the point of collapse, interrupting the respiratory process, a phenomenon that is termed *obstructive apnea*. Snoring of loud intensity, persistent occurrence, and irregular quality may be a marker of the obstructive sleep apnea disorder. Apneas are defined as episodes of cessation or near-cessation (>70% reduction) of airflow lasting 10 seconds or more, whereas hypopneas are defined as episodes of 30% or greater reduction of amplitude in thoracoabdominal movements or airflow as compared to baseline, with a greater than 4% oxygen desaturation, lasting 10 seconds or more. Central or nonobstructive apneas are characterized by a transient inhibition of the respiratory function with a duration of 10 to 60 seconds. These events are more common in patients with central nervous system disease and indicate a central alteration of the respiratory process. Earlier studies reported an increased frequency of obstructive and central sleep apneas along with arterial desaturation events in patients with PD.[23] However, more recent investigations have challenged that concept when showing that rates of obstructive sleep apnea in PD are similar to those seen in the general population.[24]

MOTOR EPIDODES OF SLEEP

Motor events in sleep may be aperiodic as exemplified by hypnic jerks, periodic as in PLMD, and rhythmic as in head banging.[25] Sleep motor activity ranges from occasional jerks to incessant restlessness, to episodic complex behaviors that unwillingly drive the patient out of bed. Such phenomena may disturb the sleep of the patient and others but more important create a risk of injury to the patient and bedmate. Often times, nonepileptic motor phenomena of sleep have been confused with seizure episodes, creating a vexing clinical problem that can only be resolved with proper testing in the sleep laboratory. Subjective recollections offered by the patient, along with possible descriptions by others, are always important. These reports may be complemented at a later time with polygraphic objective findings and nocturnal videotape recordings. Patients may have no remembrance of what happened at night but may exhibit indirect evidence from bruises, painful injuries, or disturbed bedroom furniture. Episodes occurring during REM sleep are usually attached to a dream, whereas events appearing in other stages of sleep are not remembered or associated only with imprecise static images. Thus,

dream content suggests an REM sleep-related episode, whereas no dream association is more likely an event of non–REM sleep. The time of night when the episode occurred gives a clue to the relationship with stages of sleep. Episodes occurring repeatedly during the first third of the night strongly suggest a link to slow-wave sleep, whereas events appearing in the last third suggest an association with REM sleep. The age of onset is likewise important. Episodes commencing in childhood tend to be related to slow-wave sleep, such as nocturnal terrors and sleep walking; paroxysmal dystonia, nocturnal wandering, and seizures, commonly associated with light non-REM sleep, are more frequent in youth and middle age, whereas REM-sleep related behavior disorder is usually a disorder of old age. PLMD may appear at any age but is more common as age advances. A family history may have additional diagnostic value; sleep-walking and nocturnal terrors are typically familial, whereas REM sleep behavior disorder is usually acquired. Rhythmic movements of the head or body at onset of sleep are almost exclusively seen in childhood.

Predisposing and precipitating factors of motor events are varied but identifiable if searched for. Sleep deprivation is a well-known precipitating factor of seizures. Unusually deep slow-wave sleep following sleep deprivation may predispose to nocturnal terrors and sleepwalking in children, as well as confusional episodes in adults. REM sleep deprivation followed by REM sleep rebound may trigger nightmares, hallucinations, and prolonged episodes of REM sleep behavior disorder. Factors modifying the quality, duration, and distribution of sleep architecture such as alcohol, psychoactive medications, dopaminergic agents, stress, and fever and environmental factors like noise, heat, and cold may facilitate the occurrence of motor episodes through varied mechanisms. Other disorders such as sleep apnea could precipitate sleep-walking events in children and should be investigated because successful treatment of sleep apnea may reduce sleep-walking behaviors.

The video-polysomnographic study is necessary to document visually and electrographically episodes of motor activity—should they occur on the night of testing—and serves to identify the stage of sleep wherein the event appears, as well as to reveal allied signs of pathologic conditions. Interictal phenomena such as epileptiform discharges in seizure disorders or

REM sleep without atonia in REM sleep behavior disorder have diagnostic value even in the absence of events. The videotaped registration is useful to analyze in detail the motor behavior during the episode, while procuring a correlation with electrographic phenomena. There is good specificity between certain events and stages of sleep. Thus, REM sleep behavior disorder occurs by definition during REM sleep; nightmares are also associated with REM sleep, whereas seizure activity generally vanishes during REM stage. Night terrors, somnambulism, confusional episodes, and paroxysmal awakenings are linked to slow-wave sleep. Nocturnal wanderings and paroxysmal dystonia are more common in stage II, whereas hypnic jerks and rhythmic head banging are typical of stage I of sleep. Epileptiform discharges characteristically appear in light non-REM sleep, diminish in deep non-REM sleep, and disappear in REM sleep. PLMD occurs in light non-REM sleep and tends to disappear in deep non-REM and REM sleep. Movements typical of the wake stage in PD may be observed in stage I and in the transitions of sleep stages. As sleep depth advances, movements are increasingly rare.[26] Tremors may be observed in REM sleep.

The polysomnographic study is also helpful to assess sleep spindles. Sleep spindle density is decreased in PD, whereas in Huntington's disease, sleep spindles are significantly increased in amplitude and density.[27] This observation may aid in the diagnosis of early Huntington's disease.

The response to treatment has additional diagnostic value. Episodes responding to anticonvulsants like carbamazepine are usually epileptic in nature. REM sleep behavior disorder specifically responds to clonazepam; slow-wave-sleep-associated events like somnambulism and nocturnal terrors disappear with low doses of benzodiazepines. Arousals linked to motor events may disappear differentially with benzodiazepines, improving the quality of sleep while having no effect over the motor event. This phenomenon is illustrated by the ameliorating effects of clonazepam on sleep of patients with periodic limb movements and fragmented sleep resulting from arousals. Clonazepam eliminates event-associated cortical arousals but leaves unaffected the leg movements.

The clinician should be cognizant of medication-induced sleep-related movement disorders. Dystonic dyskinesias may impact sleep or appear in the early morning, causing painful plantar flexion of the feet and curling of the toes. Early-morning dystonia in PD may resolve by changing medication or the time of its administration.[28]

Levodopa-induced myoclonus involving axial and proximal muscles occurs almost always at night during non-REM sleep.[29]

REM SLEEP PARASOMNIAS AND ABNORMAL DREAMING

Nightmares are dream-anxiety attacks that generally end in an awakening without motor enactment. They are more prevalent in younger patients, often familiar, and tend to occur in persons with borderline personality disorders. In REM sleep without atonia, inhibition of motoneurons prevalent during REM sleep fails to occur and patients are free to enact their dreams. This abnormal phenomenon may lead to REM sleep behavior disorder with punching, screaming, running, and other behaviors that translate dream content into a physical response. In some individuals lesions are found in the brainstem in the region of the peri-locus coeruleus,[30] an area responsible for generation of REM sleep–related muscle atonia.

Parasomnia overlap disorder is a variant of REM sleep behavior disorder. *ICSD-2* defines parasomnia overlap disorder as a combination of REM sleep behavior disorder and a disorder of arousal (sleep walking, confusional arousal, or sleep terror). Parasomnia overlap disorder has a male predominance with most cases occurring in adolescence.

In one series,[31] one third of subjects had a symptomatic form associated with neurological conditions such as multiple sclerosis, Möbius syndrome, Harlequin syndrome, and traumatic brain injury, all of them suggestive of brainstem pathology.

Abnormal generation of dream experiences during wakefulness may underlie some hallucinatory phenomena. Ponto-geniculo-occipital waves that originate in the pontine area travel to lateral geniculate nuclei and forebrain systems, providing nonrandom excitation of the forebrain. This input may represent the substrate for dream visual experiences and provides a rationale to comprehend partial or dissociated generation of dream phenomena outside REM sleep. PD patients with hallucinatory phenomena may be partially REM sleep deprived as a result of dopaminergic medication effect.[32] *Peduncular hallucinosis* is the term given to a condition in which intense dream-like experiences appear during wakefulness in patients with midbrain lesions usually of vascular origin[33]; excessive sleepiness is commonly found in association with peduncular hallucinosis.

DISSOCIATED STATES

Dissociated states are intrusions of one state of being (wakefulness, non-REM sleep, and REM sleep) into another, resulting in mixed states, poorly defined states, or only partially developed states.[34] These phenomena are relatively common in patients with sleep disorders and may result in extraordinarily bizarre behaviors that are otherwise difficult to explain. Pathologic dissociated states occur commonly in patients with narcolepsy, such as cataplexy, hypnagogic hallucinations, and sleep paralysis. Intense dream mentation following REM sleep deprivation may explain the vivid hallucinations encountered in the withdrawal phase of drugs that suppress REM sleep, like anticholinergic medication, dopaminergic agents, alcohol (i.e., delirium tremens), or conditions that inhibit REM sleep, like metabolic and hepatic coma.

ACUTE CONFUSIONAL STATE DELIRIUM

Delirium is defined as a transient mental alteration characterized by a global disorder of cognition and attention, a reduced level of consciousness, psychomotor agitation, and sleep-wake disturbance.[35] Older adults are specially prone to develop delirium as a consequence of a variety of predisposing and precipitating factors that include dementia, structural brain disease, medical illness, use of drugs, sensory deprivation, psychosocial factors, and sleep loss. Delirium is often superimposed on dementia, and 25% of those who are delirious have dementia.[36] Delirium is a transient disorder, usually lasting less than 1 month. Symptoms fluctuate during the daytime and reach a peak at night. The sleep-wake cycle disturbance is an essential disturbance of delirium. During daytime hours, patients are lethargic and tend to nap, whereas at night sleep is short, fragmented, and punctuated with hallucinations. Agitation, restlessness, and wakefulness dominate the nocturnal period in clear contrast with the subdued and drowsy state that prevails during the day. Cholinergic deficiency seems to be a major mechanism in delirium, and, thus, patients with Alzheimer's disease or patients with PD who are toxic with central anticholinergic medication are particularly vulnerable.

REFERENCES

1. Nausieda PA, Weiner WJ, Kaplan LR, et al. Sleep disruption in the course of chronic levodopa therapy: an early feature of the levodopa psychosis. *Clin Neuropharm* 1982;5:183.
2. Lees AJ, Blackburn NA, Campbell VL. The nighttime problems of Parkinson's disease. *Clin Neuropharm* 1988;11:512.
3. Bixler EO, Kales A, Vela-Bueno A, et al. Nocturnal myoclonus and nocturnal myoclonic activity in a normal population. *Res Commun Chem Pathol Pharmacol* 1982;36:129–40.
4. Ferri R, Manconi M, Lanuzza B, et al. Age-related changes in periodic leg movements during sleep in patients with restless legs syndrome. *Sleep Med* 2008;9:790–8.
5. Picchietti MA, Picchietti DL, England SJ, et al. Children show individual night-to-night variability of periodic limb movements in sleep. *Sleep* 2009;32:530–5.
6. Crabtree VM, Ivanenko A, O'Brien LM, et al. Periodic limb movement disorder of sleep in children. *J Sleep Res* 2003;12(1):73–81.
7. Norlinah MI, Afidah KN, Noradina AT, et al. Sleep disturbances in Malaysian patients with Parkinson's disease using polysomnography and PDSS. *Parkinsonism Relat Disord* 2009;15:670–4.
8. Lavault S, Bloch F, Houeto JL, et al. Periodic leg movements and REM sleep without atonia in Parkinson's disease with camptocormia. *Mov Disord* 2009;24:2419–23.
9. Frucht S, Rogers JD, Greene PE, et al. Falling asleep at the wheel: motor vehicle mishaps in persons taking pramipexole and ropinirole. *Neurology* 1999;52:1908.
10. Carskadon MA, Dement WC. Daytime sleepiness: quantification of a behavioral state. *Neurosci Behav Rev* 1987;11:307.
11. *Report of the New York State Governor's Task Force on Sleepiness/Fatigue and Driving.* Albany, NY: 1994.
12. Akerstedt T. Sleepiness as a consequence of shift work. *Sleep* 1988;11:17.

13. Thannickal TC, Moore RY, Nienhuis R, et al. Reduced number of hypocretin neurons in human narcolepsy. *Neuron* 2000;27:469–74.

14. Nishino S, Ripley B, Overeem S, et al. Hypocretin (orexin) deficiency in human narcolepsy. *Lancet* 2000;355:39–40.

15. Mignot E, Lammers GJ, Ripley B, et al. The role of cerebrospinal fluid hypocretin measurement in the diagnosis of narcolepsy and other hypersomnias. *Arch Neurol* 2002;59(10):1553–62.

16. Compta Y, Santamaria J, Ratti L, et al. Cerebrospinal hypocretin, daytime sleepiness and sleep architecture in Parkinson's disease dementia. *Brain* 2009;132:3308–17.

17. Hoddes E, Zarcone V, Smythe H, et al. Quantification of sleepiness: a new approach. *Psychophysiology* 1973;10:431.

18. Johns MW. A new model for measuring daytime sleepiness: the Epworth Sleepiness Scale. *Sleep* 1991;14:540.

19. Carskadon MA, Dement WC, Mitler MM, et al. Guidelines for the multiple sleep latency test (MSLT): a standard measure of sleepiness. *Sleep* 1986;9:519.

20. American Academy of Sleep Medicine. *International Classification of Sleep Disorders. Diagnostic and Coding Manual.* 2nd ed. Westchester, IL. American Academy of Sleep Medicine; 2005.

21. Allen R, Barker PB, Horská A. RLS: a hyperarousal disorder with a thalamic glutamate abnormality. *Neurology* 2011;76(Suppl 4):A369.

22. von Hilten B, Hoff JI, Middelkoop HA, et al. Sleep disruption in Parkinson's disease. *Arch Neurol* 1994;51:922.

23. Hardie RJ, Efthimiou J, Stern GM. Respiration and sleep in Parkinson's disease. *J Neurol Neurosurg Psychiatry* 1986;49:1326.

24. Trotti LM, Bliwise DL. No increased risk of obstructive sleep apnea in Parkinson's disease. *Mov Disord* 2010;25(13):2246–9.

25. Montagna P. Motor disorders of sleep. Periodic, aperiodic, and rhythmic motor disorders and parasomnias. In: Culebras A, ed. *Sleep Disorders and Neurological Disease.* New York: Marcel Dekker; 2000:193.

26. Fish DR, Sawyers D, Allen PJ, et al. The effect of sleep on the dyskinetic movements of Parkinson's disease, Gilles de la Tourette syndrome, Huntington's disease, and torsion dystonia. *Arch Neurol* 1991;48:210.

27. Emser W, Brenner M, Stober T, et al. Changes in nocturnal sleep in Huntington's and Parkinson's disease. *J Neurol* 1988;235:177.

28. Pahwa R, Busenbark K, Huber SJ, et al. Clinical experience with controlled-release carbidopa/levodopa in Parkinson's disease. *Neurology* 1993;43:677.

29. Klawans H, Goetz C, Bergen D. Levodopa-induced myoclonus. *Arch Neurol* 1975;32:331.

30. Culebras A, Moore JT. Magnetic resonance findings in REM sleep behavior disorder. *Neurology* 1989;39:1519–23.

31. Schenck CH, Boyd JL, Mahowald MW. A parasomnia overlap disorder involving sleepwalking, sleep terrors, and REM sleep behavior disorder in 33 polysomnographically confirmed cases. *Sleep* 1997;20:972–81.

32. Comella CL, Tanner CM, Ristanovic RK. Polysomnographic sleep measures in Parkinson's disease with treatment-induced hallucinations. *Ann Neurol* 1993;34:710.

33. McKee AC, Levine DN, Kowall NW, et al. Peduncular hallucinosis associated with isolated infarction of the substantia nigra pars reticulata. *Ann Neurol* 1990;27:500.

34. Mahowald MW, Schenck CH. Dissociated states of wakefulness and sleep. *Neurology* 1992;42(Suppl 6):44.

35. Lipowski ZJ. Delirium in the elderly patient. *N Engl J Med* 1989;320:578.

36. Erkinjuntti T, Wilkstrom J, Palo J, et al. Dementia among medical inpatients: evaluation of 2000 consecutive admissions. *Arch Int Med* 1986;146:1923–6.

25

Differential Diagnosis and Evaluation of Unknown Motor Disorders during Sleep

MARCO ZUCCONI

THE MAJORITY of motor episodes occurring during sleep can now be classified, according to the *ICSD-2*,[1] in the chapter on sleep-related movement disorders and a minority in the chapters of parasomnias and isolated symptoms apparently normal variants. The most important category includes the main motor disorders in sleep (restless legs syndrome [RLS], periodic limb movement disorder [PLMD], sleep-related cramps, sleep-related bruxism, sleep-related rhythmic movement disorders [SRRMD], and other unspecified). This category should also include isolated or normal variants, that is, sleep starts, benign myoclonus of infancy, hypnagogic foot tremor (HFT) and alternating leg muscle activation (ALMA) during sleep, propriospinal myoclonus (PSM), and excessive fragmentary myoclonus (EFM). Parasomnias, defined as clinical disorders characterized by undesirable physical phenomena that occur predominantly during sleep, include some motor phenomena,listed with arousal disorders (sleepwalking, sleep terrors, confusional

arousals) and parasomnias usually associated with rapid eye movement (REM) sleep (REM sleep behavior disorder [RBD]).

In the last couple of decades the clinical practice of sleep medicine has commonly reported other motor phenomona of sleep that usually take the form of unusual behavioral, motor, experiential, and autonomic episodes emerging only or almost exclusively during sleep. These phenomena have attracted research in the sleep field to understand better whether these "bumps in the night" are already correctly diagnosed and categorized in parasomnias or other well-known sleep disorders, or may represent some unidentified conditions often misdiagnosed or inappropriately forced to be considered as "known sleep disorders" with atypical features.[2]

In this chapter we try to summarize these more frequent unusual motor sleep disorders recently described by clinicians that do fit into the standard, sleep-related movement disorder categorizations. This chapter addresses the methods of evaluation and the possible differential diagnoses with other disorders belonging to sleep, movement, or seizure diagnostic categories.

METHOD OF EVALUATION

The methodology considered as the gold standard for studying abnormal motor events occurring during sleep is still video-polysomnography (PSG), which combines classic PSG recording with simultaneous audiovisual monitoring and recording of the patient in the sleep laboratory. In the past, the descriptions, on the one hand, of classical parasomnias such as sleepwalking and sleep terrors, and, on the other hand, of physiologic body movements or physiologic motor activity during sleep were done only on the basis of some PSG leads (i.e. incomplete electroencephalographic [EEG] montage or absence of autonomic and large electromyographic [EMG] monitoring), with only clinical reports of motor behavior.[1-6] Also for normal motor activity the pioneer studies were based on paper-speed recording and direct observation of the phenomena: only a few significant studies considered gross body movements[7,8] or segmental motor activity during sleep, largely because of the difficulties in both observation and categorization of the activity.[9-11] The first description of motor activity during sleep utilized the muscle artifacts on the EEG[9,12] with some evident limitations or EMG activity of different muscles[10] with many leads on PSG that produced some discomfort for the subject tested. Some studies considered minimal motor activity (hypnic myoclonus or jerks at sleep onset, fasciculations, myoclonic jerks during sleep)[13] without the aid of controlling body posture or movements. Studies considering body posture and movements in normal sleep or after sleep loss[14-16] are more numerous but once again without video recording. We also made, some years ago, a detailed analysis of motor pattern during sleep in normal young volunteers, in comparison with patients with abnormal motor behaviors, and utilized the videotapes with split-screen audiovisual circuit.[17-19] The characteristics of motor arousals or awakenings (magnitude, duration) can be masked by some sleeping postures so that the beginning or ending of the movement may not be clear, thus complicating the classification. Only the utilization of a detailed freeze-frame video review together with the presence of muscular artifact on the polygraphic traces may allow one to count and categorize the doubtful episodes and clarify the type of motor behaviors.[17]

Moreover, only the classification of motor episodes or attacks into categories, depending not only on the duration but also on the semiology and complexity may permit comparison of different types of behavior between patients and controls.[17-21] The split-screen technique of video-PSG allows the simultaneous evaluation of the sleeping subject and of the PSG recording[22] and proves useful both in analysis of normal motor patterns and disorders of motor control during sleep. The high cost and the great time spent to record and review or analyze the data are the major limits on this very useful and reliable technique, both in research and clinical fields. However, especially in the last decade, numerous video-PSG studies with detailed analysis and counting of motor phenomena have been carried out both for well-known motor disorders/parasomnias (as RBD, PLMS/RLS, PSM, ALMA, HFT, SRRMD, sleep bruxism) as well as for some new or uncommon forms of motor behaviors not necessarily pathological in definition (high-frequency leg movements [HFLMs], EFM, neck myoclonus during sleep, and sleep starts).[23-37]

Some other methods of investigation have been developed to study motor components during sleep: bed temperature monitoring, recorded with temperature sensors and a data logger inserted into the mattress,[38] actigraphy,[39,40] pressure transducers, the static-charge-sensitive bed (SCSB),[41] off body video actigraphy system,[42] and the time-lapse video recording (TLVR),[43] all permitting the recording of motor activity at home or in any other nonlaboratory condition and therefore less costly than the PSG, but these approaches have probles with reproducibilty of data and comparison with PSG.

The SCSB is a system to detect and quantify movement s during sleep through two iron plaques put into the mattress, which, on the basis of recording an electrical potential (different from different movements), provoked by the charge of the mattress (static charge), can detect, recognize, and quantify (on a logarithmic scale) the different types of movements. There are some problems with the calibration of the movements before sleep and with the electromagnetic fields in the room recording; however, the method is ecological (the subject is without electrodes and is recorded at home). It is feasible to record segmental movements,[44,45] differentiate quiet from active sleep, REM from non-REM sleep, and also sleep from wakefulness[30]; but it is difficult to recognize physiologic from pathologic motor activity.[44,46,47] Recently, it has been reappraised for movements, respiration, and heart rate variability during sleep.[48,49]

Actigraphy is a very well-known technology to study sleep-wake rhythm and pathologies and for experimental studies of physiological or peculiar motor patterns. It is attached to the wrist or ankle, where it detects motor activity in any direction. It stores the data in a memory that can transmit the results, by means of an interface, to a personal computer for the analysis. The modality of sampling may be "threshold" or "reference," indicating the frequency of the activity (with respect to the time domain) or the frequency and the amplitude to evaluate the rest-activity cycle, respectively. This technique is useful for identifying or evaluating sleep during the night (from an algorithm that has been validated in humans) both in normal subjects and in patients with sleep disorders (insomnia, sleep-wake rhythm disturbances) instead of the laboratory or ambulatory PSG, and in association with the sleep diary. The advantages of actigraphy are its practicality, ecology, and low-cost monitoring in all environments (excluding water) and its reliability in all patients (also demented ones or ones not compliant with PSG). Moreover, it may be useful in field or epidemiological study of sleep habits and rhythms in selected populations or to study motor habits during sleep.[50] However, the limits on the specific detection of movements and the lack of a means to quantify the intensity of the movements and the different patterns do not permit one to utilize actigraphy to evaluate particular body or abnormal movements. It has been applied in the field of PLMs and RLS with good internight correlation in detecting leg movements (i.e., epidemiological and genetic studies),[51,52] but with a low agreement and different absolute indices in comparison to PSG data[53] (see Chapter 15 on ambulatory monitoring for more details).

The TLVR evaluates body position with serial photographs. It consists of the only video recording during sleep in real time and successive analysis in compact (speed) or freeze-frame (slow) fashions. The advantages of this method are its simplicity, the relatively low cost, and the possibility of studying the subject or the patient in his or her habitual environment (home or other particular conditions) or when PSG is not available or is not indicated. Its limits are the lack of a means for recording any single biological parameter (EEG, EMG, ECG, respiration) with no information on cerebral state (sleep and sleep stages, wake, and transitions).

In any case, without the use of video-PSG, differential diagnosis of normal movements, abnormal behavior, seizures, or any other disorder is not feasible.

Video recordings are actually the most reliable method of obtaining the best information on motor episodes (both normal and pathologic), but they present technical complications, require high-quality video recorders and large memory capacities, and they require a circuit with infrared light to avoid problems of quality.[27-29]

NOCTURNAL FRONTAL LOBE EPILEPSY AND MOTOR BEHAVIORS OF EPILEPTIC ORIGIN

Frontal lobe epilepsy is very well known and a large series of patients have been published in the past literature[54-58]: seizures are characterized by a wide spectrum of clinical features but the motor manifestations and the nocturnal (sleep) preponderance are the main and common aspects of these seizures. Supplementary motor area (assumption of postures, rhythmic movements, and rapid uncoordinated movements), cingulate gyrus (complex repetitive movements involving arms and legs, vocalization), or orbito-frontal (pelvic thrusting, wandering) origins are difficult to evaluate with a conventional EEG. Only the dorsolateral regions of the frontal lobe are detectable with surface electrodes. Moreover, during attacks, motor artifacts often cover electrical abnormalities and only intracranial or, in some cases, sphenoidal and zygomatic leads may disclose epileptic ictal and interictal paroxysmal abnormalities.[55,58,59] For these reasons, frontal seizures, when evaluated during wakefulness, can be misdiagnosed as pseudoseizures[60,61] and, when observed during sleep, are often misdiagnosed as movement disorders or sleep disturbances.[62-66] Before video recording, the epileptic origin of paroxysmal arousals with atypical motor behaviors and, in some cases, of more pronounced complex dystonic-dyskinetic motor attacks was only postulated but not confirmed.[67,68] Only since the mid-1980s and in the last two decades, with the aid of detailed analysis of video-PSG recordings[17,18,20,59,65,69,70] and intracranial or sphenoidal electrodes,[71–73] was the epileptic origin of some unusual motor manifestations from mesial and orbital regions of the frontal lobes clearly demonstrated. These motor attacks, known as nocturnal paroxysmal dystonia, paroxysmal awakenings or arousals, paroxysmal nightmares, and episodic nocturnal wanderings, represent a spectrum of the same epileptic syndrome, with a heterogeneous group of sleep-related complex motor attacks, originating in the deep frontal lobe foci and emerging almost always from non-REM sleep. Moreover, the description of a number of family history cases have led to the delineation of an autosomal dominant form of NFLE (ADNFLE, autosomal dominant nocturnal frontal lobe epilepsy), which has been linked to chromosome 20q13 in a large Australian family,[74,75] to chromosome 15q24 in an English family,[76] and more recently to chromosome 1 in one Italian family.[77] Genetic results in European pedigrees showed autosomal dominant inheritance with reduced penetrance; however, locus heterogeneity has been hypothesized because of the absence of linkage on chromosomes 20q13 and 15q24.[78,79] Recent clinical genetic studies confirm this heterogeneity in families with NFLE.[80,81]

The electroclinical picture of ADNFLE is not different from sporadic forms: motor and/or behavioral phenomena mainly during sleep starting in childhood-adolescence (mean age 10–12 years) with interictal and ictal EEG during sleep often normal or uninformative; absence of lesions from neuroimaging (only 10%–14% with some abnormalities at brain computed tomography [CT] or magnetic resonance imaging [MRI]); normal development in the majority of the cases; frequently misdiagnosis with classical parasomnias (sleepwalking and sleep terrors) or other pathologies (psychiatric disorders); a generally good response to antiepileptic drugs (carbamazepine), although in around 30% of the cases the motor attacks are resistant to drug treatment; and persistence during adulthood.[18,19,82,83]

Recent evidence seems to indicate a nonhomogeneous disease, since some sleep-related seizures clinically indistinguishable from frontal lobe seizures may have an extrafrontal origin (temporal or insular) and may otherwise mimic sleep-related parasomnias.[84–86]

Patients may present with different sleep-related motor events of increasing complexity and duration, with possible different duration and propagation of the epileptic discharges. Studies with intracerebral electrodes in drug-resistant cases indicate the onset in the supplemetary motor area, but, on the other hand, short lasting motor events may have the relationship with epileptic discharges and the clinical manifestation not different from other sleep-related motor events (PLMS, bruxism, or sleeptalking). Moreover, the deep epileptic discharge may increase arousal fluctuations and enhance the gate mechanisms both for seizure and nonseizure events.[87]

The classification of paroxysmal arousals, *nocturnal paroxysmal dystonia*, and epileptic nocturnal wanderings as different clinical aspects of one heterogeneous syndrome is still valid and characterizes the different aspects of the epileptic syndrome, with a few problems of recognition of the epileptic nature for paroxysmal nocturnal dystonia but more difficulties for wanderings and paroxysmal arousals. This phenotypical characterization reflects a disorder not completely known and understood from a phatogenetic point of view.[87] For example, we do not know the reason of the almost always relationship of the seizures with sleep and in particular non-REM sleep. Thalamo-cortical and intracortical synchronizing functions may explain this relationship as well as a possible alteration (genetic?) of the arousal mechanism during non-REM sleep. Probably the therapeutic response and therefore the prognosis are different among the subtypes of seizures, but we must wait for a long-term follow-up of the NFLE patients to resolve its classification and semiology.

Differential Diagnosis

After the complete delineation of both the sporadic and familial NFLE, the main problems so far unresolved are (1) the differentiation and the differential diagnosis between epileptic forms and some types of parasomnias emerging from delta or non-REM sleep (sleepwalking, sleep terrors, and confusional arousals) and (2) which criteria are to be considered to distinguish paroxysmal arousal with atypical motor behaviors from normal and physiologic body or segmental movements?

Concerning the differentiation between arousal disorders and NFLE, there are some clinical/anamnestic and video-PSG features leading to differential diagnosis. On the basis of clinical history, although some overlap may exist, the start of episodes during preschool age (from 3 to 6 years), the rare frequency (usually less than one per month, with some clustering), the long duration of episodes (usually more than 5 minutes), and the disappearance before the ages of 16 to 18 are the main features characterizing arousal disorders (sleepwalking and sleep terror). The motor pattern and the semiology of the attacks are more intriguing but more revealing of NFLE when the motor episodes are stereotypic and repetitive in the same subject, in different recording or in the same PSG; the continuity and the spreading from minimal or minor attacks to the more rapidly and typical major episode (sudden elevation of head and trunk with fear expression and dystonic posture of head or limbs, diskinetic agitation of arms, vocalization or screaming) and to the more complex and prolonged dystonia involving arms, legs, and trunk or to so-called agitated somnambulism (with a sort of repetitive jump or a disordered and grotesque dance); and the elevated number of episodes, both minimal, minor and major attacks, with in some cases sleep disruption and daytime symptoms (difficulty with waking up, daytime fatigue or sleepiness). These features are different from the rare episodes of parasomnias and the absence of sleep complaints in arousal disorders (Table 25.1).[83,88,89]

The motor pattern shows characteristics belonging to one or to the other disorders, but the wake-EEG is often normal in both, and the interictal sleep-EEG shows some epileptiform abnormalities frontally dominant in about 50% of the cases of NFLE.[18,19] Concerning ictal-EEG or EEG during parasomnia episodes, the data in arousal disorders are uncertain, due to the limited number of EEG leads during the recording or to the absence of video-PSG simultaneous recording.[83,89] Thus, the differences are not so striking: prevalence of background flattening of EEG or focal rhythmic activity of delta or theta bands, burst of delta activity preceding or initiating the episode may be recorded in both types of motor episodes.[17-19,90] They were described in typical arousal disorders and in frontal lobe seizures as ictal or postictal phenomena.[91] Only less than 10% of the cases show typical epileptic discharges during the attacks and only with sphenoidal or zygomatic leads in some cases have clear-cut paroxysms of epileptic origin been shown.[72,92] Not even the great activation of vegetative parameters may be useful because

of the presence both in arousal disorders and NFLE.[3,82]

Thus, the diagnosis of NFLE and the differential diagnosis with other motor agitation episodes is a challenge, more from an EEG point of view than from motor activity evaluation.

The differential diagnosis of NFLE or motor behaviors with atypical and epileptic features may also involve nocturnal panic attacks, REM behavior disorders, prolonged episodes of non-contact during sleep or dissociated status, prolonged and violent behavior of undetermined origin, and psychiatric or psychogenic spells.

Daytime panic disorder favors a diagnosis of nocturnal panic attacks as do the strong subjective feeling of intensive fear, apprehension or imminent death during the nocturnal episode, the ease and intensity with which it is recalled, and the long duration of the attacks.[93,94] However, in some cases the diagnosis is difficult due to the lack of epileptiform abnormalities.

REM behavior disorders are different and easily distinguished from NFLE by their relation with REM sleep (less than one fourth of the patients with abnormal motor behavior presented rare episodes of NFLE that were REM related),[95] the difference in the age of the patients, the patient's recall of a dream-like content after the episodes, and the characteristics of the PSG (REM without EMG atonia, great motor periodic subtle activity also in non-REM).

Dissociative disorders are rare but characterized by some personality disturbances, or clinical and anamnestic history of early-life psychic trauma. The PSG findings include the possibility of identifying the wakefulness emerging episode without seizure activity and the absence of video-PSG features of other sleep-related attacks. Also *posttraumatic stress disorder* has some characteristics such as poor sleep continuity, nightmares during REM or non-REM sleep, and waking symptoms (heightened startle reflex and flashbacks), which may help in differentiation with epileptic attacks.[101,102]

Dystonic-dyskinetic attacks of different origin, arising from sleep and exercise, have been described in a few cases, with episodes of 2–4 minutes in duration and different morphological characteristics from typical NFLE.[103,104] The first cases described (of two children) resembled paroxysmal dystonic coreoathetosis or paroxysmal kinesigenic coreoathetosis for the sudden appearance of the motor attacks, the duration, and the dystonic components (without impairment of consciousness) but differ

Table 25.1 Clinical and Video-Polysomnographic Features of Nocturnal Frontal Lobe Epilepsy (NFLE) and Non-REM Parasomnias (Arousal Disorders)

	NFLE	AROUSAL DISORDERS
Age at onset (years)	>10 (generally during or after adolescence but any age is possible)	<10 (generally during scholar age, 3 to 8)
Attacks/month (n)	Sporadic (1 to 4 or less)	Almost every night (>30) but with possible variation
Attack distribution in the night	Generally first third	At any time
Sleep stage onset attack	Non-REM (>60% in stage 2)	Non-REM stage 3–4
Duration of the attacks	Less than 1 minute (excluding the complex prolonged dystonic or wandering seizures)	Some minutes (1 to 10)
Attacks per night	Generally one	Several
Repeated and stereotypic attacks	Generally absent	Generally present
Vocalization	Generally present (brief and unintelligible or comprehensible and prolonged)	Maybe present, generally very rapid and loud (screaming or shouting)
Dystonic or tonic posturing	Very common	Uncommon
Brief burst of running or jumping in the bed or little out of the bed	Characteristic of some complex seizures (nocturnal epileptic wanderings, even though of possible extrafrontal origin)	Generally absent (calm or quiet deambulation even out of the room or of the house)
Awareness	May be present in a proportion of seizure. Typical aura: breath is stuck in the throat	Generally absent

Recall	May be present in a proportion of attacks	Generally absent
Consciousness if awakened	Present and normal	Impaired and slower
Sleep fragmentation	Maybe present; sometimes related only to slow-wave sleep microstructure instability	Present and important
Daytime sleepiness	Infrequent	Common (often related to the high number of seizures and sleep fragmentation)
Family history	Frequent (for parasomnias)	Frequent (both for seizures and parasomnias, sometimes clinically undistinguishable)
Response to treatment	Not known (improvement with sleep stabilization)	Good response to AEDs (carbamazepine, topiramate, etc.) in at least 60%–70% of the cases
Follow-up and clinical course	Generally with decreasing or disappearing of symptoms	Stable or increasing (unknown)

for the "puppet-like" quality of the movements (brief, segmental, and repetitive), the fact they are triggered by repeated physical exercises, and by arousal from non-REM sleep (either spontaneous or provoked). The lack of epileptiform ictal and interitcal abnormalities, also during sleep, and the scarce response to antiepileptic drugs were in favor of the nonepileptic origin (different from NFLE), with possible involvement of cortical-subcortical motor circuits. Some years ago we had the chance to observe a similar case of a young girl of 15 years of age, with a slight anoxic-asphyxic insult after birth and dystonic-dyskinetic short attacks both in wakefulness and sleep, involving mainly the upper limbs and the head. The attacks were present for many years almost every day and night but after 10 years of age only after awakening or spontaneous arousals during sleep. We recorded the attacks during video-PSG recording several times during a 2-year period, considering the episodes as NFLE, sporadic form, but all the antiepileptic drugs failed to control the episodes. The episodes (5–6 per night) were all stereotypic, both for morphology and duration, arising from non-REM sleep preceded by an arousal or awakening, some poor vocalizations, and concluding with an almost immediate return to sleep. Neuroimaging was inconclusive. The morphology, the preserved consciousness during the motor attacks (i.e., she said that she was aware of the episodes and could hear the voices of people around her), the sudden start, and the dystonic but uncoordinated (almost segmental) movements together with a resistance to drugs such as carbamazepine, phenytoin, barbiturate, gabapentin, lamotrigine, and benzodiazepines (clonazepam or diazepam) led us to consider this case to be different from frontal lobe epilepsy (unpublished observation).

ATYPICAL FORMS OF MYOCLONUS (IDIOPATHIC MYOCLONUS, PROPRIOSPINAL MYOCLONUS, FRAGMENTARY MYOCLONUS)

Periodic legs movement in sleep (PLMS), originally termed *nocturnal myoclonus*, is a well-known phenomenon characterized physiologically mainly by dystonic movements but sometimes associated with myoclonic components. PLMS is characteristic of sleep in RLS patients or present in other sleep disorders (narcolepsy, sleep apnea, RBD), in aged normal subjects, and in some neurologic or nonneurologic diseases. It is well recognized in video-PSG for the periodic phasic activity in legs and (less frequently) arms with flexion of up to 5 seconds in the limbs (feet, finger, and knee). It appears during non-REM sleep usually during the unstable and light stage 1–2 non-REM.[1,105] Recently the criteria and rules for PLMS and PLMW scoring have been rearranged and redefined by the World Association of Sleep Medicine (WASM)—International Restless Legs Syndrome Study Group (IRLSSG)[106] and substantiually confirmed by the American Academy of Sleep Medicine (AASM). [107] These new criteria were based on the development of algorithms for automatic detection and mathematical handling of the different leg movement parameters: amplitude, duration, intervals, periodicity, and distribution across the night.[108]

Other atypical and rare forms of periodic or pseudoperiodic phasic activities have recently been described as resembling PLMS in some features but also differing in others.

Oromandibular myoclonus is an idiopathic form of myoclonus affecting the oromandibular region during sleep with EMG burst of less than 0.25 seconds in duration, isolated or in cluster-like fashion.[109] This activity, although found in screening for sleep bruxism, is different from phasic sleep bruxism episodes (shorter and nonperiodic) and is sometimes associated with EEG arousals but rarely if ever associated with EEG abnormalities.[110] It is different from the asymmetric and asynchronous twitching activity found, for example, in RBD (in which it is present also in other limb muscles).[111] This oromandibular myclonus should be distinguished by other lesional orfacial myoclonic jerks that are also observed or prevalent during wakefulness (palatal or lingual myoclonus, oculo-facial-skeletal myorhythmia).[112,113] Only in some cases may oromandibular myoclonus coexist with bruxism, and EEG investigation may be helpful to distinguish this activity from epileptic-related activity.[114]

Propriospinal myoclonus (PSM) is characterized by myoclonic jerks arising in the spinal cord and mainly affecting axial (trunkal) muscles sustained by an intrinsic spinal pattern generator.[115,116] One of the characteristic features is exacerbation by the horizontal position and in some cases by relaxed wakefulness before falling asleep.[117] Despite its disappearance with sleep initiation, it may provoke difficulties in sleep onset or maintenance (reappearance during the awakenings).[117] The propriospinal myclonus is generally idiopathic but may be associated with some spinal lesions (cervical trauma, tumors, demyelinating plaques). The pattern of propagation is very peculiar. It excludes the cranial muscles and spreads only gradually. It is different from cortical and reticular myoclonus and from spinal myoclonus, which are usually restricted to a single or a few segments. Mental activation or movements may provoke a relief of the symptom, but the more striking criteria to differentiate it from other forms of myoclonus (e.g., hypnic jerks) and PLMS is the very clear-cut disappearance with all sleep stages. Nevertheless, it can be a cause of insomnia.[33,34] PSM should be also differentiated from periodic limb movements during wakefulness (PLMW), which are present in the legs during quiescence before sleep onset, longer in duration, and generally not associated with extension to the trunk or arms, present in RLS, and associated with an urge to move the legs.

Sleep starts and physiological hypnic jerks or massive hypnic jerks differ in that they take place during sleep onset or light (stage 1–2 non-REM) sleep. They are related somehow to K-complexes or EEG arousals, and they usually occur in isolation; however, they sometimes occur repetitively but never periodically. They involve the whole body and not just the abdominal or axial muscles.[118,119] In these cases only polygraphy with wide and detailed EMG recordings associated with a freeze-frame videotaped analysis may be helpful in diagnosing and identifying the movement disorder during the pre-sleep period.

Neck myoclonus is a recently described phenomenon of movements associated with a short striped-shaped artifact on PSG (EEG leads), corresponding to very brief head jerks, frequent in routine PSG (>50% of patients recorded for different sleep disorders), but predominantly in REM sleep. The frequency decreases with age and may be considered a variant of some myoclonic activity, present in REM sleep also in healthy people.[27]

Excessive fragmentary myoclonus is pathologic fragmentary myoclonus characterized by a brief and phasic potential on surface EMG leads (>200 msec) in the limb, trunk, and axial muscles, but it is asymmetrical and asynchronous, and appears in relaxed wakefulness but is activated by non-REM and REM sleep.[120] The jerks

are similar in morphology to physiologic bursts of REM sleep but not in clusters. It has been described in different sleep disorders with no specific relationship to them. The only specific feature of excessive fragmentary myoclonus is some degree of sleep fragmentation in all the cases described. It seems different from fasciculations or fibrillations and resembles an accentuation of the physiological myoclonic jerks of sleep onset, present and described during all the sleep stages.[121] The index of this activity, calculated as number of 3-second mini-epochs for each 30-second epoch, is increased in different sleep disorders and with age, and seems to correlate with sleep-related breathing disorder.[30] The treatment is not specific but clonazepam may provide some results.

A similar phenomenon of sleep onset is the hypnic jerks or sleep starts that in some cases may be intensified to cause a problem in sleep onset and continuity.[118,119]

SLEEP-RELATED VIOLENT BEHAVIORS

Sleep-related violence has been described for many years in terms of isolated cases or case reports, but it has only recently received attention from sleep researchers. Despite the rare occurrence of wanderings with violence in the history of patients with nocturnal motor episodes, they are the main reason for referring a patient to a Sleep Center or for consulting sleep specialists. Moreover, the episodes have been emphasized also in the forensic sleep medicine because of some relevant aggressive behaviors perpetrated during the night in a putative "confusional state" (homicide, accidents, and injuries toward people). The defense of these acts considers the violent and aggressive behavior to be committed while the person is asleep or in a state of confusional arousal and, consequently, not accountable or responsible for this action. The debate between prosecution and defense, and the different theses in the penal processes concerning these acts, are, although very interesting, beyond the scope of this chapter.

Violence during sleep or aggressive behavior during sleep has been reported in 2% of the general population,[96] and it may occur in the course of a parasomnia and in NFLE or nocturnal temporal lobe epilepsy, but it has been described during the nocturnal period (but generally in a state of wakefulness) in dementia or cognitive decline, and in malingering and confusional states or psychiatric dissociative states. Dreamlike mentation associated with sleepwalking often may result in aggressive and violent behaviors[97]; some drugs (e.g., zolpidem or benzodiazepines) can potentially provoke complex and aggressive sleep-related behaviors.[98] In general, in arousal disorders the violence may be evoked by the touch or the action of other persons in an attempt to awake the subject and to end the parasomniac episode (noise, touch, or close proximity).[99] Dysfunction in medial prefrontal and orbitofrontal area, and thalamocortical pathway, is probably the substrate for the violence also in sleep, with demonstrated activation of the latter and hypoactivation of the projections to the frontal lobes.[100] This mechanism is modulated at different levels and the arousal disorder with its dissociative state (mixed sleep and wakefulness characteristics) is one of the factors together with genetic predisposition and provocative agents to develop violent behavior during sleep; it is difficult to video-record and to demonstrate also for forensic issues.[99,100]

Sleep-related violence appears to be a type of behavior rather than a definite diagnosis,[122] and it can be seen in relationship with essentially all the main parasomnias: from arousal disorders (confusional arousals, sleepwalking) to REM behavior disorder, from sleep-related epileptic seizures (NFLE) to some forms of wandering related to hallucinations and delirium as in "sundowning" of demented people. So a large spectrum of parasomnias may be the predisposition disorder for this type of behavior, indicating a concept of state-dependent motor control abnormality and of state dissociation.[123] The physiologic state of wake, non-REM sleep, and REM sleep may occur simultaneously in incomplete or mixed form, with oscillation from one state to another state and resulting in unclear episodes emerging from sleep but with characteristics of a subwakefulness state.

Moldofsky and collaborators[124] suggest that certain characteristics both in the subject or the subject's environment predispose this violence during sleep, for example, genetic predisposition, psychological distress, abuse of drugs or substances, sleep disruption or sleep-wake rhythm disorders, and increased sleep pressure (recovery from sleep deprivation). Moreover, some macro- and microstructure modifications, in particular of non-REM sleep, may be another trigger factor. The increase in macro- and microarousals (as delta burst during slow-wave sleep) and in sleep instability (like more cyclic alternating pattern during non-REM sleep), as found in arousal disorders (sleepwalking, sleep terror, and confusional arousal), is frequently associated with sleep-related violence. Also, sleep fragmentation, as observed in obstructive sleep apnea, may be an important trigger for the episodes.

In any case, there is some overlap between violence of a supposed ictal (epileptic) nature and episodes of uncertain origin. Both may be violent against themselves or others, the ictal EEG lacks epileptiform abnormalities, and in the family there are often siblings with similar motor behaviors (clinically defined as parasomnias) and temporal or frontal lobe interictal abnormalities. However, in some forms of complex motor activity during the night emerging from non-REM sleep, the resulting epileptic ictal and interictal paroxysms (sometimes revealed by deep electrodes), the clinical (audio-video recorded) phenomenon of the motor pattern resembling orbitofrontal seizures, and the response to anticonvulsants clearly indicated a probable (or in some cases certain) epileptic origin belonging to the group of NFLE.[73] Another kind of manifestation of violence during sleep may be the postictal phenomenon: the ictal manifestation of a seizure may precede the EEG arousal and may not be detectable by surface EEG, as illustrated by Malow and Varma[94] or during stereotatic recording in epileptic patients candidate to surgery.[91] The awareness of the subjects during the episodes is questionable and, as in NFLE, in some episodes the sensation of consciousness is incomplete but in general preserved, while in the majority of the attacks there are mental confusion, vocalization but not a comprehensible language, and no contact and oriented response to external stimulation.

Concerning the investigative approach to these phenomena, classical PSG with video recording is useful but not extremely sensitive to the episodes. They are often rare, complex, and more frequent in the usual environment of the patients. Therefore, some other diagnostic procedures such as telemetry,[125] video-screen telemetry,[126] or in some cases ambulatory monitoring (with repeated nights of recording) associated with possible home video recordings may allow the objective evaluation of sleep-related violence.[127] Other procedures such as quantitative EEG analysis; EEG mapping; and special electrodes like zygomatic, sphenoidal, or nasopharyngeal are not always useful to discriminate the etiology of the episodes. The epileptic origin should be suspected and researched independently of the duration (sometimes very long), the morphology (bizarre), and the rarity of the episodes.

REFERENCES

1. American Academy of Sleep Medicine. *International Classification of Sleep Disorders. Diagnostic and Coding Manual.* 2nd ed. Westchester, IL: American Academy of Sleep Medicine; 2005.
2. Mahowald MW, Shenck CH. Things that go bump in the night: the parasomnias revisited. *J Clin Neurophysiol* 1990;7:119–43.
3. Gastaut H, Broughton RJ. A clinical and poly-graphic study of episodic phenomena during sleep. In: Wortis J, ed. *Recent advances in biology and psychiatry.* Vol. 7. New York: Plenum Press' 1965:197–221.
4. Jacobson A, Kales A, Lehmann D, et al. Somnambulism: all-night EEGic studies. *Science* 1965;148:975–7.
5. Kales A, Jacobson A, Paulson MJ, et al. Somnambulism: psychophysiological correlates: I. All-night EEG studies. *Arc Gen Psychiatry* 1966;14:585–94.
6. Broughton RJ. Sleep diosrders: disorders of arousals? *Science* 1968;159:1070–8.
7. Oswald I, Taylor AM, Treisman M. Discriminative responses to stimulation during human sleep. *Brain* 1960;83:440–53.
8. Moses J, Lubin A, Naitoh P, et al. Reliability of sleep measures. *Psychophysiology* 1972;9:78–82.
9. Gardner R, Grossman WL. Normal motor patterns in sleep in man. In: Weitzman ED, ed. *Advances in Sleep Research.* Vol. 2. New York: Spectrum Publications; 1975:67–107.
10. Alihanka J, Vaahtoranta K. A static charge sensitive bed. A new method for recording body movements during sleep. *Electroencephalogr Clin Neurophysiol* 1979;46:731–4.
11. Aaronson ST, Rashed S, Biber MP, et al. Brain state and body position: a time-lapse video study of sleep. *Arch Gen Psychiatry* 1982;39:330–5.
12. Rechtschaffen A, Kales A. *A Manual of Standardized Terminology, Techniques and Scoring System for Sleep Stages of Human Subjects.* Los Angeles: Brain Information Service, Brain Research Institute; 1968.
13. Dagnino N, Loeb C, Masazza G, et al. Hypnic physiological myoclonus in man: an EEG-EMG study in normal and neurological patients. *Eur Neurol* 1969;2:47–58.
14. Muzet A, Naitoh P, Townsend RE, et al. Body movements during sleep as a predictor of stage change. *Psychon Sci* 1972;29(1):7–10.
15. Muzet AG, Naitoh P, Johnson C, et al. Body movements in sleep during 30-day exposure to tone pulse. *Psychophysiology* 1974;11(1):27–34.
16. Naitoh P, Muzet A, Johnson LC, et al. Body movements during sleep after sleep loss. *Psychophysiology* 1973;10(4):363–8.
17. Zucconi M, Oldani A, Ferini-Strambi L, et al. Nocturnal paroxysmal arousals with motor behaviors during sleep: frontal lobe epilepsy or parasomnia? *J Clin Neurophysiol* 1997;14(6):513–22.
18. Oldani A, Zucconi M, Ferini-Strambi L, et al. Autosomal dominant nocturnal frontal lobe epilepsy: electroclinical picture. *Epilepsia* 1996;37:964–76.
19. Oldani A, Zucconi M, Asselta R, et al. Autosomal dominant nocturnal frontal lobe epilepsy. A video-polysomnographic and genetic appraisal of 40 patients and delineation of the epileptic syndrome. *Brain* 1998;12:205–23.
20. Sforza E, Montagna P, Rinaldi R, et al. Paroxysmal periodic motor attacks during sleep: clinical and polygraphic features. *Electroencephalogr Clin Neurophysiol* 1993;86:161–6.
21. Terzano MG, Monge-Strauss F, Mikold F, et al. Cyclic alternating pattern as a provocative factor in nocturnal paroxysmal dystonia. *Epilepsia* 1997;38(9):1015–25.
22. Aldrich MS, Jahnke B. Diagnostic value of video-EEG polysomnography. *Neurology* 1991;41:1060–6.
23. Chervin RD, Consens FB, Kutluay E. Alternating leg muscle activation during sleep and arousals: a new sleep-related motor phenomenon? *Mov Disord* 2003;18:551–9.
24. Cosentino FI, Iero I, Lanuzza B, et al. The neurophysiology of the alternating leg muscle activation (ALMA) during sleep: study of one patient before and after treatment with pramipexole. *Sleep Med* 2006;7:63–71.
25. Ferri R, Zucconi M, Manconi M, et al. Computer-assisted detection of nocturnal leg motor activity in patients with restless legs

syndrome and periodic leg movements during sleep. *Sleep* 2005;28:998–1004.

26. Ferri R, Zucconi M, Manconi M, et al. New approaches to the study of periodic leg movements during sleep in restless legs syndrome. *Sleep* 2006;29:759–69.

27. Frauscher B, Brandauer E, Gschliesser V, et al. A descriptive analysis of neck myoclonus during routine polysomnography. *Sleep* 2010;33:1091–6.

28. Frauscher B, Gschliesser V, Brandauer E, et al. Video analysis of motor events in REM sleep behavior disorder. *Mov Disord* 2007;22:1464–70.

29. Frauscher B, Gschliesser V, Brandauer E, et al. The relation between abnormal behaviors and REM sleep microstructure in patients with REM sleep behavior disorder. *Sleep Med* 2009;10:174–81.

30. Frauscher B, Kunz A, Brandauer E, et al. Fragmentary myoclonus in sleep revisited: a polysomnographic study in 62 patients. *Sleep Med* 2011;12:410–15.

31. Hoban T. Sleep-related rhythmic movements disorder. In: Thorpy M, Plazzi G, eds. *The Parasomnias and Other Sleep-Related Movement Disorders*. New York: Cambridge University Press; 2010: 270–7.

32. Huynh N. Sleep-related bruxism. In: Thorpy M, Plazzi G, eds. *The Parasomnias and Other Sleep-Related Movement Disorders*. New York: Cambridge University Press; 2010:252–60.

33. Manconi M, Sferrazza B, Iannaccone S, et al. Case of symptomatic propriospinal myoclonus evolving toward acute "myoclonic status." *Mov Disord* 2005;20:1646–50.

34. Montagna P, Provini F, Vetrugno R. Propriospinal myoclonus at sleep onset. *Neurophysiol Clin* 2006;36:351–5.

35. Oudiette D, Leclair-Visonneau L, Arnulf I. Video-clinical corners. Snoring, penile erection and loss of reflexive consciousness during REM sleep behavior disorder. *Sleep Med* 2010;11:953–5.

36. Walters AS, Lavigne G, Hening W, et al. The scoring of movements in sleep. *J Clin Sleep Med* 2007;3:155–67.

37. Yang C, Winkelman JW. Clinical and polysomnographic characteristics of high frequency leg movements. *J Clin Sleep Med* 2010;6:431–8.

38. Tamura T, Miyasako S, Ogawa M, et al. Assessment of bed temperature monitoring for detecting body movement during sleep: comparison with simultaneous video image recording and actigraphy. *Med Engin Phys* 1999;21:1–8.

39. Sadeh A, Hauri P, Kripke D, et al. The role of actigraphy in the evaluation of sleep disorders. *Sleep* 1995;18:288–302.

40. Hayes MJ, Mitchell D. Spontaneous movements during sleep in children: temporal organization and changes with age. *Dev Psychobiol* 1998;32:13–21.

41. Tallila T, Polo O, Aantaa R, et al. Nocturnal body movements nad hypoxemia in middle-aged females after lower abdominal surgery under general anesthesia: a study with the static-charge-sensitive bed (SCSB). *J Clin Monit Comput* 1998;14(4):239–44.

42. Heinrich A, van Vugt H. A new video actigraphy method for non-contact analysis of body movement during sleep. *J Sleep Res* 2010;19(Suppl 2):83–4.

43. Hobson J, Spagna T,Malenka R. Ethology of sleep studied with time-lapse photography: postural immobility and sleep cycle phase in humans. *Science* 1978;201:1251–3.

44. Kronholm E, Alanen E, Hyyppa MT. Nocturnal movement activity in a conmmunity sample. *Sleep* 1993;16:565–71.

45. Kaartinen J, Erkinjuntti M, Rauhala E. Sleep stages and static charge sensitive bed (SCSB) analysisi of autonomic motor activity. *J Psychophysiol* 1996;10:1–16.

46. Jansen B, Shankar K. Sleep staging with movement related signals. *Int J Biom Comp* 1993;32:289–97.

47. Alihanka J. Basic principles for analysing and scoring Bio-Matt (SCSB) recordings. *Ann Univ Turk, D, Medica-Odontologica* 1987:26.

48. Anttalainen U, Polo O, Vahlberg T, et al. Reimbursed drugs in patients with sleep-disordered breathing: a static-charge-sensitive bed study. *Sleep Med* 2010;11:49–55.

49. Kirjavainen J, Ojala T, Huhtala V, et al. Heart rate variability in response to the sleep-related movements in infants with and without colic. *Early Hum Dev* 2004;79:17–30.

50. Reyner A, Horne J. Gender- and age-related differences in sleep determined by home-recorded sleep logs and actimetry from 400 adults. *Sleep* 1994;18(2):127–34.

51. Stefansson H, Rye DB, Hicks A, et al. A genetic risk factor for periodic limb movements in sleep. *N Engl J Med* 2007:357:639–47.

52. Trotti LM, Bliwise DL, Greer SA, et al. Correlates of PLMs variability over multiple

nights and impact upon RLS diagnosis. *Sleep Med* 2009;10:668–71.

53. Gschliesser V, Frauscher B, Brandauer E, et al. PLM detection by actigraphy compared to polysomnography: a validation and comparison of two actigraphs. *Sleep Med* 2009;10:306–11.

54. Tharp BR. Orbital frontal seizures. An unique EEGic and clinical syndrome. *Epilepsia* 1972;13:627–42.

55. Williamson PD, Spencer DD, Spencer SS, et al. Complex partial seizures of frontal lobe origin. *Ann Neurol* 1985;18:497–504.

56. Bancaud J, Talairach J. Clinical semiology of frontal lobe seizures. In: Chauvel P, Delgado-Escueta AV, Halgren E, Bancaud J, eds. *Frontal Lobe Seizures and Epilepsies. Advances in Neurology.* Vol. 57. New York: Raven Press; 1992:3–58.

57. Williamson PD. Frontal lobe epilepsy: some clinical characteristics. In: Jasper HH, Riggio S, Goldman-Rakic PS, eds. *Epilepsy and Functional Anatomy of the Frontal Lobe. Advances in Neurolgy.* Vol. 66. New York: Raven Press; 1995:127–52.

58. Chauvel P, Kliemann F, Vignal JP, et al. The clinical signs and symptoms of frontal lobe seizures: phenomenology and classification. In: Jasper HH, Riggio S, Goldman-Rakic PS, eds. *Epilepsy and the Functional Anatomy of the Frontal Lobe. Advances in Neurology.* Vol. 66. New York: Raven Press; 1995;115–26.

59. Riggio S, Harner R. Repetitive motor activity in frontal lobe epilepsy. In: Jasper HH, Riggio S, Goldman-Rakic PS eds. *Epilepsy and the Functional Anatomy of the Frontal Lobe. Advances in Neurlogy.* Vol. 66. New York: Raven Press; 1995:153–6.

60. Fusco L, Iani C, Faedda MT, et al. Mesial frontal lobe epilepsy: a clinical entity not sufficiently described. *J Epilepsy* 1990;3:123–35.

61. Kanner AM, Morris HH, Luders H, et al. Supplementary motor seizures mimicking pseudoseizures: some clinical differences. *Neurology* 1990;40:1404–7.

62. Lugaresi E, Cirignotta F. Hypnogenic paroxysmal dystonia: epileptic seizures or a new syndrome? *Sleep* 1981;4:129–38.

63. Lugaresi E, Cirignotta F,Montagna P. Nocturnal paroxysmal dystonia. *J Neurol Neurosurg Psychiatry* 1986;49:375–80.

64. Boller F, Wright DG, Cavalieri R, et al. Paroxysmal nightmares. *Neurology* 1975;25:1026–8.

65. Maselli RA, Rosemberg RS, Spire SP. Episodic nocturnal wanderings in non-epileptic young patients. *Sleep* 1988;11:156–61.

66. Meierkord H, Fish DR, Smith SJ, et al. Is nocturnal paroxysmal dystonia a form of frontal lobe epilepsy? *Mov Dis* 1993;8:252–3.

67. Pedley Ta, Guilleminault C. Episodic nocturnal wanderings responsive to anticonvulsant drug therapy. *Ann Neurol* 1977;2:30–5.

68. Peled R, Lavie P. Paroxysmal awakenings from sleep associated with excessive daytime somnolence. A form of nocturnal epilepsy. *Neurology* 1986;36:95–8.

69. Montagna P, Sforza E, Tinuper P, et al. Paroxismal arousals during sleep. *Neurology* 1990;40:1063–7.

70. Hirsch E, Sellal F, Maton B, et al. Nocturnal paroxysmal dystonia: a clinical form of focal epilepsy. *Neurophysiol Clin* 1994;24:207–17.

71. Godbout R, Montplaisir J, Rouleau I. Hypnogenic paroxysmal dystonia: epilepsy or sleep disorder? A case report. *Clin Electroencephalogr* 1985;16:136–42.

72. Tinuper P, Cerullo A, Cirignotta F, et al. Nocturnal paroxysmal dystonia with short-lasting attacks: three cases with evidence for an epileptic frontal lobe origin of seizures. *Epilepsia* 1990;31:549–56.

73. Plazzi G, Tinuper P, Montagna P, et al. Epileptic nocturnal wanderings. *Sleep* 1995;18:749–56.

74. Phillips Ha, Scheffer IE, Berkovic SF, et al. Localization of a gene for autosomal dominant nocturnal frontal lobe epilepsy to chromosome 20q13.2. *Nat Genet* 1995;10:117–18.

75. Steinlein O, Mulley JC, Propping P, et al. A missense mutation in the neural nicotinic acetylcholine receptor 4 subunit is associated with autosomal dominant nocturnal frontal lobe epilepsy. *Nat Genet* 1995;11:201–3

76. Phillips HA, Scheffer IE, Crossland KM, et al. Autosomal dominant nocturnal frontal-lobe epilepsy: genetic heterogeneity and evidence for a second locus at 15q24. *Am J Hum Genet* 1998;63:1108–16.

77. De Fusco M, Becchetti A, Patrignani A, et al. The nicotinic receptor β2 subunit is mutant in nocturnal frontal lobe epilepsy. *Nat Genet* 2000;26:275–6.

78. Mochi M, Provini F, Plazzi G, et al. Genetic heterogeneity in autosomal dominant nocturnal frontal lobe epilepsy. *Ital J Neurol Sci* 1997;18:183.

79. Tenchini ML, Duga S, Bonati MT, et al. SER252PHE and 776INS3 mutations in the CHRNA4 gene are rare in the italian ADNFLE population. *Sleep* 1999;22:637–9.

80. De Marco EV, Gambardella A, Annesi F, et al. Further evidence of genetic heterogeneity in families with autosomal dominant nocturnal frontal lobe epilepsy. *Epilepsy Res* 2007;74:70–3.

81. Aridon P, Marini C, Di Resta C. Increased sensitivity of the neural nicotinic receptor alpha 2 subunit causes familial epilepsy with norcturnal wandering and ictal fear. *Am J Hum genet* 2006;79:342–50.

82. Provini F, Plazzi G, Tinuper P, et al. Nocturnal frontal lobe epilepsy. A clinical and polygraphic overview of 100 consecutives cases. *Brain* 1999;122:1017–31.

83. Soldatos CR, Vela-Bueno A, Bixler EO, et al. Sleepwalking and night terrors in adulthood: clinical EEG findings. *Clin Electroencephalogr* 1980;11:136–9.

84. Nobili L, Cossu M, Mai R, et al. Sleep related hyperkinetic seizures of temporal lobe origin. *Neurology* 2004;62:482–5.

85. Ryvlin P, Minotti L, Demarquay G, et al. Nocturnal hypermotor seizures, suggesting frontal lobe epilepsy, can originate in the insula. *Epilepsia* 2006;47:755–65.

86. Silvestri R, Bromfield E. Recurrent nightmares and disorders of arousals in temporal lobe epilepsy. *Brain Res Bull* 2004;63:369–76.

87. Nobili L. Nocturnal frontal lobe epilepsy and non-rapid eye movement sleep parasomnias: differences and similarities. *Sleep Med Rev* 2007;11:251–4.

88. Halasz P, Ujszaszi J, Gadoros J. Are microarousals preceded by EEGic slow wave synchronization precursors of confusional awakenings? *Sleep* 1985;8:231–8.

89. Blatt I, Peled R, Gadoth N, et al. The value of sleep recording in evaluating somnambulism in young adults. *Electroencephalogr Clin Neurophysiol* 1991;78:407–12.

90. Zucconi M, Oldani A, Ferini-Strambi L, et al. Arousal fluctuations in non-rapid eye movement parasomnias: the role of cyclic alternating pattern as a measure of sleep instability. *J Clin Neurophysiol* 1995;12(2):147–54.

91. Munari C, Tassi L, Di Leo M, et al. Video-stereo electroencephalographic investigation of orbitofrontal cortex. Ictal electroclinical patterns. In: Jasper HH, Riggio S, Goldman-Rakic PS, eds. *Epilepsy and the Functional Anatomy of the Frontal Lobe. Advances in Neurlogy.* Vol. 66. New York: Raven Press; 1995;273–95.

92. Malow BA, Varma NK. Seizures and arousals from sleep-which came first? *Sleep* 1995;18:783–6.

93. Dantendorfer K, Frey R, Maierhofer D, et al. Sudden arousals from slow wave sleep and panic disorder: successfull treatment with anticonvulsants—a case report. *Sleep* 1996;19:744–6.

94. Plazzi G, Montagna P, Provini F, et al. Sudden arousals from slow-wave sleep and panic disorder. *Sleep* 1998;21:548.

95. Shenck CH, Bundlie SR, Patterson A, et al. Rapid eye movement sleep behavior disorder. A treatable parasomnia affecting older adults. *JAMA* 1987;257:1786–9.

96. Ohayon MM, Caulet M, Priest RG. Violet behavior during sleep. *J Clin Psychiatry* 1997;58:369–76.

97. Oudiette D, Leu S, Pottier M, et al. Dreamlike mentations during sleepwalking and sleep terrors in adults. *Sleep* 2009;32:1621–7.

98. Hwang TJ, Ni HC, Chen HC, et al. Risk predictors for hypnosedative-related complex sleep behaviors: a pilot study. *J Clin Psychiatry* 2010;71:1331–5.

99. Pressman MR. Disorders of arousal from sleep and violent behavior: the role of physical contact and proximity. *Sleep* 2007;30:1039–47.

100. Siclari V, Khatami R, Urbaniok F, et al. Violence in sleep. *Brain* 2010;133:3494–509.

101. Shenck CH, Milner DM, Hurwitz TD, et al. Dissociative diosrders presenting as somnambulism: polysomnographic, video, and clinical documentation (8 cases). *Dissociation* 1989;2:194–204.

102. Stewart JT, Bartucci RJ. Posttraumatic stress disorder and partial complex seizures. *Am J Psychiatry* 1986;143:113–14.

103. Montagna P, Cirignotta F, Giovanardi Rossi, et al. Dystonic attacks related to sleep and exercise. *Eur Neurol* 1992;32:185–9.

104. De Saint-Martin A, Badinand N, Picard F, et al. Dyskinesie paroxystique diurne et nocturne du jeune enfant: une nouvelle entité? *Rev Neurol* 1997;153:262–7.

105. Lugaresi E, Cirignotta F, Coccagna G, Montagna P. Nocturnal myoclonus and restless legs syndrome. *Adv Neurol* 1986;43:295–307.

106. Zucconi M, Ferri R, Allen R, et al. The official World Association of Sleep Medicine (WASM) standards for recording and scoring periodic leg movements in sleep (PLMS) and wakefulness (PLMW) developed in collaboration with a task force from the International Restless Legs Syndrome Study Group (IRLSSG). *Sleep Med* 2006;7:175–83.

107. Iber C, Ancoli-Israel S, Chesson AL, et al. *The AASM Manual for the Scoring of Sleep and Associated Events: Rules, Terminology, and Technical Specifications.* Westchester, IL: American Academy of Sleep Medicine; 2007.

108. Ferri R. The time structure of leg movement activity during sleep: the theory behind the practice. *Sleep Med* 2012;13(4):433–41.

109. Kato T, Montplaisir J, Blanchet PJ, et al. Idiopathic myoclonus in the oromandibular region during sleep: a possible source of confusion in sleep bruxism diagnosis. *Mov Disord* 1999;14(5):865–84.

110. Velly Miguel AM, Montplaisir J, Romprè PH, et al. Bruxism and other oro-facial movements during sleep. *J Craniomandib Disord Facial Oral Pain* 1992;6:71–81.

111. Aguglia U, Gambardella A, Quattrone A. Sleep-induced masticatory myoclonus: a rare parasomnia associated with insomnia. *Sleep* 1991;14:80–2.

112. Deuschl G, Toro C, Valls-Solè J, et al. Symptomatic and essential palatal tremor. 1: clinical, physiological and MRI analysis. *Brain* 1994;117:775–88.

113. Gobernado JM, Galarreta M, De Blas G, et al. Isolated continuous rhythmic lingual myoclonus. *Mov Disord* 1992;7:367–9.

114. Simpson DA, Wishnow R, Gargulinski RB, et al. Oculo-facial-skeletal myorhythmia in central nervous system Whipple's disease: additional case and review of the literature. *Mov Disord* 1995;10:195–200.

115. Brown P, Thompson PD, Rothwell JC, et al. Axial myoclonus of propriospinal origin. *Brain* 1991;114:197–214.

116. Brown P, Rothwell JC, Thompson PD, et al. Propriospinal myoclonus: evidence for spinal "pattern" generators in humans. *Mov Disord* 1994;9:571–6.

117. Montagna P, Provini F, Plazzi G, et al. Propriospinal myoclonus upon relaxation and drowsiness: a cause of severe insomnia. *Mov Disord* 1997;12:66–72.

118. Oswald I. Experimental studies of rhythm, anxiety and cerebral vigilance. *J Mental Sci* 1959;105:269–74.

119. Broughton R. Pathological fragmentary myoclonus, intensified "hypnic jerks" and hypnagogic foot tremor: three unusual sleep-related movement disorders. In: Koella WP, Obal F, Schulz H, Visser P, eds. *SLEEP '88.* Stuttgart, Germany: Gustav Fischer Verlag; 1988:240–3.

120. Broughton R, Tolentino MA, Krelina M. Excessive fragmentary myoclonus in NREM sleep: a report of 38 cases. *Electroencephalogr Clin Neurophysiol* 1985;61:123–33.

121. Montagna P, Liguori R, Zucconi M, et al. Physiological hypnic myoclonus. *Electroencephalogr Clin Neurophysiol* 1988;70:172–6.

122. Broughton RJ, Shimizu T. Sleep-related violence: a medical and forensic challenge. *Sleep* 1995;18:727–30.

123. Mahowald MW, Shenck CH. Complex motor behavior arising during sleep period: forensic science implications. *Sleep* 1985;18:724–7.

124. Moldofsky H, Gilbert R, Lue FA, et al. Sleep-related violence. *Sleep* 1985;18:731–9.

125. Gastaut H, Broughton RJ. A clinical and polygraphic study of episodic phenomena during sleep. *Rec Adv Biol Psychiatry* 1965;7:197–222.

126. Porter RJ, Sato S. Prolonged EEG and video monitoring in the diagnosis of seizure disorders. In: Niedermeyer E, Lopes da Silva M, eds. *Electroencephalography: Basic Principles, Clinical Applications and Related fields.* Baltimore, MD: Williams & Wilkins; 1993:729–46.

127. Guilleminault C, Moscovitch A, Leger D. Forensic sleep medicine: nocturnal wandering and violence. *Sleep* 1985;18:740–8.

B

Sleep Related Movements: Normal
and Abnormal

26

General Introduction and Historical Review

ELIO LUGARESI AND SUDHANSU CHOKROVERTY

THE OBJECTIVE study of body motility during sleep started in the first decades of the last century when rudimentary actigraphs became available (Szymanski quoted by Kleitman).[1,2] In humans, these devices offered the first evidence that the overall muscular rest of sleep is periodically interrupted by gross body movements. Hypnic jerks (sleep starts) were first described in the late 19th century by Weir Mitchell,[3] who emphasized that in some cases they may be so intense as to provoke insomnia. Looking at sleeping humans and domestic animals, De Lisi[4] noted that the skeletal muscles are animated by partial short-lasting muscular contractions that he named physiologic hypnic myoclonus (PHM). Investigating sleep behavior in a large population of children, De Toni[5] observed slow pendular ocular movements appearing under the eyelids at sleep onset. The discovery of bursts of rapid eye movements (REMs) characterizing REM sleep[6] marked a milestone in sleep research. However, it was the work of Dement and Kleitman,[7] showing that sleep evolves across the night following a complex but more or less consistent pattern, that offered the essential tool for the objective study of human sleep.

EARLY CLINICAL STUDIES

After this historic paper, many laboratories around the world embarked on sleep disorder studies. In Europe, Henri Gastaut and his coworkers[8] were among the first to study sleep-related normal movement patterns and movement disorders using polygraphic techniques with multiple peripheral electromyographic leads. They divided physiologic sleep movements into three groups:

1. Movements not associated with electroencephalographic changes and, thus, deemed an integral part of sleep proper (this group includes PHM and chewing, swallowing, and mimicking automatisms)

2. Movements associated with a physiologic lightening of sleep (postural changes and complex gestures)

3. Movements associated with an arousal (sleep starts and sleep paralysis)

Gastaut, Batini, Broughton, et al.[8] also described the polysomnographic features of sleep terrors and sleep walking. They deemed these nocturnal motor manifestations a consequence of partial awakening from deep sleep (stage 3 [N3] non–rapid eye movement [non-REM]) or, as Broughton[9] later suggested, a disorder of arousal. Similar findings were reported for sleepwalking by Kales and coworkers[10] around the same years·[11] and for sleep terrors considerably later by Fisher, Kahn, Edwards, et al.[12]

Gastaut and coworkers also carried out the first polysomnographic research on the evolution of abnormal movements during sleep. They showed that parkinsonian and cerebellar tremors and choreoathetoid movements disappear at sleep onset (Stage I non-REM) but can reappear during the postural changes and awakenings provoked by other stimuli.[13]

In the early 1960s, studying the evolution of epileptic and nonepileptic movements during sleep, we observed that epileptic myoclonus linked to cortical lesions, that is, Jacksonian status and epilepsia partialis continua, persist, albeit attenuated, throughout all sleep stages.[14] By comparison, myoclonic jerks linked to subcortical lesions (e.g., degenerative myoclonic epilepsies) disappear at sleep onset, thereby behaving like parkinsonian tremors and choreoathetoid movements.[14] We also showed that abnormal movements linked to peripheral lesions, for instance, fasciculations in amyotrophic lateral sclerosis and idiopathic and symptomatic facial spasms, persist throughout all sleep stages.[14] As a whole, these findings provided evidence that the evolution of abnormal sleep movements is in some way linked to the location of the underlying lesion.

We were later to show that physiologic positive motor events like the enhanced muscle tone and H reflex following a sudden noise, as well as muscular jerks related to an epileptic spike, can cause negative motor phenomena, for example, muscle atonia and inhibition of the H reflex, during slow-wave sleep.[15] Earlier our group from Bologna showed that the polysomnographic study of restless legs syndrome disclosed periodic limb movements linked to

light sleep, which at the time were referred to as nocturnal myoclonus.[16]

MECHANISMS OF MOTOR CONTROL IN SLEEP

Alongside these clinical studies on sleep disorders, the 1960s also saw the development of physiologic studies of motor control during sleep. Following Jouvet, Michel, and Courjon's[17] discovery that skeletal muscles become atonic during REM sleep, Morrison and Pompeiano[18] and Gassell, Marchiafava, and Pompeiano[19] demonstrated that monosynaptic and polysynaptic spinal reflexes are suppressed during REM sleep and that during bursts of REMs further depression may occur. The depression of monosynaptic reflexes during REM bursts depends on presynaptic inhibition of primary afferents from muscle spindles. The results of direct stimulation of motor neurons in the lumbar spinal cord suggested that postsynaptic inhibition of motor neurons causes muscle atonia.

Direct evidence that the inhibition of motor neurons during REM sleep depends on a postsynaptic mechanism was obtained a decade later when, using intracellular recordings in naturally sleeping cats, it was demonstrated that the motor neuronal membrane was hyperpolarized during REM sleep.[20] More recently, postsynaptic inhibition was shown to depend on a glycinergic[21] as well as a GABA-ergic[22] mechanism. In addition, there is disfacilitation of aminergic neurons as well as inhibition of lateral hypothalamic hypocretinergic neurons causing disfacilitation (inhibition) of brainstem and spinal motor neurons.[23,24]

At this point, mention should be made of the experimental contribution of Jouvet and Delorme[25] and subsequent studies by Henly and Morrison.[26] Twenty years before the disorder was identified in people,[27] they found that selective lesions in the pontine tegmentum reproduced the behavioral features of REM sleep without atonia. Physiologic research into motor control during sleep has clarified most of the mechanisms responsible for physiologic and pathologic motor events during REM sleep. In contrast, few studies have addressed the changes in motor control characterizing non-REM sleep, even though motor disorders can be related to the wake-to-non-REM sleep-transition period (e.g., restless legs syndrome and propriospinal myoclonus) or to slow-wave sleep (e.g., nocturnal frontal lobe epilepsy [NFLE]). It is important that future studies investigate motor control in these sleep stages.

MORE RECENT CLINICAL ADVANCES

From the 1970s, polysomnographic recordings under audiovisual control yielded important information on movement disorders related to sleep. This dual technique disclosed two important clinical conditions, REM behavior disorder (RBD) and NFLE.

RBD mainly occurs in relatively older men. In more than half of the cases the disorder appears in patients with neurodegenerative diseases, even heralding the symptoms of these conditions. Despite the fact that a similar pattern was experimentally provoked in animals more than 20 years earlier by selective pontine lesions,[25] a number of aspects remain unsettled in the physiopathogenesis of RBD. These include the remarkable male prevalence and the therapeutic effects of clonazepam.[27]

NFLE (also called nocturnal paroxysmal dystonia) may be expressed as paroxysmal awakenings, choreoathetoid or ballismic movements, or agitated somnambulism.[28-34] These different types of seizure expression are stereotyped and often overlap in a single individual. Diagnosis is based on video recordings because interictal and ictal electroencephalograms are often inconclusive. An important feature, given its implications for the molecular mechanisms of epilepsy, is the fact that NFLE can be inherited as an autosomal dominant trait.[35] Some mutations have been linked to an autosomal dominant mode of inheritance, but this has not been confirmed in other families, indicating that autosomal dominant NFLE presents genetic heterogeneity.[36-38]

A singular aspect of NFLE is that patients and their relatives also report episodes of pavor nocturnus and somnambulism much more often than the general population. This unexpected finding, confirmed in all published studies, may indicate that the functional abnormality, linked to a molecular genetic alteration favoring the onset of an epileptogenic focus in the frontal lobe, may also promote the appearance of nonepileptic motor disorders linked to non-REM sleep.

It is noteworthy that some movement disorders like periodic limb movements in sleep, restless legs syndrome (recently renamed Willis-Ekbom disease), and propriospinal myoclonus[39,40] typically arise on falling asleep, whereas they seldom occur on awakening in the morning. Unspecified circadian factors are often implicated to account for this sleep-related behavior.[41] However, a recent study of regional brain blood flow in humans[42] has suggested another possible explanation. On awakening in the morning (post-sleep wakefulness), blood flow in the brain cortical regions is markedly and consistently reduced with respect to presleep wakefulness. This different functional situation in cortical blood flow, and hence in metabolic and synaptic activities, may be responsible for the different motor control present during presleep and postsleep wakefulness. This may account for the fact that certain motor events, like periodic limb movements in wakefulness and propriospinal myoclonus, are mainly confined to presleep wakefulness and are absent on awakening, whereas parkinsonian patients have a so-called sleep benefit in postsleep wakefulness.[43]

Other motor phenomena and cognitive disturbances such as sleep inertia and sleep drunkenness may also be explained by the different functional status of the cerebral cortex in wake following, as opposed to preceding, sleep.[40] The pathophysiology of certain other motility disturbances (e.g., alternating leg muscle activation [ALMA][44] hypnagogic foot tremor,[45] and rhythmic movement disorder[46]) remains undetermined.

CONCLUSION

Over 40 years of physiologic and clinical research into normal and abnormal sleep-related movements have disclosed the complexity of this topic and allowed the definition of the clinical and physiopathologic features of some sleep-related movement disorders. However, much remains to be done to clarify the many still unresolved issues.

REFERENCES

1. Szymanski JS. Eine Methode zur Untersuchung der Ruhe und Akitivitaetsperioden bei Tieren. *Pfluegers Arch* 1914;158:343.
2. Kleitman N. Motility during sleep. In: *Sleep and Wakefulness*. Chicago, IL: University of Chicago Press; 1963:81.
3. Mitchell W. Some disorders of sleep. *Am J Med Sci* 1890;100:190.

4. De Lisi L. Su di un fenomeno motorio costante del sonno normale: le mioclonie ipniche fisiologiche. *Riv Pat Ment* 1932;39:481.

5. De Toni G. I movimenti pendolari dei bulbi oculari dei bambini durante il sonno fisiologico, ed in alcuni stati morbosi. *Pediatria* 1931;41:489.

6. Aserinsky E, Kleitman N. Regularly occurring periods of eye motility and concomitant phenomena during sleep. *Science* 1953;118:273.

7. Dement W, Kleitman N. Cyclic variations in EEG during sleep and their relation to eyes movements, body motility, and dreaming. *Electroencephalogr Clin Neurophysiol* 1957;9:673.

8. Gastaut H, Batini C, Broughton R, et al. Etude electroencephalographique des phenomenes episodiques non epileptiques au cours du sommeil. In: Fischgold H, ed. *Le sommeil de nuit normal et pathologique.* Paris: Masson & Cie Editeurs; 1965:214.

9. Broughton RJ. Sleep disorders: disorders of arousal? *Science* 1968;159:1070.

10. Kales A, Jacobson A, Paulson M, et al. Somnambulism: psychophysiological correlates: I. All-night EEG studies. *Arch Gen Psychiatry* 1966;14:585.

11. Jacobson A, Kales A, Lehmann D, et al. Somnambulism: all night electroencephalography studies. *Science* 1965;148:975.

12. Fisher C, Kahn E, Edwards A, et al. A psychophysiological study of nightmares and night terrors. *J Nerv Ment Dis* 1973;157:75.

13. Tassinari CA, Broughton R, Poire R, et al. An electroclinical study of nocturnal sleep in patients presenting abnormal movements. *Electroencephalogr Clin Neurophysiol* 1965;18:95.

14. Lugaresi E, Coccagna G, Mantovani M, et al. The evolution of different types of myoclonus during sleep. *Eur Neurol* 1970;4:321.

15. Cirignotta F, Montagna P, Mondini S, et al. Inhibitory phenomena during NREM sleep related to auditory stimuli and epileptic spikes. *Electroenceph Clin Neurophysiol* 1983;55:165.

16. Lugaresi E, Coccagna G, Tassinari CA, et al. Rilievi poligrafici sui fenomeni motori nella syndrome delle gambe senza riposo. *Riv Neurol* 1965;34:550.

17. Jouvet M, Michel F, Courjon J. Sur un stade d'activité électrique cérébrale rapide au cours du sommeil physiologique. *Compt Ren Soc Biol* 1959;153:1024.

18. Morrison AR, Pompeiano O. An analysis of the supraspinal influences acting on motoneurons during sleep in the unrestrained cat. Responses of the alpha motoneurons to direct electrical stimulation during sleep. *Arch Ital Biol* 1965;103:497.

19. Gassel MM, Marchiafava PL, Pompeiano D. An analysis of the supraspinal influences acting on motoneurons during sleep in the unrestrained cat. Modification of the recurrent discharge of the alpha motoneurons during sleep. *Arch Ital Biol* 1965;103:25.

20. Morales FR, Boxer P, Chase MH. Behavioral state-specific inhibitory post-synaptic potentials impinging on cat lumbar motoneurons during active sleep. *Exp Neurol* 1987;98:418.

21. Chase MH. Confirmation of the consensus that glycinergic postsynaptic inhibition is responsible for the atonia of REM sleep. *Sleep* 2008;31:1487–91.

22. Brooks PL, Peever JH. Impaired GABA and glycine transmission triggers cardinal features of rapid eye movement sleep disorder in mice. *J Neurosci* 2011;31(19):7111–21.

23. Fenik VB, Davies RO, Kubin L. REM sleep-like atonia of hypoglossal (xii) motoneurons is caused by loss of noradrenergic and serotenergic inputs. *Am J Respir Crit Care Med* 2005;172:1322–30.

24. Taheri S, Zeitzer JM, Mignot E. The role of hypocretins (orexins) in sleep regulation and narcolepsy. *Annu Rev Neruol* 2002;25:283–313.

25. Jouvet M, Delorme F. Locus coeruleus et somneil paradoxal. *CR Soc Biol* 1965l159:895.

26. Henly K, Morrison AR. A re-evaluation of the effects of lesions of the pontine tegmentum and locus coeruleus on phenomena of paradoxical sleep in the cat. *Acta Neurobiol Exp* 1974;34:215.

27. Schenck CH, Bundlie SR, Ettinger MG, et al. Chronic behavioral disorders of human REM sleep: a new category of parasomnia. *Sleep* 1986;9:293.

28. Pedley TA, Guilleminault C. Episodic nocturnal wanderings responsive to anticonvulsant drug therapy. *Ann Neurol* 1977;2:30.

29. Lugaresi E, Cirignotta F. Hypnogenic paroxysmal dystonia; epileptic seizures or a new syndrome? *Sleep* 1981;4:129.

30. Lugaresi E, Cirignotta F, Montagna P. Nocturnal paroxysmal dystonia. *J Neurol Neurosurg Psychiatry* 1986;49:375.

31. Peled R, Lavie P. Paroxysmal awakenings from sleep associated with excessive daytime

somnolence: a form of nocturnal epilepsy. *Neurology* 1986;36:95.

32. Montagna P, Sforza E, Tinuper P, et al. Paroxysmal arousals during sleep. *Neurology* 1990;40:1063.

33. Plazzi G, Tinuper P, Montagna P, et al. Epileptic nocturnal wanderings. *Sleep* 1995;18:749.

34. Provini F, Plazzi G, Tinuper P, et al. Nocturnal frontal lobe epilepsy. A clinical and polygraphic overview of 100 consecutive cases. *Brain* 1999;122:1017.

35. Scheffer IE, Bhatia KP, Lopes-Cendes I, et al. Autosomal dominant nocturnal frontal lobe epilepsy. A distinctive clinical disorder. *Brain* 1995;118:61.

36. Steinlein OK, Mulley JC, Propping P, et al. A missense mutation in the neuronal nicotinic acetylcholine receptor alpha 4 subunit is associated with autosomal dominant nocturnal frontal lobe epilepsy. *Nat Genet* 1995;11:201.

37. Steinlein OK, Magnusson A, Stoodt J, et al. An insertion mutation of the CHRNA4 gene in a family with autosomal dominant nocturnal frontal lobe epilepsy. *Hum Mol Genet* 1997;6:943.

38. Phillips HA, Scheffer IE, Crossland M, et al. Autosomal dominant nocturnal frontal-lobe epilepsy: genetic heterogeneity and evidence for a second locus at 15q24. *Am J Hum Genet* 1998;63:1108.

39. Brown P, Thompson PD, Rothwell JC, et al. Axial myoclonus of propriospinal origin. *Brain* 1991;114:197.

40. Montagna P, Provini F, Plazzi G, et al. Propriospinal myoclonus upon relaxation and drowsiness: a cause of severe insomnia. *Mov Disord* 1997;12:66.

41. Trenkwalder C, Hening WA, Walters AS, et al. Circadian rhythm of periodic limb movements and sensory symptoms of restless legs syndrome. *Mov Disord* 1999;14:102.

42. Braun AR, Balkin TJ, Wesenten HJ, et al. Regional cerebral blood flow throughout the sleep-wake cycle. An H2(15)O PET study. *Brain* 1997;120:1173.

43. Montagna P, Lugaresi E. Sleep benefit in Parkinson's disease. *Mov Disord* 1998;13:751.

44. Chervin RD, Consens FB, Kutluay E. Alternating leg muscle activation during sleep and arousals: a new sleep-related motor phenomenon? *Mov Disord* 2003;18:551–9.

45. Broughton R. Pathological fragmentary myoclonus, intensified sleep starts and hypnagogic foot tremor: three unusual sleep-related disorders. In: Koella W, ed. *Sleep 1986*. New York: Fischer-Verlag; 1988:240–3.

46. Mayer G, Wilde-Frenz J, Kurella B. Sleep related rhythmic movement disorder revisited. *J Sleep Res* 2007;16:110–16.

27

Physiologic Body Jerks and Movements at Sleep Onset and during Sleep

GIOVANNA CALANDRA-BUONAURA AND FEDERICA PROVINI

SLEEP IS commonly considered a time of physical and mental inactivity. Behavior and mentation, however, do not cease in the different sleep stages; they only undergo state-dependent physiologic modifications. Motor phenomena peculiar to sleep onset and during sleep, the concern of this chapter, are known, but their precise delineation had to await the development of electrophysiologic and audiovisual monitoring techniques. Their mechanisms remain predominantly unknown because of the lack of understanding of the basic physiology of sleep. Therefore, clinical information on these phenomena is usually confined to a simple description. Polysomnogram (PSG) recordings under audiovisual monitoring are the techniques that provide significant diagnostic help. However, uncertainties remain, and even the precise boundaries between physiologic and pathologic motor activity during sleep are not completely clear.

THE TRANSITION FROM WAKEFULNESS TO SLEEP: A PECULIAR NEUROPHYSIOLOGIC STATE

A more or less gradual transition leads from quiet wakefulness to sleep and vice versa. Such transitional periods are complex and autonomous neurophysiologic states, a view pioneered by Critchley,[1] who emphasized that falling asleep—a period that he termed the *predormitum*—and awakening (also called the postdormitum) should be kept distinct from wakefulness and sleep proper. The predormitum differs widely in different people. On transition from wakefulness to sleep, consciousness is reduced and afferent information inhibited. The stream of consciousness gradually changes in the predormital stage, with reflections wandering and "passing like a pageant across one's sensorium," the process of volition gradually weakening, and free associations growing into fantasies and reveries and becoming more and more unreal and even grotesque.[1] Deliberate control, up to a certain point, may check these imageries and bring back reality and rationality, or instead the subject may quietly slip into sleep. During falling asleep, responses to auditory cues are decreased but not abolished, and response time is lengthened.[2] This is also a time for illusions and hallucinations: the feeling of the body becomes distorted, blurred, and disproportionate. Visual illusions and distortions of time perception on falling asleep are reported by 25% of normal teenagers[3] and hypnagogic hallucinations by 37% of normal adults[4]; violent and abrupt sensory phenomena may occur, such as a hallucinatory crash, a bang, or explosion within the head or a flash of light (the so-called exploding head syndrome).[5]

These modifications of the mental contents and their spatiotemporal patterning are accompanied by specific electroencephalographic, autonomic, and somatic changes. On the electroencephalogram (EEG), sleep-onset period is marked at first by increased theta and reduced alpha activity over the central regions[6] and spindles marking the onset of sleep proper. This transitional period may be seen to extend over about 3 minutes; direct current negative potential shifts are seen over the midline cerebral regions, reflecting increased cortical excitability.[7] Event-related potentials and contingent negative variation show specific changes and inversion of polarity.[8] Muscle tone in the antigravity muscles is diminished, spontaneous motor activity reduced, and tendon jerks and electrically evoked monosynaptic H reflexes progressively attenuated. Slow eye movements (with a time constant longer than 3 seconds) typify the sleep-onset period, declining then with deepening of sleep and disappearing in slow-wave sleep (SWS); they are linked to decreased firing and changes in eye velocity coding of oculomotor and vestibular neurons.[9] Autonomic changes are indicated by a significant decline in brain and core temperature before falling asleep[10] and by a progressive slowing of heart rate (beginning 30 seconds before stage 1 non–rapid eye movement sleep [non-REM1]) and decreased ventilation, resulting from a fall in upper airway dilator muscle and respiratory pump muscle activity and a switch to homeostatic control.[11]

The individuality of the wake-sleep transitional states is brought about not only by the specificity of their mental, motor, and autonomic features but also by the relevant clinical phenomena that remain restricted to these sleep phases. In the predormital stage, these include physiologic sleep starts or sudden bodily jerks that accompany falling asleep; propriospinal myoclonus (PSM) at the transition from wakefulness to sleep (see later); and periodic limb movements in sleep (PLMS) that appear during quiet wakefulness, persist into light sleep, and are greatly reduced during deep and rapid eye movement (REM) sleep. In the postdormitum, these include the jerks of juvenile myoclonic epilepsy, usually confined to the first half hour after awakening, and the so-called sleep benefit reported by parkinsonian patients for the first 85 minutes after awakening[12]; from a metabolic point of view, this postdormitum period, commonly known under the term "sleep inertia," is attended by reduced cerebral blood flow in the cortex with values intermediate between wakefulness and the deep-sleep phases.[13]

The current chapter will focus on the description of those wake-sleep transition motor phenomena included in the category of Isolated Symptoms, Apparently Normal Variants and Unresolved Issues of the newly revised *International Classification of Sleep Disorders*.[14] This section comprises sleep-related symptoms that either lie at the borderline between normal and abnormal sleep or that exist on the continuum of normal to abnormal sleep and hence may appropriately be evaluated by the sleep clinician without necessarily constituting a sleep pathology.

PHYSIOLOGIC MOTOR ACTIVITY AT THE ONSET OF AND DURING SLEEP

Sleep onset is characterized by a peculiar type of motor activity typified by brief shock-like activity of the muscles or parts thereof, the so-called physiologic hypnic myoclonus, and more sporadic and diffuse axial jerks, so-called sleep starts; both may extend also into light-sleep or REM-sleep stages. Both activities retain a myoclonic character. Gross body movements, slower and displaying "normal" motor patterns, are absent on falling asleep and become evident as sleep develops.

Physiologic Hypnic Myoclonus

Physiologic hypnic myoclonias was the term by which De Lisi[15] in 1932 first described the sudden brief twitches that he observed during sleep in humans and domestic animals such as cats and dogs. These twitches resembled fasciculation potentials when they remained confined to the muscle belly and assumed a myoclonic aspect when large enough to displace the segment involved, such as the lip or fingers. They were particularly prominent in small babies and children and in muscles of acral or distal body parts such as the face and lips and the hands. This physiologic motor activity of sleep has since been variously termed *partial hypnic myoclonus* or *physiological fragmentary hypnic myoclonus*; the term *physiologic hypnic myoclonus* (PHM) is used here.

On electromyogram (EMG) recordings, PHM appears as random phasic bursts of one or several motor unit potentials, which may discharge asynchronously or in brief clusters that usually last less than 1 second. When isolated, PHM clearly resembles fasciculation potentials. These EMG potentials may appear over any body muscles but are more evident in distal muscles, especially of the hands and over facial muscles. They may occur synchronously in antagonistic muscles of the same limb.

Dagnino et al.[16] performed a quantitative study of PHM to calculate its incidence in the different sleep stages, by means of a myoclonic index in the opponens pollicis muscle of 29 normal volunteers. They also examined 18 patients with various neurologic diseases of neural, spinal, or pyramidal and extrapyramidal origin. They found the greatest value of their myoclonic index in non-REM1 sleep, decreasing progressively in REM, non-REM2, and non-REM3 stages. PHM, therefore, correlated inversely with electroencephalographic synchronization. They noted, moreover, that PHM value in non-REM3 stage was not significantly different from zero and that there was no difference between REM periods associated with or without bursts of eye movements. There was no significant variation across the different parts of the night. No PHM could be recorded from those patients with peripheral nerve complete lesions or with spinal paraplegia, whereas completely normal findings were observed in two patients with tabes dorsalis, in whom muscle proprioceptive input was probably completely abolished. In six patients with chronic ischemic hemiparesis, PHM was uniformly absent on the affected side, whereas it was greatly increased in six patients with Parkinson's disease and in one patient with Wilson's disease. Five parkinsonian patients subsequently underwent thalamotomy,

without any change in the amount of the PHM. Therefore, PHM seems to represent a universal phenomenon in normal subjects and is most apparent during non-REM1 sleep; this is in contrast to animal studies, which document that the highest peak in hypnic myoclonic activity in the cat is reached during REM sleep.[17] Finally, PHM must have a supraspinal origin, because it does not occur in muscles that are completely paralyzed because of a peripheral nerve, spinal, or pyramidal lesion; is increased in extrapyramidal diseases; and remains unaffected by changes in muscle spindle afferents.

Another quantitative analysis of PHM[18] in seven healthy volunteers led to similar results. PHM was more frequent during non-REM1 and during REM sleep stages and remained at wakefulness levels during non-REM2 and 3 sleep. Values of myoclonic activity were, however, highest during REM sleep, in keeping with the experimental studies in animals; there was again no difference between phasic and tonic (e.g., associated or not with bursts of REMs) REM sleep periods. Potentials identical to the PHM could also be recorded during quiet wakefulness, making the term *hypnic* somewhat inaccurate, and there was no difference among the first, second, or third part of the night. Comparison of different muscle groups showed that PHM was especially abundant in muscles such as the tibialis anterior and the triangularis labii, rather than in more proximal muscles such as the deltoideus.

The origin of the physiologic motor activity of sleep has been studied in the cat. Gassel and coauthors[17] concluded that the hypnic twitches in the cat were probably caused by descending volleys within the reticulospinal system, impinging on the spinal alpha motoneurons. Destruction of the fibers of the reticulospinal tract abolished the myoclonic activity, which was left unchanged by lesioning of the dorsal roots, red nucleus, or pyramidal tract (although the latter's lesions had a temporary inhibiting effect). These authors hypothesized that the volleys originate in the facilitatory descending reticular substance and that the PHM represents the motor accompaniment of tonic electroencephalographic desynchronization transmitted from the reticular substance to the spinal cord. Gastaut[19] proposed the pontine tegmentum as their site of origin. During REM sleep, hypnic myoclonus again became well evident, unassociated, however, with these cortical discharges. They speculated that hypnic myoclonus cannot be tightly linked to the cortical discharges but is rather coupled to them during light sleep by a subcortical pacemaker, which is still hypothetical. The data collected by Dagnino et al.,[16] however, point to a role of the corticospinal tract in the transmission of the excitatory volleys, which is clearly in keeping with the spatial distribution of the PHM; for example, myoclonic activity is especially evident in distal and facial muscles. Thus, the precise mechanisms responsible for PHM in humans remain controversial; however, they do appear to be particularly active at the transition from quiet wakefulness to sleep.

Sleep Starts (Hypnic Jerks)

Sleep starts (also termed *hypnic jerks*, *hypnagogic jerks*, or *predormital myoclonus*) are physiological phenomena characterized by sudden short intense myoclonic jerks of the whole body or parts of it occurring at the transition from wakefulness to sleep, mainly at the beginning of sleep. They represent a nearly universal accompaniment of sleep with a prevalence of about 60% to 70% among the general population and therefore have to be considered pathologic only when reaching abnormal proportions in frequency and magnitude that impede falling or staying asleep. Such a definitely pathological condition characterized by excessive sleep starts has been termed *intensified hypnic jerks* and was recognized anecdotally as a cause of insomnia as early as 1890 by Mitchell.[20] In 1959 Oswald[21] described, under the term of *sudden bodily jerks on falling asleep*, the sudden myoclonic jerkings of the whole body or some body parts in subjects trying to fall asleep. These sudden myoclonic jerks were not stereotyped and occurred occasionally during quiet wakefulness when the patients tried to fall asleep and also during light sleep, without any relation to external events.

Sleep starts are characteristically accompanied by subjective impressions like a feeling of falling into the void or through space, unexplained alarm or fear, or some other indistinct sensory feelings (like an electric shock or a light flash) or even by perceptions, usually frightening, or by a dream. An outcry could occasionally accompany the jerks.

Forty-three out of fifty people interviewed by Oswald[21] reported sleep starts; however, spouses described a much higher frequency than the affected individuals, suggesting that only the more violent jerks causing full awakening were recalled. The intake of stimulants such as caffeine, and anxiety and physical or mental stress before going to sleep have been reported to increase the frequency and severity of sleep starts.

On PSG, sleep starts occur singly or repeatedly, mainly during drowsiness and non-REM1 sleep, as a myoclonic contraction of all or most body muscles lasting less than a second and often associated with K-complexes or vertex sharp waves on the EEG (Fig. 27.1) and autonomic activation (tachycardia, irregular breathing with apnea followed by tachypnea, and sudomotor activation). Sleep starts are often followed by a more or less transient lightening of sleep, for instance, from non-REM2 to non-REM1 or even from non-REM1 to wakefulness. Sleep starts can occur during SWS and REM sleep, particularly in young children. The motor pattern involved in sleep starts, as well as the causative mechanism of this phenomenon, remains unclear.

According to Gastaut,[19] sleep starts are closely akin to the physiologic startle reaction during wakefulness, except they are spontaneous and not evoked by novel unexpected stimuli.

In 1996, Clouston[22] studied the polygraphic characteristics of spontaneous and induced myoclonic jerks occurring during both wakefulness and sleep in a patient with a parkinsonian syndrome and found an earlier involvement of axial muscles in the absence of cortical EEG activity preceding the jerks. These findings are more in accordance with a subcortical origin of the sleep starts.[22,23] This hypothesis is also endorsed by experimental data in decerebrate cats, which developed myoclonic jerks after lesions of the ventral mesopontine and retrorubral nucleus.[24]

Purely "sensory" sleep starts have been described by Sander et al.[25] as a perceptual phenomenon that in two subjects accompanied falling asleep and was characterized by a more or less localized sensory feeling (such as a nonradiating shock-like sensation in the chest or arm and finger numbness or itchy pinprick-like sensations anywhere in the body) occurring when falling asleep, sometimes in spells of a few minutes and in the absence of any involuntary motor contraction. The exploding head syndrome may also represent a variety of these purely sensory sleep starts.[5]

Sleep starts may be occasionally mistaken for epileptic myoclonus, for the startle reaction that accompanies hyperekplexia in children, or

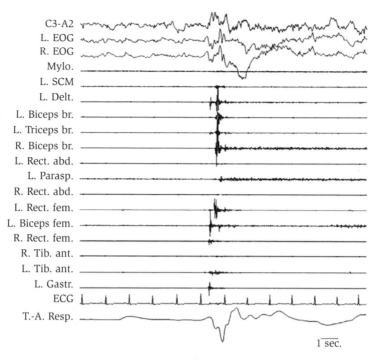

C3-A2
L. EOG
R. EOG
Mylo.
L. SCM
L. Delt.
L. Biceps br.
L. Triceps br.
R. Biceps br.
L. Rect. abd.
L. Parasp.
R. Rect. abd.
L. Rect. fem.
L. Biceps fem.
R. Rect. fem.
R. Tib. ant.
L. Tib. ant.
L. Gastr.
ECG
T.-A. Resp.

1 sec.

FIGURE 27.1   Sleep start. A short myoclonic contraction mainly involving limb muscles occurs during non-REM2 sleep associated with a K-complex on electroencephalogram. L, left; R, right; EOG, electrooculogram; Muscles: Mylo, mylohyoideus; SCM, sternocleidomastoideus; Delt., deltoideus; br., brachii; Rect., rectus; abd., abdominis; Parasp., paraspinalis; fem., femoris; Tib. ant., tibialis anterior; Gastr., gastrocnemius; T.-A. Resp., thoracic-abdominal respirogram.

even for PLMS or other parasomnias when they are repeated during light sleep. When purely sensory, sleep starts may prompt an erroneous diagnosis of epileptic seizures or psychiatric disorders. A PSG recording in such cases sets the record right.

Gross Body and Other Complex Movements during Sleep

These are complex movements that usually involve the whole musculature in a physiologic pattern that results in a change in body position. These gross body movements vary from person to person in a highly individual pattern, some people being more "shifty" than others, and remain largely independent from environmental influences.[26] Their purpose is unknown, but they evidently prevent compression and injury of relevant vascular and nervous structures because of the atonia during sleep. Indeed, peripheral nerve compression syndromes may occur in comatose patients who lack these movements.

Furthermore, drunk individuals who fall asleep with the head reclining on one arm could experience a transitory paralysis of the radial nerve (the so-called Saturday night palsy). Gross body movements may occur anytime throughout sleep but display on the whole a pattern of immobility soon after the initiation of sleep, followed by a progressive slow buildup throughout the night, especially during the second part of the night, and particularly before awakening. Deep-sleep stages are usually a time of complete immobility, when body movements are rare, mainly occurring at the end of these sleep stages. Body movements are more frequent during light sleep and at the beginning and end of REM sleep, often marking the transition from one sleep stage to another. Therefore, the distribution of body movements during the night simply reflects the patterning of sleep, deep sleep prevailing in the first half and light and REM sleep stages in the second half of the night, and may represent an indirect indicator of the quality of sleep. Body movements also appear more gross and shifting during non-REM sleep phases, when the whole body changes position, whereas distal limbs are more involved and in a more fragmentary and ineffectual fashion during REM sleep. Gross body movements show a temporal relationship to EEG signs of arousal such as K-complexes, which usually precede them by 2 to 3 seconds,[27,28] and are associated with autonomic activation in the form of tachycardia, tachypnea, and increased arterial pressure. Whereas the normal adult averages four or five gross body movements per hour, the frequency is much higher in the infant, in whom gross body movements occur also without any particular pattern. This irregular organization of the gross body movements in the infant reflects the pattern of sleep that is still not cyclic at this age. Moreover, gross and more localized movements (all lasting more than 0.5 seconds) and twitch movements (also called PHM, see previous discussion) behave differently during the night in infants, probably because they are controlled by different organization levels within the central nervous system.[29] With increasing age, there is a progressive decrease in frequency and a progressively more regular patterning of the gross body movements. The adult pattern of body motility is reached at around 1 year of life. This indicates that maturational events influence motor activity of sleep, which, therefore, may be a good detector of abnormal central nervous system development.[29] Body position changes during sleep also seem to influence the occurrence of other abnormal motor phenomena of sleep such as the PLMS, which abate immediately before and restart immediately after 90-degree body position changes.

Other motor activities commonly encountered in every sleep stage but particularly so during light sleep are represented by mimic gestures such as smiling, sighing, chewing, swallowing, and scratching.[30] Normal semipurposeful movements are occasionally seen during sleep, especially after awakenings or lightenings of sleep and in non-REM1 sleep.[31] Itching during sleep is particularly prominent in a variety of dermatologic conditions and when troublesome may cause severe insomnia and nocturnal awakenings.[32] In such patients, scratching movements occur particularly during non-REM1, non-REM2, and REM sleep.

PATHOLOGIC MOTOR ACTIVITY AT SLEEP ONSET AND DURING SLEEP

Excessive Fragmentary Myoclonus

Fragmentary pathologic myoclonus in non-REM sleep was reported for the first time by Broughton and Tolentino in 1984 in a 42-year-old patient investigated for marked daytime sleepiness.[33] This patient underwent PSG, which was otherwise unremarkable except for intense partial myoclonus sustained throughout all of the non-REM sleep stages and characterized by short (less than 150 milliseconds) contractions occurring over the leg, arm, and even face muscles in an aperiodic and asynchronous fashion. The EMG contractions often corresponded to visible brief leg twitches and were quite dissimilar from any physiologic motor activity or from the jerks of PLMS (Fig. 27.2). There was some degree of sleep fragmentation. Although the motor activity persisted unchanged throughout the non-REM sleep stages, unlike PHM described earlier,[15,16] the authors stated that it could conceivably represent an abnormal intensification of that entity. Because other possible conditions such as sleep apnea, narcolepsy, or restless legs syndrome (RLS) with PLMS were all absent, the authors associated the daytime sleepiness with this abnormal motor activity during non-REM sleep. Later, Broughton and coauthors[34] reported on 38 consecutive patients with what they termed "excessive fragmentary hypnic myoclonus" (EFHM). Almost all of the patients (36/38) were males and had a variety of primary diagnoses (sleep apnea obstructive or central in 12, narcolepsy in 6, PLMS in 11, insomnia in 2, hypersomnia or excessive daytime sleepiness in 6). On PSG, the motor activity consisted of brief sharp EMG potentials recorded asynchronously and randomly over the two sides that, when of larger magnitude, were accompanied by visible brief local twitches; sometimes polymyoclonic bursts at 2 to 3 per second were recorded. The twitches were absent in presleep wakefulness, increased abruptly at sleep onset, and persisted unchanged throughout non-REM sleep, including stage 3. They remained unassociated with any specific EEG changes and showed no relationship to nocturnal hypoxemia as recorded by continuous transcutaneous oxygen tension monitoring, even though in some cases the twitches intensified during periods of decreased oxygen saturation.

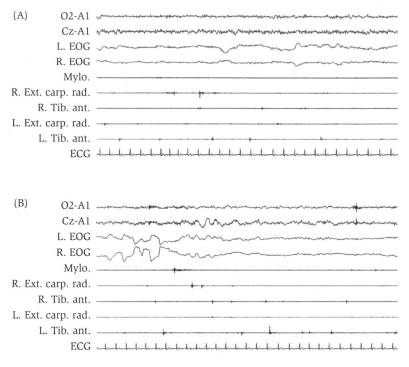

(A) O2-A1
Cz-A1
L. EOG
R. EOG
Mylo.
R. Ext. carp. rad.
R. Tib. ant.
L. Ext. carp. rad.
L. Tib. ant.
ECG

(B) O2-A1
Cz-A1
L. EOG
R. EOG
Mylo.
R. Ext. carp. rad.
R. Tib. ant.
L. Ext. carp. rad.
L. Tib. ant.
ECG

FIGURE 27.2 Excessive fragmentary myoclonus in a 58-year-old man during non-REM1 (*A*) and REM sleep (*B*). Polysomnogram recordings documented isolated and clustered abundant, asynchronous and irregular twitches in the explored muscles. L, left; R, right; EOG, electrooculogram; Muscles: Mylo., mylohyoideus; Ext. carp. rad., extensor carpi radialis; Tib. ant., tibialis anterior.

The authors went on to study a control group of 10 subjects, 4 of whom displayed similar EMG patterns in non-REM1 and 2 sleep; however, in no control subjects did the activity persist into non-REM3 nor did it reach the minimum frequency characterizing the patients' group, for example, 5 per minute sustained over 20 minutes of non-REM2 and 3 sleep. Thus, it appeared that EFHM represented a distinct abnormality, which is associated with conditions of excessive daytime sleepiness and insomnia and possibly facilitated by nocturnal hypoxemia. In the authors' view, EFHM is a deviant enhancement of the fragmentary physiologic myoclonus sometimes encountered during light sleep in normal subjects, occurring nearly always and for unclear reasons only in males.

A detailed study of the pathologic significance and distribution of EFHM during sleep was performed by Lins et al.[35] in 1993, who introduced a new quantification technique, the fragmentary myoclonus index (FMI), defined as the calculated mean of the 3-second epochs with one or more myoclonic potentials exceeding 50 microV averaged for each 30-second scoring epoch and across sleep stages. In 11 patients, the FMI was significantly higher than in a control group during all sleep stages. FMI reached the highest score during REM sleep and showed no relationship to the age of the patients. However, it tended to decrease in the first hour after sleep onset and had a somewhat lower score during SWS, findings that are attributable to a suppressive effect within SWS. There was no significant difference between patients and controls in sleep structure and specifically in SWS characteristics, making it unlikely that EFHM alone might keep patients awake during the night by lightening of sleep.

The pathophysiology of EFHM is still debated. EFHM could occur either isolated or associated with other sleep disorders, particularly REM sleep behavior disorder (RBD). In both cases, polygraphic recordings and back-averaging analysis fail to disclose any cortical EEG activity preceding the movement, suggesting a subcortical origin of this motor phenomenon.[36] The abolition in animal models of the myoclonic activity by destruction of the reticulo-spinal tract suggests that the hypnic twitches of EFHM are probably caused by descending volleys within the reticulo-spinal system modulating spinal alpha motoneuron activity. Furthermore, the observed association of EFHM and RBD in humans suggests that the interconnected brainstem regions implicated in motor control during sleep, namely the pontine nucleus oralis and the medullary nucleus reticularis gigantocellularis, are involved in EFHM pathophysiology.[23,36] However, it remains unsettled whether a similar mechanism is also responsible for the occurrence of EFHM during non-REM sleep.

The overall evidence concerning EFHM remains flimsy. Although EFHM seems to represent a somewhat pathologic phenomenon, as indicated by the quantitative findings of Lins et al.,[35] the pathogenetic relationship between EFHM and the associated sleep disturbances, especially excessive daytime sleepiness, remains murky and cannot be explained by changes in sleep structure. Likewise, the causative mechanisms of the phenomenon have yet to be definitively clarified.

Excessive Sleep Starts (Intensified Hypnic Jerks)

In some patients, sleep starts, otherwise a physiologic accompaniment of light sleep, may assume such an intensity and frequent recurrence as to markedly impede falling asleep and cause sleep-onset insomnia. This pathologic enhancement of a normal phenomenon was termed *intensified hypnic jerks* by Broughton.[37] Whether it is the pattern or frequency of the phenomenon that is abnormal or whether it is especially anxious patients who experience these physiologic motor events as pathologic remains unknown.

Excessive sleep starts have been reported in association with different pathological conditions such as patients with postpolio syndrome,[38] parkinsonism,[22] and children with migraine.[39] Furthermore, they were described to occur in clusters in children with epilepsy, mental retardation, and spastic dystonia due to birth asphyxia.[40]

When sleep starts cause sleep-onset insomnia, benzodiazepines (especially Clonazepam) could be effective in curtailing the jerks.

Propriospinal Myoclonus at the Transition from Wakefulness to Sleep

Myoclonic activity, which originates within the spinal cord, is characterized by jerks restricted to muscles innervated in one or a few adjacent myotomes and recurs usually, although not always, arhythmically on average one to three times per second. It is unaffected by peripheral sensory stimulations and is persistent throughout sleep.[41,42] In such instances, the spinal myoclonus has the characteristics of a segmental myoclonus.

More recently, however, another type of spinal myoclonic activity has been described, known under the term of *propriospinal myoclonus* (PSM). In 1991, Brown et al.[43] reported the case of a 55-year-old man with paroxysmal bouts of axial flexion jerks of the trunk and hips, lasting up to 3 hours and repeated every minute; the jerks, usually spontaneous, could be evoked by taps to the abdominal wall. Because EMG analysis documented the involvement of muscles with segmental innervations representing virtually the whole length of the cord, it appeared that the discharges originated in a spinal generator whose activity became propagated up and down the spinal cord via propriospinal pathways. Three such patients underwent back-averaging studies of the myoclonic jerks, which documented the absence of any cortical premovement EEG activity. Instead, the abnormal activity originates in the midthoracic or upper cervical cord and spreads to more rostral and caudal levels at a slow velocity of about 5 meters/second.[44]

In a detailed neurophysiologic analysis of two patients with PSM, Chokroverty et al.[45] confirmed that the activity was predominantly rhythmic, lasted 225 to 441 milliseconds, and involved only the thoracoabdominal muscles, with a rostrocaudal propagation at a velocity of 8 to 11 meters/second, without spread to the facial or limb muscles. The generator in these cases was probably located at the T5 to T8 segments.

The peculiar clinical and electrophysiologic features of PSM, confirmed by subsequent case reports,[46–48] have led to the hypothesis that PSM is due to a spinal generator, partially released by lesions to the cord which recruits muscles through long slowly conducting propriospinal pathways into a complex rhythmic activity resembling stepping.[49,50] Hypothetically, such a spinal generator may be physiologically involved in locomotion. A recent study analyzed 10 patients diagnosed with PSM and revised the cases previously reported in the literature, confirming that the typical motor pattern of PSM consists of myoclonic jerks constantly involving abdominal wall muscles, with the majority of patients showing EMG features suggestive of a "myoclonic generator" at thoracic level.[51] In addition, the 10 patients included in the study underwent a detailed neuroradiological evaluation comprising magnetic resonance (MR) diffusion tensor imaging with fiber tracking, an accurate technique for examining spinal cord structural integrity. This MR investigation disclosed abnormalities of the spinal cord in all the patients evaluated. The fiber tract abnormalities included the myoclonus generator center in seven patients and were located more rostrally in the other three. The authors suggested that the release of spinal pattern generators in patients with PSM could be associated with abnormalities in the spinal cord not detectable by standard neuroradiological investigations.

Most patients with PSM have no recognizable cause for this abnormal motor activity, but symptomatic forms have also been observed (cervical hemangioblastoma, mild cervical myeloradiculopathy or trauma,[52] posttraumatic tetraplegia,[53] multiple sclerosis,[54] Lyme neuroborreliosis,[55] HIV infection[56]).

Furthermore, the motor pattern and the electrophysiological findings typical of PSM could be mimicked voluntarily,[57] and the possibility of a psychogenic origin of the phenomenon has to be taken into account.[58]

Following the description of PSM, which remains a rare phenomenon, a propriospinal pattern of propagation was found on neurophysiologic studies of other motor activities apparently of spinal origin, such as the spasms of the stiff-man syndrome,[59] some involuntary movements encountered in syringomyelia and syringobulbia,[60] and even the involuntary movements seen in association with the RLS.[61]

Therefore, propriospinal mechanisms may underlie different clinical phenomena beside PSM; the latter moreover is probably a heterogeneous neurologic condition.

In 1997, three patients with PSM presented with myoclonic activity arising only in the period of quiet wakefulness and relaxation preceding sleep onset.[62] They were observed because of severe sleep-onset insomnia caused by the jerks. The patients had no structural lesion causing the abnormal myoclonic activity, except possibly an arachnoid cyst at the T8 root level in one. Wire EMG studies documented that the jerks arose first in the rectus abdominis, sternocleidomastoid, and thoracolumbar paraspinal muscles, propagating thereafter to more rostral and caudal axial muscles at a velocity calculated at 2 to 16 meters/second (Fig. 27.3). The jerks, therefore, conformed to a propriospinal pattern of propagation. However, in all of the patients the jerks were present only during relaxed wakefulness, especially before falling asleep.

Brown et al.[43] had previously observed that PSM was influenced by the posture of the patients, especially brought about by reclining or lying down. However, PSM at the transition from wakefulness to sleep did not seem to relate to posture[62] because the jerks could be promptly abolished by mental activation (e.g., by asking the patient to talk or to perform mental arithmetic or simply to make a fist or think) even with the patient sitting comfortably in an armchair or lying down. The myoclonus immediately restarted when the patients were left alone undisturbed and lying down. EEG-EMG correlations indeed documented that the jerks were present only with alpha activity on the EEG, a feature of the relaxed wakefulness stage, and disappeared with EEG desynchronization, a feature of mental activation. PSG recordings also showed that the jerks did not extend into sleep because they were abolished whenever the patient had fallen asleep and were never observed during either light or deep non-REM or REM sleep stages. The sleep structure in all patients was abnormal, with increased light-sleep stages and arousals and decreased sleep efficiency, thus, in accord with the subjective complaint of insomnia.

A similar case of PSM arising in the thoracic muscles only during mental relaxation and drowsiness and causing insomnia was reported by Tison et al.[63] in a 52-year-old woman. In a subsequent paper, Vetrugno et al.[64] described PSM of wake-sleep transition in another five patients complaining of insomnia and confirmed the clinical and electrophysiological characteristics of the motor phenomenon previously reported. More recently, PSM has also been described in patients with RLS,[65] associated with PLMS. The two kinds of movements (PSM and PLMS) were clearly distinguished according to peculiar polygraphic features. Axial myoclonic jerks resembling PSM occurred concurrently with the motor restlessness and sensory discomfort in the limbs typical of RLS during relaxed wakefulness preceding falling asleep and disappeared with sleep onset progressively replaced by PLMS, whose EMG pattern of activity was limited to the legs, especially

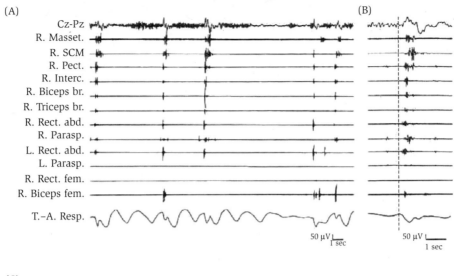

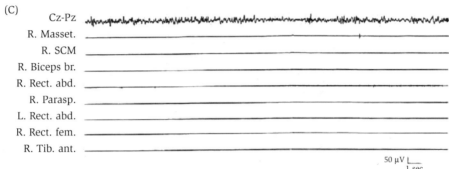

FIGURE 27.3 Excerpts from polysomnogram recording showing propriospinal myoclonus. (A) Repetitive myoclonic jerks involving axial and limb muscles occur during relaxed wakefulness characterized by diffuse alpha electroencephalographic (EEG) activity. (B) At faster recording velocity, the electromyographic activity of a single jerk is seen to originate in the rectus abdominis muscles (vertical marker) and propagate to the rostral and caudal muscles with slow velocity (2–16 m/second). (C) Propriospinal myoclonic jerks disappear when non-REM2 sleep begins and spindles become evident on EEG trace. R, right; L, left; Muscles: Masset., Masseter; SCM, sternocleidomastoideus; Pect., pectoralis; Interc., intercostalis; br., brachii; Rect., rectus; abd., abdominis; Parasp., paraspinalis; fem., femoris; T.-A. Resp., thoracic-abdominal respirogram.

the tibialis anterior muscles, and did not show a propriospinal propagation. This time relationship between the two motor phenomena led to the hypothesis that one movement is transformed into the other following the evolution from wake-sleep transition to light sleep.

Thus, it appears that PSM, unlike other pathologic motor activity of sleep (periodic limb movements, sleep starts, excessive fragmentary myoclonus), may remain restricted to the particular neurophysiologic state of transition from wakefulness to sleep and is usually absent during alert wakefulness and sleep.

This pattern endorses the seminal observations of Critchley,[1] who remarked how the wake-sleep transition state represents an independent stage, with peculiar neurophysiological, neuropsychological, and clinical characteristics (see previous discussion).

In all patients PSM is proven to be a chronic disorder, usually refractory to treatment and causing severe disability due to sleep-onset insomnia. Recently, Manconi et al.[66] described a severe and uncommon case of PSM appearing after a vertebral fracture of T11. Two polysomnographic investigations in this patient disclosed several spontaneous massive jerks with features of PSM during wake-sleep transition, awakenings, or arousals and focal myoclonic activity in the axial muscles during stable sleep. At the end of the second polysomnographic study, after awakening during a change in body position, this condition acutely evolved into a propriospinal myoclonic status also involving respiratory muscles, and leading to respiratory failure and loss of consciousness. The occurrence of focal myoclonic activity during stable sleep and the progression into a myoclonic status indicates a particularly high spinal excitability in this patient.

As explained earlier, hyperexcitability of a specific myelomere, which becomes active and thereafter spreads this excitability to the other myelomeres through propriospinal polysynaptic pathways, has been hypothesized as a possible pathophysiological mechanism causing PSM.

As proposed by Brown et al.,[49] this focal spinal pattern generator is set into motion by the lack of supraspinal inhibitory control. In the case of PSM at the transition from wakefulness to sleep, it is the supraspinal influences typifying drowsiness and sleep onset that must be involved. From a purely nosologic point of view, PSM in some cases constitutes a wake-sleep transition disorder and a cause of sleep-onset insomnia. Its relationship with the excessive sleep starts (see previous) deserves further study.

Hypnagogic Foot Tremor

Hypnagogic foot tremor (HFT) is a motor phenomenon mainly occurring on drowsiness and at sleep onset, originally described by Broughton.[37] Affected individuals display series of rhythmic oscillating movements of the whole foot or of the toes generally bilaterally but asynchronous upon falling asleep and during light non-REM sleep. PSG recordings document short series (10–15 seconds duration) of EMG bursts of leg muscles at a frequency of 1–2 per second (range: 0.5–3) with single burst duration between 300 and 700 milliseconds. Most cases have been described in patients suffering from other sleep disorders like RLS or sleep-related respiratory disorders; however, HFT was also observed in individuals with otherwise normal sleep. A single study that directly investigated HFT in 355 patients undergoing PSG for other sleep problems and 20 control subjects found a prevalence of 7.5% (27 patients and 1 control subject) with equal gender distribution and a wide age range of occurrence (from 14 to 72 years).[67] Patients were generally unaware of the movements, which did not impede falling asleep or disturb sleep, as documented by PSG.

HFT is frequently asymptomatic, being an incidental benign finding during evaluation of other sleep complaints. As a result, the prevalence of this motor phenomenon in the general population and its frequency in affected individuals remain uncertain. In view of its benign nature, HFT is considered a quasi-physiological condition, not warranting therapy, even if pathological forms, sufficiently prolonged and severe to cause sleep-onset insomnia and sleep disruption, have also been observed.

CONCLUSION

Many advances in the understanding of the motor physiology of sleep and the delineation and characterization of several motor phenomena at sleep onset and during sleep have occurred in recent decades. PSG techniques have proved invaluable means in the description of these diverse phenomena; useful as they are for diagnostic ends, however, they provide scant clues to the site of origin and pathogenetic mechanisms. One can anticipate that the future application of neuroimaging techniques and other functional investigations will give indications of origin and mechanisms for the most serious clinical conditions that are of interest to patient and clinician alike.

ACKNOWLEDGMENTS

This chapter is largely inspired by the studies carried out by Professor Pasquale Montagna over the last 15 years. It benefits from his deep insight into the topic, his many suggestions, and the scientific discussions we had with him. We consider it a great privilege to have been among his collaborators, to have shared his vast knowledge, and to have enjoyed his friendship and human qualities.

REFERENCES

1. Critchley M. The pre-dormitum. *Rev Neurol (Paris)* 1955;93:101–6.
2. Ogilvie RD, Wilkinson RT, Allison S. The detection of sleep onset: behavioral, physiological, and subjective convergence. *Sleep* 1989;12:458–74.

3. Abe K, Oda N, Araki R, et al. Macropsia, micropsia, and episodic illusions in Japanese adolescents. *J Am Acad Child Adolesc Psychiatry* 1989;28:493–6.

4. Ohayon MM, Priest RG, Caulet M, et al. Hypnagogic and hypnopompic hallucinations: pathological phenomena? *Br J Psychiatry* 1996;169:459–67.

5. Sachs C, Svanborg E. The exploding head syndrome: polysomnographic recordings and therapeutic suggestions. *Sleep* 1991;14:263–6.

6. Wright KP, Jr., Badia P, Wauquier A. Topographical and temporal patterns of brain activity during the transition from wakefulness to sleep. *Sleep* 1995;18:880–9.

7. Marshall L, Mölle M, Schreiber H, et al. Scalp recorded direct current potential shifts associated with the transition to sleep in man. *Electroencephalogr Clin Neurophysiol* 1994;91:346–52.

8. Harsh J, Voss U, Hull J, et al. ERP and behavioral changes during the wake/sleep transition. *Psychophysiology* 1994;31:244–52.

9. Henn V, Baloh RW, Hepp K. The sleep-wake transition in the oculomotor system. *Exp Brain Res* 1984;54:166–76.

10. Obál F, Jr., Rubicsek G, Alfoldi P, et al. Changes in the brain and core temperatures in relation to the various arousal states in rats in the light and dark periods of the day. *Pflugers Arch* 1985;404:73–9.

11. Worsnop C, Kay A, Pierce R, et al. Activity of respiratory pump and upper airway muscles during sleep onset. *J Appl Physiol* 1998;85:908–20.

12. Montagna P, Lugaresi E. Sleep benefit in Parkinson's disease [letter]. *Mov Disord* 1998;13:751–2.

13. Braun AR, Balkin TJ, Wesensten NJ, et al. Regional cerebral blood flow throughout the wake-sleep cycle. An H2 15O PET study. *Brain* 1997;120:1173–97.

14. American Academy of Sleep Medicine. *The International Classification of Sleep Disorders. Diagnostic and Coding Manual.* 2nd ed. Westchester, IL: American Academy of Sleep Medicine; 2005.

15. De Lisi L. Su di un fenomeno motorio costante del sonno normale: le mioclonie ipniche fisiologiche. *Riv Pat Ment* 1932;39:481–96.

16. Dagnino N, Loeb C, Massazza G, et al. Hypnic physiological myoclonias in man: an EEG-EMG study in normals and neurological patients. *Eur Neurol* 1969;2:47–58.

17. Gassel MM, Marchiafava PL, Pompeiano O. Phasic changes in muscular activity during desynchronized sleep in unrestrained cats. An analysis of the pattern and organization of myoclonic twitches. *Arch Ital Biol* 1964;102:449–70.

18. Montagna P, Liguori R, Zucconi M, et al. Physiological hypnic myoclonus. *Electroencephalogr Clin Neurophysiol* 1988;70:172–6.

19. Gastaut H. Les myoclonies—Séméiologie des myoclonies et nosologie analytique des syndromes myocloniques. *Rev Neurol* 1968;119:1–30.

20. Mitchell SW. Some disorders of sleep. *Int J Med Sci* 1890;100:109–27.

21. Oswald I. Sudden bodily jerks on falling asleep. *Brain* 1959;82:92–103.

22. Clouston PD, Lim CL, Fung V, et al. Brainstem myoclonus in a patient with non-dopa-responsive parkinsonism. *Mov Disord* 1996;11:404–10.

23. Montagna P. Sleep-related non epileptic motor disorders. *J Neurol* 2004;251:781–94.

24. Lai YY, Siegel JM. Brainstem-mediated locomotion and myoclonic jerks. I. Neural substrates. *Brain Res* 1997;745:257–64.

25. Sander HW, Geisse H, Quinto C, et al. Sensory sleep starts [letter]. *J Neurol Neurosurg Psychiatry* 1998;64:690.

26. Gardner R, Grossman WI. Normal motor patterns in sleep in man. In: Weitzman ED, ed. *Advances in Sleep Research.* New York: Spectrum; 1976:67–107.

27. Sassin JF, Johnson LC. Body motility during sleep and its relation to the K-complex. *Exp Neurol* 1968;22:133–44.

28. Sassin JF, Johnson LC. EEG correlates of body movements during sleep. *Electroencephalogr Clin Neurophysiol* 1969;26:237.

29. Fukumoto M, Mochizuki N, Takeishi M, et al. Studies of body movements during night sleep in infancy. *Brain Dev* 1981;3:37–43.

30. Savin JA, Paterson WD, Oswald I. Scratching during sleep. *Lancet* 1973;2:296–7.

31. Fish DR, Sawyers D, Allen PJ, et al. The effect of sleep on the dyskinetic movements of Parkinson's disease, Gilles de la Tourette syndrome, Huntington's disease, and torsion dystonia. *Arch Neurol* 1991;48:210–4.

32. Savin JA, Adam K, Oswald I, et al. Pruritus and nocturnal wakenings. *J Am Acad Dermatol* 1990;23:767–8.

33. Broughton R, Tolentino MA. Fragmentary pathological myoclonus in NREM sleep.

Electroencephalogr Clin Neurophysiol 1984;57:303–9.

34. Broughton R, Tolentino MA, Krelina M. Excessive fragmentary myoclonus in NREM sleep: a report of 38 cases. *Electroencephalogr Clin Neurophysiol* 1985;61:123–33.

35. Lins O, Castonguay M, Dunham W, et al. Excessive fragmentary myoclonus: time of night and sleep stage distributions. *Can J Neurol Sci* 1993;20:142–6.

36. Vetrugno R, Plazzi G, Provini F, et al. Excessive fragmentary hypnic myoclonus: clinical and neurophysiological findings. *Sleep Med* 2002;3:73–6.

37. Broughton R. Pathological fragmentary myoclonus, intensified hypnic jerks and hypnagogic foot tremor: three unusual sleep-related movement disorders. In Koella WP, Obàl F, Schulz H, Visser P, eds. *Sleep 1986*. Stuttgart, Germany: Fischer Verlag; 1988:240–3.

38. Bruno RL. Abnormal movements in sleep as a post-polio sequelae. *Am J Phys Med Rehabil* 1998;77:339–43.

39. Bruni O, Galli F, Guidetti V. Sleep hygiene and migraine in children and adolescents. *Cephalalgia* 1999;19(Suppl 25):57–9.

40. Fusco L, Pachatz C, Cusmai R, et al. Repetitive sleep starts in neurologically impaired children: an unusual non-epileptic manifestation in otherwise epileptic subjects. *Epileptic Disord* 1999;1:63–7.

41. Hopkins AP, Michael WF. Spinal myoclonus. *J Neurol Neurosurg Psychiatry* 1974;37:1112–15.

42. Frenken CWGM, Korten JJ, Gabreëls FJM, et al. Spinal myoclonus. *Clin Neurol Neurosurg* 1974;77:44–53.

43. Brown P, Thompson PD, Rothwell JC, et al. Paroxysmal axial spasms of spinal origin. *Mov Disord* 1991;6:43–8.

44. Brown P, Thompson PD, Rothwell JC, et al. Axial myoclonus of propriospinal origin. *Brain* 1991;114:197–214.

45. Chokroverty S, Walters A, Zimmerman T, et al. Propriospinal myoclonus: a neurophysiological analysis. *Neurology* 1992;42:1591–5.

46. Nishiyama K, Ugawa Y, Takeda K, et al. Axial myoclonus mediated by the propriospinal tract: a case report. *Eur Neurol* 1994;34:48–50.

47. Pisano F, Miscio G, Romorini A, et al. Abdominal propriospinal myoclonus of unknown etiology. *Rev Neurol (Paris)* 1995;151:209–11.

48. Schulze-Bonhage A, Knott H, Ferbert A. Pure stimulus-sensitive truncal myoclonus of propriospinal origin. *Mov Disord* 1996;11:87–90.

49. Brown P, Rothwell JC, Thompson PD, et al. Propriospinal myoclonus: evidence for spinal "pattern" generators in humans. *Mov Disord* 1994;9:571–6.

50. Chokroverty S. Propriospinal myoclonus. *Clin Neurosci* 1996;3:219–22.

51. Roze E, Bounolleau P, Ducreux D, et al. Propriospinal myoclonus revisited: clinical, neurophysiologic, and neuroradiologic findings. *Neurology* 2009;72:1301–9.

52. Brown P. Spinal myoclonus. In: Marsden CD, Fahn S, eds. *Movement Disorders*. 3rd ed. Oxford, England: Butterworth-Heinemann; 1994:459–76.

53. Fouillet N, Wiart L, Arne P, et al. Propriospinal myoclonus in tetraplegic patients: clinical, electrophysiological and therapeutic aspects. *Paraplegia* 1995;33:678–81.

54. Kapoor R, Brown P, Thompson PD, et al. Propriospinal myoclonus in multiple sclerosis. *J Neurol Neurosurg Psychiatry* 1992;55:1086–8.

55. de la Sayette V, Schaeffer S, Queruel C, et al. Lyme neuroborreliosis presenting with propriospinal myoclonus [letter]. *J Neurol Neurosurg Psychiatry* 1996;61:420.

56. Lubetzki C, Vidailhet M, Jedynak CP, et al. Propriospinal myoclonus in a patient seropositive for human immunodeficiency virus. *Rev Neurol (Paris)* 1994;150:70–2.

57. Kang SY, Sohn YH. Electromyography patterns of propriospinal myoclonus can be mimicked voluntarily. *Mov Disord* 2006;21:1241–4.

58. Williams DR, Cowey M, Tuck K, et al. Psychogenic propriospinal myoclonus. *Mov Disord* 2008;23:1312–3.

59. Meinck HM, Ricker K, Hülser PJ, et al. Stiff man syndrome: neurophysiological findings in eight patients. *J Neurol* 1995;242:134–42.

60. Nogués MA, Leiguarda RC, Rivero AD, et al. Involuntary movements and abnormal spontaneous EMG activity in syringomyelia and syringobulbia. *Neurology* 1999;52:823–34.

61. Trenkwalder C, Bucher SF, Oertel WH. Electrophysiological pattern of involuntary limb movements in the restless legs syndrome. *Muscle Nerve* 1996;19:155–62.

62. Montagna P, Provini F, Plazzi G, et al. Propriospinal myoclonus upon relaxation and drowsiness: a cause of severe insomnia. *Mov Disord* 1997;12:66–72.

63. Tison F, Arné P, Dousset V, et al. Myoclonies propriospinales induites par la relaxation

et l'endormissement. *Rev Neurol (Paris)* 1998;154:423–5.

64. Vetrugno R, Provini F, Meletti S, et al. Propriospinal myoclonus at the sleep-wake transition: a new type of parasomnia. *Sleep* 2001;24:835–43.

65. Vetrugno R, Provini F, Plazzi G, et al. Propriospinal myoclonus: a motor phenomenon found in restless legs syndrome different from periodic limb movements during sleep. *Mov Disord* 2005;20:1323–9.

66. Manconi M, Sferrazza B, Iannaccone S, et al. Case of symptomatic propriospinal myoclonus evolving toward acute "myoclonic status." *Mov Disord* 2005;20:1646–50.

67. Wichniak A, Tracik F, Geisler P, et al. Rhythmic feet movements while falling asleep. *Mov Disord* 2001;16:1164–70.

28

Disorders of Arousal
from Non-REM Sleep

SHANNON SULLIVAN AND CHRISTIAN GUILLEMINAULT

DISORDERS OF arousal from non–rapid eye movement (non-REM) sleep classically include sleepwalking, sleep terrors, and confusional arousals. These fascinating entities, the non-REM "arousal disorders," are thought to be related to one another, or to exist on a continuum, typically occurring from a disturbance or incomplete arousal in slow-wave (N3) sleep, though they may occur out of stage 2 sleep. In general, arousal disorders occur in the first third or half of the night, are more common in children than adults, and may be triggered by a host of disturbances such as sleep deprivation, a full bladder, fever, alcohol, emotional stress, and central nervous system depressants such as alcohol, sedative hypnotics, and antihistamines.[1] While these entities are hypothesized to be triggered by similar phenomena, may coexist in individuals and within episodes, and may respond to similar interventions, the three classic non-REM arousal parasomnias are nonetheless distinct.

The diagnosis of non-REM parasomnias may be made based on a detailed history, but some patients may require more extensive evaluation, including polysomnographic study with an expanded electroencephalographic (EEG) montage to rule out other disorders—such as seizure disorder, REM sleep behavior disorder—that are not possible to distinguish by history alone. Having more than one disorder of arousal is not uncommon; for example, sleepwalking may share characteristics of confusional arousal, but it involves mobilization/walking; and it may coexist with confusional arousal. Likewise, sleep terrors, which involve a high degree of autonomic stimulation, may coexist with sleepwalking. These disorders are inextricably linked in timing, trigger, and co-occurrence in individuals, but they may be distinguished by elemental features of the behaviors themselves as well as epidemiological differences in age and prevalence.

Additionally, disorders of arousal are commonly thought to predominate in childhood;

in a recently published, longitudinal, prospective study of 1000 children in Quebec between the ages of 2.5 and 6 years, 88% manifested at least one parasomnia during the study period, with an overall prevalence rate of 14.5% for sleepwalking and 39.8% for sleep terrors.[2] Such disorders may be seen in children during daytime naps as well as nocturnal sleep. Despite a strong predominance in childhood, disorders of arousal may persist, or start, in adulthood; for example, disorders of arousal in adults have been reported to occur in 3% to 4% of all adults and to occur weekly in 0.4% of all adults.[3,4]

CONFUSIONAL AROUSALS

Definition and Clinical Presentation

Confusional arousals may go by several names, including "sleep drunkenness." According to the *International Classification of Sleep Disorders*, second edition (*ICSD-2*),[5] confusional arousals involve mental confusion or confusional behavior during or following arousals from sleep, typically SWS in the first part of the night but also upon awakening in the morning. Specific features include disorientation in time and space, diminished responsiveness, slowed responsiveness and/or mental processing, unusual or inappropriate behavior, and poor memory recall of the event.[5] Confusional arousal alone is not accompanied by autonomic hyperactivity as in sleep terrors, or by notable wandering as in sleepwalking.[6] Behavior may be inappropriate, resistive, even violent; it may be augmented by forced awakenings. The individual may give the appearance of being awake despite reduced vigilance and impaired responsiveness. As the disorder is most common in children,[7] a typical confusional arousal might include a child sitting up in bed, muttering, whimpering, or moaning, who is difficult to soothe but is not exhibiting the sweating, flushing, and tachycardia seen in sleep terrors. The individual may be staring without responding. These episodes typically last several to 15 minutes, but they can be much longer. The following morning there is no recollection of the event, and the subject typically feels refreshed and reports an uneventful night of sleep. In the pediatric population, confusional arousals may not be as well recognized as sleepwalking and sleep terrors, since events can be short lived and may be milder in presentation. Regarding adolescents and adults, *ICSD-2* briefly describes an "adult variant form" of confusional arousals, which is characterized by severe morning sleep inertia which can be associated with injury to self or others.[5] Such "sleep drunkenness" is persistent, hard to treat, and may affect work performance, safety behind the wheel, and other safety, social, and work function.

Epidemiology and Genetics

The age of onset, time of occurrence at night, and the frequency of spells are similar in confusional arousals, sleepwalking, and sleep terrors, all of which can start in early childhood. As noted previously, confusional arousals are especially prevalent in pediatric populations and have even been described as "almost universal" in children less than 5 years of age.[1] Other studies cite prevalence ranges from 2.9% to 4% in adults to 17.3% in children (aged 3–13 years).[8,9] Typically prevalence of this disorder wanes by middle childhood, but in some cases, as with all non-REM parasomnias, confusional arousals may persist from childhood into adulthood or less commonly, they may start in adolescence or adulthood. There is no sex difference with confusional arousals.[5]

Pathophysiology

A genetic predisposition and acquired and/or environmental disturbances that alter arousability or trigger an increase in shifts from slow-wave sleep to lighter stages of sleep (such as sleep-disordered breathing, shift work/circadian rhythm disorders, periodic limb movements, gastroesophageal reflux), combined with other vulnerabilities such as age (generally 2–12 years), sleep deprivation, fever, and sedative-hypnotics seem to precipitate arousal parasomnias.[10] Central nervous system lesions and central hypersomnias have been noted to trigger confusional arousals, especially if the arousal systems are affected.[11,12]

Diagnosis

The diagnosis of confusional arousals can be strongly suggested by a careful clinical history, and an exam can help evaluate for possible triggers. Like all the non-REM disorders of arousal, these episodes typically occur from stage N3 sleep. If polysomnography is performed, it is ideal to record such a confusional arousal arising from slow-wave sleep. At the time of the confusional arousal, a simultaneously recorded EEG may show generalized, high-amplitude rhythmic delta or stage 1 theta activity or a diffuse and poorly reactive alpha rhythm. However, more commonly polysomnography does not capture a confusional arousal itself, but there may be evidence of multiple arousals from slow-wave sleep without confusional behaviors. In any case, normal nocturnal polysomnography does not rule out the diagnosis. As discussed later, there are no polysomnographic findings for which a scientific consensus has been developed that serve as reliable markers of disorders of arousal.

Treatment

Regular and adequate sleep routines to prevent sleep loss and disturbance are important, as are addressing other potential triggers such as full bladder, stress, sleep deprivation, illness, and coexisting sleep disorders such as obstructive sleep apnea and, to a lesser extent, periodic limb movements or restless legs syndrome.[13] Along with an adequate evaluation of possible triggers and predisposing factors, reassurance in children with confusional arousals is the first-line treatment because they often disappear by later childhood.[14] Despite this, it is necessary to explore the possible social consequences of this as well as all disorders of arousal, such as difficulty sleeping with peers away from home (e.g., camp, sleepovers, school).

Anticipatory or scheduled awakening is a behavioral technique used to prevent confusional arousals. Because the occurrence of these events is often tied to the first third of the night, awakening the child 15 to 20 minutes before the usual time of occurrence may alter the sleep state and therefore abort the event. During the scheduled awakening, the parent should comfort the child.[8] It should be noted, though, that forced awakenings can precipitate a confusional arousal, particularly early in the sleep period. Persistent or frequent confusional arousals, or those seen in combination with other disorders of arousal, may give rise to suspicion for comorbid obstructive sleep apnea, for which workup and treatment should be initiated. Treatment of underlying abnormal nocturnal breathing can frequently ameliorate or resolve symptoms.[13]

During the episodes themselves, efforts to curtail the behavior may lead to aggression and should therefore be avoided; the episode should be allowed to run its course unless intervention is required to maintain safety of the individual.[15,16] Every effort should be made to avoid an individual's known triggers such as sleep deprivation or irregular sleep pattern[9]; and awareness of unavoidable triggers (such as fever) may also help family members anticipate when an event may occur. In all the arousal parasomnias, given the frequency of sleep deprivation in the general population, it is advisable to especially emphasize avoidance of sleep deprivation. In toddlers and young children in particular, the importance of maintaining adequate daytime naps should be emphasized.

There is no specific pharmacologic management for confusional arousals, and it is not commonly needed in pediatric patients. With significant, persistent, frequent, severe symptoms, however, tricyclic antidepressants such as imipramine and clomipramine have been suggested to be effective, as well as the benzodiazepine clonazepam.[16] Longer term use of such agents necessitates clear communication with patients about drug side effects, risks, and possible dependence; it is possible that withdrawal could result in rebound of arousal episodes.[11]

SLEEPWALKING (SOMNAMBULISM)

Definition and Clinical Presentation

Sleepwalking is a disorder of arousal characterized by complex purposeless tasks and wandering episodes of variable duration (from a minute to greater than half an hour), with memory impairment or amnesia for the event. According to ICSD-2,[5] sleepwalking must consist of (1) ambulation which occurs during sleep; with (2) persistence of sleep, altered consciousness, or impaired judgment as demonstrated by difficulty arousing the person, mental confusion when awakened, amnesia (complete or partial) for the episode, routine behaviors occurring at inappropriate times, inappropriate or nonsensical behaviors, and/or dangerous or potentially dangerous behaviors.[5] Sleepwalking behaviors may range from simple to complex, starting with sitting up in bed in confusion before initiating walking, though subjects may start walking immediately. Sleepwalking may be relatively subdued and calm, and terminate spontaneously (sometimes not back in bed); however, individuals may also bolt from bed or make frantic attempts to escape. There is difficulty awakening the individual, but when awakened, the sleepwalker is confused and amnestic, though fragments of the episode may be remembered. Dreaming during sleepwalking may be reported, making it difficult to distinguish clinically from REM sleep behavior disorder. It has been proposed that in adults, multiple influences may play a role in the sleepwalker's subjective experience of sleepwalking.[17] During the episode, sleep talking or shouting may also occur. Eyes are usually open in sleepwalking and may be reported to "stare," as compared to REM sleep behavior disorder, in which the eyes are reportedly more likely to be closed.[5]

Sleepwalking can also involve inappropriate behaviors, such as driving or climbing through a window; this can lead to dangerous and serious consequences for subjects and bed partners or housemates. Violence may occur spontaneously or be provoked during an attempt to awaken the sleepwalker. Homicide, pseudo-suicide, and abnormal sexual behaviors have been reported during sleepwalking.[5] Abnormal sexual behaviors, termed "sexsomnia" by some, and sleep-related eating disorder are examples of variants of sleepwalking featuring inappropriate activity with potentially serious or disastrous consequences.

Epidemiology and Genetics

Episodes may occur as soon as and as long as the individual can walk, but sleepwalking is perhaps most common in children, particularly prepubertal children. Reports of the prevalence of sleepwalking vary from up to 4% in adults to 17% in children younger than 13 years of age.[18,19] In the general population, prevalence has been estimated to be 1%–17%.[9] When considering the possible violent manifestations of sleepwalking, in a multi-country population-based study of nearly 20,000 respondents, violent behaviors during sleep were found in 1.6% of the sample, and in nearly 73% of these cases, other parasomnias such as sleepwalking and sleep terrors were reported. Family history of violent behaviors during sleep, sleepwalking, and sleep terrors was reported more frequently in those with violent behaviors during sleep than in those without, with odds ratio of 9.3, 2.0, and 4.2, respectively.[20]

Adult sleepwalkers usually, but not always, report a positive pediatric history. In one large cohort study, among adult men sleepwalkers 88.9% had a positive history of sleepwalking in childhood, while in women, 84.5% had a positive history of sleepwalking in childhood.[3] In adults, violent sleepwalking is more commonly reported in men. In another smaller series, one third of adult patients with injurious sleepwalking began somnambulism after the age of 16 years.[5]

Sleepwalking has a familial pattern and is based on genetic susceptibility.[21,22] Prevalence of sleepwalking in first-degree relatives of an affected individual is reported to be at least 10 times greater than that in the general population.[23] About 80% of sleepwalking patients are reported to have at least one family member with this parasomnia.[24] In the Finnish Twin Cohort, a study of 11,220 subjects aged 33 to 60 years, including 1045 monozygotic and 1899 dizygotic twin pairs, sleepwalking in childhood had a probandwise concordance rate of 0.55 for monozygotic and 0.35 for dizygotic pairs; adult sleepwalking had a probandwaise concordance that was five times as high in monozygotic pairs compared to dyzygotic.[3] One study of 60 Caucasian sleepwalking subjects and matched controls of HLA DQB1 typing revealed significant excess transmission for DQB1*05 and *04 alleles in familial cases, suggesting that specific DQB1 genes may also play role.[25] It has been proposed that the patient with a genetic predisposition to sleepwalking and priming factors still requires a precipitating factor or trigger to set the sleepwalking episode in motion.[22]

Pathophysiology

Sleepwalking, like other arousal parasomnias, typically involves slow-wave sleep instability with disordered arousals. However, the exact pathophysiological mechanisms of sleepwalking remain unknown. It tends to arise from stage N3 sleep but may arise out of N2 sleep. It has been suggested that sleepwalkers may be more likely to have a somnambulistic episode when factors that deepen sleep (like sleep deprivation) are combined with factors that fragment sleep (like environmental stimuli).[24] A host of triggers for sleepwalking have been reported, mostly summarized as physiologic disturbance (e.g., sleep deprivation, fever) or emotional stress (e.g., separation anxiety in children[2]), underlying medical conditions (obstructive sleep apnea (OSA),[13,26] hyperthyroidism, migraines, stroke, encephalitis), centrally acting medications and substances (alcohol, sedative hypnotics, anticholinergics, lithium), internal or physiologic stimuli (e.g., full bladder, peri-menstrual timing), or external stimuli (noise or light). These "triggers" are hypothesized to lower the threshold for sleepwalking if other factors are also present; but there is no direct experimental evidence that alcohol, for example, predisposes or triggers sleepwalking or related disorders.[27] It has been proposed that sleepwalkers are especially vulnerable to increased homeostatic sleep pressure following sleep deprivation, especially when recovery sleep is initiated when the circadian wake signal is strong.[24] Serotonin has been hypothesized to play a role in the pathophysiology of sleepwalking based on observations that sleepwalking is four to nine times more common in disorders involving serotonin abnormalities such as migraine headaches; the serotonergic system has also been suggested to be a bridge between sleepwalking and one of its triggers, OSA.[28] Despite the association between sleep walking and OSA, it has been reported that a majority of adult sleepwalkers referred to a sleep clinic did not have comorbid sleep disorders.[29]

Diagnosis

The diagnosis may again be suspected clinically, with a detailed clinical history, including that from bed partners, family members, and housemates. In recent times, advances in technology have made it possible for patients' families to record episodes at home, and such recordings may be helpful during the evaluation. Polysomnography studies may be of value in evaluating for alternative diagnoses such as REM sleep behavior disorder, nocturnal wandering, or nocturnal seizures. Sleepwalking events themselves do not often occur in the clinical sleep laboratory, but 25–40 hours of sleep deprivation have been shown to increase the number of somnambulistic episodes seen in the lab.[29,30] However, such sleep deprivation may be difficult or dangerous for patients to achieve.

Normal polysomnography cannot rule out the diagnosis of sleepwalking. Unfortunately, there are no EEG or polysomnographic markers for which a consensus has been developed to serve as reliable markers of disorders of arousal. Nonetheless, several findings such as heart rate acceleration, EEG "delta wave buildup" (also called hypersynchronous delta or HSD), and EMG activation have been proposed with conflicting evidence.[4,31–33] In a systematic study of 38 patients with injurious sleepwalking or sleep

terrors, in which events were captured during polysomnography, before nonbehavioral and behavioral arousals from SWS, neither EEG, nor heart rate, nor tonic/phasic EMG findings could be identified. However, the postarousal EEG could be divided into several categories: (a) diffuse, rhythmic, delta activity with a typical frequency (2.2 Hz), amplitude (85 μV), and duration (20 seconds); (b) diffuse delta and theta activity intermixed with alpha and beta activity; and (c) prominent alpha and beta activity.[31] Others have reported that rarely, delta wave buildup may be visually detected prior to event; however, this is not specific for sleepwalking and may occur in other conditions. In other work, EEG spectral analysis of sleepwalkers has revealed high slow-wave sleep fragmentation[34,35]; abnormal cyclic alternating patterns, which are periodic EEG events of non-REM sleep that are characterized by repeated and spontaneous high-voltage EEG periods that recur at regular intervals of up to 2 minutes in duration[36]; and reduced slow-wave activity.[22] These findings have led some to suggest that non-REM sleep microstructure is disturbed in these patients even on nonsleepwalking nights.

Treatment

Like the other arousal parasomnias, first-line treatment of sleepwalking is supportive and involves systematic consideration of triggers, including comorbid disorders such as obstructive sleep apnea or other sleep disorders, which should be treated if found.[37] There is evidence that treating comorbid OSA can ameliorate or eliminate sleepwalking.[38,39] Avoiding sleep deprivation and alcohol and treating other apparent predisposing factors such as stress or illness/fever are important. Addressing safety concerns and creating a safe environment for the sleepwalker are also key.

Unintentional injury to self or others is always a concern in arousal parasomnias, in particular in sleepwalking, in which subjects usually move beyond the bed. This has been shown to be especially true of chronic adult sleepwalkers.[38,40] Recommendations such as locating the patient's bedroom on the ground floor, providing special locks or alarms for windows and doors and heavy window coverings, removing obstructions in the bedroom, removing objects potentially in the sleepwalkers' path, and securing keys may be appropriate.[41] Environmental safety and risk of harm to self

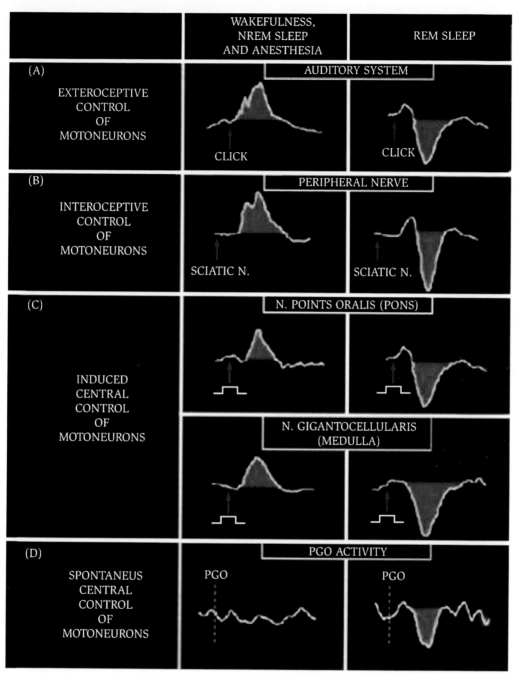

FIGURE 5.9 Patterns of state-dependent motor control based upon the phenomenon of reticular response-reversal. Motor inhibition during REM sleep replaces motor excitation during either wakefulness or non-REM sleep. Various excitatory stimuli that are accompanied by arousal or enhanced wakefulness result in the generation of depolarizing (i.e., excitation; upward cross-hatched deflection) postsynaptic activity in motoneurons during wakefulness, non-REM sleep, or anesthesia. On the other hand, when identical stimuli are present during REM sleep, motoneurons exhibit prominent hyperpolarizing (i.e., inhibitory; downward cross-hatched deflection) postsynaptic activity. However, the depolarizing drives that characterize the periods of wakefulness or NREM sleep are still present during REM sleep, as evidenced by the depolarizing potentials that immediately precede the onset of the more dominant hyperpolarizing potentials.

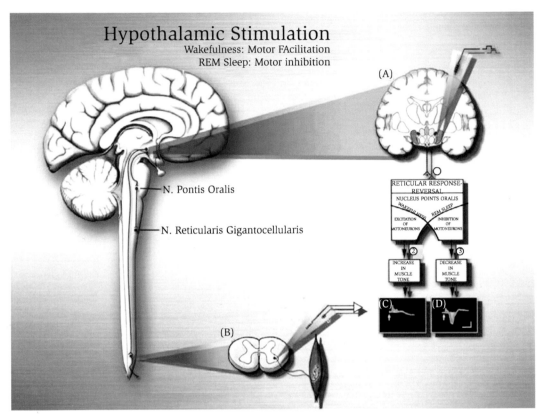

FIGURE 5.10 Stimulation of the hypocretinergic system promotes motoneuron excitation or inhibition according to the behavioral state of the individual. During wakefulness, intracellular recordings reveal that an excitatory potential (upward cross-hatched deflection) is induced in lumbar motoneurons. During carbachol-induced REM sleep, the same hypothalamic stimulus produces a large amplitude inhibitory (i.e., downward cross-hatched deflection) response (D). Note, however, that a short-latency depolarizing (excitatory) potential is still present during REM sleep, which is typical of reticular response-reversal. During wakefulness, the hypocretinergic system promotes an increase in motor activity by direct projections to brainstem nuclei such as the NPO and also to motoneurons. During REM sleep, these excitatory actions are superseded by hypocretinergically induced inhibitory drives. Cataplexy may be due to the absence of hypocretinergic directives, which would result in a decrease in motor activity during wakefulness and an increase during REM sleep. (See Yamuy et al., 2010.)

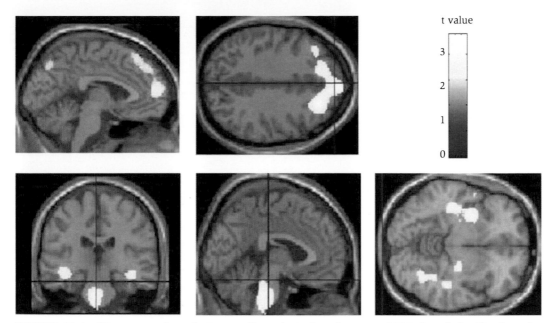

FIGURE 19.1   Hippocampal perfusion predicts clinical evolution in REM sleep behavior disorder (RBD). (Upper panels) Brain perfusion increases at baseline in RBD patients who would convert to neurodegenerative disease (RBDEv), compared to those who would not (RBDSt), were located in the hippocampus. The panels show the peak hyperperfusion, centered on the left hippocampus, and represented on sagittal, coronal and transverse sections (from left to right panels) ($P^{corr} < 0.05$). The level of section is indicated on the top of each panel (x, y, and z coordinates, in mm). The color scale indicates the range of t values for this contrast.

(Lower panel) Plot of the adjusted regional cerebral blood flow values (arbitrary units) in the left hippocampus ($x=-30$mm, $y=-30$mm, $z=-14$mm), showing the distinct distribution in RBDEv and RBDSt patients. Each circle represents one subject. Horizontal bars represent mean values. This figure shows results from a ^{99m}Tc-ECD SPECT study. (Reproduced from Dang-Vu et al.,[link to Dang-Vu 2012] with permission.)

FIGURE 19.2   Brain glucose metabolism in fatal familial insomnia (FFI). Decrease of glucose metabolism in the thalamus has been consistently shown in FFI. Thalamic hypometabolism is manifest in this patient with symptomatic FFI, along with metabolic decrease in the basal ganglia (*right*), as compared to controls (*left*). A milder decrease of glucose metabolism in the thalamus was already detected in that FFI patient more than 1 year before the onset of symptoms (*middle*). This figure shows results from an ^{18}F-FDG PET study. (Reproduced from Cortelli et al.,[104] with permission.)

2-[^{18}F]-F-A-85380   [^{18}F]-FDG

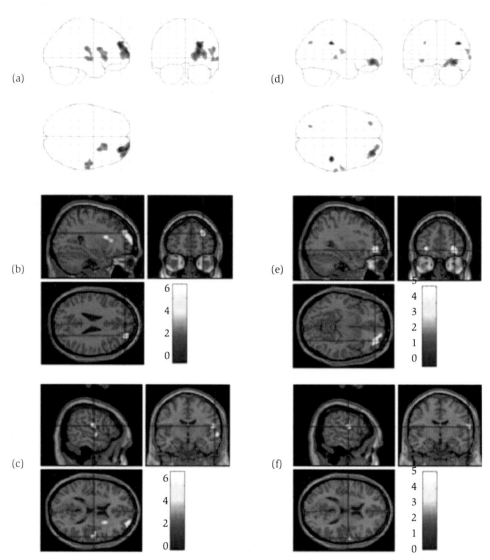

FIGURE 19.3   Brain glucose metabolism and nicotinic acetycholine receptor density in autosomal dominant nocturnal frontal lobe epilepsy. The right panels (D–F) illustrate the decrease of glucose metabolism in the right prefrontal region (E) and right opercular cortex (F), in ADNFLE as compared to controls, during the interictal period (^{18}F-FDG PET study). Given that ADNFLE is associated with mutations in the genes encoding subunits α4 and β2 of nAChR, the brain regional density of nAChR has also been investigated. As shown in the left panels (A–C), ADNFLE is associated with a lower nAChR density in the right prefontal region (B) and right opercular cortex (C), as compared to controls (^{18}F-A-85380 PET study). Note the similarity between glucose metabolism and nAChR distributions, both of which being in agreement with the frontal origin of ADNFLE. (Reproduced from Picard et al.,[114] with permission.)

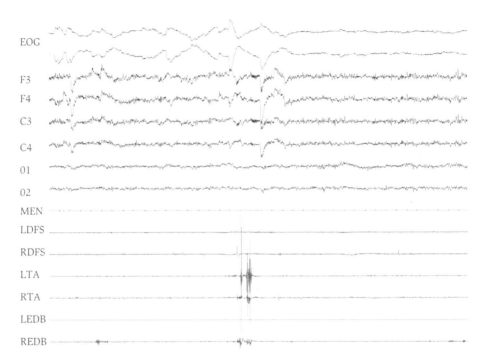

FIGURE 30.6 Polysomnographic representation of normal REM sleep in a healthy human. This figure represents 30 seconds of a normal human during REM sleep undergoing polysomnography. The recording shows physiological muscle atonia in the mentalis and an isolated burst of phasic electromyographic activity only in the lower limbs during REM sleep in a normal person. EOG, electrooculogram; F3,F4,C3,C4, O1, and O2, electroencephalographic electrode positions (frontal, central, and occipital of each side) according to the 10/20 International system referenced to combined ears; LDFS, left flexor digitorum superficialis muscle in the upper limb; LEDB, left extensor digitorum brevis muscle in the lower limb; LTA, left tibialis anterior muscle in the lower limb; MEN, mentalis muscle; RDFS, right flexor digitorum superficialis muscle in the upper limb; REDB, right extensor digitorum brevis muscle in the lower limb; RTA, right tibialis anterior muscle in the lower limb.

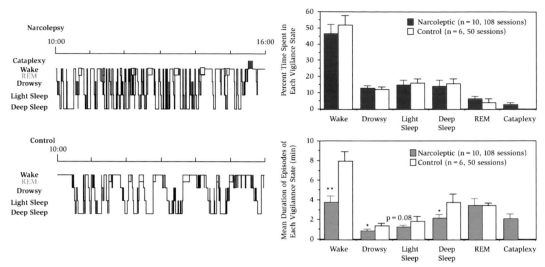

FIGURE 34.3　(*A*) Typical hyponograms from a narcoleptic and a control Doberman. (*B* and *C*) Percent of time spent in, mean frequency of, and mean duration for each vigilance state of narcoleptic and control Dobermans during daytime 6-hour recordings (10:00 to 16:00). No significant difference was found in the percentage of time spent in each vigilance state between narcoleptic and control dogs. However, the mean duration of waking, drowsy, and deep-sleep episodes was significantly shorter in the narcoleptics, suggesting a fragmentation of the vigilance states (wake and sleep) in these animals. To compensate for the influence of cataplectic episodes on wake and drowsiness, those episodes interrupted by the occurrence of cataplexy were excluded.

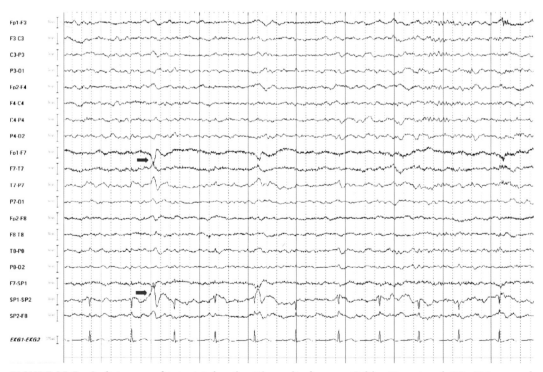

FIGURE 35.5　Left temporal interictal epileptiform discharges. Calibration signal: 35 μV, 1 second.

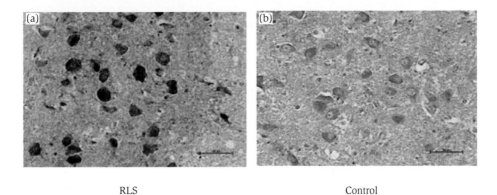

RLS   Control

FIGURE 44.4   HIF-1 alpha immunostaining in substantia nigra of control and restless legs syndrome (RLS) patients. This figure demonstrates inducible factor (HIF-1 alpha) staining is much increased in RLS compared to control tissue from the substantia nigra. (Reproduced from Patton et al.[64])

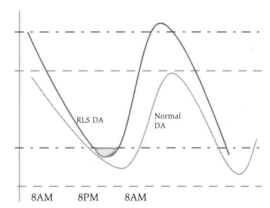

        8AM   8PM   8AM

FIGURE 44.7   Concept of effects of restless legs syndrome (RLS) chronic increase in dopaminergic (DA) activity (solid red line) producing desensitized postsynaptic response (dashed red lines), which leaves a period at the low point of the dopamine cycle with inadequate dopamine activation corresponding to periods with RLS symptoms. Adding small amounts of dopamine stimulation during the symptomatic period will initially correct the problem but then lead to further postsynaptic desensitization and RLS augmentation with symptoms starting earlier in the day. Circadian dopamine cycle for normal (blue) and moderate RLS (red). Dashed lines indicate range for normal postsynaptic dopamine activity for normal (blue) and RLS (red). Filled pink indicates time with RLS symptoms. Dopamine falls below level needed to produce normal postsynaptic response.

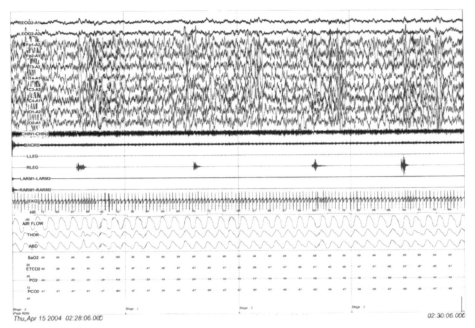

FIGURE 46.1   This 30-second recording shows periodic limb movement in sleep in children with restless legs syndrome and attention-deficit/hyperactivity disorder. There are four periodic bursts of electromyographic activity with 0.5- to 2-second duration and an interval of less than 90 seconds.

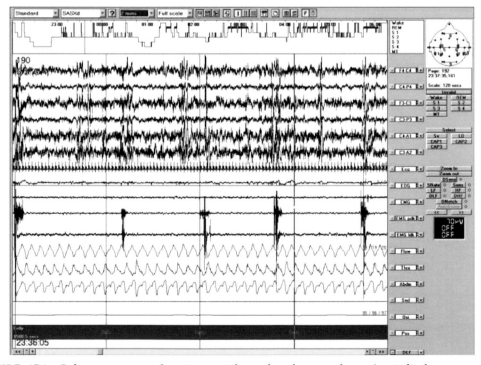

FIGURE 47.1   Polysomnogram of patients with restless legs syndrome/periodic leg movements during sleep. Duration of the hypnogram is 2 minutes. From the top to bottom: hypnogram (blue), EEG (six black leads), ECG (purple), EOG (two black leads), EMG (two black leads), with periodic leg movements (arrows indicate a periodicity of 20–30 seconds).

or others must be addressed with all patients, and parents in the case of pediatric patients.

As with other arousal parasomnias, bed partner or family member instructions regarding not waking the patient but rather quietly guiding the patient back to bed may be helpful. Generally, some reassurance may be given to parents of pediatric patients regarding the drop in prevalence of these disorders with age; however, as has been mentioned, the disorders can persist into adulthood. Reassurance that underlying psychiatric illness is generally not the cause of the sleepwalking may also be indicated.

Beyond management of sleep deprivation and avoidance of substance use, behavioral nonpharmacologic methods have been suggested, including stress management psychotherapy[16] and hypnosis,[42-44] though data are limited, anecdotal, and with mixed results.[6,45] Anticipatory/scheduled awakenings were shown to be effective in pediatric sleepwalking in one publication, with maintained benefits for some time after treatment.[46] If the patient and/or family are determined to be at risk for injury, or if events are frequent or disruptive, then pharmacologic approaches should be considered. Controlled clinical trials for sleepwalking treatment are lacking. Benzodiazepines are typically first-line agents, though data are relatively limited. Clonazepam 0.5 to 2 mg has been shown to be effective in larger case series,[40,47] though diazepam, triazolam, and flurazepam have all been reported in smaller numbers.[43,48,49] Imipramine[50] and paroxetine[51] have also been reported to be helpful. Melatonin in a child with sleep walking has been successful in a case report.[52]

SLEEP TERRORS

Definition and Presentation

Sleep terrors, the third in the triad of non-REM parasomnias, is characterized by an explosive onset that typically consists of an abrupt arousal from stage N3 sleep, accompanied by a high degree of agitation such as a piercing scream or incoherent speech. The individual is classically in a state characterized by autonomic hyperactivity and may exhibit behavioral manifestations of intense fear, panic, confusion, or an apparent desire to escape. There is no response to soothing from others. Prominent motor activity may occur, and while it is not entirely usual for patients to leave the bed, bodily displacement or jumping out of bed could occur, which may result in bodily injury.[53] Episodes may become violent, with potential forensic implications in some patients.[54] A typical pediatric scenario would be a young child between 3 and 10 years who awakens abruptly from sleep with a blood-curdling scream and is agitated, flushed, sweating, tachypneic, and tachycardic. The episodes are typically followed by amnesia and disorientation.

Epidemiology and Genetics

Sleep terrors have been estimated to occur in about 3%–6.5% of children from early childhood to preadolescence/adolescence, 1% in the elderly, and to have a higher male predilection.[1,55-57] The genetic predisposition to sleep terrors has been studied and found to be strong. Using maternal report in 18-month-old and 30-month-old twins, recent evidence supports the notion of a strong pattern of heritability in sleep terrors. In that study, the prevalence of sleep terrors was 36.9% at 18 months and 19.7% at 30 months; 49% of affected children were boys, and 51% were girls. The polychoric correlations were 0.63 for monozygotic and 0.36 for the dizygotic twins at 18 months, and 0.68 and 0.24, respectively, at 30 months. A model generated showed an approximately 40% additive genetic effect.[55] Older evidence also supports a strong genetic contribution: in a cohort of 27 patients with sleep terrors, analysis of family pedigree revealed that 26 had one or more family members with sleepwalking and/or sleep terrors.[23]

Pathophysiology and Diagnosis

Like the other disorders of arousal, arousal from slow-wave sleep and environmental, acquired, or intrinsic sleep disturbances have been implicated in the genesis of sleep terrors. Psychopathology is often rare in affected children, but it has been proposed to have a more significant role in adult sufferers.[1]

Similar to other non-REM arousal disorders, a careful clinical history can strongly suggest or make the diagnosis. Nightmares, which occur during REM sleep, may be difficult to clinically distinguish from sleep terrors. A key difference is the vivid recollection of dream content in the case of nightmares, as compared to amnesia in sleep terrors; nightmares are also more likely to occur later during the sleep period; both may be precipitated by daytime stress. In some cases, it may be clinically appropriate to perform a polysomnogram to rule out other disorders that may contribute to or mimic sleep terrors such as nocturnal seizure. An EEG during a sleep terror may show high-amplitude, rhythmic delta or theta activity.[10] As in sleepwalking, abnormal rate of cyclic alternating patterns has been proposed to be one marker of unstable sleep and as such are increased during the slow-wave sleep of children with sleep terrors.[58]

Treatment

As with the other arousal parasomnias, patients should be counseled to avoid sleep deprivation and other precipitants, such as drugs, alcohol, stress, and so on.[59] Psychotherapy, relaxation therapy, and autogenic training or hypnosis have all been proposed in the treatment of sleep terrors.[44,60,61] Like other arousal parasomnias, scheduled awakenings may be attempted to reduce sleep terrors. Once an episode is under way, attempts to interrupt the episode are discouraged because it may lead to injury; it is preferable to wait until the spell is over and then guide the person gently back to bed.[41] As with all disorders of arousal, safety precautions to prevent injury must be discussed.

Reassurance is often enough in children with a low burden of frequency of sleep terrors, as they tend to disappear by late adolescence.[14] Pharmacologic therapies may be considered if episodes are self-injurious, frequent, or especially disruptive, though careful consideration should be given to using polysomnography to rule out comorbid conditions first.

Proposed pharmacologic therapy for sleep terrors has included benzodiazepines such as diazepam[62] or clonazepam, and tricyclics such as imipramine[63] or clomipramine.[6] Trazodone, paroxetine, melatonin in children, and L-5-hydroxytryptophan have all been reported as helpful in some patients with sleep terrors.[6,52,64]

DIFFERENTIAL DIAGNOSIS FOR DISORDERS OF AROUSAL

Nocturnal seizures can mimic the arousal parasomnias—disorganized bodily movements, staring, unresponsiveness, vocalizations, and confused behavior are common to both groups of disorders.[10] Nocturnal frontal lobe epilepsy (NFLE) in particular may present in varied ways, including with a confusional state; most recently it has been proposed that increased frequency of arousal parasomnias among families with NFLE suggests a common etiologic link.[65,66] A full EEG montage should be used along with polysomnography to investigate suspicion for nocturnal seizure. Age of onset may be anytime from infancy through adulthood, unlike arousal disorders, which more commonly start in childhood. Seizures may occur at any time during the night at random (compared to the first third of the night for arousal parasomnias); they occur from stages N1 or N2 sleep (often at stage transitions), and events may be similar in duration or shorter lived than typical arousal parasomnias. Subjects may exhibit irritability or sleepiness during the day in nocturnal seizure, and events may exhibit stereotypy of behavior.[67] If seizures are generalized, there is no recall of the event; however, there may be partial recall if a simple seizure has occurred.[1]

REM sleep behavior disorder (RBD) must also be considered in some cases of parasomnia, particularly where limb movements are prominent. RBD occurs during REM sleep and may also feature kicking, grabbing or punching, talking or utterances, or violence. If awakened, the patient may have very detailed dream recall and dream content that provides context for the behaviors observed during sleep. The potential for self or bed partner injury is high in this disorder, which may lead to the initial evaluation. The condition has an estimated prevalence of 0.38% of the general population, with a predilection in elderly males.[68] Importantly, polysomnography reveals abnormal EMG tone during REM sleep ("loss of muscle atonia"). This condition has an association with neurodegenerative disease, the synucleinopathies, but may be seen with certain drugs (often serotonergic medications such as serotonin reuptake inhibitors and other antidepressants); RBD-type presentation has also been reported in severe OSA.[69] Parasomnia overlap syndrome has been presented as a subtype of RBD and is defined as the co-occurrence of RBD and non-REM parasomnia, usually sleepwalking or confusional arousal.

Sleep-related dissociative disorder is a psychiatric condition that can mimic any parasomnia and almost always is accompanied by anxiety disorders or dissociative disorder during wakefulness. The key feature of this parasomnia is that, despite behaviorally appearing asleep during the event, the person is awake by electrographic criteria. In one study, out of 100 consecutive patients referred to a tertiary sleep center, 7 had sleep-related dissociative disorder.[70]

RISKS AND IMPLICATIONS OF DISORDERS OF AROUSAL

Some have argued that disorders of arousal are common enough that they ought to be considered part of the normal human condition, not the manifestation of underlying disease, psychiatric or otherwise.[71] Nonetheless, non-REM disorders of arousal have serious implications: they may lead to serious injury; they can be disturbing and disconcerting to bed partners and family members, and they may reflect underlying sleep disturbances such as obstructive sleep apnea that require diagnosis and treatment. They may also be mistaken for, or misdiagnosed as, nocturnal seizure or other conditions.

Beyond uncomplicated childhood non-REM parasomnias, in older or adult individuals, an increasing number of criminal cases have claimed the defendant to be in a state of sleepwalking or other non-REM parasomnia, sometimes induced by excessive alcohol intake or stress. This is an intriguing defense, as sleepwalkers who commit violent acts or assaults are thought to be in a state of automatism, without conscious awareness or criminal intent. Acquittal is possible in criminal trials. This is to be distinguished from criminal acts performed as a result of alcohol intoxication alone. Claims that direct alcohol provocation tests can assist in the forensic assessment of these cases found no support of any kind in the medical literature. There are no reports of alcohol testing in normative or patient groups nor of validation testing of any sort.[27] The legal precedents and considerations regarding somnambulism as a sane automatism defense in violent nocturnal behaviors leading to tragic outcomes are reviewed elsewhere, and they are exemplified in the Canadian Supreme Court case *Regina vs Parks* and in the State Supreme Court case *State of Arizona v. Scott Falater*.[4]

REFERENCES

1. Avidan A. Parasomnias and movement disorders of sleep. *Sem Neurol* 2009;29(4):372–92.
2. Petit D, Touchette E, Tremblay RE, et al. Dyssomnias and parasomnias in early childhood. *Pediatrics* 2007;119:e1016–25.
3. Hublin, C, Kaprio, J, Partinen, M, et al. Prevalence and genetics of sleepwalking: a population-based twin study. *Neurology* 1997;48,177–81.
4. Bornemann MA, Mahowald MW, Schenck CH. Parasomnias: clinical features and forensic implications. *Chest* 2006;130(2):605–10.
5. American Academy of Sleep Medicine. *International Classification of Sleep Disorders. Diagnostic and Coding Manual.* 2nd ed. Westchester IL: American Academy of Sleep Medicine; 2005.
6. Attarian H. Treatment options for parasomnias. *Neurol Clin* 2010;28(4):1089–106.
7. Stores G. Parasomnias of childhood and adolescence. *Sleep Med Clin* 2007;2:405–17.
8. Kotagal S. Parasomnias in childhood. *Sleep Med Rev* 2009;13(2):157–68.
9. Ohayon MM, Guilleminault C, Priest RG. Night terrors, sleepwalking, and confusional arousals in the general population: their frequency and relationship to other sleep and mental disorders. *J Clin Psychiatry* 1999;60(4):268–77.
10. Kotagal S. Parasomnias of childhood. *Curr Opin Ped* 2008;20:659–65.
11. Stores G. Confusional arousals. In: Thorpy MJ, Plazzi G, eds. The Parasomnias and Other sleep disorders. Cambridge, England: Cambridge University Press; 2010:103.
12. Billiard M, Dauvilliers Y. Idiopathic hypersomnia. *Sleep Med Rev* 2001;5:351–60.
13. Guilleminault C, Palombini L, Pelayo R, et al. Sleepwalking and sleep terrors in prepubertal children: what triggers them? *Pediatrics* 2003;111(1):e17–25.
14. Mason TB, 2nd, Pack AI. Pediatric parasomnias. *Sleep* 2007;30(2):141–51.
15. Pressman MR. Disorders of arousal from sleep and violent behavior: the role of physical contact and proximity. *Sleep* 2007;30(8):1039–47.
16. Mahowald MW, Schenck CH. Non-rapid eye movement sleep parasomnias. *Neurol Clin* 2005;23(4):1077–106, vii.
17. Zadra A, Pilon M, Montplaisir J. Phenomenology of somnambulism. *Sleep* 2006;29:A269.
18. Plazzi G, Vetrugno R, Provini F, et al. Sleepwalking and other ambulatory behaviours during sleep. *Neurol Sci* 2005;26(Suppl 3):S193–8.
19. Klackenberg G. Somnambulism in childhood—prevalence, course and behavioral correlations. A prospective longitudinal

study (6–16 years). *Acta Paediatr Scand* 1982;71(3):495–9.

20. Ohayon MM, Schenck CH. Violent behavior during sleep: prevalence, comorbidity and consequences. *Sleep Med* 2010;11(9):941–6.

21. Cao M, Guilleminault C. Families with sleepwalking. *Sleep Med* 2010;11(7):726–34.

22. Pressman MR. Factors that predispose, prime and precipitate NREM parasomnias in adults: clinical and forensic implications. *Sleep Med Rev* 2007;11(1):5–30.

23. Kales A, Soldatos CR, Bixler EO, et al. Hereditary factors in sleepwalking and nightmares. *Br J Psychiatry* 1980;137:111–18.

24. Zadra A, Montplaisir J. Sleepwalking. In: Thorpy MJ, Plazzi G, eds. *The Parasomnias and Other Sleep Disorders*. Cambrige, England: Cambridge Univeristy Press; 2010:115.

25. Lecendreux M, Bassetti C, Dauvilliers Y, et al. HLA and genetic susceptibility to sleepwalking. *Mol Psychiatry* 2003;8(1):114–7.

26. Goodwin JL, Kaemingk KL, Fregosi RF, et al. Parasomnias and sleep-disordered breathing in Caucasian and Hispanic children—the Tucson children's assessment of sleep apnea study. *BMC Med* 2004;2:14.

27. Pressman MR, Mahowald MW, Schenck CH, et al. Alcohol-induced sleepwalking or confusional arousal as a defense to criminal behavior: a review of scientific evidence, methods and forensic considerations. *J Sleep Res* 2007;16(2):198–212.

28. Juszczak GR, Swiergiel AH. Serotonergic hypothesis of sleepwalking. *Med Hypotheses* 2005;64(1):28–32.

29. Zadra A, Pilon M, Montplaisir J. Polysomnographic diagnosis of sleepwalking: effects of sleep deprivation. *Ann Neurol* 2008;63(4):513–19.

30. Blatt I, Peled R, Gadoth N. The value of sleep recording in evaluating somnambulism in young adults. *Electroencephalogr Clin Neurophysiol* 1991;78(6):407–12.

31. Schenck CH, Pareja JA, Patterson AL, et al. An analysis of polysomnographic events surrounding 252 slow-wave sleep arousals in 38 adults with injurious sleepwalking and sleep terrors. *J Clin Neurophysiol* 1998;15:159–66.

32. Pressman, MR. Hypersynchronous delta sleep EEG activity and sudden arousals from slow-wave sleep in adults without a history of parasomnias: clinical and forensic implications. *Sleep* 2004;27:706–10

33. Pilon, M, Zadra, A, Joncas, S, et al. Hypersynchronous delta waves and somnambulism: brain topography and effect of sleep deprivation. *Sleep* 2006;29:77–84

34. Espa F, Ondze B, Deglise P, et al. Sleep architecture, slow wave activity, and sleep spindles in adult patients with sleepwalking and sleep terrors. *Clin Neurophysiol* 2000;111(5):929–39.

35. Guilleminault C, Poyares D, Aftab FA, et al. Sleep and wakefulness in somnambulism: a spectral analysis study. *J Psychosom Res* 2001;51(2):411–16.

36. Guilleminault C, Kirisoglu C, da Rosa AC, et al. Sleepwalking, a disorder of NREM sleep instability. *Sleep Med* 2006;7(2):163–70.

37. Espa F, Dauvilliers Y, Ondze B, et al. Arousal reactions in sleepwalking and night terrors in adults: the role of respiratory events. *Sleep* 2002;25:871–5.

38. Guilleminault C, Kirisoglu C, Bao G, et al. Adult chronic sleepwalking and its treatment based on polysomnography. *Brain* 2005;128:1062–9.

39. Pirelli P, Saponara M, Guilleminault C. Rapid maxillary expansion in children with obstructive sleep apnea syndrome. *Sleep* 2004;27(4):761–5.

40. Schenck CH, Milner DM, Hurwitz TD, et al. A polysomnographic and clinical report on sleep-related injury in 100 adult patients. *Am J Psychiatry* 1989;146(9):1166–73.

41. Stores G. Clinical diagnosis and misdiagnosis of sleep disorders. *J Neurol Neurosurg Psychiatry* 2007;78(12):1293–7.

42. Hauri PJ, Silber MH, Boeve BF. The treatment of parasomnias with hypnosis: a 5-year follow-up study. *J Clin Sleep Med* 2007;3(4):369–73.

43. Remulla A, Guilleminault C. Somnambulism (sleepwalking). *Expert Opin Pharmacother* 2004;5(10):2069–74.

44. Hurwitz TD, Mahowald MW, Schenck CH, et al. A retrospective outcome study and review of hypnosis as treatment of adults with sleepwalking and sleep terror. *J Nerv Ment Dis* 1991;179(4):228–33.

45. Reid WH, Ahmed I, Levie CA. Treatment of sleepwalking: a controlled study. *Am J Psychother* 1981;35(1):27–37.

46. Tobin JD, Jr. Treatment of somnambulism with anticipatory awakening. *J Pediatr* 1993;122(3):426–7.

47. Schenck CH, Mahowald MW. Long-term, nightly benzodiazepine treatment of injurious parasomnias and other disorders of disrupted nocturnal sleep in 170 adults. *Am J Med* 1996;100(3):333–7.

48. Berlin RM, Qayyum U. Sleepwalking: diagnosis and treatment through the life cycle. *Psychosomatics* 1986;27(11):755–60.

49. Kavey NB, Whyte J, Resor SR, Jr., et al. Somnambulism in adults. *Neurology* 1990;40(5):749–52.

50. Cooper AJ. Treatment of coexistent night-terrors and somnambulism in adults with imipramine and diazepam. *J Clin Psychiatry* 1987;48(5):209–10.

51. Lillywhite AR, Wilson SJ, Nutt DJ. Successful treatment of night terrors and somnambulism with paroxetine. *Br J Psychiatry* 1994;164(4):551–4.

52. Jan JE, Freeman RD, Wasdell MB, et al. A child with severe night terrors and sleep-walking responds to melatonin therapy. *Dev Med Child Neurol* 2004; 46(11):789.

53. Rosen GM, Mahowald MW. Disorders of arousal in children. In: Sheldon SH, Ferber R, Kryger MH, eds. *Principles and Practice of Pediatric Sleep Medicine*. Philadelphia, PA: Elsevier Saunders; 2005:293–304.

54. Mahowald MW, Bundlie SR, Hurwitz TD, et al. Sleep violence—forensic science implications: polygraphic and video documentation. *J Forensic Sci* 1990;35(2):413–32.

55. Nguyen BH, Perusse D, Paquet J, et al. Sleep terrors in children: a prospective study of twins. *Pediatrics* 2008;122(6):e1164–7.

56. Laberge L, Tremblay RE, Vitaro F, et al. Development of parasomnias from childhood to early adolescence. *Pediatrics* 2000;106(1 Pt 1):67–74.

57. Kales A, Beall GN, Berger RJ, et al. Sleep and dreams. Recent research on clinical aspects. *Ann Intern Med* 196868(5):1078–104.

58. Bruni O, Ferri R, Novelli L, et al. NREM sleep instability in children with sleep terrors: the role of slow wave interruptions. *Clin Neurophysiol* 2008;119:985–92.

59. Heussler HS. 9. Common causes of sleep disruption and daytime sleepiness: childhood sleep disorders II. *Med J Aust* 2005;182(9):484–9.

60. Kales JC, Cadieux RJ, Soldatos CR, et al. Psychotherapy with night-terror patients. *Am J Psychother* 1982;36(3):399–407.

61. Kellerman J. Behavioral treatment of night terrors in a child with acute leukemia. *J Nerv Ment Dis* 1979;167(3):182–5.

62. Allen RM. Attenuation of drug-induced anxiety dreams and pavor nocturnus by benzodiazepines. *J Clin Psychiatry* 1983;44(3):106–8.

63. Burstein A, Burstein A. Treatment of night terrors with imipramine. *J Clin Psychiatry* 1983;44(2):82.

64. Bruni O, Ferri R, Miano S, et al. L-5-Hydroxytryptophan treatment of sleep terrors in children. *Eur J Pediatr* 2004;163(7):402–7.

65. Provini F, Plazzi G, Montagna P, et al. The wide clinical spectrum of nocturnal frontal lobe epilepsy. *Sleep Med Rev* 2000;4(4):375–86

66. Bisulli F, Vignatelli L, Naldi I, et al. ncreased frequency of arousal parasomnias in families with nocturnal frontal lobe epilepsy: a common mechanism? *Epilepsia* 2010;51(9):1852–60.

67. Tinuper P, Provini F, Bisulli F, et al. Movement disorders in sleep: guidelines for differentiating epileptic from nonepileptic motor phenomena arising from sleep. *Sleep Med Rev* 2007; 11:255–67.

68. Schenck CH, Mahowald MW. Rapid eye movement sleep parasomnias. *Neurol Clin* 2005;23(4):1107–26.

69. Iranzo A, Santamaría J. Severe obstructive sleep apnea/hypopnea mimicking REM sleep behavior disorder. *Sleep* 2005;28(2):203–6.

70. Turkus JA, Kahler JA. Therapeutic interventions in the treatment of dissociative disorders. *Psychiatr Clin North Am* 2006;29(1):245–62, xi.

71. Mahowald MW, Schenk CH, Cramer Bornemann MA. Violent parasomnias forensic implications. *Handb Clin Neurol* 2011;99:1149–59.

29

REM Sleep Behavior Disorder

Discovery of REM Sleep Behavior Disorder, Clinical and Laboratory Diagnosis, and Treatment

BIRGIT FRAUSCHER AND BIRGIT HÖGL

IN 1965, Jouvet and Delorme reported for the first time on persistent loss of physiological muscle atonia in cats with symmetrical, dorsolateral pontine tegmental lesions.[1] These cats also exhibited new onset of hallucinatory behaviors during rapid eye movement (REM) sleep, in absence of external stimuli, with attack-like behavior being the most characteristic feature.[2] Four different patterns of behaviors, which depended on the size and site of the experimental lesion, were identified. A "minimal syndrome" of increased proximal limb and head movements resulted from selective destruction of the tegmento-reticular pathway, orienting and exploratory behaviors from a destruction of the superior colliculus, episodic attack behaviors from damage extending rostroventrally into the midbrain, and locomotion from more ventral lesions.[3]

In humans, the possible first anecdotal clinical description of RBD features was reported long before the detection of REM sleep[4] by Lasègue[5] in patients with delirium tremens. Reported features that may correspond to REM sleep behavior disorder (RBD) are "agitated nocturnal sleep," "vividly talking while being asleep," and "rampaging in the bed." Lasègue concludes from his observations that "le délir alcoolique n'est pas un délire, mais un rêve" (the alcoholic delirium is not a delirium, but a dream). First polysomnographic reports on RBD (persistence of tonic electromyographic [EMG] activity during REM sleep, abnormal or delirious behaviors during sleep) were published by scientists from Asia, Europe, and the United States in the 1960s and 1970s.[6-24] Cases described were either patients with extrapyramidal motor system disorders such as Parkinson's disease or multiple-system atrophy[6,8,11,13,21]; brainstem tumors[12,20]; amyotrophic lateral sclerosis[23]; subacute sclerosing panencephalitis[7]; patients undergoing alcohol, meprobamate, barbiturate, or pentazocine withdrawal (see also recent review on RBD history by Tachibana[25])[14,17,18,24]; patients treated with MAO inhibitors, biperiden, or clomipramine[9,10,15,16,19]; or elderly patients without associated comorbidity.[22]

In patients with Parkinson's disease, REM sleep without atonia was first described in the late 1960s. In 1969, Traczynska-Kubin and collegues[8] reported on sleep parameters of 14 Parkinson patients, of whom 12 were diagnosed with idiopathic Parkinson's disease. Concerning electromyographic activity during sleep, the authors described that "le tonus musculaire au niveau des muscles de la houppe du menton peut persister au cours de la phase de mouvement oculaires rapides" (the muscle tone derived from the chin muscles can persist during the phase with rapid eye movements).[8] Two years earlier, a US group led by Stern investigated tremor during sleep in seven patients with Parkinson's disease.[6] They found that when "tremor" occurred in REM sleep, "it was closely associated with REM bursts and that it varied in its amplitude which sometimes altered from deflection to deflection." By looking, however, at the polysomnographic example given by the authors, the earlier described "irregular manifestation of tremor" could also be REM sleep without atonia (Fig. 29.1).

In 1975, the presence of REM sleep without atonia was further confirmed in 23 untreated patients with Parkinson's disease.[13] Mouret stated that "the abnormal behavior of the chin muscles during paradoxical sleep consisted in either a clear persistence of EMG activity, with or without short-lasting inhibitions, or of the reappearance of tonic EMG activity without any concomitant phasic events."[13]

A very interesting case report providing to the best of our knowledge the first quantitative assessment of REM sleep without atonia is that from de Barros-Ferreira,[12] who reported on an 8-year old child with a pontine tumor. Chin EMG muscle tone did lack atonia in 87.3% of total time of REM sleep (Figs. 29.2 and 29.3). In addition, the authors described an association between phasic discharges of EMG activity

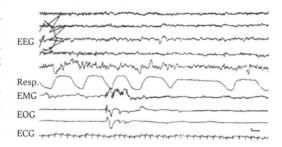

FIGURE 29.2 Complex phasic discharge, including eye movements and peribuccal movements, starting on a ground of muscular atonia but followed by persistent axial tone (from de Barros-Ferreira[12]). ECG, electrocardiogram; EEG, electroencephalogram; EMG, electromyogram; EOG, electrooculogram.

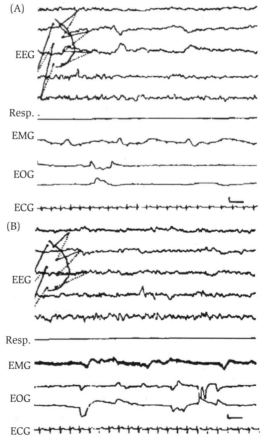

FIGURE 29.3 (A) Burst of rapid eye movements with muscular atonia (from de Barros-Ferreira[12]). (B) A few minutes later, burst of rapid eye movements with conservation of muscle tone (from de Barros-Ferreira[12]). ECG, electrocardiogram; EEG, electroencephalogram; EMG, electromyogram; EOG, electrooculogram.

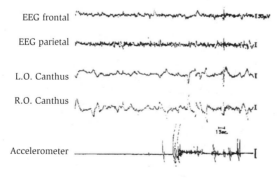

FIGURE 29.1 Polysomnographic example of a burst of phasic muscle activity during REM sleep (from Stern[6]). EEG, electroencephalogram.

and rapid eye movements (Fig. 29.2) as well as an occurrence of REM sleep without atonia irrespective of the presence of rapid eye movements (Fig. 29.3).

Apart from the EMG characteristics in the chin muscles, de Barros-Ferreira described behavioral phenomena with episodes of laughing, sleep talking, or "body or facial agitation."[12]

Of note, REM sleep without atonia was named differently according to the various investigators. In the Japanese literature REM sleep without atonia was called "stage 1-REM with tonic EMG activity." This term was chosen by Tachibana M. and describes the concomitant appearance of a low-voltage, mixed-frequency EEG, rapid eye movements, and tonic EMG in the mentalis muscle.[14] Another term, found in the literature, which described exactly the same phenomenon was coined by Guilleminault and colleagues as "sleep stage 7."[15] According to Guilleminault, "sleep stage 7" describes the presence of rapid eye movements in conjunction with a low-amplitude, mixed-frequency EEG and a tonically elevated EMG (Fig. 29.4).

Only in 1986, human REM sleep behavior disorder was first formally described in a series of five patients by Schenck and collegues.[26] The five very well-characterized patients (four men, one woman) whose detailed illustrative histories of RBD episodes are provided in the milestone paper were between 60 and 72 years of age. Four of the five patients had neurological comorbidities (Guillain-Barré syndrome, olivo-ponto-cerebellar degeneration, atypical dementia, and subarachnoid hemorrhage).[26] The authors put special emphasis on the behavioral manifestations of this "new category of parasomnia," which may lead to injuries to the patient or spouse due to aggressive REM

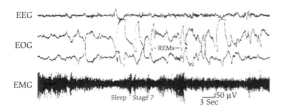

FIGURE 29.4 Sleep stage 7 was scored when a predominance of rapid eye movements was seen in conjunction with a low-amplitude, mixed-frequency electroencephalogram (ECG) and a tonically elevated electromyogram (EMG). EOG, electrooculogram. (From Guilleminault.[15])

sleep–related behavior often during attempted dream enactment.[26]

As a diagnosis, RBD was introduced into the *International Classification of Sleep Disorders* (*ICSD*) in 1990,[27] and since the current *ICSD-2*, polysomnographic confirmation of REM sleep without atonia is required.[28]

The first large RBD series of 96 patients was also published by Schenck and Mahowald in 1993.[29] In this article, the authors not only reported on their own case series but also summarized 70 cases of the world literature, which were published after its formal description in 1986. From this description, it became common knowledge that RBD affects predominantly elderly men and is associated with various neurological diseases.[29] Moreover, in 1996, the same group first demonstrated in a prospective follow-up of their original sample of 29 patients that 38% of idiopathic RBD patients progressed into a neurodegenerative disease.[30] In the following decade, further follow-up studies of several groups revealed even higher progression rates up to 65% depending on the observational period.[31-34] Nowadays it is common knowledge that RBD is a potential early nonmotor marker of a neurodegenerative disease.

SLEEP LABORATORY DIAGNOSIS OF REM SLEEP BEHAVIOR DISORDER

The *ICSD-2* established that the diagnosis of RBD requires demonstration of REM sleep without atonia (RWA) or excessive phasic muscle bursts by polysomnography.[28] In addition, patients need to have either a history of sleep-related injurious, potentially injurious, or disruptive behaviors by history or documentation of abnormal REM sleep behaviors during polysomnographic monitoring.[28] Possible scenarios allowing for an RBD diagnosis are provided in Table 29.1.

Only video-polysomnographic recording in the sleep laboratory allows for a sufficiently sensitive and specific diagnosis of RBD. Sleep history alone leads to a considerable number of false-positive and false-negative RBD cases since (1) nocturnal behaviors associated with obstructive sleep apnea or sleep-related seizures mimic RBD[35-37,38] and (2) a significant number of "true" RBD cases is missed by clinical interview alone.[39] This is even more pronounced in patients with Parkinson's disease.[40] Reasons for "history alone false negatives" may

Table 29.1 Possible Minimal Scenarios Allowing for a Definite Diagnosis of RBD According to ICSD-2 Criteria

SCENARIO	RBD BEHAVIORS		EMG ACTIVITY	
	History of sleep-related injurious, potentially injurious, or disruptive behaviors by history	Documentation of RBD behaviors during PSG monitoring	Excessive phasic muscle activity during REM in the chin or limb EMG	Excessive sustained muscle activity during REM in the chin EMG
A	+	–	+	–
B	+	–	–	+
C	–	+	+	–
D	–	+	–	+

Note that a substantial proportion of RBD patients fulfill both categories in the sections "RBD behaviors" and/or "EMG activity".

be milder disease severity, rare manifestations, the patient's unawareness, or lack of an attentive bed partner. A correct diagnosis of RBD by both history and video-polysomnography is of utmost importance given the risk for injury, including life-threatening injury to patient and spouse,[41] and also because of considerably increased risk for the future emergence of a parkinsonian disorder in older adults.[31,32,34,42] During the last several years, considerable progress in quantitative video-polysomnography methods for RBD has been made to improve diagnostic accuracy.

Analysis of Polysomnography in REM Sleep Behavior Disorder

A correct sleep laboratory diagnosis of RBD involves specific analysis of video-polysomnography. This includes quantitative EMG analysis of RWA and detailed analysis and classification of abnormal REM sleep behaviors in the video. RWA is defined as the "EMG finding of excessive amounts of sustained or intermittent elevation of submental EMG tone or excessive phasic submental or (upper or lower) limb EMG twitching."[28] Except in research settings, objective quantification of muscle activity is not performed and definition of "excessive" is arbitrarily chosen by each scorer. Moreover, no rules or at least consensus on scoring of muscle activity in RBD exists. In addition, up to now, different recommendations have been made for EMG montages to detect EMG muscle activity

related or unrelated to RBD behavioral episodes, but it has not been specifically studied, which is the most appropriate EMG montage for RBD detection. Another important issue is that "abnormal" or "excessive" EMG activity is not adequately defined.

Manual Scoring Methods for REM Sleep without Atonia

The first manual scoring method for quantification of EMG activity has been published by Lapierre and Montplaisir in 1992.[43] The authors differentiated between phasic and tonic EMG activity measured in the submental EMG. Phasic EMG activity was rated for each 2-second mini-epoch and was defined as any EMG increase with an amplitude exceeding four times the background EMG activity lasting between 0.1 and 5 seconds. Each 20-second epoch was scored as tonic or atonic depending on whether tonic chin EMG activity was present for more or less than 50% of the epoch. The percentage of phasic EMG activity was calculated as the percentage of mini-epochs containing phasic EMG activity divided by the total number of mini-epochs. The percentage of REM atonia was defined as percentage of epochs with REM atonia divided by all REM epochs.[43] This scoring method was used in only a slightly modified manner over the last years by various groups focusing on analysis of EMG activity in RBD.[44–48] Most authors outside Canada used 3-second mini-epochs and 30-second epochs instead of 2-second mini-epochs and 20-second epochs.[44–47] Moreover, definition of the amplitude criterion for phasic EMG activity slightly varied between two and four times the background EMG activity.[45,46] In 2007, the Montplaisir scoring system was introduced into the AASM manual for the scoring of sleep and associated events.[49] It is an easily applicable and reliable manual scoring system. Increased tonic EMG activity is scored in the chin, whereas excessive phasic EMG activity can be scored either in the chin or the limb muscles. One potential drawback is that it does not account for the absolute number of phasic EMG potentials per mini-epoch but categorizes phasic EMG activity in 3-second mini-epochs as either positive meaning this mini-epoch contains phasic EMG activity or negative meaning this mini-epoch contains no phasic EMG activity. In addition, differentiation into phasic and tonic EMG activity sometimes turns out to be challenging. To account for this issue, and to account for muscle activity with a duration between 5 and 15 seconds, which is disregarded/ignored in most other scoring systems for REM muscle activity, the SINBAR group[50] introduced the new measure "any" EMG activity to simplify the scoring process of chin EMG activity. "Any" comprises all EMG activity exceeding 0.1 milliseconds with an amplitude of at least twice the background EMG irrespective of the total EMG event duration. Apart from this classification system, two different classification systems[51–55] have been published. In contrast to the Montplaisir system,[43] Eisensehr et al. differentiated between what they denominated "short-lasting" and "long-lasting" muscle activity. They defined a 10-second epoch as containing short-lasting muscle activity when 10 or more short-lasting EMG events between 0.1 and 0.5 seconds duration were present within this epoch. Long-lasting muscle activity was scored for each 10-second epoch in which persistently increased muscle activity was present for at least 1 second cumulatively (duration of each single long-lasting event was defined to be at least 0.5 second).[51] Eisensehr et al. chose the terms "short-lasting" and "long-lasting" for simplification, because the otherwise used terms "phasic" and "tonic" have been applied differently in different contexts. Puzzlingly, the duration of long-lasting EMG activity is defined to be very short with 1 second. Apart from this, the Eisensehr system uses 10-second epochs (and not 20- or 30-second epochs and 2- and

3-second mini-epochs as most other systems) and could be seen as arbitrary due to a rough categorization because, for example, eight phasic events per 10-second epoch are scored as "0" when interpreting muscle activity, whereas 10 phasic events per 10-second epoch are scored as "1."[51] Another method was introduced by Bliwise et al., who examined exclusively phasic EMG activity, which the authors called "phasic electromyographic metric (PEM)." Phasic EMG metric was defined for each 2.5-second mini-epoch as any EMG increase of more than four times the background EMG lasting ≥ 0.1 second with a detectable return to baseline within the 2.5-second mini-epoch.[52–54] The Bliwise method is another approach focusing on phasic EMG activity. This system may lead to false-negative results since it arbitrarily demands a detectable return to baseline within the individual 2.5-second mini-epoch independent of the total duration to count this mini-epoch as "1." For further details of the published manual scoring methods, see Table 29.2.

Since manual scoring of RWA is very time consuming, computer-assisted algorithms for scoring of RWA in the chin have been developed.[55–59] Up to now, this software is only used for research purposes and has not entered clinical routine. Moreover, introduction of these scoring algorithms for scoring of RWA in the limb muscles, which seems to be a necessary further step, has not been performed so far.

Electromyographic Derivations

There is some controversy on which is the most appropriate combination of EMG derivations to investigate RBD in a clinical or research setting. In previous studies, EMG montages varied from using the chin EMG alone,[43,44] over chin and lower-extremity muscles,[48,51] to montages containing chin as well as upper- and lower-extremity muscles.[45–47,52–54] The SINBAR group undertook a study to investigate which combination of muscles provided the highest rates of phasic EMG activity by still acceptable number of EMG channels.[45] In this study, 13 different muscles of the body were investigated.[45] Results suggested that a combination of the chin (mentalis muscle), one muscle of the upper extremities (flexor digitorum superficialis), and one muscle of the lower extremities (extensor digitorum brevis) provided the highest rates of phasic EMG activity and therefore seems to be the most appropriate montage for

Table 29.2 Summary of Scoring Methods for Quantification of EMG Activity during REM Sleep

STUDIES	MUSCLES WHICH WERE INVESTIGATED	TYPE OF MUSCLE ACTIVITY	DEFINITION OF EVENTS FOR ANALYSIS		EPOCH
			DURATION	AMPLITUDE	
Bliwise 2006, 2008, 2010[52-54]	Mental, biceps, tibialis anterior	"Phasic electromyographic metric" (PEM)	≥ 0.1 s and detectable return to baseline within 2.5 s mini-epoch	> 4× background	2.5 s
Consens 2005[44]	Chin	Phasic Tonic RBD score	0.1-5 s 50% tonic Phasic + tonic score / 2	> 4× background not indicated	3/30 s
Eisensehr 2003[51]	Mental, submental, tibialis anterior	Short-lasting Long lasting	> 10 short-lasting events with a duration between 0.1 and 5 s > 0.5 s for more than 1 s of epoch	50% amplitude increase 50% amplitude increase	10 s
Frauscher 2008[45]	Mental, sternocleidomastoid, deltoid, biceps, flexor dig. sup., abductor pollicis brev, thoracolumbar paraspinal, rectus femoris, gastrocnemius, tibialis anterior, extensor dig. brevis	Phasic	0.1-5 s	> 2× background	3 s
Iranzo 2011[46]	Mental, flexor dig. sup., tibialis anterior, extensor dig. brevis	Phasic	0.1-5 s	> 2× background	3 s
Frauscher 2012[43]	Mental, sternocleidomastoid, biceps, flexor dig. sup, tibialis anterior, extensor dig. brevis	Phasic Tonic Any	0.1-5 s > 50% tonic EMG ≥ 0.1 s	> 2× background > 2× background /10 μV > 2× background	3/30 s
Lapierre & Montplaisier 1992[48]	Submental	Phasic Tonic	0.1-5 s > 50% tonic EMG	> 4× background not indicated	2/20 s
Montplaisir 2010	Submental, tibialis anterior	Phasic Tonic LMSI	0.1-10 s > 50% tonic EMG 0.1-10 s	> 4× background > 2× background /10 μV > 4× background	2/20 s
Zhang 2008[47]	Chin, extensor forearm, tibialis anterior	Phasic Tonic 0.1-5 s REMREEA	0.1-5 s > 50% tonic % of phasic and tonic MA	> 4× background > 4× background	3/30 s

s, second; MA muscle activity; dig, digitorum; sup, superficialis; LMSI, leg movement in sleep index; REMREA, REM related EMG activity

RBD detection.[45] A modified version of the original SINBAR montage consists of the mentalis, the flexor digitorum superficialis, and the tibialis anterior instead of the extensor digitorum brevis muscles. In a second step, the authors showed that by using the SINBAR montage the majority of motor events in the video are captured.[46]

Normative Studies on Quantitative Electromyographic Analysis

For a sensitive and specific diagnosis of RBD, cutoff values for quantification of muscle activity are a prerequisite. Since RBD is a potential premotor sign of a neurodegenerative disease[31,32,34,42] and false-positive diagnosis therefore has a substantial negative impact, high specificity is of much more impact than sensitivity. In a controlled bicentric study of 60 patients, the SINBAR group[50] investigated cutoff values for phasic, tonic, and "any" EMG activity in 11 different body muscles, which were selected according to a prior study on EMG activity rates in RBD.[45] The authors demonstrated that the measure "any" EMG activity, which is very easy to apply in clinical routine, shows similar discriminative power to phasic and tonic EMG activity, which is sometimes challenging to distinguish. When choosing a specificity of 100%, the 3-second mini-epoch cutoff for a diagnosis of RBD was 18% for "any" EMG activity in the mentalis (AUC 0.990). Discriminative power was higher in upper limbs (100% specificity, AUC 0.987–9.997) than in lower limb muscles (100% specificity, AUC 0.813–0.852), which may be due to overlapping motor phenomena such as fragmentary myoclonus and periodic leg movements in sleep. Since the chin is very prone to artifacts and RBD abnormal movements typically correspond to movements of the limbs, we combined "any" EMG activity in the mentalis with both phasic flexor digitorum superficialis muscles for the detection of RBD and found a cutoff of 32% (AUC 0.998). This cutoff value was true for both subjects with iRBD and PD-RBD. Another study by Montplaisir et al. investigated cutoff values for phasic and tonic EMG activity in the chin gathered from 80 idiopathic RBD patients and compared them to sex- and age-matched controls.[48] In contrast to their previous paper,[43] they used a duration criterion for phasic EMG activity between 0.1 and 10 seconds. The authors demonstrated a total correct classification of 82% for a percentage of ≥30% of 20-second epochs containing tonic chin EMG activity, and a total correct classification of 84% for a percentage of ≥15% of 2-second mini-epochs containing phasic EMG activity.[48] The latter is very similar to that of the measure of "any" EMG activity in the mentalis muscle for 3-second mini-epochs. Concerning night-to-night variability, Zhang et al. examined how many nights have to be recorded for detection of RBD.[47] They demonstrated that a single night of video-PSG was adequate for the diagnosis of RBD in most clinical patients and that the combination of PSG and video analysis further enhanced the detection rate of RBD.[47]

Videographic Analysis of REM Sleep Behavior Disorder

Studies of video event classification in RBD range from investigations aiming to perform a detailed video characterization in order to develop a motor event classification system[46,60,61] to studies using ad-hoc sytems for video analysis for specific research purposes.[47,62–65] In addition to this descriptive approach, there are studies aiming to rate RBD severity based on videographic analysis.[66,67]

Our group conducted several studies to classify video events in RBD.[46,60,61] In a time-synchronized video-polysomnographic analysis of a total of 1392 motor events, Frauscher et al. scored every single motor event according to the type of movement, the topographical distribution, and the duration. Motor events were frequent in RBD and consisted of predominantly minor motor activity. Violent behaviors only made 3.6% of all behaviors.[60] Based on this meticulous analysis, the authors developed an easy-to-use scoring system of motor activity in RBD, the Innsbruck video classification system for RBD.[61] This system differentiates between minor motor activity (small jerky or nonjerky excursions that include not more than one body region and usually would not be noticed by a sleeping bed partner) and major jerks/movements (simple movements of larger excursion of the body being mostly of myoclonic nature that typically involve the trunk), scenic/complex behaviors (apparent "acting out" of dream contents or movements different from elementary simple events in terms of complexity of action), as well as violent behaviors (forceful and vehement movements that could potentially injure a bed partner). In REM sleep, REMs occur in bursts alternating with REM sleep without REMs. Based on our clinical experience that major motor activity in RBD is associated with REM sleep with REMs, we investigated the association between REM sleep with REMs, phasic and tonic EMG activity, and motor events. Major motor activity of RBD was closely associated with REM sleep with REMs, whereas background jerking occurred throughout REM sleep.[61] This finding could point to a potential gate control mechanism of REM sleep with REMs for the manifestation of elaborate or violent behaviors in RBD.[61] Results of this study were later confirmed by Manni et al.,[65] who differentiated between primitive motor episodes (simple jerky movements with no apparent purpose) and purposeful motor episodes (e.g., gesturing, punching, fighting-like behavior), with verbalizations.[65] All aforementioned studies contributed to a better understanding of the broad spectrum of motor events in RBD and helped to develop a simple easy-to-apply video classification system. Moreover, they demonstrated a close temporal association between major motor activity and REM sleep with REMs.

The first polysomnographic study in RBD incorporating preliminary video results for RBD characterization dates back to the late 1990s.[62] The authors differentiated between simple events (e.g., twitches, grimaces, chewing automatisms) and complex events (e.g., gesticulations, searching movements, aggressive behavior).[62] This elementary classification system was also applied by Fantini et al., who investigated the therapeutic effect of pramipexole in RBD.[63]

Based on reports of spouses of Parkinson's disease patients, de Cock et al. investigated the hypothesis that restoration of motor control occurs during REM sleep in patients with both Parkinson's disease and REM sleep behavior disorder.[64] They performed a videographic analysis of RBD behavioral episodes and classified movements according to the nature, the body location, body side, and the dynamics of the movements. They reported that in contrast to waking movements, RBD-related movements were "surprisingly fast, although jerky, coordinated and symmetrical, without obvious sign of parkinsonism." The authors speculated that this may be due to cortical generation of RBD motor behaviors that bypass the extrapyramidial motor system.[64] Similar motor improvement was also shown for RBD in multiple-system atrophy.[68]

The Innsbruck video classification for RBD was slightly modified by Arnulf's group.[69,70] Leclair-Visonneau et al. demonstrated that the direction of gaze and the direction of action taken during RBD behavioral manifestations are highly correlated.[69] Cygan performed a night-to-night comparison of video-polysomnographic results[70] and found in agreement with other groups [60,66] significant night-to-night variability in motor events in RBD.[69] Zhang et al. used a similar system differentiating between simple motor events, significant movements, other unclassified movements, and vocalizations.[47] They replicated that significant movements occur rarely in a sleep laboratory setting. In addition, they showed that night-to-night variability of motor events is high.[47] Other studies focused on RBD severity or how to translate RBD-related movements into severity. Iranzo et al. rated RBD severity according to videographic manifestation of RBD in the sleep laboratory.[66] They differentiated between mild (e.g., excessive limb jerking with minimal separation from the body, quiet vocalizations), moderate (e.g., gesturing, raising the arms, vocalizations), and severe RBD severity (e.g., waving the arms vigorously, kicking, punching, loud vocalizations).[66] A new time-efficient approach to score RBD severity is from Sixel-Döring et al., who developed an RBD severity scale for routine use.[67] They differentiated between slight movements or jerks (rated as "1"), movements involving proximal extremities (rated as "2"), and movements involving axial involvement (rated as "3"), as well as the presence or absence of vocalizations.[67] For further details of the studies reported, see Table 29.3. In contrast to studies translating RBD behaviors into RBD severity, other severity measures are solely based on history. Consens et al.[44] designed a questionnaire rating the severity of RBD by including basically the former *ICSD* criteria. It comprised seven items, which had to be rated according to the symptom frequency as well as symptom severity. The average score (each question was rated from 0 to 1) was then used as the overall RBD symptom score. Another severity scale was developed and validated by the Hong Kong group.[71] This scale included 13 items. Severity was measured according to the recent 1-year item frequency and ranged from 0 to 5 for each item. The authors suggested using this scale to monitor the disease course of RBD in clinical follow-up investigations.[71]

Table 29.3 Studies Involving Videographic Analysis in REM Sleep Behavior Disorder

AUTHOR	N (P/C)	AIM OF THE STUDY	VIDEOGRAPHIC METHODS	VIDEOGRAPHIC OUTCOME
Cygan[70]	7	To investigate night-to-night variability of phasic, tonic EMG activity, and motor events	Real-time video analysis (minor, major, complex, scenic events, vocalizations)	In contrast to tonic EMG activity, phasic EMG activity/motor events show significant night-to-night variability
De Cock[64]	51	To investigate the abnormal RBD movements in PD	Video-analysis of behavioral episodes were rated by several scorers	RBD movements may be generated in the cortex bypassing the EPMS
De Cock[68]	22	To investigate motor improvement during RBD in MSA	Video movement analysis, rating by several scorers	Surprising transient disappearance of Parkinsonism during RBD in MSA
Fantini[63]	5	To evaluate the effect of PPX on RBD	Video-PSG analysis (simple vs. complex)	Significant reduction of simple, but not complex motor events under PPX therapy
Frauscher[60]	5/5	To systematically describe motor events in RBD	Real-time video analysis	High number of motor events (majority: small movements, rare: scenic, violent behaviors)
Frauscher[61]	8/8	To systematically analyze the association between REM sleep with REMs, phasic EMG activity, and motor events in RBD	Combined analysis of EMG activity and time synchronous videographic analysis	Association of major motor activity in RBD and phasic REM sleep
Iranzo 2005[66]	110	To compare clinical and video-PSG features of iRBD vs. RBD due to PD/MSA	RBD severity classification (mild, moderate, severe)	iRBD patients had more severe RBD than patient PD and MSA patients
Iranzo & Frauscher[46]	11	To evaluate the SINBAR EMG montage for detection of RBD episodes	Combined analysis of phasic EMG activity and time synchronous video analysis	Detection of majority of motor activity in RBD by the SINBAR EMG montage

(Continued)

Table 29.3 Continued

AUTHOR	N (P/C)	AIM OF THE STUDY	VIDEOGRAPHIC METHODS	VIDEOGRAPHIC OUTCOME
Leclair-Visonneau[69]	56/17	To use the model of RBD to investigate if the eyes scan dream images during REM sleep	Combined analysis of REMs and behavior during PSG according to Frauscher et al. 2007	Tough link between the dream action during RBD and the direction of the gaze
Manni[65]	12	To investigate if sudden-onset motor behavioral episodes in RBD are associated with phasic events of REM sleep	Combined analysis of EMG activity and time synchroneous videographic analysis	Association of RBD behavioral episodes and phasic REM sleep
Oudiette[97]	24	To report non-violent RBD behaviors and to evaluate their frequency by interview	Description of video-behavioral episodes	Nonviolent elaborative behaviors may also occur in RBD
Sforza[62]	6	To report PSG findings in RBD	PSG under video-tape monitoring (simple vs. complex events)	Presence of behavioral episodes during REM sleep
Sixel-Döring[67]	20	To develop a PSG video-based scale for RBD severity	Rating of movements (1–3) and presence of vocalizations (0,1)	RBD severity scale is reliable and easy-to-use
Zhang[47]	55	To assess whether one night is enough for RBD diagnosis	Video analysis (simple, significant, unclassified, vocalization)	1 night of PSG is adequate for RBD diagnosis Diagnostic accuracy is increased by video

EMG, electromyography; i, idiopathic; MSA, multiple-system atrophy; PD, Parkinson's disease, PPX, pramipexole; PSG, polysomnography; RBD, REM sleep behavior disorder.

TREATMENT OF REM SLEEP BEHAVIOR DISORDER

Symptomatic Treatment of REM Sleep Behavior Disorder

Except for a single very small study, no randomized controlled trials for treatment of RBD have been performed. Current treatment options are based on case series, and the comparatively best evidence still exists for low-dose clonazepam and melatonin. Other treatment options that have been reported in the literature, partly in single case reports, will also be discussed. Apart from clonazepam and melatonin, levodopa and dopamine agonists, cholinesterase inhibitors, and atypical neuroleptics have been proposed by some authors for the treatment of RBD, but the evidence is controversial, as will be discussed.

Clonazepam

Clonazepam is generally considered "highly effective for the treatment of RBD." It is estimated that 90% of the patients respond to a dose of 0.5–1 mg.[72] Schenck and Mahowald also note that the response to clonazepam is usually within the first week, and the development of tolerance to the beneficial effects on RBD is infrequent, so that sustained benefit of treatment can be expected. On the other hand, they note that there is a "hierarchical benefit" with initial suppression of sleep motor activity, then reoccurrence of twitching, talking, and more complex behavior but still persisting control of problematic, vigorous behaviors and nightmares. Relapse usually occurs after discontinuation of clonazepam.[72] The authors reported the first small case series ($n = 5$) with clonazepam treatment of RBD as early as 1986, with a good response.[26] In an update of their patient cohort, they reported that 90% of 67 patients responded completely or at least partially to clonazepam.[29] In the meantime, this finding was confirmed by various groups.[73,74] Data on dose increase of clonazepam over time are conflicting.[30,74] A series from Turkey on 35 patients with RBD also reported a preponderantly positive response, but exact numbers were not given, and apparently "a few patients" took the medication only occasionally due to daytime effects. Polysomnography was not performed in that study.[75] Despite these excellent treatment results, some patients do not respond, and side effects of clonazepam treatment have been reported in up to 50% by Anderson and Shneerson.[76] In case of clonazepam administration, patients should be carefully monitored for the potential development or aggravation of sleep apnea,[77] which is a frequent comorbid condition in patients with Parkinson's disease.

Melatonin

The first RBD patient treated with melatonin was reported by Kunz in 1997.[78] He had a positive response and a gradual return of symptoms after discontinuation.

Two years later, the same author reported six patients with RBD, five of whom had dramatic clinical improvement with reduction of REM sleep without atonia and movement time during REM sleep in polysomnography.[79] Takeuchi reported in 2001 a larger series of 25 patients treated with melatonin[80]; 13 of them improved,

10 had even a marked improvement in polysomnography with doses from 3–9 mg, and partial restoration of REM atonia in polysomnography. It must be noted, that five of the patients were co-treated with clonazepam. In 2003, Boeve and coworkers[81] reported on an RBD patient series of 14 (seven dementia with Lewy bodies, three parkinsonism, two multiple-system atrophy, two narcolepsy). Six had an incomplete response to clonazepam previously, and cognitive impairment was present in five; two had side effects with clonazepam, one had sleep apnea, and one had narcolepsy and was therefore not treated with clonazepam. RBD was controlled in six patients, significantly improved in further four and relapsed in two, unchanged in one and worse in one. Seven of these patients were on co-treatment with clonazepam (0.5–1 mg). Eight patients had continuous benefit after 1 year. The mean doses used were 3–9 mg.

Kunz and coworkers also reported the first double-blind crossover study of melatonin treatment versus placebo in eight patients with RBD. Compared to placebo, melatonin improved subjective (Clinical Global Impression) and objective (REM muscle atonia) correlates of RBD.[82]

Levodopa and Dopamine Agonists

Tan and coworkers reported in 1996 three patients with RBD preceding the clinical onset of PD. After levodopa treatment they noted a significant improvement or complete abolition of complex, vigorous movements in all patients and reduction of vivid dreams in one.[83] Polysomnography was not performed and so patients with only occasional behaviors might have been misclassified as improved. A Brazilian report on a patient with severe head trauma 10 years ago with multiple lesions in cortical and cerebellar areas was reported to have RBD in polysomnography with agitated and aggressive behavior during REM sleep. When treatment with levodopa 100/25 mg was initiated, the behavior was thought to improve, and also no more periodic leg movements were observed.[84]

In 2003 Fantini et al. performed a careful study with detailed analysis of muscle activity during REM sleep in eight patients with idiopathic RBD who were treated with pramipexole.[63] All patients underwent two polysomnographic recordings (baseline and after treatment). Fantini found a sustained reduction in the frequency or intensity of behaviors as well as a reduction of tonic EMG activity, but no change in phasic EMG activity and periodic limb movement index.[63] Schmidt and coworkers reported a case series of 10 RBD, who had a sustained reduction of "frequency and severity" of RBD on pramipexole.[85] This study did not include polysomnographic evaluation. In contrast to these studies, Kumru and coworkers did not find an improvement in tonic or phasic EMG activity or behaviors in a consecutive study on pramipexole treatment in 11 Parkinson patients with RBD.[86]

Cholinesterase Inhibitors

In a single case report it was reported that rivastigmine improved the sleep profile in dementia with Lewy bodies with RBD.[87] Ringman and coworkers reported on three patients (one possible Alzheimer's disease, one iRBD, one RBD with memory impairment) treated with donepezil; one was said to have a marked decrease in dreams and agitation, one was found to have a long-term benefit, and the other one was said to have a long-lasting reduction in parasomnic spells. Doses up to 15 mg were used.[88] Massironi and coworkers reported on drug treatment of RBD in dementia with Lewy bodies. They had three patients with RBD, treated with clonazepam or donepezil. One patient was unresponsive to clonazepam but was found to respond well to donepezil; two were unresponsive to donepezil but responded well to clonazepam. The study did not include polysomnography, and it is difficult to judge from the report whether all had definite RBD (e.g., one patient was said to have called "fire, fire," covered with sweat and begged to leave the home, which would possibly not correspond to a classical RBD manifestation).[89] In summary, there is weak evidence for a possible beneficial effect of cholinesterase inhibitors on RBD. On the contrary, a recent case suggests reversible induction of RBD by rivastigimine.[90]

Others

In previous years some antidepressants have also been used. One patient with RBD improved with desipramine.[91] Bush and coworkers used tricyclic antidepressants in a dog diagnosed with RBD, but the dog also had seizures and generalized anxiety disorder.[92] A single case report exists on successful treatment of RBD with sodium oxybate,[93] which remains to be confirmed in future studies. Further anecdotal reports of improvement of RBD exist for benzodiazepines other than clonazepam, carbamazepine, clonidine, and zopiclone.[94]

REM Sleep Behavior Disorder Exacerbated or Aggravated by Drugs

Several drugs have been reported to induce, exacerbate, aggravate, or unmask RBD: tricyclic antidepressants (amitryptiline, clomipramine, desipramine, imipramine, nortriptyline, trimipramine), selective serotonin reuptake inhibitors (citalopram, fluoxetine, paroxetine, sertraline), monoamine oxidase inhibitors (phenelzine), serotonin–norepinephrine reuptake inhibitors (mirtazapine, venlafaxine), and bisoprolol and selegiline.[95] The strongest evidence for drug-induced RBD exists for clomipramine, selegiline, and phenelzine.[95] Some of the other studies were single case reports without polysomnographic confirmation of RBD diagnosis. The beta blocker bisoprolol was reported to induce RBD in two cases.[96] On the other hand, in a large case series of 703 sleep laboratory patients, beta blocker intake was not associated with RBD in 34 RBD cases.[39] If the time course of RBD occurrence suggests any possible relationship with drug intake, the potentially inducing agent should be withdrawn. Buproprion is thought by some experts to be the antidepressant of choice to treat depression in RBD subjects.

REM Sleep Behavior Disorder Treatment: Conclusions and Sleep Environment

In summary, the evidence for treatment of RBD is still limited and largely empirical. If the RBD behaviors are very mild and occur only sporadically, and do not bother or endanger the patient or bed partner, initiation of drug treatment may be delayed. In most cases, low-dose clonazepam (0.5–1 mg) will be the first step in RBD treatment. As an alternative, or if clonazepam is ineffective, or contraindicated, melatonin (mostly 3–5 mg) can be tried. Potentially aggravating substances should be discontinued. The evidence for all other drugs that have been tried is limited, and sometimes contradictory. In cases with advanced PD, drug-induced psychosis, and severe RBD, atypical neuroleptics (quetiapine and clozapine) may prove useful, but there are no studies that have adequately addressed behaviors due to drug-induced psychosis and RBD behaviors.

On a behavioral level, the importance of measures to create and maintain a safe sleep environment cannot be overemphasized. Patients and bed partners need to understand that the dangers in RBD arise from the mismatch between enacted dream content and real environment. At home, the bed should be low, or even the mattress should be placed on the floor. The head of the bed (and if present, other parts) should be covered with sponge or cushions. Any objects with sharp edges should be removed far enough from the bed (bedside tables, bedside glass lamps) as should furniture which may be unwillingly torn down such as bookshelves. Patients with iRBD should also know that they need to inform any new bed partner about the condition.

REM Sleep Behavior Disorder: Candidate Disorder for Neuroprotection

On a final note: In the future, RBD will not only be a target of symptomatic treatment. The fact, that RBD can occur decades before manifestation of a neurodegenerative disease[31,34,42] opens a window into an early otherwise presymptomatic state of neurodegeneration. It makes also a rewarding target for neuroprotective treatment once that becomes available.

REFERENCES

1. Jouvet M, Delorme F. [Locus coeruleus et sommeil paradoxal]. *CR Soc Biol* 1965;159:895–9.
2. Sastre JP, Jouvet M. [Le comportement onirique du chat]. *Physiol Behav* 1979;22:979–89.
3. Hendricks JC, Morrison AR, Mann GL. Different behaviors during paradoxical sleep without atonia depend on pontine lesion site. *Brain Res* 1982;239:81–105.
4. Aserinsky E, Kleitman N. Regularly occurring periods of eye motility, and concomitant phenomena, during sleep. *Science* 1953;118:273–4.
5. Lasègue, C. [Le délire alcoolique n'est pas un délir, mais un rêve]. *Arch Gen Med* 1881;88:513–86.
6. Stern M, Roffwarg H, Duvoisin R. The Parkinsonian tremor in sleep. *J Nerves Mental Dis* 1968;147:202–10.

7. Petre-Quadens O, Sfaello Z, van Bogaert L, et al. Sleep study in SSPE (first results). *Neurology* 1968;18:60–8.
8. Traczynska-Kubin D, Atzef E, Petre-Quandens O. [Le somneil dans la maladie de Parkinson]. *Acta Neurol Psychiatr Belg* 1969;69:727–33.
9. Akindele MO, Evans JI, Oswald I. Mono-amine oxidase inhibitors, sleep and mood. *EEG Clin Neurophysiol* 1970;29:47–56.
10. Passouant P, Cadilhac J, Ribstein M. [Les privations de sommeil avec mouvements oculaires par les anti-depresseurs]. *Rev Neurol* 1972;127:173–92.
11. Schott B, Michel D, Mouret J, et al. Monoamines et regulation de la vigilance II—syndromes lésionnels du système nerveux central. *Rev Neurol (Paris)* 1972;127:157–71.
12. De Barros-Ferreira BDM, Chodkiewicz J, Lairy GC, et al. Disorganized relations of tonic and phasic events of REM sleep in a case of brain stem tumor. *Electroenceph Clin Neurophysiol* 1975;38:203–71.
13. Mouret J. Difference in sleep in patients with Parkinson's disease. *Electroenceph Clin Neurophysiol* 1975;38:653–7.
14. Tachibana M, Tanaka K, Hishikawa Y, et al. A sleep study of acute psychotic states due to alcohol and meprobamate addiction. In: Weitzman ED, ed. *Advances in Sleep Research.* New York: Spectrum; 1975:175–205.
15. Guilleminault C, Raynal D, Takahashi S, et al. Evaluation of short-term and long-term treatment of the narcolepsy syndrome with clomipramine hydrochloride. *Acta Neurol Scand* 1976;54:71–87.
16. Atsumi Y, Kojima T, Matsu'ura M, et al. [Polygraphic study of altered consciousness—effect of biperiden on EEG and EOG.] *Annu Rep Res Psychotrop Drugs* 1977;9:171–8.
17. Sugita Y, Tanaka K, Teshima Y, et al. [A study on the physiopathological mechanism of withdrawal delirium in patients with chronic drug intoxication.] *Clin Electroenceph (Osaka)* 1978;20:606–14.
18. Tanaka, K. [Polygraphic study of nocturnal sleep in patients with acute alcoholic psychosis.] *Med J Osaka Univ* 1978;30:287–308.
19. Bental E, Lavie P, Sharf B. Severe hypermobility during sleep in treatment of cataplexy with clomipramine. *Israel J Med Sci* 1979;15:607–9.
20. Isono G, Ishii K, Shibata Y, et al. [REM sleep without muscle atonia in a case of bilateral accoustic tumor.] *Seishin Igaku* 1979;21:1221–8.

21. Laffont F, Autret A, Minz M, et al. [Polygraphic study of nocturnal sleep in three degenerative diseases: ALS, olivo-ponto-cerebellar atrophy, and progressive supranuclear palsy.] *Waking Sleeping* 1979;3:17–30.

22. Minami R, Harada M. [The relationship between nocturnal delirium and REM sleep.] *Clin Electroenceph (Osaka)* 1979;21:315–23.

23. Minz M, Autret A, Laffont F, et al. A study on sleep in amyotrophic lateral sclerosis. *Biomedicine* 1979;30:40–6.

24. Tanaka K, Kameda H, Sugity Y, et al. [A case with pentazocine dependence developing delirium on withdrawal.] *Seishin Shinkeigaku Zasshi* 1979;81:289–99.

25. Tachibana N. [Historical overview of REM sleep behavior disorder in relation to its pathophysiology.] *Brain Nerve* 2009;61:558–68.

26. Schenck CH, Bundlie SR, Ettinger MG, et al. Chronic behavioral disorders of human REM sleep: a new category of parasomnia. *Sleep* 1986;9:293–308.

27. Diagnostic Classification Steering Committee, Thorpy MJ. *International Classification of Sleep Disorders: Diagnostic and Coding Manual.* Rochester, MN: American Sleep Disorders Assocation; 1990.

28. American Academy of Sleep Medicine. *International Classification of Sleep Disorders. Diagnostic and Coding Manual.* 2nd ed. Westchester, IL: American Academy of Sleep Medicine; 2005.

29. Schenck CH, Hurwitz TD, Mahowald MW. REM sleep behaviour disorder: an update on a series of 96 patients and a review of the world literature. *J Sleep Res* 1993;2:224–31.

30. Schenck CH, Bundlie SR, Mahowald MW. Delayed emergence of a Parkinsonian disorder in 38% of 29 older men initially diagnosed with idiopathic rapid eye movement sleep behavior disorder. *Neurology* 1996;46:388–93.

31. Schenck CH, Bundlie SR, Mahowald MW. (2003) REM behavior disorder (RBD): delayed emergence of parkinsonism and/or dementia in 65% of older men initially diagnosed with idiopathic RBD, and an analysis of the minimum and maximum tonic and/or phasic electromyographic abnormalities found during REM sleep. *Sleep* 2004;26(Suppl):A316.

32. Iranzo A, Molinuevo JL, Santamaría J, et al. Rapid eye movement sleep behaviour disorder as an early marker for a neurodegenerative disorder: a descriptive study. *Lancet Neurol* 2006;5:572–7.

33. Tippmann Peikert M, Olson EJ, Boeve B, et al. Idiopathic REM sleep behavior disorder: a follow-up of 39 patients. *Sleep* 2006;29(Suppl):A272.

34. Postuma RB, Gagnon JF, Vendette M, et al. Quantifying the risk of neurodegenerative disease in idiopathic REM sleep behavior disorder. *Neurology* 2009;72:1296–300.

35. Nalamalapu U, Goldberg R, DiPhillipo M, et al. Behaviors simulating REM behavior disorder in patients with severe obstructive sleep apnea. *Sleep Res* 1996;25:311.

36. D'Cruz OF, Vaughn BV. Nocturnal seizures mimic REM sleep behavior disorder. *Am J Electroneurodiagn Technol* 1997;37:258–64.

37. Guilleminault C, Leger D, Philip P, et al. Nocturnal wandering and violence: review of a sleep clinic population. *J Forensic Sci* 1998;43:158–63.

38. Iranzo A, Santamaría J. Severe obstructive sleep apnea/hypopnea mimicking REM sleep behavior disorder. *Sleep* 2005;28:203–6.

39. Frauscher B, Gschliesser V, Brandauer E, et al. REM sleep behavior disorder in 703 sleep-disorder patients: the importance of eliciting a comprehensive sleep history. *Sleep Med* 2010;11:167–71.

40. Eisensehr I, v Lindeiner H, Jäger M, et al. REM sleep behavior disorder in sleep-disordered patients with versus without Parkinson's disease: is there a need for polysomnography? *J Neurol Sci* 2001;186:7–11.

41. Schenck CH, Lee SA, Bornemann MA, et al. Potentially lethal behaviors associated with rapid eye movement sleep behavior disorder: review of the literature and forensic implications. *J Forensic Sci* 2009;54:1475–84.

42. Claassen DO, Josephs KA, Ahlskog JE, et al. REM sleep behavior disorder preceding other aspects of synucleinopathies by up to half a century. *Neurology* 2010;75:494–9.

43. Lapierre O, Montplaisir J. Polysomnographic features of REM sleep behavior disorder: development of a scoring method. *Neurology* 1992;42:1371–4.

44. Consens FB, Chervin RD, Koeppe RA, et al. Validation of a polysomnographic score for REM sleep behavior disorder. *Sleep* 2005;28:993–7.

45. Frauscher B, Iranzo A, Högl B, et al. Quantification of electromyographic activity

during REM sleep in multiple muscles in REM sleep behavior disorder. *Sleep* 2008;31:724–31.

46. Iranzo A, Frauscher B, Santos H, et al. Usefulness of the SINBAR electromyographic montage to detect the motor and vocal manifestations occurring in REM sleep behavior disorder. *Sleep Med* 2011;12:284–8.

47. Zhang J, Lam SP, Ho CK, et al. Diagnosis of REM sleep behavior disorder by video-polysomnographic study: is one night enough? *Sleep* 2008;31:1179–85.

48. Montplaisir J, Gagnon JF, Fantini ML, et al. Polysomnographic diagnosis of idiopathic REM sleep behavior disorder. *Mov Disord* 2010;25:2044–51.

49. Iber C, Ancoli-Israel C, Chesson A, et al. *The AASM Manual for the Scoring of Sleep and Associated Events: Rules, Terminology and Technical Specifications.* Westchester, IL: American Academy of Sleep Medicine; 2007.

50. Frauscher B, Iranzo A, Gaig C, et al. Normative EMG values during REM sleep in REM sleep behavior disorder. *Sleep* 2012;35(6):835–47.

51. Eisensehr I, Linke R, Tatsch K, et al. Increased muscle activity during rapid eye movement sleep correlates with decrease of striatal presynaptic dopamine transporters. IPT and IBZM SPECT imaging in subclinical and clinically manifest idiopathic REM sleep behavior disorder, Parkinson's disease, and controls. *Sleep* 2003;26:507–12.

52. Bliwise DL, He L, Ansari FP, et al. Quantification of electromyographic activity during sleep: a phasic electromyographic metric. *J Clin Neurophysiol* 2006;23:59–67.

53. Bliwise DL, Rye DB. Elevated PEM (phasic electromyographic metric) rates identify rapid eye movement behavior disorder patients on nights without behavioral abnormalities. *Sleep* 2008;31:853–7.

54. Bliwise DL, Trotti LM, Greer SA, et al. Phasic muscle activity in sleep and clinical features of Parkinson disease. *Ann Neurol* 2010;68:353–9.

55. Burns JW, Consens F, Little RJ, et al. EMG variance during polysomnography as an assessment for REM sleep behavior disorder. *Sleep* 2007;30:1771–8.

56. Mayer G, Kesper K, Ploch T, et al. Quantification of tonic and phasic muscle activity in REM sleep behavior disorder. *J Clin Neurophysiol* 2008;25:48–55.

57. Ferri R, Manconi M, Plazzi G, et al. A quantitative statistical analysis of the submental muscle EMG amplitude during sleep in normal controls and patients with REM sleep behavior disorder. *J Sleep Res* 2008;17:89–100.

58. Ferri R, Rundo F, Manconi M, et al. Improved computation of the atonia index in normal controls and patients with REM sleep behavior disorder. *Sleep Med* 2010;11:947–9.

59. Kempfner J, Sorensen G, Zoetmulder M, et al. REM behaviour disorder detection associated with neurodegenerative diseases. *Conf Proc IEEE Eng Med Biol Soc* 2010;2010:5093–6.

60. Frauscher B, Gschliesser V, Brandauer E, et al. Video analysis of motor events in REM sleep behavior disorder. *Mov Disord* 2007;22:1464–70.

61. Frauscher B, Gschliesser V, Brandauer E, et al. The relation between abnormal behaviors and REM sleep microstructure in patients with REM sleep behavior disorder. *Sleep Med* 2009;10:174–81.

62. Sforza E, Zucconi M, Petronelli R, et al. REM sleep behavioral disorders. *Eur Neurol* 1988;28:295–300.

63. Fantini ML, Gagnon JF, Filipini D, et al. The effects of pramipexole in REM sleep behavior disorder. *Neurology* 2003;61:1418–20.

64. De Cock VC, Vidailhet M, Leu S, et al. Restoration of normal motor control in Parkinson's disease during REM sleep. *Brain* 2007;130:450–6.

65. Manni R, Terzaghi M, Glorioso M. Motor-behavioral episodes in REM sleep behavior disorder and phasic events during REM sleep. *Sleep* 2009;32:241–5.

66. Iranzo A, Santamaria J, Rya DB, et al. Characteristics of idiopathic REM sleep behavior disorder and that associated with MSA and PD. Neurology 2005;65:247–52.

67. Sixel-Döring F, Schweitzer M, Mollenhauer B, et al. Intraindividual variability of REM sleep behavior disorder in Parkinson's disease: a comparative assessment using a new REM sleep behavior disorder severity scale (RBDSS) for clinical routine. *J Clin Sleep Med* 2011;7:75–80.

68. De Cock VC, Debs R, Oudiette D, et al. The improvement of movement and speech during rapid eye movement sleep behaviour disorder in multiple system atrophy. *Brain* 2011;134:856–62.

69. Leclair-Visonneau L, Oudiette D, Gaymard B, et al. Do the eyes scan dream images during rapid eye movement sleep? Evidence from the

rapid eye movement sleep behaviour disorder model. *Brain* 2010;133:1737–46.

70. Cygan F, Oudiette D, Leclair-Visonneau L, et al. Night-to-night variability of muscle tone, movements, and vocalizations in patients with REM sleep behavior disorder. *J Clin Sleep Med* 2010;6:551–5.

71. Li SX, Wing YK, Lam SP, et al. Validation of a new REM sleep behavior disorder questionnaire (RBDQ-HK). *Sleep Med* 2010;11:43–8.

72. Mahowald MW, Schenck CH. REM sleep parasomnias. In: Kryger MH, Roth T, Dement WC, editors. *Principles and Practice of Sleep Medicine.* Philadelphia, PA: Elsevier Saunders; 2005:897–916.

73. Olson EJ, Boeve BF, Silber MH. Rapid eye movement sleep behaviour disorder: demographic, clinical and laboratory findings in 93 cases. *Brain* 2000;123:331–9.

74. Wing YK, Lam SP, Li SX, et al. REM sleep behaviour disorder in Hong Kong Chinese: clinical outcome and gender comparison. *J Neurol Neurosurg Psychiatry* 2008;79:1415–16.

75. Ozekmekçi S, Apaydin H, Kiliç E. Clinical features of 35 patients with Parkinson's disease displaying REM behavior disorder. *Clin Neurol Neurosurg* 2005;107:306–9.

76. Anderson KN, Shneerson JM. Drug treatment of REM sleep behavior disorder: the use of drug therapies other than clonazepam. *J Clin Sleep Med* 2009;5:235–9.

77. Schuld A, Kraus T, Haack M, et al. Obstructive sleep apnea syndrome induced by clonazepam in a narcoleptic patient with REM-sleep-behavior disorder. *J Sleep Res* 1999;8:321–2.

78. Kunz D, Bes F. Melatonin effects in a patient with severe REM sleep behavior disorder: case report and theoretical considerations. *Neuropsychobiology* 1997;36:211–14.

79. Kunz D, Bes F. Melatonin as a therapy in REM sleep behavior disorder patients: an open-labeled pilot study on the possible influence of melatonin on REM-sleep regulation. *Mov Disord* 1999;14:507–11.

80. Takeuchi N, Uchimura N, Hashizume Y, et al. Melatonin therapy for REM sleep behavior disorder. *Psychiatry Clin Neurosci* 2001;55:267–9.

81. Boeve BF, Silber MH, Ferman TJ. Melatonin for treatment of REM sleep behavior disorder in neurologic disorders: results in 14 patients. *Sleep Med* 2003;4:281–4.

82. Kunz D, Mahlberg R. A two-part, double-blind, placebo-controlled trial of exogenous melatonin in REM sleep behaviour disorder. *J Sleep Res* 2010;19:591–6.

83. Tan A, Salgado M, Fahn S. Rapid eye movement sleep behavior disorder preceding Parkinson's disease with therapeutic response to levodopa. *Mov Disord* 1996;11:214–16.

84. Rodrigues RN, Silva AA. [Excessive daytime sleepiness after traumatic brain injury: association with periodic limb movements and REM behavior disorder: case report]. *Arq Neuropsiquiatr* 2002;60:656–60.

85. Schmidt MH, Koshal VB, Schmidt HS. Use of pramipexole in REM sleep behavior disorder: results from a case series. *Sleep Med* 2006;7:418–23.

86. Kumru H, Iranzo A, Carrasco E, et al. Lack of effects of pramipexole on REM sleep behavior disorder in Parkinson disease. *Sleep* 2008;31:1418–21.

87. Grace JB, Walker MP, McKeith IG. A comparison of sleep profiles in patients with dementia with lewy bodies and Alzheimer's disease. *Int J Geriatr Psychiatry* 2000;15:1028–33.

88. Ringman JM, Simmons JH. Treatment of REM sleep behavior disorder with donepezil: a report of three cases. *Neurology* 2000;55:870–1.

89. Massironi G, Galluzzi S, Frisoni GB. Drug treatment of REM sleep behavior disorders in dementia with Lewy bodies. *Int Psychogeriatr* 2003;15:377–83.

90. Yeh SB, Yeh PY, Schenck CH. Rivastigmine-induced REM sleep behavior disorder (RBD) in a 88-year-old man with Alzheimer's disease. *J Clin Sleep Med* 2010;6:192–5.

91. Schenck CH, Boyd JL, Mahowald MW. A parasomnia overlap disorder involving sleepwalking, sleep terrors, and REM sleep behavior disorder in 33 polysomnographically confirmed cases. *Sleep* 1997;20:972–81.

92. Bush WW, Barr CS, Stecker MM, et al. Diagnosis of rapid eye movement sleep disorder with electroencephalography and treatment with tricyclic antidepressants in a dog. *J Am Anim Hosp Assoc* 2004;40:495–500.

93. Shneerson JM. Successful treatment of REM sleep behavior disorder with sodium oxybate. *Clin Neuropharmacol* 2009;32:158–9.

94. Aurora RN, Zak RS, Maganti RK, et al. Best practice guide for the treatment of REM sleep behavior disorder (RBD). *J Clin Sleep Med* 2010;6:85–95.
95. Hoque R, Chesson AL, Jr. Pharmacologically induced/exacerbated restless legs syndrome, periodic limb movements of sleep, and REM behavior disorder/REM sleep without atonia: literature review, qualitative scoring, and comparative analysis. *J Clin Sleep Med* 2010;6:79–83.
96. Iranzo A, Santamaria J. Bisoprolol-induced rapid eye movement sleep behavior disorder. *Am J Med* 1999;107:390–2.
97. Oudiette D, De Cock VC, Lavault S, et al. Nonviolent elaborate behaviors may also occur in REM sleep behavior disorder. *Neurology* 2009;72:551–7.

30

Pathophysiology of REM Sleep Behavior Disorder, Including Its Relationship with Neurodegenerative Diseases, Evolving Concepts, and Controversies

ALEX IRANZO AND JUN LU

REM SLEEP behavior disorder (RBD) is a parasomnia characterized by abnormal motor and vocal behaviors (e.g., jerking, punching, yelling, crying, laughing), unpleasant dreams (e.g., being attacked or chased by unknown people or animals), and excessive electromyographic activity during rapid eye movement (REM) sleep. RBD may be idiopathic or secondary to neurodegenerative diseases, narcolepsy, focal structural lesions in the brain, and the use of some medications.[1,30] If one aims to learn the pathophysiology of RBD, one must first attempt to understand the mechanisms that generate and modulate REM sleep in normal conditions and identify the anatomic structures, pathways, and neurotransmitter systems that regulate muscle atonia during this sleep stage. The neuronal network responsible for REM sleep and REM sleep atonia and their underlying abnormalities causing RBD are under discussion and have been reviewed recently by leading investigators in the field.[2-6]

NEURAL NETWORK RESPONSIBLE FOR REM SLEEP

The neural network that generates REM sleep is responsible for REM sleep polysomnographic parameters such as REM sleep onset latency, percentage of REM sleep across the night, and number of REM sleep periods (see Fig. 30.1).

REM sleep generation mechanisms are complex, unclear, and still under debate. REM sleep is characterized by rapid eye movements, skeletal muscle atonia, desynchronized electroencephalographic activity, and dreams that can have an emotional content. A large number of anatomic structures are directly or indirectly implicated in the generation and maintenance of the sleep-wake cycle, where REM sleep is one of the main components. These structures are mainly located in the brainstem, limbic system, thalamus, hypothalamus, and cortex. Such a large number of different structures explain why many neurotransmitters have

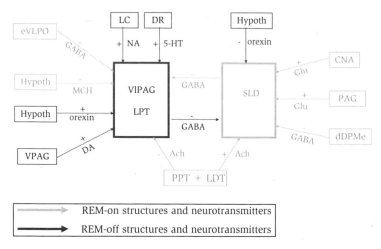

FIGURE 30.1   REM sleep flip-flop model. In this flip-flop model the REM-on structures promote REM sleep inhibiting the REM-off structures, while the REM-off nuclei inhibit REM sleep through inhibition of the REM-on structures. REM-on structures are in gray and REM-off structures are in black. −, inhibition; +, activation; ACh, acetylcholine; CNA, central nucleus of the amygdala; DA, dopamine; dDpME, dorsal deep mesencephalic reticular nucleus; DR, dorsal raphe nucleus; eVLPO, extended ventrolateral preoptic nucleus; GABA, gamma-aminobutyric acid; Glut, glutamate; hypoth, hypothalamus; LC, locus coeruleus nucleus; LDT, lateral dorsal tegmentum; LPT, lateral pontine tegmentum; MCH, melanin concentrating hormone; NA, noradrenaline; PAG, periaqueductal gray matter; PPT, pedunculopontine tegmentum nucleus; SLD, sublaterodorsal nucleus; VlPAG, ventrolateral part of the periaqueductal gray matter; VPAG, ventral part of the periaqueductal gray matter; 5-HT, serotonin.

been implicated in sleep regulation, including glutamate, gamma-aminobutyric acid (GABA), glycine, hypocretin/orexin, melanin concentrating hormone (MCH), melatonin, histamine, acetylcholine, dopamine, serotonin, and noradrenaline.[2,4–6]

The critical structures for REM sleep generation and REM sleep muscle atonia are located in the mesopontine tegmentum and the ventral medial medulla (VMM). In these regions there exist a large number of nuclei that send projections inhibiting or activating nearby nuclei in the brainstem or other distant brain regions. For the basic researcher, working in such a tiny region is a challenge as some nuclei can be difficult to identify. When trying to damage a specific brainstem nucleus with a cytotoxic injection, the lesion

may expand to surrounding nuclei or unintended neurons within the nucleus, producing unexpected results. More clean and accurate results can be obtained using c-Fos labelling, retrograde and anterograde tracing, administration of neurotransmitters agonists and antagonists (Table 30.1), selective electric stimulation, and genetic manipulation with knockout animals of neurotransmitters and receptors. Experimental studies in animals have provided a great amount of knowledge on the generation of REM sleep and several models of RBD. However, results in animals may depend on the species studied (rats, mice, felines, dogs, nonhuman primates, and humans) because the location of some nuclei and configurations of REM sleep control neurons may be different. [2,4–6]

Table 30.1 Chemical Compounds Inducing Normal REM Sleep Atonia with Short Latency

1) Injection of $GABA_A$ antagonists (bicuculine and gabazine) into the rat sublaterodorsal nucleus
2) Injection of NMDA glutamate agonists (kainic acid) into the rat sublaterodorsal nucleus
3) Injection of cholinergic agonists (carbachol) in the cat peri-locus coeruleus alpha

For the clinician, REM sleep generation and RBD pathophysiology are very difficult to understand not only because of their complexity and the changing nature of the field but also because different terminology is used to label the same structures across species and across different group of investigators. The subcoeruleus nucleus in humans is the equivalent to peri-locus coeruleus alpha nucleus (peri-LCa) in cats and to the sublaterodorsal tegmental nucleus (SLD) in rats and mice. The subcoeruleus nucleus in humans is located ventral to the locus coeruleus, and the SLD in rodents is ventral to the laterodorsal tegmental nucleus (LDT). The seemingly different location of the subcoeruleus and SLD is due to the fact that the locus coeruleus in primates and humans and even cats extends very rostrally. This REM sleep control structure is also named pontine inhibitor area (PIA), dorsal nucleus pontis oralis (PnO), and dorsal rostral pontine reticular nucleus, depending on the investigators.[2,4,5,7,8] In the VMM, the ventral gigantocellular nucleus in rodents corresponds to the nucleus magnocellularis in cats and in humans. The VMM also contains medium- and small-sized neurons as well. As expected, the larger neurons have longer projections than medium and small neurons. Thus, large neurons in the VMM may regulate REM sleep atonia when reaching the spinal cord. REM sleep is also called paradoxical sleep[5] and active sleep.[8]

Although it was first reported that central mechanisms regulating REM sleep were cholinergic and monoaminergic in nature, recent evidence indicates that the system responsible for REM sleep is more complex, involving critical GABA-ergic and glutamatergic neurotransmission in the brainstem.[2,9–13] Early pharmacological and electrophysiological experiments in the mesopontine tegmentum of animals showed that cholinergic administration promotes REM sleep, whereas serotonin and noradrenaline application suppresses REM sleep. However, selective lesions of the mesopontine cholinergic nuclei (pedunculopontine tegmentum nucleus [PPT] and lateral dorsal tegmentum nucleus [LDT]), serotonergic nuclei (dorsal raphe nucleus [DR]), and noradrenergic nuclei (locus coeruleus nucleus [LC]) did not change the amount of REM sleep or have an effect on the muscular activity during REM sleep. This suggested that there were additional brain regions and neurotransmitter systems that are more critically involved in REM sleep.[5,6,12]

Recent studies in rodents have revealed the presence of nonmonoaminergic and noncholinergic REM-on and REM-off structures in the mesopontine tegmentum that form the basis of a REM sleep generation model, which is analogous to an electronic flip-flop switch. This flip-flop switch consists of a rapid and complete transition from REM sleep to non-REM sleep and back. In this model, REM-on neurons inhibit REM-off neurons, and vice versa. This mutually inhibitory relationship ensures fast transitions from one state to another. REM-on neurons fire during REM sleep and enhance this sleep stage. During non-REM sleep and wakefulness, REM-on neurons do not fire because they are inhibited by REM-off cells. REM-on neurons are GABA-ergic in nature, are located in the SLD, and inhibit REM-off neurons. REM-off cells are also GABA-ergic and are located in the lateral pontine tegmentum (LPT) and ventrolateral periaqueductal gray matter (vlPAG).[2,5,12]

The flip-flop model, however, is much more complex. It has been shown that other structures and neurotransmitters modulate the REM-on cells of the SLD, and also the REM-off cells of the LPT and vlPAG. These structures and their corresponding neurotransmitters have an important role in the modulation, but not generation, of the flip-flop switch model. The following structures are thought to promote REM sleep either activating the REM-on neurons of the SLD or inhibiting the REM-off cells of the LPT and vlPAG: the GABA-ergic extended ventrolateral preoptic nucleus (eVLPO) in the hypothalamus, the MCH cells in the hypothalamus, the glutamatergic cells from the central nucleus of the amygdala (CAN), the cholinergic PPT and LDT in the mesopontine tegmentum, the GABA-ergic projections from the dorsal deep mesencephalic reticular nucleus (dDpME) in the midbrain, and the glutamatergic cells from the periaqudeductual gray matter (PAG). Conversely, the following structures activate the REM-off sleep neurons of the LPT and vlPAG: the hypocretinergic/orexinergic cells in the dorsolateral hypothalamus, and several brainstem nuclei such as the serotonergic DRN, noradrenergic LC, and dopaminergic ventral periaqueductal gray matter (vPAG).[12] Interestingly, the neurons in the core of the VLPO regulate non-REM sleep while the dorsal and medial neurons (the extended VLPO [eVLPO]) are involved in REM sleep.[12] Of note, the cholinergic PPT and LDT nuclei promote REM sleep through (1) activation of the inhibitory M2 and M4 receptors of the VlPAG and LPT, and (2) activation of the excitatory M3 receptors of the SLD.

The importance of these modulators is seen in narcolepsy, a disease characterized by selective loss of hypocretin/orexin cells in the dorsolateral hypothalamus, leading to increased REM sleep pressure causing hypersomnia and episodes of muscle atonia during wakefulness triggered by emotional stimuli (cataplexy).[14] Moreover, antidepressants with serotonergic, noradrenergic, and anticholinergic activity increase REM sleep latency and reduce the amount of REM sleep.[15]

The GABA-ergic dorsal deep mesencephalic reticular nucleus (dDpMe) in the LPT is also proposed to be an REM-off structure.[5,167] It is also speculated that the REM-on neurons in the SLD are glutamatergic and probably not GABA-ergic.[16]

Neuronal activation during REM sleep generation is not confined to nuclei located in the brainstem. Functional neuroimaging studies in humans during REM sleep have shown activation of not only the pontine tegmentum but also the thalamus, basal forebrain, limbic areas (amygdala, hippocampus, anterior cingulate cortex), and temporo-occipital cortices. Functional neuroimaging during REM sleep also shows deactivation of the dorsolateral prefrontal cortex, inferior parietal cortex, precuneus, and posterior cingulate gyrus.[17] The characteristic electroencephalographic activity of REM sleep is mediated by glutamatergic inputs from the precoeruleus area (PC, which is located in the pons rostral to the LC) and parabrachial nucleus (PB, which is located in the basal forebrain)[12,18] and cholinergic inputs from the PPT and LDT[5,12] that reach the intralaminar and reticular thalamic nuclei, lateral hypothalamus, basal forebrain, and prefrontal cortex. These structures send cholinergic, glutamatergic, and GABA-ergic projections that reach the cortex and hippocampus, producing cortical activation. This REM sleep cortical activation is also mediated by decreased noradrenergic activity in the LC, reduced serotonergic activity in the DRN, decreased histaminergic activity in the tuberomammillary nucleus, and reduced hypocretinergic/orexinergic activity in the lateral hypothalamus.[6] The characteristic rapid eye movements seen in REM sleep are mediated by brainstem structures involved in ocular motility, such as the para-abducens nucleus and medial pontine reticular formation.[7]

NEURAL NETWORK RESPONSIBLE FOR REM SLEEP MUSCLE ATONIA

The precise neuronal network responsible for muscle atonia during REM sleep is not entirely understood and is still under debate. REM sleep muscle atonia is characterized by (1) continuous sustained absence of muscle tone and (2) few intermittent bursts of phasic muscular activity, which can be associated with minimal muscle twitches and rapid eye movements.[19,20] REM sleep atonia requires (1) sustained inhibition throughout the REM sleep period of the tonic electromyographic activity that underlies the postural tone, and (2) disfacilitation of the phasic electromyographic activity that influences movements and locomotion. In other words, muscle tone in REM sleep is reduced by linked activation of inhibitory systems and inactivation of facilitatory systems.[4] The final result is inhibition of the lower motoneurons of the cranial nerves in the brainstem and of the ventral spinal cord, both resulting in skeletal muscle atonia (see Figs. 30.2 and 30.3).

Neural inhibition of generators for tonic and phasic muscular components are thought to be different but located in the pontine tegmentum and VMM. Neurons generating REM sleep atonia are glutamatergic cells localized in the ventral region of the SLD (vSLD).[9,12,16,21] The vSLD lies in the pons and is ventral to the LC. Muscle atonia is ultimately the result of glycine and GABA that hyperpolarize the motoneurons of the cranial nerve nuclei in the lower brainstem and of the motoneurons of the ventral horn in the spinal cord.[22]

The vSLD generates muscle atonia by two different pathways (Fig. 30.2). There is a direct pathway of excitatory vSLD glutamatergic projections to the ventral horn interneurons of the spinal cord, which in turn inhibit the ventral horn motoneurons with GABA/glycinergic inputs.[12] An indirect polysynaptic pathway consists of other descending glutamatergic vSLD neurons that send their projections to the VMM,[4,23] which in turn inhibits the motoneurons of the ventral horn of the spinal cord, resulting in muscle atonia. It is possible that the neurons of the VMM release GABA/glycine to the ventral horn motoneurons[5,24] and glutamate[25,26] to the spinal cord GABA-ergic/glycinergic interneurons, which in turn inhibit the motoneurons of the ventral horn. The neurons of the VMM that promote REM sleep atonia are thought to

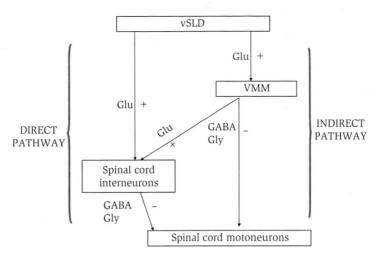

FIGURE 30.2   Schematic diagram of REM sleep atonia circuitry. The vSLD in the mesopontine tegmentum is the main structure that promotes REM sleep atonia. It inhibits the spinal cord motoneurons through a direct pathway and also through an indirect pathway that relies on the VMM. The
direct pathway inhibits the tonic electromyographic activity. The indirect pathway defacilitates the
phasic electromyographic activity. Damage to the vSLD and VMM results in REM sleep behavior disorder. Transgenic mice with deficient glycine and GABA receptors also result in REM sleep behavior
disorder. –, inhibition; +, activation; GABA, gamma-aminobutyric acid; Gly, glycine; VMM, ventral
medial medulla; vSLD, ventral sublaterodorsal nucleus.

be located in the supraolivary medulla (SOM),
which is the rostro-caudal segment of the
gigantocellular reticular field and corresponds
to what has been called the gigantocellular
reticular nucleus (GiV), the ventral gigantocellularis nucleus, the nucleus magnocellularis,
and to the "medullary inhibiting area" proposed
by Magoun and Rhines in 1946.[26]

It has been speculated that the direct pathway that reaches the ventral horn from the
vSLD is responsible for inhibiting the tonic
muscular activity,[12] whereas the indirect pathway is responsible for disfacilitating the phasic muscular activity.[26] Other investigators
have hypothesized that sustained tonic muscle
activity during REM sleep represents inhibition of centers within the VMM controlling
normal REM sleep-related atonia[27] and that the
high neuronal firing rates within the substantia nigra pars reticulata can mediate the phasic
electromyographic activity seen in REM sleep
through inhibitory descending influences to the
pedunculopontine region, subcoeruleus, and/or
magnocellularis nucleus.[28]

The glutamatergic descending neurons from
the vSLD that decrease REM sleep electromyographic activity are modulated by direct and
indirect projections from the brainstem and

from supratentorial structures (Fig. 30.3). They
include inhibitory GABA-ergic projections from
the dorsal deep mesencephalic reticular nuclei
(dDpMe) and excitatory glutamatergic projections from the primary motor area of the frontal
cortex, supplementary somatosensory area, central nucleus of the amygdala, and the midbrain
periaqueductal gray matter.[10] The glutamatergic
neurons of the vSLD also receive afferents from
cholinergic neurons from the PPT and LDT,
serotonergic neurons from the DR, noradrenergic neurons from the LC and medullary A1 and
A2 cell groups, and hypocretinergic/orexinergic
neurons from the dorsolateral hypothalamus.[10]
The substantia nigra pars reticulata and the
internal segment of the globus pallidum send
GABA-ergic projections to the PPN, which in
turn excites the neurons of the VMM with glutamatergic and cholinergic inputs.[29]

On the other hand, the ventral mesopontine junction (VMPJ) is a region that includes
the substantia nigra pars reticulata, the caudal
portion of the retrorubral nucleus (RRN), and
the ventral tegmental area (VTA). The VMPJ
is also involved in the control of muscle tone
since glutamatergic neurons from this region
activate the vSLD and VMM, promoting REM
sleep atonia.[4]

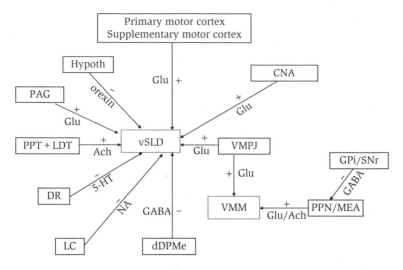

FIGURE 30.3 Afferents of the ventral sublaterodorsal nucleus and ventral medial medulla. During REM sleep (1) the vSLD is activated through excitatory inputs from the cortex, VMPJ, amygdala, PPT, and LDT, and (2) the VMM is activated through excitatory inputs from the VMPJ and PPN/MEA. The inhibitory activity of the hypocretinergic hypothalamus, serotonergic DR, and noradrenergic LC nuclei allow promoting REM sleep atonia due to activation of the vSLD. –, inhibition; +, activation; ACh, acetylcholine; CNA, central nucleus of the amygdala; dDpME, dorsal deep mesencephalic reticular nucleus; DR, dorsal raphe nucleus; GABA, gamma-aminobutyric acid; Glu, glutamate; GPi, internal segment of the globus pallidus; hypoth, hypothalamus; LC, locus coeruleus nucleus; LDT, lateral dorsal tegmentum; MEA, midbrain extrapiramydal area; NA, noradrenaline; PAG, periaquedeductual gray matter; PPN, pedunculopontine nucleus; PPT, pedunculopontine tegmentum nucleus; SNr, sunstantia nigra pars reticulata; VMM, ventral medial medulla; VMPJ, ventral mesopontine junction; vSLD, ventral sublaterodorsal nucleus; 5-HT, serotonin.

PATHOPHYSIOLOGY OF REM SLEEP BEHAVIOR DISORDER

Patients with RBD exhibit increased electromyographic activity during REM sleep. Other components of REM sleep are normal such as density of rapid eye movements, REM sleep onset latency, percentage of REM sleep across the night, and number of REM sleep periods.[30] Electroencephalographic activity is apparently normal, but spectral analysis in subjects with idiopathic RBD (IRBD) may show subtle slowing that may predict the future development of cognitive abnormalities.[31,32]

Available data indicate that RBD in humans is caused by damage of the nuclei that generates REM sleep atonia, namely the subcoeruleus nucleus in the pons and the nucleus magnocellularis in the medulla. Therefore, impairment of glutamatergic neurotransmission from the subcoeruleus nucleus, and GABA-ergic and glycinergic neurotransmission from the nucleus magnocellularis, underlie the pathophysiology of RBD. Alternatively, it is plausible that RBD can also be caused by damage of the anatomical connections of the SLD and

VMM with other structures such as the dorsolateral hypothalamus and the amygdala. Our knowledge on the pathophysiology of RBD is based on (1) the existence of animal models of RBD and (2) the occurrence of RBD in subjects with neurodegenerative diseases, narcolepsy, focal structural lesions in the brain, and with the use of some medications.

Animal Models of REM Sleep Behavior Disorder

Normal domestic dogs may display physiological facial and tail-muscle twitching, subtle rhythmic paddling movements, and whining sounds during sleep.[32a] Domestic dogs have also been documented to have RBD, with violent movements of the head, trunk, and extremities; running-like movements of the limbs; vocalizations emerging in association with REM sleep without atonia; and absence of electroencephalographic epileptiform activity. Dogs with RBD may propel themselves long distances and displace objects during apparent dream enactment. RBD has been described in both young and old dogs, in females and males, and across breeds (e.g., boxers, Labradors, mongrels).[33-35] This has been shown in some Disney shorts and films like in *Lady and the Tramp* (1955),[35a] 10 years before animal models of RBD were first described.[36] RBD in domestic dogs can be apparently idiopathic or associated with waking neurological abnormalities such as seizures or myoclonus.[32-35]

Experimental localized lesions in cats and rodents confined to the dorsolateral pontine tegmentum involving the SLD and also to the VMM impairing the nucleus magnocellularis produce REM sleep without atonia associated with what looks like dream-enacting behaviors during unequivocal REM sleep. These observations emphasized that the lower brainstem is the critical area for inducing muscle atonia during REM sleep and provided animal models for human RBD. About 20 years before the formal description of human RBD by Schenck and Mahowald in 1986[37] Jouvet and Delrome showed in 1965 that electrolytic lesions of the subcoeruleus region in cats resulted in REM sleep without atonia associated with simple and complex motor behaviors such as orienting, walking, and attacking.[36] This observation was confirmed by many other investigators.[38-40] It was shown that the site and extent of the lesions in the pontine tegmentum determine the severity of the behaviors that the cat releases, ranging from prominent limb jerks to locomotion and attack behaviors.[39] Asymmetrical or unilateral electrolytic lesions in the subcoerulus region or caudally projecting fibers resulted in minimal release of proximal limb movements and rocking head and neck movements. Orienting and searching movements of the eyes and head were associated with damage of pontine afferents to the superior colliculus, a midbrain visual center controlling eye movements during wakefulness that plays a critical role in the ability to direct behaviors toward specific moving objects and generating spatially directed head turns and arm-reaching movements. Cats with larger lesions extending rostrally and ventrally in the pons showed more elaborate behaviors, including raising the head, searching, and walking. Some of the cats that showed violent attacking behaviors had damage to the pathway arising from the central nucleus of the amygdala.[39] In a different study with rats, small unilateral lesions in the subcoeruleus region were sufficient to remove the atonia of REM sleep, but larger and bilateral lesions were required to release abnormal behaviors.[41] In another study

in cats, REM sleep atonia was intact after selective electrolytic or radio frequency lesions of the cholinergic nuclei PPT and LDT and of the noradrenergic LC nucleus. In contrast, lesions confined to the subcoeruleus nucleus eliminated atonia during REM sleep. These findings indicate that selective cholinergic and noradrenergic damage does not play a major role in the pathogenesis of RBD.[40]

In rodents, recent studies have revealed that selective damage of the glutamatergic neurons of the vSLD produce REM sleep with increased muscular activity, prominent jerks, and locomotion.[12] In rats, ibotenic acid (a GABA$_A$ agonist) lesions in the vSLD also cause loss of REM sleep atonia associated with jerks and complex movements such as walking (Fig. 30.4).[12]

On the other hand, selective experimental lesions in the VMM also produce REM sleep without atonia associated with abnormal behaviors. In cats, cytotoxic glutamate-induced lesions of the VMM that included the nucleus magnocellularis, the caudal nucleus gigantocellularis, and the rostral nucleus paramedianus result in REM sleep without atonia associated with a variety of behaviors such as lifting the head, slow lateral movements of the head to both sides, chewing-like movements, pawing at the air, extension and alternating movements of all limbs, but not locomotion. In this experiment, REM sleep without atonia and abnormal movements in REM sleep were not observed after acetylcholine induced-lesions in the VMM.[42] Restricted glutamatergic lesions in the SOM of rodents also produce increased tonic and phasic muscular activity linked to whole-body movements during REM sleep.[26] In rodents, selective loss of glutamate release from the VMM, but not GABA/glycine release from the VMM, produces increased phasic muscular activity and movements in REM sleep that are similar to those observed after restricted glutamatergic SOM lesions.[26] However, in general, the degree of motor movements with the VMM lesions is much less than that of SLD lesions.[26]

Neurotoxic lesions in the caudal VMPJ of cats produce increased tonic and phasic electromyographic activity in the neck and limbs and RBD-like behaviors such as jerking, kicking, raising and moving the head, and lifting of the body. These behaviors were not significantly correlated with the number of dopaminergic losses at the VMPJ. The authors speculated that impairment of the glutamatergic projections from the VMPJ to the SLD and to the VMM

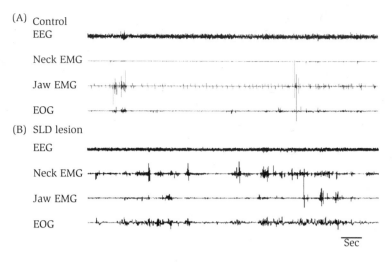

(A) Control
EEG

Neck EMG

Jaw EMG

EOG

(B) SLD lesion
EEG

Neck EMG

Jaw EMG

EOG

Sec

FIGURE 30.4   The effects of the sublaterodorsal nucleus in rats on cortical electroencephalography and electromyographic activity of neck, jaw, and eye muscle (electrooculography) during REM sleep. In (A), a control rat (sham lesion) shows a 10-second duration of REM sleep, in which high theta electroencephalographic activity (hippocampal activation, upper trace) and electromyographic atonia of neck muscle, phasic jaw, and eye muscles are observed. In (B), a rat with ibotenic acid lesions of the sublaterodorsal nucleus shows high theta EEG and loss of neck muscle atonia during REM sleep. However, muscle activity of jaw and eyes is not altered, and moreover the phasic electromyographic activity of jaw and eyes is not synchronized. Thus, lesion of the sublaterodorsal nucleus in rats produces REM sleep without atonia but does not increase the phasic electromyographic activity. These data suggest that the sublaterodorsal nucleus is involved in control of postural muscles (such as neck muscles) but has a limited role in control of cranial (jaw and eye) muscle phasic activity during REM sleep. EEG, electroencephalography; EMG, electromyography; EOG, electrooculogram; SLD, sublaterodorsal nucleus.

could explain the occurrence of an animal model of RBD caused by damage of the VMPJ.[43]

In rodents, increased electromyography activity in REM sleep can be obtained after knockout of the vesicular glutamate transporter 2 gene in the sublaterodorsal nucleus and in the ventral medial medulla.[12] This suggests that decreased glutamate release from both SLD and VMM to the spinal cord is a model of RBD.

A recent study has shown that transgenic mice with deficient glycine receptor α_1 and GABA$_A$ receptor resulted in a model of RBD characterized by increased phasic electromyographic activity in REM sleep linked to abnormal movements, including chewing, jerking and running, normal absence of tonic electromyographic activity in REM sleep, jerking in non-REM sleep, sleep fragmentation, subtle EEG slowing in the spectral analysis, and normal REM sleep percentage. The increased phasic electromyographic activity was recorded in the masseter, neck, and limbs. Interestingly, clonazepam and melatonin, the two drugs of choice in human RBD, decreased the phasic electromyographic

activity and the abnormal behaviors seen in REM sleep. This study provided the first genetic model of RBD and indicates that GABA-ergic and glycinergic impairment may also underlie RBD.[44] However, one major difference compared to many patients with idiopathic RBD is that these mice also showed significant phasic movements during non-REM sleep. It is not clear, but we suspect that glycine-GABA receptors in the spinal cord motor neurons are altered. If this is true, GABA and glycine may also involve muscle tone control during non-REM sleep (see Table 30.2).

REM Sleep Behavior Disorder in Neurodegenerative Diseases

In humans, idiopathic RBD (IRBD) is diagnosed when a patient with video-polysomnographic confirmation of RBD has no evidence of a neurological disease or other possible causes (for review, see Iranzo et al.[30]).

In IRBD, diffusion-tensor neuroimaging during wakefulness shows evidence of

Table 30.2 Animal Models of REM Sleep Behavior Disorder

1) Unilateral or bilateral lesions of the subcoeruleus region in cats
2) Lesions of the glutamatergic cells in the sublaterodorsal nucleus in rats
3) Lesions in the ventral medial medulla in cats and rats
4) Selective damage of the cells in the ventral medial medulla in rats
5) Lesions in the caudal ventral mesopontine junction in cats
6) Knockout of the vesicular glutamate transporter 2 gene in the sublaterodorsal nucleus in mice (personal observation)
7) Knockout of the vesicular glutamate transporter 2 gene in the ventral medial medulla in mice
8) Injection of $GABA_A$A agonists (ibotenic acid and muscimol) into the sublaterodorsal nucleus in rats
9) Injection of NMDA glutamate antagonists (kynuenic acid) into the sublaterodorsal nucleus in rats
10) Transgenic mice with deficient glycine receptor α_1 and $GABA_A$ receptor

neuronal and axonal damage in mesopontine structures known to regulate REM sleep atonia, including the SLD, PPT, LC, and PAG, and no apparent damage in the medulla, amygdala, or substantia nigra.[45] Longitudinal follow-up of IRBD patients seen at sleep centers has shown the frequent development of the classical motor and cognitive symptoms of three neurodegenerative diseases, namely Parkinson disease (PD), dementia with Lewy bodies (DLB), and multiple-system atrophy (MSA).[46-48] In some IRBD patients, though, subclinical abnormalities can be detected, such as olfactory deficits,[49] color vision impairment,[50] cognitive deficits on neuropsychological tests,[51] subtle cortical electroencephalographic slowing,[31,51a] dysautonomic abnormalities,[52] reduced cardiac 123-I MBIG scintigraphy,[53] decreased dopamine transporter imaging,[32] and increased substantia nigra echogenicity.[54] All these features are common in patients with the established classic motor and cognitive features of PD, DLB, and MSA. None of these features are the cause or the consequence of RBD. They are epiphenomena caused by damage of several brain areas that are not associated with the regulation of REM sleep like the olfactory system and the nigrostriatal system. Neuropathological examination in two IRBD patients showed the hallmarks of PD, namely neuronal cell loss and Lewy bodies in the brainstem.[55,56] Thus, available data indicate that in IRBD, this parasomnia can be considered part of the degenerative process damaging the structures that regulate REM sleep atonia. It is still unknown, however, how many IRBD patients will develop PD, DLB, or MSA, and how many will remain disease-free.

This has led to looking for biomarkers of disease progression[32,57] which can be used to monitor the effect of potential neuroprotective drugs in future clinical trials in IRBD.[58]

RBD occurs in 30%–50% of patients with PD, in 70%–80% of patients with DLB, and in 90%–100% of patients with MSA. RBD precedes the classical symptoms of PD in 18%–22% of the cases, in 44%–52% of the cases of MSA, and in 90%–100% of the cases with DLB.[30,59-62] In PD, RBD is more frequent in the akinetic-rigid subtype than in the tremoric subtype, probably because the akinetic-rigid subtype is associated with more severe and widespread pathologic process.[63] RBD-associated motor behaviors, vocalizations, and nightmares are the same in PD, DLB, MSA, and IRBD.[30,64] RBD may occur, but it is very rare in the setting of other neurodegenerative diseases such as Alzheimer disease,[65] progressive supranuclear palsy,[66] Huntington disease[67] frontotemporal dementia (unpublished observations), corticobasal degeneration (unpublished observations), and amyotrophic lateral sclerosis (unpublished observations). In neurodegenerative diseases where RBD is frequent, such as PD, DLB, and MSA, pathological changes are common in the brainstem structures modulating REM sleep atonia (e.g., locus subcoeruleus, nucleus magnocellularis, PPN, LC, and DR) and in the amygdala.[68-71] In contrast, full-blown expression of RBD is uncommon in diseases associated with widespread brainstem cell loss but little limbic system damage, such as in progressive supranuclear palsy, as well as in diseases with no marked brainstem cell loss like Alzheimer disease and frontotemporal dementia. Taken together, it is tempting to speculate that RBD when occurring in neurodegenerative diseases can be explained by regional distribution and severity of neuronal dysfunction in the brainstem structures that regulate REM sleep, and their anatomic connections, particularly with the limbic system. PD, DLB, and MSA subjects without RBD are probably those in whom the pathological threshold for RBD symptomatology is not exceeded in the brainstem nuclei that modulate REM sleep atonia.

REM Sleep Behavior Disorder in Narcolepsy

Narcolepsy is believed to be an autoimmune disorder characterized by intrusion of REM sleep into wakefulness leading to hypersomnia and cataplexy. This is due to selective loss of hypocretin/orexin-producing neurons in the dorsolateral hypothalamus.[14] RBD can occur in both children and adults with narcolepsy. In a very few patients, RBD can even be the first manifestation of the disease.[72-75] In a series of 44 patients with narcolepsy and cataplexy, 61% reported symptoms suggestive of RBD and 43% had an RBD episode at video-polysomnography regardless of the frequency of cataplectic attacks or gender.[76] It is our experience that RBD symptoms in narcolepsy are much less severe than hypersomnia and cataplexy. It is also our experience that RBD is much more frequent in narcoleptics with cataplexy than without cataplexy. Treatment of cataplexy with antidepressants may trigger or exacerbate RBD symptoms. The effect of sodium oxybate (a $GABA_B$ agonist) on RBD in patients with narcolepsy is not known. Like in all forms of RBD, clonazepam improves RBD symptoms in patients with narcolepsy.

Patients with narcolepsy and RBD do not develop a neurodegenerative disease like PD, DLB, and MSA. In narcolepsy, there is no neurodegeneration of the brainstem and limbic structures that regulate REM sleep. The neuronal loss is confined to the hypothalamic cells that produce hypocretin/orexin, probably due to an acute or subacute autoimmune process. The occurrence of RBD in narcolepsy may be explained by hypocretin/orexin deficiency since hypocretinergic/orexinergic neurons have wide projections to several nuclei that regulate REM sleep atonia (e.g., subcoeruleus nucleus) and the emotional content of dreams (e.g., central nucleus of the amygdala) (Fig. 30.5).[77,78]

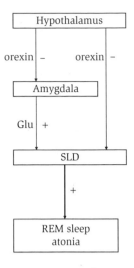

FIGURE 30.5 Major orexin (hypocretin) projections to brain structures involved in REM sleep atonia generation. In narcolepsy, the occurrence of REM sleep behavior disorder can be explained by loss of orexin (hypocretin) cells that results in dreams with fearful content due to amygdalar dysfunction and REM sleep without atonia caused by dysfunction of the sublaterodorsal nucleus. −, inhibition; +, activation; Glu, glutamate; SLD, sublaterodorsal nucleus.

REM Sleep Behavior Disorder Associated with Focal Lesions in Humans

In humans, RBD has been reported to be caused by a structural unilateral lesion[80] or bilateral focal lesions confined to the mesopontine tegmentum,[81-86,168,169] and much less frequently to the medulla.[79] (For review, see Iranzo and Aparicio.[79]) The nature of lesions can be ischemic,[81,86,168] hemorrhages from vascular malformations,[83] tumors,[87] demyelinating plaques,[169] and inflammatory.[80,82,84,88] These patients had nightmares suggesting the occurrence of functional dysregulation of those supratentorial structures that modulate intense emotions and that are anatomically connected with the mesopontine tegmentum such as the limbic system. RBD has also been reported to occur in neurological disorders involving the amygdala (limbic encephalitis)[88] or anterior thalamus (familial fatal insomnia)[89] with no apparent primary brainstem damage. RBD has been described in disorders with combined lesions of the amygdala and the mesopontine tegmentum, where some narcoleptic features were also present.[90]

REM Sleep Behavior Disorder and Medications

Clonazepam and melatonin improve RBD symptoms, whereas other drugs such as antidepressants and beta-blockers can induce or aggravate RBD. These data reveal some neurochemical aspects of the underlying mechanisms of RBD that may involve GABA-ergic, serotonergic, noradrenergic, and anticholinergic neurotransmission. (For review, see Gagnon et al.[166])

Clinical experience shows that in any form of human RBD (idiopathic or associated with neurodegenerative diseases, narcolepsy, and structural lesions) nightmares and motor and vocal dream-enacting behaviors usually respond to small doses of clonazepam (0.25–4 mg) at bedtime. This suggests that different forms of RBD share similar pathophysiologic mechanisms, perhaps mainly involving GABA-ergic transmission. However, for unknown reasons, a few patients do not respond to clonazepam, particularly those with IRBD.[30] Clonazepam does not protect IRBD patients from developing a neurodegenerative disease with time.[47] One study involving five IRBD patients showed that clonazepam decreases phasic, but not tonic, electromyographic activity in the mentalis muscle during REM sleep.[91] The beneficial effect of clonazepam might be related to its GABA-ergic activity inhibiting the lower motoneurons. However, this does not explain why other benzodiazepines with GABA-ergic activity do not ameliorate RBD symptoms.

Melatonin (3–12 mg at bedtime or 30 minutes before bedtime) is also effective in patients with idiopathic and secondary RBD. Unlike clonazepam, melatonin decreases the tonic, but not the phasic, electromyographic activity in the mentalis muscle in subjects with RBD. It has been speculated that melatonin improves RBD due to restoration of the REM sleep circadian rhythm[92,93] or due to its GABA-ergic activity.[44]

In a genetic animal model of RBD lacking GABA-ergic and glycinergic neurotransmission, both clonazepam and melatonin restored muscle atonia in REM sleep and decreased abnormal behaviors.[44] There is no strong evidence indicating that anticholinergics or dopaminergics improve RBD symptoms and decrease the excessive electromyographic activity in REM sleep.[95-97]

Some medications have been described to induce RBD. It is possible that these medications are capable of unmasking RBD in subjects destined to develop this parasomnia at a later time.[98] Several antidepressants, including tricyclics, selective serotonin reuptake inhibitors, and selective noradrenaline reuptake inhibitors, have been described to trigger or aggravate RBD.[99,100] We have seen patients reporting a temporal association between onset of RBD and the introduction of sertraline ($n = 8$), fluoxetine ($n = 4$), venlafaxine ($n = 3$), clomipramine ($n = 3$), paroxetine ($n = 2$), escitalopram ($n = 2$), and citalopram ($n = 2$).[30] Overall, these medications increase serotonin and noradrenergic activity, and decrease cholinergic activity. Of note, in subjects without RBD undergoing polysomnography, increased tonic, but not phasic, electromyographic activity during REM sleep is seen in those taking antidepressants.[101] For unknown reasons lipophilic beta blockers such as bisoprolol can cause RBD.[102] Interestingly, the first description of "REM sleep without atonia" in humans came from patients during delirium tremens episodes after alcohol withdrawal.[103]

EVOLVING CONCEPTS IN REM SLEEP BEHAVIOR DISORDER

What Is the Significance of Excessive Tonic and Phasic Electromyographic Activity in REM Sleep Behavior Disorder?

In normal humans there is almost no sustained tonic electromyographic activity and only minimal phasic electromyographic activity during REM sleep. The minimal phasic activity is usually seen in the mentalis, other peri-bucal muscles, and distal muscles of the lower limbs.[20] It is much less common in the upper extremities in normal humans. This normal phasic electromyographic activity may or may not coincide with rapid eye movements and sometimes it is associated with brief and fast bursts of twitches producing little body jerks and small repetitive movements of the feet (Fig. 30.6).[104] These are asymptomatic causing no arousals or awakenings. These twitches and small movements are much more prominent in normal newborns,[105] particularly in the face (unpublished observations).

Patients with RBD have increased phasic and/or tonic electromyographic activity during REM sleep (Fig. 30.7). In RBD, severity of excessive tonic electromyographic activity during REM sleep is stable across two consecutive nights. In contrast,

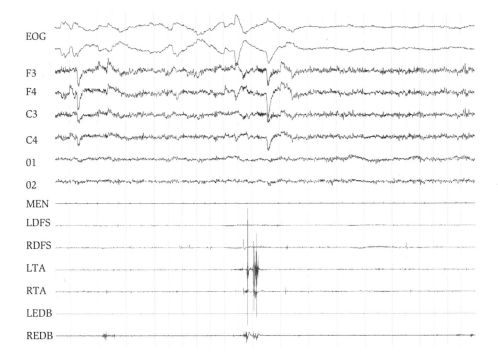

FIGURE 30.6   Polysomnographic representation of normal REM sleep in a healthy human. This figure represents 30 seconds of a normal human during REM sleep undergoing polysomnography. The recording shows physiological muscle atonia in the mentalis and an isolated burst of phasic electromyographic activity only in the lower limbs during REM sleep in a normal person. EOG, electrooculogram; F3,F4,C3,C4, O1, and O2, electroencephalographic electrode positions (frontal, central, and occipital of each side) according to the 10/20 International system referenced to combined ears; LDFS, left flexor digitorum superficialis muscle in the upper limb; LEDB, left extensor digitorum brevis muscle in the lower limb; LTA, left tibialis anterior muscle in the lower limb; MEN, mentalis muscle; RDFS, right flexor digitorum superficialis muscle in the upper limb; REDB, right extensor digitorum brevis muscle in the lower limb; RTA, right tibialis anterior muscle in the lower limb. (*See* color insert.)

severity of phasic electromyographic activity and the frequency and complexity of behaviors and vocalizations in REM sleep are variable between two consecutive nights. This led to the speculation that the atonia system is permanently damaged, whereas impairment of the phasic motor system may depend on the intensity of dream processing occurring each night, if one assumes that dreams in RBD can be translated into movements and vocalizations.[98,106] One study in IRBD showed that after a mean follow-up of 5 years, both tonic and phasic excessive electromyographic activity during REM sleep increased over time. This suggests that in IRBD there is an underlying progressive pathological process damaging the brainstem structures that suppress both REM sleep tonic and phasic electromyographic activity. This finding reflects a greater extent of brainstem dysfunction occurring with

the passage of time in subjects with IRBD.[107] In another study, both tonic and phasic excessive electromyographic activity were similar between IRBD patients and patients with RBD linked to PD. In contrast, tonic electromyographic activity, but not phasic, was higher in RBD linked to MSA than in IRBD and RBD linked to PD.[64] This difference may have a basis in different direct or indirect effects of disease-specific pathology upon brainstem structures that modulate REM sleep. Pathological involvement in MSA is more severe and diffuse, and clinically MSA is characterized by faster progression and poorer prognosis than PD and IRBD. Thus, a more widespread and severe dysfunction in the brainstem structures that regulate REM sleep probably accounted for higher proportions of REM sleep without atonia in MSA. This is in agreement with the finding that in PD the excessive electromyographic

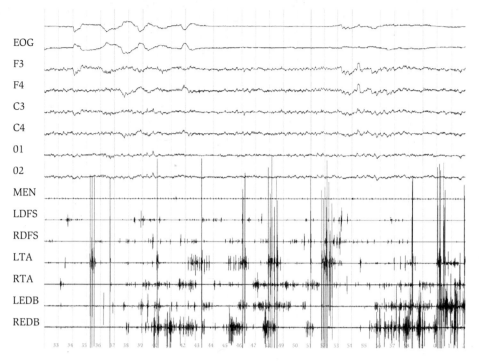

FIGURE 30.7   Polysomnographic representation of abnormal normal REM sleep in a patient with idiopathic REM sleep behavior disorder. This figure represents 30 seconds showing normal muscle atonia in the mentalis but excessive phasic electromyographic activity in the upper and lower limb muscles of both sides that was clinically associated with prominent jerks in the limbs. EOG, electrooculogram; F3, F4, C3, C4, O1, and O2, electroencephalographic electrode positions (frontal, central, and occipital of each side) according to the 10/20 International system referenced to combined ears; LDFS, left flexor digitorum superficialis muscle in the upper limb; LEDB, left extensor digitorum brevis muscle in the lower limb; LTA, left tibialis anterior muscle in the lower limb; MEN, mentalis muscle; RDFS, right flexor digitorum superficialis muscle in the upper limb; REDB, right extensor digitorum brevis muscle in the lower limb; RTA, right tibialis anterior muscle in the lower limb.

activity is more marked in the akinetic-rigid form and in the symmetric form, two subtypes of PD linked to widespread and severe pathological damage[163] and more likely to be associated with the occurrence of RBD.[63] One study reported that in patients with IRBD the severity of increased tonic electromyographic activity at baseline in the mentalis muscle was a marker for the future development of PD. In this study, the reason for the link between the severity of REM atonia loss and development of PD was not clear, particularly because the tonic activity did not predict the development of dementia and because phasic activity did not predict the development of either PD or dementia.[57] This study needs to be replicated.

In RBD, the excessive tonic electromyographic activity can be continuous or intermittent throughout REM sleep. Excessive tonic electromyographic activity is asymptomatic. In RBD, the increased tonic electromyographic activity is prominent in the cranially innervated muscles like the mentalis and the sternocleidomastoid, and it is almost absent in the trunk and limbs (unpublished observations). If tonic electromyographic activity is seen in the limbs, it is usually observed in the proximal upper-limb muscles such as the deltoid (unpublished observations).

In IRBD, increased phasic electromyographic activity may be asymptomatic or linked to simple or complex behaviors. In RBD, excessive phasic electromyographic activity in the mentalis and upper- and lower-extremity muscles is still evident in those polysomnographic studies where overt dream enactment is not captured by video analysis.[164] In one study in IRBD, 65% of REM sleep time had phasic electromyographic activity in the mentalis and limb muscles, and only 28% of REM sleep time was associated with movements or vocalizations. The majority of the increased phasic electromyographic activity seen in the mentalis is asymptomatic, but sometimes it may be associated with repetitive opening of the mouth, grimacing, and vocalizations. Isolated electromyographic recording of the mentalis muscle does not show phasic electromyographic activity in 35% of the behaviors displayed by RBD patients.[129] In patients with RBD, the greatest amount of phasic electromyographic activity is detected in the mentalis, followed in descending order by the flexor digitorum superficialis, extensor digitorum brevis, abductor pollicis brevis, sternocleidomastoid, deltoid, biceps brachii, gastrocnemius, anterior tibialis, rectus femoris, and thoraco-lumbar paraspinal muscles. The greatest amount of phasic electromyographic activity is detected in cranially innervated muscles (mentalis and sternocleidomastoid), followed by muscles of the upper and then the lower limbs. Phasic electromyographic activity is much less prominent in the axial paraspinal muscles in the trunk than in the limbs. Phasic electromyographic activity is detected more frequently in distal than in proximal muscles in both upper and lower extremities. Phasic electromyographic activity in proximal limb muscles tends to appear simultaneously with distal limb activity, whereas phasic electromyographic activity in distal limb muscles tends to appear independently from proximal limb muscles, both in upper and lower limbs. The mentalis muscle provides higher rates of excessive phasic electromyographic activity than all other muscles but only detects 55% of the mini-epochs with phasic electromyographic activity. This suggests that for the diagnosis of RBD, assessment of additional muscles in the limbs is needed when using routine polysomnography. Simultaneous recording of the mentalis, flexor digitorum superficialis, and extensor digitorum brevis muscles detects 82% of all mini-epochs containing phasic electromyographic activity.[124] This combination of muscles detects more than 90% of the motor and vocal manifestations occurring in RBD subjects and can be useful for the routine diagnosis of RBD in sleep centers.[129] For the clinical practice, the distinction between healthy controls and RBD patients can be obtained quantifying "any" (either tonic or phasic) electromyographic activity in the mentalis and phasic electromyographic activity in the right and left flexor digitorum superficialis in the upper limbs with a cutoff of 32%.[165] Individuals exceeding this cutoff are likely to have RBD. This is important since there are conditions that may resemble the clinical picture of RBD (e.g., obstructive sleep apnea, confusional arousals, epilepsy, etc.).

Some RBD patients have both increased tonic and phasic activity in the mentalis and limb muscles. Another group of RBD patients exhibits only increased phasic electromyographic activity in the limbs and normal atonia in the mentalis. In few RBD cases the increased phasic activity may only involve the upper or only the lower limbs. Another group of RBD patients has only increased tonic activity in the mentalis and not excessive phasic activity in the limbs (this is possibly a subclinical form of RBD that may later evolve to clinical RBD if phasic electromyographic activity appears with time). These different presentations of muscle activity in RBD may underlie different degrees and extent of dysfunction in the brainstem structures that modulate REM sleep tonic and phasic electromyographic activity.[30] It has been suggested that the direct pathway that originates from the SLD and reaches directly the spinal cord regulates tonic electromyographic activity, whereas the indirect pathway that originates in the SLD and reaches first the VMM and then the spinal cord regulates the phasic electromyographic activity.[26] This is in line with the observation in rats that SLD lesions produce loss of atonia in neck muscle but appear to have no significant effect on phasic electromyographic activity of the jaw (Fig. 30.4).[123]

Is There a Motor Somatotopic Representation in the Brainstem Nuclei That Generate REM Sleep Atonia?

In the primary motor cortex there are distinct subpopulations of neurons that innervate specific skeletal muscles through the corticospinal pyramidal tract. The muscles of one side of the face, arm, and leg are represented in the contralateral primary motor cortex. The cortical representation is not homogeneous since the parts of the body capable of the most delicate and elaborate movements have the largest cortical representation. The face, lips, and tongue are overrepresented followed by the hand and the foot in what has been called the Penfield's homunculus. Muscles in the trunk and in the proximal upper and lower limbs have a much smaller cortical representation.

To the best of our knowledge, a motor somatotopic distribution in the brainstem nuclei that modulate REM sleep has not been evaluated. Unlike primary motor cortex, it is unknown if the vSLD and the nucleus magnocellularis have a somatotopic representation where different subregions of cells modulate the activity of specific skeletal muscles in the face, trunk, and limbs. Projections from these different subgroups of neurons within the brainstem nuclei would reach either the cranial nerve nuclei in the brainstem or the cervical, thoracic, or lumbar segments of the spinal cord. It is also uncertain whether in these nuclei some body parts are overrepresented (e.g., upper limbs versus lower limbs, and flexors versus extensors). Such a topographic microstructure would explain the observation that in some RBD patients the increased phasic electromyographic activity is more marked in the upper limbs than in the lower limbs, or the contrary. In cats,[19] healthy people,[20] and RBD subjects,[124] phasic electromyographic activity is more frequent in distal muscles than in proximal muscles and more prominent in flexor muscles than in extensor muscles. Thus, it can be speculated that the excessive electromyographic expression of RBD seen in distal and flexor limb muscles represents an abnormal increase of a physiological tendency occurring in REM sleep.

Can REM Sleep Behavior Disorder Be Caused by Unilateral or Nondominant Lesions?

It has never been evaluated whether RBD can be caused by unilateral damage to the structures that regulate REM sleep, or whether it is necessary to have a bilateral damage for the development of this parasomnia. To the best of our knowledge, there are no descriptions of RBD patients having abnormal behaviors in only one hemi-body.

The SLD and nucleus magnocellularis are paired symmetric structures located in the two different sides of the brainstem. The SLD sends bilateral projections with ipsilateral dominance to the layer VII-VIII ventral horn of the spinal cord. The SLD from one side of the brainstem sends projections to the SLD of the other side, and vice versa.[10] In one study

performed with cats, unilateral electrolytic lesions in the SLD or caudally projecting fibers resulted in REM sleep without atonia associated with minimal release of proximal limb movements and rocking head and neck movements. More complex behaviors were seen when the lesions were larger and bilateral.[39] In another study, small unilateral lesions in the subcoeruleus region of cats were sufficient to remove the atonia of REM sleep, whereas larger and bilateral lesions were required to release abnormal behaviors.[41] Similar to cats, unilateral lesion of the SLD in rats results in REM sleep without atonia (unpublished observation).

In humans, RBD can be caused by a structural unilateral[80] or bilateral focal lesion (e.g., stroke, tumor, demyelinating plaque) confined to the brainstem.[80–86,168,169] We have seen a patient who developed RBD after an acute unilateral hemorrhage in the medulla who showed abnormal behaviors in the four limbs on videopolysomnography.[79] This indicates that a unilateral brainstem lesion may be sufficient to cause RBD. There is not a single description of RBD in humans and experimental animals where only one side of the body was involved. It has not been studied whether the abnormal movements seen in human RBD can be unilateral or predominate in the dominant or nondominant hemibody. In PD subjects with asymmetrical parkinsonism when awake, RBD behaviors are more common in the most disabled arm, hand, and leg.[113]

Neurons from the primary cortex innervate the contralateral SLD. Most of the glutamatergic descending neurons from the SLD that inhibit the spinal cord are ipsilateral.[12] Thus, neurons from the dominant left motor cortex innervate the right SLD, which inhibits the right lower motor neuron in the spinal cord, resulting in muscle atonia of the right hemibody. In normal people, when nonpathological unilateral movements are made during REM sleep, they are more prominent (70%) in the nondominant hand. Thus, it seems that in normal conditions the dominant hand is less responsive during sleep than during wakefulness.[125] The amount of phasic electromyographic activity is similar between both sides of the body in both RBD patients and healthy controls (personal observations). However, it has never been investigated whether RBD behaviors are more prominent in the dominant or nondominant hemibody.

ARE REM SLEEP ONSET AND CONTINUITY PARAMETERS AFFECTED IN REM SLEEP BEHAVIOR DISORDER?

In rats, the ventral part of SLD contains a mixed population of glutamatergic and GABA-ergic cells; glutamatergic neurons modulate the muscle tone, whereas GABA-ergic cells modulate REM sleep onset and continuity parameters (REM sleep latency, percentage of REM sleep, and number of REM sleep periods).[21] The dorsal part of the SLD also contains glutamatergic and GABA-ergic cells that modulate REM sleep onset and continuity parameters [5,12] but not REM sleep atonia. The VMM modulates REM sleep atonia and not REM sleep onset and continuity. Patients with IRBD have increased phasic and tonic electromyographic activity in REM sleep, but parameters of REM sleep onset and continuity are normal.[30] REM sleep onset and continuity parameters remain stable across consecutive nights.[106] A longitudinal follow-up study of 5 years showed that in patients with the IRBD both excessive tonic and phasic electromyographic activity increase with time, whereas REM sleep parameters of onset and continuity remain normal with the passage of time.[107] This finding suggests that in IRBD there is a progressive pathologic process damaging the structures that generate REM sleep atonia (the ventral subcoeruleus, the VMM) but sparing those that modulate REM sleep continuity (the dorsal subcoeruleus, LPT, and vlPAG). Large experimental lesions of the mesopontine tegmentum in rodents produce not only REM sleep without atonia but also a decrease in REM sleep percentage.[12] It is possible that these large lesions are also damaging some brainstem nuclei that regulate REM sleep onset and continuity such as the LPT and vlPAG. Taken together, it seems that IRBD patients have restricted lesions in the brainstem that selectively impair the structures that generate REM sleep atonia, preserving those that modulate REM sleep onset and continuity.[5]

What Is the Origin of Motor Behaviors in REM Sleep Behavior Disorder

Patients with RBD display two types of motor behaviors during REM sleep[108]:

1. *Simple motor behaviors.* They are primitive jerky movements of the head, face, limbs, or the whole body. They are exaggerated expressions of those small movements and jerks seen in normal people during normal REM sleep linked to bursts of phasic electromyographic activity. Some RBD patients occasionally may display these movements in non-REM sleep.

2. *Complex motor behaviors.* These are classical dream-enacting behaviors that represent elaborated purposeful movements that can be violent (punching, kicking, biting, pulling hair) or nonviolent (mimicking eating, drinking, kissing, dancing, smoking, clapping, spitting, inspecting the army, pointing, searching for something). They resemble very much the movements that are displayed during wakefulness in normal people, with the exception that RBD patients have their eyes closed.[109]

In IRBD, simple motor behaviors (69%) are more frequent than complex motor behaviors (31%).[104,108] Both types of movements are usually displayed by the same person. Simple motor behaviors may occur while the patient mutters, groans, moans, or shouts. Complex behaviors can be associated with shouts, swearing, singing, or giving long instructions or speeches.

It is thought that simple motor behaviors, particularly those fast myoclonic body or limb jerks, are primitive movements that arise from the activation of central pattern generators at the level of the brainstem.[110]

In contrast, the presence of complex, elaborated, and purposeful motor behaviors is indicative of the participation of motor neocortical areas. There are no reports of RBD linked to cortical lesions (e.g., stroke, tumors) or neurodegenerative diseases selectively damaging the cortex (e.g., pure Alzheimer disease without Lewy body pathology). Bilateral lesions of the parieto-occipital cortex can prevent dreaming, but REM sleep is still characterized by muscle atonia.[111] Thus, it can be speculated that complex behaviors in RBD are mediated by abnormal activation of motor cortical areas rather than their damage. This is in line with a recent report on functional neuroimaging that showed activation of the supplementary motor area during an RBD episode in a man with MSA who was gesturing while dreaming that he was searching for something.[112] The supplementary area is implicated in the planning of motor actions. In normal conditions, the supplementary motor area is anatomically connected with the SLD[9] and promotes REM sleep. Therefore, it is possible that in

RBD the activation of the supplementary motor area reaches the spinal cord directly, bypassing a damaged brainstem, resulting in elaborated dream-enacting behaviors. This speculation is in agreement with the observations that during RBD episodes PD and MSA patients show purposeful movements that are faster, stronger, and smoother than during wakefulness.[113,114] The authors of these studies in PD and MSA proposed the following hypothesis to explain the restoration of normal motor control seen in patients during RBD: the complex movements are generated by the motor areas and follow the pyramidal tract bypassing the basal ganglia, which is damaged by the disease. The inputs from the cortex are transmitted directly to lower motor neurons, resulting in dream-enacting behaviors since the brainstem structures that produce REM sleep atonia are impaired by the disease. Thus, in this model the motoneurons of the spinal cord during REM sleep are not submitted to the influence of the brainstem structures that regulate REM sleep and basal ganglia, resulting in dream-enacting behaviors without parkinsonian features.

In summary, it is possible that the origin of the simple motor behaviors in RBD arise from a primary damage of the brainstem, leading to increased phasic electromyographic activity. The origin of the complex behaviors probably lies in the abnormal activation of the motor cortex that reaches the spinal cord directly.

What Is the Origin of Vocalizations in REM Sleep Behavior Disorder?

There are two types of vocalizations in RBD[115]:

1. *Simple vocalizations.* These elementary and primitive vocalizations include groaning, muttering, catcall, moaning, shouts, swearing, crying, and laughing. They are primitive, brief, and usually include an emotional component.

2. *Complex vocalizations.* They are much less common than simple vocalizations. They include singing, whistling, arguing, complaining, and giving short or long speeches. They can be intelligible or have normal prosody. They are linked to a negative emotional component (arguing) and less frequently to a pleasant component (singing). Few patients may use foreign languages or combine two different mother-tongue languages like Spanish and Catalán (unpublished observations).

An elementary model of normal vocal control during wakefulness, based mainly on research in the squirrel monkey, consists of two different pathways.[116,117]

1. In the first pathway the anterior cingulate gyrus and the supplementary motor area project to the PAG in the midbrain, and the PAG projects to an extensive area in the reticular formation of the pons and medulla that includes the retroambiguus nucleus and the gigantocellularis nucleus. Finally, these lower brainstem nuclei project bilaterally to the phonatory motoneurons of the nucleus ambiguus and hypoglossal nucleus. The anterior cingulate cortex, supplementary motor area, and PAG are responsible for voluntary initiation of vocal behavior. In this same pathway the pontine and medullar nuclei of the reticular formation modulate innate vocal reactions such as nonverbal emotional vocal utterances (crying, laughing, screaming). Electrical stimulation of the anterior cingulate gyrus, PAG, and reticular formation in the lower brainstem induces vocalizations such as screaming and laughing. PAG stimulation with glutamate, with acetylcholine, and with GABA antagonists also results in vocalizations. Lesions in the anterior cingulate gyrus, supplementary motor area, and PAG cause mutism.

2. The second pathway runs from the primary motor cortex via the reticular formation in the pons and medulla to the phonatory motoneurons. This pathway is modulated by basal ganglia and cerebellar inputs. It is responsible for the production of learned vocal patterns. Lesions of the primary motor cortex produce mutism and lack of singing, but patients are still able to moan, cry, and laugh.

This anatomic model of vocalizations should be inactive during sleep, particularly during REM sleep. It is tempting to speculate that in RBD simple vocalizations arise from abnormal activation of the first pathway at the level of the brainstem nuclei, including the PAG, whereas complex vocalizations may result from abnormal activation of the primary motor cortex and cortical language areas.

The speech of patients with PD and MSA is more intelligible, louder, and better articulated during RBD episodes than during wakefulness.[113,114] This may be explained by impairment of the basal ganglia and cerebellum by the disease that does not inhibit the activity of motor and cortical language areas to reproduce learned vocal patterns during REM sleep.

Does the Limbic System Have a Role in the Pathophysiology of REM Sleep Behavior Disorder?

The limbic system is a set of brain structures, including the amygdala, hippocampus, cingulate gyrus, mammillary bodies, and nucleus accumbens, that modulates a variety of functions, including emotion, behavior, reward, long-term memory, and autonomic function. In particular, the amygdala regulates intense emotions (pleasure and fear) during wakefulness.[118,119]

In RBD, the characteristic emotional component of the dream-enacting behaviors and vocalizations (e.g., punching, screaming, groaning) and the common occurrence of nightmares (e.g., being attacked, being chased) have led to the hypothesis that the limbic system, and particularly the amygdala, is involved in the pathogenesis of this parasomnia. The following lines of evidence indicate that the amygdala participates in the generation of REM sleep and that its dysfunction can lead to the occurrence of RBD.

1. Positron emission tomography studies have demonstrated that the amygdala shows an intense metabolic activation during REM sleep that has been related to the affective content of dreams.[17]

2. The central nucleus of the amygdala sends direct excitatory glutamatergic projections to the subcoeruleus nucleus, resulting in REM sleep.[8,10]

3. Amygdala damage is linked to some forms of epilepsy during wakefulness characterized by violence.[120]

4. In patients with narcolepsy, abnormal activation of the amygdala occurs during cataplexy, a symptom characterized by the acute occurrence of REM sleep atonia triggered by emotional stimuli (e.g., laughing, anger).[121]

5. Cats with unilateral damage to the central nucleus of the amygdala preceded by bilateral pontine lesions exhibit attack behaviors associated with increased electromyographic activity during REM sleep.[122]

6. In cats, pontine lesions damaging the pathway arising from the central nucleus of the amygdala results in violent attacking behaviors during REM sleep.[39]

7. Pathological changes in the limbic structures are common in neurodegenerative diseases where RBD is very frequent such as PD, MSA, and DLB.[126]

8. RBD occurs in limbic encephalitis associated with raised antibodies to voltage-gated potassium channels (VGKC-LE). This disorder spares the brainstem and is characterized by prominent amygdalar-hippocampal damage leading to RBD, memory problems, confusion, and seizures.[88,127] In VGKC-LE the origin of RBD may be explained by primary damage to the limbic system leading to functional dysregulation of the brainstem REM sleep atonia–related structures. It should be noted, though, that RBD does not occur in patients with chronic epilepsy secondary to bilateral amygdalar-hippocampal sclerosis without brainstem impairment. This might indicate that the limbic damage occurring in epileptic patients with chronic bilateral mesial temporal sclerosis is not severe enough to damage the REM sleep atonia network.[128]

CONTROVERSIES IN REM SLEEP BEHAVIOR DISORDER

Do the Experimental Animal Models of REM Sleep Behavior Disorder Represent the Exact Equivalent to Human REM Sleep Behavior Disorder?

Overall, experiments with rodents and felines have provided a large amount of knowledge on the normal REM sleep control and on the pathophysiology of RBD. However, one should question whether these animal models showing increased electromyographic activity in REM sleep are the exact paradigm of the pathophysiology of human RBD. The human brain is not exactly the same as the brain of rodents and cats. Size, localization, and the role of some nuclei may vary across species. Vocalization is another issue that may distinguish RBD patients from experimental animals with RBD. Published articles on animal models of RBD have some limitations. Early studies did not distinguished tonic from phasic electromyographic activity and they only used the term "REM sleep without atonia." In many papers, video analysis was not used, and subsequently we had no information about whether the excessive electromyographic activity was sufficient to cause movements. In humans with RBD, the mentalis, the flexor digitorum superficialis in the upper limbs, and the extensor digitorum brevis in the lower limbs are the muscles where the increased phasic electromyographic activity is more prominent.[124] Simultaneous electromyographic recording of these three muscles detects 95% of the motor and vocal manifestations occurring in patients with RBD.[129] Electromyographic activity in animal models of RBD has always been recorded in the neck (analogous with the mentalis muscle in humans), but only recently it has been investigated in the limbs where the manifestations of human RBD are characteristic and very prominent.[44]

Although SLD lesions in rats trigger prominent tonic and phasic electromyographic activity of postural muscles (neck and limbs), it appears not to increase significantly phasic activity of cranial muscles of jaw and eyes (Fig. 30.4).[123] This observation is consistent with the finding that direct stimulation of the SLD induces RBD-like sleep behavior disorder but without inducing more rapid eye movements.[9] Thus, neurons that regulate phasic movements of cranial motor neurons may locate in the SLD. Assumed strong phasic activity of the cranial motor neurons of RBD suggests that the animal model of SLD lesions does not capture the full spectrum of RBD. It is likely that the neural degeneration of RBD spreads further than the subcoeruleus nucleus.

Is REM Sleep Behavior Disorder More Frequent in Men?

More than 80% of the patients presenting to sleep centers with IRBD are men.[46-48] A strong male predominance is also observed in DLB patients with RBD.[30] In PD, the male predominance has been observed in most but not all series.[11,13] The male predominance, however, is not evident in MSA, probably because RBD occurs in most, if not all, patients with MSA, and this disease has no gender predominance.[59,64]

The origin of the male preponderance in RBD is unknown. It has been hypothesized that sex hormone abnormalities might account for this male predominance and for the violent nature of the RBD-associated behaviors.[130] Two studies, however, in male patients with IRBD[131] and in RBD linked to PD[132] showed no differences in morning circulating sex hormone levels between patients and controls.

Aside from potential hormonal issues, there are other possible explanations for the male predominance of patients with RBD. First, RBD may be milder in females and may produce less vigorous and disruptive behaviors, thereby making female patients less prone to seek medical help. This hypothesis is supported by (1) the finding that in PD the mildest form of RBD (subclinical increased submental tonic electromyographic activity in REM sleep) is equally frequent in men and women, whereas clinically evident RBD is more common in men[62]; (2) the result of an epidemiological study showing that subjects with a milder clinical form of RBD do not seek medical attention[133]; and (3) the fact that unpleasant dream content in RBD is somewhat different between males and females. RBD-related dream content in men usually compromises physical and vocal self-defense against unknown attackers. In contrast, dream content in women includes sensation of threat and fear and being chased, while physical aggression against someone is rarely reported.[134] A different explanation for the male predominance is a referral bias. RBD may manifest similarly in women and men, but women may be more embarrassed by their condition and ashamed to seek medical consultation. It is also possible that women are more capable than men in detecting sleep disorders of their bed partners (such as snoring, apneas, and abnormal sleep behaviors) and are more prompt to seek medical attention for them.

Does Alpha-Synuclein Pathology Cause REM Sleep Behavior Disorder?

Alpha-synuclein is a normal brain protein that is thought to be involved in synaptic vesicle transport. Diseases characterized by abnormal alpha-synuclein aggregates in the nervous system include PD, MSA, and DLB and pure autonomic failure, which are termed *synucleinopathies*.[126]

It has been speculated that RBD is linked to accumulation of alpha-synuclein aggregates.[135] This conclusion is based on the following observations. First, Lewy bodies (neuronal inclusions containing abnormal deposition of alpha-synuclein) were found in the autopsied brains of the only two published IRBD patients with no clinical evidence of a neurodegenerative disease.[55,136] Second, pathology in RBD subjects with comorbid parkinsonism and/or dementia demonstrates widespread Lewy bodies in the brain.[94] Third, RBD is very frequent in those neurodegenerative disorders characterized by deposition of alpha-synuclein, such as PD, MSA, and DLB.[30] Conversely, RBD is not described, absent, or uncommon in several neurodegenerative disorders lacking alpha-synuclein inclusions, including pallido-ponto-nigral degeneration,[56] Alzheimer disease, frontotemporal dementia, corticobasal degeneration, Wilson disease, and amyotrophic lateral sclerosis.[30]

Available data, though, indicate that RBD in the setting of a neurodegenerative disease is not an exclusive finding of a synucleinopathy. RBD occurs in several disorders involving intracellular accumulation of other abnormal proteins such as ataxins, parkin, and tau. RBD has been found in disorders in which synuclein pathology is generally lacking such as spinocerebellar ataxias,[137–139] parkinsonism with *Parkin* mutations,[115] progressive supranuclear palsy,[140] Guadeloupean parkinsonism,[141] and Huntington disease.[142] Conversely, RBD is uncommon in patients with pure autonomic failure, a disorder where Lewy bodies are found in the central and autonomic nervous systems.[143] Taken together, we believe that there is no strong evidence indicating that RBD is caused by the abnormal deposition of a single protein like alpha-synuclein. Moreover, it is unclear whether Lewy bodies are a toxic aggregation contributing to neuronal death or have a neuroprotective role.[144]

Does Nigrostriatal Dopaminergic Deficiency Play a Central Role in REM Sleep Behavior Disorder?

It has been hypothesized that dysfunction of the dopaminergic nigrostriatal system plays an important role in the pathogenesis of RBD.[145] RBD occurs frequently in PD, MSA, and DLB, three neurodegenerative diseases where substantia nigra neuronal loss is prominent.[47,48] There are published reports of a few patients who experienced subjective improvement of RBD symptoms after the administration of dopaminergic agents.[96,146] In about 40%–50% of patients with IRBD, FP-CIT-SPECT shows reduced striatal dopamine transporters.[32,58] However, this observation may alternatively represent a comorbid finding and not the primary pathogenic determinant of RBD, as subjects with IRBD frequently develop a neurodegenerative disorder associated with substantia nigra cell loss (e.g., PD, MSA, and DLB).[47,48] In PD,

parkinsonism only manifests when the substantia nigra pars compacta reaches a 50%–60% of cell loss. Thus, it is possible that FP-CIT-SPECT in IRBD is detecting subjects close to 50%–60% substantia nigra neuronal loss at a high risk for developing parkinsonism, rather than explaining the pathophysiology of RBD. Moreover, dopamine transporter FP-CIT-SPECT is abnormal in idiopathic PD regardless of the presence or absence of RBD.

There are many lines of evidence suggesting that dopaminergic deficiency is not directly responsible for RBD pathogenesis:

1. RBD or REM sleep without atonia does not occur in about half of the PD patients.[60,62]

2. In some PD patients with RBD, the parasomnia onset clearly antedates the onset of parkinsonism.[64]

3. In PD, longer duration of parkinsonism is linked to higher dopaminergic deficit and to a decrease in the percentage of subjects suffering from RBD [61,62]

4. Total levodopa equivalent dose and the use of dopamine agonists are not different between PD patients with and without RBD.[64,113]

5. In PD patients with RBD, total levodopa equivalent dose is not associated with measures of RBD severity, such as tonic electromyographic activity in the mentalis, phasic electromyographic activity in the mentalis and limbs, self-reported severity of the RBD symptoms, and severity of the behaviors detected on video-polysomnography.[64]

6. The use of dopaminergic agents usually does not improve RBD. In PD, pramipexole, a dopamine agonist, does not improve RBD symptoms and video-polysomnographic RBD-related measures.[97] Dopaminergic agents in subjects with IRBD [95] and RBD secondary to PD[147] increase the tonic electromyographic activity during REM sleep. Moreover, in some PD patients, RBD onset was temporarily associated with the initiation of levodopa,[147] dopamine agonists,[148] and selegiline.[149]

7. In PD, surgical techniques (e.g., deep brain subthalamic stimulation) do not ameliorate RBD while they provide effective control of the parkinsonian dopaminergic motor symptoms.[150–152]

8. In RBD cases secondary to structural brainstem lesions (stroke, tumors) the substantia nigra is habitually spared ().[79–86,168,169]

9. Two conditions that respond to dopaminergic agents, restless legs syndrome and periodic

leg movements in sleep, are not more common in PD patients with RBD than without RBD.[113]

10. Although not systematically studied, there are neither published reports of RBD precipitated by antipsychotic drugs blocking dopaminergic receptors nor descriptions of RBD occurring in subjects with drug-induced parkinsonism.

11. Animals studies in rats and cats with lesions of substantia nigra dopaminergic and GABA-ergic cells did not show REM sleep without atonia.[153,154]

In contrast, one study has shown that in monkeys treated with MPTP (the nonhuman primate model for PD characterized by toxic nigrostriatal dopaminergic deficit), there is increased tonic, but not phasic, electromyographic activity in the chin and neck muscles.[155] Other author, however, found that increased REM sleep electromyographic activity and abnormal behaviors during REM sleep do not occur in the chronic MPTP-treated primate.[29]

Does the Braak et al. Ascending Hypothesis for Parkinson's Disease Fit with the Time of Appearance of REM Sleep Behavior Disorder?

Braak and collegues[156] reported that in sporadic PD, Lewy pathology (Lewy bodies and Lewy neurites containing alpha-synuclein aggregates) begins in the dorsal motor nucleus of the vagus nerve in the medulla (stage 1) and advances upward through the magnocellularis reticular nucleus and the subcoeruleus-coeruleus complex (stage 2), the substantia nigra, the pedunculopontine nucleus, and the amygdala (stage 3), the temporal mesocortex (stage 4), and finally reaches the neocortex (stages 5 and 6). Braak et al. postulated that stages 1 and 2 correspond to a pre-motor state of PD, stages 3 and 4 to the development of parkinsonism, and stages 5 and 6 to parkinsonism associated with cognitive impairment.[156] This temporal sequence of Lewy pathology in PD may account for the finding that in some patients, RBD (stage 2) antedates the clinical onset of parkinsonism (stage 3).[46–48] This temporal sequence, however, does not explain why some PD patients do not develop RBD[60] and why parkinsonism precedes RBD onset in most PD subjects.[64] One possible explanation is that in these situations severity of neuronal dysfunction in the brainstem structures modulating REM sleep does not reach a

critical threshold for the clinical expression of RBD. Alternatively, it is possible that the Braak et al. staging system in sporadic PD may not be valid in all instances. A study evaluating 71 PD cases showed that the caudo-rostral spreading described by Braak et al. did not occur in 47% of the cases.[157] The clinical significance of the Braak et al. staging system in PD is debatable because (1) the patients that based the Braak et al. original hypothesis were not clinically phenotyped, (2) inclusion criteria may have biased the results since only cases with Lewy pathology in the medulla were studied, (3) cell loss was not assessed, and (4) it is unknown whether Lewy pathology is directly responsible for neurological symptoms. Several studies have shown that in PD and DLB, Lewy pathology may be found in multiple sites sparing the medulla.[126,158,159] Moreover, Lewy pathology is found in 2%–20% of the normal aged population,[160] and 10% of the healthy aged people exhibit Lewy bodies in the substantia nigra.[161] It may be that the severity of cell loss in the nuclei that modulate REM sleep, rather than the presence of Lewy bodies in surviving neurons, is necessary for the development of RBD.

The caudo-rostral topographical sequence for PD described by Braak et al.[156] has not been found in DLB, a neurodegenerative disorder commonly associated with RBD where dementia antedates parkinsonism onset. It has been suggested that in DLB a neuropathological regional pattern of Lewy pathology exists that progresses downward from the neocortex to the amygdala, diencephalon, and finally reaches the brainstem (substantia nigra, locus coeruleus, reticular formation, and dorsal vagal nucleus).[162] This stage system, however, does not fit with the common observation that RBD usually precedes dementia in DLB.[30]

REFERENCES

1. Boeve B. REM sleep behavior disorder. *Ann NY Acad Sci* 2010;1184:15–54.
2. Fuller PM, Saper CB, Lu J. The pontine REM switch: past and present. *J Physiol* 2007;584–3:735–41.
3. Boeve B, Silber M, Saper C, et al. Pathpphysiology of REM sleep behaviour disorder and relevance to neurodegenerative disease. *Brain* 2007;130:2770–88.
4. Siegel JM. The neurobiology of sleep. *Sem Neurol* 2009;29:277–96.

5. Luppi PH, Clement O, Sapin E, et al. The neuronal network responsble for paradoxical sleep and its dysfunctions causing narcolepsy and rapid eye movement (REM) behavior disorder. *Sleep Med Rev* 2011;15:153–63.

6. Saper CB, Fuller PM, Pedersen NP, et al. Sleep state switching. *Neuron* 2010;68:1023–42.

7. Reinoso-Suárez F, de Andrés I, Rodrigo-Angulo ML, et al. Brain structures and mechanisms involved in the generation of REM sleep. *Sleep Med Rev* 2001;5:67–77.

8. Fung SJ, Xi M, Zhang J, et al. Projection neurons from the central nucleus of the amygdala to the nucleus pontis oralis. *J Neurosci Res* 2011;89:429–36.

9. Boissard R, Gervasoni D, Scmidt MH, et al. The rat ponto-medullary network responsible for paradoxical sleep onset and maintenance: a combined microinjection and functional neuroanatomical study. *Eur J Neurosci* 2002;16:1959–73.

10. Boissard R, Fort P, Gervasoni D, et al. Localization of the GABAergic and non-GABAergic neurons projecting to the sublaterodorsal nucleus and potentially gating of paradoxical sleep. *Eur J Neurosci* 2003;18:1627–39.

11. Crochet S, Onoe H, Sakai K. A potent non-monoaminergic paradoxical system: a reverse microdyalisis and single-unit recording study. *Eur J Neurosci* 2006;24:1404–12.

12. Lu J, Sherman D, Devor M, et al. A putative flip-flop switch for control of REM sleep. *Nature* 2006;441:589–94.

13. Luppi PH, Gervasono D, Verret L, et al. Paradoxical (REM) sleep genesis: The switch from an aminergic-cholinergic to a GABAergic-glutamatergic hypothesis. *J Phsiol* 2007;100:271–83.

14. Thannickal TC, Moore RY, Nienhuis R, et al. Reduced number of hypocretin neurons in human narcolepsy. *Neuron* 2000;27:469–74.

15. Blanchard AR, Chaudhary BA. Neuropharmacology of sleep and wakefulness. In: Lee-Chiong TL, Jr., Sateia MJ, Carskadon MA, eds. *Sleep Medicine.* Philadelphia, PA: Hanley and Belfus; 2002:565–674.

16. Clément O, Sapin E, Bérod A, et al. Evidence that neurons of the sublaterodorsal tegmental nucleus triggering paradoxical (REM) sleep are glutamatergic. *Sleep* 2011;34:419–23.

17. Dang-Vu TT, Schabaus M, Desseilles M, et al. Functional neuroimaging insights into the physiology of human sleep. *Sleep* 2010;33:1589–603.

18. Fuller P, Sherman D, Pedersen N, et al. Reassessment of the structural basis of the ascending arousal system. *J Comp Neurol* 2011; 519:933–56.

19. Gassel MM, Marchiafava PL, Pompeiano O. Phasic changes in muscular activity during desynchronized sleep in unrestrained cats. An analysis of the pattern and organization of myoclonic twitches. *Arch Ital Biol* 1964;102:449–70.

20. Gardner R, Jr., Grossman WI. Normal patterns in sleep in man. *Adv Sleep Res* 1975;2:67–107.

21. Krenzer M, Anaclet C, Vetrivelan R, et al. Brainstem and spinal cord circruity regulating REM sleep and muscle atonia. *PLoS One* 2011;6(10):e24998.

22. Chase MH, Soja PJ, Morales FR. Evidence that glycine mediates the post-synaptic potentials that inhibit lumbar motoneurons during the atonia of active sleep. *J Neurosci* 1989;9:743–51.

23. Sakai K, Kanamori N, Jouvet M. Neuronal activity specific to paardoxical sleep in the bulbar reticular formation in the unrestrained cat. *C R Seances Acad Sci D* 1979;289:557–61.

24. Chase MH. Confirmation of the consensus that glycinergic postsynaptic inhibition is responsible for the atonia of REM sleep. *Sleep* 2008;31:1487–91.

25. Brooks PL, Peever JH. Glycinercic and GABAA-mediated inhibition of somatic motoneurons does not mediate rapid eye movement sleep motor atonia. *J Neurosci* 2008;28:3535–45.

26. Vetrivelan R, Fuller PM, Tong Q, et al. Medullary circuitry regulating rapid eye movement sleep and motor atonia. *J Neurosci* 2009;29:9361–9.

27. Rye DB. Contributions of the pedunculopontine region to normal and altered REM sleep. *Sleep* 1997;20:855–90.

28. Data S, Curro Dossi R, Pare D, et al. Substantia nigra reticulata neurons during sleep-wake states: relation with ponto-geniculo-occipital waves. *Brain Res* 1991;566:344–7.

29. Rye DB, Bliwise DL. Movement disorders specific to sleep and the nocturnal manifestations of waking movement disorders. In: Watts RL, Koller WC, eds. *Movement Disorders: Neurologic Principles and Practice.* 2nd ed. New York: McGraw Hill; 2004:855–90.

30. Iranzo A, Santamaria L, Tolosa E. The clinical and pathophysiological relevance of REM

sleep behavior disorder in neurodegenerative diseases. *Sleep Med Rev* 2009;13:385–401.

31. Massicotte-Marquez J, Carrier J, Décary A, et al. Slow-wave sleep and delta power in rapid eye movement sleep behavior disorder. *Ann Neurol* 2005;57:277–82.

32. Iranzo A, Lomeña F, Stockner H, et al. Decreased striatal dopamine transporter uptake and substantia nigra hyperechogenicity as risk markers of synucleinopathy in patients with idiopathic rapid-eye-movement sleep behaviour disorder: a prospective study. *Lancet Neurology* 2010; 9:1070–7.

32a. Hendricks JC, Morrison AR. Normal and abnormal sleep in animals. *JAVMA* 1981;178:121–6.

33. Hendricks JC, Lager A, O'Brien D, et al. Movement disorders during sleep in cats and dogs. *JAVMA* 1989;194:686–9.

34. Inada S, Nomoto H, Kawasaki Y. Canine distemper myoclonus and sleep: observation of a case. *Electromyogr Clin Neurophysiol* 1993;33:137–41.

35. Bush WW, Barr CS, Stecker MM, et al. Diagnosis of rapid eye movement sleep disorder with electroencephalography and treatment with tryciclic antidepressant in a dog. *J Am Anim Hosp Assoc* 2004;40:495–500.

35a. Iranzo A, Schenck C, Fonte J. REM sleep behavior disorder and other sleep disturbances in Disney animated films. *Sleep Medicine* 2007; 8:531–6.

36. Jouvet M, Delrome F. Locus coeruleus et sommeil paradoxal. *C R Soc Biol* 1965;159:895–9.

37. Schenck CH, Bundlie SR, Ettinger MG, et al. Chronic behavioural disorders of human REM sleep: a new category of parasomnia. *Sleep* 1986;9:293–308.

38. Morrison AR, Mann GL, Hendrijks JC. The relationship of excessive exploratory behavior in wakefulness to paradoxical sleep without atonia. *Sleep* 1981;4:247–57.

39. Hendricks JC, Morrison AR, Mann GL. Different behaviors during paradoxical sleep without atonia depend on pontine lesion site. *Brain Res* 1982;239:81–105.

40. Shouse MN, Siegel JM. Pontine regulation of REM sleep components in cats: integrity of the pedunculopontine tegmentum (PPT) is important for phasic events but unnecessary for atonia during REM lseep. *Brain Res* 1992;571:50–63.

41. Sandford LD, Cheng CS, Sivestri AJ, et al. Sleep and behavior in rats with pontine

lesions producing REM without atonia. *Sleep Research Online* 2001;4:1–5.

42. Schenckel E, Siegel JM. REM sleep without atonia after lesions of the medial medulla. *Neursci Letters* 1989;98:159–65.

43. Lai YY, Hsieh KC, Nguyen D, et al. Neurotoxic lesions at the ventral mesopontine junction change sleep time and muscle activity during sleep: an animal model of motor disorders in sleep. *Neuroscience* 2008;154:431–43.

44. Brooks PL, Peever JH. Impaired GABA and glycine transmission triggers cardinal features of rapid eye movement sleep disorder in mice. *J Neurosci* 2011;31(19):7111–21.

45. Scherfler C, Frauscher B, Schocke M, et al. With and gray matter abnormalities in idiopathic rapid eye movement disorder: a diffusion-tensor imaging and voxel-based morphometry study. *Ann Neurol* 2011;12:284–8.

46. Schenck CH, Bundlie SR, Mahowald MW. Delayed emergence of a parkinsonian disorder in 38% of 29 older men initially diagnosed with idiopathic rapid eye movement sleep behavior disorder: *Neurology* 1996;46:388–92.

47. Iranzo A, Molinuevo JL, Santamaria J, et al. Rapid-eye-movement sleep behaviour disorder as an early marker for a neurodegenerative disease: a descriptive study. *Lancet Neurol* 2006;5:572–7.

48. Postuma RB, Gagnon JF, Vendette M, et al. Quantifying the risk of neurodegenerative disease in idiopathic REM sleep behavior disorder. *Neurology* 2009;72:1296–300.

49. Fantini ML, Postuma RB, Montplaisir J, et al. Olfactory deficit in idiopathic rapid eye movements sleep behavior disorder. *Brain Res Bull* 2006;70:386–90.

50. Postuma RB, Lang AE, Massicotte-Marquez J, et al. Potential early markers of Parkinson disease in idiopathic REM sleep behavior disorder. *Neurology* 2006;66:845–51.

51. Ferini-Strambi L, Di Gioia MR, Castronovo V, et al. Neuropsychological assessment in idiopathic REM sleep behavior disorder. *Neurology* 2004;62:41–5.

51a. Iranzo A, Isetta V, Molinuevo JL et al. Electroencephalographic slowing heralds mild cognitive impairment in idiopathic REM sleep behavior disorder. *Sleep Med* 2010b;11:534–9.

52. Ferini-Strambi L, Oldani A, Zucconi M, et al. Cardiac autonomic activity during wakefulness and sleep in REM sleep behavior disorder. *Sleep* 1996;19:367–9.

53. Miyamoto T, Miyamoto M, Inoue Y, et al. Reduced cardiac 123I-MBIG scintagrophy in idiopathic REM sleep behavior disorder. *Neurology* 2006;67:2236–8.

54. Stockner H, Iranzo A, Seppi K, et al. Midbrain hyperechogenicity in idiopathic REM sleep behavior disorder. *Mov Disord* 2009;24:1906–9.

55. Uchiyama M, Isse K, Tanaka K, et al. Incidental Lewy body disease in a patient with REM sleep behavior disorder. *Neurology* 1995;45:709–12.

56. Boeve BF, Lin SC, Strongosky A, et al. Absence of rapid eye movement sleep behavior disorder in 11 memebers of the pallidopontonigral degeneration kindred. *Arch Neurol* 2006;63:268–72.

57. Postuma RB, Gagnon JF, Rompré S, et al. Severity of REM atonia loss in idiopathic REM sleep behaviour disorder predicts Parkinson disease. *Neurology* 2010;74:239–44.

58. Iranzo A, Valldeoriola F, Lomeña F, et al. Serial dopamine transporter imaging of nigrostriatal function in patients with idiopathic rapid-eye-movement sleep behaviour disorder: a prospective study. *Lancet Neurol* 2011;10:797–805.

59. Plazzi G, Corsini R, Provini F, et al. REM sleep behavior disorders in multiple system atrophy. *Neurology* 1997;48:1094–7.

60. Gagnon JF, Bédard MA, Fantini ML, et al. REM sleep behavior disorder and REM sleep without atonia in Parkinson's disease. *Neurology* 2002;59:585–9.

61. Gjestard MD, Boeve B, Wentzel-Larsen, et al. Prevalence of restless legs syndrome and REM sleep behavior disorder in multiple sclerosis. *Multiple Sclerosis* 2007;13:805–8.

62. Sixel-Döring F, Trauttman E, Mollenhauer B, et al. Associated factors for REM sleep behavior disorder in Parkinson disease. *Neurology* 2011;77:1048–54.

63. Kumru H, Santamaria J, Tolosa E, et al. Relation between subtype of Parkinson's disease and REM sleep behavior disorder. *Sleep Medicine* 2007;8:779–83.

64. Iranzo A, Santamaria J, Rye DB, et al. Characteristics of idiopathic REM sleep behavior disorder and that associated with MSA and PD. *Neurology* 2005; 65:247–52.

65. Gagnon F, Petit F, Fantini ML, et al. REM sleep behavior and REM sleep without atonia in probable Alzheimer disease. *Sleep* 2006;29:1321–5.

66. Arnulf I, Merino-Andreu M, Bloch F, et al. REM sleep behavior disorder and REM sleep without atonia in progressive supranuclear palsy. *Sleep* 2005;28:349–54.

67. Arnulf I, Nielsen J, Lehman E, et al. Rapid eye movement sleep disturbances in Huntington disease. *Arch Neurol* 2008;68:482–8.

68. Arima K, Murayama S, Mukoyama M, et al. Immunocytochemical and ultrastructural studies of neuronal and oligodendroglial cytoplasmic inclusions in multiple system atrophy. *Acta Neuropathol* 1992;83:453–60.

69. Braak H, Rüb U, Sandmann-Keil D; et al. Parkinson's disease: affection of brain stem nuclei controlling premotor and motor neurons of the somatomotor system. *Acta Neuropathol* 2000;99:489–95.

70. Pahapill PA, Lozano AM. The pedunculopontine nucleus and Parkinson's disease. *Brain* 2000;123:1767–83.

71. Harding AJ, Broe AJ, Halliday GM. Visual hallucinations in Lewy body disease relate to Lewy bodies in the temporal lobe. *Brain* 2002;125:391–403.

72. Schenck CH, Mahowald MW. Motor dyscontrol in narcolepsy: rapid-eye-movement (REM) sleep without atonia and REM sleep behaviour disorder. *Ann Neurol* 1992;32:3–10.

73. Nightingale S, Orgill JC, Ebrahim IO, et al. The association between narcolepsy and REM behavior disorder (RBD). *Sleep Med* 2005;6:253–8.

74. Nevismalova S, Prihodova I, Kemlink D, et al. REM behavior disorder (RBD) can be one of the first symptoms of childhood narcolepsy. *Sleep Med* 2007;8:784–6.

75. Cipolli C, Franceschini C, Mattarozzi K, et al. Overnight distribution and motor characteristics of REM sleep behaviour disorder episodes in patients with narcolepsy-cataplexy. *Sleep Med* 2011;12(7):635–40.

76. Mattarozzi K, Belluci C, Campi C, et al. Clinical, behavioural and polysomnographic correlates of cataplexy in patients with narcolepsy/cataplexy. *Sleep Med* 2008;9:425–33.

77. Kiyaschenko LI, Mileykovskiy BY, Lai YY, et al. Increased and decreased muscle tone with orexin (hypocretin) microinjections in the locus coeruleus and pontine inhibitory area. *J Neurophysiol* 2001;85:2008–16.

78. Knudsen S, Gammeltoft S, Jennum PJ. Rapid eye movement sleep behaviour disorder in patients with narcolepsy is associated with hypocretin-1 deficiency. *Brain* 2010;133:568–79.

79. Iranzo A, Aparicio J. A lesson from anatomy: focal brain lesions causing REM sleep behavior disorder. *Sleep Med* 2009;10:9–12.

80. Limousin N, Dehais C, Gout O, et al. A brainstem inflammatory lesion causing REM sleep behavior disorder and sleepwalking (parasomnia overlap disorder). *Sleep Med* 2009;10:1059–62.

81. Kimura K, Tachibana N, Kohyama J, et al. A discrete pontine ischemic lesion could cause REM sleep behavior disorder. *Neurology* 2000;55:894–5.

82. Plazzi G, Montagna P. Remitting REM sleep behavior disorder as the initial sign of multiple sclerosis. *Sleep Med* 2002;3:437–9.

83. Provini F, Vertugno R, Pastorelli F, et al. Status dissociatus after surgery for tegmental ponto-mesencephalic cavernoma: a state dependent disorder of motor control during sleep. *Mov Disord* 2004;19:719–23.

84. Tippmann-Peikert M, Boeve BB, Keegan BM. REM sleep behavior disorder initiated by acute brainstem multiple sclerosis. *Neurology* 2006;66:1277–9.

85. Tippmann-Peikert M, Boeve BF, Silber MH. Structural lesions associated with REM sleep behavior disorder. *Sleep* 2008;31(Suppl):A264.

86. Xi Z, Luning W. REM sleep behavior disorder in a patient with a pontine stroke. *Sleep Med* 2009;10:143–6.

87. Zambelis T, Paparrigopoulos T, Soldatos CR. REM sleep behaviour disorder associated with a neurinoma of the left pontocerebellar angle. *J Neurol Neurosurg Psychiatry* 2002;72:821–2.

88. Iranzo A, Graus F, Clover L, et al. Rapid eye movement sleep behavior disorder and potassium channel antibody-associated limbic encephalitis. *Ann Neurol* 2006b;59:178–82.

89. Lugaresi E, Provini F. Agrypinia excitata: clinical features and pathophysiologic implications. *Sleep Med Reviews* 2001;5:313–22.

90. Compta Y, Iranzo A, Santamaría J, et al. REM sleep behavior disorder and narcoleptic features in anti-Ma2-asociated encephalitis. *Sleep* 2007;30:767–9.

91. Lapierre O, Montplaisir J. Polysomnographic features of REM sleep behavior disorder: development of a scoring method. *Neurology* 1992;42:1371–4.

92. Kunz D, Bes F. Melatonin as a therapy in REM sleep behavior disorder patients: an open-labeled pilot study on the possible influence of melatonin on REM-sleep regulation. *Mov Disord* 1999;14:507–11.

93. Boeve BF, Silber MH, Ferman TJ. Melatonin for treatment of REM sleep behavior disorder in neurological disorders: results in 14 patients. *Sleep Med* 2003;4:281–4.

94. Boeve BF, Silber MH, Parisi JE. Synucleinopathy pathology and REM sleep behavior disorder plus dementia or parkinsonism. *Neurology* 2003;61:40–5.

95. Fantini ML, Gagnon JF, Filipini D, et al. The effects of pramipexole in REM sleep behavior disorder. *Neurology* 2003;61:1418–20.

96. Schmidt MH, Koshal VB, Schmidt HS. Use of pramipexole in REM sleep behavior disorder: results from a case series. *Sleep Med* 2006;7:418–23.

97. Kumru H, Iranzo A, Carrasco E, et al. Lack of effects of pramipexole on REM sleep behavior disorder in Parkinson's disease. *Sleep* 2008;31:1418–21.

98. Schenck CH. The REM sleep behavior disorder odyssey. *Sleep Med* 2009;13:381–4.

99. Schenck CH, Mahowald MW, Kim SW, et al. Prominent eye movements during NREM sleep and REM sleep behaviour disorder associated with fluoxetine treatment of depression and obsessive-compulsive disorder. *Sleep* 1992;15:226–35.

100. Onofrj, Luciano AL, Thomas A, et al. Mirtazapine induces REM sleep behavior disorder (RBD) in parkinsonism. *Neurology* 2003;60:113–15.

101. Winkelman JW, James L. Serotonergic antidepressants are associated with REM sleep without atonia. *Sleep* 2004;27:2:317–21.

102. Iranzo A, Santamaría J. Bisoprolol-induced REM sleep behavior disorder. *Am J Med* 1999:107:390–2.

103. Tachibana M, Tanaka K, Hishikawa Y, et al. A sleep study of acute psychotic states due to alcohol and meprobate addiction. *Adv Sleep Res* 1975;2:177–205.

104. Frauscher B, Gschkliesser, Brandauer E, et al. The relationship between abnormal behaviors in patients with REM sleep behavior disorder. *Sleep Med* 2009;10:174–81.

105. Cecchini M, Baroni E, Di Vito C, et al. Smiling newborns during comminicative wake and active sleep. *Infant Behav Dev* 2011;34:417–23.

106. Cygan F, Oudiette D, Leclair-Visonneau L, et al. Night to night variability of muscle tone, movements and vocalizatons in patients with REM sleep behavior disorder. *J Clin Sleep Med* 2010;6:551–5.

107. Iranzo A, Ratti PL, Casanova-Molla J, et al. Excessive muscle activity increases over time in idiopathic REM sleep behavior disorder. *Sleep* 2009;32:1149–53.

108. Manni R, Terzaghi M, Glorioso M. Motor-behavioral episodes in REM sleep behavior disorder and phasic events during sleep. *Sleep* 2009;32:241–5.

109. Oudiette D, De Cock VC, Lavault S, et al. Nonviolent elaborate behaviors may also occur in REM sleep behavior disorder. *Neurology* 2009;72:551–7.

110. Tassinari CA, Rubboli G, Gardella E, et al. Central pattern generators for a common semiology in fronto-limbic seizures and parasomnias: a neuroethologic approach. *Neurol Sci* 2005; 26(Suppl 3):225–32.

111. Bischof M, Bassetti CL. Total dream loss: a distinct neuropsychological dysfunction after bilateral PCA stroke. *Ann Neurol* 2004;56:583–6.

112. Dauvilliers Y, Boudousq V, Lopez R, et al. Increased perfusion in supplementary area during a REM sleep behaviour episode. *Sleep Med* 2011;531–2.

113. De Cock VC, Vidailhet M, Leu S, et al. Restoration of motor control in Parkinson's disease during REM sleep. *Brain* 2007;130:450–6.

114. De Cock VC, Debs R, Oudiette D, et al. The improvement of movement and speech during rapid eye movement sleep behaviour disorder in multiple system atrophy. *Brain* 2011;134:856–62.

115. Kumru H, Santamaria J, Tolosa E, et al. Rapid eye movement disorder in Parkinsonism with PARKIN mutations. *Ann Neurol* 2004;56:599–603.

116. Jürgens U. Neural pathways underlying vocal control. *Neurosci Biobehav Reviews* 2002;26:235–58.

117. Jürgens U. The neural control of vocalization in mammals: a review. *J Voice* 2009;23:1–10.

118. Davis M. The role of the amygdala in conditioned and unconditioned fear and anxiety. In: Aggleton JP, ed. *The Amygdala.* New York: Oxford University Press; 2000:213–88.

119. Phelps EA. The human amygdala and control of fear. In: Whalen PJ, Phelps EA, eds. *The human amygdale.* New York: Guilford Press; 2009:204–19.

120. van Elst LT, Woermann FG, Lemieux L, et al. Affective aggression in patients with temporal lobe epilepsy: a quantitative MRI study of the amygdala. *Brain* 2000;123:234–43.

121. Schwartz S, Ponz A, Poryazova R, et al. Abnormal activity in hypothalamus and amygdala durinh humour processing in human narcolepsy with cataplexy. *Brain* 2008;131:514–22.

122. Zagrodzka J, Hedberg CE, Mann GL, et al. Contrasting expressions of aggressive behavior related by lesions of the central nucleus of the amygdala during wakefulness and rapid eye movement sleep without atonia in cats. *Behav Neuroscience* 1998;112:589–602.

123. Anaclet C, Pedersen NP, Fuller PM, et al. Brain circuitry regulating phasic activity in the trigeminal motor nucleus (Mo5) during REM sleep. *PLoS One* 2010;5:e878.

124. Frauscher B, Iranzo A, Höghl, et al. Quantification of electromyographic activity during REM sleep in multiple muscles in REM sleep behaviour disorder. *Sleep* 2008;31:724–31.

125. Jovanovic U. Normal sleep in man. *Hippokrates Verlag, Stutgart,* 1971:99–124.

126. Jellinger KA. Neuropathological spectrum of synucleinopathies. *Mov Disord* 2003;18(Suppl6);S2–12.

127. Cornelius JR, Pittock SJ, McKeon A, et al. Sleep manifestations of voltage-gated potassium channel complex autoimmunity. *Arch Neurol* 2011;68:733–8.

128. Iranzo A, Carreño M. Absence of REM sleep behavior disorder in epileptic patients with bilateral mesial temporal sclerosis not due to autoimmune encephalitis. Abstract number 2.075.Americam Epilepsy Society Annual Meeting. http://www.aesnet.org.

129. Iranzo A, Frauscher B, Santos H, et al. Usefulness of the SINBAR electromyographic montage to detect the motor and vocal manifestations occurring in REM sleep behaviour disorder. *Sleep Med* 2011;12:284–8.

130. Schenck CH, Mahowald MW. REM sleep behavior disorder: clinical, developmental, and neuroscience perspectives 16 years after its formal identification in SLEEP. *Sleep* 2002;25:120–38.

131. Iranzo A, Santamaria J, Vilaseca I, et al. Absence of alterations in serum sex hormones levels in idiopathic REM sleep behavior disorder. *Sleep* 2007;30:803–6.

132. Chou KL, Moro-De-Casillas, Amick MM, et al. Testosterone not associated with violent dreams or REM sleep behavior disorder in men with Parkinson's. *Mov Disord* 2007;22:411–14.

133. Chiu HFK, Wing YK, Lam LCW, et al. Sleep-related injury in the elderly. An epidemiological study in Hong Kong. *Sleep* 2000;23:513–17.

134. Borek LL, Kohn R, Friedman JH. Phenomenology of dreams in Parkinson's disease. *Mov Disord* 2007;22:198–202.

135. Boeve BF, Silber MH, Ferman TJ, et al. Association of REM sleep behavior disorder and neurodegenerative disease nay reflect an underlying synucleionopathy. *Mov Disord* 2001;16:622–30.

136. Boeve BF, Dickson DW, Olson EJ, et al. Insights into REM sleep behavior disorder pathophysiology in brainstem-predominant Lewy body disease. *Sleep Med* 2007;8:60–4.

137. Friedman JH, Fernandez HH, Sudarsky L. REM behavior disorder and excessive daytime somnolence in Machado-Joseph disease (SCA-3): *Mov Disord* 2003;18:1520–2.

138. Syed BH, Rye DB, Singh G. REM sleep behavior disorder and SCA-3 (Machado-Joseph disease). *Neurology* 2003;60:148.

139. Iranzo A, Muñoz E, Santamaria J, et al. REM sleep behavior disorder and vocal cord paralysis in Machado-Joseph disease. *Mov Disord* 2003;18:1179–83.

140. Arnulf I, Merino-Andreu M, Bloch F, et al. REM sleep behavior disorder and REM sleep without atonia in progressive supranuclear palsy. *Sleep* 2005;28:349–54.

141. De Cock VC, Lannuzel A, Verhaeghe S, et al. REM sleep behavior disorder in patients with Guadeloupean parkinsonism, a taupathy. *Sleep* 2007;30:1026–32.

142. Arnulf I, Nielsen J, Lehman E, et al. Rapid eye movement sleep disturbances in Huntington disease. *Arch Neurol* 2008;68:482–8.

143. Plazzi G, Cortelli P, Montagna P, et al. REM sleep behaviour disorder differentiates pure autonomic failure from multiple system atrophy with autonomic failure. *J Neurol Neurosurg Psychiatry* 1998;64:683–5.

144. Jellinger KA. Lewy body-related alpha-synucleionopathy in the aged human brain. *J Neural Transm* 2004;11:1219–35.

145. Eisensehr I, Linke R, Tatsch K et al. Increased muscle activity during rapid eye movement sleep correlates with decrease of striatal presynaptic dopamine transporters. IPT and IBZM SPECT imaging in subclinical and clinically manifest idiopathic REM sleep behavior disorder, Parkinson's disease, and controls. *Sleep* 2003;26:507–12.

146. Tan A, Salgado M, Fahn S. Rapid eye movement sleep behavior disorder preceding Parkinson's disease with therapeutic response to levodopa. *Mov Disord* 1996;11:214–16.

147. García-Borreguero D, Caminero AB, de la Llave Y, et al. Decreased phasic EMG activity during rapad eye movement sleep in treatment-naïve Parkinson's disease: effects of treatment with levodopa and progression of illness. *Mov Disord* 2002;17:934–41.

148. Kanyak D, Kiziltan H, Benbir G, et al. Sleep and sleepiness in patients with Parkinson's disease before and after dopaminergic treatment. *Eur J Neurol* 2005;12:199–207.

149. Louden MB, Morehead MA, Schmidt MS. Activation by selegiline of REM sleep behavior in parkinsonism. *W V Med J* 1995;91:101.

150. Arnulf I, Bejjani BP, Garma L, et al. Improvement of sleep architecture in PD with subthalamic stimulation. *Neurology* 2000;55:1732–4.

151. Cicolin A, Lopiano L, Zibetti M, et al. Effects of deep brain stimulation of the subthalamic nucleus on sleep architecture in Parkinsonian patients. *Sleep Med* 2004;5:207–10.

152. Iranzo A, Valldeoriola F, Santamaria J, et al. Sleep symptoms and polysomnographic architecture in advanced Parkinson's disease after chronic bilateral subthalamic stimulation. *J Neurol Neurosurg Psychiatry* 2002;72:661–4.

153. Lai YY, Hsieh KC, Nguyen D, et al. Neurotoxic lesions at the ventral mesopotime junction change in sleep time and muscle activity during sleep: an animal model of motor disorders in sleep. *Neuroscience* 2008;154:431–43.

154. Gerashchenko D, Blanco-Centurion CA, Miller JD, et al. Insomnia following hypocretin2-saporin lesions of the substantia nigra. *Neuroscience* 2006;137:29–36.

155. Verhave PS, Jongsma MJ, Van der Berg RM, et al. REM sleep behaviour disorder in the marmoset MPTP model of early Parkinson disease. *Sleep* 2011;34:119–25.

156. Braak H, Del Tredici K, Rub U, et al. Staging of brain pathology related to sporadic Parkinson's disease. *Neurobiol Aging* 2003;24:197–211.

157. Kalaitzakis ME, Graeber MB, Gemtelmen SM, et al. The dorsal motor nucleus of the vagus is not an obligatory trigger site of Parkinson's disease: a critical analysis of

alpha-synuclein staging. *Neuropathol Appl Neurobiol* 2008;34:284–95.

158. Ozawa T, Paviour D, Quinn NP, et al. The spectrum of pathological involvement of the striatonigral and olivopontocerebellar systems in multiple system atrophy: clinicopathological correlations. *Brain* 2004;127:2657–71.

159. Parkkinen L, Kauppinen T, Pirttilä, et al. Alpha-synuclein pathology does not predict extrapyramidal symptoms or dementia. *Ann Neurol* 2005;57:82–91.

160. Lindboe CF, Hansen HB. The frequency of Lewy bodies in a consecutive autopsy series. *Clin Neuropathol* 1998;17:2004–9.

161. Parkkinen L, Soininen H, Laasko M, et al. Alpha-synuclein pathology is highly dependent on the case selection. *Neuropathol Appl Neurobiol* 2001;27:314–25.

162. Yamamoto R, Iseki E, Marui W, et al. Non-uniformity in the regional pattern of Lewy pathology in brains of dementia with Lewy bodies. *Neuropathology* 2005;25:188–94.

163. Bliwise DL, Trotti LM, Greer SA, et al. Phasic muscle activity in sleep and clinical features of Parkinson disease. *Ann Neurol* 2010;68:353–9.

164. Bliwise DL, Rye DB. Elevated PEM (phasic electromyographic metric) rates identify rapid eye movementbehavior disorder patients on nights without behavioral abnormalities. *Sleep* 2008;31:853–7.

165. Frauscher B, Iranzo A, Gaig C. Normative EMG values for the diagnosis of REM sleep behavior disorder. *Sleep* 2012;35(6):835–47.

166. Gagnon JF, Postuma RB, Montplaisir J. Update on the pharmacology of REM sleep behavior disorder. *Neurology* 2006;67:742–7.

167. Sapin E, Lapray D, Bérod A, et al. Localization of brainstem GABAergic neurons controlling paradoxical (REM) sleep. *PloS ONE* 2009;4:e4274.

168. Condurso R, Aricò I, Romanello G, Gervasi G, Silvestri R. Status dissociatus in multilacunar encephalopathy with median pontine lesion: a video-polygraphic presentation. *J Sleep Res* 2006;15 (Suppl 1): 212.

169. Gomez-Choco M, Iranzo A, Blanco Y, Graus F, Santamaria J, Saiz A. Prevalence of Restless Legs Syndrome and REM Sleep Behavior Disorder in Multiple Sclerosis. *Multiple Sclerosis* 2007; 13:805–808.

31

Neurodegenerative Disease in Idiopathic REM Sleep Behavior Disorder
Quantifying Risk and Measuring Preclinical Markers of Disease

RONALD B. POSTUMA, JEAN-FRANCOIS GAGNON,
AND JACQUES Y. MONTPLAISIR

AS DISCUSSED in the previous chapter, REM sleep behavior disorder (RBD) is most often caused by synuclein-associated degeneration of brainstem structures (i.e., Parkinson's disease [PD], Lewy body dementia [LBD], and multiple-system atrophy [MSA]). Whereas RBD is often a relatively benign syndrome that can generally be successfully treated with medications, the other aspects of degenerative synucleinopathies are devastating to patients and their families. Therefore, the most important clinical implications of RBD stem from its relation with synuclein-mediated neurodegenerative disease. In particular, the ability of RBD to predict future disease by years or even decades in advance of their clinical presentation has the potential to lead to breakthroughs in disease treatment. This chapter outlines the evidence that RBD predicts disease and discusses how study of RBD patients can help us predict neurodegeneration and even perhaps lead to the development of neuroprotective therapy.

WHAT IS THE RISK OF NEURODEGENERATIVE DISEASE IN IDIOPATHIC REM SLEEP BEHAVIOR DISORDER?

It is clear that many (if not most) patients who present to sleep clinics with idiopathic RBD will eventually develop a neurodegenerative syndrome. In the vast majority of cases, this will be PD, LBD, or MSA. Information as to the outcome of RBD has come mainly from three studies.

In 1996 Schenck et al. reported that after a median follow-up of 5 years, 11 of their original 29 (38%) male patients with idiopathic RBD had developed a parkinsonian disorder.[1] The diagnosis was "definite PD" in 8 (of whom 7 had rest tremor) and "probable PD" in the remaining 3. Two patients with PD later developed PD dementia. A twelfth patient developed dementia and was given a diagnosis of Alzheimer's disease (given subsequent studies, the disease may have in fact been LBD). Neurodegenerative disease developed on average 4 years after diagnosis of RBD, but more than *12 years* after developing RBD symptoms. Subsequent follow-up of this cohort (reported in abstract form only) has found that risk of disease continues to increase; at 10 years follow-up, 65% have developed a defined neurodegenerative disease.[2]

In 2006, Iranzo and colleagues reported outcome of a larger series of 44 idiopathic RBD patients.[3] This follow-up included neuropsychological evaluation, which likely increased sensitivity to identify dementia. Sixteen of 44 (36%) patients developed a defined neurodegenerative disorder, and an additional 4 patients developed mild cognitive impairment. Strikingly similar to the Schenck's study, the mean latency between diagnosis of RBD and development of degenerative disease was 5.1 years, with 13.4 years between symptom onset and disease. Of the 16 patients, 9 developed PD (2 with PD dementia), 1 developed MSA, and 6 developed LBD. Subsequent follow-up of this cohort (reported in abstract form only) also found that 64% of patients developed a neurodegenerative disease (including mild cognitive impairment) by 7 years.[4]

In 2009, our group examined risk of disease in a cohort of 93 patients with idiopathic RBD5 (Fig. 31.1). Using a Kaplan-Meier analysis, we estimated a disease risk of 17.7% at 5 years in patients with idiopathic RBD, which increased to 40.6% at 10 years and 52.4% at 12 years. Although these estimates are somewhat lower than the previous two studies, they are not as divergent as they initially appear; if we had calculated using the same method as the previous studies, estimated conversion rate would be 28% for a mean 5.2-year follow-up (calculation of mean years follow-up can "overestimate" disease risk by equally weighting patients with short and long follow-up, a problem corrected by Kaplan-Meier analysis). At the time of disease onset, the primary diagnosis was parkinsonism in 15 (14 PD, 1 MSA) and dementia in 11; however, we found substantial overlap between conditions,[6] which suggests that boundaries between disease states are not clear (see discussion that follows).

On review of these studies, several key findings emerge:

1. The risk of neurodegeneration is high. With estimates as high as 65% at 10 years, RBD is by far the strongest clinical predictor of neurodegenerative disease available.[7] However, important caveats must be noted. Of critical importance, the aforementioned studies were all performed on patients in sleep clinics who were presenting with clinical RBD; this implies they were on the severe end of the disease spectrum. Results may not apply as well to those with milder or occasional symptoms, who could have lower disease risk.[8] We commonly encounter persons (most often young-adult males) who recall having had one or a few episodes of

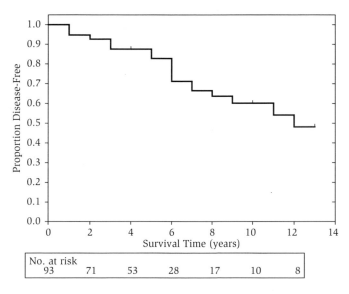

FIGURE 31.1 The survival curve of patients with idiopathic REM sleep behavior disorder over a 12-year follow-up duration. Disease outcome is defined as the development of parkinsonism or dementia. (Reprinted from Postuma et al., 2009.[5])

infrequent dream enactment behavior; occasional dream-enactment behavior can perhaps be normal.[9] As RBD becomes more readily recognized, it is likely that milder cases will come to medical attention, and disease risk may not be the same in these cases. Similarly, the risk of medication-induced RBD may be different than in those with idiopathic RBD; if antidepressants unmask a latent synucleinopathy, disease risk would presumably still be present, but lower. On the other hand, if antidepressants can cause RBD in the absence of preclinical degeneration, risk may be similar to the general population. Therefore, it will be essential to find methods to stratify disease risk in different patient groups, perhaps using other markers of neurodegeneration (see later).

2. Latency to clinical disease is long. In the three major series, mean interval between RBD symptom onset and neurodegenerative disease exceeded 10 years. This is in contrast to positron emission tomography (PET) studies of the substantia nigra, which have estimated preclinical PD phases of 4–7 years before clinical symptoms.[10-12] A recent report has suggested that some cases of RBD have extremely long latency; of 550 patients with clinical RBD and neurodegenerative disease, 27 had latencies of more than 15 years between symptom onset and disease (mean interval = 25 years).[13] (Note that interpretation of extremely long latencies depends critically upon understanding the prevalence of RBD—there may be a relatively common young-onset form of RBD unrelated to synucleinopathy of whom some would coincidentally develop neurodegenerative disease.)

An interval >10 years has major implications for our concept of disease pathogenesis. Do synucleinopathies really "start" at advanced age, or do the initial processes "hit" at a very young age but are kept in check for decades by robust compensatory mechanisms? If synucleinopathies start very early, must the search for epidemiologic variables be expanded to early-life factors (e.g., early-life "single hits" such as infections or toxin exposures)?

The other major implication to this prolonged RBD-disease interval is the existence of a very promising window of opportunity for intervention. One of the major unmet needs in the field of neurodegeneration is the absence of a neuroprotective therapy, that is, a therapy that can slow down the underlying degenerative process. Despite decades of research, no clear successful treatment has been developed. Perhaps an important clue about why comes from the long disease latency with idiopathic RBD; if a neurodegenerative disease has a prodrome of a decade or longer, perhaps it is too late to intervene if we wait until clinical signs of parkinsonism or dementia start. Potentially, a partially effective neuroprotective agent with minor utility in established disease could, if given before symptoms, slow or even prevent the onset of clinical disease.

In this regard, idiopathic RBD may help considerably. First, patients with idiopathic RBD are the ideal test subjects for a neuroprotective trial—using patients in preclinical disease provides the maximum opportunity for benefit and provides a potential "hard" endpoint, that is, "conversion" to clinical neurodegeneration (note that such trials are by definition of long duration, a major consideration for pharmaceutical companies who might otherwise wish to sponsor such a trial). Second, RBD patients are the ideal candidates for therapy once neuroprotection is developed. Conversion rates of over 50% to neurodegenerative disease imply that if a safe and effective neuroprotective agent were ever developed, all idiopathic RBD patients might consider taking it. Finally, as discussed later, study of RBD can help us find other potential predictors of disease.

WHAT DISEASE DO REM BEHAVIOR DISORDER PATIENTS REALLY DEVELOP?

In clinical follow-up studies, the vast majority of patients who developed neurodegenerative disease developed a synucleinopathy. However, it is important to note that RBD does not occur exclusively in synuclein-mediated diseases; RBD has been documented in diverse conditions such as progressive supranuclear palsy, spinocerebellar ataxias, amyotrophic lateral sclerosis, Huntington disease, and even in Guillain-Barré syndrome. Given that there have been no reported cases of these diseases emerging out of idiopathic RBD, the RBD in other neurodegenerative diseases is probably a late feature in most.

One notable condition in which RBD appears to be uncommon is Alzheimer disease (AD). AD is by far the commonest neurodegenerative disease, affecting up to 30% of the population over 85. Despite this, descriptions of RBD in AD are strikingly uncommon, and in all described cases, diagnoses were only clinical.[14] In a descriptive analysis of the neurodegenerative disease emerging from idiopathic RBD, we found that patients with dementia, regardless of whether they met criteria for LBD (i.e., had hallucinations or fluctuations), had motor, olfactory, and autonomic abnormalities typical of what is seen in LBD and a cognitive profile that resembled LBD rather than AD.[6] In a prospective study of 12 patients with dementia and RBD who did not have hallucinations or parkinsonism, nine developed these features on follow-up evaluation, suggesting that the classical criteria for LBD are insensitive in early stages.[15] Finally, pathological examination in an autopsy study of 12 patients with RBD and dementia found synuclein deposition in 100% of patients examined.[16] This suggests that the presence of RBD in dementia is a very strong indication of an underlying synucleinopathy. As a clinical rule of thumb, presence of RBD in a patient with a diagnosis of AD signals a need to rethink the diagnosis.

Although the vast majority of patients who develop neurodegeneration from idiopathic RBD will develop a synucleinopathy, it is often surprisingly difficult to determine which synucleinopathy is present. In a recent prospective follow-up study that included a comprehensive annual examination, 16 of 21 patients who developed neurodegeneration had evidence of both parkinsonism and cognitive impairment at disease onset.[17] The majority of those with a primary diagnosis of dementia developed defined parkinsonism within a year of onset, and vice versa. This suggests a generalized advancing synuclein-mediated neurodegeneration, the presentation of which may depend upon subtle individual differences in brainstem versus cortical vulnerability. This is a profile unlike that seen in most cases of PD, in which dementia is a later feature. This has important implications for testing predictors of disease and for eventual neuroprotection trials—trials that may, for example, use RBD patients to test an agent to protect against PD must consider dementia as an important outcome (perhaps prioritizing agents that have potential utility against both diseases, such as synuclein-based targets).

Observation of overlap between dementia and parkinsonism suggests RBD in PD may mark a specific type of PD—in other words, PD patients with RBD may have a different disease process than those without. Numerous studies have suggested that RBD in PD is associated with diverse features, such as akinetic-rigid rather than tremor-predominant subtype, more clinical autonomic dysfunction and degeneration of cardiac sympathetic neurons, hallucinations, waking electroencephalogram (EEG) slowing, and cognitive impairment.[18-26] Similarly, studies suggest that autonomic dysfunction markers such as MIBG scintigraphy are worse in patients with RBD than in PD.[27] Understanding the link between RBD and these disease features may have implications for our understanding of heterogeneous disease mechanisms in PD.

PREDICTING OUTCOMES— MARKERS FOR DISEASE OUTCOME

As discussed earlier, a major limitation to the development of neuroprotective therapy is that disease is well established by the time a patient presents with classical clinical symptoms. Currently, there are no reliable ways to identify patients at high risk for PD or other synucleinopathies. Several centers have commenced prospective studies to predict the outcome in idiopathic RBD, mainly to determine who will develop disease and who will not. Being able to predict disease in idiopathic RBD has two major implications:

1. *Implications for RBD patients.* Ability to predict which RBD patients will develop disease can be of critical importance. At present, it can help patients plan for the future, arranging retirement planning, insurance, and so on (although potential insurance implications and distress at receiving higher risk diagnosis must be considered). Second, it can help stratify patients for neuroprotective trials, in order to select those at sufficiently high risk for disease conversion. And finally, once disease-modifying therapy is developed, it will help select patients for therapy.

2. *Implications for the general population.* Idiopathic RBD patients rarely present to sleep centers; so far, the largest series of idiopathic RBD ever reported is only 93 patients.[5] Therefore, the principal implications from studies of idiopathic RBD come from generalization to neurodegenerative disease as a whole, from the realization that idiopathic RBD gives a unique window into preclinical stages of neurodegeneration. There are many potential predictors of neurodegeneration that have been

proposed; unfortunately, testing is difficult, mainly because of difficulties in identifying sufficiently high-risk patients (for a study to have sufficient power to test a potential predictor of PD, it would need a minimum of 3000 patients followed for 5 years). In this regard, idiopathic RBD patients are the ideal "high-risk" group who can be used as test subjects to examine whether and how other potential predictors of disease can be markers for disease risk in the general population.

Potential markers of neurodegeneration in idiopathic RBD are very diverse. Most of these factors have been assessed in PD; research into prediction of LBD and MSA is less developed. Generally, potential markers have been proposed based on either of two principles: redundancy (the ability of the organism to compensate for mild losses of neuronal function) or the presence of nonmotor manifestations of PD early in disease, which may therefore precede disease. The most important potential predictors are discussed in the following sections.

MARKERS OF SUBSTANTIA NIGRA DYSFUNCTION

Motor manifestations of PD are classically related to degeneration of the substantia nigra pars compacta (SNpc). Pathologic and neuroimaging studies suggest that motor signs of PD only develop once 30%–70% of SNpc neurons have degenerated.[10] Therefore, there is presumably an opportunity to identify milder stages of SNpc degeneration. One potential marker of subtle dopaminergic denervation is dopaminergic PET and single-photon emission computed tomography (SPECT) imaging—this uses radiolabeled ligands to label either pre- or postsynaptic dopaminergic terminals[28] and therefore directly measure innervation from the SNpc. Dopaminergic PET and SPECT have very high sensitivity and specificity for parkinsonism, regardless of cause (i.e., they may also detect MSA and LBD).[28] Since they directly measure dopaminergic function, evidence of dopaminergic tracer uptake is strong evidence for a state of preclinical parkinsonism. Abnormalities on dopaminergic imaging have been well described in idiopathic RBD.[29,30] However, these abnormalities are clearly identifiable only in a minority of patients, consistent with staging systems of PD that suggest that SNpc is a later "Stage 3" feature of PD.

A second potential marker of preclinical PD is transcranial ultrasound (TCS). Approximately 80%–90% of PD patients have abnormal hyperechogenicity of the SN.[31] Hyperechogenicity is found early in disease course. It is normal in MSA and other parkinsonian conditions, so it may help in differential diagnosis of equivocal parkinsonian signs.[31] Studies finding that transcranial ultrasound abnormalities are found in 9% of young healthy adults,[32] that hyperechogenicity does not progress as disease progresses,[33] and that there is no correlation between the degree of hyperechogenicity and severity of dopaminergic degeneration[34] suggest that hyperechogenicity, rather than being a direct marker of preclinical PD, may indicate an at-risk state for PD. Recent studies have suggested that approximately 40% of patients with idiopathic RBD have abnormalities on TCS.[35,36]

Recently, an important prospective study has shown that indeed, TCS and dopaminergic PET/SPECT can predict neurodegenerative outcome in RBD. In a cohort of 43 idiopathic RBD patients, 40% had abnormal B-CIT SPECT, and 36% had abnormal TCS (63% had abnormalities on either modality). Over a 2.5-year prospective follow-up, 8 (19%) patients developed disease. Six of eight patients with disease had had abnormal SPECT at baseline, and five of eight had had abnormal TCS; all patients had an abnormality of at least one modality. This is the first study to directly confirm in a prospective manner that abnormalities of SNpc are detectible before clinical PD. As such, there is very strong evidence to support these modalities as predictive markers. However, caveats should be noted. First, neither imaging procedure on its own was capable of predicting disease; it required both examinations with an either/or determination. Second, prospective follow-up duration was limited to 2.5 years, and interval between procedure and development of disease was 21 months. The utility of a predictive marker depends entirely upon the lead time that can be gained by its use; clearly, future studies should be able to assess predictive utility at intervals of 5 years, 10 years, or longer. Third, B-CIT SPECT, and TCS were disconcordant in most patients; this is hard to understand if we presume that they are measuring the same function. Finally, in a future age of neuroprotection, screening for degenerative disease will probably need to be population-wide—PET/SPECT are relatively expensive and require injection of radiotracer, and transcranial ultrasound requires specialized training. This implies that these modalities will probably be especially useful in identified high-risk populations (e.g., idiopathic RBD patients, persons who screen positive on simpler inexpensive modalities, etc.).

OTHER NONMOTOR MEASURES

Sleep Measures

Although disease processes such as RBD are commonly conceived of as homogenous, there is of course variability between patients in severity, presentation, and underlying etiology. In a clinical follow-up study, we recently examined baseline sleep variables compared between idiopathic RBD patients who eventually developed a defined neurodegenerative disease, compared with those who had remained disease-free. There were no clear differences in sleep stages between groups, except for a slight increase in Stage 1 sleep in those who eventually developed disease, and a slight reduction in slow-wave sleep in those destined to develop dementia (consistent with known abnormalities in patients with early-stage neurodegeneration). The most prominent abnormality was that patients who would eventually develop disease had more severe loss of REM atonia at baseline (63 +/− 6% tonic REM) than those who remained disease-free (42 +/− 6%). This change was most prominent in those destined to develop PD (73 +/− 6%). This effect was present after controlling follow-up duration (important since REM atonia loss may progress with time).[37] This suggests that there may be a "milder" subtype of idiopathic RBD who could have a lower progression risk. Although this finding would obviously have little clinical significance for the general population (for whom no such data would be available), it is relevant in RBD patients and may be useful in clinical counseling and in stratification of patients for clinical trials.

Olfaction

There have been compelling suggestions that olfaction can predict PD. The large majority of PD patients have severe olfactory loss at disease onset.[38] Olfaction is usually normal in other parkinsonian disorders.[38] Olfactory loss may also be an important preclinical marker of AD and particularly LBD.[39] Impaired olfaction was associated with a 5.2-fold increased risk of developing incident PD in a prospective pathological study.[40]

Recently, we were able to confirm that olfaction can indeed predict synucleinopathies such as PD and LBD in patients with idiopathic RBD. In a 5-year prospective follow-up study of 62 patients with idiopathic RBD, those with impaired olfaction had a 65% 5-year risk of developing a defined neurodegenerative disease, whereas those with normal olfaction had only a 14% risk (Fig. 31.2a). The strength of this association is also encouraging for potential clinical utility. Additionally, olfactory abnormalities appeared to be present up to 5 years before diagnosis—a long lead time that implies potential for neuroprotective intervention. However, sensitivity is not 100%; a clear subset of tremor-predominant PD patients were identified who developed olfactory abnormalities only at time of diagnosis. Also, specificity is likely limited; up to 25% of the elderly population has hyposmia,[40] suggesting olfactory testing will be insufficient to indicate a need for neuroprotective therapy in the general population (although probably not in patients with idiopathic RBD). Olfaction may have particular potential as a general population screen for preclinical dementia, which could be followed by more specific/ expensive tests for screen positives.

Visual Changes

Numerous visual changes occur in PD, often early in the course of the disease. Loss of color vision is found early in PD and may be due either to retinal degeneration[41] or to subtle visual perceptual dysfunction. Reduced contrast sensitivity (the ability to distinguish shades of gray) is also found early in PD,[41] suggesting potential as a predictor. We recently explored color vision, as assessed by the Farnsworth-Munsell 100-Hue test, in prospective studies of idiopathic RBD, and found considerable predictive value of color vision (Fig. 31.2b). Those with impaired color vision had an estimated 74% risk of developing a defined neurodegenerative disease at 5 years follow-up, compared to 26% of those with normal vision. As with olfaction, abnormalities were present as much as 5 years before diagnosis and predicted both parkinsonism and dementia. It is unclear whether these results were due to retinal changes, or perhaps to subtle

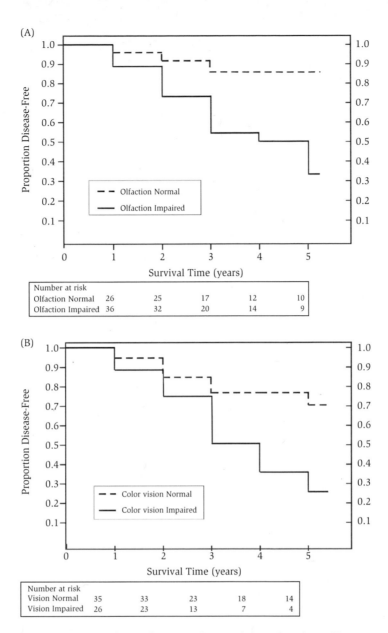

FIGURE 31.2 (A) Kaplan Meier plot of disease risk according to baseline olfaction in patients with idiopathic REM sleep behavior disorder. For illustration, values are dichotomized—olfaction is defined as abnormal if University of Pennsylvania Smell Identification test scores are <80% expected for age and sex. p value for difference = .029 (Cox proportional hazards). (Reprinted from Postuma et al., 2011.[8]) (B) Kaplan Meier plot of disease risk according to baseline color vision testing in patients with idiopathic REM sleep behavior disorder. For illustration, values are dichotomized; vision is defined as abnormal if Farnsworth-Munsell 100 Hue scores are >125% expected for age and sex. p value for difference = .009 (Cox proportional hazards). (Reprinted from Postuma et al., 2011.[8])

visuoperceptive changes present in preclinical dementia, since those with normal cognition demonstrated relatively preserved color vision even at disease onset.

Autonomic Dysfunction

Staging systems of PD have described synuclein deposition of unmyelinated projection neurons of the dorsal motor nucleus of the vagus,[42] and postganglionic sympathetic denervation at earliest stages of the degeneration of PD.[43,44] These abnormalities are also often seen in LBD, and cardiac denervation may even be more severe in LBD than PD.[45,46] There has been some evidence that autonomic dysfunction can predict PD. For example, in a prospective pathologic study, those who reported a bowel movement frequency of <1/day had a 4.8-fold increased odds ratio for PD compared to those with frequency >2 per day.[47]

Numerous groups have found evidence of autonomic dysfunction in RBD, as measured by orthostatic blood pressure drop,[25, 48] symptoms of constipation,[25] decreased beat-to-beat variability in cardiac rhythm,[49] and decreased MIBG tracer uptake on scintigraphy, a marker of cardiac sympathetic innervation.[50,51] Interestingly, however, in the only prospective follow-up that examined autonomic dysfunction as a predictor of disease, cardiac denervation on electrocardiogram trace was unable to distinguish between idiopathic RBD patients who were destined to develop neurodegenerative disease from those who remained disease-free, despite clear ability to distinguish patients from controls.[49] This could be consistent with the concept that essentially *all* RBD patients are in "Stage 2" Braak PD and have near-complete cardiac denervation by the time they present to a sleep clinic. If so, autonomic dysfunction may be the ideal predictor of disease. On the other hand, it could also be consistent with a more direct connection—that is, autonomic dysfunction as a generator of RBD, perhaps via alteration of dream content (similar to informal observations that large meals commonly trigger intense dreams), disturbance in cerebral autoregulation (increased cerebral perfusion at night when patients are supine), and so on. This counterintuitive concept is supported by descriptions of RBD occurring with a Guillain-Barré syndrome, a peripheral nervous system disorder unrelated to synucleinopathy which exclusively affected those with autonomic dysfunction.[52] Also, in patients with established PD, we noted a striking connection between orthostatic blood pressure drop and RBD; PD patients without RBD were indistinguishable from controls on orthostatic changes, whereas those with RBD dropped and average of 24 mmHg when standing.[25] In other words, autonomic dysfunction is more linked to RBD than to PD. Long-term prospective follow-up studies using more sensitive measures will be essential to clarify the true predictive value of autonomic dysfunction as a predictor of disease.

OTHER POTENTIAL PREDICTORS IN IDIOPATHIC REM BEHAVIOR DISORDER

Numerous groups have also found other potential markers of disease in patients with idiopathic RBD, including subtle motor dysfunction on clinical examination,[25] motor slowing on quantitative tests of movement speed,[25,48] anxiety and depression symptoms, personality changes (similar to the putative "Parkinson personality"),[25] subtle cognitive dysfunction,[53,54] waking EEG slowing,[55] volumetric magnetic resonance imaging changes,[56] cerebral blood flow changes,[57] and diffusion tensor imaging.[56,58] These markers are abnormal in clinical synucleinopathies, often early in the disease course, suggesting that they will be able to identify patients in preclinical stages of disease. However, confirmation of their predictive value will require prospective studies that correlate abnormalities at baseline with eventual disease risk.

CONCLUSION

Patients with idiopathic RBD are at a very high risk of developing neurodegenerative disease, a risk that continues for decades after the first symptoms develop. This has profound implications for our understanding of etiology and pathology of neurodegenerative disease, for predicting disease even in the general population, and hopefully for the future development of neuroprotective therapy. The rare window into preclinical neurodegeneration provided by RBD has the potential to lead to important breakthroughs in diagnosis and treatment of disease.

REFERENCES

1. Schenck CH, Bundlie SR, Mahowald MW. Delayed emergence of a Parkinsonian disorder in 38% of 29 older men initially diagnosed with idiopathic rapid eye movement sleep behaviour disorder. *Neurology* 1996;46(2):388–93.
2. Schenck CH, Mahowald MW. REM behavior disorder (RBD): delayed emergence of parkinsonism and/or dementia in 65% of older

men initially diagnosed with idiopathic RBD, and an analysis of the minimum & maximum tonic and/or phasic electromyographic abnormalities found during REM sleep. *Sleep* 2003;26:A316.

3. Iranzo A, Molinuevo JL, Santamaria J et al. Rapid-eye-movement sleep behaviour disorder as an early marker for a neurodegenerative disorder: a descriptive study. *Lancet Neurol* 2006;5(7):572–7.

4. Iranzo A, Molinuevo J, Santamaria J, et al. Sixty-four percent of patients with idiopathic REM sleep behavior disorder developed a neurological disorder after a mean clinical follow-up of seven years. *Sleep* 2008;31:A280.

5. Postuma RB, Gagnon JF, Vendette M, et al. Quantifying the risk of neurodegenerative disease in idiopathic REM sleep behavior disorder. *Neurology* 2009;72(15):1296–300.

6. Postuma RB, Gagnon JF, Vendette M, et al. Idiopathic REM sleep behavior disorder in the transition to degenerative disease. *Mov Disord* 2009;24(15):2225–32.

7. Postuma RB, Gagnon JF, Montplaisir J. Clinical prediction of Parkinson's disease—planning for the age of neuroprotection. *J Neurol Neurosurg Psychiatry* 2010;81(9):1008–13.

8. Postuma RB, Gagnon JF, Rompre S, et al. Severity of REM atonia loss in idiopathic REM sleep behavior disorder predicts Parkinson disease. *Neurology* 2010;74:239–44.

9. Nielsen T, Svob C, Kuiken D. Dream-enacting behaviors in a normal population. *Sleep* 2009;32(12):1629–36.

10. Morrish PK, Rakshi JS, Bailey DL, et al. Measuring the rate of progression and estimating the preclinical period of Parkinson's disease with [18F]dopa PET. *J Neurol Neurosurg Psychiatry* 1998;64(3):314–19.

11. Hilker R, Schweitzer K, Coburger S, et al. Nonlinear progression of Parkinson disease as determined by serial positron emission tomographic imaging of striatal fluorodopa F 18 activity. *Arch Neurol* 2005;62(3):378–82.

12. Vingerhoets FJ, Snow BJ, Lee CS, et al. Longitudinal fluorodopa positron emission tomographic studies of the evolution of idiopathic parkinsonism. *Ann Neurol* 1994;36(5):759–64.

13. Claassen DO, Josephs KA, Ahlskog JE, et al. REM sleep behavior disorder preceding other aspects of synucleinopathies by up to half a century. *Neurology* 2010;75(6):494–9.

14. Gagnon JF, Petit D, Fantini ML, et al. REM sleep behavior disorder and REM sleep without atonia in probable Alzheimer disease. *Sleep* 2006;29(10):1321–5.

15. Ferman TJ, Boeve BF, Smith GE, et al. Dementia with Lewy bodies may present as dementia and REM sleep behavior disorder without parkinsonism or hallucinations. *J Int Neuropsychol Soc* 2002;8(7):907–14.

16. Boeve BF, Silber MH, Parisi JE, et al. Synucleinopathy pathology and REM sleep behavior disorder plus dementia or parkinsonism. *Neurology* 2003;61(1):40–5.

17. Postuma RB, Gagnon JF, Vendette M, et al. Olfaction and color vision identify impending neurodegeneration in REM behavior disorder. *Ann Neurol* 2011;69(5):811–8.

18. Postuma RB, Montplaisir J, Lanfranchi PA, et al. Cardiac autonomic denervation in Parkinson's disease is linked to REM sleep behavior disorder. *Mov Disord* 2011;26(8):1529–33.

19. Lee JE, Kim KS, Shin HW, et al. Factors related to clinically probable REM sleep behavior disorder in Parkinson disease. *Parkinsonism Relat Disord* 2010;16(2):105–8.

20. Postuma RB, Gagnon JF, Vendette M, et al. Manifestations of Parkinson disease differ in association with REM sleep behavior disorder. *Mov Disord* 2008;23(12):1665–72.

21. Postuma RB, Gagnon JF, Vendette M, et al. REM sleep behavior disorder in Parkinson's disease is associated with specific motor features. *J Neurol Neurosurg Psychiatry* 2008;79(10):1117–21.

22. Kumru H, Santamaria J, Tolosa E, et al. Relation between subtype of Parkinson's disease and REM sleep behavior disorder. *Sleep Med* 2007;8(7–8):779–83.

23. Gagnon JF, Fantini ML, Bedard MA, et al. Association between waking EEG slowing and REM sleep behavior disorder in PD without dementia. *Neurology* 2004;62(3):401–6.

24. Gagnon JF, Vendette M, Postuma RB, et al. Mild cognitive impairment in rapid eye movement sleep behavior disorder and Parkinson's disease. *Ann Neurol* 2009;66(1):39–47.

25. Postuma RB, Gagnon JF, Vendette M, et al. Markers of neurodegeneration in idiopathic REM sleep behavior disorder and Parkinson disease. *Brain* 2009;132(12):2298–307.

26. Sinforiani E, Zangaglia R, Manni R, et al. REM sleep behavior disorder, hallucinations, and cognitive impairment in Parkinson's disease. *Lost Data* 2006;21(4):462–6.

27. Nomura T, Inoue Y, Hogl B, et al. Relationship between (123)I-MIBG scintigrams and REM sleep behavior disorder in Parkinson's disease. *Parkinsonism Relat Disord* 2010;16(10):683–5.

28. Ravina B, Eidelberg D, Ahlskog JE, et al. The role of radiotracer imaging in Parkinson disease. *Neurology* 2005;64(2):208–15.

29. Eisensehr I, Linke R, Noachtar S, et al. Reduced striatal dopamine transporters in idiopathic rapid eye movement sleep behaviour disorder. Comparison with Parkinson's disease and controls. *Brain* 2000;123(Pt 6):1155–60.

30. Albin RL, Koeppe RA, Chervin RD, et al. Decreased striatal dopaminergic innervation in REM sleep behavior disorder. *Neurology* 2000;55(9):1410–12.

31. Gaenslen A, Unmuth B, Godau J, et al. The specificity and sensitivity of transcranial ultrasound in the differential diagnosis of Parkinson's disease: a prospective blinded study. *Lancet Neurol* 2008;7(5):417–24.

32. Berg D, Becker G, Zeiler B, et al. Vulnerability of the nigrostriatal system as detected by transcranial ultrasound. *Neurology* 1999;53(5):1026–31.

33. Berg D, Merz B, Reiners K, et al. Five-year follow-up study of hyperechogenicity of the substantia nigra in Parkinson's disease. *Lost Data* 2005;20(3):383–5.

34. Spiegel J, Hellwig D, Mollers MO, et al. Transcranial sonography and [123I] FP-CIT SPECT disclose complementary aspects of Parkinson's disease. *Brain* 2006;129(Pt 5):1188–93.

35. Unger MM, Moller JC, Stiasny-Kolster K, et al. Assessment of idiopathic rapid-eye-movement sleep behavior disorder by transcranial sonography, olfactory function test, and FP-CIT-SPECT. *Lost Data* 2008;23(4):596–9.

36. Stockner H, Iranzo A, Seppi K, et al. Midbrain hyperechogenicity in idiopathic REM sleep behavior disorder. *Mov Disord* 2009;24(13):1906–9.

37. Iranzo A, Ratti P, Casanova-Molla J, et al. Excessive muscular activity increases over time in idiopathic REM sleep behavior disorder. *Sleep* 2009;32(9):1149–53.

38. Hawkes C. Olfaction in neurodegenerative disorder. *Lost Data* 2003;18(4):364–72.

39. Olichney JM, Murphy C, Hofstetter CR, et al. Anosmia is very common in the Lewy body variant of Alzheimer's disease. *J Neurol Neurosurg Psychiatry* 2005;76(10):1342–7.

40. Ross GW, Petrovitch H, Abbott RD, et al. Association of olfactory dysfunction with risk for future Parkinson's disease. *Ann Neurol* 2008;63(2):167–73.

41. Price MJ, Feldman RG, Adelberg D, et al. Abnormalities in color vision and contrast sensitivity in Parkinson's disease. *Neurology* 1992;42(4):887–90.

42. Braak H, Del Tredici K, Rub U, et al. Staging of brain pathology related to sporadic Parkinson's disease. *Neurobiol Aging* 2003;24(2):197–211.

43. Orimo S, Takahashi A, Uchihara T, et al. Degeneration of cardiac sympathetic nerve begins in the early disease process of Parkinson's disease. *Brain Pathol* 2007;17(1):24–30.

44. Braak H, Sastre M, Bohl JR, et al. Parkinson's disease: lesions in dorsal horn layer I, involvement of parasympathetic and sympathetic pre- and postganglionic neurons. *Acta Neuropathol* 2007;113(4):421–9.

45. Yoshita M, Taki J, Yokoyama K, et al. Value of 123I-MIBG radioactivity in the differential diagnosis of DLB from AD. *Neurology* 2006;66(12):1850–4.

46. Oka H, Morita M, Onouchi K, et al. Cardiovascular autonomic dysfunction in dementia with Lewy bodies and Parkinson's disease. *J Neurol Sci* 2007;254(1–2):72–7.

47. Abbott RD, Petrovitch H, White LR, et al. Frequency of bowel movements and the future risk of Parkinson's disease. *Neurology* 2001;57(3):456–62.

48. Postuma RB, Lang AE, Massicotte-Marquez J, et al. Potential early markers of Parkinson disease in idiopathic REM sleep behavior disorder. *Neurology* 2006;66(6):845–51.

49. Postuma RB, Lanfranchi PA, Blais H, et al. Cardiac autonomic dysfunction in idiopathic REM sleep behavior disorder. *Mov Disord* 2010;25(14):2304–10.

50. Miyamoto T, Miyamoto M, Inoue Y, et al. Reduced cardiac 123I-MIBG scintigraphy in idiopathic REM sleep behavior disorder. *Neurology* 2006;67(12):2236–8.

51. Oka H, Yoshioka M, Onouchi K, et al. Characteristics of orthostatic hypotension in Parkinson's disease. *Brain* 2007;130(Pt 9):2425–32.

52. Cochen V, Arnulf I, Demeret S, et al. Vivid dreams, hallucinations, psychosis and REM sleep in Guillain-Barre syndrome. *Brain* 2005;128(Pt 11):2535–45.

53. Massicotte-Marquez J, Decary A, Gagnon JF, et al. Executive dysfunction and memory impairment in idiopathic REM sleep behavior disorder. *Neurology* 2008;70(15):1250–7.

54. Ferini-Strambi L, Di Gioia MR, Castronovo V, et al. Neuropsychological assessment in idiopathic REM sleep behavior disorder (RBD): does the idiopathic form of RBD really exist? *Neurology* 2004;62(1):41–5.

55. Fantini ML, Gagnon JF, Petit D, et al. Slowing of electroencephalogram in rapid eye movement sleep behavior disorder. *Ann Neurol* 2003;53(6):774–80.

56. Scherfler C, Frauscher B, Schocke M, et al. White and gray matter abnormalities in idiopathic rapid eye movement sleep behavior disorder: a diffusion-tensor imaging and voxel-based morphometry study. *Ann Neurol* 2011;69(2):400–7.

57. Mazza S, Soucy JP, Gravel P, et al. Assessing whole brain perfusion changes in patients with REM sleep behavior disorder. *Neurology* 2006;67(9):1618–22.

58. Unger MM, Belke M, Menzler K, et al. Diffusion tensor imaging in idiopathic REM sleep behavior disorder reveals microstructural changes in the brainstem, substantia nigra, olfactory region, and other brain regions. *Sleep* 2010;33(6):767–73.

32

Sleep-Related Eating Disorders

FEDERICA PROVINI

THE EXISTENCE of nocturnal sleep-related eating disorders that usually are distinct from daytime eating disorders (e.g., bulimia nervosa) has been known for a number of years. The disorders are readily recognized by persons who suffer from them and are becoming more widely known in medical circles.

In 1955, Stunkard et al. described a particular nocturnal eating pattern, the night eating syndrome (NES), in a group of 25 severe obese patients referred to a special clinic for the treatment of obesity. NES is characterized by morning anorexia, evening hyperphagia, and insomnia.[1] During the episodes the patients are conscious and fully aware of their eating behaviors. The disorder was particularly prominent in these patients during the period of weight gain and could represent a response to life-stressing factors.

Some decades later, Schenck et al. reported on 19 consecutive adult patients who presented to a sleep disorders center with histories of involuntary nocturnal sleep-related eating, usually occurring in combination with other nocturnal behaviors (mainly sleepwalking and periodic limb movements in sleep).[2] They termed the condition "sleep-related eating disorder" (SRED).[2] SRED is characterized by a compulsive behavior of food seeking associated with an absence of real hunger, and a prompt return to sleep after food intake. During the episodes, the level of consciousness spans the range from virtual unconsciousness to various levels of partial consciousness to full alertness.

Another diagnostic category, "nocturnal eating (drinking) syndrome,"[3] including "frequent and recurrent awakenings to eat and/or drink and normal sleep onset following the ingestion of the desired foods," initially defined as an extrinsic sleep disorder primarily affecting nursing young infants, is now described as a variant of a sleep-onset association disorder.[4]

This condition is primarily a problem of infancy or early childhood, and it is characterized by recurrent awakenings with an inability to resume sleep without eating or drinking. The disorder is more likely to occur if the mother feeds the child each time he awakens because the child learns that it needs to eat to go back to sleep and cries each time it awakens until the mother feeds it.[4]

This chapter describes the major findings of the different night-eating behaviors that might serve to distinguish the different patterns of eating. Although the relationship between NES and SRED remains unclear, two basic drive states, sleep and eating, appear to be pathologically intertwined.

The growing awareness and interest in nocturnal eating behaviors and their serious adverse effects are an increasing matter of concern to the medical community and should promote convergent investigations from diverse research fields, such as sleep medicine, circadian rhythms, endocrinology, eating disorders, psychiatry, and obesity.

NIGHT EATING SYNDROME

Night eating syndrome (NES) is characterized by evening hyperphagia, insomnia, and morning anorexia.[1] Since this first definition of NES was proposed, its diagnostic criteria have been debated and a variety of changes have been introduced into the literature. In particular, the criterion of night awakenings was added as an inclusion criterion, and the presence of bulimia nervosa (BN) or binge eating disorder (BED) was deemed an exclusionary criterion in 1999.[5]

Evening hyperphagia is described as the consumption of a large portion of the total daily caloric intake (at least 25% of total daily calories), after the evening meal, a time when the food intake of nonobese people is negligible.[6,7] Compared to controls, the cumulative caloric intake of night eaters lagged far behind, so that at 18.00 they had consumed only 30% of their daily caloric intake, compared to 74% of the control subjects.[8] The food intake of the controls then slowed, while that of the night eaters continued at a rapid pace until after midnight.[5]

The night eaters awakened far more often than did the control subjects, and more than half of their awakenings were associated with ingestion of food, usually in modest amounts. The patients often believe that they must eat in order to get to sleep.[9]

The second feature of NES is insomnia, an anxious or irritable sleeplessness, that persists until at least midnight (often until 2–3 am), usually occurring three or more times a week.

Morning anorexia (a negligible intake at breakfast) varies widely and is defined in the literature from "no appetite for breakfast" to a "delay of eating for several hours after awakening."[10]

Some studies considered mood disturbance a diagnostic feature of NES,[1,11] while others found mood disturbances (especially depression, minimal in the morning and increasing during the evening and night, anxiety, and lower self-esteem scores compared to controls) a comorbid feature of NES.[7,12–14]

The last proposal for diagnostic criteria for NES stipulated that nocturnal awakenings with ingestion of food must occur at least twice a week, NES must have lasted a minimum of 3 months, and that the disorder is not secondary to another medical or psychiatric disorder.[9]

NES affects adult patients (mean age was 36.1 years), especially females, with or without obesity, with a striking similarity in the characteristics.[13] Obese patients manifesting NES had more difficulty losing weight than obese patients without NES and experienced a high incidence of complications in their attempts.[1]

Polysomnographic and actigraphic studies documented that NES subjects did not differ from controls in timing of sleep onset or offset, but 93% of them ate on awakening while the same percentage of controls did not eat.[8]

The maintenance of normal timing for sleep-wake behavior in the presence of a phase delay in the timing of caloric intake suggests NES reflects a state of internal circadian desynchrony associated with significant sleep complaints. NES is now considered a circadian disorder with a dissociation of the circadian control of eating relative to sleep.[8,15–17]

Both in overweight and normal weight individuals NES is associated with an attenuation of the usual nighttime increase in plasma levels of melatonin (contribute to the sleep maintenance insomnia) and leptin, limiting its usual time suppression of appetite.[5,18] Confirming the earlier clinical impression that NES was associated with stress, beginning in more than half the cases during a period of life stress,[19] plasma cortisol levels of the NES subjects were higher than those of control subjects for most of the 24 hours.[5]

The etiology of the NES syndrome has not been determined.

There is an open discussion on NES in the literature. Some authors are convinced that there are sufficient reasons for recognizing this disorder in the official diagnostic nomenclature (until now the disorder has not been included in the *International Classification of Sleep Disorders*). Others discuss the utility of NES as a new nosological entity because data to determine whether NES is distinct from other eating disorders are lacking,[20] also considering the limitations of the literature, including small cohorts, retrospective and often questionnaire-based assessments, varying lengths of follow-up, and differing definitions of NES to define the clinical course of NES.

SLEEP-RELATED EATING DISORDER

According to the *International Classification of Sleep Disorders*,[4] sleep-related-eating disorder (SRED), classified in the "other parasomnia" section, is characterized by recurrent episodes of involuntary eating and drinking during arousal from sleep in an absence of real hunger (Fig. 32.1). The behavior consists of partial arousals from sleep, usually within the first 1–4 hours after sleep onset, and subsequent compulsive food seeking, occurring in an "out of control" manner with a sequence of rapid, "automatic" behavior of arising from bed and immediate entry into the kitchen. Patients almost never experienced hunger or thirst despite their compulsive and immediate urge to eat and drink; there was no complaint of

abdominal pain, nausea, heartburn, or hypoglycemic symptoms. Some patients binged on high-calorie foods (e.g., sweets, peanut butter, chips) or performed elaborate food preparations; others ate modest snacks such as cold cereal. Impaired judgment and sloppiness were described, such as food dropped on the floor or items taken out of the freezer or large quantities of sugar or salt put on food. Ingestion of no-edible or toxic items is also occasionally reported. Alcoholic beverages were not consumed, despite the availability of alcohol in most kitchens.[21] The majority of patients ate nightly, manifesting more than one episode per night. After each episode of food intake they subsequently went back to sleep.

The episodes can occur along a spectrum of consciousness level, from partial and/or confusional awakening from sleep, with subsequent partial recollection of the event, to full awareness during the episode, with substantial clear recall in the morning.[2,4,22]

In some patients the nocturnal eating behavior did not appear if they slept away from home.

Patients may report negative consequences of the recurrent eating nocturnal behavior, including complaints of nonrestorative sleep or morning anorexia (due to the distension caused by excessive nocturnal eating). In nearly three quarters of the patients the major patient concern is weight gain.[4,21]

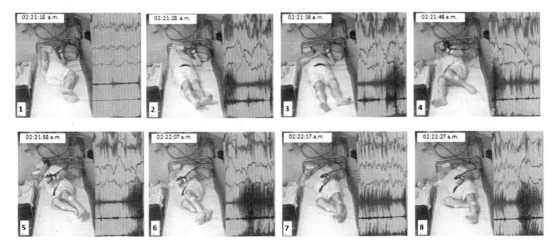

FIGURE 32.1 Nocturnal eating episode. The patient is sleeping (stage 2; picture 1). The sudden awakening from sleep is briefly followed by eating: the patient turned his body to the right, where there is the food brought with him to the sleep laboratory according to his nocturnal eating habits (picture 3), then grasped his bread (picture 4) and ate it (pictures 5–8) before going back to sleep.

SRED can affect both sexes and all ages, but it is most common in young adult women.[21] It is generally a long-standing disorder.[2,21,23]

SRED can be idiopathic or associated with a variety of underlying sleep disorders (i.e., restless legs syndrome [RLS], obstructive sleep apnea), the most frequent of which is sleepwalking.[4,21,23,24] The association of RLS with SRED, first identified in 1993,[21] was recently confirmed both in a large case control-study[25] and in a single case.[26] In our study, compared to controls living in the same place, SRED was more prevalent in RLS patients (33% vs. 1%, $p < .001$). RLS patients with SRED compared with RLS patients without SRED had more pathological Maudsley Obsessive-Compulsive Inventory (MOCI) scores and used significantly more drugs for other concomitant diseases. Patients did not report any use of dopaminergic or hypnotic drugs for RLS correlated with the presence of SRED. The association between the RLS and sleep-related eating disorder was tentatively attributed to an underlying common abnormality in dopaminergic metabolism.[25] Indeed, eating as a compulsive symptom was found to be induced by dopaminergic medications in patients with RLS and psychiatric comorbidity.[27]

In some patients, not only in heavy daytime smokers, the compulsion to eat during the night can be associated with a nocturnal compulsion to smoke.[28, 29] The patients reported that they are conscious and fully aware during the episodes but that they had no control over the compulsive behavior to smoke and they were unable to return to sleep without smoking and/or eating.[28,29]

SRED has also been reported in association with medical (autoimmune hepatitis), neurological (narcolepsy, encephalitis) or psychiatric disorders,[2] or with administration of medications such as zolpidem,[30,31] zaleplon,[32] triazolam,[2] or antipsychotic medications, especially in schizophrenic patients.[33,34]

In some cases, the onset of SRED could be sudden after the cessation of long-standing alcohol or opiates/cocaine abuse or a permanent cessation of cigarette smoking. In other patients the onset of SRED was associated with acute psychological stress in which patients reported arousals associated with worry (the health of the mother, the safety of a newborn child, the problem of living alone after a relationship break-up, etc.) resulted in going to the kitchen to eat.[21]

Although SRED is usually not associated with the presence of waking eating disorder, a minority of patients present a history of current or past anorexia nervosa or bulimia.[2,23]

SRED video-polysomnographic (VPSG) studies have documented that multiple complex feeding behaviors (up to eight times) often occur each night, throughout the sleep cycle, more frequently during the first third of the night, arising abruptly from non-REM sleep.[21] The interval between awakening and chewing start was very short (Fig. 32.2). In some cases, despite the prompt emergence of a wakeful electroencephalogram (EEG), the patient did not appear to be fully awake and was somewhat disinhibited in his or her mannerisms while eating.[21]

PSG recordings in another series of 35 SRED patients showed eating episodes occurred after complete awakening usually from non-REM sleep, without mental confusion and exhibiting an appropriate behavior during the nocturnal eating.[22]

More than 70% of patients presented with RLS or increased periodic limb movements in sleep.[22] In addition, VPSG documented frequently repetitive chewing and swallowing movements during sleep in many cases, especially during light sleep, with trigeminal and facial muscle electromyographic involvement[22,24] (Fig. 32.3).

SRED shares pathogenetic mechanisms with the disorders of arousal within the parasomnias, but its etiology remains unclear.

SLEEP-ONSET ASSOCIATION DISORDER: NOCTURNAL EATING/DRINKING SYNDROME SUBTYPE

Nocturnal eating-drinking syndrome is described in the *International Classification of Sleep Disorders*[4] as a behavioral insomnia (sleep-onset association type). The essential feature of the disease is the difficulty to fall asleep as the result of inappropriate sleep associations.[4] These phenomena are highly prevalent in the childhood population, and they are characterized by recurrent awakenings with inability to resume sleep without eating or drinking. The child is unable to fall asleep within a reasonable time in the absence of these conditions and a caregiver intervention is always required to aid the onset or resumption of sleep.[4] This condition may have its onset at any time during late infancy, and the course of the disease is strongly

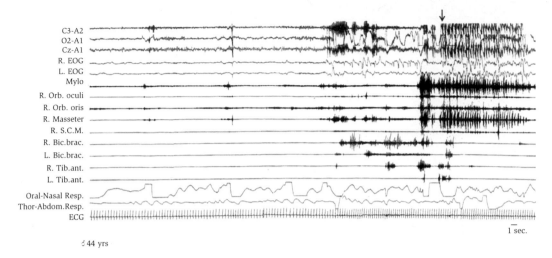

C3-A2
O2-A1
Cz-A1
R. EOG
L. EOG
Mylo
R. Orb. oculi
R. Orb. oris
R. Masseter
R. S.C.M.
R. Bic.brac.
L. Bic.brac.
R. Tib.ant.
L. Tib.ant.
Oral-Nasal Resp.
Thor-Abdom.Resp.
ECG

1 sec.

♀ 44 yrs

FIGURE 32.2   Sleep-related eating episode from sleep (stage 2). Polysomnographic excerpt shows an awakening from sleep stage 2: after about 15 seconds the patient begins to eat (see chewing movements corresponding to the rhythmic artefact on EEG leads). EEG, electroencephalogram (C3-A2; O2-A1; Cz-A1); R, right; L, left; EOG, electrooculogram; Mylo, mylohyoideus muscle; Orb. Oculi, orbicularis oculi muscle; Orb. Oris, orbicularis oris muscle; S.C.M., sternocleidomastoideus muscle; Bic. Brac., biceps brachii muscle; Tib. ant., tibialis anterior muscle; Resp., respirogram; Thor-Abdom: thoraco-abdominal.

related to caregivers' behaviors, bedtime interactions, culture, and environmental factors.[4]

EPIDEMIOLOGY

NES is more common among obese persons, but it is also present in nonobese subjects. However, its prevalence increases with increasing weight varying from 1.5% in the general population[11] to 1.6% in a community study among young women,[35] to 6% to 8.9% among obesity clinic patients,[6,36] to 12.3% in psychiatric outpatients.[37]

The prevalence of SRED has not well studied. The first large series of 19 subjects constituted 0.5% of all adult referrals to a sleep disorder

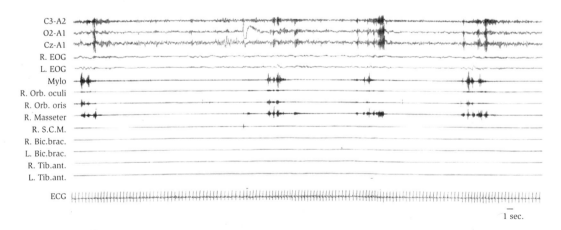

C3-A2
O2-A1
Cz-A1
R. EOG
L. EOG
Mylo
R. Orb. oculi
R. Orb. oris
R. Masseter
R. S.C.M.
R. Bic.brac.
L. Bic.brac.
R. Tib.ant.
L. Tib.ant.
ECG

1 sec.

FIGURE 32.3   Repetitive masticatory movements during sleep stage 2 in a patient with nocturnal eating episodes, involving mylohyoideus, orbicularis oculi, orbicularis oris, and masseter muscles. EEG, electroencephalogram (C3-A2; O2-A1; Cz-A1); R, right; L, left; EOG, electrooculogram; Mylo, mylohyoideus muscle; Orb. Oculi, orbicularis oculi muscle; Orb. Oris, orbicularis oris muscle; S.C.M., sternocleidomastoideus muscle; Bic. Brac., biceps brachii muscle; Tib. ant., tibialis anterior muscle.

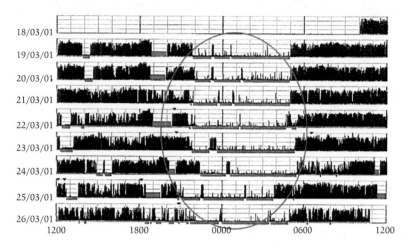

FIGURE 32.4   An example of actigraphic monitoring in a nocturnal eater (each row represents a 24-hour period). Actigraphy associated with a sleep diary, in this case for 8 days, showed the frequent nighttime awakenings (stronger black lines with greater amplitude similar to those during the day) associated with eating (information obtained from associated sleep diary).

center.[2] Another study found about 6% of a total of 120 insomniacs referred to a sleep center had a sleep-related eating disorder.[38] A prevalence of almost 5% with a much higher rate among patients with eating disorders (8.7%–16.7%) or healthy college students (4.6%) has been reported.[39] A family history of SRED was described in 26% of affected individuals,[23] also in fraternal twins,[40] suggesting a genetic predisposition.

The prevalence of nocturnal eating/drinking syndrome is not known, but approximately 5% to 10% of the childhood population could manifest the syndrome, without any sex prevalence.[4]

ASSESSMENT OF NOCTURNAL EATING BEHAVIOR AND DIFFERENTIAL DIAGNOSIS

There are no consistently used, well-designed instruments to determine the presence and severity of NES. Most studies used self-report questionnaires, clinical interviews or the Night Eating Questionnaire (NEQ), a 14-item screening instrument that assesses appetite, craving, nighttime awake nights, and mood, using Likert scores of 0–4.[41] The NEQ has been modified a number of times since its initial use, and there is no consensus on how the NEQ performs in terms of establishing a diagnosis of NES.[20] Other studies used food diaries to evaluate intake or structured clinical interviews to assess

eating disorders and/or mood. Actigraphy and sleep diary, including all food intake and bedtime and morning rising times, are useful in the evaluation of the entity of the syndrome and its follow-up (Fig. 32.4).

In SRED, data from extensive video-PSG monitoring were crucial in evaluating complaints of sleep-relating eating and in guiding treatment selection. Particular attention should be paid to symptoms suggestive of other parasomnias or sleep disorders (particularly sleepwalking, restless legs and periodic limb movements during sleep) present in more than half of the cases.

The precise boundaries between NES and SRED are not clear: some authors prefer to consider them as two distinct nocturnal eating disorders; others prefer a continuum of severity. The fact that SRED and NES share some overlapping features (the near-nightly frequency of eating in most patients, and the excessive weight gain and obesity in many of them) suggests that the two disorders may exist along a shared spectrum of pathophysiology.

According to Stunkard and Allison, the main feature differentiating NES from SRED is the lack of any consciousness impairment during eating in NES,[18] but wakeful and appropriate behavior during the episodes was indeed possible[24] or even the rule.[17,22]

SRED appears to be more female predominant than NES and less likely to be associated with a mood disorder. Unlike NES, none of the

SRED patients described had problematic eating in the evening between dinner and bedtime. Patients with NES rarely have an identified sleep disorder associated apart from sleep-onset insomnia. In SRED patients, sleep latency is usually brief, apart from patients with RLS.

Differential diagnosis with the daytime eating behavior disorders (bulimia nervosa and binge eating disorder) may be difficult, especially because daytime bulimia nervosa at times may extend to nocturnal hours. SRED and NES lack associated compensatory behaviors such as purging and induced vomiting and the food ingestions are small, amounting to repeated snacks rather than true binges.[18] Moreover, in NES and SRED the timing of food intake remains restricted to the evening and/or the night, whereas in binge-eating disorder or bulimia nervosa with nocturnal eating, nocturnal eating with full alertness is combined with a daytime eating disorder.

TREATMENT

Treatments for NES are limited, and very little has been published to date. Some case series reported efficacy with selective serotonin reuptake inhibitors, such as paroxetine and fluvoxamine[42] and, in particular, sertraline (50–200 mg/day).[43–45] Other treatments, such as the anticonvulsant topiramate and d-fenfluramine (a potent serotoninergic agent) (15–30 mg daily at bedtime), determine a drastic reduction in the number of nocturnal episodes in the few patients treated.[24,38,46,47]

The efficacy of brief progressive muscle relaxation training[12] and long-term psychodynamic psychotherapy[18] is controversial. Cognitive-behavioral therapy in NES patients could significantly decrease caloric intake, the number of nocturnal ingestions, and weight, improving mood and quality of life.[48]

A number of potential treatments of SRED have been described, but it should be noted that all such reports have been retrospective, unblended, and not placebo controlled.

The etiology of SRED may affect the treatment of patients because if a patient is considered to have an underlying sleep disorder, treatment will be primarily directed toward that aspect. Monotherapy with clonazepam (0.5–2 mg at bedtime) could be efficacious in controlling nocturnal eating associated with somnambulism; nasal continuous positive airway pressure is the choice treatment for patients suffering from nocturnal eating and obstructive sleep apnea; dopaminergic agonists/benzodiazepines are indicated for RLS.[21] If SRED is thought to be primarily an eating disorder, treatment would be more likely initiated with behavioral measures or antidepressants.[21] Schenck and Mahowald reported success with a combination of dopaminergic agonists or precursors, either alone or in combination with opioids or sedative-hypnotics.[21,49] In general, hypnotics alone have been less successful at treating SRED. Dopaminergic agents, including bromocriptine, can reduce food intake and induce weight loss.[2] Fluoxetine monotherapy (or combined with a dopaminergic agent) may be effective in sleep-related eating patients with major depression/dysthymia or a history of substance abuse for whom a benzodiazepine or opiate agent may be contraindicated.[21]

Topiramate, at a dose range of 100–400 mg at night, reduced night eating, improved nocturnal sleep, and led to substantial weight loss.[46,50,51] Other antiepileptic medications such as zonisamide or carbamazepine might have a role in the treatment of eating disorders, but controlled trials are still lacking.[52] Low doses of pramipexole (0.18–0.36 mg at bedtime) were reported effective in a randomized, double-blind, placebo-controlled trial in 11 patients with SRED.[53] Pramipexole improved the quality of sleep and reduced motor activity during the night without a clear effect on the eating behavior per se.[53]

REFERENCES

1. Stunkard AJ, Grace WJ, Wolff HG. The night-eating syndrome: a pattern of food intake among certain obese patients. *Am J Med* 1955;19:78–86.
2. Schenck CH, Hurwitz TD, Bundlie SR, et al. Sleep-related eating disorders: polysomnographic correlates of a heterogeneous syndrome distinct from daytime eating disorders. *Sleep* 1991;14:419–31.
3. Diagnostic Classification Steering Committee. *International Classification of Sleep Disorders: Diagnostic and Coding Manual.* Rochester, MN: American Sleep Disorders Association; 1990.
4. American Academy of Sleep Medicine. *The International classification of sleep disorders. Diagnostic and Coding Manual.* 2nd ed. Westchester, IL: American Academy of Sleep Medicine; 2005.
5. Birketvedt GS, Florholmen J, Sundsfjord J, et al. Behavioral and neuroendocrine

characteristics of the night-eating syndrome. *JAMA* 1999;282:657–63.

6. Stunkard AJ, Berkowitz R, Wadden T, et al. Binge eating disorder and the night eating syndrome. *Int J Obes* 1996;20:1–6.

7. Gluck ME, Geliebter A, Satov T. Night eating syndrome is associated with depression, low self-esteem, reduced daytime hunger, and less weight loss in obese outpatients. *Obes Res* 2001;9:264–7.

8. O'Reardon JP, Ringel BL, Dinges DF, et al. Circadian eating and sleeping patterns in the night eating syndrome. *Obes Res* 2004;12:1789–96.

9. Allison KC, Lundgren JD, O'Reardon JP, et al. Proposed diagnostic criteria for night eating syndrome. *Int J Eat Disord* 2010;43:241–7.

10. Striegel-Moore RH, Franko DL, May A, et al. Should night eating syndrome be included in the DSM? *Int J Eat Disord* 2006;39:544–9.

11. Rand CS, Macgregor AM, Stunkard AJ. The night eating syndrome in the general population and among postoperative obesity surgery patients. *Int J Eat Disord* 1997;22:65–9.

12. Pawlow LA, O'Neil PM, Malcolm RJ. Night eating syndrome: effects of brief relaxation training on stress, mood, hunger, and eating patterns. *Int J Obes Relat Metab Disord* 2003;27:970–8.

13. Marshall HM, Allison KC, O'Reardon JP, et al. Night eating syndrome among nonobese persons. *Int J Eat Disord* 2004;35:217–22.

14. Vinai P, Allison KC, Cardetti S, et al. Psychopathology and treatment of night eating syndrome: a review. *Eat Weight Disord* 2008;13:54–63.

15. Allen RP. Behavioral and neuroendocrine characteristics of the night-eating syndrome. *Sleep Med* 2000;1:67–8.

16. O'Reardon JP, Peshek A, Allison KC. Night eating syndrome: diagnosis, epidemiology and management. *CNS Drugs* 2005;19:997–1008.

17. Rogers NL, Dinges DF, Allison KC, et al. Assessment of sleep in women with night eating syndrome. *Sleep* 2006;29:814–9.

18. Stunkard AJ, Allison KC. Two forms of disordered eating in obesity: binge eating and night eating. *Int J Obes Relat Metab Disord* 2003;27:1–12.

19. Allison KC, Ahima RS, O'Reardon JP, et al. Neuroendocrine profiles associated with energy intake, sleep, and stress in the night eating syndrome. *J Clin Endocrinol Metab* 2005;90:6214–7.

20. Striegel-Moore RH, Franko DL, Garcia J. The validity and clinical utility of night eating syndrome. *Int J Eat Disord* 2009;42:720–38.

21. Schenck CH, Hurwitz TD, O'Connor KA, et al. Additional categories of sleep-related eating disorders and the current status of treatment. *Sleep* 1993;16:457–66.

22. Vetrugno R, Manconi M, Ferini-Strambi L, et al. Nocturnal eating: sleep-related eating disorder or night eating syndrome? A videopolysomnographic study. *Sleep* 2006;29:949–54.

23. Winkelman JW. Clinical and polysomnographic features of sleep-related eating disorder. *J Clin Psychiatry* 1998;59:14–9.

24. Spaggiari MC, Granella F, Parrino L, et al. Nocturnal eating syndrome in adults. *Sleep* 1994;17:339–44.

25. Provini F, Antelmi E, Vignatelli L, et al. Association of restless legs syndrome with nocturnal eating: a case-control study. *Mov Disord* 2009;24:871–7.

26. Mahowald MW, Cramer Bornemann MA, et al. A case of reversible restless legs syndrome (RLS) and sleep-related eating disorder relapse triggered by acute right leg herpes zoster infection: literature review of spinal cord and peripheral nervous system contributions to RLS. *Sleep Med* 2010;11:583–5.

27. Pourcher E, Rémillard S, Cohen H. Compulsive habits in restless legs syndrome patients under dopaminergic treatment. *J Neurol Sci* 2010;290:52–6.

28. Provini F, Vetrugno R, Montagna P. Sleep-related smoking syndrome. *Sleep Med* 2008;9:903–5.

29. Provini F, Antelmi E, Vignatelli L, et al. Increased prevalence of nocturnal smoking in restless legs syndrome (RLS). *Sleep Med* 2010;11:218–20.

30. Morgenthaler TI, Silber MH. Amnestic sleep-related eating disorder associated with zolpidem. *Sleep Med* 2002;3:323–7.

31. Hoque R, Chesson AL, Jr. Zolpidem-induced sleepwalking, sleep related eating disorder, and sleep-driving: fluorine-18-flourodeoxyglucose positron emission tomography analysis, and a literature review of other unexpected clinical effects of zolpidem. *J Clin Sleep Med* 2009;5:471–6.

32. Molina SM, Joshi KG. A case of zaleplon-induced amnestic sleep-related eating disorder. *J Clin Psychiatry* 2010;71:210–1.

33. Paquet V, Strul J, Servais L, et al. Sleep-related eating disorder induced by olanzapine. *J Clin Psychiatry* 2002;63:597.

34. Cohrs S. Sleep disturbances in patients with schizophrenia: impact and effect of antipsychotics. *CNS Drugs* 2008;22:939–62.

35. Striegel-Moore RH, Franko DL, Thompson D, et al. Night eating: prevalence and demographic correlates. *Obesity (Silver Spring)* 2006;14:139–47.

36. Ceru-Bjork C, Andersson I, Rossner S. Night eating and nocturnal eating—two different or similar syndromes among obese patients? *Int J Obes Relat Metab Disord* 2001;25:365–72.

37. Lundgren JD, Allison KC, Crow S, et al. Prevalence of the night eating syndrome in a psychiatric population. *Am J Psychiatry* 2006;163:156–8.

38. Manni R, Ratti MT, Tartara A. Nocturnal eating: prevalence and features in 120 insomniac referrals. *Sleep* 1997;20:734–8.

39. Winkelman JW, Herzog DB, Fava M. The prevalence of sleep-related eating disorder in psychiatric and non-psychiatric populations. *Psychol Med* 1999;29:1461–6.

40. De Ocampo J, Foldvary N, Dinner DS, et al. Sleep-related eating disorder in fraternal twins. *Sleep Med* 2002;3:525–6.

41. Allison KC, Lundgren JD, O'Reardon JP, et al; The Night Eating Questionnaire (NEQ): psychometric properties of a measure of severity of the night eating syndrome. *Eat Behav* 2008;9:62–72.

42. Miyaoka T, Yasukawa R, Tsubouchi K, et al. Successful treatment of nocturnal eating/drinking syndrome with selective serotonin reuptake inhibitors. *Int Clin Psychopharmacol* 2003;18:175–7.

43. O'Reardon JP, Stunkard AJ, Allison KC. Clinical trial of sertraline in the treatment of night eating syndrome. *Int J Eat Disord* 2004;35:16–26.

44. O'Reardon JP, Allison KC, Martino NS, et al. A randomized, placebo-controlled trial of sertraline in the treatment of night eating syndrome. *Am J Psychiatry* 2006;163:893–8.

45. Stunkard AJ, Allison KC, Lundgren JD, et al. A paradigm for facilitating pharmacotherapy at a distance: sertraline treatment of the night eating syndrome. *J Clin Psychiatry* 2006;67:1568–72.

46. Winkelman JW. Treatment of nocturnal eating syndrome and sleep-related eating disorder with topiramate. *Sleep Med* 2003;4:243–6.

47. Aloe F, Mancini M, Araujo LA, et al. Nocturnal eating syndrome: a case report with therapeutic response to dexfenfluramine. *Sleep Res* 1995;24A:279.

48. Allison KC, Lundgren JD, Moore RH, et al. Cognitive behavior therapy for night eating syndrome: a pilot study. *Am J Psychother* 2010;64:91–106.

49. Schenck CH, Mahowald MW. Combined bupropion-levodopa-trazodone therapy of sleep-related eating and sleep disruption in two adults with chemical dependency. *Sleep* 2000;23:587–8.

50. Martinez-Salio A, Soler-Algarra S, Calvo-Garcia I, et al. Nocturnal sleep-related eating disorder that responds to topiramate. *Rev Neurol* 2007;45:276–9.

51. Howell MJ, Schenck CH. Treatment of nocturnal eating disorders. *Curr Treat Options Neurol* 2009;11:333–9.

52. McElroy SL, Guerdjikova AI, Martens B, et al. Role of antiepileptic drugs in the management of eating disorders. *CNS Drugs* 2009;23:139–56.

53. Provini F, Albani F, Vetrugno R, et al. A pilot double-blind placebo-controlled trial of low-dose pramipexole in sleep-related eating disorder. *Eur J Neurol* 2005;12:432–6.

33

Fatal Familial Insomnia

FEDERICA PROVINI, ELIO LUGARESI,
AND PIETRO CORTELLI

THE CLINICAL and neuropathologic features of fatal familial insomnia (FFI) were first reported in 1986 by Lugaresi et al.[1]

Subsequent reports from Lugaresi and his group examined in detail the alterations of the wake-sleep cycle,[2,3] the dysautonomic and hormonal characteristics,[4-9] and the neuropsychological traits[10,11] that clinically typify FFI. In the meantime, Gambetti and his collaborators demonstrated that FFI is a genetic prion disease characterized by a mutation in the prion protein (PrP) gene (*PRNP*), established the neuropathologic features, and defined the peculiar genotype linked to FFI, as well as the characteristics of the protease-resistant scrapie prion protein (PrPSc) present in FFI.[12-17]

Additional studies examined the metabolic [18F]fluorodeoxyglucose positron emission tomography (18F-PET)[18,19] and showed that FFI can be transmitted to experimental animals, thus placing FFI within the group of transmissible prion diseases.[20-22] Currently, FFI has been definitely established as a distinct disease entity

with worldwide distribution.[23-30] It represents the third most frequent hereditary prion disease worldwide, and more than 40 apparently unrelated families are known to be affected. Although rare, FFI is an important disease on several accounts: it has widened the phenotypic spectrum of prion diseases, it has led to the discovery of a novel mechanism of phenotypic heterogeneity in human genetic diseases, and it has led to the identification of the two major forms of scrapie PrP in human prion diseases. Moreover, it is the first disease characterized by peculiar alterations in the wake-sleep cycle and other circadian rhythms that, together with the preferential pathologic involvement of the dorsomedial and anteroventral thalamic nuclei, emphasize the role that the limbic portion of the thalamus plays in the regulation of sleep. FFI therefore represents a model disease for the investigation of the integrative role of the limbic thalamus.

This chapter focuses on the description of the circadian sleep-wake and hormonal and dysautonomic alterations in FFI and their pathologic correlates.

GENETIC FEATURES

FFI is linked to a missense mutation at codon 178 of *PRNP* that results in the substitution of aspartic acid with asparagine in PrP (D178N).[12] The same D178N mutation is linked to another familial prion disease that is different from FFI and carries a clinical and pathologic disease phenotype similar to that of Creutzfeldt-Jakob disease (CJD).[13] Allele-specific sequencing demonstrated that codon 129 of the PrP gene, the site of a common methionine/valine polymorphism, is the determinant of the disease phenotypes linked to the D178N mutation. In patients affected by CJD linked to the D178N mutation (CJD[178]), codon 129 located on the mutated allele is valine, whereas in patients with FFI, codon 129 is methionine.[13]

Furthermore, because codon 129 located on the normal allele can be either methionine or valine, each of the FFI and CJD[178] group of patient populations comprises patients that are homozygotes and patients that are heterozygotes at codon 129.[13] The homozygote (methionine/methionine) FFI patients have on average a shorter disease duration than the heterozygote (methionine/valine) patients, whereas the age at onset is not significantly different in the two patient populations.[13] Subsequent studies have also shown that the clinical and pathologic features differ slightly in homozygote and heterozygote subjects.[31]

CLINICAL FEATURES

FFI affects men and women equally and is transmitted as an autosomal dominant trait. It is a disorder of middle age, presenting at a mean of 51 ± 7.1 years but with a range of 36 to 62 years in 14 pathologically verified patients.[31] FFI uniformly ends in death of the patient, after a variable disease duration and course (ranging from 8 to 72 months, mean 18.4 ± 17.3 months, according to Montagna et al.[31]). As mentioned previously, the variability of disease duration and clinical and pathologic features, but not the age at onset, are related to the *PRNP* codon 129. In a series of 45 FFI patients, the homozygote subjects ($N = 30$) had a disease duration of 12 ± 4 months, whereas in the heterozygote subjects ($N = 15$) the duration was 21 ± 15 months.[27] Clinical symptoms and signs in FFI patients

fall within three major categories: disturbances of wake and sleep, disturbances of autonomic functioning, and behavioral abnormalities. Insomnia represents an often-neglected symptom, which is frequently missing from standard clinical history but is reported by patients or relatives when it is specifically sought. Insomnia indeed is often considered trivial by attending physicians and attributed to environmental or psychological conditions. It is often an early symptom, with patients complaining of unrefreshing sleep and frequent arousals during the night. In the course of the disease, falling asleep and maintaining nocturnal sleep or daytime naps become progressively harder, and sleep may be completely lost, resulting in complete agrypnia (organic insomnia). Patients are unable to initiate and maintain sleep, passing their time in an uncomfortable state of no wake–no sleep. From disease onset, patients appear apathetic, indifferent to their surroundings, and drowsy, giving the false impression that the problem is hypersomnolence. As insomnia worsens, daytime somnolence becomes increasingly pronounced. When sitting, patients close their eyes and drop their heads, but they cannot fall asleep; when lying down, they keep their eyes closed, but if touched or called, they open their eyes and immediately reply, although in monosyllables. Later in the course of the disease, patients display additional peculiar oneiric disturbances (oneiric stupor [OS]), where upon "wake" is abruptly interrupted by episodes of dreaming activity, which increase in frequency and duration. During these episodes, patients perform automatic gestures mimicking daily-life activities (dressing, combing their hair, drinking, eating, washing hands, manipulating nonexistent objects) and are unresponsive to their environment. At first, patients may be easily awakened from such drowsy condition and, if questioned, report a single oneiric scene more than a dream to which the complex gestures seem to closely correspond. However, gesturing progressively becomes coarser and interspersed with tremor-like and spontaneous and evoked jerks; patients become confused and have increasing difficulties in reporting any dreaming content. Speech becomes increasingly slurred and weakens to the point of being incomprehensible. Gait becomes ever more uncertain and ultimately impossible unaided. Death is sudden, especially in 129 homozygote patients, or is preceded by an ever-increasing stupor state and an akinetic mutism. Sleep disturbances are usually associated from the beginning with autonomic alterations, in the form of subtle pyrexia, especially in the evening; increased salivation and diaphoresis; and mild elevation of blood pressure, heart rate, and irregular breathing. Impotence may occur early in men, and sphincter control may be lost in the later stages of the disease, especially in the heterozygote patients. From disease onset there may be episodes of diplopia varying in duration.

Wake-Sleep and Other Circadian Autonomic and Hormonal Changes

POLYSOMNOGRAPHY

The electroencephalographic (EEG) background activity becomes progressively reduced in amplitude and slow and then unreactive and monomorphic in the advanced stages. The periodic activity characteristic of CJD is usually absent throughout the course of FFI, even though bursts of repetitive, diffuse 1- to 2-Hz

sharp waves may appear in advanced stages of long-duration cases. These bursts are associated with diffuse and focal myoclonus.

The 24-hour EEG recordings are characterized by a continuous oscillation between the EEG activity associated with normal, relaxed wakefulness and that associated with diffuse theta activity. In more advanced stages, EEG patterns typical of synchronized sleep (spindling and delta activity) are completely absent throughout the 24 hours. Patients spend most of the recorded time in a non-wake/non-sleep-like state, characterized by a combination of alpha and theta EEG activity, similar to stage 1 sleep or better defined as "subwakefulness" (Fig. 33.1A). Synchronized sleep progressively attenuates and even intravenous administration of barbiturates or benzodiazepines at dosages inducing coma fails to evoke spindle-like or delta activities (Fig. 33.1B). Sleep spindles and K-complexes are better preserved in patients who display a prolonged disease course, but they tend to become altered and eventually disappear in these patients, too. Rapid eye

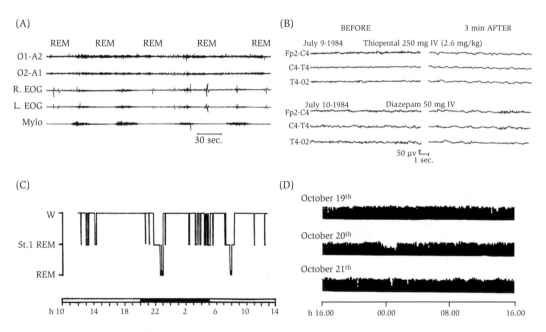

FIGURE 33.1   (A) Polysomnographic excerpted recordings of a 57-year-old male fatal familial insomnia patient. Electroencephalographic tracings show transitions between rapid eye movement (REM) and subwakefulness stage recurring in a quasiperiodic fashion. (B) Intravenous administration of barbiturates or benzodiazepines at dosages inducing coma fails to evoke spindle-like or delta activities. (C) The 24-hour wake-sleep histogram demonstrates reduced total sleep time (TST), progressive loss of synchronized sleep and rapid eye movement (REM) sleep stages, and abnormal cyclic organization of sleep. (D) Actigraphic recordings in a fatal familial insomnia patient. Each line represents 24 hours (16:00 to 16:00). Motor activity is indicated by the black spikes. Grossly increased motor activity is evident throughout the 24 hours, without consistent circadian rhythmicity.

movement (REM) sleep initially may remain normal or display a pathologically preserved muscle tone on antigravity muscles (chin muscles) associated with increased myoclonic activity in limb muscles, similar to the patterns observed during REM sleep behavior disorder (RBD). Notably, the cyclic organization of sleep is lost with absence of the orderly transition between sleep stages and abrupt passages between wake and synchronized and REM sleep stages (Fig. 33.1C). Unlike synchronized sleep, REM sleep persists until the most advanced disease stages, appearing in isolated or clustered short-lasting (no longer than 20–30 second) episodes (Fig. 33.1A). However, these abnormal REM stages do not always lack physiologic atonia and are associated with oneiric behavior. Total sleep time is drastically reduced and sleep efficiency severely impaired. Actigraphic recordings throughout 52 days in an FFI patient[3] showed an 80% increase in motor activity (Fig. 33.1D). Furthermore, indirect calorimetry in a closed respiratory chamber demonstrated that in this patient the 24-hour energy expenditure was increased by an astonishing 60%, which may explain the wasting and emaciation typical of FFI.[3]

AUTONOMIC AND HORMONAL FINDINGS

Autonomic studies in FFI have shown higher blood pressure and heart rate in the resting state with elevated levels of noradrenaline, which further increase on postural challenge or Valsalva maneuver. Baroreflex pathways remain unimpaired, indicating overall unbalanced autonomic control with preserved parasympathetic function but increased background and stimulated orthosympathetic activity.[4] Sympathetic skin response was abolished in four FFI patients that we tested.[32] Muscle sympathetic nerve activity during resting wakefulness was abnormally high in a FFI patient recently examined.[33]

Circadian rhythms of blood pressure and heart rate are present but with decreasing amplitude of the oscillations, until they disappear entirely in the late stages of the disease. Blood pressure mean values and body core temperature are persistently mildly elevated throughout the 24 hours (Fig. 33.2A). Plasma cortisol is also persistently high in the presence of remarkably normal or even reduced corticotropin levels. Eventually secondary hypertension develops paralleled by increasing catecholamine levels and heart rate.[6] These abnormalities of autonomic functions are also associated with noncatecholaminergic hormonal changes. The nocturnal physiologic elevation of somatotropin disappears in parallel with the loss of deep sleep, but prolactin maintains a normal circadian rhythmicity, which is lost only in the final stages of the disease.[5,8] Melatonin concentrations gradually decrease, showing a circadian oscillation in the early stages of the disease, which is subsequently lost (Fig. 33.2B).[7] Moreover, there is an increased sympathetic activation of central origin, associated with hypercortisolism and elevated catecholamine levels. Diurnal and nocturnal norepinephrine (NE) secretion was constantly elevated, invariably two or three times higher than normal in all (Fig. 33.2B).[9] The two- to three-fold increase in serum NE level and the absence of the physiological nocturnal peak of melatonin secretion are the most prominent hormonal markers of the disease.

Movement Disorders in Fatal Familial Insomnia

Somatomotor abnormalities regularly occur in FFI patients, especially in patients with a prolonged disease course.[1,31] Patients in the early stages of the disease may report transient diplopia, but the most striking motor abnormality in FFI consists of myoclonus, arising in the middle stages of the disease and usually persisting until death. Myoclonus is both spontaneous and evoked by somesthetic stimuli, such as tapping or stroking of the skin, in particular with the patient keeping the eyes closed. Evoked myoclonus is usually diffuse, involving the large proximal muscles of the neck, trunk, and limbs. Spontaneous myoclonus is either diffuse, or segmental, in such cases especially involving the distal muscles of the upper and lower limbs. Fragmentary myoclonic activity is regularly found in facial and limb muscles whenever patients lapse into an oneiric stupor state and forms part of the complex gesturing that accompanies the sleep disturbances of FFI. Such activity, however, disappears immediately whenever patients are awakened and able to remain in a normal, although transitory, waking state. Another somatomotor abnormality typical of FFI, although by no means present in all cases, is ataxia or gait apraxia. Patients have difficulty in standing and walking and are unable to run. When standing, they tend to fall statue-like to the ground and, when walking, are unable to propel the lower limbs forward,

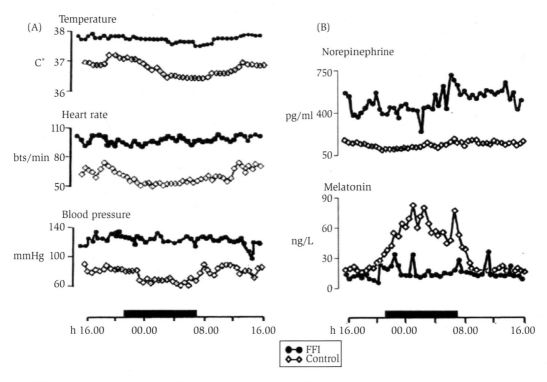

(A) Temperature

(B) Norepinephrine

Heart rate

Melatonin

Blood pressure

FFI
Control

FIGURE 33.2 (*A*) The 24-hour body core temperature (°C), heart rate (HR), and mean arterial pressure (BP) in a 53-year-old 129 codon *PRNP* homozygote fatal familial insomnia patient and in a control subject (black bar indicates lights-out time). In the FFI patient °C, HR, and BP are elevated without circadian fluctuations. (*B*) Twenty-four hour recordings of norepinephrine and melatonin concentrations in a patient with FFI and in a control individual. Norepinephrine secretion is higher than normal throughout the 24 hours. The nocturnal peak of melatonin secretion is lost.

their feet "glued" to the ground. Such combination of ataxic and apraxic abnormalities may be described as astasia-abasia and is not observed at disease onset but in more advanced stages. Speech becomes slurred and feeble, and dysphagia may finally necessitate artificial feeding. Neurologic examination discloses brisk tendon jerks and Babinski signs. Only a few patients display sporadic epileptic, tonic-clonic seizures and only in the very late, terminal stages of the disease.[31,34]

Neuropsychological Features

Detailed neuropsychological studies of the cognitive and behavioral abnormalities carried out by the original investigators in Bologna in seven FFI patients[10,11] documented a progressive disturbance of attention and vigilance associated with a deficit of working memory characterized by difficulty in the manipulation and temporal ordering of events and a defect of frontal functions (planning and forecast of events). IQ and

general intelligence, however, remain remarkably normal, as far as patients can be tested. These findings are considered to be distinctive within the group of neurodegenerative disorders characterized by cognitive decline and to differ also from the features of Wernicke-Korsakoff syndrome. The preservation of global intelligence and the presence of persistent and prominent disturbances of vigilance, as clearly shown by the polysomnographic studies, challenge the concept of thalamic dementia, because dementia implies by definition a normal vigilance state. Therefore, FFI is best defined as a confusional oneiric state, rather than a dementing illness.

Neuroradiologic and Metabolic Features

Routine imaging studies of the brain in FFI by means of computed tomography (CT) or magnetic resonance imaging (MRI) are usually unrevealing or at best show diffuse cerebral and cerebellar atrophy and ventricular dilatation, without specific characteristics. Studies with 18F-PET of regional cerebral glucose utilization have been performed in a series of FFI patients.[18,19] A prominent and nearly selective hypometabolism of the thalami and, to a lesser extent, of the cingulate cortex is observed in patients with a short-lasting disease course. In cases with longer disease duration, the cerebral cortex (except for the occipital region), basal ganglia, and cerebellum are also involved. Postmortem brain examination documented that the cortical areas most affected are invariably the limbic areas (the anterior cyngulate gyrus and the orbitofrontal cortex) also in longer evolution cases.[35] Thalamic hypometabolism is, therefore, the metabolic hallmark of FFI. Furthermore, the distribution of the hypometabolism in patients with different disease duration suggests that the hypometabolism starts in the thalamus and cingulate cortex but subsequently spreads to the other cortical and subcortical regions.

Longitudinal PET (18 FDG-PET) studies in carriers of FFI mutation have shown that thalamic hypometabolism may precede the disease onset by several months.[36]

Neuropathology of Fatal Familial Insomnia

The neuropathologic hallmark of FFI[1,37,38] is severe atrophy of the anterior ventral and mediodorsal thalamic nuclei with loss of 80% to 90% of the neurons and two- to threefold increase in astroglial cells, whereas spongiosis is conspicuously absent. The other thalamic nuclei are less and inconsistently affected. Atrophy of the inferior olives is also commonly found. The involvement of other brain regions is a function of the disease duration, which, in turn, as mentioned previously, is largely related to the genotype at codon 129 PRNP. Although the mesio-orbital frontal cortex and attendant substantia innominata (ventral pallidum and extended amygdala) may show spongiosis also in cases of short duration, the neocortex is affected by spongiosis, gliosis, and to a lesser extent neuronal loss only in cases of more than 18 months' disease duration.[38] Abundant apoptotic neurons have been found in the brains of FFI patients with a distribution that correlates closely with the distribution of the neuronal loss.[39]

Prion Protein Characteristics

Most human prion diseases are characterized by the presence of protease-resistant PrP (PrP^{Sc}) fragments of two major sizes, types 1 and 2, which migrate at approximately 21 kDa and 19 kDa on gel electrophoresis.[40] The different sizes are likely to reflect the different conformation of the two PrP^{Sc} species, which in turn may cause different pathologies. FFI is characterized by the presence in the brain tissue of PrP^{Sc} of 19 kDa, whereas CJD[178] is associated with PrP^{Sc} of 21 kDa. Therefore, the different codons at position 129, methionine in FFI and valine in CJD[178], appear to act as determinants of the PrP^{Sc} conformation. Furthermore, the PrP^{Sc} associated with FFI is present in very low quantities, 6 to 10 times less than most other human prion diseases.[41] FFI has been transmitted to receptive transgenic mice expressing a "humanized" PrP by intracerebral injection of brain homogenate from subjects affected by FFI.[22] This important experiment has demonstrated that FFI is transmissible like most prion diseases.

The Sporadic Form of Fatal Familial Insomnia or Sporadic Fatal Insomnia

Sporadic cases displaying clinical and pathologic features indistinguishable from those of FFI, including the polysomnographic findings, have also been reported[41–45] under the term *sporadic fatal insomnia* (sFI).[41] It is notable that little more than 10 cases of proven sFI are methionine homozygotes at codon 129.[41,44] Furthermore, all sFI cases examined have PrP^{Sc} in very low amounts as in FFI. In one case, sFI was transmitted to "humanized" transgenic mice that developed a disease characterized by a PrP^{Sc} of 19 kDa as in the human disease and histologic lesions similar to those of sFI and FFI.[44]

The co-occurrence of both sporadic and genetic forms of FFI within the same family was recently described.[46]

Fatal Familial Insomnia as a Model Disease: Implications for the Study of Sleep and Circadian Functions

It is important that the insomnia of FFI not be equated with the "trivial" insomnia so frequent in the general population; rather, it can be more aptly defined as an example of organic insomnia, or agrypnia. The complex and sustained sleep abnormality of FFI consists primarily of an inability to initiate and maintain synchronized (spindle and delta) sleep. Transition from wakefulness to sleep is impaired, and the sleep EEG patterns that exemplify the initiation of sleep, that is, sleep spindles and K-complexes, are affected early and in full-blown and advanced disease stages disappear completely. REM sleep is also affected, giving rise to complex and, especially in early disease stages, purposeful motor activities associated with dreaming mentation, we named oneiric stupor (OS). OS is reminiscent of but different from RBD, as are the polysomnographic features of the episodes, with persisting electromyographic tone and prominent limb twitching. OS episodes occur during day and night, arising from an abnormally disorganized sleep structure, and are characterized by a quiet motor pattern mimicking daily-life activities and by a neutral dream content. When questioned, patients report a single oneiric scene rather than a structured dream.

All of these symptoms and signs, when correlated to the striking hypometabolism of the thalamus shown in vivo[18,19] and the severe neuronal loss and gliosis on postmortem verification,[1,37,38] point to the thalamus as the central structure in the organization of circadian activities.[47,48] The thalamus, especially its dorsomedian part, was originally considered by Hess to be a structure favoring sleep. Hess[49] induced sleep behaviors in cats on electrical stimulation of the antero-median thalamus. Parmeggiani obtained similar results stimulating the cortico-limbic (rhinencephalic) formations with the same technique.[50] Moreover, severe and persistent insomnia appeared in cats with ablation of the thalamus, the so-called athalamic cats,[51] and bilateral lesions of the dorsomedian thalamic nuclei caused insomnia in the experimental animal, in contrast to lesions of the anterior nuclei that left sleep structure unaffected.[52] Clinical studies in patients with chronic ischemic or hemorrhagic lesions of the thalamus, especially its medial part (the so-called paramedian thalamic syndrome), have demonstrated a complex sleep disorder with daytime somnolence but inability to fall asleep and to maintain sustained sleep with polysomnographic features similar to those of FFI.[53,54] The experimental and clinical evidence combined definitely points to the thalamus, especially its dorsomedian portion, as the structure generating and organizing behavior aimed at maintaining the body homeostasis.

The regulative role of the medial thalamus is best understood if one bears in mind that the anteromedial nuclei, also called "visceral thalamus," is prominently connected with the limbic cortex, especially the cingulate gyrus and the orbital frontal cortex. Furthermore, the medio-dorsal thalamic nucleus functions as a relay between the mesio-orbital cortex and the basal forebrain, hypothalamic and upper brainstem regions that also regulate sleep behavior. An interaction of the abnormal PrP with gamma-aminobutyric acid (GABA)ergic synapses[55] or with protein receptors constitutive of the system[56] has been proposed. The peculiar polysomnographic features of FFI and the several other sleep abnormalities reported in CJD[57–60] spurred studies on the possible role of PrP in sleep regulation. Mice devoid of PrP show abnormalities in circadian activity rhythms and patterns.[61] They exhibit a larger, almost double, amount of sleep fragmentation than wild-type mice and smaller power in the spectrum of EEG slow waves.[62] These findings led to the suggestion that PrP plays a role in promoting sleep continuity.[62] All of these findings have to be confirmed, especially because the precise function of the PrP remains unknown. Indeed, even though FFI has already provided a useful model for clinical and pathologic correlations and revolutionary insights into the regulation of sleep and the integrative function of the thalamus, several questions, especially pertaining to the pathogenesis of the disease, remain unanswered. Unfortunately, therapy, the most pressing need, is currently unavailable and FFI remains an untreatable disease.

FATAL FAMILIAL INSOMNIA AND THE CONCEPT OF AGRYPNIA EXCITATA

The cardinal features of FFI are shared by other clinical conditions such as Morvan Syndrome (MS) and delirium tremens (DT), in which the apparent site of lesion resides in the limbic thalamus and connected cortical regions.[63] The term *agrypnia excitata* aptly defines these peculiar behavioral and polysomnographic pictures.[63–66] All of these conditions are characterized by severe disturbances of sleep (*agrypnia*), whereby deep sleep is lacking and oneiric behaviors with hallucinations and pathologic dreaming activity are associated with autonomic hyperfunction (hypertension, tachycardia, tachypnea, pyrexia, and perspiration) and motor agitation with irregular jerky movements and tremors (*excitata*). In all of these conditions, the brunt of the pathologic condition, whether degenerative as in FFI, autoimmune as in MS, or toxic as in DT, bears on the thalamus and limbic regions (limbic encephalitis in MS[67,68]; the anterior thalamus, cingulate cortex, and mammillary bodies in DT[69,70]). Agrypnia excitata represents, therefore, a distinct and useful cliniconeurophysiologic concept, with a pathologic correlate in the function of the thalamolimbic system.[63–66]

ACKNOWLEDGMENTS

We thank Ms. A. Laffi for assistance with the manuscript, and Ms. A. Collins for revising the English.

REFERENCES

1. Lugaresi E, Medori R, Montagna P, et al. Fatal familial insomnia and dysautonomia with selective degeneration of thalamic nuclei. *N Engl J Med* 1986;315:997–1003.
2. Sforza E, Montagna P, Tinuper P, et al. Sleep-wake cycle abnormalities in fatal familial insomnia. Evidence of the role of the thalamus in sleep regulation. *Electroencephalogr Clin Neurophysiol* 1995;94:398–405.
3. Plazzi G, Schutz Y, Cortelli P, et al. Motor overactivity and loss of motor circadian rhythm in fatal familial insomnia: an actigraphic study. *Sleep* 1997;20:739–42.
4. Cortelli P, Parchi P, Contin M, et al. Cardiovascular dysautonomia in fatal familial insomnia. *Clin Auton Res* 1991;1:15–21.
5. Avoni P, Cortelli P, Montagna P, et al. Circadian hormonal rhythms in two new cases of fatal familial insomnia. *Acta Neurol* 1991;13:574–6.
6. Portaluppi F, Cortelli P, Avoni P, et al. Diurnal blood pressure variation and hormonal correlates in fatal familial insomnia. *Hypertension* 1994;23:569–76.
7. Portaluppi F, Cortelli P, Avoni P, et al. Progressive disruption of the circadian rhythm of melatonin in fatal familial insomnia. *J Clin Endocrinol Metab* 1994;78:1075–8.
8. Portaluppi F, Cortelli P, Avoni P, et al. Dissociated 24-hour patterns of somatotropin and prolactin in fatal familial insomnia. *Neuroendocrinology* 1995;61:731–7.
9. Montagna P, Cortelli P, Gambetti P, et al. Fatal familial insomnia: sleep, neuroendocrine and vegetative alterations. *Adv Neuroimmunol* 1995;5:13–21.
10. Gallassi R, Morreale A, Montagna P, et al. "Fatal familial insomnia": neuropsychological study of a disease with thalamic degeneration. *Cortex* 1992;28:175–87.
11. Gallassi R, Morreale A, Montagna P, et al. Fatal familial insomnia: behavioral and cognitive features. *Neurology* 1996;46:935–9.
12. Medori R, Tritschler HJ, LeBlanc A, et al. Fatal familial insomnia, a prion disease with a mutation at codon 178 of the prion protein gene. *N Engl J Med* 1992;326:444–9.
13. Goldfarb LG, Petersen RB, Tabaton M, et al. Fatal familial insomnia and familial Creutzfeldt-Jakob disease: disease phenotype determined by a DNA polymorphism. *Science* 1992;258:806–8.
14. Monari L, Chen SG, Brown P, et al. Fatal familial insomnia and familial Creutzfeldt-Jakob disease: different prion proteins determined by a DNA polymorphism. *Proc Natl Acad Sci USA* 1994;91:2839–42.
15. Petersen RB, Goldfarb LG, Tabaton M, et al. A novel mechanism of phenotypic heterogeneity demonstrated by the effect of a polymorphism on a pathogenic mutation in the PRNP (prion protein gene). *Mol Neurobiol* 1994;8:99–103.
16. Gambetti P, Parchi P, Petersen RB, et al. Fatal familial insomnia and familial Creutzfeldt-Jakob disease: clinical, pathological and molecular features. *Brain Pathol* 1995;5:43–51.
17. Parchi P, Capellari S, Gambetti P. Intracerebral distribution of the abnormal isoform of the prion protein in sporadic Creutzfeldt-Jakob disease and fatal insomnia. *Microsc Res Tech* 2000;50:16–25.
18. Perani D, Cortelli P, Lucignani G, et al. [18F] FDG PET in fatal familial insomnia: the functional effects of thalamic lesions. *Neurology* 1993;43:2565–9.
19. Cortelli P, Perani D, Parchi P, et al. Cerebral metabolism in fatal familial insomnia: relation to duration, neuropathology, and distribution of protease-resistant prion protein. *Neurology* 1997;49:126–33.
20. Collinge J, Palmer MS, Sidle KC, et al. Transmission of fatal familial insomnia to laboratory animals. *Lancet* 1995;346:569–70.
21. Tateishi J, Brown P, Kitamoto T, et al. First experimental transmission of fatal familial insomnia. *Nature* 1995;376:434–5.
22. Telling GC, Parchi P, DeArmond SJ, et al. Evidence for the conformation of the

pathologic isoform of the prion protein enciphering and propagating prion diversity. *Science* 1996;274:2079–82.

23. Silburn P, Cervenakova L, Varghese P, et al. Fatal familial insomnia: a seventh family. *Neurology* 1996;47:1326–8.

24. Nagayama M, Shinohara Y, Furukawa H, et al. Fatal familial insomnia with a mutation at codon 178 of the prion protein gene: first report from Japan. *Neurology* 1996;47:1313–6.

25. McLean CA, Storey E, Gardner RJ, et al. The D178N (cis-129M) "fatal familial insomnia" mutation associated with diverse clinicopathologic phenotypes in an Australian kindred. *Neurology* 1997;49:552–8.

26. Kretzschmar H, Giese A, Zerr I, et al. The German FFI cases. *Brain Pathol* 1998;8:559–61.

27. Padovani A, D'Alessandro M, Parchi P, et al. Fatal familial insomnia in a new Italian kindred. *Neurology* 1998;51:1491–4.

28. Almer G, Hainfellner JA, Brucke T, et al. Fatal familial insomnia: a new Austrian family. *Brain* 1999;122:5–16.

29. Harder A, Jendroska K, Kreuz F, et al. Novel twelve-generation kindred of fatal familial insomnia from Germany representing the entire spectrum of disease expression. *Am J Med Genet* 1999;87:311–6.

30. Tabernero C, Polo JM, Sevillano MD, et al. Fatal familial insomnia: clinical, neuropathological, and gene description of a Spanish family. *J Neurol Neurosurg Psychiatry* 2000;68:774–7.

31. Montagna P, Cortelli P, Avoni P, et al. Clinical features of fatal familial insomnia: phenotypic variability in relation to a polymorphism at codon 129 of the prion protein gene. *Brain Pathol* 1998;8:515–20.

32. Montagna P, Cortelli P, Avoni P, et al. Abnormal sympathetic skin responses in thalamic lesions. *Electroencephalogr Clin Neurophysiol* 1992;85:225–7.

33. Donadio V, Montagna P, Pennisi M, et al. Agrypnia excitata: a microneurographic study of muscle sympathetic nerve activity. *Clin Neurophysiol* 2009;120:1139–42.

34. Montagna P, Gambetti P, Cortelli P, et al. Familial and sporadic fatal insomnia. *Lancet Neurol* 2003;2:167–76.

35. Kong Q, Surewicz WK, Petersen RB, et al. Inherited prion diseases. In: Prusiner SB, ed. *Prion Biology and Diseases*. 2nd ed. New York: Cold Springs Harbor Laboratory Press; 2004:673–775.

36. Cortelli P, Perani D, Montagna P, et al. Pre-symptomatic diagnosis in fatal familial insomnia: serial neurophysiological and 18FDG-PET studies. *Brain* 2006;129:668–75.

37. Manetto V, Medori R, Cortelli P, et al. Fatal familial insomnia: clinical and pathologic study of five new cases. *Neurology* 1992;42:312–9.

38. Parchi P, Petersen RB, Chen SG, et al. Molecular pathology of fatal familial insomnia. *Brain Pathol* 1998;8:539–48.

39. Dorandeu A, Wingertsmann L, Chrétien F, et al. Neuronal apoptosis in fatal familial insomnia. *Brain Pathol* 1998;8:531–7.

40. Parchi P, Capellari S, Chen SG, et al. Typing prion isoforms. *Nature* 1997;386:232–4.

41. Parchi P, Capellari S, Chin S, et al. A subtype of sporadic prion disease mimicking fatal familial insomnia. *Neurology* 1999;52:1757–63.

42. Gambetti P, Petersen R, Monari L, et al. Fatal familial insomnia and the widening spectrum of prion diseases. In: Allen I, ed. *Spongiform Encephalopathies. Br Med Bull* 1993;49:980–94.

43. Kawasaki K, Wakabayashi K, Kawakami A, et al. Thalamic form of Creutzfeldt-Jakob disease or fatal insomnia? Report of a sporadic case with normal prion protein genotype. *Acta Neuropathol (Berl)* 1997;93:317–22.

44. Mastrianni JA, Nixon R, Layzer R, et al. Prion protein conformation in a patient with sporadic fatal insomnia. *N Engl J Med* 1999;340:1630–8.

45. Scaravilli F, Cordery RJ, Kretzschmar H, et al. Sporadic fatal insomnia: a case study. *Ann Neurol* 2000;48:665–8.

46. Capellari S, Parchi P, Cortelli P, et al. Sporadic fatal insomnia in a fatal familial insomnia pedigree. *Neurology* 2008;70:884–5.

47. Montagna P. Fatal familial insomnia: a model disease in sleep physiopathology. *Sleep Med Rev* 2005;9:339–53.

48. Montagna P. Fatal familial insomnia and the role of the thalamus in sleep regulation. *Handb Clin Neurol* 2011;99:981–96.

49. Hess WR. Das Schlafsyndrom als Folge diencephaler Reizung. *Helv Physiol Pharmacol Acta* 1944;2:305–44.

50. Parmeggiani PL. Telencephalo-diencephalic aspects of sleep mechanisms. *Brain Res* 1968;7:350–9.

51. Villablanca J. Behavioral and polygraphic study of "sleep" and "wakefulness" in chronic decerebrate cats. *Electroencephalogr Clin Neurophysiol* 1966;21:562–77.

52. Marini G, Imeri L, Mancia M. Changes in sleep-waking cycle induced by lesions of medialis dorsalis thalamic nuclei in the cat. *Neurosci Lett* 1988;85:223–7.

53. Bassetti C, Mathis J, Gugger M, et al. Hypersomnia following paramedian thalamic stroke: a report of 12 patients. *Ann Neurol* 1996;39:471–80.

54. Guilleminault C, Quera-Salva M-A, Goldberg MP. Pseudo-hypersomnia and pre-sleep behaviour with bilateral paramedian thalamic lesions. *Brain* 1993;116:1549–63.

55. Autret A, Henry-Le Bras F, Duvelleroy-Hommet C, et al. Agrypnia. *Neurophysiol Clin* 1995 ;25:360–6.

56. Cortelli P, Gambetti P, Montagna P, et al. Fatal familial insomnia: clinical features and molecular genetics. *J Sleep Res* 1999;8:23–9.

57. Donnet A, Farnarier G, Gambarelli D, et al. Sleep electroencephalogram at the early stage of Creutzfeldt-Jakob disease. *Clin Electroencephalogr* 1992;23:118–25.

58. Terzano MG, Parrino L, Pietrini V, et al. Precocious loss of physiological sleep in a case of Creutzfeldt Jakob disease: a serial polygraphic study. *Sleep* 1995;18:849–58.

59. Chapman J, Arlazoroff A, Goldfarb LG, et al. Fatal insomnia in a case of familial Creutzfeldt-Jakob disease with the codon 200(Lys) mutation. *Neurology* 1996;46:758–61.

60. Carpizo MR. Sleep and dementias. *Rev Neurol (Paris)* 2000;30:586–90.

61. Tobler I, Gaus SE, Deboer T, et al. Altered circadian activity rhythms and sleep in mice devoid of prion protein. *Nature* 1996;380:639–42.

62. Tobler I, Deboer T, Fischer M. Sleep and sleep regulation in normal and prion protein-deficient mice. *J Neurosci* 1997;17:1869–79.

63. Lugaresi E, Provini F. Agrypnia excitata: clinical features and pathophysiological implications. *Sleep Med Rev* 2001;5:313–22.

64. Montagna P, Lugaresi E. Agrypnia excitata: a generalized overactivity syndrome and a useful concept in the neurophysiopathology of sleep. *Clin Neurophysiol* 2002;113:552–60.

65. Lugaresi E, Provini F. Fatal familial insomnia and agrypnia excitata. *Rev Neurol Dis* 2007;4:145–52.

66. Provini F, Cortelli P, Montagna P, et al. Fatal insomnia and agrypnia excitata: sleep and the limbic system. *Rev Neurol (Paris)* 2008;164:692–700.

67. Barber PA, Anderson NE, Vincent A. Morvan's syndrome associated with voltage-gated K+ channel antibodies. *Neurology* 2000;54:771–2.

68. Liguori R, Vincent A, Clover L, et al. Morvan's syndrome: peripheral and central nervous system and cardiac involvement with antibodies to voltage-gated potassium channels. *Brain* 2001;124:2417–26.

69. Eckardt MJ, Campbell GA, Marietta CA, et al. Ethanol dependence and withdrawal selectively alter localized cerebral glucose utilization. *Brain Res* 1992;584:244–50.

70. Plazzi G, Montagna P, Meletti S, et al. Polysomnographic study of sleeplessness and oneiricisms in the alcohol withdrawal syndrome. *Sleep Med* 2002;3:279–82.

34

Narcolepsy, Cataplexy, and Sleep Paralysis

MASASHI OKURO AND SEIJI NISHINO

NARCOLEPSY IS a chronic hypersomnia, but the disease also exhibits unique sleep associated-movement impairments, such as cataplexy and sleep paralysis. Gélineáu first coined the term "narcolepsy" in 1880 when describing a patient with excessive daytime sleepiness (EDS), sleep attacks, and episodes of muscle weakness triggered by emotions.[1] In the current international classification, narcolepsy is characterized by "excessive daytime sleepiness that is typically associated with cataplexy (i.e., narcolepsy with cataplexy) and/or with abnormal rapid eye movement (REM) sleep phenomena such as sleep paralysis and hypnagogic hallucinations".[2]

After the discovery of sleep-onset REM sleep,[3-5] narcolepsy has often been referred to as a "REM sleep disorder." It was interpreted that REM sleep can intrude in active wake or at sleep onset, resulting in cataplexy, sleep paralysis, and hypnagogic hallucinations, and these three symptoms are often categorized as "dissociated manifestations of REM sleep" (see Nishino and Mignot[6]).

The major pathophysiology of human narcolepsy has been recently elucidated based on the discovery of narcolepsy genes in animals; mutations in hypocretin-related genes are rare in humans, but hypocretin-ligand deficiency is found in many cases.[7-9]

It is therefore conceivable that impairments of the hypocretin system result in EDS, cataplexy, and other REM sleep abnormalities. In this chapter, sleep and movement abnormalities characteristic of narcolepsy are described followed by discussions on the possible mechanisms involved. Since the abnormalities seen in narcolepsy cannot be explained independently from occurrences of EDS and sleep fragmentations, pathophysiological aspects of these symptoms are also discussed.

CLINICAL CHARACTERISTICS OF NARCOLEPSY

EDS and cataplexy are considered to be the two primary symptoms of narcolepsy, with EDS often being the more disabling symptom.[6] EDS in narcolepsy is most often relieved by short naps (15–30 minutes), but in most cases, the refreshed sensation only lasts a short time after waking. Sleepiness also occurs in irresistible waves in these patients, a phenomenon best described as "sleep attacks."

EDS is usually the first symptom to appear, followed by cataplexy, sleep paralysis, and hypnagogic hallucinations.[10–14] These are often referred to as the narcolepsy tetrad.

Although some people confuse cataplexy with sleep attacks, cataplexy is distinct from sleep attacks (and EDS) and is pathognomonic of the disease.[15] Cataplexy is defined as a sudden episode of muscle weakness triggered by emotional factors, most often in the context of positive emotions (such as laughter), and less frequently by negative emotions (most typically anger or frustration; see sequences of cataplectic attacks in a narcoleptic Doberman [Fig. 34.1]). All antigravity muscles can be affected, leading to a progressive collapse of the subject, but respiratory and eye muscles are not affected.

The patient is typically awake at the onset of the attack but may experience blurred vision or ptosis. The attack is almost always bilateral and usually lasts a few seconds. Neurological examination performed at the time of attack shows suppression of the patellar reflex and sometimes of Babinski's sign.

Sleep paralysis is present in 20%–50% of all narcoleptic subjects[12,16–18] and is often associated with hypnagogic hallucinations. Sleep paralysis is best described as a brief inability to perform voluntary movements at the onset of sleep, upon awakening during the night, or in the morning. Contrary to simple fatigue or locomotion inhibition, the patient is unable to perform even a small movement, such as lifting a finger. Sleep paralysis may last a few minutes and is often finally interrupted by noise or other external stimuli. The symptom is occasionally bothersome in narcoleptic subjects, especially when associated with frightening hallucinations.[19]

Abnormal visual (most often) or auditory perceptions that occur while falling asleep (hypnagogic) or upon waking up (hypnopompic) are

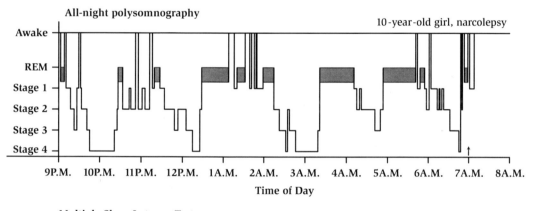

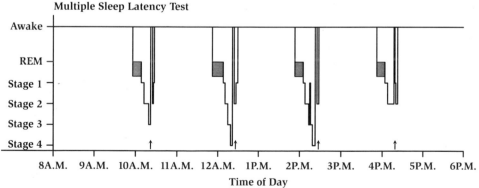

FIGURE 34.1   All-night polysomnography and multiple sleep latency test of a narcoleptic patient. (Adapted from Honda.[14])

frequently observed in narcoleptic subjects.[20] These hallucinations are often unpleasant and are typically associated with a feeling of fear or threat.[18,19] Polygraphic studies indicate that these hallucinations occur most often during REM sleep.[18,21] These episodes are often difficult to distinguish from nightmares or unpleasant dreams, which also occur frequently in narcolepsy.

These hallucinations are usually easy to distinguish from hallucinations observed in schizophrenia or related psychotic conditions.

One of the most frequently associated symptoms is insomnia, best characterized as a difficulty to maintain nighttime sleep.[6] Typically, narcoleptic patients fall asleep easily, only to wake up after a short nap and are unable to fall asleep again for an hour or so.

Other frequently associated problems are REM behavior disorders, other parasomnias,[22,23] periodic leg movements during sleep (PLMS),[24,25] and obstructive sleep apnea.[24,26,27]

OBJECTIVE MEASURES OF SLEEP ABNORMALITIES IN NARCOLEPSY

The primary sleep abnormalities observed in narcoleptic subjects is extremely short sleep latency during REM sleep. In addition, the patients have an abnormal tendency to fall into REM sleep very quickly, a phenomenon called sleep-onset REM periods (SOREMPs).[3-6] SOREMPs are initially found during nighttime polysomnography (PSG), but they are also seen during daytime naps (Fig. 34.1). REM sleep usually appears 90–110 minutes after the onset of sleep and reappears every 90–110 minutes in humans, but if the first REM sleep episode occurs within 15 minutes after the onset of sleep, these episodes are defined as SOREMPs (Fig. 34.2).

These sleep abnormalities in narcoleptic subjects are objectively evaluated with multiple sleep latency tests (MSLTs). The PSG nap test consists of four or five 20-minute nap opportunities that are scheduled 2 hours apart.[28] A mean sleep latency of less than 8 minutes on the MSLT is usually considered indicative of excessive sleepiness.[29] A total of more than two transitions to REM sleep out of the four to five naps (SOREMPs) is usually considered diagnostic for narcolepsy (Fig. 34.2).

Despite the tendency to sleep during the daytime (frequent sleep episodes) in narcolepsy, narcoleptic patients do not usually sleep more than normal individuals over the 24-hour cycle[30-32] and frequently have a very disrupted nighttime sleep.[30-32] Sleep efficiency during nocturnal PSG may also be normal or low due to the frequent waking episodes at night.

SLEEP ABNORMALITIES IN ANIMAL MODELS OF NARCOLEPSY

Just as animal models of narcolepsy significantly contribute to the discovery of narcolepsy genes and major pathophysiology of human narcolepsy (i.e., hypocretin ligand deficiency), animal models also contribute to understanding physiological and pathophysiological mechanisms involved in sleep abnormalities in human narcolepsy.[6,33,34] These researches were initiated by detailed characterizations of sleep phenotypes in narcoleptic dogs, followed by those in rodent models.

Narcoleptic Dobermans showed shortened sleep latency and reduced latency to REM sleep during multiple daytime naps according to the canine version of MSLT,[35] suggesting that these dogs have a very similar phenotype to those in human narcolepsy. A series of polygraphic studies clearly demonstrated a difference in sleep patterns between narcoleptic dogs and control dogs. Compared to age- and breed-matched dogs, narcoleptic dogs exhibit an increased frequency in sleep state changes, their sleep-wake pattern is shorter and more fragmented, and their wake-sleep bouts are much shorter than those of the control dogs (Fig. 34.3).[35-37]

Abnormal sleep patterns of prepro-orexin (preprohypocretin) gene knockout (KO) mice and hypocretin neuron-ablated (orexin/ataxin-3 transgenic) mice were also characterized, and these mice exhibit highly fragmented vigilance states, occasional direct transition to REM sleep from wakefulness, and behavioral arrest similar to cataplexy.[33,34]

It appears that sleep-wake fragmentation is therefore the primary symptom of narcolepsy across different species. In other words, narcoleptic subjects could not maintain long bouts of both wakefulness and sleep, which also explains why most narcoleptic humans are insomniac at night while they have EDS during the daytime (see Nishino and Mignot[6]).

Interestingly, however, animal studies demonstrated that REM sleep in narcoleptic subjects is not fragmented and the mean bout length of REM sleep is the same or slightly longer that

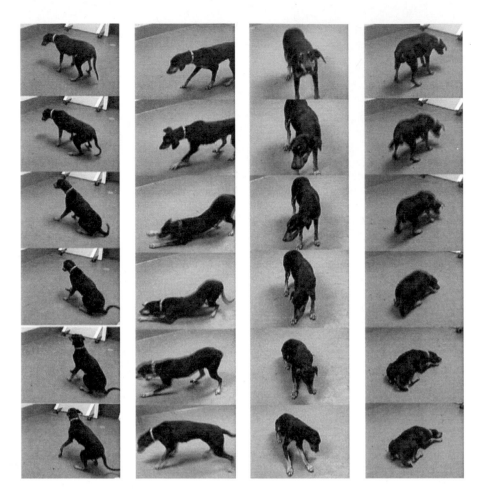

FIGURE 34.2   Cataplectic attacks in Doberman pinschers. Emotional excitations, appetizing food, or playing readily elicits multiple cataplectic attacks in these animals, mostly bilateral (97.9%). Atonia initiated partially in the hind legs (79.8%), front legs (7.8%), neck/face (6.2%), or whole body/complete attacks (6.2%). Progression of attacks was also seen (49% of all attacks) (Fujiki et al., 2002).

those of controls (Fig. 34.3) (see also Chemelli et al.[33] and Hara et al.[34]), suggesting that REM sleep maintenance is not affected in a similar way to the wake and slow-wave sleep (SWS) maintenance.

PATHOPHYSIOLOGICAL CONSIDERATIONS OF SLEEP ABNORMALITIES IN NARCOLEPSY

Several authors have proposed the pathophysiological aspect of sleep abnormalities and sleep-related symptoms in hypocretin-deficient narcoleptics. These include (1) unstable sleep-wake circuits, (2) abnormal timing of circadian distribution of sleep and wakefulness, (3) insufficient

non–rapid eye movement sleep (non-REM sleep) intensity, and (4) enhanced strength of the REM oscillator. The former two theories are from the results of animal studies, while the latter two theories are from human studies, and these concepts are introduced and discussed.

Unstable Sleep-Wake Switch

No apparent abnormalities have been found in sleep homeostasis and the suprachiasmatic nucleus (SCN) function in human narcoleptics (i.e., they show compensatory responses to sleep loss and show normal entrainment to light-dark cycles).[32,38–40] Thus, loss of hypocretin signaling itself may directly contribute to the instability of vigilance states independent

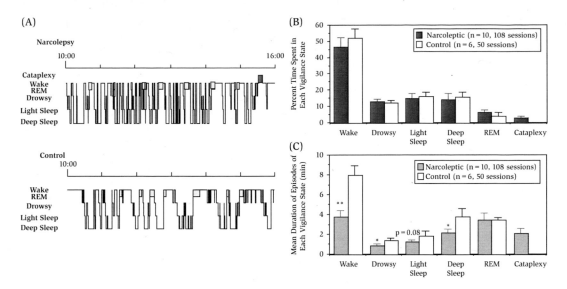

FIGURE 34.3   (*A*) Typical hyponograms from a narcoleptic and a control Doberman. (*B* and *C*) Percent of time spent in, mean frequency of, and mean duration for each vigilance state of narcoleptic and control Dobermans during daytime 6-hour recordings (10:00 to 16:00). No significant difference was found in the percentage of time spent in each vigilance state between narcoleptic and control dogs. However, the mean duration of waking, drowsy, and deep-sleep episodes was significantly shorter in the narcoleptics, suggesting a fragmentation of the vigilance states (wake and sleep) in these animals. To compensate for the influence of cataplectic episodes on wake and drowsiness, those episodes interrupted by the occurrence of cataplexy were excluded. (*See* color insert.)

from the circadian and homeostasis regulatory mechanisms of sleep. In this regard, hypocretin may stabilize the sleep-wake switch, and loss of hypocretin signaling may induce abnormally unstable sleep-wake transitions.[41]

The hypocretin neurons are mainly active during wakefulness and especially during motor activity when animals actively explore their environment.[42-44] They have ascending projections to the cerebral cortex, as well as descending projections to all the monoaminergic and cholinergic cell groups of the arousal systems.[45] There are mutual projections between the ventrolateral preoptic (VLPO) sleep active neurons and the hypocretin neurons, directly or indirectly.[46-48] The sleep-producing neurons of the VLPO receive substantial aminergic inputs[49] and are inhibited by norephinephrine, acetylcholine, and serotonin.[46] During wakefulness, high monoaminergic activity likely inhibits the VLPO, thus reducing inhibition of the arousal regions, which further enhances their activity. Conversely, during sleep, VLPO neurons are active and inhibit the arousal regions, thus disinhibiting and reinforcing their own firing. This mutual inhibitory relationship may create a bistable feedback loop that avoids intermediate

states and inappropriate transitions between states when input signals to the VLPO or the arousal regions transiently fluctuate. This asymmetric relationship could help stabilize the flip-flop switch (circuits familiar to electrical engineers) like a "finger" on the switch that might prevent unwanted transitions into sleep. The increase in the homeostatic sleep drive due to consolidated wakefulness might, in turn, help produce consolidated sleep. When animals switch between behavioral states, they spend little time in intermediate states. This is adaptive for survival since an animal performing daily tasks in a state of muddled drowsiness, neither fully awake nor asleep, would be in danger from predators and would be unable to carry out essential tasks. Narcoleptic people and animals lacking the hypocretin inputs may behave as if their sleep flip-flop switch has been destabilized.[50] They do not sleep more than normal individuals but easily doze off during the day and wake more often from sleep at night,[51] as the flip-flop model would also predict.

Although this hypothesis by Saper et al. explains well the mechanisms of the sleep fragmentation in narcoleptic animals whose sleep-wake is not consolidated, it is uncertain whether this mechanism can also explain the sleep abnormalities in human narcolepsy, since normal subjects can stay awake over 16 hours without naps.

Hypocretin injection promotes wakefulness,[52,53] and hypocretin levels stay high during forced wakefulness in experimental animals.[54] Hypocretin levels in the cerebrospinal fluid are also correlated with locomotor activity in normal and the SCN lesioned animals.[55] The hypocretin system may thus generate a positive feedback loop for maintaining active wakefulness, and thus a lack of this system may also contribute to the difficulties of maintaining the wakefulness during active period in narcoleptic subjects. Of note, it is recently reported that the hypocretin system has a positive feedforward system through hypocretin receptor 2, and this system may be important for maintaining prolonged active wakefulness.[56]

Loss of Circadian Wake Signal

The circadian process sets the time for sleep and wakefulness to occur and helps to consolidate wakefulness during the active period and sleep during the rest period.[57,58] It achieves this by opposing or compensating the homeostatic process; toward the end of the active period, despite a strong drive to initiate sleep (i.e., high levels of "S"), wakefulness can remain consolidated through an "alerting" circadian signal that reaches peak levels at this time of the day.[58] This circadian signal originates from the SCN, since consolidated episodes of sleep and wakefulness were absent in SCN lesioned animals.[57] Thus, both circadian and homeostatic processes likely contribute to the ability to maintain wakefulness throughout the active period (and sleep throughout the rest period).

As stated earlier, the hypocretin system is at least partially activated by a circadian-independent reactive homeostatic mechanism. In addition, it is likely that the hypocretin system is also regulated by the circadian pacemaker. Hypocretin levels in the brain extracellular fluids and in the cerebrospinal fluid (CSF) increase during the active period, with highest levels at the end of the active period, declining with the onset of sleep.[59] Fluctuation of hypocretin levels in the CSF disappeared in the SCN lesioned rats, while a weak (but significant) fluctuation in activity and temperature was still observed in these rats, suggesting that a daily oscillation of hypocretin tonus is also controlled by a circadian clock.[55]

Unstable sleep-wake behavior is the hallmark of narcolepsy, but narcoleptic subjects also have disturbed circadian timing of sleep and wakefulness.[40,60] In normal individuals, wakefulness is strongly promoted through much of the day, and REM sleep occurs mainly between 2 and 8 am.[61] Narcoleptic subjects have difficulty maintaining wakefulness, and their naps often include bouts of REM sleep, regardless of the time of day.[40,62] As stated before, this marked attenuation of the normal sleep-wake rhythm in narcolepsy is not caused by an underlying defect in the generation of circadian rhythms because the rhythms of body temperature, cortisol, and melatonin under the constant dark condition are essentially normal.[63-65] Altered circadian distribution of sleep and wakefulness is also not caused by a simple disinhibition of sleep because narcoleptic subjects have normal amounts of sleep over 24 hours.[32,40,60] The hypocretin neurons may thus play a critical role in diurnal distributions of sleep and wakefulness.

Animal studies demonstrated that diurnal non-REM sleep distribution in hypocretin-deficient narcolepsy seems to be intact,[34,66] while distribution of REM sleep is impaired significantly (the animals have a large amount of REM sleep during the active phase). It thus appears that the distribution patterns of REM sleep are highly dependent on the availability of the hypocretin system and on the changes in the neuronal activities. Hypocretin deficiency may therefore result in disinhibition of REM sleep, especially during the active phase; therefore, narcoleptic subjects may have various REM sleep–related abnormalities during the daytime (such as frequent REM sleep episodes during daytime naps) as well as sleep onset and offset (if the SCN function is intact).

Insufficient Non–Rapid Eye Movement Sleep Intensity

From the results of human PSG studies, Khatami et al.[67] proposed that insufficient non-REM sleep intensity contributes to disturbed nocturnal sleep in patients with narcolepsy. The authors addressed the changes in homeostatic sleep regulation as a possible mechanism underlying nocturnal sleep fragmentation in narcolepsy. These authors reported that REM sleep cycles were longer in patients with narcolepsy than in those of the controls. Mean slow-wave activity (SWA) declined in both groups across the first three non-REM sleep episodes. The rate of decline, however, appeared to be steeper in patients with narcolepsy-cataplexy than in those of the controls. The steeper decline of SWA in narcolepsy-cataplexy compared to those of the controls was related to an impaired buildup of SWA in the second cycle. Buildup of SWA after sleep deprivation in narcolepsy was normal, suggesting that their sleep homeostasis is intact. Since the increased non-REM sleep intensity in recovery sleep postpones sleep fragmentation, these authors speculate that sleep fragmentation in narcolepsy is directly related to insufficient non-REM sleep. Sleep deprivation in narcoleptic subjects also increased SOREMP duration, and the authors also suggest an abnormal interaction between non-REM sleep and REM sleep regulatory processes in narcolepsy.[68]

Altered REM-on/REM-off Interaction

Another human study by Ferrillo et al.[69] presented a mathematical model of sleep-electroencephalographic (EEG) structure applied to the analysis of sleep patterns in narcoleptics by combining the two-process model of sleep regulation and the reciprocal interaction model of REM. The REM oscillator, characterized by two coupled differential equations (Lotka-Volterra type), has been added on the basis of the reciprocal interaction model suggested by McCarley and Hobson.[70] It consists of two coupled, nonlinear differential equations describing the dynamics of REM-on and REM-off variables, where the strength of the interactions is denoted by the coupling parameters. The mathematical model was fit to quantitative EEG data by an optimization procedure. The sleep model was fit to the SWA profile for each recording and to the averaged SWA profile for each group. The Bartlett and Kolmogorov-Smirnov tests were used to evaluate the goodness of the fit and the accuracy of model predictions. In both controls and narcoleptics, the optimization procedure produced a good fit for SWA raw data, but significant differences in the REM-on/REM-off coupling parameters between the groups were observed, suggesting an enhanced strength of the REM oscillator in narcoleptics. The authors suggested that this difference can explain the occurrence of SOREMPs and variations of REM–non-REM sleep cycle duration

in narcoleptic subjects, also reported by other authors.

PATHOPHYSIOLOGICAL CONSIDERATIONS OF CATAPLEXY

After the discoveries of SOREMs in narcolepsy,[3-6] it was thought that in narcolepsy, REM sleep can intrude in active wakefulness or at sleep onset, resulting in cataplexy, sleep paralysis, and hypnagogic hallucinations, and these three symptoms are often categorized as "dissociated manifestations of REM sleep" (see Nishino and Mignot[6]).

The similarity between cataplexy and REM sleep atonia (the presence of frequent episodes of hypnagogic hallucinations and of sleep paralysis, and the propensity for narcoleptics to go directly from wakefulness into REM sleep [i.e., SOREMs]), suggests that narcolepsy is primarily a "disease of REM sleep."[5] This hypothesis may, however, be too simplistic and does not explain the presence of sleepiness during the day and the short latency to both non-REM and REM sleep during nocturnal and nap recordings. Another complementary hypothesis is that narcolepsy results from the disruption of the control mechanisms of both sleep and wakefulness or, in other words, of the vigilance-state boundary problems.[71] According to this hypothesis, a cataplectic attack represents an intrusion of REM sleep atonia during wakefulness, while the hypnagogic hallucinations appear as dream-like imagery taking place in the waking state, especially at sleep onset in patients who frequently have SOREMs.

Another important pathophysiological consideration of cataplexy is that chronic hypocretin deficiency is likely required for the occurrence of narcolepsy. In other words, acute hypocretin deficiency is not sufficient to cause cataplexy.

EDS is the first symptom to occur in most narcolepsy cases, and hypocretin deficiency is already evident at the onset of EDS even before the onset of cataplexy (Arii et al., 2004).[72] Cataplexy most typically occurs several months after the onset of EDS.[10-14] This suggests that chronic loss of hypocretin neurotransmission may be required for the occurrence of cataplexy. In addition, we have experienced several symptomatic cases of EDS associated with multiple sclerosis and neuromyelitica optica. In some of these cases, CSF hypocretin levels became undetectably low during the course of the disease, but they never developed cataplexy (but displayed SOREMs). This contrasts with symptomatic narcolepsy-cataplexy cases associated with a dozen multiple sclerosis cases appearing in the old literature. Of note, most recent multiple sclerosis/neuromyelitica optica cases are treated with steroids at the early stage of the disease, and EDS and hypocretin levels are completely recovered in most cases.

The reason for the delays in the cataplexy onset (after that of EDS) is not known, and an additional pathologic process secondary to hypocretin deficiency may possibly be involved.

To understand mechanisms of cataplexy and REM sleep abnormalities in narcolepsy, it is essential to examine whether REM sleep generation in narcolepsy is impaired. We have first analyzed the REM sleep and cataplexy cyclicity in narcoleptic and control canines to observe whether the cyclicity at which REM sleep occurs is disturbed in narcoleptic canines.[35] Interval histograms for REM sleep episodes revealed that a clear 30-minute cyclicity exists in both narcoleptic and control animals, suggesting that the system controlling REM sleep generation is intact in narcoleptic dogs. In contrast to REM sleep, cataplexy can be elicited anytime upon emotional stimulation (i.e., no 30-minute cyclicity is observed)[35] (Fig. 34.4).

These results, together with the results of extensive human studies, show that cataplexy is tightly associated with hypocretin deficiency status (cataplexy appears now to be a unique pathological condition caused by a loss of hypocretin neurotransmission),[73] suggesting that the mechanisms for the triggering of cataplexy and REM sleep are distinct.

The fact that patients with other sleep disorders, such as sleep apnea, and even healthy controls can manifest SOREMs, hypnagogic hallucinations, and sleep paralysis when their sleep-wake patterns are sufficiently disturbed, yet these subjects never develop cataplexy, provides further support to the proposal that cataplexy may be unrelated to other REM-associated symptoms.[74-77]

However, previous electrophysiological data have also demonstrated various similarities between REM sleep atonia and cataplexy.[26] Since H-reflex activity (one of the monosynaptic spinal electrically induced reflexes) profoundly diminishes or disappears during both REM sleep and cataplexy, it is likely that the motor inhibitory components of REM sleep are also responsible for the atonia during cataplexy.[26]

Thus, the executive systems for the induction of muscle atonia during cataplexy and REM sleep are likely to be the same. This interpretation is also supported by the pharmacological findings that most compounds that significantly reduce or enhance REM sleep reduce and enhance cataplexy, respectively. However, some exceptions, such as discrepant effects of dopamine D2/D3 antagonists on REM sleep and cataplexy, also exist.[78] Similarly, the mechanisms of emotional induction of cataplexy are completely unknown, and this should be elucidated.

PATHOPHYSIOLOGICAL CONSIDERATIONS OF SLEEP PARALYSIS

Whereas EDS and cataplexy are cardinal symptoms of narcolepsy, sleep paralysis occurs frequently as an isolated phenomenon (i.e., isolated sleep paralysis, affecting 5%–40% of the general population.[74,79,80] Occasional episodes of sleep paralysis are often seen in adolescence and after sleep deprivation; thus, prevalence for single episodes is high. Sleep paralysis is often seen in a familial context [80-82] and may be more frequent in some ethnic groups,[18] especially with African ancestry.[82]

If the episodes occur recurrently in the absence of a diagnosis of narcolepsy, the diagnosis of recurrent isolated sleep paralysis (RISP) can be made.[2] According to the *International Classifications of Sleep Disorders*,[2] the criteria for the RISP are as follows: (1) the patient complains of an inability to move the trunk and all limbs at sleep onset or on waking from sleep; (2) each episode lasts seconds to a few minutes; and (c) the sleep disturbance is not better explained by another sleep disorder (particularly narcolepsy), a medical or neurological disorder, mental disorder, medication use, or substance use disorder.

In sleep paralysis in narcolepsy, Hishikawa et al. [18,30] have used polygraphic recordings to show that sleep paralysis occurs only at the SOREMP. Takeuchi and Fukuda had intensively studied occurrence of sleep paralysis in normal subjects with the sleep interruption technique at night.[83,84] These authors reported that their sleep interruption method elicited SOREMP on about 30% of the interrupted nights in normal subjects.[85] The authors succeeded to elicit isolated sleep paralysis with their modified multiphasic sleep-wake schedule and found that isolated sleep paralysis was caused specifically by SOREMPs,[86] and early-onset REM sleep after

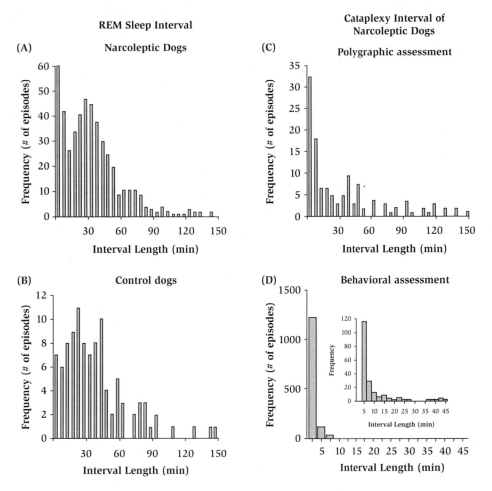

FIGURE 34.4 Frequency of interval lengths between consecutive REM sleep episodes in narcoleptic and control dogs and cataplexy interval lengths in narcoleptic canines. (A) REM sleep intervals are shown in 5-minute bins, while cataplexy intervals are shown in 2.5-minute bins. (B) A clear 30-minute interval between consecutive REM sleep episodes is present in both narcoleptic and control animals. (C) No such cyclicity is present for spontaneous cataplectic attacks that occurred during daytime 6-hour sleep recordings. (D) Cyclicity of emotionally stimulated cataplectic attacks was also evaluated during a separate behavioral assay session, the Play Elicited Cataplexy Test. Two dogs were brought into a procedure room (3 x 6 m), and dogs were allowed to play freely with each other and with toys provided. These interactions resulted in multiple cataplectic attacks. The occurrence of cataplexy was continuously monitored for 2 hours. More than 90% of cataplectic attacks occurred within short intervals of each other (f5 minutes), suggesting that cataplexy can be elicited anytime with emotional excitation. The frequencies that occurred at intervals of more than 5 minutes are magnified and replotted inside the frame; no 30-minute cyclicity was observed. (Adapted from Nishino et al.[35])

forced awakenings has been shown to predispose an individual to having sleep paralysis. It may be that subjects with less tolerance to sleep disruption are more likely to experience the phenomenon.

Of note, SOREMPs are required for occurrence sleep paralysis. SOREMSs are, however, not sufficient for sleep paralysis, since not all SOREMs cause sleep paralysis.[83,84] PSGs recorded during sleep paralysis of narcoleptic subjects showed the simultaneous appearance of indices of wakefulness and REM sleep at sleep onset, as this has also been reported in isolated sleep paralysis associated with narcolepsy.[18,87] Therefore, it was suggested that isolated sleep paralysis shares a common physiological background with narcoleptic sleep paralysis. Since isolated sleep paralysis (and hypnagogic hallucinations) is observed in normal subjects (without hypocretin deficiency), sleep paralysis is an example of state dissociation with elements of REM sleep persisting into wakefulness under frequent sleep fragmentations and REM sleep intrusions in normal and hypocretin-deficient narcoleptic subjects.

TREATMENT OF CATAPLEXY, SLEEP PARALYSIS, AND HYPNOGOGIC HALLUCINATIONS

EDS of narcolepsy has been treated with amphetamine, amphetamine-like compounds, and modafinil.[88-90] These wake-promoting compounds have little effect on cataplexy and other REM sleep abnormalities, and additional treatments are often required.

Tricyclic antidepressants potently reduce REM sleep and have been used as treatments of cataplexy and other REM sleep abnormalities, but these classes of compounds induce various sides effects (anticholinergic and antihistaminergic).[88,90] The second-generation antidepressants, selective serotonin re-uptake inhibitors, are also very commonly used as anticataplectics in humans. This is mostly due to their better side-effect profiles, but the anticataplectic effects of these compounds are rather modest. Recently, selective NE and NE/5-HT reuptake inhibitors, such as atomoxetine and venlafaxine, were introduced, and evaluations of these are in progress and may bring profound beneficial insights.

GHB, a compound with remarkable REM- and SWS-inducing properties, has also been used for consolidating nighttime sleep, an effect that leads to decreased sleepiness and cataplexy the following day.[88,91] Recent large-scale, double-blind, placebo-controlled clinical trials in the United States led to the reestablishment of sodium oxybate (sodium salt of GHB) as a first-line treatment for narcolepsy-cataplexy.[92] The mechanism of action of GHB in treating these symptoms is unknown.[90] It should be noted that the therapeutic window for the compound is narrow, and overdose may induce fatal side effects.

The treatment of sleep paralysis and hypnagogic hallucinations is much less well codified. Hypnagogic hallucinations can be quite bothersome and often occur in patients who also suffer from frequent nightmares. As they are a manifestation of sleep-onset REM sleep, the compounds that suppress REM sleep are usually helpful in alleviating this symptom, and tricyclic antidepressant treatment has been reported to have some beneficial effects.[93] Sleep paralysis only rarely requires treatment, but tricyclic antidepressants are also very effective in preventing this symptom. Recently, high doses (60 mg qd) of fluoxetine have been advocated as a very active treatment for isolated sleep paralysis.[94] GHB is also effective in suppressing both hypnagogic hallucinations and sleep paralysis.[95]

PERIODIC LIMB MOVEMENTS DURING SLEEP/RESTLESS LEGS SYNDROME IN NARCOLEPSY

Other frequently associated movement disorders associated with narcolepsy include REM behavior disorder, other parasomnias,[22,23] periodic leg movements during sleep (PLMS),[24,25] and PLMS in narcolepsy; these may require special attention, nosologically and pharmacologically. Involuntary leg movements during sleep are often associated with restless leg syndrome (RLS) and disturbed nighttime sleep. The disease is pharmacologically treated with dopaminergic agonists (i.e. D2/D3 agonists) and opiates. PLMS often occur in narcoleptic patients. Epidemiological studies demonstrated up to 50% of prevalence of PLMS in narcolepsy compared to 6% in general populations.[96,97]

Although earlier studies reported that the prevalence of RSL in narcolepsy is not increased,[22,23] a recent larger scale study pointed out increase in RLS in narcolepsy-cataplexy subjects,[98] suggesting common pathophysiological mechanisms between narcolepsy-cataplexy and RLS/PLMS.

Narcoleptic canines, like narcoleptic humans, also exhibit jerky, unilateral or bilateral slow leg movements during sleep. Interestingly, compounds that aggravate canine cataplexy, such as dopaminergic D2/D3 agonists, improve PLMS in humans and PLMS-like movements in narcoleptic dogs, which suggests that altered dopaminergic regulation in canine narcolepsy may play a critical role in both cataplexy and PLMS. Whether these animals exhibit RLS-like symptoms is not known. Hypocretin deficiency may thus primarily affect dopaminergic regulation of motor components of involuntary leg movements during sleep.

CONCLUSIONS

Narcolepsy is a chronic hypersomnia, but the disease also exhibits unique sleep-associated movement impairments, such as cataplexy and sleep paralysis. The major pathophysiology of human narcolepsy (i.e., postnatal loss of hypocretin/orexin neurons) has been recently elucidated based on the discovery of narcolepsy genes in animals. It is now conceived that impairments of hypocretin system result in EDS, cataplexy, and other REM sleep abnormalities, but precise mechanisms involved are still largely unknown.

Although REM sleep abnormalities were initially emphasized as the major characteristics of narcolepsy, these abnormalities cannot be discussed separately from other sleep abnormalities, namely EDS and sleep-wake fragmentation.

Since the hypoceretin system is likely involved in both sleep homeostasis and circadian control of occurrences of sleep and wake, complex mechanisms are likely involved for pathological manipulations of sleep and its related phenomena.

Even more complexly, cataplexy is likely to be distinct from other dissociated manifestations of REM sleep (i.e., sleep paralysis and hypnagogic hallucinations). The observation that prepubertal narcolepsy-cataplexy cases are almost always hypocretin deficient suggests that hypocretin deficiency occurs at the onset of cataplexy. Studies in symptomatic cases of EDS, however, suggest that acute hypocretin deficiency induces EDS, but not cataplexy. Chronic and selective loss of the hypocretin ligands may be required to exhibit cataplexy. The consequence of the chronic and selective loss of the hypocretin ligand (vs. acute loss of hypocretin neurotransmission) involved in the induction of cataplexy is not known. The mechanisms of emotional induction of cataplexy remain to be studied.

The occurrences of sleep paralysis also require some discussion. It is not known whether hypocretin deficiency is directly involved in the occurrences of sleep paralysis (and hypnagogic hallucinations). Isolated sleep paralysis occurs in nonnarcoleptic general populations, especially when their sleep-wake rhythms are disturbed, sharing a common physiological background with narcoleptic sleep paralysis. This suggests that sleep fragmentation, due to hypocretin deficiency, contributes to the occurrences of sleep paralysis in narcolepsy. SOREMPs are necessary for the occurrences of sleep paralysis, but are not sufficient, and it is proposed that sleep paralysis is a state dissociation with elements of REM sleep persisting to wakefulness under frequent sleep fragmentations and REM sleep intrusions. This may explain why hypocretin-deficient narcoleptic subjects frequently exhibit sleep paralysis.

Narcoleptic subjects are reported to often exhibit RLS/PLMS, another frequent movement disorder associated with sleep. Thus, common pathophysiological mechanisms between narcolepsy-cataplexy and RLS/PLMS may exist. Altered dopaminergic systems are reported in human and canine narcolepsy and, thus, hypocretin deficiency may affect the dopaminergic system and predispose RLS/PLMS.

REFERENCES

1. Gélineau JBE. De la narcolepsie. *Gazette des hôpitaux* 1880;53:626–8.
2. American Academy of Sleep Medicine. *International Classification of Sleep Disorders. Diagnostic and Coding Manual.* 2nd ed.Westchester, IL: American Academy of Sleep Medicine; 2005.
3. Vogel G. Studies in psychophysiology of dreams III. The dream of narcolepsy. *Arch Gen Psychiatry* 1960;3:421–8.
4. Takahashi Y, Jimbo M. Polygraphic study of narcoleptic syndrome, with special reference to hypnagogic hallucinations and cataplexy. *Folia Psychiatr Neurol Jpn Suppl* 1963;7:343–7.
5. Dement W, Rechtschaffen A, Gulevich G. The nature of the narcoleptic sleep attack. *Neurology* 1966;16:18–33.
6. Nishino S, Mignot E. Pharmacological aspects of human and canine narcolepsy. *Prog Neurobiol* 1997;52:27–78.
7. Nishino S, Ripley B, Overeem S, et al. Hypocretin (orexin) deficiency in human narcolepsy. *Lancet* 2000;355:39–40.
8. Peyron C, Faraco J, Rogers W, et al. A mutation in a case of early onset narcolepsy and a generalized absence of hypocretin peptides in human narcoleptic brains. *Nat Med* 2000;6:991–7.
9. Nishino S, Ripley B, Overeem S, et al. Low CSF hypocretin (orexin) and altered energy homeostasis in human narcolepsy. *Ann Neurol* 2001;50:381–8.

10. Yoss RE, Daly DD. Criteria for the diagnosis of the narcoleptic syndrome. *Proc Staff Meet Mayo* 1957;32:320–8.

11. Parkes JD, Baraitser M, Marsden CD, Asselman P. Natural history, symptoms and treatment of the narcoleptic syndrome. *Acta Neurol Scand* 1975;52:337–53.

12. Roth B. *Narcolepsy and Hypersomnia.* Basel, Switzerland: Karger; 1980.

13. Billiard M, Besset A, Cadilhac J. The clinical and polygraphic development of narcolepsy. In: Guilleminault C, Lugaresi E, eds *Sleep/Wake Disorders: Natural History, Epidemiology and Longterm Evolution.* New York: Raven Press; 1983:171–85.

14. Honda Y. Clinical features of narcolepsy. In: Honda Y, Juji T, eds *HLA in Narcolepsy.* Berlin: Springer-Verlag; 1988:24–57.

15. Guilleminault C, Wilson RA, Dement WC. A study on cataplexy. *Arch Neurol* 1974;31:255–61.

16. Yoss RE, Daly DD. Narcolepsy. *Med Clin North Am* 1960;44:953–67.

17. Parkes JD, Fenton G, Struthers G, et al. Narcolepsy and cataplexy. Clinical features, treatment and cerebrospinal fluid findings. *Q J Med* 1974;172:525–36.

18. Hishikawa Y. Sleep paralysis. In: Guilleminault C, Dement WC, Passouant P, eds. *Narcolepsy.* New York: Spectrum; 1976:97–124.

19. Rosenthal C. Uber das aufreten von halluzinatorisch-kataplektischem angstsyndrom, wachanfallen und ahnlichen storungen bei schizophrenen. *Mschr Psychiat* 1939;102:11.

20. Ribstein M. Hypnagogic hallucinations. In: Guilleminault C, et al., eds. *Narcolepsy.* New York: Spectrum; 1976:145–60.

21. Chetrit M, Besset A, Damci D, Lelarge C, Billiard M. Hypnogogic hallucinations associated with sleep onset REM period in narcolepsy-cataplexy. *J Sleep Res* 1994;3:43

22. Schenck CH, Mahowald MW. Motor dyscontrol in narcolepsy: rapid-eye-movement (REM) sleep without atonia and REM sleep behavior disorder. *Annals of Neurology* 1992;32:3–10.

23. Mayer G, Pollmächer T, Meier-Ewert K, et al. Zur Einschätzung des Behinderungsgrades bei Narkolepsie. *Gesundh-Wes* 1993;55:337–42.

24. Mosko SS, Shampain DS, Sassin JF, et al. Nocturnal REM latency and sleep disturbance in narcolepsy. *Sleep* 1984;7:115–25.

25. Godbout R, Montplaisir J. Comparison of sleep parameters in narcoleptics with and without periodic movements of sleep. In: Koella WP, et al., eds. *Sleep 1984* Gustav: Fischer Verlag; 1985:380–2.

26. Guilleminault C. Cataplexy. Narcolepsy. *Adv Sleep Res* 1976;3:125–43.

27. Chokroverty S. Sleep apnea in narcolepsy. *Sleep* 1986;9:250–3.

28. Carskadon MA, Dement WC. Daytime sleepiness: quantification of a behavioral state. *Neurosci Biobehav Rev* 1987;11:307–17.

29. Moscovitch A, Partinen M, Guilleminault C. The positive diagnosis of narcolepsy and narcolepsy's borderland. *Neurology* 1993;43:55–60.

30. Hishikawa Y, Wakamatsu H, Furuya E, et al. Sleep satiation in narcoleptic patients. *Electroencephalogr Clin Neurophysiol* 1976;41:1–18.

31. Montplaisir J, Billard M, Takahashi S, et al. Twenty-four-hour recording in REM-narcoleptics with special reference to nocturnal sleep disruption. *Biol Psych* 1978;13:78–89.

32. Broughton R, Dunham W, Newman J, et al. Ambulatory 24 hour sleep-wake monitoring in narcolepsy-cataplexy compared to matched control. *Electroenceph Clin Neurophysiol* 1988;70:473–81.

33. Chemelli RM, Willie JT, Sinton CM, et al. Narcolepsy in orexin knockout mice: molecular genetics of sleep regulation. *Cell* 1999;98:437–51.

34. Hara J, Beuckmann CT, Nambu T, et al. Genetic ablation of orexin neurons in mice results in narcolepsy, hypophagia, and obesity. *Neuron* 2001;30:345–54.

35. Nishino S, Riehl J, Hong J, et al. Is narcolepsy REM sleep disorder? Analysis of sleep abnormalities in narcoleptic Dobermans. *Neurosci Res* 2000;38:437–46.

36. Kaitin KI, Kilduff TS, Dement WC. Evidence for excessive sleepiness in canine narcoleptics. *Electroencephalogr Clin Neurophysiol* 1986;64:447–54.

37. Kaitin KI, Kilduff TS, Dement WC. Sleep fragmentation in genetically narcoleptic dogs. *Sleep* 1986;9:116–19.

38. Tafti M, Rondouin G, Basset A, et al. Sleep deprevation in narcoleptic subjects: effect on sleep stages and EEG power density. *Electroencephalogr Clin Neurophysiol* 1992;83:339–49.

39. Tafti M, Villemin E, Carlander B, et al. Sleep onset rapid-eye-movement episodes in narcolepsy: REM sleep pressure or nonrem-rem sleep dysregulation? *J Sleep Res* 1992;1:245–50.

40. Dantz B, Edgar DM, Dement WC. Circadian rhythms in narcolepsy: studies on a 90 minute day. *Electroceph Clin Neurophy* 1994;90:24–35.

41. Saper CB, Chou TC, Scammell TE. The sleep switch: hypothalamic control of sleep and wakefulness. *Trends Neurosci* 2001;24:726–31.

42. Estabrooke IV, McCarthy MT, Ko E, et al. Fos expression in orexin neurons varies with behavioral state. *J Neurosci* 2001;21:1656–62.

43. Lee MG, Hassani OK, Jones BE. Discharge of identified orexin/hypocretin neurons across the sleep-waking cycle. *J Neurosci* 2005;25:6716–20.

44. Mileykovskiy BY, Kiyashchenko LI, Siegel JM. Behavioral correlates of activity in identified hypocretin/orexin neurons. *Neuron* 2005;46:787–98.

45. Peyron C, Tighe DK, van den Pol AN, et al. Neurons containing hypocretin (orexin) project to multiple neuronal systems. *J Neurosci* 1998;18:9996–10015.

46. Gallopin T, Fort P, Eggermann E, et al. Identification of sleep-promoting neurons in vitro. *Nature* 2000;404:992–5.

47. Sakurai T, Nagata R, Yamanaka A, et al. Input of orexin/hypocretin neurons revealed by a genetically encoded tracer in mice. *Neuron* 2005;46:297–308.

48. Yoshida K, McCormack S, Espana RA, et al. Afferents to the orexin neurons of the rat brain. *J Comp Neurol* 2006;494:845–61.

49. Chou TC, Bjorkum AA, Gaus SE, et al. Afferents to the ventrolateral preoptic nucleus. *J Neurosci* 2002;22:977–90.

50. Mochizuki T, Crocker A, McCormack S, et al. Behavioral state instability in orexin knock-out mice. *J Neurosci* 2004;24:6291–300.

51. Scammell TE. The neurobiology, diagnosis, and treatment of narcolepsy. *Ann Neurol* 2003;53:154–66.

52. Hagan JJ, Leslie RA, Patel S, et al. Orexin A activates locus coeruleus cell firing and increases arousal in the rat. *Proc Natl Acad Sci USA* 1999;96:10911–16.

53. Haynes AC, Jackson B, Overend P, et al. Effects of single and chronic intracerebroventricular administration of the orexins on feeding in the rat. *Peptides* 1999;20:1099–105.

54. Fujiki N, Yoshida Y, Ripley B, et al. Changes in CSF hypocretin-1 (orexin A) levels in rats across 24 hours and in response to food deprivation. *NeuroReport* 2001;12:993–7.

55. Zhang S, Zeitzer JM, Yoshida Y, et al. Lesions of the suprachiasmatic nucleus eliminate the daily rhythm of hypocretin-1 release. *Sleep* 2004;27:619–27.

56. Yamanaka A, Tabuchi S, Tsunematsu T, et al. Orexin directly excites orexin neurons through orexin 2 receptor. *J Neurosci* 2010;30:12642–52.

57. Edgar DM, Dement WC, Fuller CA. Effect of SCN-lesions on sleep in squirrel monkeys: evidence for opponent processes in sleep-wake regulation. *J Neureosci* 1993;13:1065–79.

58. Dijk DJ, Czeisler CA. Paradoxical timing of the circadian rhythm of sleep propensity serves to consolidate sleep and wakefulness in humans. *Neurosci Lett* 1994;166:63–8.

59. Yoshida Y, Fujiki N, Nakajima T, et al. Fluctuation of extracellular hypocretin-1 (orexin A) levels in the rat in relation to the light-dark cycle and sleep-wake activities. *Eur J Neurosci* 2001;14:1075–81.

60. Broughton R, Krupa S, Boucher B, et al. Impaired circadian waking arousal in narcolepsy-cataplexy. *Sleep Research Online* 1998;1:159–65.

61. Dijk DJ, Czeisler CA. Contribution of the circadian pacemaker and the sleep homeostat to sleep propensity, sleep structure, electroencephalographic slow waves, and sleep spindle activity in humans. *J Neurosci* 1995;15:3526–38.

62. Lavie P. REM periodicity under ultrashort sleep/wake cycle in narcoleptic patients. *Can J Psychol* 1991;45:185–93.

63. Weitzman E. Twenty-four hour neuroendocrine secretory patterns: observations on patients with narcolepsy. In: Guilleminault C, et al., eds. *Narcolepsy. Advances in Sleep Research.* Vol 3. New York: Spectrum Publications; 1976:521–42.

64. Bourgine N, Claustrat B, Besset A, et al. Melatonin plasma concentrations during day-time and night-time in narcoleptic subjects and controls. *Sleep Res* 1986;15:46.

65. Mayer G, Hellmann F, Leonhard E, et al. Circadian temperature and activity rhythms in unmedicated narcoleptic patients. *Pharmacol Biochem Behav* 1997;58:395–402.

66. Beuckmann CT, Sinton CM, Williams SC, et al. Expression of a poly-glutamine-ataxin-3 transgene in orexin neurons induces

narcolepsy-cataplexy in the rat. *J Neurosci* 2004;24:4469–77.

67. Khatami R, Landolt HP, Achermann P, et al. Insufficient non-REM sleep intensity in narcolepsy-cataplexy. *Sleep* 2007;30:980–9.

68. Khatami R, Landolt HP, Achermann P, et al. Challenging sleep homeostasis in narcolepsy-cataplexy: implications for non-REM and REM sleep regulation. *Sleep* 2008;31:859–67.

69. Ferrillo F, Donadio S, De Carli F, et al. A model-based approach to homeostatic and ultradian aspects of nocturnal sleep structure in narcolepsy. *Sleep* 2007;30:157–65.

70. Hobson JA, McCarley RW, Wyzinski PW. Sleep cycle oscillation: reciprocal discharge by two brainstem neuronal groups. *Science* 1975;189:55–8.

71. Broughton R, Valley V, Aguirre M, et al. Excessive daytime sleepiness and pathophysiology of narcolepsy-cataplexy: a laboratory perspective. *Sleep* 1986;9:205–15.

72. Arii J, Kanbayashi T, Tanabe Y, et al. CSF hypocretin-1 (orexin-A) levels in childhood narcolepsy and neurologic disorders. *Neurology* 2004;63:2440–2.

73. Mignot E, Lammers GJ, Ripley B, et al. The role of cerebrospinal fluid hypocretin measurement in the diagnosis of narcolepsy and other hypersomnias. *Arch Neurol* 2002;59:1553–62.

74. Fukuda K, Miyasita A, Inugami M, et al. High prevalence of isolated sleep paralysis: Kanashibari phenomenon in Japan. *Sleep* 1987;10:279–86.

75. Bishop C, Rosenthal L, Helmus T, et al. The frequency of multiple sleep onset REM periods among subjects with no excessive daytime sleepiness. *Sleep* 1996;19:727–30.

76. Ohayon MM, Priest RG, Caulet M, et al. Hypnagogic and hypnopompic hallucinations: pathological phenomena? *Br J Psychiatry* 1996;169:459–67.

77. Aldrich MS, Chervin RD, Malow BA. Value of the multiple sleep latency test (MSLT) for the diagnosis of narcolepsy. *Sleep* 1997;20:620–9.

78. Okura M, Riehl J, Mignot E, et al. Sulpiride, a D2/D3 blocker, reduces cataplexy but not REM sleep in canine narcolepsy. *Neuropsychopharmacology* 2000;23:528–38.

79. Goode B. Sleep paralysis. *Arch Neurol* 1962;6:228–34.

80. Dahlitz M, Parkes JD. Sleep paralysis. *Lancet* 1993;341:406–7.

81. Roth B, Bruhová S, Berková L. Familial sleep paralysis. *Archiv für Neuro,Neurch und Psychiatry* 1968;102:321–30.

82. Bell C, Dixie-Bell D, Thompson B. Further studies on the prevalence of isolated sleep paraylsis in black subjects. *J Natl Med Assoc* 1986;78:649–59.

83. Takeuchi T, Miyasita A, Sasaki Y, et al. Isolated sleep paralysis elicited by sleep interruption. *Sleep* 1992;15:217–25.

84. Takeuchi T, Fukuda K, Sasaki Y, et al. Factors related to the occurrence of isolated sleep paralysis elicited during a multi-phasic sleep-wake schedule. *Sleep* 2002;25:89–96.

85. Miyasita A, Fukuda K, Inugami M. Effects of sleep interruption on REM-NREM cycle in nocturnal human sleep. *Electroencephalogr Clin Neurophysiol* 1989;73:107–16.

86. Miyasita A, Fukuda K, Inugami M, et al. Appearancerate ofsleep onset REM period and pre-awakening NREM duration. *Sleep Res Online* 1989;18:141.

87. Hishikawa Y, Koida H, Yoshino K, et al. Characteristics of REM sleep accompanied by sleep paralysis and hypnogogic hallucinations in narcoleptic patients. *Waking Sleeping* 1978;2:113–23.

88. Nishino S, Kotorii N. Overview of management of narcolepsy. In: Goswami M, et al., eds *Narcolepsy.*Totowa, NY: Humana; 2010:251–65.

89. Nishino S, Mignot E. CNS stimulants in Sleep Medicine: Basic Mechanisms and Pharmacology. In: Kryger MH, Roth T, Dement WC. eds. *Principles and Practice of Sleep Medicine.* 4th ed. Philadelphia, PA: Elsvier Saunders; 2005:468–98.

90. Nishino S. Modes of action of drugs related to narcolepsy: pharmacology of wake-promoting compounds and anticataplectics. In: Goswami M, et al., eds.*Narcolepsy.* Totowa, NY: Humana; 2010:267–86.

91. Robinson DM, Keating GM. Sodium oxybate: a review of its use in the management of narcolepsy. *CNS Drugs* 2007;21:337–54.

92. Morgenthaler TI, Kapur VK, Brown T, et al. Practice parameters for the treatment of narcolepsy and other hypersomnias of central origin. *Sleep* 2007;30:1705–11.

93. Takahashi S. The action of tricyclics (alone or in combination with methylphenidate) upon several symptoms of narcolepsy. In: Guilleminault C, Dement WC, Passouant P. eds *Narcolepsy.* New York: Spectrum; 1976:625–38.

94. Koran L, Raghavan S. Fluoxetine for isolated sleep paralysis. *Psychomatics* 1993;34:184–7.

95. Mamelak M, Scharf MB, Woods M. Treatment of narcolepsy with γ-hydroxybutyrate. A review of clinical and sleep laboratory findings. *Sleep* 1986;9:285–9.

96. Wittig R, Zorick F, Piccione P, et al. Narcolepsy and disturbed nocturnal sleep. *Clin Electroencephalogr* 1983;14:130–4.

97. Dauvilliers Y, Pennestri MH, Petit D, et al. Periodic leg movements during sleep and wakefulness in narcolepsy. *J Sleep Res* 2007;16:333–9.

98. Plazzi G, Ferri R, Antelmi E, et al. Restless legs syndrome is frequent in narcolepsy with cataplexy patients. *Sleep* 2010;33:689–94.

35

Nocturnal Seizures

LANA JERADEH BOURSOULIAN, GIUSEPPE PLAZZI,
AND BETH A. MALOW

Sleep is an essential, a health-giving restorative....Yet, darkness is also a cloak for hob-goblins and evildoers....Seizures are probably more common in sleep than in waking. Phenomena such as extreme restlessness, excessive swallowing movements, nightmares, and sleepwalking may possibly be seizures, masked and disguised by the altered physical and mental state of sleep.

—Lennox and Lennox, 1960[1]

SINCE ANTIQUITY, when Aristotle compared sleep to epilepsy,[2] the occurrence of seizures during sleep has intrigued clinicians and researchers alike. In the late 19th century, Gowers documented that 21% of epilepsy patients had seizures exclusively during sleep and 37% had a combination of diurnal and nocturnal epilepsies.[3] Gowers's contemporary Féré reported that 1285 out of 1985 seizures recorded in hospitalized epilepsy patients occurred between 8 pm and 8 am and described that a shortened duration of sleep facilitated seizures. In 1929, several decades before the discovery of non–rapid eye movement–rapid eye movement (non-REM–REM) sleep cycles, Langdon-Down and Brain[4] were impressed by the occurrence of "time peaks" for seizure activity. For example, "peak N1" was described as occurring "in the second hour after retiring to bed ... it seems probable that the peak N1 is the response of certain patients, either to the act of falling asleep or to the early stages of sleep itself." In 1962, Janz[5] reported that 45% of subjects with generalized tonic-clonic seizures (GTCSs) had seizures predominantly during sleep. Subsequent studies of subjects with either partial or generalized seizures, or both, have estimated the relative occurrence of seizures during sleep to be 7.5% to 30%.[6]

Why certain types of seizures are facilitated preferentially by sleep remains uncertain, although several theories have been proposed. The first theory is that non-REM sleep is a physiologic state of relative neuronal synchronization, in which recruitment of a critical mass of neurons needed to initiate and sustain a seizure is more likely to occur.[7] Using simultaneous recordings from thalamus, thalamocortical projection neurons, and pyramidal neurons in anesthetized cats, Steriade and McCarley[8] have characterized non-REM sleep as a state of relative hyperpolarization or synchronization within thalamocortical neurons resulting from a progressive reduction in the firing rates of brainstem (midbrain and pontine reticular) cholinergic and monoaminergic afferents. This synchronization is apparent in the electroencephalogram (EEG) of non-REM sleep, characterized by sleep spindles and high-amplitude delta waves. In contrast, REM sleep is associated with increased brainstem cholinergic input to thalamocortical neurons, producing a relative state of cortical activation. Support for this theory of state-varying synchronization comes from the penicillin model of generalized epilepsy, in which spindle oscillations are transformed into bilaterally synchronous spike-wave complexes.[9] Steriade and Contreras[10] have shown that similar thalamic and cortical physiologic events underlie the generation of sleep spindles and spike-wave discharges. Further support for the facilitating role of non-REM sleep in activation of epileptic cortex comes from the study of interictal epileptiform discharges, which become more prevalent in non-REM sleep and, at least in temporal lobe epilepsy (TLE), predominate during delta (stages III and IV) non-REM sleep.[11,12]

Arousal mechanisms may also be important in facilitating sleep-related seizures. Shouse and Martins da Silva[13] have proposed that sudden synchronous excitatory input from waking-active neurons in the posterior hypothalamus (e.g., histaminergic), which project to the neocortical mantle, may facilitate seizures via exacerbation of cortical hyperexcitability. The strongest clinical examples supporting this theory come from syndromes in which seizures occur shortly after awakening (e.g., juvenile myoclonic epilepsy [JME] and GTCSs on awakening). Finally, anatomic substrate is certain to be an important factor. Several of the sleep-related epilepsy syndromes discussed in this chapter involve seizures of frontal lobe origin.[14] Crespel, Baldy-Moulinier, and Coubes[15] compared patients with frontal lobe and mesial TLE and found significant differences between the two groups in the occurrence of seizures. In frontal lobe epilepsy patients, most seizures occurred during sleep, whereas in TLE patients, most seizures occurred while the patients were awake.

Herman et al.[16] analyzed 613 seizures in 133 patients with complex partial seizures; they found that 43% of all partial seizures began during sleep. Most seizures began in stages N1 and N2. No seizures occurred during REM sleep. Frontal seizures were more likely to occur during sleep; however, temporal lobe seizures were more likely to generalize secondarily during sleep.

These findings suggest that changes in neuronal excitability associated with sleep are different in frontal and temporal structures. The frontal lobe receives ascending input from the thalamus and has rich interconnections,[17] which may explain its propensity to the facilitation of seizures during sleep.

EPILEPSY SYNDROMES ASSOCIATED WITH SLEEP

The proportion of patients who have seizures that occur either exclusively or predominantly during sleep has been estimated between 7.5% and 45%.[6] This wide prevalence range most likely reflects the heterogeneity of nocturnal seizures. The International League Against Epilepsy (ILAE) classification of epileptic seizures defines a variety of epileptic syndromes primarily on the basis of clinical characteristics, epidemiology, and EEG and neuroimaging studies.[18] The description of sleep-related epilepsy syndromes discussed later follows the ILAE classification. Features distinguishing each sleep-related epilepsy syndrome from other nocturnal movements and behaviors are highlighted.

A major distinguishing feature in the ILAE classification is whether seizures originate in a group of neurons within one hemisphere (focal, partial, or localization-related) or within neurons throughout both hemispheres (generalized). For several reasons, it is not always possible to classify seizures that occur during sleep. First, the patient may sleep alone and be unwitnessed, or the bed partner may not be fully awake and coherent during the seizure to give an adequate description. Second, the patient may not experience or remember an aura, the first sign of a seizure before loss of consciousness occurs. Third, the interictal EEG and brain magnetic resonance imaging (MRI) may be normal. When seizures cannot be defined as partial or generalized, they are classified as "epilepsies and syndromes undetermined as to whether focal or generalized." This category includes epilepsy with continuous spike-waves during slow-wave sleep (CSWS) and acquired epileptic aphasia (Landau-Kleffner syndrome).

Within these categories of focal, generalized, and undetermined, epileptic syndromes are classified as symptomatic, cryptogenic, or idiopathic. Symptomatic epilepsies are the consequence of a known or suspected disorder of the nervous system, with cryptogenic epilepsies presumed to be symptomatic but of unknown etiology. Idiopathic syndromes imply that there is no underlying cause other than a possible hereditary predisposition and are defined by age-related onset, clinical and EEG characteristics, and a presumed genetic etiology.[18]

GENERALIZED EPILEPSIES: IDIOPATHIC

Juvenile Myoclonic Epilepsy

JME is one of the most common forms of idiopathic generalized epilepsy, consisting of a triad of three seizure types: myoclonic jerks, GTCSs, and absence seizures.[19] Myoclonic jerks occur predominantly after awakening. GTCSs often occur after awakening but may also occur during sleep or randomly during the day. Absence seizures are present in 10% to 33% of JME patients. The typical presentation is of GTCSs; the patient may not acknowledge that myoclonic jerks are present unless specifically asked. However, jerks or absence seizures may precede GTCSs or predominate throughout a patient's life span with only rare GTCSs.

Sleep deprivation is a common and important precipitant of the seizures. Photosensitivity is present in one third of patients.[20]

Until recently, valproate was considered the usual first-line treatment in both men and women. However, frequent adverse effects, such as weight gain and the risk of teratogenicity, have resulted in decrease in its use in women. Other antiepileptic drugs (AEDs) used to treat this syndrome include lamotrigine, topiramate, levetiracetam, and zonisamide. These drugs have been used as monotherapy or adjunctive therapy in small patient series with JME. Those new AEDs, however, may not be effective for all the seizure types of JME, and clinical correlation is usually recommended.[21] Therapy is usually lifelong.

The mean age of onset of JME is 14 years, with most presenting between 12 and 18 years of age. The percentage of JME patients with a family history of epilepsy has been estimated at between 17% and 49%.[22] A gene locus linked to the human leukocyte antigen (HLA) region on the short arm of chromosome 6 has been identified.[23] However, this disorder appears to be genetically heterogeneous in that not all syndromes resembling JME have been localized genetically to chromosome 6.[24]

The epileptic myoclonic jerks of JME may mimic nonepileptic myoclonus seen in other neurologic disorders, including movement disorders. These bilateral irregular arrhythmic jerks, usually of the shoulders and arms, may be manifested dramatically by throwing objects out of the hands. Differentiating features include that the jerks of JME always affect limbs rather than isolated muscles, with videotape analysis showing either distal or proximal muscles predominating.[26] The jerks of JME are most prominent in the early morning and are often accompanied by a history of GTCSs and possibly absence seizures. In addition, an EEG demonstrates polyspike-wave discharges, with photoparoxysmal responses common. These EEG discharges may be seen either during myoclonic jerks or in the interictal (between seizure) state.

GENERALIZED TONIC-CLONIC SEIZURES ON AWAKENING

Another idiopathic generalized epilepsy syndrome associated with the sleep-wake cycle is GTCSs on awakening (or epilepsy with grand mal on awakening [EGMA]).[26] Similar to JME, this syndrome typically begins in the second decade of life, may consist of absence and myoclonic seizures in addition to GTCSs, has a genetic component, and has an EEG pattern seen in idiopathic generalized epilepsy, including a photoparoxysmal response. As with JME, the seizures respond well to treatment, but lifelong therapy is often necessary. A wide prevalence range is reported (10% to 53%), which varies depending on the number of GTCSs required for diagnosis, the presence of other seizure types, and the time of occurrence of GTCSs. Janz's prevalence of 10% included only patients with GTCSs on awakening (e.g., no other seizure types, GTCSs were exclusively on awakening, and subjects had at least six GTCSs).

When myoclonus is a prominent feature of this disorder, GTCSs on awakening may be confused with a movement disorder. However, as with JME, the characteristic EEG patterns and presence of GTCSs should allow differentiation from a movement disorder without difficulty.

The syndromes of GTCSs on awakening and JME show overlap, especially in seizure type and age of onset. In fact, JME may appear with GTCSs on awakening but, in this case, rhythmic myoclonic jerks often precede the tonic-clonic seizures. In general, a useful distinguishing feature is that relatively frequent myoclonic jerks and infrequent GTCSs characterize JME.

Patients with "pure" GTCSs on awakening have had at least six GTCSs.[26]

Although several gene mutations were found to be associated with the some familiar types of idiopathic generalized epilepsies, only mutations of the *EFHC* gene are associated with classical JME.[27] Mutations of the *CLCN2* gene were found to be associated with JME, the generalized tonic clonic seizures on awakening (EGMA), and other generalized epilepsy syndromes.[26]

Some observational studies propose that these syndromes may represent a biological continuum.[29] However, additional data will be needed to further explore the overlap between these various epileptic syndromes.

GENERALIZED EPILEPSIES: SYMPTOMATIC AND CRYPTOGENIC

Lennox-Gastaut Syndrome

This symptomatic generalized epilepsy has been defined by (1) mixed type of epileptic seizures, with mainly atypical absence, which is a more prolonged absence seizure and is usually associated with generalized spike and wave discharges at less than 3 Hz on EEG, axial tonic, and atonic seizures; (2) a static encephalopathy; and (3) a characteristic EEG pattern.[30] Tonic seizures are more common during sleep. They are characterized by neck and body flexion, with raising of the arms in either a semiflexed or extended position and leg extension. It typically lasts for 30 seconds or less, and there is no postictal confusion.

Electrographically, tonic seizures consist of either a flattening or a bilateral discharge of rapid rhythms (10 to 12 Hz), occasionally preceded by a generalized burst of slow spike-waves.

When they occur during sleep, they may resemble other types of seizures, including those of frontal lobe origin or psychogenic spells. These tonic seizures can be diagnosed by the characteristic ictal pattern described previously.

Between seizures, the EEG shows a distinctive EEG pattern, which is a slow background and multifocal or diffuse slow spike-wave discharges with frequency of 2.5 Hz per second. During sleep, bursts of 10 Hz activity may occur with or without tonic seizures. Other epilepsy types seen in Lennox-Gastaut syndrome (LGS) include myoclonic, partial, and GTCS. In LGS, seizures are frequent and are typically refractory to medications. There are two forms, a symptomatic form and a cryptogenic form. The symptomatic form is associated with a variety of etiologies, including cerebral malformations and antenatal, perinatal, or postnatal ischemia or infections. The cryptogenic form has no known etiology. The onset of LGS is usually before age 8, with a peak between 3 and 5 years. Medications used to treat this syndrome include lamotrigine, valproate, and topiramate. Carbamazepine and oxcarbazepine can worsen seizures and are to be avoided. Approximately 25% of Lennox-Gastaut syndrome cases evolve from infantile spasms or West syndrome.

West Syndrome

West syndrome is a form of epilepsy that is associated with many underlying conditions and often has a poor developmental outcome. The most common etiologies are perinatal asphyxia and tuberous sclerosis. West syndrome refers to the triad of infantile spasms, mental retardation, and a characteristic EEG pattern called hypsarrythmia. Infantile spasms are considered the main clinical feature. They typically occur in clusters, usually during the first 2 years of life.[31] The clustering of spasms usually occurs during sleep transition. The movements may be flexor or extensor or a combination of both flexor and extensor movements and may be asymmetrical.

The classic electrographic pattern of hypsarrhythmia consists of very high voltage (200 microvolts), asynchronous, random, and typically independent, spike and sharp wave discharges. During clinical spasms, periods of electrodecrements lasting several seconds can be identified.[31] The discharges are worse during non-REM sleep and may improve significantly during REM sleep.

The most common treatment options include ACTH and vigabatrin. The latest has shown to be useful, especially in the cases of tuberous sclerosis. Other treatment options may include topiramate, zonisamide, levetriacetam, benzodiazepine, and ketogenic diet.

PARTIAL EPILEPSIES: IDIOPATHIC

Benign Epilepsy of Childhood with Centrotemporal Spikes

Benign epilepsy of childhood with centrotemporal spikes (BECT) is the most common form of partial epilepsy in children.[32, 33] BECT displays a strong genetic predisposition and appears in healthy subjects, with no evidence of brain lesion. Spontaneous remission of epilepsy occurs in more than 97%.[34]

Seizure onset is around 7 years of age, ranging between 3 and 13 years. Sleep is an important activating state of seizures; in 70% to 80% of cases seizures are confined to sleep. Seizures are often rare and tend to occur in clusters with prolonged seizure-free intervals. Because of their rarity and their occurrence exclusively or predominantly during sleep, seizures may remain unnoticed by parents for years. Typical seizures are characterized by paresthesias in one half of the face, sometimes involving the tongue and lips, followed by clonic jerks involving the face, tongue, lips, larynx, and pharynx. These clonic jerks may provoke speech impairment. Clonic movements cause a feeling of suffocation and dysphagia with hypersalivation. Consciousness is usually preserved. Patients may be awakened by the seizures. The typical hemifacial seizure may spread to the ipsilateral arm (brachiofacial convulsion) and rarely to the leg, producing a hemiconvulsive seizure, which may involve loss of consciousness. A postictal Todd's paresis is observed in 7% to 16% of cases.[35] GTCSs are rare. The EEG reveals characteristic high-amplitude interictal spikes followed by slow waves in the centrotemporal areas (Fig. 35.1). The EEG spike activity is enhanced during sleep and, in about 30% of cases, appears only during sleep. Spikes can remain unilateral or can spread to the contralateral hemisphere (50% of the cases). Epileptiform discharges sometimes occur outside the centrotemporal region in children exhibiting symptoms consistent with BECT.[36]

The prognosis is excellent, with response to antiepileptic medications the rule. If there are atypical features or examination abnormalities, a brain MRI is mandatory to exclude an underlying lesion.[37]

The neuropsychomotor development is normal; seizures usually disappear by the age of 15, with normalization of the EEG. However, in recent decades, cognitive deficits, alterations in specific neuropsychological tests, learning difficulties, and worsening of school performance have been found in children with BECT. The deficits were mostly related to language, memory, and execution functions.[38,39] The seizures of BECT are usually easily distinguishable from movement disorders and psychogenic disorders on the basis of the history, EEG, and the response to medications. Treatment of choice usually includes cabamazepine or oxcarbazepine.

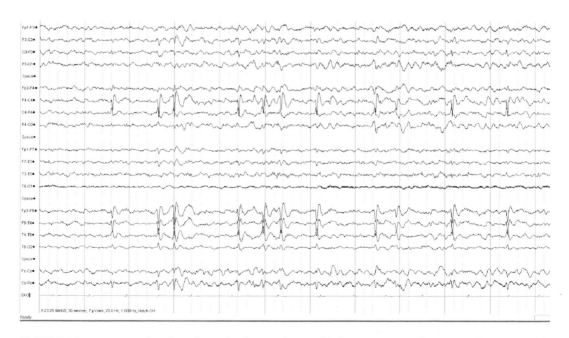

FIGURE 35.1   Interictal epileptiform discharges (asterisk) characteristic of benign epilepsy of childhood with centrotemporal spikes. Calibration signal: 150 μV, 3 seconds.

PARTIAL EPILEPSIES: SYMPTOMATIC AND CRYPTOGENIC

Nocturnal Frontal Lobe Epilepsy

Nocturnal frontal lobe epilepsy (NFLE) has become clinically relevant in recent years.[40] NFLE represents a spectrum of clinical manifestations, with seizures varying in intensity and duration. Autosomal dominant nocturnal frontal lobe epilepsy (ADNFLE), a familial form of NFLE, is clinically and biologically heterogeneous.[41] In a large series studied by video-polysomnographic recording, three types of seizures have been described, differing in intensity and duration: (1) minor motor events, called paroxysmal arousals (PAs); (2) major attacks, with more complex motor behavior, called nocturnal paroxysmal dystonia (NPD); and (3) episodic nocturnal wanderings (ENWs), which can mimic sleepwalking episodes.[38] Although seizure patterns differ, there is marked intraindividual stereotypy over the years. Few patients presented with only one type of seizure and different seizures tend to overlap in the same patient, the briefest episodes being the initial fragment of more prolonged attacks.[42]

PAs are abrupt, frequently recurring arousals from non-REM sleep with a stereotyped sequence of movements, lasting from 2 to 20 seconds.

The most common pattern consists of a sudden arousal during which patients raise their heads, sit on the bed with a frightened expression, look around, and scream (Fig. 35.2). They often present a dystonic posture of the upper limbs.

A minority of cases display an atypical pattern: slow bizarre asymmetric dystonic posture with choreoathetoid, vermicular movements of the fingers and toes. Sometimes the attacks are violent

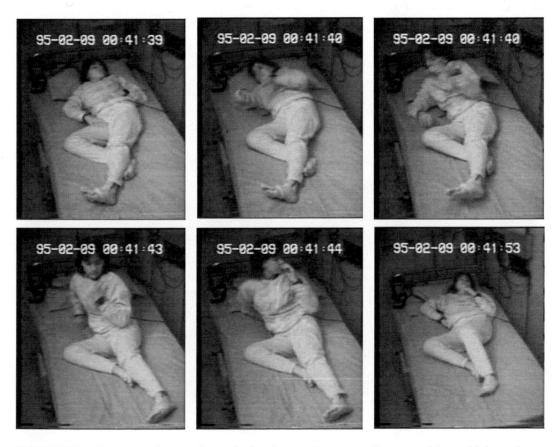

FIGURE 35.2   Paroxysmal arousals are the briefer manifestation of nocturnal frontal lobe epilepsy seizures. The episodes arise from non–rapid eye movement sleep with a stereotyped sequence of movements, lasting 14 seconds. The patient abruptly raises her head, sits on the bed with a frightened expression, looks around and screams. A dystonic posture of the upper limbs is present.

enough to wake the patient, but many patients remain unaware of their seizures. Patients with PA alone are rare but share some peculiar characteristics (lack of daytime seizures or personal antecedents and normal neuroradiologic findings).

NPD is characterized by a sudden arousal associated with a complex sequence of movements, lasting from 25 to 100 seconds on average.[40] Patients move their legs and arms with cycling or kicking movements, rock their trunks, and present a tonic asymmetric or dystonic posture of the limbs (Fig. 35.3). Clonic asymmetric jerks may also appear. A few cases are characterized by a violent ballistic pattern with flailing of the limbs.

ENWs are the longest episodes (lasting up to 3 minutes) during which patients jump out of bed, move around, talk unintelligibly, or scream with a terrified expression (Fig. 35.4). Dystonic postures may involve the face, trunk, and limbs. The events may last longer if patients were confused in the postictal phase. The agitated and violent motor behavior may lead to severe injuries to the patient and is different from the calmer "physiologic" motor pattern of walking in the sleepwalking patient. The motor pattern of ENW is characterized by an extreme intraindividual stereotypy, often including a dystonic posture or other typical motor behaviors of frontal lobe seizures and can be distinguished from sleep terrors, which are less stereotyped and influenced by the environment.

Some of those events may result in violent behavior causing self-injury or injury to others

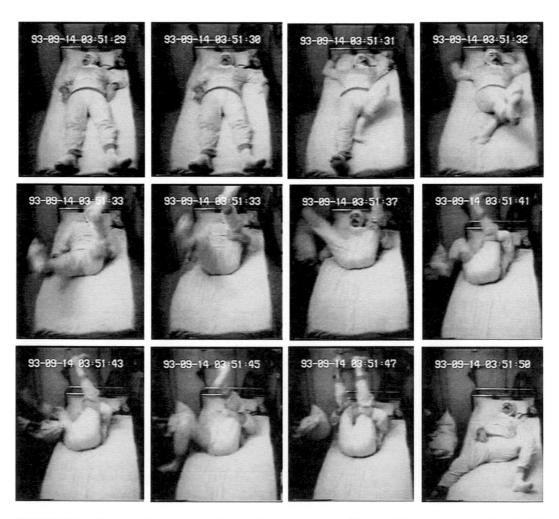

FIGURE 35.3 Nocturnal paroxysmal dystonia is characterized by a sudden arousal associated with a complex sequence of movements. This patient moves his legs with cycling and kicking movements and violently rocks his trunk. The seizure lasts 21 seconds.

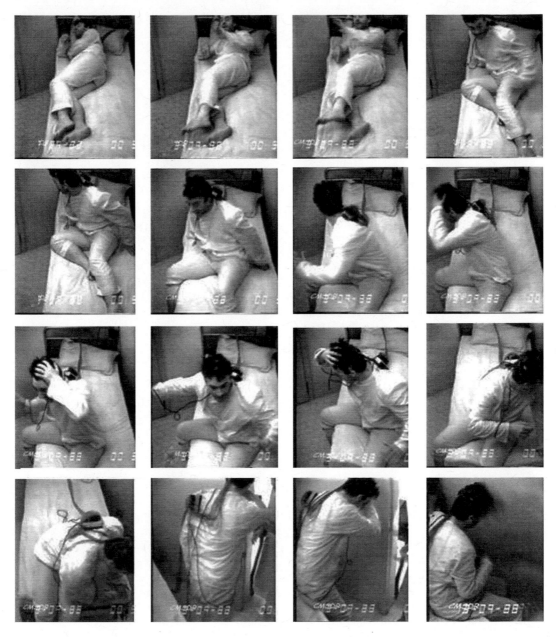

FIGURE 35.4   Episodic nocturnal wanderings are the longest episodes. In this case the patient jumps out of bed, moves around, and screams with a terrified expression. Seizures are again stereotyped within the same patient.

during sleep. Although this phenomenon is most likely to occur during a parasomnia, it may also be seen in the setting of epilepsy especially during ENW.

To protect patient and partner during those events, security measures are indicated. For example: sleeping in separate beds; sleeping on the ground floor; locking the windows or covering them with heavy drapes; removing mirrors and furniture from the room; removing sharp objects and objects with sharp corners. In more severe cases, the patient should sleep in a sleeping bag closed with a zip.

The syndrome of ADNFLE was initially described in 47 individuals from five families. These individuals exhibited clusters of brief nocturnal motor seizures with hyperkinetic or tonic manifestations indistinguishable from NPD.[43] In addition to NPD, sleepwalking and sudden awakenings with fear and tachycardia were also exhibited. One large Australian kindred with frontal lobe epilepsy (FLE) showed a missense mutation in the A4 subunit of the neuronal nicotinic acetylcholine receptor gene, located on chromosome 20q.[44] Oldani, Zucconi, Asselta, et al.[41] reported on ADNFLE in 40 subjects from 30 unrelated Italian families. This group of investigators also determined that ADNFLE is a genetically heterogeneous disorder, in that their five families undergoing genetic sequencing did not show linkage to the long arm of chromosome 20.

Currently, it is known that mutations in two nicotinic acetylcholine receptor genes (n AChR alpha4 and beta2 subunits) are associated with ADNFLE, with a third potential locus identified.[45,46] The seizures usually respond well to carabamazepine. In addition, the use of nicotine has been reported with decreased seizure frequency.[47]

NFLE affects both sexes with a higher prevalence for men, is often cryptogenic, and displays a strong familial trait for parasomnias and epilepsy.[38] One fourth of patients have a positive family history for epilepsy, but only a few families had two or more members with the same seizure type, consistent with a possible autosomal dominant pattern (ADNFLE). Kindreds reported are phenotypically and genetically heterogeneous. Nearly 40% of the patients have a positive family history for one or more parasomnias. This frequency is much higher than that reported for large control populations in which the prevalence for sleep terrors and sleepwalking ranges from 1% to 6% of the entire population.[48,49] In addition, history-taking disclosed parasomnia in a third of cases. This may represent a bias or it may mean that epileptic seizures appearing during childhood were mistaken for night terrors and sleepwalking. If this is the case, the familial recurrence would be higher, and this may also explain the wide range of incidence of ADNFLE reported in NFLE populations.[37,38] Alternative explanations are (1) both epileptic and nonepileptic nocturnal motor attacks may share a common genetic predisposition or (2) sleep fragmentation and sleep disruption as a result of nocturnal seizures may facilitate the occurrence of parasomnias.

Stress, sleep deprivation, and menstruation are triggering factors. A third of the patients present with occasional secondarily generalized seizures or rare seizures during wakefulness.[40,50] Neurologic examination is almost always normal. A few cases present positive risk factors for epilepsy (e.g., birth anoxia, febrile convulsions, or head injury) or focal brain computed tomography (CT) or MRI abnormalities. Seizures are most common between ages 14 and 20 years, although they can affect any age and tend to increase in frequency during life.

Virtually all attacks arise from non-REM sleep, in particular during light (non-REM stages I and II) sleep. In one fourth of patients, seizures of different intensity recurred periodically every 20 seconds to 2 minutes during sleep, mostly during light sleep. A K-complex often coincides or immediately precedes the ictal EEG and autonomic modifications on the recordings, suggesting that they are correlated. K-complexes seem to trigger the onset of NFLE seizures; seizures tend to cluster with a quasiperiodic repetition at a rate similar to that of the K-complexes.[40,51,52] These findings suggest that the epileptic discharges diffuse to limbic cortical and subcortical circuits, provoking sudden vigilance and autonomic changes and peculiar motor patterns. Awake and sleep interictal EEG recordings are normal during the seizures in more than half of the patients, with very few EEGs displaying unequivocal interictal discharges.

Numerous arguments suggest that NPD is a result of epilepsy. Normal EEG during the seizures suggests that these seizures involve the mesial frontal regions.[50]

Carbamazepine or oxcarbazepine taken at night is often effective, but one third of patients are resistant to AED treatment. Patients often report a marked improvement in daytime symptoms (e.g., tiredness) after AED introduction.[40]

Diagnosis remains a challenge in NFLE. NFLE is often misdiagnosed as an arousal disorder, especially in children.[53,54] Subjects with ADNFLE were also commonly misdiagnosed with parasomnias and psychiatric disorders, including non-REM arousal disorders and conversion disorders.[55] Even though NPD was initially described as a motor disorder of sleep of uncertain etiology, it is now generally accepted as a form of FLE.[56,57] The reason why it was originally thought to be nonepileptic is that the EEG was often normal during the events.

Evidence supporting the epileptic etiology of NPD are (1) the stereotyped nature of the spells; (2) the observation that seizures originating in deep mesial frontal generators often lack interictal and ictal correlates and require invasive monitoring for definitive diagnosis[54,55]; (3) the occurrence of cases in which convulsive seizures, with epileptiform EEG patterns, have followed typical NPD episodes[40,56]; (4) the presence of daytime dystonic events; and (5) the similarity in clinical features between patients with NPD, daytime frontal lobe seizures, and nocturnal epilepsy.[57] A similar argument of an epileptic etiology can be made for the other manifestations of FLE, including PA and ENW, especially in that patients with coexisting PA, NPD, and ENW often present with the same motor pattern at seizure onset.

Most NFLE attacks occur during the night and may be unwitnessed or witnessed by groggy bed partners. The lack of clear-cut epileptic EEG abnormalities on surface recordings is another major shortcoming in diagnosing FLE.

Workup for the diagnosis of NFLE usually includes the standard 21-lead EEG; however, this can be normal during the ictal event. In a series of 100 consecutive patients with FLE studied by Provini, Plazzi, Tinuper, et al.,[40] the ictal EEG failed to reveal epileptic activity in 44%. In some of these patients, muscle artifact interfered with interpretation of the recording. In a series of 47 individuals with ADNFLE studied by Scheffer, Bhatia, Lopes-Cendes, et al.,[43] only 4 of 10 subjects (40%) had ictal correlates to their seizures. In a series of 40 subjects with ADNFLE studied by Oldani, Zucconi, Asselta, et al., 32% showed ictal correlates and an additional 47% showed ictal rhythmic slow activity. In cases in which ictal correlates are either lacking or obscured, the stereotyped nature of the spells and their occurrence from sleep (rather than from wakefulness, as occurs in psychogenic seizures)[59] support an epileptic etiology.

Other clinical features can also help differentiate NFLE from other disorders, such as t the duration of the events; parasomnias are usually relatively prolonged events, whereas epileptic seizures, especially frontal lobe seizures, are usually very brief lasting less than 2 minutes on average.[60] In addition, non-REM arousal disorders usually appear in childhood and often resolve, whereas NFLE usually persists into adulthood. Nevertheless, disorders of partial arousal present more isolated attacks once or twice per night, whereas seizures usually cluster during the night[60] (Table 35.1). REM sleep behavior disorder starts much later than NFLE (around 60 years of age); it is associated with less stereotyped behavior, an intense vivid dream mentation, and the typical polygraphic finding of REM sleep without atonia.[61] Nocturnal panic attacks may also mimic NFLE, occurring with a sudden, often fearful, awakening from sleep with dramatic autonomic activation.[62] Other subjective complaints in panic attacks include tachycardia, constriction around the chest and neck,[63] and a sensation of imminent death. Age at onset of panic attacks is in adolescence (15 to 19 years) or middle age[64]; they are usually vividly recalled and seldom recur more than once per night. Their mean duration is usually prolonged, 24 minutes as a mean,[53] but very brief episodes have also been described.[65]

Panic attacks might also be confused with paroxysmal arousals, but they are not confused usually with NPD or ENW, since dystonia and nocturnal wondering are not usually present in panic attacks.

Sleep-related psychogenic dissociative disorders are also in the differential diagnosis. They are defined as intermittent disruption in consciousness, and memory without the conscious awareness of the part of the individual. It typically affects females subjected to physical and/or sexual abuse. However, episodes occur during EEG wakefulness after sustained arousals from sleep, and the behaviors are not stereotypical.[66]

Differential diagnosis of NFLE must also include attacks described under the terms NPD of intermediate and long duration.[67-68] NPD with intermediate duration (3 to 5 minutes) was observed in two children who had attacks triggered by arousal during sleep and by protracted exercise during wakefulness. Attacks were characterized by asynchronous jerks of the head, trunk, and limbs resembling a puppet on strings, not associated with epileptic EEG activity, and not responding to AEDs. This aspect, coupled with the triggering effect of prolonged exercise, suggests a paroxysmal motor disorder.[68] NPD with long-lasting (2 to 50 minutes) dystonic-dyskinetic attacks, arising from light sleep, recurring several times per night, and resistant to AEDs, was observed in two patients. One of them developed Huntington's disease 20 years after onset of the nocturnal attacks. The long duration of the attacks, the inefficacy of anticonvulsants, and the link with Huntington's disease in one patient suggest that these events are not epileptic in nature and are probably related to basal ganglia involvement.[69,70]

Table 35.1 Distinguishing Features of Non–Rapid Eye Movement Arousal Disorders versus Nocturnal Frontal Lobe Epilepsy

CHARACTERISTICS	NON-REM AROUSAL DISORDERS	NOCTURNAL FRONTAL LOBE EPILEPSY
Disorders of arousal in the family	~80%	~40%
Age at onset	Childhood	Adolescence (or any age)
Episodes per night	1–2	Usually >2
Episode semiology	Complex and nonstereotypic (calm)	Stereotypic (violent)
Episode duration	On average >2 minutes	On average: seconds to 2 minutes
Time of occurrence	First third of the night	Random
Sleep stage of appearance	Non-REM stages III and IV	Non-REM stage II
Ictal electroencephalogram	High-amplitude delta activity	Rare epileptic activity
Autonomic activation	Yes	Yes
Triggers (sleep deprivation, febrile illness, stress, alcohol consumption)	Yes	Rarely
Natural history	Spontaneous remission	Persist

Nocturnal Temporal Lobe Epilepsy

Although frontal lobe seizures have a predilection for occurring during sleep, a subset of patients with TLE may also have sleep-related seizures.[71] Although temporal lobe complex partial seizures are most commonly encountered during wakefulness,[16] Bernasconi and colleagues identified a group of 26 patients with nonlesional refractory TLE in whom seizures occurred exclusively or predominantly (90%) after they fell asleep or before they awakened. Simple partial seizures occurred in 69% of patients and were responsible for waking the patient; they consisted of experiential, autonomic, or special sensory components. Brief periods of impaired consciousness with motionless staring or automatisms dominated, although sleepwalking was reported in five patients. Eighty-one percent had secondary generalization of the partial attacks. These patients were compared to an age-matched group of patients with nonlesional TLE and predominantly diurnal seizures and were found to differ in having infrequent and nonclustered seizures, a rare family history of epilepsy, and a low prevalence of childhood febrile convulsions. All eight patients undergoing epilepsy surgery became seizure-free for at least 1 year. This subset of patients with nocturnal TLE is especially important to recognize because of their favorable surgical outcome. As with the other nocturnal seizure types listed previously, nocturnal TLE may occasionally be mistaken for a non-REM arousal disorder, REM sleep behavior disorder, panic disorder, or psychogenic seizure.

UNDETERMINED EPILEPSIES

Continuous Spike-Waves during Non-REM Sleep and Landau-Kleffner Syndrome

CSWS and Landau-Kleffner syndrome are both classified under the undetermined epilepsies because it is not clear whether they are focal or generalized. Epilepsy with CSWS has a heterogeneous clinical presentation.[72] Some patients have rare partial motor or GTCSs in sleep, whereas others may lack seizures during sleep. Still others may not have clinically apparent seizures at all. Clinical epileptic seizures are sometimes seen in the daytime.

The defining feature of CSWS is an EEG pattern consisting of generalized slow-spike-wave discharges, which are present for 85% to 90% of slow-wave sleep, less likely to be present in light non-REM sleep, and relatively suppressed during REM sleep and wakefulness. The syndrome used to be called electrical status epilepticus of sleep (ESES), but the name was changed because ESES implied frequent seizures, which may be absent in this syndrome. The seizures are usually responsive to AEDs and remit by the middle teenage years. Cognitive disturbances do not remit and are not improved by AEDs. A recent report emphasizes the etiologic heterogeneity of this disorder, which may be cryptogenic or result from a variety of central nervous system insults, including posthemorrhagic hydrocephalus, focal cortical dysplasia, or perinatal occlusion of the middle cerebral artery.[73]

Landau-Kleffner syndrome or "acquired epileptiform aphasia" is a syndrome of acquired aphasia and paroxysmal, sleep-activated EEG abnormalities predominantly from the temporal or parieto-occipital regions in a previously normal child. Secondary symptoms include seizures, which are present in 70% to 80%, and behavioral abnormalities.[74] Clinical manifestations of seizures usually are eye-blinking or brief ocular deviation, head drop, and minor automatisms with occasional secondary generalization.

Electrographically, several abnormalities have been described; temporal slowing and generalized, multifocal, or unilateral discharges. Those discharges are activated by sleep, especially sleep onset. CSWS is usually seen during non-REM sleep.

Outcomes range from complete recovery to permanent severe aphasia, with most experiencing improvement and residual moderate language deficits.[75]

AED therapy has been confounding, and several agents were found to be ineffective. Corticosteroids have been an efficacious treatment for both clinical and EEG abnormalities[73]; however, recurrence of epileptiform EEG followed by an aphasic relapse has been described after tapering steroids.[76]

These two disorders are mentioned here primarily because they illustrate the tendency of non-REM sleep to facilitate epileptic activity. They are rarely confused with other types of nocturnal seizures or nocturnal movement disorders. In cases of diagnostic uncertainty, the EEG pattern is diagnostic.

CASE EXAMPLES

Vignette 1

A 34-year-old woman with a remote history of daytime complex partial seizures presented with nocturnal spells occurring several times weekly. According to her husband, within 15 minutes of falling asleep she would sit up, appear frightened, breathe rapidly, and look around the room with a blank, wide-eyed stare, then return to sleep. The episodes lasted less than a minute. She responded almost immediately to observers and did not recall the episodes. Many EEGs, including those recorded during spells, had been normal. She underwent video-EEG-polysomnography and multiple spells from all stages of sleep were recorded. Although none showed ictal EEG changes, all were stereotyped. She was treated for presumed epilepsy and switched from treatment with three antiepileptic medications to CBZ monotherapy. At medium levels of CBZ, she experienced a daytime seizure resembling her nocturnal spells, preceded by an aura of "butterflies in her stomach." This aura was the same aura she had experienced in her childhood daytime complex partial seizures. At high levels of CBZ, her nocturnal spells and daytime seizures resolved.

This case illustrates that the diagnosis of nocturnal seizures is not always straightforward, especially if the spells lack EEG changes and share features with other sleep disorders, such as nocturnal panic disorder. The stereotyped nature of the spells prompted an adjustment in her medication regimen, which resulted in a seizure during the day, with an aura consistent with her prior history of epileptic seizures. When the medication regimen was optimized, her events resolved, supporting their epileptic etiology.

Vignette 2

This 18-year-old man had daytime complex partial seizures since age 5, well controlled on CBZ. At age 10, he developed episodes of heavy breathing and moving around in bed, followed by "sleepwalking." He had walked out of motel rooms and unlatched doors and windows. He was frequently able to be led back to bed and would end up going back to sleep. He did not recall the sleepwalking attacks. Attacks occurred approximately two nights a week, approximately 60 to 90 minutes after falling asleep. He had several spells during naps. He had one daytime spell of disorientation and agitation after a busy day of travel, associated with being sleep deprived and missing a dose of CBZ. EEG studies were normal between spells.

Because of the daytime spell, he was admitted for long-term video-EEG monitoring and a typical nocturnal seizure was captured. The seizure was characterized by an arousal from non-REM sleep in which he sat up, turned his head to the right, and postured his right hand. He then tried to walk around and was combative and confused. The EEG during the seizure showed myogenic and movement artifact initially, with subsequent left anterior and midtemporal alpha activity, then delta activity. Between seizures, left temporal sharp waves were recorded (Fig. 35.5). When this seizure was reviewed with his parents, they confirmed his activity before the sleepwalking (i.e., arousal from sleep, head turning, right hand posturing) as typical and stereotyped. His spells persisted despite the addition of other medications.

This case illustrates that the most prominent feature of his spells, the sleepwalking, may be preceded by a stereotyped phase of posturing, head turning, or other complex behavior. This stereotyped phase is highly suggestive of epilepsy. The daytime event prompted the consideration that his spells represented an epileptic disorder instead of a non-REM arousal disorder with prominent sleepwalking. In this case, the EEG was diagnostic.

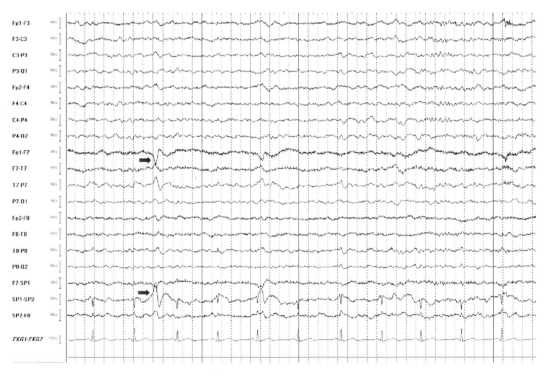

FIGURE 35.5   Left temporal interictal epileptiform discharges. Calibration signal: 35 μV, 1 second. (*See* color insert.)

PROGNOSIS

The prognosis of nocturnal seizures depends on the seizure type. Certain epilepsy syndromes, such as BECT and JME, typically respond to AEDs. Remission by the early adult years is the rule. Other partial epilepsy syndromes predominating during sleep do not carry as favorable a prognosis. Partial seizures that are limited to sleep often develop into waking seizures. Park, Lee, Park, et al.[77] retrospectively identified 63 patients with pure sleep epilepsy, 21 of whom had GTCSs during sleep and 42 of whom had partial seizures during sleep. Two years later, 17 (81%) of the patients with GTCSs were seizure-free as compared with 15 (36%) of the patients with partial seizures. Eleven patients (26%) with partial seizures developed seizures during wakefulness as compared with one patient with GTCSs (5%). In NFLE, CBZ abolished seizures in 20% of cases and reduced seizures by at least 50% in another 48% of cases.[40] In approximately one third of patients, however, seizures were refractory to AEDs. Cases responding to treatment relapsed when AEDs were withdrawn.

REFERENCES

1. Lennox W, Lennox M. *Epilepsy and Related Disorders*. Boston, MA: Little, Brown; 1960.
2. Temkin O. *The Falling Sickness: A History of Epilepsy from the Greeks to the Beginning of Modern Neurology*. Baltimore, MD: Johns Hopkins Press; 1971.
3. Passouant P. Historical aspects of sleep and epilepsy. In: Rodin EA, Degen R, eds. *Epilepsy, Sleep and Sleep Deprivation*. 2nd ed. Amsterdam, The Netherlands: Elsevier; 1991:19.
4. Langdon-Down M, Brain WR. Time of day in relation to convulsions in epilepsy. *Lancet* 1929;1:1029.
5. Janz D. The grand mal epilepsies and the sleeping-waking cycle. *Epilepsia* 1962;3:69.
6. Young GB, Blume WT, Wells GA, et al. Differential aspects of sleep epilepsy. 1985;*Can J Neurol Sciences* 12:317.
7. Steriade M, Conteras D, Amzica F. Synchronized sleep oscillations and their paroxysmal developments. *Trends Neurosci* 1994;17:199.
8. Steriade M, McCarley R. *Brainstem Control of Wakefulness and Sleep*. New York: Plenum; 1990.
9. Prince D, Farrell D. Centrencephalic spike-wave discharges following parenteral penicillin injection in the cat. *Neurology* 1963;19:309.
10. Steriade M, Contreras D. Relations between cortical and thalamic cellular events during transition from sleep patterns to paroxysmal activity. *J Neurosci* 1995;15:623.
11. Sammaritano M, Gigli GL, Gotman J. Interictal spiking during wakefulness and sleep and the localization of foci in temporal lobe epilepsy. *Neurology* 1991;41:290.
12. Malow B, Lin X, Kushwaha R, et al. Interictal spiking increases with sleep depth in temporal lobe epilepsy. *Epilepsia* 1998;39:1309.
13. Shouse MN. *Martins da Silva A: Chronobiology*. In: Engel J, Jr., Pedley TA, eds. *Epilepsy: A Comprehensive Textbook*. Philadelphia, PA: Lippincott-Raven; 1997:1917.
14. Commission on Classification and Terminology of the International League Against Epilepsy. Proposal for revised classification of epilepsies and epilepsy syndromes. *Epilepsia* 1989;30:389.
15. Crespel A, Baldy-Moulinier M, Coubes P. The relationship between sleep and epilepsy in frontal and temporal lobe epilepsies: practical and physiopathologic considerations. *Epilepsia* 1998;39:150.
16. Herman ST, Walczak TS, Bazil CW. Distribution of partial seizures during the sleep—wake cycle: differences by seizure onset site. *Neurology* 2001;56(11):1453–9
17. Lamarche M, Menini C, Silva-Barrat C, et al. Experimental models of frontal lobe epilepsy. In: Chauvel P, Delgado-Escueta A, eds. *Frontal Lobe Seizures and Epilepsies*. New York, Raven Press; 1992:159.
18. Commission on Classification and Terminology of the International League Against Epilepsy. Proposal for revised clinical and electroencephalographic classification of epileptic seizures. *Epilepsia* 1989;26:268.
19. Grunewald R, Panayiotopoulos C. Juvenile myoclonic epilepsy: a review. *Arch Neurol* 1993;50:594–8.
20. Appelton R, Beirne M, Acomb B. Photosensitivity in juvenile myoclonic epilepsy. *Seizure* 2000;9:108–11.
21. Montouris G, Abou-Khalil B. The first line of therapy in a girl with juvenile myoclonic epilepsy: should it be valproate or a new agent? *Epilepsia* 2009;50(Suppl 8):16–20.

22. Janz D. Epilepsy with impulsive petit mal (juvenile myoclonic epilepsy). *Acta Neurol Scand* 1985;72:449.
23. Durner M, Sander T, Greenberg D, et al. Localization of idiopathic generalized epilepsy on chromosome 6p in families of juvenile myoclonic epilepsy patients. *Neurology* 1991;41:1651.
24. Whitehouse W, Rees M, Curtis D, et al. Linkage analysis of idiopathic generalized epilepsy (IGE) and marker loci on chromosome 6p in families of patients with juvenile myoclonic epilepsy: no evidence for an epilepsy locus in the HLA region. *Am J Hum Genet* 1993;53:652.
25. Oguni H, Mukahira K, Oguni M, et al. Video-polygraphic analysis of myoclonic seizures in juvenile myoclonic epilepsy. *Epilepsia* 1994;35:305.
26. Janz D, Wolf P. Epilepsy with grand mal on awakening. In: Engel J, Jr., Pedley T, eds. *Epilepsy: A Comprehensive Textbook.* Philadelphia, PA: Lippincott-Raven; 1997:2347.
27. Suzuki T, Delgado-Escueta AV, Aguan K, et al. Mutations in EFHC1 cause juvenile myoclonic epilepsy. *Nat Genet* 2004;36:842–9.
28. Haug K, Warnstedt M, Alekov AK, et al. Mutations in CLCN2 encoding a voltage-gated chloride channel are associated with idiopathic generalized epilepsies. *Nat Genet* 2003;33:527–32.
29. Berkovic SF, Andermann F, Andermann E, et al. Concepts of absence epilepsies: discrete syndromes or biological continuum? *Neurology* 1987;37:993–1000.
30. Roger J, Dravet C, Bureau M. The Lennox-Gastaut syndrome. *Cleve Clin J Med* 1989;56:S172.
31. Gibbs FA, Gibbs EL. *Atlas of Electroencephalography*, Vol. 2. *Epilepsy.* Reading, MA: Addison-Wesley; 1952.
32. Loiseau P, Duche B. Benign childhood epilepsy with centrotemporal spikes. *Cleve Clin J Med* 1989;56:17.
33. Wirrel E. Benign epilepsy of childhood with centrotemporal spikes. *Epilepsia* 1998;39:S32.
34. Bouma PA, Bovenkerk AC, Westendorp RG, et al. The course of benign partial epilepsy of childhood with centrotemporal spikes: a meta-analysis. *Neurology* 1997; 48: 430–7.
35. Wirrel E, Camfield P, Gordon K, et al. Benign rolandic epilepsy: atypical features are very common. *J Child Neurol* 1995;10:455.
36. Drury I, Beydoun A. Benign partial epilepsy of childhood with monomorphic sharp waves in centrotemporal and other locations. *Epilepsia* 1991;32:662.
37. Santanelli P, Bureau M, Magaudda A, et al. Benign partial epilepsy with centrotemporal (or rolandic) spikes and brain lesions. *Epilepsia* 1989;30:182.
38. Vinayan KP, Biji V, Thomas SV. Educational problems with underlying neuropsychological impairment are common in children with benign epilepsy of childhood with centrotemporal spikes. *Seizure* 2005;14:207–12.
39. Lindgren A, Kihlgren M, Melin L, et al. Development of cognitive functions in children with rolandic epilepsy. *Epilepsy Behav* 2004;5:903–10.
40. Provini F, Plazzi G, Tinuper P, et al. Nocturnal frontal lobe epilepsy. A clinical and polygraphic overview of 100 consecutive cases. *Brain* 1999;122:1017.
41. Oldani A, Zucconi M, Asselta R, et al. Autosomal dominant nocturnal frontal lobe epilepsy. A video-polysomnographic and genetic appraisal of 40 patients and delineation of the epileptic syndrome. *Brain* 1998;121:205.
42. Sforza E, Montagna P, Rinaldi R, et al. Paroxysmal periodic motor attacks during sleep: clinical and polygraphic features. *Electroencephalogr Clin Neurophysiol* 1993;86:161.
43. Scheffer IE, Bhatia KP, Lopes-Cendes I, et al. Autosomal dominant nocturnal frontal lobe epilepsy—a distinctive clinical disorder. *Brain* 1995;118:61.
44. Phillips H, Scheffer I, Berkovic S, et al. Localization of a gene for autosomal dominant nocturnal frontal lobe epilepsy to chromosome 20q 13.2. *Nat Genet* 1995;10:117.
45. Steinlein OK. Nicotinic receptor mutations in human epilepsy. *Prog Brain Res* 2004;145:275–85.
46. Picard F, Bruel D, Servent D, et al. Alteration of the in vivo nicotinic receptor density in ADNFLE patients: a PET study. *Brain* 2006;129(Pt 8):2047–60.
47. Brodtkorb E, Picard F. Tobacco habits modulate autosomal dominant nocturnal frontal lobe epilepsy. *Epilepsy Behav* 2006;9(3):515–20.
48. Hublin C, Kaprio J, Partinen M. Prevalence and genetics of sleepwalking: a population-based twin study. *Neurology* 1997;48:177.

49. Partinen M. Epidemiology of sleep disorders. In: Kryger M, Roth T, Dement W, eds. *Principles and Practice of Sleep Medicine*. Philadelphia, PA: WB Saunders; 1994:437.

50. Hirsh E, Sellal F, Maton B, et al. Nocturnal paroxysmal dystonia: a clinical form of focal epilepsy. *Neurophysiol Clin* 1994;24:207.

51. Talairach J, Bancaud J, Geier S. The cingulate gyrus and human behaviour. *Electroencephalogr Clin Neurophysiol* 1973;34:45.

52. Lugaresi E, Coccagna G, Mantovani M, et al. Some periodic phenomena arising during drowsiness and sleep in man. *Electroencephalogr Clin Neurophysiol* 1972;32:701.

53. Pedley TA, Guilleminault C. Episodic nocturnal wanderings responsive to anticonvulsant drug therapy. *Ann Neurol* 1977;2:30.

54. Plazzi G, Tinuper P, Montagna P. Epileptic nocturnal wanderings. *Sleep* 1995;18:749.

55. Scheffer IE, Bhatia KP, Lopes-Cendes I, et al. Autosomal dominant frontal epilepsy misdiagnosed as sleep disorder. *Lancet* 1994;343:515.

56. Tinuper P, Cerullo A, Cirignotta F, et al. Nocturnal paroxysmal dystonia with short-lasting attacks: three cases with evidence for an epileptic frontal lobe origin of seizures. *Epilepsia* 1990;31:549.

57. Meierkord H, Fish D, Smith S. Is nocturnal paroxysmal dystonia a form of frontal lobe epilepsy. *Mov Disord* 1992;7:38.

58. Williamson PD, Spencer SS. Clinical and EEG features of complex partial seizures of extratemporal origin. *Epilepsia* 1986;27:S46.

59. Thacker K, Devinsky O, Perrine K, et al. Nonepileptic seizures during apparent sleep. *Ann Neurol* 1993;33:414.

60. Provini F, Plazzi G, Lugaresi E. From nocturnal paroxysmal dystonia to nocturnal frontal lobe epilepsy. *Clin Neurophysiol* 2000;111(Suppl 2):S2–8.

61. Mahowald M, Schenck C. REM sleep parasomnias. In: Kryger M, Roth T, Dement W, eds. *Principles and Practice of Sleep Medicine*. 3rd ed. Philadelphia, PA: WB Saunders; 2000:724.

62. Plazzi G, Montagna P, Provini F, et al. Sudden arousals from slow-wave sleep and panic disorder. *Sleep* 1998;21:548.

63. Craske M, Barlow D. Nocturnal panic. *J Nerv Ment Dis* 1989;177:160.

64. Von Korff MR, Eaton W, Key PM. The epidemiology of panic attacks and panic disorders. Results of three community surveys. *Am J Epidemiol* 1985;122:970.

65. Dantendorfer K, Frey R, Maierhofer D, et al. Sudden arousals from slow wave sleep and panic disorders: successful treatment with anticonvulsants—a case report. *Sleep* 1996;19:744.

66. Schenck CH, Milner DM, Huwitz TD, et al. Dissociative disorders presenting as somnambulism. Polysomnographic video and clinical documentation (8 cases). *Dissociation* 1989b; 11:194–204.

67. Montagna P. Nocturnal paroxysmal dystonia and nocturnal wandering. *Neurology* 1992;42:61.

68. Lugaresi E, Cirignotta F. Two variants of nocturnal paroxysmal dystonia with attacks of short and long duration. In Degen R, Niedermeyer E, eds. *Epilepsy, Sleep, and Sleep Deprivation*. Amsterdam, The Netherlands: Elsevier;1984:169.

69. Montagna P, Cirignotta F, Giovanardi Rossi P, et al. Dystonic attacks related to sleep and exercise. *Eur Neurol* 1992;32:185.

70. Lugaresi E, Cirignotta F, Montagna P. Nocturnal paroxysmal dystonia. *J Neurol Neurosurg Psychiatry* 1986;49:375.

71. Bernasconi A, Andermann F, Cendes F, et al. Nocturnal temporal lobe epilepsy. *Neurology* 1998;50:1772.

72. Jayakar P, Seshia S. Electrical status epilepticus during slow-wave sleep: a review. *J Clin Neurophysiol* 1991;8:299.

73. Veggiotti P, Beccaria F, Guerrini R, et al. Continuous spike-and-wave activity during slow-wave sleep: syndrome or EEG pattern? *Epilepsia* 1999;40:1593.

74. Mouridsen SE. The Landau-Kleffner syndrome: a review. *Eur Adolesc Psychiatry* 1995;4:223–8.

75. McKinney W, McGreal DA. An aphasic syndrome in children. *Can Med Assoc J* 1974;110:637–9.

76. Marescaux C, Hirsch E, Finck P, et al. Landau-Kleffner syndrome: a pharmacologic study of five cases. *Epilepsia* 1990;31:768–72.

77. Park SA, Lee BI, Park SC, et al. Clinical course of the pure sleep epilepsies. *Seizure* 1998;7:369.

36

Complex (Including Violent) Sleep Behavior

MARK R. PRESSMAN

PARASOMNIAS ARE behaviors that occur during sleep or come out of sleep.[1] Parasomnias may occur during deep non–rapid eye movement (non-REM) sleep, rapid eye movement (REM) sleep, or in the transitions to and between REM and non-REM sleep and/or wakefulness. During deep non-REM sleep, behaviors may vary from minor movements to complex movements and behaviors. During REM sleep, behaviors may vary from minor movements to complex behaviors associated with the enactment of ongoing dreams. Complex behaviors occurring during REM and non-REM sleep may appear similar but actually differ in significant ways, including underlying pathophysiology.

NON-REM PARASOMNIAS

Pathophysiology of Disorders of Arousal during Non-REM Sleep

Until the advent of the modern sleep laboratory in the early 1960s, sleepwalking was thought to be a result of the enactment of dreams. However, the first sleep laboratory studies showed that sleepwalking and related disorders instead occur following a sudden arousal during deep non-REM sleep.[2] It is now generally accepted that most parasomnias occurring during non-REM typically arise from deep or slow-wave sleep (SWS). As most SWS occurs during the first 2–4 hours of the sleep period, non-REM parasomnias most often occur early in the sleep period. As these non-REM parasomnias—sleepwalking, confusional arousals, and night or sleep terrors—all follow a sudden arousal from sleep, these disorders have been labeled Disorders of Arousal.[3]

The occurrence of disorders of arousal is hypothesized to require the simultaneous presence of three different factors[4]:

1. *Genetic predisposition.* Disorders of arousal have a clear familiar pattern. A clinical history of a disorder of arousal in a first-degree relative increases the chances of a disorder of arousal

some 40 times. Several studies have identified DNA markers for disorders of arousal.[4a] However, these markers have not been noted in the majority of patients studied. Furthermore, it is not known just what the DNA might code for.

2. *Priming factors*. Disorders of arousal have been noted to occur more frequently following acute or partial sleep deprivation.[5] Following sleep deprivation there is often an increase—rebound—in deep non-REM sleep. The threshold for arousal is highest during deep non-REM sleep, and during a rebound the arousal threshold may be very high. Sleep deprivation is often associated with situational stress in these patients.

3. *Precipitating factors*. Even when a genetic predisposition and priming factors are present, a disorder of arousal may not occur. A proximal trigger is required. This trigger could be a sound or touch—something that might result in an arousal. In both children and adults it has been noted that sleep-disordered breathing—apneas, hypopneas, snoring, —are often the trigger for disorders of arousal.[6] This is more than a theory as effective treatment of the sleep-disordered breathing by continuous positive air pressure (CPAP) or by surgery often results in elimination of the disorder of arousal as well.[7]

Organic Changes in Brain Function That May Underlie Complex Behaviors in Non-REM Sleep

There is no evidence that disorders of arousal are caused by any organic brain disorder. Neuroimaging studies have never reported any tumors, lesions, or other visible changes in the brains of these patients. However, disorders of arousal are occasionally observed in patients who also have a diagnosis of epilepsy, and a similar pathophysiology in response to arousal has been suggested.

Functional Changes in Brain Function That May Underlie Complex Behaviors in Non-REM Sleep

Bassetti and colleagues[8] are the only research group to capture an episode of a sleepwalking-related behavior—night terrors—from SWS during neuroimaging—using a single-photon emission computed tomography (SPECT). An increase of 25% in regional cerebral blood flow in the posterior cingulate cortex and anterior cerebellum was noted when this scan was compared to a group of 24 normal waking control subjects. Furthermore, regional cerebral blood flow decreased in the frontal and parietal association cortexes. Thalamocortical circuits that are typically deactivated were found to remain active.[9] Bassetti and colleagues hypothesize that sleepwalking results from the specific activation of the thalamocingulate circuits, while other thalamocortical arousal pathways remain inhibited and the frontal cortex remains deactivated.

General Limitation on Complex Behaviors in Non-REM Sleep

Due to the fact that disorders of arousal arise from deep sleep, almost all higher cognitive functions are absent or greatly diminished. Planning, memory, attention, intent, and social interaction are not available to the sleeping or sleepwalking individual. Thus, complex behaviors that require these cognitive functions should not—cannot—be present during an episode.

Non-REM Disorder of Arousal Characteristics

Disorders of arousal have a number of features in common[10,11]:

1. Follow an arousal from deep sleep
2. Occur in first half of the sleep period
3. Have eyes open
4. May be able to navigate in familiar areas
5. Difficult to arouse
6. No social skills
7. Amnesia for episode
8. High pain threshold
9. Failure to recognize family or friends
10. No concern for modesty or social graces

CONFUSIONAL AROUSALS

Confusional arousal differs from sleepwalking only insofar as where the behavior occurs. All confusional arousals occur in bed. When the patient's foot hits the floor, it becomes sleepwalking.[1]

Common behaviors occurring during confusional arousals include the following:

• Thrashing around
• Sudden movement of the head

- Sudden sitting up
- Vocalizations
  - Sleep talking may occur during REM or non-REM sleep. Most often words are not spoken clearly and the meaning of the utterance cannot be deciphered. However, there are reports of individuals holding conversations of sorts while in the midst of a confusional arousal. Initially it may not be clear to the other individual that the person is asleep. However, responses in these types of conversations are often bizarre and nonresponsive.
- Injury to self[12,13]
  - Unintentional striking of furniture
  - Unintentional breaking of lamp shades, mirrors, and so on
- Injury to others[12-14]
  - Accidental hitting or kicking of bed partner
  - Defensive and violent reaction to someone in close proximity or to someone who is attempting to awaken or restrain them—most often by touch (see later section on "Sleep Violence")
- Sexual behavior in sleep[15,16]
  - As this behavior most often occurs in bed and individuals rarely walk to other locations before initiating sexual behavior, it is considered a variant of confusional arousal (see later discussion)

NIGHT OR SLEEP TERRORS

The night of sleep terror occurs in two stages. Initially, the night terror is identical to a confusional arousal. It is triggered by a partial arousal from deep sleep. The same triggers that precede confusional arousals and sleepwalking may also trigger night terrors. The night terror differs from the confusional arousal because of the significant autonomic activation that accompany the episode. When occurring in the sleep laboratory, a doubling of the heart rate may be noted. The patient with a night terror often appears frightened, if not terrified. The night terror is often associated with a specific frightening image—house on fire, intruder in bedroom, and so on—and the patient may react to that image in a variety of ways. This has led to suggestions that the frightening image is the trigger for night terrors. Most often—especially in children—night terror may result in the following:

1. Sudden piercing scream
2. Sudden sitting up

3. Lack of responsiveness to others
4. Thrashing about
5. Other vocalizations

After the initial appearance of behaviors the patient may simply lay back down and return to sleep. The patient typically has no memory of the episode.

However, in a minority of episodes, the patient may react to the frightening image with more complex movements and behavior. This results in the patient leaving the bed in a state often described as "agitated sleepwalking." The behaviors noted during this time are often related to the nature of the image. Common complex behaviors related to night terrors include the following[17]:

- Jumping out of bed
- Falling out of bed
- Running
- Jumping out of windows
- Crashing through windows or doors
- Injuring oneself—running with diminished cognitive and perceptual abilities is likely to result in crashes and falls
- Injuring another (see later section on "Sleep Violence")
- Screaming

Anecdotal reports of complex behaviors often appear to require higher cognitive function than are usually attributed to patients with night terrors. One report describes an adult patient who experienced a frightening night terror in which there was an image of his house on fire.[18] The patient jumped out of bed and went to his children's rooms one by one and carried them out of the house to the sidewalk. Only later did he realize there actually was no fire. This sequence of behavior is reported to have occurred more than once. An alternate theory suggests that the patient was having a vivid dream and awakened suddenly not realizing he had been dreaming and was actually awake when he saved his family.

There are numerous other anecdotal reports of such complex behavior. As with other disorders of arousal, they are very unlikely to occur in the sleep laboratory and attempts to provoke them in the research setting have been unsuccessful. Thus, we are left with anecdotal reports—sometimes months or years—after the incident.

SLEEPWALKING

"Sleepwalking" is something of a misnomer.[1] This term is often applied to a wide variety of behaviors that occur out of bed in addition to walking. All sleepwalking episodes start with a confusional arousal. However, the diagnostic label of sleepwalking or somnambulism is not applied until the patient has left the bed. On some occasions, an arousal triggers a confusional arousal with high levels of autonomic activation (night terrors), which then lead to agitated sleepwalking-related behaviors.

Sleepwalking behaviors often include the following:

1. Standing
2. Walking
3. Running
4. Climbing
5. Eating
6. Violence
7. Sexual behaviors

There are several hypotheses regarding the cause of sleepwalking behaviors.

Automatic Behaviors. The phrase "I have done it so often I could do it in my sleep" suggests that behaviors that can be performed without conscious input and control might be a behavior that could be triggered during sleep. Why one behavior occurs and not another is unknown. For instance, a common complex behavior reported by men is that they arouse, get out of bed, and move toward the bathroom, apparently with the intent to urinate. However, in the sleepwalking state they are unable to perform this common behavior properly. They typically enter a room other than the bathroom and discover later that they have urinated in a trash basket or other circular receptacle.

It has been suggested that sleepwalkers may incorporate memories or elements of behaviors or actions from the prior waking period. This has found no support in the scientific sleep literature and appears to run counter to what we know about the pathophysiology of sleepwalking and the nature of deep sleep. The severe limitations on memory and other higher cognitive functions make retrieval and response to earlier memories or intents highly unlikely.

Two more complex apparently automatic behaviors that can occur during sleep are as follows:

1. *Sleep driving.*[19,20] Sleep driving is most often reported to be a sleepwalking variant that is often associated with hypnotic/sedative use, in particular zolpidem and zopiclone. However, there is limited scientific evidence that sleep driving requires a genetic predisposition, priming factors, or trigger as with sleepwalking. Sleep driving has rarely been reported in the absence of sleeping medication, alcohol, or other central nervous system (CNS) depressants. Furthermore, the description of the sleep driver following accidents or police stops does not represent the expected behaviors of a sleepwalker. Sleep drivers typically have trouble standing up but may be able to answer police questions and requests with difficulty. Sleepwalkers, on the other hand, generally have no trouble standing but are unable to socially interact. Supposed sleep drivers sometimes are able to complete part or all of a field sobriety test. A sleepwalker would not be able to understand or respond to police requests. It has been proposed that sleep driving may be composed of an initial sleepwalking-like behavior, which is self-limited to minutes. After that the sleep driver would be driving with a significant blood level of the sedative hypnotic causing CNS depression. However, in most cases reported, there is little if any scientific evidence that sleep drivers are in a true sleepwalking state.

1. *Sleep texting or e-mailing.*[21] There have been several reports, for the most part in the popular media, of teenagers or young adults apparently texting or sending e-mails while they were asleep. All reports are anecdotal, and there is some doubt whether these complex behaviors occurred during a true sleepwalking state. Did these individuals fall asleep only to be aroused 50–90 minutes later from deep sleep? Did they then proceed to their computers or use their phones? In terms of an automatic behavior resulting from frequent performance of that behavior, texting and e-mailing would appear to fulfill these criteria. However, addressing the text or mail to a particular individual and then typing in a meaningful message appears inconsistent with the very limited cognitive function typical of the sleepwalking state.

Automatic behaviors may also result from activation of locomotor centers, which are present in many areas of the CNS.[22] These locomotor centers connect with central pattern generators in the spinal cord. These generators are preprogrammed and do not require wakefulness or consciousness. Thus, basic behaviors such as sitting up, walking, or running would not require input from the cortex. The proverbial chicken with his head cut off can still run.

RELEASE OF PRIMITIVE DRIVES

There are several common forms or variants of sleepwalking that appear to be related to the release of basic human drives: hunger, sex, and violence. In the absence of higher cognitive functions, especially frontal lobe functions, these drives may be disinhibited.

Sleep Eating

Sleep eating[23,24] is a well-described and established variant of sleepwalking. In this disorder, the patient arouses and navigates to the kitchen. Once in the kitchen, the patient may remove food from the refrigerator and cabinets. Food is often combined in ways that would not be typical for a waking person. He or she may light the stove or burners in an attempt at cooking. Burnt food and even kitchen fires may result. Other damage to the kitchen may occur, such as damage to cabinet doors. Most often the patient leaves the kitchen and returns to sleep at some other location. The patient may later discover the kitchen in a state of disarray and have no clue as to how this occurred. Sleep eating has been associated with use of sedative/hypnotic drugs, especially zolpidem, often taken along with antidepressant medications.

Sleep Sex

Sleep sex[15,16] (sexual behavior in sleep, sexsomnia) is generally classified as a variant of confusional arousal because it occurs in bed. Sleep sex along with sleep eating appears to be a manifestation of a basic human drive released from high-level cognitive control during sleep. Sleep sex is reported to involve all types of sexual activities and most often occurs between individuals who are already consenting sexual partners and share the same bed. Occasionally, sexual behavior in sleep is directed at individuals who are not otherwise consenting adults. Sometimes the nonconsenting individual is in the same bed or comes into bed with the patient, perhaps accidentally triggering

sexual behavior. Alternately, the patient may leave the bed and bedroom, and walk to an area where another individual is sleeping and initiate sexual behavior. Cases of sexual behavior in sleep with a nonconsenting partner have resulted in criminal charges. Amnesia for the sexual behavior is typical.

Sleep Violence

Apparent sleep-related violence is not a rare occurrence. At least one episode of violence during sleep was reported by 1.6% of a large population surveyed in Europe.[25] Not all of this violence was sleepwalking related. However, sleep-related violence reported in this survey as well as elsewhere included hitting, kicking, assaults, attempted killings, killings, and violent sexual assaults. There are well over 100 cases reported in medical/legal literature.[14,26,27] However, the medical literature on sleep violence relies almost exclusively on anecdotal reports often months or years after their date of occurrence. Anecdotal reports are an important starting point for scientific research but occupy the lowest level of scientific evidence.

However, the manner in which these violent acts are hypothesized to have occurred is supported by the unplanned actions of sleepwalkers in a research study reported by Guilleminault and colleagues.[15] They describe sleep studies conducted in patients with a history of sleepwalking-related violence. Technical staff reported that on occasion when they approached the patient and attempted to block or restrain the patient for his or her safety, they were met by aggression and violence. Some members of the technical staff were hit or pushed. Pieces of equipment within arm's reach were thrown at the technical staff. Some staff members were injured.

The occurrence of sleepwalking violence appears to require one or more factors in additional to genetic predisposition, priming factors, and triggers:

1. *Provocation.* As noted by Guilleminault and in a recent review by Pressman, sleepwalkers do not seek out their victims.[14,18] In the unusual brain state of the sleepwalker, the individual would have no knowledge of perceived slights, insults, or feelings of anger or revenge directed against another person. The sleepwalker has no access to long-term memory and lives in the moment without the cognitive resources to evaluate a situation. A sleepwalker sees an

unknown individual walking toward him or her and reacts defensively. The sleepwalker cannot process the fact that this individual is a family member and means no harm. Sleepwalking violence is simply a defensive act resulting from the most basic and primitive of instincts.

2. *Proximity.* Sleepwalkers do not leave the bed and bedroom and then wander the house in search of victims. Victims are almost always within arm's reach or the victims themselves seek out the sleepwalker. A common scenario is when a family member leaves the bedroom in a sleepwalking state. Another family member hears a door open or footsteps and goes in search of the source. If the family member approaches the sleepwalker or grabs, blocks, or touches the sleepwalker, a violent defensive response may occur.

Violence to other individuals may occur as a result of the patient responding to a frightening image inappropriately, especially in cases of night terrors or agitated sleepwalking. As noted earlier, while in a sleepwalking or night terror state, the individual does not have access to abilities to properly evaluate a situation. Is the house really on fire? Is there actually an intruder in the house? In a classic 19th-century case, the sleeping father of an infant reported he saw a wild beast come up through the floor.[28,29] He grabbed at the wild beast and flung it away. Unfortunately, he had instead grabbed his baby and thrown it against the wall, killing him. More recently a man from Wales was found to have choked his wife to death while asleep while responding inappropriately to a frightening image of an intruder attacking her.

Sleep-related violence may involve fists, legs, feet, and so on. It may also involve use of primitive tools or weapons such as knives, axes, and more rarely guns. Other objects found close by may also be used. The sleepwalking individual does not retrieve objects or weapons from a closet or shelf and then seek out the victim.

There are a number of theories regarding the occurrence of sleep-related violence.

Fight or Flight

Violent behavior against others by sleepwalkers has in the past been ascribed to the "fight or flight reflex." Recent research has suggested that the sequence of events first described by Canon in 1929 is not accurate. Rather, the response to a threat is actually (1) freeze, (2) attempt to flee, (3) attempt to fight, or (4) fright or tonic immobility.[30] Violent sleepwalkers are not reported to freeze before engaging in violent behaviors. Additionally, fight or flight does not account for the violent behavior of someone who is suddenly awakened from sleep or who became violent in the midst of a sleep terror. The patient in the midst of a sleep terror is initially acting in response to frightening imagery, not to the threat of another person. Thus, the original concept of fight or flight or the updated freeze-flee-fight-fright concept does not appear to account for the violent behaviors.

Reaction to Imagery

Reports of imagery by patients diagnosed with disorders of arousal other than night terrors are quite infrequent due to the presence of amnesia. However, when a patient does report an image, it may incorrectly give the appearance that he or she is enacting a dream. However, a close examination of these reports suggests this imagery lacks the details and complexity of typical dreaming. Instead, patients with a diagnosis of disorders of arousal most often appear to be reacting to a frightening scene.

Pressman and colleagues described a patient being treated for sleep apnea with CPAP.[31] The CPAP was quite effective, and as a result a significant rebound of deep non-REM sleep occurred. A single apnea occurred during the deep non-REM sleep followed by an arousal. The patient immediately sat up and then jumped from the bed screaming. His heart rate more than doubled. He ripped off all electrodes and sensors. However, most important for the issue of sleep violence, he then turned around, saw a framed picture on the wall, and with one big slap, knocked it down. When questioned later, he reported only that he thought someone was chasing him. This episode thus appeared to involve a night terror, followed by agitated sleepwalking that included a violent behavior. It was hypothesized that the patient mistook the picture for the individual who was chasing him. He then reacted with defensive aggressiveness. Thus, the proximity to the picture as well as inappropriate perception of it led to the violent act.

Complete amnesia may not be typical of all episodes of disorders of arousal. Questioning of the patient soon after the episode may result in some description by patients of their experiences. Zadra and colleagues questioned 34 diagnosed sleepwalkers about their perceptions and experiences.[32] A minority of patients reported perceptual elements from the sleeper's actual environment during a somnambulistic episode. Seventy-four percent of patients reported that various forms of mental content or sleep mentation such as images, thoughts, and emotions were present or accompanied their episodes. Emotions such as fear, panic, confusion, anger, frustration, and helplessness were described by 65% as being often or always experienced during their episodes. These data remain to be replicated but suggest that in some patients with a disorder of arousal the observed behavior may not be "automatic" but instead a reaction to the content of the mentation or image. This is clearly true in cases of sleep terrors when the stimulus is a frightening but static image that contains no plot or other dream-like aspects.

VIOLENCE, THE FRONTAL LOBE, AND SLEEPWALKING

The neurophysiology and neuroanatomy of violence and that of SWS and sleepwalking have many points in common. The frontal lobes and the limbic system are reported to have extensive interconnections[33] and are also the two major centers most often implicated in violent behavior.[34] Additionally, the frontal lobes contain centers for higher cognitive functions, including alertness, attention, decision making, planning, and exercise of judgment in social situations.[35] There is a substantial scientific literature documenting the consequences of frontal lobe damage to waking behavior, including (1) inability to control anger, (2) deficits in inhibitory control, (3) exaggerated emotional responses, (4) deficits in attention and planning, and (5) deficits in social skills.[34-35]

Neuroimaging studies have demonstrated that reduced prefrontal cortical size or prefrontal cortical activity is related to increased aggression and violence.[34,36] Damage to the frontal lobe in combat veterans has been found to be associated with an increased risk for violent behavior. Violent behaviors in schizophrenia as well as with chronic alcohol intoxication have been reported to be associated with frontal lobe dysfunction.

Slow-Wave Sleep and the Frontal Lobes

Neuroimaging studies of humans during SWS sleep have reported that there is a general deactivation of the frontal lobes and that total sleep deprivation[9, 37]—a common priming factor for sleepwalking—is also reported to result in a significant decrease in metabolism in the frontal lobe that is not reversed by a full night of recovery sleep.[38-40] With increasing SWS activity there is a highly significant reduction in rCBF associated with direct inhibition of thalamocortical neurons and pathways. The loss of consciousness and sensory awareness during SWS has been hypothesized to result from closing off of afferent pathways to the cortex.

At the same time the frontal lobe is deactivated during SWS, activation of primary and secondary auditory and visual cortical occurs. This could explain reports of dream-like imagery during non-REM or the vivid visual imagery reported in sleep terrors.[39]

There are interesting points of comparison between the neurophysiology of SWS and violence. Frontal lobe deactivation is a typical finding in normal controls during SWS as well as in a single clinically diagnosed night terror patient studied during SWS.[8,9] Reports of sleepwalking are frequently associated with acute sleep deprivation. An increased degree of SWS deactivation of the frontal lobe, possibly as a consequence of sleep deprivation, could underlie the pathophysiology of sleepwalking. With the frontal lobes in a state of deactivation, inhibition of the limbic system may be incomplete and aggressive, or violent impulses originating in the limbic system may not be suppressed.

Defensive Aggressiveness

Defensive aggressiveness is a violent response to minor provocations or to close proximity to others.[41] Defensive aggressiveness has been extensively studied in the rat. It can be elicited in response to perceived threats from an attacker or to the experimenter—even when no real threat is actually present.[42] Defensive aggression in humans has been reported to be elicited by frustration, perceived threat, and interruption of an activity. Many reported episodes of sleepwalking violence are associated with interruption of an activity—often by family members.

Sleepwalking Violence versus *DSM-IV* Disorders Characterized by Violence or Aggression

Aggressive or violent patients diagnosed with *DSM-IV*-defined disorders—severe conduct disorder, antisocial personality disorder, and intermittent explosive disorder—may have certain neurophysiological elements in common with violent sleepwalkers. These groups have frontal lobe dysfunctions of various types on neurophysiological tests, and SWS quantity and percentage are reported to be significantly elevated compared to normal controls.[43–45] Violence while awake due to reduced inhibition of limbic impulses could be a result of reduced frontal lobe size and/or activity. Increased SWS activity could also be related.[46,47]

A synthesis of the neurophysiological literature suggests that the functional deactivation of the frontal lobes during SWS has distinct similarities to changes in frontal lobe size and activity that are reported in aggressive or violent individuals. The failure of the thalamus to completely gate afferent impulses in sleepwalkers allows these impulses to reach the cortex in the absence of frontal lobe inhibitions.

There is no evidence that violent sleepwalkers differ from nonviolent sleepwalkers in any way. Theoretically, any sleepwalker might respond to a perceived threat or close proximity with violence. Aggression or violence is not reported in the overwhelming majority of sleepwalking, confusional arousal, and sleep terror episodes. Sleepwalkers are not inherently violent. Furthermore, when episodes of sleepwalking violence do occur, they are almost never repeated.[48] Violent sleepwalking episodes appear to require not only a "perfect storm" of genetic predisposition, priming factors such as sleep deprivation and situational stress, and a proximal trigger but also provocation and/or close proximity.

Injury to Self

In addition to deaths of others attributed to sleepwalking-related violence, deaths of sleepwalkers as a result of their own behavior have been noted. In a number of cases, deaths ruled as suicides have been later shown to have resulted from night terrors, sleepwalking, or agitated sleepwalking.[49] In these cases patients fell out of windows or ran through glass doors. In one case a sleepwalker left his home in 30 degree weather in his underpants and then suddenly entered a local highway, where he was hit and killed by a car.

Schenck and colleagues surveyed a large group of patients with a diagnosis of sleepwalking or night terrors and found the following:[13]

- 53.7% reported running into walls or furniture or falling out of bed.
- 18.5% reported falling out of windows.
- 18.5% had left their homes. Behaviors included driving, climbing ladders, and walking into lakes.
- 7.4% reported they had handled loaded guns.

Their injuries included the following:

- 98.1% bruises
- 18.5% lacerations
- 5.6% fractures

There are also two reports of patients who jumped out of windows and suffered severe injuries leading to paraplegia.

REM SLEEP-RELATED PARASOMNIAS

REM sleep is a neurophysiologically distinct state of being. REM sleep is characterized by a low-voltage, mixed-frequency pattern of brain waves similar in many ways to that of wakefulness. Bursts of rapid eye movements are noted. Additionally, there is an active inhibition of somatic musculature. During REM sleep almost all voluntary muscles are atonic. REM sleep is also highly correlated with dreaming.

The inhibition of voluntary muscles during REM sleep is controlled by areas of the pons and medulla. Destruction of these centers in animals results in REM sleep without atonia. In this state animals are physically active and appear to be enacting common locomotor scenarios such as attacking imaginary objects.

REM sleep without atonia has also been reported in human beings most often in the form of REM sleep behavior disorder (RBD). First described in 1986, the pathophysiology of RBD is well described. Behaviors in RBD may superficially resemble those of disorders of arousal, but they are distinctly different in many ways.

Organic Changes in Brain Function That May Underlie Complex Behaviors in REM Sleep

While there is no evidence of neuropathology in disorders of arousal, RBD has been clearly linked to numerous degenerative brain diseases, including synucleinopathies, for example, Parkinson's disease, dementia with Lewy bodies, and multiple-system atrophy. Symptoms of RBD have been shown to precede the development of symptoms of parkinsonism and neurodegenerative diseases and to coexist in >50% of patients.[50, 51]

Functional Changes in Brain Function That May Underlie Complex Behaviors in REM Sleep

PATHOPHYSIOLOGY OF REM BEHAVIORS: ENACTING VERSUS REACTING

Complex behaviors due to RBD do not occur in all REM periods. Polysomnographic signs such as bursts of tonic electromyographic (EMG) activity may be present, but in most patients more complex behaviors occur intermittently or even rarely. What determines when a complex behavior will occur during RBD is unknown. It is true that the tonic EMG activity during REM in many patients is not continuous. Short periods of tonic EMG activity may limit the complexity of the behavior.

GENERAL LIMITATION ON COMPLEX BEHAVIORS IN REM SLEEP

RBD patients exist within their own dream world. They are not aware of the external environment, including the presence of bed partners or nearby furniture or windows. Their actions, movements, and behaviors are those of an actor in the dream. They may move their legs as they ride a bicycle in a dream, move their arms as if sword fighting as if repealing pirates in a dream, or get into a three-point position of a football player and launch themselves into space if playing football in a dream. While the trigger for a complex behavior in patients with a disorder of arousal is a partial arousal from sleep when a "perfect storm" of factors is present, the RBD patient enacts dreams. This is identical to what has been hypothesized for the cat with a brainstem lesion who during REM sleep without atonia appears to be stalking and attacking a dream mouse. Theoretically, there is no limitation to what behaviors might occur in REM sleep without atonia.

REM SLEEP BEHAVIOR DISORDER–RELATED VIOLENCE

There are numerous reported incidents of violent behaviors reported by patients during REM sleep without atonia. These resulted in injury to others as well as injury to themselves.

Injury to others has been reported in a recent review in 45.3% of men with RBD and and 45% of women.[51] RBD behaviors included the following:

1. Choking bed partner
2. Headlock on bed partner
3. Hitting, punching, and kicking
4. Pushing bed partner from bed
5. Throwing bed partner from bed

Injury to self has been reported in a recent review[52] in 47.3% of females and 55% of males. The most common behaviors resulting in self-injury from RBD were as follows:

1. Diving from the bed
2. Hitting or kicking furniture

Injuries include the following:

1. Bruises
2. Lacerations
3. Broken bones
4. Subdural hematomas

There have been no reports of deaths attributed to complex behaviors during RBD, but the complex behavior reported during RBD clearly has the potential for deadly consequences.

DISORDERS OF AROUSAL VERSUS REM BEHAVIOR DISORDER

Complex behaviors associated with disorders of arousal (DOAs) and RBD may appear similar. They may be differentiated in most cases as follows:

1. *Time of night.* DOAs occur early in the night when SWS is more likely to be present. RBD more often occurs later in the night when REM sleep is more likely to be present.
2. *Eyes.* DOA patients are reported to have eyes open; RBD patients are reported to have eyes closed.
3. *Memory.* Most DOA patients report complete amnesia for their episodes; RBD patients can describe the content of the dream they were enacting—often in great detail—and correlate their complex behaviors with dream content.

4. *Location.* Sleepwalkers and night terror patients may leave the bed, bedroom, and even the house. RBD patients almost never leave the bed. On occasion it has been reported that an RBD patient who dove out of bed serendipitously exited the door instead of hitting a wall.

5. *Trigger for violence.* DOA patients often react defensively to another individual who approaches them or who may try to block or touch them. DOA patients do not seek out their victims. RBD patients are not reacting defensively to the object of violence and are not seeking out victims. Rather, their violent actions are part of the dream sequence and those injured just happen to be in the path of the physical action.

6. *Medication effects.* Both DOA and RBD have been associated with medication effects. DOA has been associated with the use of sedative/hypnotic medications, especially when taken together with other psychotropic medications or CNS depressants. RBD has been associated with selective serotonin reuptake inhibitor antidepressants. RBD-like symptoms may also occur following sudden withdrawal of REM-suppressing medications or withdrawal from severe alcohol intoxication.

7. *Age.* DOAs are much more common in children and decrease significantly with age. RBD is rare in children and young adults and is much more common in older individuals.

8. *Concurrent medical disorders.* DOAs are not related to or are secondary to any medical disorder. RBD precedes and is often associated with serious degenerative brain disorders.

9. *Psychological disorders.* Neither DOA nor RBD is secondary to psychological disorders. However, the occurrence of a DOA is often associated with presence of situational stress.

ALCOHOL INTOXICATION VERSUS DISORDER OF AROUSAL/REM SLEEP BEHAVIOR DISORDER

Despite the generally held opinions of the lay public and out-of-date textbooks, there is no scientific evidence to support alcohol as a trigger or cause of DOA.[53] Alcohol intoxication has been frequently associated with disinhibition and violent behaviors.

As noted earlier, alcohol is not related to RBD, except in cases where severe alcoholics stop drinking suddenly. Alcohol is a potent suppressor of REM sleep, and an active alcoholic may have little or no REM sleep on a nightly basis. When the alcohol is withdrawn, a massive rebound of REM sleep may occur. During this rebound, a dissociation of the elements of REM sleep may occur. Presence of tonic EMG during REM sleep is a common finding. However, less use of alcohol has not been shown to have any relationship to RBD.

SUMMARY

Sleep-related complex behaviors are not uncommon. They can result in injury to the sleeper as well as others. The underlying pathophysiology and behaviors differ significantly between deep non-REM sleep and REM sleep.

REFERENCES

1. American Academy of Sleep Medicine. *International Classification of Sleep Disorders. Diagnostic and Coding Manual.* 2nd ed. Westchester, IL: American Academy of Sleep Medicine; 2005.
2. Jacobson A, Kales A, Lehmann D, et al. Somnambulism: all-night electroencephalographic studies. *Science* 1965:975–7.
3. Broughton RJ. Sleep disorders: disorders of arousal? *Science* 1968;159:1070–8.
4. Pressman MR. Factors that predispose, prime and precipitate NREM parasomnias in adults: clinical and forensic implications. *Sleep Medicine Reviews* 2007;11:5–30.
4a. Lecendreux M, Bassetti C, Dauvilliers Y, et al. HLA and genetic susceptibility to sleepwalking. *Mol Psychiatr* 2003;8:114–17.
5. Pilon M, Zadra A, Gosselin N, et al. Experimentally induced somnambulistic episodes in adult sleepwalkers: effects of forced arousal and sleep deprivation. *Sleep* 2005;28:A258.
6. Guilleminault C, Palombini L, Pelayo R, et al. Sleepwalking and sleep terrors in prepubertal children: what triggers them? *Pediatrics* 2003;111:e17-e25.
7. Guillemiault C, Kirisoglu C, Bao G, et al. Adult chronic sleepwalking and its treatment based on polysomnography. *Brain* 2005;128:1062–9.
8. Bassetti C, Vella S, Donati F, et al. SPECT during sleepwalking. *Lancet* 2000;356:484–5.
9. Braun A, Balkin T, Wesensten N, et al. Regional cerebral blood flow throughout the sleepwake cycle: an H2150 study. *Brain* 1997;120:1173–97.

10. Broughton RJ. NREM arousal parasomnias. In: Kryger MH, Roth T, Dement WC, eds. *Principles and Practice of Sleep Medicine*. 3rd ed. Philadelphia, PA: WB Saunders Company; 2000:1336.

11. Mahowald MW, Schenck CH. NREM sleep parasomnias. *Neurol Clin* 2005;23:1077–106.

12. Schenck CH, Mahowald MW. Injurious sleep behavior disorders (parasomnias) affecting patients on intensive care units. *Int Care Med* 1991;17:219–24.

13. Schenck CH, Milner DM, Hurwitz TD, et al. A polysomnographic and clinical report on sleep-related injury in 100 adult patients. *Am J Psychiatry* 1989;146:1166–73.

14. Pressman MR. Disorders of arousal from sleep and violent behavior: the role of physical contact and proximity. *Sleep* 2007;30(8):1039–47.

15. Guilleminault C, Moscovitch A, Yuen K, et al. Atypical sexual behavior during sleep. *Psychosom Med* 2002; 64:328–36.

16. Schenck CH, Arnulf I, Mahowald MW. Sleep and sex: what can go wrong? A review of the literature on sleep related disorders and abnormal sexual behaviors and experiences. *Sleep* 2007;2007:683–702.

17. Schenck CH, Hurwitz TD, Bundlie SR, et al. Sleep-related injury in 100 adult patients: a polysomnographic and clinical report. *Am J Psychiatry* 1989; 146:1166–73.

18. Guilleminault C, Moscovitch A, Leger D. Forensic sleep medicine: nocturnal wandering and violence. *Sleep* 1995;18:740–8.

19. Pressman MR. Sleep and drug impaired driving overlap syndrome. In: Pressman MR, ed. *Sleep Med Clin* 2011;6(4): 441–6.

20. Pressman MR. Sleep driving and z-drugs: sleepwalking variant or sedative-induced impaired driving. *Sleep Med Rev* 2011;15:285–92.

21. Siddiqui F, Osuna E, Chokroverty S. Writing emails as part of sleepwalking after increase in Zolpidem. *Sleep Med* 2009;10(2):262–4.

22. Tassinari CA, Rubboli G, Gardella E, et al. Central pattern generators for a common semiology in fronto-limbic seizures and in parasomnias. A neuroethologic approach. *Neurol Sci* 2005;26:S225–32.

23. Schenck CH, Mahowald MW. Review of nocturnal sleep-related eating disorders. *Int J Eat Disord* 1994;15:343–56.

24. Winkelman JW. Clinical and polysomnographic features of sleep-related eating disorder. *J Clin Psychiatry* 1998;59:14–19.

25. Ohayon MM, Schenck CH. Violent behavior during sleep: prevalence, comorbidity and consequences. *Sleep Med* 2010;11(9):941–6.

26. Mahowald MW, Bundlie SR, Hurwitz TD, et al. Sleep violence—forensic science implications: polygraphic and video documentation. *J Forensic Sci* 1990; 35:413–32.

27. Bonkalo A. Impulsive acts and confusional states during incomplete arousal from sleep: criminological and forensic implications. *Psychiat Q* 1974;48:400–9.

28. H.M. Advocate v Simon Fraser (1878) 4 Couper 70.

29. Yellowless D. Homicide by a somnambulist. *J Ment Sci* 1878;24:451–8.

30. Bracha HS, Ralston TC, Matsukawa JM, et al. Does fight or flight need updating? *Psychosomatic Medicine* 2004;45:448–9.

31. Pressman MR, Meyer TJ, Kendrick-Mohamed J, et al. Night terrors in an adult precipitated by sleep apnea. *Sleep* 1995;18:773–5.

32. Zadra A, Pilon M, Montplaisir J. Phenomenology of somnambulism SLEEP. *Abstract Supplement* 2006;29:A269.

33. Nauta W. The problem of the frontal lobe. *J Psychiatr Res* 1971;17:367–70.

34. Filley CM, Price BH, Nell V, et al. Toward an understanding of violence: neurobehavioral aspects of unwarranted physical aggression: Aspen Neurobehavioral Conference consensus statement. *Neuropsychiatry Neuropsychol Behav Neurol* 2001;14:1–14.

35. Hawkings KA, Trobst KK. Frontal lobe dysfunction and aggression: conceptual issues and research findings. *Aggression Violent Behav* 2000;5:147–57.

36. Brower MC, Price BH. Neuropsychiatry of frontal lobe dysfunction in violent and criminal behaviour: a critical review. *J Neurol Neurosurg Psychiatry* 2001;71:720–6.

37. Kaufmann C, Wehrle R, Wetter TC, et al. Brain activation and hypothalamic functional connectivity during human non-rapid eye movement sleep: an EEG/fMRI study. *Brain* 2006;129:655–67.

38. Wu JC, Gillin JC, Buchsbaum MS, et al. Frontal lobe metabolic decreases with sleep deprivation not totally reversed by recovery sleep. *Neuropsychopharmacology* 2006;31(12):2783–92.

39. Hofle N, Paus T, Reutens D, et al. Regional cerebral blood flow changes as a function of delta and spindle activity during slow wave sleep in humans. *J Neurosci* 1997;17:4800–8.

40. Dang-Vu TT, Desseilles M, Laureys S, et al. Cerebral correlates of delta waves during non-REM sleep revisited. *Neuroimage* 2005;28:14–21.

41. Albert DJ, Walsh ML, Jonik RH. Aggression in humans: what is its biological foundation? *Neurosci Biobehav Rev* 1993;17:405–25.

42. Albert DJ, Walsh ML. The inhibitory modulation of agonistic behavior in the rat brain: a review. *Neurosci Biobehav Rev* 1982;6:125–43.

43. Lindberg N, Tani P, Appelberg B, et al. Human impulsive aggression: a sleep research perspective. *J Psychiatr Research* 2003;37:313–24.

44. Lindberg N, Tani P, Appelberg B, et al. Sleep among habitually violent offenders with antisocial personality disorder. *Neuropsychobiology* 2003;47:198–205.

45. Coble PA, Taska LS, Kupfer DJ, et al. EEG sleep "abnormalities" in preadolescent boys with a diagnosis of conduct disorder. *J Am Acad Child Psychiatry* 1984;23:438–47.

46. Kim MS, Kim JJ, Kwon JS. Frontal P300 decrement and executive dysfunction in adolescents with conduct problems. *Child Psychiatry Hum Dev* 2001;32:93–106.

47. Lueger RJ, Gill KJ. Frontal-lobe cognitive dysfunction in conduct disorder adolescents. *J Clin Psychol* 1990;46:696–706.

48. Schenck CH, Mahowald MW. A polysomnographically documented case of adult somnambulism with long-distance automobile driving and frequent nocturnal violence: parasomnia with continuing danger as a noninsane automatism? *Sleep* 1995;18:765–72.

49. Mahowald MW, Schenck CH, Goldner M, et al. Parasomnia pseudo-suicide. *J Forensic Sci* 2003;48:1158–62.

50. Boeve BF, Silber MH, Parisi JE, et al. Synucleinopathy pathology often underlies REM sleep behavior disorder and dementia or parkinsonism. *Neurology* 2003; 61:40–5.

51. Plazzi G, Corsini R, Provini F, et al. REM sleep behavior disorders in multiple system atrophy. *Neurology* 1997; 48:1094–7

52. Schenck CH, Lee SA, Cramer Bornemann MA, et al. Potentially lethal behaviors associated with rapid eye movement sleep behavior disorder. Review of the literature and forensic implications. *J Forensic Sci* 2009;54(6):1475–84.

53. Pressman MR, Mahowald MW, Schenck CH, et al. Alcohol-induced sleep-walking or confusional arousal as a defense to criminal behavior: a review of scientific evidence, methods and forensic implications. *J Sleep Res* 2007;16:198–212.

37

Benign Sleep Myoclonus of Infancy

PHILIP A. HANNA, TASNEEM PEERAULLY, NANCY GADALLAH, AND ARTHUR S. WALTERS

MYOCLONUS IS defined as sudden, brief, shock-like involuntary movements involving the face, extremities, and trunk and arising from the central nervous system.[1-3] In the neonatal period, myoclonus may raise concerns as to whether the involuntary movements reflect seizures, which may indicate underlying brain pathology such as a progressive encephalopathy.[4] Benign sleep myoclonus of infancy (BSMI), formerly known as benign neonatal sleep myoclonus (BNSM), is a nonepileptic phenomenon typically presenting between birth and 1 month of age and resolving by 6 months, although it may persist up to 1 year of age. It is characterized by repetitive myoclonic jerks involving the whole body, trunk, or limbs, which usually occur only during quiet sleep. Rocking will often precipitate these myoclonic jerks. There is consistently reproducible immediate cessation upon arousal, although it does not itself trigger arousal. In addition, there should be no electroencephalographic (EEG) abnormalities suggestive of seizures. In general, infants have normal psychomotor development, with no requirement for treatment, and a good outcome.[5-15] Thus, recognition of this benign condition is critical in order to avoid unnecessary, costly, and potentially harmful testing and treatment.

The myoclonic jerks seen in BSMI may be partial, multifocal, or generalized.[5-12] The myoclonic jerks are often bilateral and massive, typically involving large muscle groups. The myoclonic jerks last 40 to 300 milliseconds at a frequency of 1 per second,[5,8,12,16] typically with 4–5 jerks in a cluster, although clusters may last up to 60 minutes.[5] In four of the ten patients reported by Daoust-Roy and Seshia,[5] the duration and the amplitude of the myoclonic jerks simulated "convulsive status epileptics or serial convulsive seizures." The myoclonic jerks in BSMI do not remit[17] and may even worsen[5] if restraint is attempted. Although nearly one third of neonates are initially placed on anticonvulsants prior to a correct diagnosis,[12] these agents are not effective. In fact, Daoust-Roy and Seshia[5] reported worsening of myoclonus in two of their patients treated with anticonvulsants. Furthermore, Reggin and Johnson[18] reported worsening of BSMI with the use of benzodiazepines.

In a study of 18 patients (10 male, 8 female) with a diagnosis of benign neonatal sleep myoclonus who underwent EEG and video monitoring, 94% had bilateral upper- and lower-extremity myoclonus, 66.7% had lateralized features, 53% had asymmetrical jerking, and 11% had head and facial myoclonus. In addition, myoclonus during the transition from sleep to awakening was observed in two children.[19] A Slovenian study of 38 infants with BNSM found a 2:1 ratio of males to females. Jerks were noted by parents most commonly when the infant was falling asleep (9/16) and were most frequent in the first month of life (12/16).[20] A review of 24 articles, encompassing a total of 216 infants with BSMI, by Maurer et al. found reports of myoclonus occurring during all stages of sleep, but only rarely during active sleep.[21]

Although *The International Classification of Sleep Disorders* emphasizes that infants with BSMI have normal psychomotor development, Paro-Panjan and Neubauer commented that mild nonspecific neurological abnormalities may be present, predominantly in those with prenatal or perinatal risk factors. In their study of 38 infants with BNSM, hyperirritability was found in 11 and hypotonia in 5. At follow-up between 3 and 12 months of age, mild abnormalities in axial tone were found in 8 infants.[20]

DIFFERENTIAL DIAGNOSIS

The differential diagnosis for BSMI can be divided into convulsive (epileptic) and nonepileptic disorders (see Tables 37.1 and 37.2). These epileptic conditions include neonatal seizures (which may be in the context of perinatal asphyxia, metabolic disturbances, or infectious processes), pyridoxine-dependent seizures, benign neonatal seizures (familial or nonfamilial), or infantile spasms[22,23] (Table 37.1). BSMI also needs to be distinguished from nonepileptic paroxysmal conditions such as hyperekplexia,[24,25] benign myoclonus of early infancy,[26] phasic REM twitches, hypnic jerks/sleep starts,[27] excessive fragmentary myoclonus,[28–30] and withdrawal from opiates.[31]

Epileptic Conditions

The epileptic conditions listed in the previous section are relatively easily distinguished from

BSMI due to the clinical status of the newborn, EEG findings, and relationship of the observed movements to the sleep-wake cycle. In an otherwise healthy newborn, the main diagnostic challenge is differentiating BSMI from benign neonatal (familial or nonfamilial) seizures, though the presence of generalized spike-wave complexes in EEG recordings of benign neonatal seizures, compared with normal EEG findings in BSMI, is clinically important. Please refer to Table 37.1 for further details regarding these epileptic conditions.

Nonepileptic Conditions

Hyperekplexia, a nonepileptic phenonemon, is characterized by excess motor response/startle to unexpected auditory, visual, or somaesthetic stimuli.[24,25] While hyperekplexia may be secondary to brainstem pathology, it also occurs as an autosomal dominant condition linked to chromosome 5q, identified as a point mutation in the alpha-1 subunit of the glycine receptor.[32] Newborns with hyperekplexia may have prominent myoclonic jerks during the first few hours of life, which may occur either in sleep or wakefulness. In addition, they may have more prolonged tonic spasms, usually triggered by external stimulation, but may occur spontaneously, mimicking seizures.[6] Apnea, cyanosis, and bradycardia may be associated with these attacks, even resulting in sudden infant death.[33] The interictal EEG is normal and, according to Di Capua et al.,[6] the most potent stimulus for triggering a startle is tactile stimulation of the glabella, which does not evoke a response in patients with BNSM.

In contrast to BSMI, benign myoclonus of infancy has a later age of onset and the myoclonic jerks are present strictly during wakefulness, whereas myoclonus is limited to sleep in BSMI. Of note, 2 of the 21 patients with BNSM reported by Caraballos[15] later developed benign myoclonus of infancy.

BSMI also needs to be distinguished from phasic REM twitches, a normal phenomenon present is all individuals. Phasic REM twitches consist of small movements, most commonly of the digits, face, and corner of the mouth, although they can occur in any muscle group, generally without visible movement across a joint space. These small movements typically are in clusters lasting 5–15 seconds. In the neonate, brief smiles, facial grimaces, and isolated twitches are seen in REM sleep.

Table 37.1 Characteristics of the Differential Diagnosis of Benign Sleep Myoclonus of Infancy—Epileptic Disorders

ETIOLOGY	TYPE OF MOVEMENT	DURATION/ FREQUENCY	WAKE/ SLEEP	AGE OF ONSET	COURSE	FAMILIAL PATTERN	POLYSOMNOG-RAPHY/ EEG	ACCENTUATING/ INHIBITING FACTORS
Benign sleep myoclonus of infancy	Flexion/ extension or abduction/ adduction. UE>LE	Clusters of 4–5 jerks (each 40–300 ms) at 1 per second	Only during sleep	First week of life	Benign. Usually resolve by 6–7 months of age. May persist until 1 year of age.	Occ. History	Primarily in quiet sleep. 40–300 ms jerks. EEG: normal; may have increased sharp transients.	May worsen with anticonvulsants, restraint. Precipitated by rocking.
Neonatal seizures (asphyxia, infection, metabolic causes)	Variable	Variable	Both	Variable	Variable	Variable	EEG: epileptiform discharges	Treatment with anticonvulsants.
Pyridoxine-dependent seizures	Multifocal clonic jerks	Status epilepticus frequent	Both	Immed. newborn period	Psycho-motor delay; may be fatal if not treated	AR	Continuous generalized or multifocal spikes	Pyridoxine—dramatic response
Benign familial neonatal seizures	Multifocal clonic jerks	Brief, intermittent	Both	First week	Resolve within 6 weeks	AD. Chrom. 8 or 20	EEG: interictal normal. Generalized spike wave during clonic phase	N/A
Infantile spasms	Flexor or extensor spasms	Brief flexion. 2–10 second tonic phase	Primarily while awake	Peak 4–7 months	Variable	Variable	Hypsarrhythmia	ACTH, steroids, clonazepam, valproate lessen spasms

ACTH, adrenocorticotropic hormone; AD, autosomal dominant; AR, autosomal recessive; EEG, electroencephalogram; LE, lower extremity; N/A, not applicable; UE, upper extremity.

Table 37.2 Characteristics of the Differential Diagnosis of Benign Sleep Myoclonus of Infancy — Nonepileptic Disorders

ETIOLOGY	TYPE OF MOVEMENT	DURATION/ FREQUENCY	WAKE/ SLEEP	AGE OF ONSET	COURSE	FAMILIAL PATTERN	POLYSOMNOG-RAPHY/ EEG	ACCENTUATING/ INHIBITING FACTORS
Benign sleep myoclonus of infancy	Flexion/ extension or abduction/ adduction. UE>LE	Clusters of 4–5 jerks (each 40–300 ms) at 1 per second	Only during sleep	1st week of life	Benign. Usually resolve by 6–7 months of age. May persist until 1 year of age.	Occasional history	Primarily in quiet sleep. 40–300 ms jerks. EEG: normal; may have increased sharp transients	May worsen with anticonvulsants, restraint. Precipitated by rocking.
Hyperekplexia	Exaggerated startle, stiff on awakening and in sleep	Variable	Both?	At birth or infancy	May be lifelong	AD. Chrom. 5q	Infantile apnea	Valproate or clonazepam help. Triggered by external stimuli
Benign myoclonus of early infancy	Generalized contractions	Clusters	Only while awake	Early infancy	3 months duration; stop by 2 years	N/A	Normal EEG	?
Phasic REM twitches	Small focal twitches of digits, face, mouth, or small muscle groups	5–15 second clusters	During REM sleep	Any age	Normal event	N/A	Few second clusters of EMG potentials. Similar in duration to excessive fragmentary myoclonus	?

(Continued)

Table 37.2 Continued

ETIOLOGY	TYPE OF MOVEMENT	DURATION/ FREQUENCY	WAKE/ SLEEP	AGE OF ONSET	COURSE	FAMILIAL PATTERN	POLYSOMNOG- RAPHY/ EEG	ACCENTUATING/ INHIBITING FACTORS
Hypnic jerks/ sleep starts	Single contraction LE>UE	Single	Sleep onset	Any age	Benign	N/A	Transition from wake to sleep. Brief, high-amplitude muscle potentials	?
Excessive fragmentary myoclonus	Small focal twitches of digits, face, mouth, or small muscle groups	irregular for 10 min to >60 min	Sleep; all stages	Usually older males	Benign	N/A	Recurrent brief 75–150 ms EMG potentials	?
Opiate withdrawal	Tremor, myoclonus	May be continual	Only during wake	First 48 hours	Variable	None	Disrupted sleep architecture	Phenobarbital for seizures; clonidine for autonomic symptoms.

EEG, electroencephalogram; EMG, electromyogram; LE, lower extremity; N/A, not applicable; REM, rapid eye movement sleep; UE, upper extremity.

Another phenomenon with similar appearance to phasic REM twitches is excessive fragmentary myoclonus,[28-30] where brief (<150-millisecond), fine twitches of distal limbs and face occur at irregular frequencies, typically lasting 10 to 60 minutes. Similar to phasic REM twitches, the movements in excessive fragmentary myoclonus can occur in any muscle group, sometimes without visible movement across a joint space. Unlike phasic REM twitches, which are present only during REM sleep, the movements in excessive fragmentary myoclonus may be present in any stage of sleep, and during REM they are not easily distinguished from phasic REM twitches.

Hypnic jerks (sleep starts) are characterized by single, brief, large-amplitude movements across large joint spaces such as elbows, hips, and knees and occur at sleep onset. While hypnic jerks are a common phenomenon, not all individuals will have sleep starts during their lifetime. Like phasic REM twitches, hypnic jerks are considered a normal phenomenon. (See Table 37.2.)

ELECTROENCEPHALOGRAPHY

With regard to the EEG findings in patients with BSMI, Daoust-Roy and Seshia[5] found an increased frequency of sharp transients in four of their ten patients compared with normal neonates as reported by Karbowski and Nencka.[34] Scher[35] concluded that the clinical importance of spikes and sharp waves in neonates has not been clearly established; thus, Daoust-Roy and Seshia[5] suggested that frequent sharp transients in neonatal EEGs "on an otherwise normal background, can be associated with subsequent normalcy," given the good neurodevelopmental outcome in their patients. A limitation of the study by Caraballo[15] is that in only five patients were EEGs performed during the events and only two patients had video-EEG monitoring, unlike studies by Daoust-Roy and Seshia[5] and Di Capua et al.[6] in which EEG studies were done during the myoclonic episodes. In fact, in Daost-Roy and Seshia, for example, neonates were excluded if events did not occur during EEG recording.

PATHOGENESIS INCLUDING FAMILY HISTORY

The pathogenesis of BSMI is not well understood. Coulter and Allen[7] postulated that BSMI may represent a disturbance of the reticular activating system. Resnick et al.[11] suggested the possibility of a transient imbalance of serotonin as patients with posthypoxic myoclonus have low cerebrospinal fluid levels of 5-hydroxyindoleacetic acid.

BSMI may be related to the incomplete maturation of sleep patterns in infancy, in particular suppression of body movements during quiet sleep mediated by thalamocortical networks, which requires complex feedback mechanisms.[36]

In reference to family history data, Tardieu et al.[10] suggested that a genetic factor was likely in that one of their four patients had a family history of sleep myoclonus. Daoust-Roy and Seshia[5] also reported a family history of sleep myoclonus in the parents of a few of their patients but warned that objective data in the form of polysomnography are needed in order to more precisely ascertain the true familial incidence and prevalence.

There have been several reports of familial cases described in the literature. Vaccario et al. reported on five siblings, two male and three female with typical BNSM with a negative parental history, suggestive of an autosomal recessive inheritance pattern.[37]

More recently, Cohen et al reported on three patients from the same family (a brother, sister, and female cousin) affected with BSMI. The authors postulated autosomal recessive inheritance versus autosomal dominant inheritance with incomplete penetrance.[36]

TRIGGERING FACTORS AND TREATMENT CONSIDERATIONS

Alfonso et al.[12] reported four neonates with BNSM in whom rocking motion precipitated the repetitive myoclonic jerks. All of these patients underwent continuous video-EEG telemetry, and the myoclonic jerks were triggered by rocking of the mattress in a head-to-toe direction, particularly during quiet sleep. They initiated the rocking motion at low frequency, which was increased until either the neonate awakened or had a "paroxysmal motor event." The events described were "low-frequency repetitive limb jerks without concomitant EEG changes."

Neonatal abstinence syndrome (NAS) occurs in newborns exposed to opiates before birth and is characterized by poor feeding, gastrointestinal disorders, and abnormal sleep patterns as well as jitteriness and tremors. Held-Egli et al. found a 26-fold increased incidence of BNSM in infants with NAS compared with controls.[38] They identified 78 infants with NAS and 78 age-matched controls. BNSM was diagnosed in 67% of infants with NAS compared to 2.6% of controls. The myoclonus was noted to appear as early as day 2 and as late as day 56 of life, lasting between 1 and 93 days. Ninety-seven percent of infants with NAS were treated with, either morphine (30 infants) or chlorpromazine. Those treated with chlorpromazine alone had an 82% incidence of BNSM compared to a 47% incidence in those treated with morphine alone, suggesting that chlorpromazine may induce myoclonus in these cases.

Similar to reports by others, restraining the limbs did not stop the myoclonic jerks, while awaking did bring cessation. They report that this rocking maneuver can help in distinguishing BNSM from seizures in that rocking does not activate neonatal seizures. As described at the beginning, no treatment is indicated for BSMI, and medications such as anticonvulsants, including benzodiazepines, have been reported to worsen the myoclonus.

CONCLUSION

In summary, benign sleep myoclonus of infancy is a nonepileptic phenomenon typically manifesting as brief (though may be prolonged), often repetitive and bilateral myoclonic jerks, most prominent in the upper limbs and usually occurring during non-REM sleep. These myoclonic jerks are not associated with EEG abnormalities suggesting seizures, may worsen with anticonvulsants and restraint, are triggered by rocking, and cease upon arousal. They tend to remit by 6 to 7 months of age, although the condition may persist up to 1 year of age as reflected by the new nomenclature, being a change from benign neonatal sleep myoclonus to benign sleep myoclonus of infancy. The pathophysiology has not been clearly established. As BSMI is in the differential diagnosis of neonatal seizures and as the early literature did not always distinguish this condition from epileptic phenomenon, recognition and understanding of these benign movements are important so as to avoid unnecessary testing and potentially harmful treatment.

REFERENCES

1. Fahn S, Marsden CD, Van Woert M. Definition and classification of myoclonus. In: Fahn S, Marsden CD, Van Woert M, eds. *Myoclonus. Advances in Neurology*, Vol. 43. New York: Raven, 1986:1–5.
2. Shibasaki J. Myoclonus and startle syndromes. In: Jankovic J, Tolosa E, eds. *Parkinson's Disease and Movement Disorders*. Baltimore, MD: Williams and Wilkins: 1998:453–66.
3. Dyken ME, Rodnitzky RL. Periodic, aperiodic, and rhythmic motor disorders of sleep. *Neurology* 1992;42(Suppl 6):68–74.
4. Aicardi J, Goutieres F. Encephalopathie myoclonique neonatale. *Rev Eeg Neurophysiol* 1978;8:99–101.
5. Daoust-Roy J, Seshia SS. Benign neonatal sleep myoclonus. A differential diagnosis of neonatal seizures. *Am J Dis Child* 1992;146:1236–41.
6. Di Capua M, Fusco L, Ricci S, et al. Benign neonatal sleep myoclonus: clinical features and video-polygraphic recordings. *Mov Disord* 1993;8:191–4.
7. Coulter DL, Allen RJ. Benign neonatal sleep myoclonus. *Arch Neurol* 1982;39:191–2.
8. Blennow G. Benign infantile nocturnal myoclonus. *Acta Paediatr Scand* 1985;74:505–7.
9. Dooley JM. Myoclonus in children. *Arch Neurol* 1984;41:138.
10. Tardieu M, Khoury W, Navelet Y, et al. A spectacular and benign syndrome of neonatal convulsions: deep sleep myoclonus. *Arch Fr Pediatr* 1986;43:259–60.
11. Resnick TJ, Moshe SL, Perotta L, et al. Benign neonatal sleep myoclonus. Relationship to sleep states. *Arch Neurol* 1986;43:266–8.
12. Alfonso I, Papazian O, Aicardi J, et al. A simple maneuver to provoke benign neonatal sleep myoclonus. *Pediatrics* 1995;96:1161–3.
13. Queralt A. Parasomnias in infants below one-year old of age. *Rev Neurol* 1998;26:476–9.
14. Noone PG, King M, Loftus BG. Benign neonatal sleep myoclonus. *Ir Med J* 1995;88:172.
15. Caraballo R, Yepez I, Cersosimo R, et al. Benign neonatal sleep myoclonus. *Rev Neurol* 1998;26:540–4.
16. Thorpy MJ and the Diagnostic Classification Steering Committee. *The International Classification of Sleep Disorders: Diagnostic and Coding Manual*. Rochester, MN: American Sleep Disorders Association; 1990.
17. Smith LJ, Thomas NH. Benign neonatal sleep myoclonus. *Am J Dis Child* 1993;147:817.

18. Reggin JD, Johnson MI. Exacerbation of benign neonatal sleep myoclonus by benzodiazepines. *Ann Neurol* 1989;26:455.

19. Kaddurah AK, Holmes GL. Benign neonatal sleep myoclonus: history and semiology. *Pediatr Neurol* 2009;40(5)343–6.

20. Paro-Panjan D, Neubauer D. Benign neonatal sleep myoclonus: experience from the study of 38 infants. *Eur J Pediatr Neurol* 2008;12:14–18.

21. Maurer VO, Rizzi M, Bianchetti MG, Ramelli GP. Benign neonatal sleep myoclonus: a review of the literature. *Pediatrics* 2010;12:e919–24.

22. Volpe JJ. Neonatal seizures. In: Volpe JJ, ed. *Neurology of the Newborn*. Philadelphia, PA: WB Saunders; 1995:172–207.

23. Fenichel GM. Paroxysmal disorders. In: Fenichel GM, ed. *Clinical Pediatric Neurology*. Philadelphia, PA: WB Saunders; 1997:1–46.

24. Andermann F, Andermann E. Excessive startle syndromes:startle disease, jumping, and startle epilepsy. *Adv Neurol* 1986;43:321–38.

25. Brown P, Rothwell JC, Thompson PD, et al. The hyperekplexias and their relationship to the normal startle reflex. *Brain* 1991;114:1903–28.

26. Lombroso CT, Fejerman N. Benign myoclonus of early infancy. *Ann Neurol* 1977;1:137–43.

27. Rechtschaffen A, Kales A, eds. *A Manual of Standardized Terminology, Techniques and Scoring System for Sleep Stages of Human Subjects*. University of California, Los Angeles: Brain Information Service/Brain Research Institute;1968.

28. Lins O, Castonguay M, Dunham W, et al. Excessive fragmentary myoclonus: time of night and sleep stage distributions. *Can J Neurol Sci* 1993;20:142–6.

29. Broughton R, Tolentino MA, Krelina M. Excessive fragmentary myoclonus in NREM sleep: a report of 38 cases. *Electroencephalogr Clin Neurophysiol* 1985;61:123–33.

30. Broughton R, Tolentino MA. Fragmentary pathological myoclonus in NREM sleep. *Electroencephalogr Clin Neurophysiol* 1984;57:303–9.

31. Lane JC, Tennison MB, Lawless ST, et al. Clinical and laboratory obsevation. Movement disorder after withdrawal of fenanyl infusion. *J Pediatr* 1991;119:649–51.

32. Shiang R, Ryan SG, Zhu YZ, et al. Mutational analysis of familial and sporadic hyperekplexia. *Ann Neurol* 1995;38:85–91.

33. Vigevano F, Di Capua M, Dalla Bernardina B. Startle disease: an avoidable cause of sudden infant death. *Lancet* 1989;1:216.

34. Karbowski K, Nencka A. Right mid-temporal sharp EEG transients in healthy newborns. *Electroencephalogr Clin Neurophysiol* 1980;48:461–9.

35. Scher MS. Pathologic myoclonus of the newborn: electrographic and clinical correlations. *Pediatr Neurol* 1985;1:342–8.

36. Cohen R, Shuper A, Straussberg R. Familial benign neonatal sleep myoclonus. *Pediatr Neurol* 2007;36:334–337.

37. Vaccario ML, Valenti MA, Carullo A, Di Bartolomeo R, Mazza S. Benign sleep myoclonus of infancy: case report and follow-up of four members of an affected family. *Clin Electroencephalogr* 2003;33(1):15–17.

38. Held-Egli K, Ruegger C, Das-Kundu S, Schmitt B, Bucher HU. Benign neonatal sleep myoclonus in newborn infants of opioid dependent mothers. *Acta Paediatrica* 2009;98:69–73.

C

Movement Disorders and Sleep

38

Movement Disorders and Sleep

Introduction

STANLEY FAHN AND SUDHANSU CHOKROVERTY

BOTH SLEEP specialists and movement disorder specialists see patients presenting with a variety of movements, some physiologic and some pathologic, which continue into or only manifest during sleep at night. At times it may be difficult to differentiate physiologic from pathologic movements. Sometimes one is not certain whether these movements are triggered by a particular state or stages of sleep or whether they simply represent reemergence or persistence of the abnormal movements that the patients may have during the daytime. What generates these abnormal movements? We are still ignorant about the ways the movements are generated by the central nervous system. We have better ideas about the genesis of the diurnal movement disorders than of sleep-related nocturnal movements. Some are hereditary, whereas others are nonfamilial. Some are drug induced or result from deficiency, excess, or other dysfunction of the neurotransmitters. Molecular neurobiology of sleep-related abnormal movements

remains an unexplored and unexplained science at present.

For the neurologist or movement disorder specialist, sleep has often formed a neglected corner of the clinical picture. However, in the last decade there has been an ever-increasing interest in the problems of sleep and their impact on quality of life and daytime symptoms, which has extended to patients with diurnal movement disorders. It has become clear that sleep is important and that its abnormalities cannot be neglected in clinical practice. This development has recently been underlined by controversies about the role of medications inducing sleepiness in patients with Parkinson's disease (PD).[1-3] The report that some of the newer dopamine agonists may induce sudden and unpredictable "sleep attacks" that might result in automobile accidents created shock waves in the movement disorder community. That initial report has led to a barrage of replies trying to define whether there is any specific role for these agents in causing unexpected sleepiness in PD and even wondering to what extent these sleep attacks have any actual validity or are even new phenomena. Although this controversy has generated much heat, it has also begun to shed a strong and useful light on the whole issue of sleep in the field of movement disorders. This has begun to extend from PD patients to other patients with akinetic disorders and even to the general field of hyperkinetic movement disorders. It is important to mention that James Parkinson in his 1817 treatise[4] clearly pointed out about two important observations, which contemporary movement disorder specialists neglected to emphasize until recently: sleep dysfunction as a prominent feature and persistence of tremor in the light stage of sleep. The following quotes from James Parkinson clearly make these points: "But as the malady proceeds ..." (p. 6). "In this stage (stooped posture with 'unwillingly a running pace' ... *most likely stage* 3), then sleep becomes much disturbed. The tremulus motion of the limbs occur[s] during sleep, and augment[s] until they awaken the patient, and frequently with much agitation and alarm" (p. 7). "... and at the last (advanced bedridden stage), constant sleepiness, with slight delirium, and other marks of extreme exhaustion, announce the wished-for release" (p. 9).

For a long time REM behavior disorder (RBD) was thought to be an idiopathic REM parasomnia until Schenck and Mahowald[5] reported delayed emergence of a parkinsonian disorder in 38% of 29 older men initially diagnosed with idiopathic RBD. It is now known that RBD may be an important nonmotor manifestation of PD preceding the disease, and, in fact, may be a preclinical marker of many neurodegenerative diseases, particularly synucleinopathies (e.g., PD, diffuse Lewy body disease, multiple-system atrophy). Intense research is currently under way globally to identify preclinical markers to diagnose and possibly in future prevent progression to or development of neurodegenerative diseases.

Another important neurological movement disorder impacting sleep is restless legs syndrome (RLS, now renamed Willis-Ekbom disease), which is slowly but surely finding its place in the diagnostic and therapeutic armamentarium of movement disorder specialists. There is also currently a hotly debated discussion about the relationship between PD and RLS that may shed light on understanding the pathophysiology of RLS, a largely undiagnosed and neglected condition. For those interested in the motor system and sleep, and its pathologies, this recent knowledge is a welcome development. It should help the clinician to take sleep seriously and the investigator to add the sleep-related aspects of movement disorders to his or her field of interest.

In this section, several experts discuss the effects of a variety of diurnal abnormal movements on sleep and the effect of sleep on these movement disorders and how the daytime and nighttime abnormal movements are modulated by sleep-wake states. The final two chapters in this section are devoted to general sleep difficulties in some psychiatric conditions that may be associated with abnormal movements, and pediatric sleep-related movement disorders.

REFERENCES

1. Frucht S, Rogers JD, Greene PE, et al. Falling asleep at the wheel: motor vehicle mishaps in persons taking pramipexole and ropinirole. *Neurology* 1999;58:1908.
2. Hobson DE, Lang AE, Martin WRW, et al. Excessive daytime sleepiness and sudden-onset sleep in Parkinson disease. *JAMA* 2002;287:455.
3. Comella CL. Daytime sleepiness, agonist therapy and driving in Parkinson disease [Editorial]. *JAMA* 2002;287:509.
4. Parkinson J. An essay on the shaking palsy. London: Whittingham and Rowland, 1817: 1–66.
5. Schenck CH, Mahowald MW. Delayed emergence of a Parkinsonian disorder in 38% of 29 older males initially diagnosed with idiopathic REM sleep behavior disorder. *Neurology* 1996;46:388.

39

Persistence of Daytime Movement Disorders during Sleep

ROSALIA C. SILVESTRI

ABNORMAL MOVEMENTS may be the consequence of different neurologic disorders, deriving either from higher center lesions, mostly cerebral cortex, basal ganglia, and the upper brainstem, or from the posterior fossa, the medulla, and the spinal cord.

The oldest literature reports based on clinical observation referred to the common disappearance of abnormal movements during sleep, with a few exceptions, including ballism.[1] This first observation was later modified by Tassinari and Broughton,[2,3] who noticed how parkinsonian and choreic patients may display occasional sleep "tremors" under selected circumstances, that is, arousals, body movements intervening during sleep and awakenings. Their report and a number of later ones included polygraphic recordings as evidence. An extensive review by Mano, Shaoizawa, and Sobu[4] in 1982 distinguished "extrapyramidal movements" by their origin from either supratentorial or lower brainstem and spinal cord. The former dyskinesias decrease constantly during sleep, maintaining the same electromyographic pattern as in waking. The latter instead increase remarkably during non–rapid eye movement (non-REM) sleep to subside early during rapid eye movement (REM). Most of the disorders, formerly presumed to be of spinal or mixed origin, are now considered idiopathic dyssomnias (periodic myoclonus, restless legs syndrome [RLS]) and are discussed elsewhere in this book.

The most common movement disorders are those involving basal ganglia pathologic condition, that is, Parkinson's disease, Huntington's disease, hemiballism, and Gilles de la Tourette's syndrome. A second group, in my view, includes cranial-facial dystonias to be distinguished from more widespread or peripheral disorders such as torsion dystonia, the extensive group of spino-cerebellar ataxias (SCAs), and finally myoclonic movements. Of the latter, only subcortical syndromes such as palatal myoclonus are included in this chapter.

PARKINSON'S DISEASE

Usually the motoric manifestations of the syndrome disappear with the occurrence of stage I sleep and are absent in slow-wave sleep (SWS) stages III to IV and REM. However, low-amplitude tremor may be occasionally present during stage II, in association with body movements, or during sleep transition to or from REM sleep[5,6] in agreement with the physiologic pattern of body movement facilitation during sleep transitions.[7] Tremor may be present overall in 30% of the time spent in bed, thus contributing to nocturnal discomfort and wakefulness. Askenasy and Yahr[8] reported that typical features of parkinsonian tremor, that is, the alternating contractions of agonist and antagonist muscles, disappear during sleep to be replaced by different muscle activities. Two types of sleep-related patterns are observed. One pattern corresponds to subclinical rhythmic contractions involving simultaneously all muscles of a joint. Frequency is constant through the same sleep stage and tends to decrease progressing to SWS, along with parallel muscle tone decrease. In addition, duration of contractions is influenced according to the same paradigm. This qualitatively different type of tremor may be compatible with the loss during sleep of a central oscillator activity, as well as loss of peripheral reciprocal inhibition. The second type of movements[5] consists of anarchic nonrhythmic muscle discharges accompanied by minimal movements only when meeting criteria for sufficient amplitude and duration (600 microseconds, 175 mV). According to Fish, Sawyers, Allen, et al.,[9] these movements, which are present during wakefulness, may intervene with decreasing frequency during arousal or shifts to lighter stages of sleep. These types of movements are the most commonly observed on polygraphic awakening and they appear to be inhibited by SWS amplitude criteria.

Conversely, nocturnal akinesia, stiffness, rigidity, and cogwheeling, albeit reduced during sleep, are often experienced as the most troublesome symptoms responsible for discomfort, if not pain, and sleep maintenance insomnia.

Abnormal tone and incoordination of the upper respiratory muscles may induce respiratory dysrhythmia often misinterpreted as sleep apnea. Careful L-dopa dosing at bedtime may relieve nocturnal akinesia as well as irregular respiration often at the price of nighttime hallucinations.

Periodic arm and leg movements during sleep and REM sleep behavior disorder (RBD), dealt with elsewhere in this book, represent other often-encountered features in parkinsonian sleep. Of notice, Kumru et al.[10] reported that RBD is definitely more common in akinetic rather than dyskinetic Parkinson's disease. RBD usually precedes Parkinson's disease onset by several years,[11] confirming Brak's theory about sleep involvement along with olfactory disturbance in the premotor phase of Parkinson's disease, stage 1 and 2, of the dorsal motor nucleus of the vagus and lower brainstem nuclei.[12]

Interestingly, beyond vocalization and violent aggressive movements, more fluent speech and unrestricted fine motor control have been noticed in RBD, leading to the concept of an ad interim REM restoration of motor control in Parkinson's disease, probably due to the unopposed direct cortical commands, bypassing the basal ganglia during this sleep phase.[13]

Besides an increased number of periodic limb movements during sleep, which are usually unassociated with arousals and therefore not responsible for sleep disruption,[14] there is an increased prevalence of RLS in Parkinson's disease, nearly 12%, often associated with initial insomnia (30%) and decreased quality of life.

Parkinson's disease diagnosis precedes RLS developments by several years in 80% of cases, but it remains unclear what contributes to RLS development in Parkinson's disease: long-term dopamine depletion, genetic and family factors, or primary striatal degeneration with presynaptic hypofunction?

In most studies, RLS was mild and predicted by low serum-ferretin levels.[15] The fact that symptoms correlated with "weaning off" at night raises the possibility of RLS mimics in patients with fluctuating control of Parkinson's disease.[16] Interestingly, the typical RLS augmentation phenomenon with L-dopa or dopamine agonists has never been reported in Parkinson's disease patients with RLS. Also, RLS alone, but not Parkinson's disease symptoms, are positively affected by opioids, gabapentin, pregabalin, and iron supplementation, whereas iron deposition in the substantia nigra pars compacta is typical of Parkinson's disease.

A distinctive, albeit rare, motor phenomenon seen in these patients' sleep is REM-onset blepharospasm.[17] Unfortunately, given the complex medical regimen in which patients are involved, it is difficult to differentiate disease from therapy and dose-related motor phenomena of sleep. Teeth grinding and nocturnal vocalization may also occur. Leg cramps and increased rigidity during REM are often reported. Sleep continuity is globally perturbed with an increased number of arousals that seem to correlate with dopaminergic therapy-induced psychiatric symptoms,[6] rather than daytime motor function variability.[18]

At a microstructural level, sleep spindle density in stage II is significantly reduced independent of age, duration of disease, or increasing functional impairment. According to Neal and Keane,[19] dopaminergic pathways are involved in the production of both spindles and slow waves. Therefore, dopamine reduction in the striatum of parkinsonian patients (also by interfering with the gamma-aminobutyric acid [GABA] ergic inhibitory system) may decrease at the same time as sleep spindling and SWS.

HUNTINGTON'S DISEASE

Nocturnal sleep in Huntington's disease is conversely characterized by increased density of sleep spindling[20-22] on a background of aspecific abnormalities, including increased sleep latency, number of awakenings, and reduced sleep efficiency. Controversial reports exist on SWS percentage, which usually is reported to be reduced[22,22] but is sometimes reported to be increased.[20]

A strong correlation between caudate atrophy on computed tomography scan, nighttime spent awake, and SWS reduction has been reported by Wiegand et al.[23] Decreased or absent REMs during paradoxical sleep have been reported not only in patients[22,24] but even in healthy offspring.[25] These offspring share with the patients reduced velocity of both vertical voluntary saccades and the fast phase of optokinetic nystagmus.

As for typical choreic movements, they tend to be suppressed at the beginning of sleep but may return during stage I or II and promptly during arousals (Fig. 39.1).[9,22,18] In several cases, they have even been recorded during REM.[2] Lugaresi, Cirignotta, and Montagna[26] reported prolonged dyskinetic bursts labeled as long-lasting attacks of nocturnal paroxysmal dystonia in one patient with Huntington's disease. However, this finding has so far remained isolated.

Initial and maintenance insomnia have both been reported in Huntington's disease, along with delayed awakening in the morning. Delayed sleep phase seems to be consistently associated with depression and lower cognitive testing.[27] A delayed onset of the diurnal melatonin rise and an increased rate of early day cortisol production in early-stage Huntington's disease might also explain such clinical symptoms. Also, excessive daytime somnolence is overtly associated with depression in Huntington's disease.

RBD has also been recently reported by several authors among night problems in Huntington's disease. Of the 25 patients reported by Morton et al.,[28] 12%, none of which were on antidepressants, had RBD, whereas some of the patients,

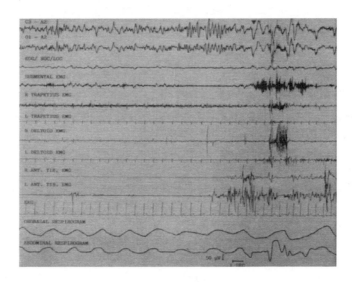

FIGURE 39.1 Huntington's disease. Movements involving the limbs precede an arousal.

23%, lately reported by Videnovic et al.[29] were on selective serotonin reuptake inhibitors.

RLS has also been described independently in Huntington's disease patients and unaffected members of the same family,[30] whereas some authors even suggested that RLS could be an early manifestation of Huntington's disease.[31]

AMYOTROPHIC CHOREOACANTHOCYTOSIS

Amyotrophic choreoacanthocytosis is a rare inherited disease of adult onset characterized by normal lipoproteinemic acanthocytosis and paroxysmal chorea complicated by tongue and lip biting, neurogenic muscle atrophy, and vocalization. Dyskinesias persist; they are decreased in amplitude, frequency, and duration during sleep and are observable in all sleep stages.[7] Vocalization is particularly prominent during REM sleep.

HEMIBALLISM

In this rare disorder, lesions caused by different etiologies impact on the subthalamic nucleus, causing typical slow, ample movements involving the proximal limbs contralaterally. Hyperkinesias, although decreased in frequency and intensity,[7] persist in light

non-REM sleep, stage I and II, but also during REM (Fig. 39.2). Other authors, however,[32,33] did not record any movements in REM sleep regardless of whether this sleep stage may have been underscored due to stroke-related absence of REMs.

GILLES DE LA TOURETTE'S SYNDROME

In Gilles de la Tourette's syndrome, a genetic disorder whose neurologic mechanisms are far from being fully understood, obsessive-compulsive disorder, motor tics, and vocalization represent the main symptoms, which fluctuate in severity for several years across a life span. Dopaminergic abnormalities in the ventral tegmental area may account for most of the symptoms,[34] including sleep abnormalities. Sleep is severely disturbed in children, who complain of severe insomnia and are also prone to parasomnias, especially night terrors and confusional arousals. These all decrease with age, and toward adolescence sleep efficiency and continuity tend to improve and converge on normal values.[35,36] SWS tends to extend at the expense of REM sleep. Tics and vocalization persist during sleep with up to 12 cluster episodes per night,[37] decreasing in frequency with increasing sleep depth

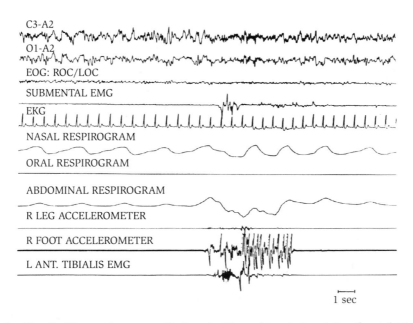

FIGURE 39.2 Hemiballism—sleep stage II. A typical hyperkinesia involving the right foot does not cause any arousal.

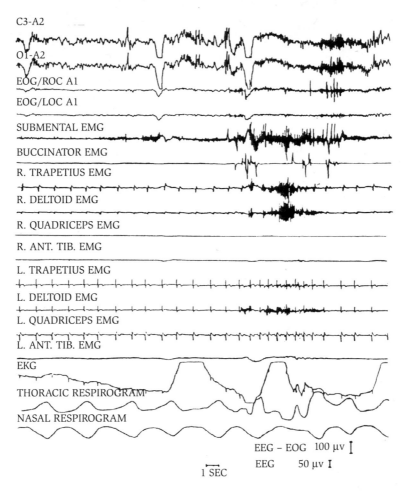

C3-A2

O1-A2

EOG/ROC A1

EOG/LOC A1

SUBMENTAL EMG

BUCCINATOR EMG

R. TRAPETIUS EMG

R. DELTOID EMG

R. QUADRICEPS EMG

R. ANT. TIB. EMG

L. TRAPETIUS EMG

L. DELTOID EMG

L. QUADRICEPS EMG

L. ANT. TIB. EMG

EKG

THORACIC RESPIROGRAM

NASAL RESPIROGRAM

EEG – EOG 100 µv

EEG   50 µv

1 SEC

FIGURE 39.3 Gilles de La Tourette's syndrome—sleep stage II. A series of complex movements determines a brief arousal (9 seconds).

(Figs. 39.3 and 39.4). They are almost absent during REM sleep, which is instead poorly defined. Movements can follow a spindle, as well as a K-complex following or preceding a subsequent arousal.[38] In addition, increased phasic motor activity and body movement, opposite to Parkinson's disease, are often reported. Also, sleep spindles are increased in severely disturbed sleep.

There seems to be a consistent age-related effect on sleep in Gilles de la Tourette's syndrome: sleep tics, vocalization, and also disorders of arousal tend to decrease with age,[39] replaced by more common periodic limb movements and RBD.[40,41]

Attention-deficit/hyperactivity disorder comorbidity impacts sleep efficiency and a hyperarousal tendency more severely,[42] whereas REM microarousals seem to be unique to Gilles de la Tourette's syndrome. Low ferritin, correlating with motor tic severity and prevalence of RLS, prompted a unifying theory on the role of iron metabolism for RLS, attention-deficit/hyperactivity disorder, and Gilles de la Tourette's syndrome.[43]

SPINAL CEREBELLAR ATAXIAS

Autosomal dominant SCAs are inherited neurodegenerative disorders characterized by progressive ataxias and various degrees of extrapyramidal symptoms, including parkinsonism, oculomotor abnormalities, Corea, dystonia, and brainstem signs. They result from mutations in different genes, leading to translated CAG repeat expansions producing abnormal protein aggregation or ion channel alterations in the central nervous system.

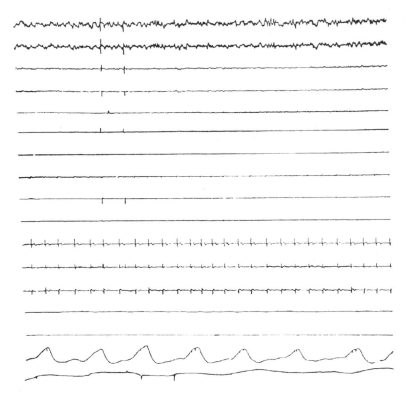

FIGURE 39.4   Gilles de La Tourette's syndrome—rapid eye movement (REM) sleep. Sample of indeterminate sleep electroencephalographic (EEG) and electromyographic (EMG) activity typical of stage REM yet total absence of eye movements.

The most common forms are SCA_1, SCA_2, SCA_3 (Machado-Joseph disease), and SCA_6. Central dopaminergic dysfunction with decreased nigro-striatal transporter binding with, but even without, extrapyramidal symptoms, is probably at the origin of most of sleep-related abnormalities in these patients.

SCA_3 patients are the ones referring most sleep abnormalities, ranging from insomnia to motor sensory dyscontrol during sleep.

Several reports described clinical and preclinical RBD in SCA3 patients[44,45] but also RLS,[46,47] with periodic limb movements index >15 usually unassociated with arousal.

Even hypnagogic/hypnopompic hallucinations were highly prevalent (38.4% vs. 9.43% in controls) in a recent cohort described by D'Abreu et al.[48]

SCA2 patients have marked cerebellar ataxia and slow eye movements as clinical key features but usually less pyramidal and extrapyramidal signs.

Despite no reported history of full-blown RBD and few recalled dreams, REM without atonia (REMWA) was observed in four out of five patients,[49] and subclinical RBD with minimal nonviolent movements during REM were also observed consisting of generalized or cranio-cervical myoclonic jerks.

The early pons involvement in SCA_2 degeneration, along with the midbrain and red nucleus,[50] may explain central dysinhibition in SCA_2.

Interestingly, even in presymptomatic subjects subtle REM sleep abnormalities, such as a decreased REM percentage and REM density, may be assessed by video-polysomnography (VPSG) along with altered muscle control during sleep, including bruxism and nocturnal leg cramps.

The REM sleep abnormalities in presymptomatic SCA_2 carriers might suggest an early neurodegeneration of REM-on neurons in the pons.

With the advancement of the disease, beyond the pons, the substantia nigra, and the cerebellum, atrophy of the locus coeruleus and the thalamus becomes prominent at later stages.[51] As subclinical RBD may be detectable along with reduction in REM density in early SCA_2 stages, progressive loss of dream recall later correlates with complete loss of REM sleep and marked increase of SWS at the expenses of light non-REM.

Interestingly, patients' reports of disturbed sleep are scanty until the latest stages of the disease and no hallucinations, nor cognitive dysfunction, parallel the loss of REM sleep.

RLS is estimated overall at 28% in SCA_1, SCA_2, and SCA_3 and the probability of developing RLS increases with age but not with CAG repeat length or higher age of ataxia onset.[52] Central dopaminergic dysfunction is one potential mechanism involved, even if normal postsynaptic striatal D2 receptor availability has been shown in SCA_1, SCA_2, and SCA_3.[53]

RLS symptoms must, in any case, be assessed since they may be severe, heavily impacting quality of life in these already frail patients; but they may electively respond to L-dopa.

DYSTONIAS

Dystonias can be symptomatic or hereditary, focal, multifocal, segmental, or generalized. The latter have been better polygraphically investigated during sleep.[9] Almost nothing is known about sleep features of focal dystonia such as writer's cramp or spasmodic torticollis. In cranial dystonias, spasms can prevail in the facial nerve territory (blepharospasm, Meige syndrome) or primarily involve the orobuccal and masticatory apparatus (idiopathic orobuccal dyskinesias, tardive dyskinesia, and rabbit syndrome).

Silvestri, De Domenico, Di Rosa, et al.[7] and Sforza, Montagna, Defazio, and Lugaresi[54] found impaired motor control during sleep in Meige syndrome; abnormal muscle activity was present mainly during light sleep of the first part of the night, although a smaller number of movements persisted during SWS. In blepharospasm alone,[7] spasms of the orbicularis oculi were observed during all stages of sleep, including REM, although decreased in frequency (e.g., occurring only once in approximately 5 minutes as opposed to twice a minute) and reduced in duration (3 to 4 seconds compared with 25 seconds during wakefulness).

A recent paper evaluated quality of sleep in primary focal dystonia through sleep questionnaires and scales without VPSG.[55] Pittsburgh Sleep Quality Index (PSQI) scores were significantly impaired both in cervical dystonia (CD) and in blepharo spasm (BSP). In BSP in particular, these results were not confounded by Beck Depression Inventory (BDI) scores. There was also no correlation between PSQI and dystonia severity scores in patients with BSP, and interestingly, despite severely disturbed sleep, no excessive daytime somnolence was reported nor emerged from the Epworth Sleepiness Scale (ESS) in either CD or BSP. These clinical data may support the hypothesis that these patients have a primary low propensity to sleep and have comorbid primary insomnia along with primary hyperexcitability of brainstem circuits.

TARDIVE DYSKINESIA

Baca-Garcia, Stanilla, Buchel, et al.[56] reported that severity of symptoms and diurnal variations of tardive dyskinesia depended on both sleeping and smoking patterns. Sleep has an inhibitory effect on dyskinesias, whereas smoking, through a nicotine-mediated dopamine release, can adversely contribute to the enhancement of dyskinetic movements.

Villeneuve, Jus, and Jus[57] have distinguished the sleep behavior of classic bucco-lingual or bucco-linguo-masticatory dyskinesia from a particular extrapyramidal effect called the *rabbit syndrome* (consisting of a fine, parkinsonian-like tremor of the lips resembling the movements of a rabbit's mouth). Although classic tardive dyskinesia disappears in all stages of sleep, rabbit syndrome persists during stage I and is the first type of dyskinesia to reappear during arousals or awakening. The authors[57] speculate that the rabbit syndrome dyskinesias are akin to parkinsonian tremor. They share a common pathogenesis, clinical mechanisms, and pharmacologic response to anticholinergic treatment. Changes in muscle tone exert a crucial role in triggering dyskinesias. The submental region muscle tone, exquisitely sensitive to sleep inhibition, is not primarily involved in the oral movements typical of rabbit syndrome. Phasic and tonic alterations of muscle tone seem to serve different roles depending on sleep stage. Although tonic changes in the transition from REM to stage I promote dyskinesias, phasic increase in muscle tone as seen during REM are not associated with triggering the dyskinesia but rather with occasional muscle twitching noted during REM in normals.

Idiopathic orobuccal dyskinesia[7] seems to follow the pattern of total disappearance during all sleep stages, as in neuroleptic-induced tardive dyskinesia.

Torsion dystonia (dystonia musculorum deformans) may be idiopathic or hereditary, starting earlier in childhood. It typically involves the head and the limbs, and severity of sleep disruption is generally comparable with severity of clinical symptoms. Specifically as in Parkinson's and Huntington's diseases, dystonic movements prevail in the following order: wake, awakening, arousals, light sleep, stages I and II.[9] Jankel, Allen, Niedermeyer, et al.[58] and Wein and Golubez[59] reported high-amplitude spindles that in one patient were reduced after unilateral ventrothalamotomy.[60] Alteration in the central nervous system monoamine distribution and functions in the dorsal raphe and the locus coeruleus nuclei may possibly account for some of the sleep abnormalities.[61]

A distinctive form of hereditary progressive dystonia with diurnal fluctuations has been reported by Segawa and coworkers.[62-64] Subjects, young female patients who exhibit fatigue, gait disturbance, and tonic posturing of one foot, respond dramatically to L-dopa therapy. Sleep (nighttime and long naps but not simple rest) produces a significant improvement of all symptoms, which has been attributed to REM sleep (on the basis of selective sleep deprivation experimental protocols). An increase of gross body movements during stage II is paralleled by a decrease of phasic twitches during REM. *Hypnogenic paroxysmal dystonia*[26] attacks are actually promoted by sleep in subjects otherwise normal between the dystonic attacks. Although most brief and extra brief attacks can now be retrospectively interpreted as partial motor seizures from the frontal lobe, some of the rare long-lasting or intermediate attacks may derive from a functional alteration of the basal ganglia akin to paroxysmal kinesigenic[65] or dystonic choreoathetosis.[66]

MYOCLONUS

Myoclonic movements of noncortical and nonepileptic origin have been rarely studied during sleep. Silvestri, De Domenico, Di Rosa, et al.[7] reported persistence of short, asynchronous, or rhythmic muscular jerks in subjects affected by Marinesco-Sjorgen syndrome, a rare autosomal recessive disease characterized by cataract, cerebellar ataxia, mental retardation, and generalized muscle jerks.

Idiopathic palatal myoclonus disappears during sleep.[67,68] However, palatal myoclonus secondary to an ischemic or anoxic or multiple sclerosis–related lesion, in the Molleret triangle[69,70] or in the medulla,[71] may persist during sleep and can be variably regulated (enhancement or disappearance) during REM, unrelated to REMs or respiratory phenomena.[72] Also, while some authors reported palato-ocular synchrony persisting from wake to sleep with the exception of SWS,[73] others reported loss of such synchrony during sleep.[74]

DISCUSSION

Persistence with decreasing frequency, amplitude, and duration across non-REM sleep is the rule for most abnormal movements during sleep. REM sleep is generally spared with some exceptions (hemiballism, Gilles de la Tourette's syndrome, amyotrophic choreoacanthocytosis), especially when the stage is significantly reduced or when its formal features are inconsistently defined, in severe clinical cases (see Huntington's disease or SCA_2). Only a few disorders show complete cessation of movements in sleep, and these include idiopathic or secondary tardive dyskinesias and idiopathic palatal myoclonus.

Stage IV and REM maintain higher threshold to the occurrence of movements because of the highest disfacilitation (stage IV) and active inhibition (REM) of muscle tone. Alteration or interruption of the long central white pathways descending to the brainstem (Parkinson's and Huntington's disease) may occasionally alter state physiology that is otherwise mostly preserved even in pathologic conditions. The emergence of sleep-related motor disorders such as bruxism, nocturnal leg cramps, periodic leg movements, RLS, and RBD contributes to further enhance motor dyscontrol during sleep but may also elucidate different stages of pathology with neuro-anatomic correlates of degeneration.

Many syndromes are yet to be polygraphically investigated at night, and conclusions are far from definitive. A clear understanding of sleep mechanisms and features is needed to help correct poor sleep, which contributes to the patient's poor quality of life in these pathologic conditions.

REFERENCES

1. De Jong RN. Abnormal movements. In: *The Neurologic Examination. Incorporating the Fundamentals of Neuroanatomy and Neurophysiology*, second ed. London: Pitman Medical; 1958:503.

2. Tassinari CA, Broughton R, Roger J, et al. A polygraphic study of the evolution of abnormal movements during sleep. *Electroencephalogr Clin Neurophysiol* 1964;17:721.

3. Tassinari CA, Broughton R, Poire R, et al. *Sur l'évolution des mouvements anormaux au cours du sommeil.* In: Fischgold H, ed. *Sommeil de Nuit Normal et Pathelogique.* Paris: Masson;1965:314.

4. Mano T, Shaoizawa Z, Sobue I. Extrapyramidal involuntary movements during sleep. In: Broughton RJ, ed. *Henry Gastaut and the Marseilles School's Contribution to the Neurosciences (EEG Suppl 35).* Amsterdam, The Netherlands: Elsevier Biochemical Press; 1982:431.

5. Autret A, Lucas B, Henry F, et al. Influence du sommeil sur les mouvements anormaux de la veille. *Neurophysiol Clin* 1994;24:218.

6. Nausieda PA. Sleep in Parkinson disease. In: Thorpy M, ed. *Handbook of Sleep Disorder.* New York: Marcel Dekker; 1990:719.

7. Silvestri R, De Domenico P, Di Rosa AE, et al. The effect of nocturnal physiological sleep on various movement disorders. *Mov Disord* 1990;5:8.

8. Askenasy JJM, Yahr MD. Parkinsonian tremor loses it alternating sleep aspect during non-REM sleep and is inhibited by REM sleep. *J Neurol Neurosurg Psychiatry* 1990;53:749.

9. Fish DR, Sawyers D, Allen PJ, et al. The effect of sleep on the dyskinetic movements of Parkinson's disease, Gilles de la Tourette Syndrome, Huntington's disease, and torsion dystonia. *Arch Neurol* 1991;48:210.

10. Kumru H, Santamaria J, Tolosa E, et al. Relation between subtype of Parkinson's disease and REM sleep behavior disorder. *Sleep Med* 2007;8(7–8):779–83.

11. Boeve BF, Silber MH, Parisi JE, et al. Synucleinopathy pathology and REM sleep behavior disorder plus dementia or parkinsonism. *Neurology* 2003;861(1):40–5.

12. Postuma RB, Gagnon JF, Montplaisir J, et al. Autonomic dysfunction in RBD—what can it teach us about disease progression? *Sleep Med* 2008;9(5):473–4.

13. De Cock VC, Vidailhet M, Leu S, et al. Restoration of normal motor control in Parkinson's disease during REM sleep. *Brain* 2007;130(Pt 2):450–6.

14. Iranzo A, Comella CL, Santamaria J et al. Restless legs syndrome in Parkinson's disease and other neurodegenerative diseases of the central nervous system. *Movement Disorders* 2007;18(22):S424–30.

15. Ondo WJ, Dat Vuong K, Jancovic H. Exploring the relationship between Parkinson's disease and restless legs syndrome. *Arc Neurol* 2002;59:421–4.

16. Peralta CM, Wolf E, Seppi K et al. Restless legs in idiopathic Parkinson's disease. *Mov Disord* 2005;20(Suppl 10):S108.

17. Mouret J. Differences in sleep in patients with Parkinson's disease. *Electroencephalogr Clin Neurophysiol* 1975;38:653.

18. Factor SA, Mc Alarney T, Sanchez-Ramos JR, et al. Sleep disorders and sleep effect in Parkinson's disease. *Mov Disord* 1990;2:280.

19. Neal H, Keane PE. Electrically and chemically induced spindling and slow waves in the encéphale isolé rat: a possible role for dopamine in the regulation of electrocortical activity. *Electroencephalogr Clin Neurophysiol* 1980;48:318.

20. Wiegand M, Moller AA, Lauer CJ, et al. Nocturnal sleep in Huntington's disease. *J Neurol* 1991;238:203.

21. Aldrich MS. Sleep and degenerative neurological disorders involving the motor system. In Thorpy M, ed. *Handbook of Sleep Disorder.* New York: Marcel Dekker; 1990:673.

22. Silvestri R, Raffaele M, De Domenico P, et al. Sleep features in Tourette's syndrome, neuroacanthocytosis and Huntington's chorea. *Neurophysiol Clin* 1995;25:66.

23. Wiegand M, Moller AA, Schreiber W, et al. Brain morphology and sleep EEG in patients with Huntington's disease. *Eur Arch Psychiatry Clin Neurosci* 1991;240:148.

24. Oepen G, Clarenbach P, Thoden U. Disturbance of eye movements in Huntington's chorea. *Arch Psychiatr Nervenkr* 1981;229:205.

25. Spire JP, Bliwise DL, Noronha AB, et al. Sleep in Huntington's disease. *Neurology* 1981;31:151.

26. Lugaresi E, Cirignotta F, Montagna P. Nocturnal paroxysmal dystonia. *J Neurol Neurosurg Psychiatry* 1986;49:375.

27. Aziz NA, Anguelova GV, Marinus J, et al. Sleep and circadian rhythm alterations correlate with depression and cognitive impairment in Huntington's disease. *Parkinsonism Rel Disord* 2010;16:345–50.

28. Morton AJ, Wood NI, Hastings MH et al. Disintegration of the sleep-wake cycle and circadian timing in Huntington's disease. *J Neuro Sci* 2005;25(1):157–63.

29. Videnovic A, Leurgans S, Fan W et al. Daytime somnolence and nocturnal sleep disturbances in Huntington's disease. *Parkinsonism Rel Disord* 2009;15:471–4.

30. Evers S, Stögbauer F. Genetic association of Huntington's disease and restless legs syndrome? A family report. *Mov Disord* 2003;18:225–7.

31. Savva E, Schnorf H, Burkhard PR. Restless legs syndrome: an early manifestation of Huntington's disease? *Acta Neurol Scand* 2009;119(4):274–6.

32. Mano T, Schozawa Z, Sobue I. Extrapyramidal involuntary movements during sleep. In Broughton RJ, ed. *Henri Gastaut and the Marseilles School's Contribution to the Neurosciences (EEG Suppl 35)*. Amsterdam, The Netherlands: Elsevier; 1982:431.

33. Dyken MD, Rodnitzky RL. Periodic, aperiodic and rhythmic motor disorders of sleep. *Neurology* 1992;42(Suppl 6):68.

34. Comings DE. A controlled study of Tourette's syndrome. VII. Summary: a common genetic disorder causing disinhibition of the limbic system. *Am J Hum Genet* 1987;41:839.

35. Comings DE, Comings BG. A controlled study of Tourette's syndrome. VI. Early development, sleep problems, allergies, and handedness. *Am J Hum Genet* 1987;41:822.

36. Erenberg G. Sleep disorders in Gilles de la Tourette's syndrome. *Neurology* 1985;35:1397.

37. Glaze DG, Frost JD, Jankovic J. Sleep in Gilles de la Tourette's syndrome: disorders of arousal. *Neurology* 1983;33:586.

38. Silvestri R, De Domenico P, Raffaele M, et al. Gilles de la Tourette syndrome: Wake and sleep electroclinical observations in four patients. In Mancia M, Marini G, eds. *The Diencephalon and Sleep*. New York: Raven Press; 1990:379.

39. Fish DR, Sawyers D, Allen PJ et al. The effect of sleep on the dyskinetic movements of Parkinson's disease, Gilled de la Tourette syndrome, Huntington's disease and torsion dystonia. *Arch Neurol* 1991;48:210.

40. Voderholzer U, Muller N, Haag C, et al. Periodic limb movements during sleep are a frequent finding in patients with Gilles de la Tourette's syndrome. *Neurol* 1997;244:521–6.

41. Trajanovic NN, Voloh I, Shapiro CM, et al. REM sleep behavior disorder in a child with Tourette's syndrome. *Can J Neurol Sci* 2004;31:572–5.

42. Kirov R, Kinkelbur J, Banaschewski T, et al. Sleep patterns in children with attention-defecit/hyperactivity disorder, tic disorder and comorbidity. *J Child Psychol Psychiatry* 2007;48(6):561–70.

43. Cortese S, Lecendreux M, Bernardina BD, et al. Attention-deficit/hyperactivity disorder, Tourette's syndrome, and restless legs syndrome: the iron hypothesis. *Med Hypotheses* 2008;70(6):1128–32.

44. D'Abreu A, Friedman J, Coskun J. Non-movement disorder heralds symptoms of Machado-Joseph disease years before ataxia. *Mov Disord* 2005;20:739–41

45. Friedman JH, Fernandez HH, Sudarsky LR. REM behavior disorder and excessive daytime somnolence in Machado-Joseph disease (SCA-3). *Mov Disord* 2003;18(12):1520–2.

46. Schöls L, Haan J, Riess O, et al. Sleep disturbances in spinal cerebellar ataxias. Is the SCA3 mutation a cause of restless legs syndrome? *Neurology* 1998;51:1603–7.

47. Iranzo A, Munoz E, Santamaria J, et al. REM sleep behavior disorder and vocal cord paralysis in Machado-Joseph disease. *Mov Disord* 2003;18:1179–83.

48. D'Abreu A, França M Jr, Conz L, et al. Sleep symptoms and their clinical correlates in Machado-Joseph disease. *Acta Neurol Scand* 2009;119(4):277–80.

49. Boesch SM, Frauscher B, Brandauer E, et al. Disturbance of rapid eye movement sleep in spinocerebellar ataxia type 2. *Mov Disord* 2006;21(10):1751–4.

50. Rüb U, Bürk K, Schöls L et al. Damage to the reticulotegmental nucleus of the pons in spinocerebellar ataxia type 1, 2, and 3. *Neurology* 2004;63(7):1258–63.

51. Tuin I, Voss U, Kang JS, et al. Stages of sleep pathology in spinocerebellar ataxia type 2 (SCA2). *Neurology* 2006;67:1966–72.

52. Abele M, Bürk K, Laccone F, et al. Restless legs syndrome in spinocerebellar ataxia types 1, 2, and 3. *J Neurol* 2001;248:311–14.

53. Reimold M, Globas C, Gleichmann M, et al. Spinocerebellar ataxia type 1, 2, and 3, and restless legs syndrome: striatal dopamine D2 receptor status investigated by [11C] raclopride, positron emission tomography. *Mov Disord* 2006;10:1667–73.

54. Sforza E, Montagna P, Defazio G, et al. Sleep and cranial dystonia. *Electroencephalogr Clin Neurophysiol* 1991;79:166.

55. Avanzino L, Martino D, Marchese R, et al. Quality of sleep in primary focal dystonia: a casa-control study. *European J of Neurol* 2010;17:576–81.

56. Baca-Garcia E, Stanilla JK, Buchel C, et al. Diurnal variability of orofacial dyskinetic movements. *Pharmacopsychiatry* 1999;32:73.

57. Villeneuve A, Jus K, Jus A. Polygraphic studies of tardive dyskinesia and of the rabbit syndrome during different stages of sleep. *Biol Psychiatry* 1973;6:259.

58. Jankel WR, Allen RP, Niedermeyer E, et al. Polysomnographic findings in dystonia musculorum deformans. *Sleep* 1983;6:281.

59. Wein A, Golubez V. Polygraphic analysis of sleep in dystonia musculorum deformans. *Waking Sleep* 1979;3:41.

60. Jankel WR, Niedermeyer E, Graf M, et al. Case report: polysomnographic effects of thalamotomy for torsion dystonia. *Neurosurgery* 1984;14:495.

61. Hornykiewicz O, Kish SJ, Becker LE, et al. Brain neurotransmitter in dystonia musculorum deformans. *N Engl J Med* 1986;31:347.

62. Segawa M, Hosaka A, Miyagawa F, et al. Hereditary progressive dystonia with marked diurnal fluctuation. In: Eldridge R, Fahn S, eds. *Dystonia. Advances in Neurology.* Vol. 14. New York: Raven Press; 1976:215.

63. Segawa M, Nomura Y, Tanaka S, et al. Hereditary progressive dystonia with marked diurnal fluctuation—Consideration on its pathophysiology based on the characteristics of clinical and polysomnographical findings. In: Fahn S, Marsden CD, Calne DB, eds. *Dystonia 2. Advances in Neurology.* Vol. 50. New York: Raven Press; 1988:367.

64. Deonna T. Dopa-sensitive progressive dystonia of childhood with fluctuations of symptoms—Segawa's syndrome and possible variants. *Neuropediatrics* 1986;17:75.

65. Hudgins RL, Corbin KB. An uncommon seizure disorder: familial paroxysmal choreoathetosis. *Brain* 1966;89:199.

66. Lance JW. Familial paroxysmal dystonic choreoathetosis and its differentiation from related syndromes. *Ann Neurol* 1977;2:285.

67. Montagna P, Cirignotta F, Lugaresi E. Disappearance of palatal myoclonus during sleep. *Sleep* 1983;6:386.

68. Yokota T, Hirashima F, Ito Y, et al. Idiopathic palatal myoclonus. *Acta Neurol Scand* 1990;81:239.

69. Chokroverty S, Barron KD. Palatal myoclonus and rhythmic ocular movements: a polygraphic study. *Neurology* 1969;19:975.

70. Kayed K, Sjaastad O, Magnussen I, et al. Palatal myoclonus during sleep. *Sleep* 1986;6:130.

71. Askenasy JJM, Brunet P, Leger JM, et al. Postradiation segmental myoclonus selectively inhibited by REM sleep (sleep-wake myoclonus). *Eur Neurol* 1988;28:317.

72. Kayed K, Sjaastad O, Marnussen I, et al. Palatal myoclonus during sleep. *Sleep* 1983;6:130.

73. Jacobs L, Bender B. Palato-occular synchrony during eyelid closure. *Arch Neurol* 1976;33:289.

74. Tahmoush AJ, Brooks JE, Keltner JL. Palatal myoclonus associated with abnormal ocular and extremity movements: a polygraphy study. *Arch Neurol* 1972;27:431.

40

Sleep-Related Leg Cramps, Sleep-Related Rhythmic Movement Disorder, and Sleep Talking

MICHAEL J. THORPY

SLEEP-RELATED LEG cramps and sleep-related rhythmic movement disorder are subcategories of the sleep-related movement disorders subsection of the *International Classification of Sleep Disorders* (*ICSD*).[1] Sleep talking is in the *ICSD* subsection entitled "Isolated symptoms, apparently normal variants and unresolved issues."

SLEEP-RELATED LEG CRAMPS

Sleep-related leg cramps, otherwise known as *nocturnal leg cramps*, describes cramping of a leg muscle or, more colloquially, a "charley horse"[1] (Table 40.1). Sleep-related leg cramps are painful muscular contractions associated with sensations of muscular tightness or tension that usually occur unilaterally in the calf but can also occur in the foot or thigh.[2,3] During the cramp, which usually lasts for a few seconds and remits spontaneously, the muscle is often visibly bulging and firm to the touch; afterward it is often sore and tender. Rarely, episodes last as long as 30 minutes. Residual tenderness in the affected muscles usually lasts about 30 minutes. Leg cramps are unilateral in 99% of cases, and the ipsilateral foot is involved in approximately 20% of cases.[4] Typically, episodes occur once or twice per night. Leg cramps can also occur during the daytime, and some patients have episodes exclusively in the daytime.

Sleep-related leg cramps should be differentiated from leg cramps that are secondary to an underlying disorder. There are many disorders and medications that have been associated with leg cramps (Table 40.2). The cause of sleep-related leg cramps is unknown, although a metabolic disturbance, such as abnormal calcium metabolism, is a possibility.[5,6] Muscle membrane overexcitability has been suggested as a cause of sleep-related leg cramps. Leg cramps are more common in the following disorders: myotonia congenita; the stiff-person syndrome; myokymia; McArdle's myophosphorylase deficiency; tetany from hypoparathyroidism and other hypocalcemic states; hypothyroidism;

Table 40.1 *ICSD-2* Diagnostic Criteria for Sleep-Related Leg Cramps

A. Painful sensation in the leg of foot associated with sudden muscle hardness or tightness indicating a strong muscle contraction.
B. The painful muscle contraction in the legs or feet occurs during the sleep period.
C. The pain is relieved by forceful stretching of the affected muscles, releasing the contraction.
D. The sleep-related leg cramps are not better explained by another sleep disorder, medical or neurological disorder, medication use, or substance use disorder.

Source: American Academy of Sleep Medicine. *The International Classification of Sleep Disorders. Diagnostic and Coding Manual*. 2nd ed. Westchester, IL: American Academy of Sleep Medicine; 2005.

hyponatremia; hypomagnesemia; tetanus; lead poisoning; diabetes mellitus; and after treatment with diuretics, renal dialysis, or clofibrate.[7] Leg cramps appear to be more common during pregnancy.[8] The use of oral contraceptives, as well as disorders of reduced mobility such as arthritis and Parkinson's disease, have also been associated with leg cramps. The most striking difference between patients with cramps and controls are with cardiovascular diseases such as peripheral vascular disease (34% versus 12%) and neurologic diseases such as peripheral neurologic deficit (12% versus 0%).[9] Leg cramps appear to be more common following vigorous exercise. Familial forms of the disorder have been reported sometimes with an autosomal dominant pattern of inheritance.[3,10,11]

Sleep-related leg cramps are believed to occur in up to 16% of healthy individuals with an increased incidence among older adults.[12] Sleep-related leg cramps are present in 7.3% of children, and they occur only in children aged 8 years or older. The incidence increases at 12 years and peaks at 16 to 18 years of age.[4] Most children (81.6%) with sleep-related leg cramps have episodes one to four times per year, and the mean duration of episodes is approximately 2 minutes.[4] The male:female ratio is 1:1, and the disorder may have a heredity factor and be autosomal dominant.

Sleep-related leg cramps should be differentiated from muscle contraction related to chronic myopathy, peripheral neuropathies, akathisia, restless legs syndrome, muscular pain-fasciculation syndromes, and disorders of calcium metabolism.[2] Usually there is no difficulty in differentiating these disorders because the nocturnal occurrence of leg cramps and lack of daytime neurologic signs and symptoms are clear distinguishing features. Metabolic disorders can be excluded by appropriate biochemical screening.

Sleep-related leg cramps are usually distinguished by the characteristic clinical features. Polysomnographic studies may reveal nonperiodic bursts of gastrocnemius

Table 40.2 Conditions Associated with Leg Cramps

Neurologic
Neuropathy, dystonia, amyotrophic lateral sclerosis, Parkinson's disease, nerve root compression, motor neuron disease, multiple sclerosis
Endocrine
Hypothyroidism, hyperthyroidism, diabetes mellitus, Addison's disease
Metabolic
Hypoglycemia, hypocalcemia, hyperkalemia, hypokalemia, hyponatremia, dialysis, diarrhea
Vascular
Peripheral vascular disease, Reynaud's disease
Drugs
Nifedipine, diuretics, ethanol, phenothiazides, penacillamine, steroids, lithium, statins, fibrates, terbutaline, cimentadine, oral contraceptives, morphine withdrawal
Toxins
Lead toxicity, strychnine poisoning, tetanus
Congenital
Autosomal dominant cramping disease, McArdle's disease

electromyographic activity, although they are not usually necessary for the diagnosis.[13] The course of sleep-related leg cramps is not well understood.

The disorder usually has a benign course, and episodes remit spontaneously. Avoidance of plantar flexion in bed may prevent episodes.[5] During an episode of sleep-related leg cramps, dorsiflexion of the foot may terminate an episode. Nonpharmacologic therapy, such as regular passive stretching of the affected muscle, may be the best first-line treatment.[14]

Medications are most useful when the cramps are frequent and very painful (Table 40.3). Quinine sulfate (325 mg) before bedtime appears to be helpful, although the benefit is not large.[14–17] Lower starting doses are appropriate for senior citizens and individuals with impaired renal function. In general, quinine in any form should be avoided by pregnant women and people with hepatic failure.[18] The only form of quinine available in the United States is qualaquin, which is not FDA approved for the treatment of leg cramps. In fact, the FDA has

Table 40.3 Medications for Sleep-Related Leg Cramps

	MEDICATION	DOSE	COMMENTS	REFERENCES
First-line Choices	Verapamil	120 mg	Limited data but may be beneficial	28
	Diltiazem	30 mg	Limited data but appears to be beneficial	29
Second-line Choices	Gabapentin	400 mg–1600 mg	May be beneficial for cramps secondary to neurologic disease	32–34
	Vitamin E	400–800 IU	May be in effective in dialysis patients	22, 23
	Vitamin B complex	–	Limited data	24
	Magnesium sulfate/ citrate	300–900 mg	May be beneficial in pregnancy	25–27
	Levetiracetam	500 mg	Limited data	31
	Orphenadrine citrate	100 mg	Limited data	37
Third-line Choices	Carisoprodol	250 mg–350 mg	Has abuse potential	30
	Naftidrofuryl	30 mg	Limited data; not available in the United States	38
	Diphenhydramine	25–50 mg	Limited data	35
	Procainamide	250 mg	Limited data	36
	Quinine sulfate	200–500 mg	Clinically appears effective. Serious but rare side effects. Should be avoided.	14–21

warned that qualaquin should not be used for leg cramps because of ocular toxicity and potentially fatal hypersensitivity reactions, including serious and life-threatening thrombocytopaenia and hemolytic-uremic syndrome.[19] A recent review by the American Academy of Neurology recommended that quinine should be avoided for routine treatment of cramps and only considered when cramps are very disabling and no other agents relieve the symptoms.[20] There are also reports of ineffectiveness of quinine.[21]

The vitamins B and E have been thought to be useful. Vitamin E (400 IU) was shown to be effective for leg cramps in patients on dialysis,[22] but not in other studies.[16] Vitamin B complex was shown to be effective in elderly patients who were vitamin deficient.[23]

Magnesium sulphate or citrate has been shown to be variably effective in helping leg cramps.[24-26] The effect is mild at best and can be associated with diarrhea.

The calcium channel blockers verapamil and diltiazem, which block neuromuscular transmission, may be the most useful in leg cramps.[27,28] Verapamil (120 mg) at bedtime was helpful in older patients refractory to quinine,[27] and diltiazem produced a significant reduction in frequency of nocturnal leg cramps without side effects.[28]

Carisoprodol, a centrally active skeletal muscle relaxant, is widely used for the treatment of acute, painful musculoskeletal disorders and has been shown to be effective for leg cramps; however, it does have abuse potential.[29]

The anticonvulsant levetiracetam has been effective for leg cramps in patients with motor neuron disease.[30] Gabapentin has shown varied results but may be useful for some patients.[31-33] Although there are very little data available, diphenhydramine (25 to 50 mg)[34] at bedtime or procainamide (250 mg three times per day) may also be beneficial.[35]

The muscle relaxant baclofen, and the anticonvulsants carbamazepine and oxcarbazepine, have been used, but there is no evidence of effectiveness.[20] Orphenadrine, a muscle relaxant, has been shown to be effective.[36] Clonazepam may be helpful, but there have been no clinical trials.[37]

Naftidrofuryl, a medication that enhances utilization of oxygen and glucose in peripheral vascular disease, has been shown to be effective, but it is not available in the United States.[38]

It would appear that the best treatment at the current time is to use a calcium blocker, such as verapamil or diltiazem, and if that is not effective, then consideration should be given to a trial of vitamin E, vitamin B complex, magnesium sulphate or citrate, orphenadrine, or levetiracetam. Third-line medications might include carisoprodol or naftidrofuryl in Europe. In very severe cases, a careful trial of quinine may be justified.

RHYTHMIC MOVEMENT DISORDER

The term *rhythmic movement disorder* was adopted by the International Classification of Sleep Disorders in 1990 to reflect the different forms of rhythmic movements that can occur during sleep. The term *jactatio capitis nocturna*, originally proposed by Zappert[39] in 1905, is still used frequently. In France at about the same time, Cruchet[40] described the disorder and gave it the name *rhythmie du sommeil*. The terms *head banging*, *head rolling*, *body rocking*, and *body rolling* have also been applied to this group of disorders.

Patients with rhythmic movement disorder have stereotyped, repetitive movements involving large muscles, usually of the head and neck.[41] The movements typically occur immediately before sleep onset and continue into light sleep, and they most commonly involve the head, which is sometimes forcibly banged into the pillow or mattress.[42] Violent head movements usually occur in the prone position and the term *head banging* is often applied. When the movements involve rocking on the hands and knees, referred to as body rocking, the frontal region of the head can be forcefully banged into a headboard or wall.[43] Other types of movements include head rolling, a side-to-side head movement that occurs when the individual is prone; body rolling; leg banging; and leg rolling. A review of epidemiological studies suggests that between 3% and 5% of children are affected with head banging, and as many as 12%–19% have body rocking.[44]

Episodes of repetitive movements typically occur at sleep onset, although they may also occur during periods of quiet relaxation. Predisposed individuals may have episodes while riding in motor vehicles or listening to music. The rhythmic movements usually occur between 0.5 and 2 oscillations per second. A cluster of movements may only last a few minutes in duration or may last up to 30 minutes or longer.[45] Patients are usually unresponsive during the events and amnestic to them on awakening.

The cause of idiopathic rhythmic movement disorders is unknown. Episodes usually begin in infancy and are more common in patients who are mentally retarded. No etiologic pathophysiologic lesion has been described, although an abnormality of the basal ganglia has been suggested.[46]

Rhythmic movement disorder has been described after head injury and in association with other disorders such as restless legs syndrome, REM behavior disorder and obstructive sleep apnea syndrome.[47-51]

Radiographic changes in severely affected patients have been reported to include enlargement of the diploic space in the parietal and occipital bones and gray matter loss adjacent to the bony changes. This pattern of injury is similar to neuronal injury seen in boxers (dementia pugilistica) and Minimata disease.[52]

Most individuals with rhythmic movement disorder are otherwise normal infants and children. Persistence of the disorder into older childhood or adulthood may be associated with mental retardation, autism, or other major psychopathologic conditions.

Rhythmic movement disorder may be confused with bruxism, thumb sucking, and rhythmic sucking of a pacifier. Rarely, periodic limb movement disorder may produce similar features. There is one report of rhythmic movement disorder associated with epilepsy.[53]

Rhythmic movement disorder typically occurs in infants and toddlers and usually resolves in the second or third year of life.[54] A study of children 9 months to 60 months shows a prevalence of any type of rhythmic activity decreasing from 66% to 6%.[54] Although persistence beyond 4 years of age is unusual, symptoms may occasionally persist into adolescence or adulthood.

Rhythmic movement disorder can be recognized by its characteristic clinical features (Table 40.4). However, in some circumstances, polysomnographic evaluation may be useful to differentiate the disorder from an epileptic disorder. Episodes typically occur in presleep drowsiness and light non–rapid eye movement (non-REM) sleep, although rarely the activity occurs in deep slow-wave sleep[55] or solely during rapid eye movement (REM) sleep.[56-58] Because the differential for rhythmic movement disorder includes a large number of disorders associated with abnormal, and at times, violent nocturnal movements, diagnosis can be greatly enhanced by documenting suspected nocturnal behaviors with thorough clinical assessment during split-screen, video-polysomnographic analysis.[59]

Several variants of idiopathic rhythmic disorder with headbanging have been described with atypical features such as quasi-rhythmic frontal head punching and head-slapping.[60] Multiple forms of rhythmic movements in the one patient have been described including bodyrocking, headbanging, body or leg rolling movements.[61,62]

The treatment of rhythmic movement disorder depends on the age of onset. Young infants or children require no treatment, because the condition usually resolves spontaneously. If the condition persists into adolescence or adulthood, behavioral treatments may rarely be helpful, such as overpracticing the activity during wakefulness. Avoidance of emotional stress and

Table 40.4 ICSD-2 Diagnostic Criteria for Sleep-Related Rhythmic Movement Disorder

1) Movements are characterized by repetitive, stereotyped, and rhythmic motor activity.
2) Movements involve large muscle groups.
3) Movements are predominantly sleep related, occurring near sleep onset or during drowsiness or sleep.
4) The movements or behaviors result in at least one referable complaint:
   a) Interference with normal sleep
   b) Significant impairment of daytime function
   c) Self-inflicted bodily injury (or risk of injury without use of protective measures)
5) Rhythmic movements are not better explained by an alternative sleep or medical disorder, neurological or psychiatric disorder, or by medication or substance use.

Source: American Academy of Sleep Medicine. *The International Classification of Sleep Disorders. Diagnostic and Coding Manual.* 2nd ed. Westchester, IL: American Academy of Sleep Medicine; 2005.

lack of environmental stimulation can prevent rhythmic movement disorder in some individuals. Hypnosis has been reported to be helpful.[63]

Two patients have been reported who had sleep-related rhythmic movement disorder in association with severe obstructive sleep apnea syndrome.[64,65] Both patients had a dramatic reduction of the rhythmic movement disorder with treatment of the sleep apnea by continuous positive airway pressure.

Short-acting benzodiazepines can be helpful in severe cases,[41] and longer acting benzodiazepines such as clonazepam and oxazepam have also been reported to be effective.[66-68] Imipramine has been helpful when benzodiazepines, such as clonazepam, have not.[69] Citalopram may be helpful.[70]

SLEEP TALKING

Sleep talking refers to a variety of utterances, moans, or spoken words that can occur during the major sleep episode.[1,71,72] The utterances may be very brief, infrequent, and devoid of any emotional stress, or they may include long speeches and hostile or angry outbursts. Sleep talking can sometimes be induced by conversation with a predisposed sleeping individual. Balanced bilinguals (those who have equal proficiency in both languages) may sleep talk in either of the two languages. Dominant bilinguals (i.e., having greater proficiency in one language) may preferentially sleep talk in their dominant language.[73]

Sleep talking in adults is sometimes associated with stress, psychopathology, or medical illness. Children are more likely to sleep talk if a parent had a parasomnia such as sleepwalking.[74] Sleep talking may be a feature of sleep terrors.

Sleep talking can be a prodrome of REM sleep behavior disorder that may herald the development of Parkinson's disease. Loud sleep talking has also been associated with dementia with Lewy bodies and may be helpful in differentiating DLB from Alzheimers disease and other forms of dementia.[75]

Sleep talking is also a common feature of disrupted sleep in patients with obstructive sleep apnea syndrome. An association with psychiatric comorbidity is found only in adult sleep talking and is highest in those with adult-onset sleep talking; however, most cases of sleep talking are not associated with serious psychopathologic conditions.[76] A case of progressive supranuclear palsy and preclinical REM sleep behavior disorder presenting as inhibition of speech during wakefulness and somniloquy with phasic muscle twitching during REM sleep has been reported.[77]

Sleep talking is common, although very loud sleep talking that is of annoyance to others may be rare. Approximately 10% of children, between 3 and 10 years of age, sleep talk on a nightly basis. The occurrence of childhood and adult sleep talking is highly correlated.[76] A gender difference is only seen in adults, with sleep talking being more common in males than in females.[76] Sleep talking should be differentiated from periods of talking during nocturnal awakenings.

Sleep talking usually does not require any diagnostic workup, unless features of other sleep disorders, such as obstructive sleep apnea syndrome or REM sleep behavior disorder, are present, in which case polysomnographic documentation may be needed. A disorder termed sleep-related groaning, or catathrenia, should be distinguished (Table 40.5). Catathrenia

Table 40.5 *ICSD-2* Diagnostic Criteria for Sleep Talking and Catathrenia

Sleep talking	A. Talking during sleep. Sleep talking is usually reported by the bed partner or someone sleeping in the same room or sleeping area as the affected individual. The sleep talker is rarely aware of his or her sleep talking.
Catathrenia	A. A history of regularly occurring groaning (or related monotonous vocalization) during sleep. or B. Polysomnography, if performed, with respiratory sound monitoring reveals a characteristic respiratory dysrhythmia predominantly or exclusively during REM sleep.

Source: American Academy of Sleep Medicine. *The International Classification of Sleep Disorders. Diagnostic and Coding Manual.* 2nd ed. Westchester, IL: American Academy of Sleep Medicine; 2005.

is a chronic, usually nightly disorder characterized by expiratory groaning during sleep, particularly during the second half of the night. Polysomnography reveals recurrent bradypneic episodes that emerge mainly during REM sleep: a deep inspiration is followed by protracted expiration when a monotonous vocalization is produced that closely resembles groaning.[1]

Sleep talking is usually a benign condition that resolves spontaneously. It may last for a few nights, several months, or years. There is no specific treatment for sleep talking, although treatment of an underlying disorder that precipitates the sleep talking is usually helpful. Avoidance of emotional stress may be helpful in preventing episodes.

REFERENCES

1. American Academy of Sleep Medicine. *The International Classification of Sleep Disorders. Diagnostic and Coding Manual.* 2nd ed. Westchester, IL: American Academy of Sleep Medicine; 2005.
2. Layzer RB, Rowland LP. Cramps. *N Engl J Med* 1971;283:31.
3. Jacobsen JH, Rosenberg RS, Huttenlocher PR, et al. Familial nocturnal cramping. *Sleep* 1986;9:54.
4. Leung AK, Wong BE, Chan PY, et al. Nocturnal leg cramps in children: Incidence and clinical characteristics. *J Natl Med Assoc* 1999;91:329.
5. Weiner IH, Weiner HL. Nocturnal leg muscle cramps. *JAMA* 1980;244:2332.
6. Hammar M, Larsson L, Tegler L. Calcium treatment of leg cramps in pregnancy. Effect on clinical symptoms and total serum and ionized serum calcium concentrations. *Acta Obstet Gynecol Scand* 1981;60(4):345–7.
7. Whitely AM. Cramps, stiffness and restless legs. *Practitioner* 1982;226:1085.
8. Hertz G, Fast A, Feinsilver SH, et al. Sleep in normal late pregnancy. *Sleep* 1992;15:246.
9. Haskell SG, Fiebach NH. Clinical epidemiology of nocturnal leg cramps in male veterans. *Am J Med Sci* 1997;313:210.
10. Lazaro RP, Rollinson RD, Fenichel GM. Familial cramps and muscle pain. *Arch Neurol* 1981;38:22.
11. Ricker K, Moxley RT. Autosomal dominant cramping disease. *Arch Neurol* 1990;47:810.
12. Norris FH. An electromyographic study of induced and spontaneous muscle cramps. *Electroenceph Clin Neurophysiol* 1957;9:139.
13. Saskin P, Whelton C, Moldofsky H, et al. Sleep and nocturnal leg cramps. *Sleep* 1988;11:307.
14. Man-Son-Hing M, Wells G, Lau A. Quinine for nocturnal leg cramps: a meta-analysis including unpublished data. *J Gen Intern Med* 1998;13:600.
15. Walton T, Kolb KW. Treatment of nocturnal leg cramps and restless leg syndrome. *Clin Pharm* 1991;10:427.
16. Connolly PS, Shirley EA, Wasson JH, et al. Treatment of nocturnal leg cramps. A crossover trial of quinine vs vitamin E. *Arch Intern Med* 1992;152:1877.
17. Man-Son-Hing M, Wells G. Meta-analysis of efficacy of quinine for treatment of nocturnal leg cramps in elderly people. *BMJ* 1995;310:13.
18. Brasic JR. Should people with nocturnal leg cramps drink tonic water and bitter lemon? *Psychol Rep* 1999;84:355.
19. Mackie MA, Davidson J, Clarke J. Quinine—acute self-poisoning and ocular toxicity. *Scott Med J* 1997;42:8.
20. Katzberg HD, Khan AH, So YT. Assessment: symptomatic treatment for muscle cramps (an evidence-based review): report of the therapeutics and technology assessment subcommittee of the American academy of neurology. *Neurology* 2010;74(8):691–6.
21. Sidorov J. Quinine sulfate for leg cramps: does it work? *J Am Geriatr Soc* 1993;41:498.
22. Roca AO, Jarjoura D, Blend D, et al. Dialysis leg cramps. Efficacy of quinine versus vitamin E. *ASAIO J* 1992;38:M481.
23. Chan P, Huang TY, Chen YJ, et al. Randomized, double-blind, placebo-controlled study of the safety and efficacy of vitamin B complex in the treatment of nocturnal leg cramps in elderly patients with hypertension. *J Clin Pharmacol* 1998;38(12):1151–4.
24. Dahle LO, Berg G, Hammar M, et al. The effect of oral magnesium substitution on pregnancy-induced leg cramps. *Am J Obstet Gynecol* 1995;173(1):175–80.
25. Frusso R, Zárate M, Augustovski F, et al. Magnesium for the treatment of nocturnal leg cramps: a crossover randomized trial. *J Fam Pract* 1999;48(11):868–71.
26. Roffe C, Sills S, Crome P, et al. Randomised, cross-over, placebo controlled trial of magnesium citrate in the treatment of

chronic persistent leg cramps. *Med Sci Monit* 2002;8(5):CR326–30.

27. Baltodano N, Ballo BV, Weidler DJ. Verapamil vs quinine in recumbent nocturnal leg cramps in the elderly. *Arch Int Med* 1988;148:1969.

28. Voon WC, Sheu SH. Diltiazem for nocturnal leg cramps. *Age Ageing* 2001;30(1):91–2.

29. Chesrow EJ, Kaplitz SE, Breme JT, et al. Use of carisprodol (Soma) for treatment of leg cramps associated with vascular, neurologic or arthritic disease. *J Am Geriatr Soc* 1963;11:1014–16.

30. Bedlack RS, Pastula DM, Hawes J, et al. Open-label pilot trial of levetiracetam for cramps and spasticity in patients with motor neuron disease. *Amyotroph Lateral Scler* 2009;10(4):210–15.

31. Miller RG, Moore DH, II, Gelinas DF, et al. Western ALS Study Group. Phase III randomized trial of gabapentin in patients with amyotrophic lateral. *Sclerosis Neurology* 2001;56(7):843–8.

32. Serrao M, Rossi P, Cardinali P, et al. Gabapentin treatment for muscle cramps: an open-label trial. *Clin Neuropharmacol* 2000;23(1):45–9.

33. Mueller ME, Gruenthal M, Olson WL, et al. Gabapentin for relief of upper motor neuron symptoms in multiple sclerosis. *Arch Phys Med Rehabil* 1997;78(5):521–4.

34. Misischia N. Treatment of leg cramps during pregnancy: use of diphenhydramine HCl. *Am Pract Dig Treat* 1960;11:1022–3.

35. Satoyoshi E. Recurrent muscle spasms of central origin. *Trans Am Neurol Assoc* 1967;92:153–7.

36. Guay DR. Are there alternatives to the use of quinine to treat nocturnal leg cramps? *Consult Pharm* 2008;23(2):141–56.

37. Mahajan S, Engel WK. Assessment: symptomatic treatment for muscle cramps (an evidence-based review): report of the Therapeutics and Technology Assessment Subcommittee of the American Academy of Neurology. *Neurology* 2010;75(15):1397–8.

38. Young G. Muscle cramps: quinine derivatives likely to be effective but not recommended for routine use due to toxicity; vitamin B complex, naftidrofuryl and calcium channel blockers possibly effective. *Evid Based Med* 2010;15(4):114–15.

39. Zappert J. Über nachtliche Kopfbewegungen bei Kindern (jactatio capitis nocturna). *Jahrb Kinderheilkd* 1905;62:70.

40. Cruchet R. Tics et sommeil. *Presse Med* 1905;13:33.

41. Thorpy MJ. Rhythmic movement disorder. In: Thorpy MJ, ed. *Handbook of Sleep Disorders.* New York: Marcel Dekker; 1990:xx–xx.

42. De Lissovoy V. Headbanging in early childhood. *Child Dev* 1962;33:43

43. Kravitz H, Rosenthal V, Teplitz Z, et al. A study of headbanging in infants and children. *Dis Nerv Syst* 1960;21:203.

44. Hoban T. Sleep-related rhythmic movement disorder. In: Thorpy MJ, Plazzi G, eds. *Parasomnias and Other Sleep-Related Movement Disorders.* Cambridge, England: Cambridge University Press; 2010:xx–xx.

45. Sallustro C, Atwell F. Jactatio capitis. *J Pediatr* 1978;93:704.

46. Freund HJ, Hefter H. The role of the basal ganglia in rhythmic movement. *Adv Neurol* 1993;60:88.

47. Drake ME. Jactatio nocturna after head injury. *Neurology* 1986;36:867.

48. Chirakalwasan N, Hassan F, Kaplish N, et al. Near resolution of sleep related rhythmic movement disorder after CPAP for OSA. *Sleep Med* 2009;10:497–500.

49. Gharagozlou P, Seyffert M, Santos R, Chokroverty S. Rhythmic movement disorder associated with respiratory arousals and improved by CPAP titration in a patient with restless legs syndrome and sleep apnea. *Sleep Med* 2009;10:501–03.

50. Lombardi C, Provini F, Vetrugno R, et al. Pelvic movements as rhythmic motor manifestation associated with restless legs syndrome. *Mov Disord* 2003;18:110–13.

51. Walters AS Frequent occurrence of myoclonus while awake and at rest, body rocking and marching in place in a subpopulation of patients with restless legs syndrome. *Acta Neurol Scand* 1988;77:418–21.

52. Carlock KS, Williams JP, Graves GC. MRI findings in headbangers. *Clin Imaging* 1997;21:411.

53. Guilleminault C, Silvestri R. Disorders of arousal and epilepsy during sleep. In: Sterman MD, Shouse MN, Passouant P, eds. *Sleep and Epilepsy.* New York: Academic Press; 1983:513.

54. Klackenberg G: Rhythmic movements in infancy and early childhood. *Acta Paediatr Scand* 1971;224(Suppl):74.

55. Thorpy MJ. Rhythmical body movements during sleep. In: Segawa M, ed. *Body Movements During Sleep.* Tokyo: Sanposha; 1987:xx–xx.

56. Regestein QR, Hartmann E, Reich P. A head movement disorder occurring in dreaming sleep. *J Neurol Nerv Ment Dis* 1977;164:432.

57. Gagnon P, DeKonick J. Repetitive head movements during REM sleep. *Biol Psychiatry* 1985;20:176.

58. Kempenaers C, Bouillon E, Mendlewicz J. A rhythmic movement disorder in REM sleep: a case report. *Sleep* 1994;17:274.

59. Dyken ME, Lin-Dyken DC, Yamada T. Diagnosing rhythmic movement disorder with video-polysomnography. *Pediatr Neurol* 1997;16:37.

60. Yeh SB, Schenck CH. Atypical headbanging presentation of idiopathic sleep related rhythmic movement disorder: three cases with video-polysomnographic documentation. *J Clin Sleep Med* 2012 Aug 15;8(4):403–11.

61. Jankovic SM, Sokic DV, Vojvodic NM, et al. Multiple rhythmic movement disorders in a teenage boy with excellent response to clonazepam. *Mov Disord* 2008;23:767–8.

62. Su C, Miao J, Liu Y, et al. Multiple forms of rhythmic movements in an adolescent boy with rhythmic movement disorder. *Clin Neurol Neurosurg* 2009;111:896–9.

63. Chirakalwasan N, Hassan F, Kaplish N, et al. Near resolution of sleep related rhythmic movement disorder after CPAP for OSA. *Sleep Med* 2009;10(4):497–500.

64. Gharagozlou P, Seyffert M, Santos R, et al. Rhythmic movement disorder associated with respiratory arousals and improved by CPAP titration in a patient with restless legs syndrome and sleep apnea. *Sleep Med* 2009;10(4):501–3.

65. Rosenberg C. Elimination of a rhythmic movement disorder with hypnosis—A case report. *Sleep* 1995;18:608.

66. Chisholm T, Morehouse RL. Adult headbanging: Sleep studies and treatment. *Sleep* 1996;19:343.

67. Merlino G, Serafini A, Dolso P, et al. Association of body rolling, leg rolling, and rhythmic feet movements in a young adult: a video-polysomnographic study performed before and after one night of clonazepam. *Mov Disord* 2008;23(4):602–7.

68. Walsh JK, Kramer M, Skinner JE. A case report of jactatio capitis nocturna. *Am J Psychiatry* 1981;138(4):524–6.

69. Alves RS, Aloe F, Silva AB, et al. Jactatio capitis nocturna with persistence in adulthood. Case report. *Arq Neuropsiquiatr* 1998;56:655.

70. Vogel W, Stein DJ. Citalopram for head-banging. *J Am Acad Child Adolesc Psychiatry* 2000;39(5):544–5.

71. Arkin AM. Sleep talking: a review. *J Nerv Ment Dis* 1966;143:101.

72. Arkin AM, Toth MF, Baker J, et al. The frequency of sleep talking in the laboratory among chronic sleep talkers and good dream recallers. *J Nerv Ment Dis* 1970;151:369.

73. Pareja JA, de Pablos E, Caminero AB, et al. Native language shifts across sleep-wake states in bilingual sleeptalkers. *Sleep* 1999;22:243.

74. Abe K, Amatoni M, Oda N. Sleepwalking and recurrent sleeptalking in children of childhood sleepwalkers. *Am J Psychiatry* 1984;141:800.

75. Honda K, Hashimoto M, Yatabe Y, et al. The usefulness of monitoring sleep talking for the diagnosis of dementia with Lewy bodies. *Int Psychogeriatr* 2013 Feb 21:1–8.

76. Hublin C, Kaprio J, Partinen M, et al. Sleeptalking in twins: epidemiology and psychiatric comorbidity. *Behav Genet* 1998;28:289.

77. Pareja JA, Caminero AB, Masa JF, et al. A first case of progressive supranuclear palsy and pre-clinical REM-sleep behavior disorder presenting as inhibition of speech during wakefulness and somniloquy with phasic muscle twitching during REM sleep. *Neurologia* 1996;11:304.

41

Sleep Bruxism and Other Disorders with Orofacial Activity during Sleep

TAKAFUMI KATO, PIERRE J. BLANCHET, NELLY T. HUYNH, JACQUES Y. MONTPLAISIR, AND GILLES J. LAVIGNE

SLEEP BRUXISM (SB) was previously defined by the *International Classification of Sleep Disorders* (ICSD) as a parasomnia.[1] In the second version of the *ICSD* (*ICSD-2*), it is defined as a sleep-related movement disorder with a stereotyped movement characterized by grinding or clenching teeth during sleep.[2] SB is produced by either phasic (rhythmic) or tonic (sustained) muscle activity in jaw-closing muscles and can be associated with tooth-grinding sounds.[2,3] Most SB patients are usually unaware of the tooth-grinding sounds they generate, although their bed partners complain that the noise disturbs their sleep. SB can also be harmful to the teeth or dental restorations; SB patients often complain of (1) tooth wear, (2) frequently fractured dental restorations, (3) hypersensitivity of the teeth to cold liquid or air, and (4) orofacial pain or discomfort that may include temporal headache.[3,4] These complications eventually lead patients to consult a physician or dentist.

Bruxism, whether it occurs during wakefulness or sleep, is classified into primary (idiopathic), secondary, or iatrogenic forms (Table 41.1).[3-5] In this section, SB refers to oromandibular motor activity related to tooth grinding and clenching during sleep regardless of the cause.

PREVALENCE

In the adult population, the prevalence of patients reporting SB with grinding is 8%.[6,7] In children younger than 11 years, the prevalence of tooth grinding as reported by parents varies from 14% to 20%.[8-10] No gender difference is observed. A linear decrease with age is noted: from 19% in ages 3 to 10 years to 13% in ages 18 to 19 years to a further 3% in people aged 60 and older.[6,7] These data should be interpreted with caution because they are based on self-reports of tooth-grinding sounds. Such reports may not be very accurate; most SB patients are not aware of the sounds. In addition, the prevalence of edentulism is higher in the older adult population. Although edentulism is a confounding factor when assessing the

Table 41.1 Classification of Sleep Bruxism

BRUXISM*

A. Primary or idiopathic

Without medical or dental causes
Sleep bruxism
Daytime clenching

B. Secondary or iatrogenic

B-1: Associated with sleep disorders, movement disorders, neurologic disorders, and psychiatric disorders
or
B-2: Associated with drug administration/withdrawal

Concomitant Sleep Disorders

Restless legs syndrome
Periodic limb movement syndrome
Sleep myoclonus
Sleep apnea
Nocturnal groaning
Enuresis
Rapid eye movement (REM) sleep behavior disorders (RBD)

Concomitant Movement Disorders

Gilles de la Tourette's syndrome
Oromandibular dystonia (cranial dystonia)

Hemifacial spasm
Huntington's disease
Tardive dyskinesia
Parkinson's disease

Concomitant Neurologic or Psychiatric Conditions

Epilepsy
Coma
Whipple's disease
Dementia
Attention-deficit/hyperactivity disorder
Anxiety disorders
Mood disorders

Drugs That May Induce Tooth Grinding during Wake or Sleep

Antidopaminergic drugs
Selective serotonin reuptake inhibitors
Calcium antagonists
Alcohol, caffeine, or cigarettes
Cocaine
Amphetamine

*With or without tooth grinding.

prevalence based on self-reports, a recent study has suggested that age is independently associated with the prevalence of SB.[11] The daytime form of bruxism, mainly characterized by clenching, is reported by 20% of the population with a gender difference (female more than male).[5] Daytime bruxism should be differentiated from SB because the two have been suggested to be different entities.[3-5] Daytime clenching is mainly reactive and frequently induced in patients under life pressure or stress and anxiety,[4] whereas SB is involuntary and could be related to sleep-regulatory processes (e.g., sleep arousal).[12-14] Patients with mild frequency of rhythmic jaw muscle activity during sleep, who also present tooth grinding related to a possible diagnostic of SB, do have more frequent self-reported awareness of daytime clenching than those with severe SB.[15] The interaction or relation between the two conditions, however, remains to be proven.

PATHOPHYSIOLOGY

The mechanisms involved in SB genesis are yet to be established. However, studies suggest that the expression of SB is likely to be multifactorial; SB may be influenced by activity in the physiologic central nervous system (oromotor, sleep-wake regulation, catecholaminergic) and autonomic nervous systems in interaction with psychosocial factors, plus a contribution from genetic factors remains possible but not dominant, as explained later in this section.

Approximately 60% of normal controls, as well as SB subjects, exhibited rhythmic masticatory muscle activity (RMMA), which is the repetition of episodes of rhythmic jaw muscle activity (see Fig. 41.1), in the absence of tooth grinding during sleep.[16-18] This masticatory muscle activity during sleep, named "chewing automatism," had been noted earlier in patients with somnambulism and rapid eye movement (REM) sleep behavior disorder.[19,20] When compared with normal controls without tooth-grinding history or SB-related clinical complaints (see section on "Clinical Diagnosis"), moderate to severe SB subjects showed three times more RMMA episodes (normal controls: 1.8 episodes/hour; SB patients: 5.8 episodes/

hour) with twice as many muscle bursts and 30% higher electromyographic (EMG) amplitude.[18] As discussed later, SB can be an extreme expression of ongoing physiologic arousal activity during the sleep of the individual.

Most of the oromotor activity related to SB occurs in sleep stages I and II.[12,16,17,21-24] The episodes occur in cluster during the ascending phase of non–rapid eye movement (non-REM) sleep within a sleep cycle.[14] Interestingly, although SB patients have a normal macrostructure of sleep,[12,16,17,21,23,24] some physiologic changes related to microarousals such as transient electroencephalographic (EEG) alpha activity,[23] a transient increase in heart rate, and frequent shifts in sleep stages have been observed in association with SB episodes.[12,13,16,21,23,25] Fewer K-complexes and K-alphas were found to occur during sleep in SB patients compared to normal subjects[24]; these EEG events were less frequently associated with RMMA episodes in SB patients (12.1%) than in normal subjects (21.2%). The number of sleep spindles did not differ between SB patients and

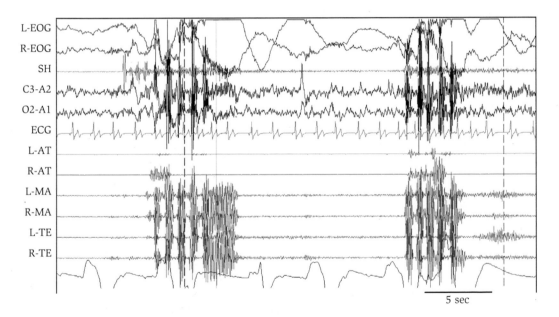

FIGURE 41.1 Polysomnographic records of two sleep bruxism episodes occurring during sleep stage II. The first episode was characterized by a rhythmic series of contractions in left (L) and right (R) masseter (MA) and temporalis (TE) muscles with tooth-grinding sounds followed by a tonic contraction of those muscles (mixed type). The second one exhibited only rhythmic contractions of MA and TE muscles with grinding sounds (rhythmic type). The shortening of R-R interval in the electrocardiogram (ECG) visibly starts after the beginning of these episodes. Bilateral anterior tibialis muscles (AT) are also active during this episode as a part of generalized body movement. Masticatory muscles contractions caused artifacts in the electrooculograms (L- and R-EOG) and the EEG (C3-A2, O2-A1). SH: EMG from suprahyoid muscles. Vertical bars, 100 µV; horizontal bar, 2 seconds.

normal subjects.[24] Studies revealed an association between SB and a transient EEG/autonomic activating pattern called the cyclic alternating pattern (CAP), which represents a period of higher cortical and microarousal activities during non-REM sleep.[12,13,16,21,23,25-29] A sequence from an increase of sympathetic activity, cortical EEG activation, to cardiac activation precedes RMMA episodes,[13,14,18,30] and RMMA episodes are associated with the augmentation of respiratory activity, and increase of blood pressure and concomitant swallowing.[31-33] RMMA episodes can be followed to experimental microarousal triggered by sensory stimulation in SB patients, while this was not obvious in normal subjects.[30] These suggest that SB is characterized by a heightened responsiveness of RMMA episodes to arousal activity in SB patients. More recently, however, micro-arousal and CAP provide a permissive window for the genesis of SB in the predisposed subjects rather than act as a direct triggering factor.[28,29]

Various neurochemicals such as catecholamines, serotonin, and GABA have been shown to modulate SB activity (see the section on "Management of Sleep Bruxism" for details). Currently, however, no single neurochemical has been determined to cause SB. In addition, these neurochemicals may interact with each other and are known to be involved in the factors contributing to SB pathophysiology (e.g., sleep-wake regulation, autonomic functions motor controls, and anxiety/stress). The specific roles of neurochemicals in SB pathophysiology need to be investigated in a future study.

Other factors contributing to SB have also been considered. Although the role of dental occlusal discrepancies has been controversial in dentistry, recent studies support that SB is of central origin.[4,34-36] The contribution of emotional factors such as psychological stress, although it seems to be clinically relevant, has not yet been fully established.[37] One study, combining self-reports of daytime stress and jaw muscle EMG recording during sleep, revealed a low correlation between self-perceived daytime stress and masseter EMG activity during sleep.[38] A recent study has shown that sleep-related EMG activity of temporalis muscles was significantly associated with trait anxiety in healthy subjects rather than acute episodes of anxiety.[39] In another study, mild SB patients reported stress more frequently than moderate to severe patients.[15] In addition, SB patients were not different from matched controls in motor reaction time, but they were more anxious to maintain a high quality of performance during the task.[40] Subjects with tooth-grinding awareness reported less positive coping strategies than those without.[41] Some recent evidence supports the influence of putative genetic factors. For example, SB is more frequently reported in monozygotic than in dizygotic twins, and when SB was present in childhood it persisted into adulthood in 90% of the subjects interviewed.[42] In our sleep laboratory sample of SB patients with confirmed tooth grinding, about one third of subjects had direct family members with a history of SB (Khoury S, unpublished observation). More recent study suggests the genetic contribution to the etiology of SB by showing that polymorphism of the gene related to serotonergic transmission was associated with SB.[43] SB genetics is an open domain for the future studies and multiple genes are likely involved.

CLINICAL FEATURES

Clinical Diagnosis

The clinical diagnosis of SB is based on a suggestive history (e.g., self-reported tooth-grinding sounds, morning masticatory muscle fatigue) and a global orofacial examination (e.g., tooth wear, masseter muscle hypertrophy) (Table 41.2).[3,5]

The history of tooth-grinding sounds reported by a sleep partner or parents is the most solid basis in recognizing a patient with SB. However, the presence of such sounds is variable over time (50%), and patients sleeping alone have no source of such history.[3,5] Tooth-grinding or -tapping sounds should be distinguished from other oral sounds during sleep such as snoring, coughing, sighing, tongue clicking, grunting, or temporomandibular clicking sound.[44,45]

The presence of tooth wear constitutes a salient observation in SB patients. Tooth wear is assessed by a direct oral examination or by an indirect observation using dental plaster models for future monitoring. Tooth wear may be found on a few teeth or the whole dentition. The presence of tooth wear is more frequently observed in SB patients than in normal subjects.[46] However, it does not necessarily reflect the severity of ongoing active bruxism, since the incidence of SB events fluctuates over time and wear may represent past SB activity.

Masseter muscle hypertrophy is another sign that appears with voluntary teeth

Table 41.2 Clinical Observations in Sleep Bruxism Patients

1. Reports of tooth grinding or tapping sounds by a sleep partner or parents (most reliable)
2. Presence of tooth wear seen within normal range of jaw movements or at eccentric position (might have happened years earlier)
3. Presence of masseter muscle hypertrophy seen on voluntary contraction (not specific to sleep bruxism; awake habit or clenching may explain such hypertrophy)
4. Complaint of masticatory muscle discomfort, fatigue, or stiffness in the morning (occasionally, transient headache in temporal muscle region in absence of breathing disorder)
5. Hypersensitive tooth (in the morning)
6. Clicking or locking of temporomandibular joint function
7. Tongue indentation (may be a concomitant awake time habit)

clenching. It should be differentiated from inflammatory swelling, the parotid-masseter syndrome that is secondary to the blockade of salivary ducts by muscle and parotid gland tumor.[3] Masseter hypertrophy is not a solid outcome for identifying current tooth grinding; again, a sleep partner's report of tooth grinding described earlier is probably the most reliable indicator.

In addition, masticatory muscle discomfort or temporomandibular joint (TMJ) pain, temporal headache, and tooth pain may coexist with SB. Many SB patients report such complaints in the morning following a night of intense SB activity.[47] It is a transient jaw muscle pain or fatigue frequently intersecting with temporal headache that is reported. A causal relationship between SB and temporomandibular disorder pain (most frequently myofascial pain reported in afternoon or evening) remains probable, but it has not yet been fully established.[48,49] It is important to record the history of temporomandibular signs and symptoms in order to further isolate predisposing factors to SB. The clinicians must distinguish transient morning pain, a possible delayed-onset muscle-soreness type of pain,

from afternoon to evening myofascial pain; these two may have different causative risk factors and physiopathology. Patients with lower frequency of RMMA episodes have a higher likelihood of reporting orofacial pain, mainly transient morning pain, and stress.[15]

Presence of possible dental problems include noncarious cervical lesions,[50] tooth fracture,[51] or the fracture of dental restorations.[52] In some patients, tooth indentation is observed on the margin of the tongue. Although this is not specific to SB, it could be associated with a habit of pushing the tongue against teeth during clenching episodes.

To summarize, the following criteria can help clinicians diagnose moderate to severe SB: recent history of tooth-grinding sounds (occurring at least three to five nights per week over the preceding 6 months), presence of tooth wear, morning masticatory muscle fatigue or pain, and masseter muscle hypertrophy.[2–5]

ELECTROPHYSIOLOGIC DIAGNOSIS

Two methods are used to document oromotor activities associated with SB: ambulatory monitoring and polysomnographic (PSG) recording in a sleep laboratory. In both methods EMG recordings from the jaw-closing muscles (e.g., masseter) should ideally be accompanied with simultaneous audio-video recordings to allow confirmation of the presence of tooth-grinding sounds.[3,5,53]

Monitoring SB with ambulatory devices is a technology that is currently available. Type 2 full PSG sleep recording is available, and it is of a comparable quality to sleep laboratory system. However, system failure is admittedly a limitation; necessary technical assistance is not available at home to overcome technical problems such as electrode displacement. Type 3 system is more limited in number of channels (EMG, breathing, and cardiac outputs collected with 4 to 6 channels) with dedicated software to make a scoring proxy of PSG. The type 4 is a minimalist system with one or two channels that do not allow assessments of sleep quality, duration, concomitant disorders, and so on. Even with such limitations ambulatory systems are advantageous because they allow patients to sleep in their own environment. The use of such systems may open opportunities for large-population based studies, patient monitoring, or follow-up.

Table 41.3 Criteria in Detection of Sleep Bruxism by Ambulatory System

1. Electromyogram (EMG) activity (acquisition at a minimum frequency of 16.7 Hz)
   - Amplitude: >10% of maximal voluntary contraction during awake with:

     >3 sec of duration

     <5 sec between EMG events
2. Heart rate
   - Increase of at least 5% in presence of an EMG rhythmic masticatory muscle activity type of event

---

It also offers an alternative to patients in rural or remote areas without access to organized sleep medicine. Nevertheless, in the absence of home audio-video recordings, it may be difficult to distinguish SB-related orofacial activities from other orofacial activities during sleep[44,45,54,55] Therefore, with these technologies, we recommend the use of audio-video recording. Some criteria have been suggested for the use of ambulatory devices in detecting SB episodes (Table 41.3).[25,56] These criteria need further validation to assess the percentage of variability in scoring in absence of audio-video recordings. The selection of an SB diagnostic recording system needs to be made while balancing the needs of recognizing possible concomitant sleep disorders such as periodic limb movement syndrome (PLMS), REM sleep behavior disorder (RBD), sleep apnea-hypopnea syndrome, or Cheney-Stoke breathing because all have significant health consequences.

Sleep laboratory recording, conducted in a highly controlled environment, makes it possible to distinguish SB from other sleep-related disorders mentioned earlier. However, it has a drawback: it has lower validity in studies on the influences from natural milieu on sleep behavior.

Owing to the limitations of ambulatory and sleep laboratory recording, we suggest, based on the literature and current criteria, the following use of full PSG systems in conducting SB analysis and scoring specific behavior or physiological activities[57]: (1) to score sleep structure and microarousal—at least two EEG (C3A2, O2A1), bilateral electrooculogram (EOG), and one EMG from chin/suprahyoid muscle; (2) to distinguish SB from other orofacial activities—EMG recordings at least from bilateral masseter muscles and possibly temporal muscles; (3) to rule out other sleep disorders (e.g., sleep apnea [SA] or periodic limb movements)—nasal air flow, respiratory belt, and EMGs from bilateral anterior tibialis muscles. Again, we strongly suggest simultaneous audio-video recordings with the use of an ambulatory device (at least when recording EMG of masseter, respiration, and heart rate outputs) and a sleep laboratory system to better distinguish SB episodes from other orofacial activities during sleep (e.g., coughing, sleep talking, and excessive swallowing).

Jaw EMG episodes (single or repetitive or rhythmic) are identified in order to score bursts from one or bilateral jaw-closing muscle (e.g., masseter) recording. In parallel with audio-video signals, SB episodes should be discriminated from oromotor events associated with swallowing, snoring, grunting, coughing, sighing, and other nonspecific jaw motor contractions. The EMG activity should be at least 10% to 20% of the maximum voluntary teeth clenching that is done before sleep. Originally, an EMG level of more than 20% of maximal voluntary clenching (MVC) during wakefulness was proposed as a minimum threshold in scoring EMG events.[17] However, we retrospectively found that, in combination with audio-video records, EMG events with a level of 10% to 20% of MVC (approximately 10% of total events) also can be scored. We have used 10% to 20% of MVC as the criterion in recent studies.

As shown in Table 41.4, each episode is further classified into a type: phasic (rhythmic), tonic (sustained), or mixed.[17] Phasic or rhythmic episodes are defined if at least three EMG bursts (duration: 0.25 to 2.0 seconds) are observed and are separated by two interburst intervals (Fig. 41.1). Tonic or sustained episodes are scored if the EMG burst is longer than 2 seconds. A mixed episode is a combination of these two patterns (Fig. 41.1). These episodes were separately counted when interburst interval was longer than 3 seconds. SB episodes occurring with tooth-grinding noise are also documented. Brief EMG bursts (duration: <0.25 second) in association with a jaw jerk or tooth-tapping movements are scored separately as myoclonic events.[54]

Again these scorings are based on the EMG activity of masseter or temporalis muscles (trigeminal nerves). On the other hand, chin EMG activity (e.g., mentalis muscle innervated by facial nerve) is the minimum requirement based on the scoring manual issued by the

Table 41.4 Polysomnographic Diagnostic Research Criteria for Sleep Bruxism

1. Electromyogram (EMG) activity in masticatory muscles (masseter, temporalis)
   - EMG level of >10%–20% of a maximum voluntary clenching in wakefulness
   - Duration of EMG bursts of >0.25 sec to exclude myoclonus
2. Types of rhythmic masticatory muscle activity (RMMA) episodes
   - Phasic (rhythmic): 3 or more EMG bursts with the duration from 0.25 to 2.0 sec, separated by two intervals less than 3.0 sec
   - Tonic (sustained): EMG bursts lasting >2.0 sec
   - Mixed: both phasic and tonic types
3. Diagnostic cutoff criteria (either a or b, with c)
   a. >4 sleep bruxism episodes per hour of sleep for frequent RMMA case OR 2–4 from light- to moderate-frequency RMMA
   b. >25 EMG bursts per hour of sleep for frequent RMMA case
   c. At least two sleep bruxism episodes with tooth-grinding sounds per night

American Academy of Sleep Medicine.[57] The same duration criteria are recommended for identifying phasic and tonic EMG bursts. The use of chin EMG is operationally convenient because this is included in a standard PSG montage. However, chin EMG, in our experience, is not reliable and specific to SB episodes. Chin EMG amplitude cannot be standardized as is done for masseter EMG (e.g., % of maximal voluntary contraction). Chin muscles are not always activated simultaneously with the masseter in response to arousal and oromandibular movements. Thus, it needed to be investigated how accurately the diagnosis based on the use of chin EMG without masseter EMG can be made.

Different PSG criteria have been used to make a diagnosis of SB in different sleep laboratories. The validated research diagnostic criteria for SB (RDC/SB) in SB patients with frequent (e.g., at least 5 nights per week) tooth grinding are as follows (Table 41.4)[17]: (1) high frequency SB in a patient with positive history of tooth grinding—more than four RMMA episodes per hour of sleep or more than 25 SB-related EMG bursts per hour of sleep, with at least two events of grinding noises per night; and (2) lower frequency SB with positive history of tooth grinding—2–4 RMMA episodes per hour of sleep.[15] The latter group was derived from the results of a recent study in which RDC/CB was reevaluated in 100 SB patients and 43 controls[15]: there was a subgroup of SB patients who did not fulfill the RDC/SB (e.g., fewer than 4 episodes per hour), although they had a history of tooth grinding. Thus, clinically, a cutoff value of 2–4 RMMA episodes per hour, instead of 4.0, is relevant. Moreover, a subgroup of SB patients (e.g., 2 to 4 episodes per hour of sleep) had a higher likelihood of reporting orofacial pain in morning compared to the moderate to severe patients (e.g., more than 4.0 episodes per hour of sleep). More recently, 55 patients with temporomandibular disorders were recorded by PSG.[58] Although 75% patients had self-reported SB, only 17% were found to fulfill the RDC/SB criteria based on PSG data (e.g., more than 4 RMMA episodes per hour of sleep). The poor concordance between the frequency of RMMA and temporomandibular disorders shown in the aforementioned studies suggests that SB and TMD are two different entities, although many studies have shown that one is a risk factor for another.[48,49]

MANAGEMENT OF SLEEP BRUXISM

Since no specific cure exists, the main goal in the management of SB lies in the prevention or reduction of complaints related to damages to orofacial structures. Behavioral (e.g., biofeedback), dental (e.g., occlusal appliances), and pharmacologic (e.g., benzodiazepines, muscle relaxants, dopaminergic drugs) strategies have been suggested for managing SB, but the efficacy of these strategies has yet to be proven scientifically.[3,5,59]

Behavioral Strategies

Two approaches have been proposed for managing SB: psychological or physiologic relaxation, including sleep hygiene and the use of biofeedback techniques.

The present-day practice of a typical behavioral approach[59,60] involves explaining the concept of SB and instructing patients (1) to avoid intense mental and physical activities during the second half of the evening and to rest for 1 hour before sleep; (2) to learn a relaxation technique such as abdominal breathing and to practice it during daytime when the patient is aware of clenching teeth and before sleep (to seek help from psychologists and physical therapists, if necessary, to master such a technique); (3) to avoid large meals as well as beverages such as coffee, tea, alcohol, and soft drinks, and to avoid smoking in the evening since it may be a risk factor for SB[7,61,62]; and (4) to create a comfortable sleeping environment by reducing external noise, adjusting room temperature, allowing fresh air ventilation, and using comfortable bed sets. Although sleep hygiene seems a reasonable approach, its therapeutic effect has not been tested in SB patients.

In an open-designed study, hypnosis has been reported to reduce EMG activity and tooth-grinding frequency.[63] However, the efficacy of hypnosis remains to be tested in a controlled study. Sound-related biofeedback paradigms, specifically activated by masticatory EMG activity, were shown to reduce SB activity. This effect, however, does not appear to persist after cessation of the treatment.[64,65] It is more appealing to the patient if alternative methods (e.g., vibration, slight electrical shock) were used in this paradigm rather than sound, which may disturb the sleep of the patient's bed partner. Recently, it was shown that nonnoxious electrical stimuli exert decreasing influence on SB activity without worsening the subjective sleep quality.[66,67] The possible influence of this paradigm on the objective sleep quality (e.g., increase in sleep arousal, effects to sleep deprivation) and, although a promising avenue, the long-term effects (e.g., habituation over the risk of sleep disturbance) need to be confirmed by any independent laboratory.[67a]

Dental Strategies

Occlusal appliances such as hard occlusal splints or soft mouth guards that prevent tooth damage have been used by dentists for years in the management of SB.[68] These appliances usually cover a full dental arch (maxillary or mandibular arch) and require intraoral adjustments by a dentist. The hard occlusal splint is made with acrylic resin and is recommended for long-term, full-night use. The soft ones are mainly made from vinyl sheet and are used for a short period. Some reports showed that the use of such appliances reduced SB-related

RMMA EMG activity, but the effects did not last more than few weeks[65,69-71] while others showed either an increase or no change in EMG activity.[72-74] It is worth noting that no difference has been observed in sleep macrostructures and microstructures.[71] The insertion of the splint may not influence the sleep process. Although occlusal appliances are widely prescribed by dentists, their mechanism of action and their efficacy in SB management remain to be further documented. Recent studies demonstrated that there was no difference in the effects of occlusal splints and a palatal splint that did not cover maxillary dentition.[70,71,74] These suggest that occlusal splint that cover teeth can be an effective technique to protect teeth from damage.[68] Prior to prescribing an occlusal splint, a dentist should screen the patient for concomitant obstructive sleep apnea (OSA) and snoring since the use of occlusal splint by patients with OSA can aggravate their respiratory events and snoring.[75] Among other types of occlusal appliance that have been tested more recently, mandibular advancement appliances for snoring and OSA were found to reduce RMMA frequency related to SB in patients with primary SB. This finding was obtained after a 2-week observation period; a longer observation period is needed to assess clinical benefit/risk (e.g., tooth displacement) of such appliances in managing SB.[76,77] Oral device that covers upper incisors only, called NTI in the market, also reduced SB activity for a short time, but the risk of posterior tooth displacement is not yet fully known.[78]

Another form of dental treatment for SB, called occlusal adjustment therapy, equilibrates the relationship between upper and lower dentitions by trimming natural teeth or dental restorations, thereby putatively stabilizing the forces at the TMJ or teeth. However, this irreversible therapy remains controversial, and its efficacy has yet to be demonstrated in a controlled study.[3,56,79,80]

Pharmacologic Strategies

Several centrally acting drugs have been suggested to reduce SB. The mechanism of action of these drugs remains elusive; it is unclear whether they act directly on SB motor mechanism or indirectly by reducing the probability of sleep arousal. Thus, the need for long-term administration of any medication mentioned in the following should be carefully assessed.

Benzodiazepines (diazepam; 5 or 10 mg/night) and centrally acting muscle relaxants (e.g., methocarbamol; 1 to 2 g/night) at bedtime have been reported to reduce SB-related oromotor activity.[81,82] These drugs were mainly used for short periods (e.g., one or two nights). Although low to modest efficacy is expected, further controlled trials are needed. The long-term efficacy of clonazepam (approximately 1 mg/night for up to 3.5 to 8 years) has been demonstrated in the treatment of injurious sleep parasomnias (e.g., sleep terror, sleepwalking, RBD).[83] In a recent placebo control trial, a short-term use of clonazepam (1 mg/night) decreased SB-related activity (EMG) by 30% in SB patients with sleep disorders (e.g., restless legs syndrome [RLS], etc.).[84] Patients should be informed that these drugs carry significant risks of dizziness or somnolence and dependence-addiction. Small doses of tricyclic antidepressants, amitriptyline (25 mg/night), failed to control SB and associated discomforts.[85,86] Selective serotonin-reuptake inhibitor (SSRI) antidepressants (e.g., fluoxetine, sertraline) should be avoided because they may increase the risk of SB.[87-89] A decrease in SSRI dosage or the administration of buspirone (serotonin [5HT]1A agonist) has been suggested as a means of reducing SSRI-related SB.[87] It may also be pathogenetically significant that SSRIs are known to induce extrapyramidal symptoms, presumably via the inhibitory effect of these drugs on dopamine transmission.[90] The interaction of several drugs with this neurotransmitter system may explain the genesis of iatrogenic SB.[4]

A placebo-controlled study has reported that dopaminergic medications such as the dopamine precursor L-dopa (two doses of 100 mg/night) moderately reduce SB activity by 30%.[91] However, another placebo-controlled study revealed that the dopamine agonist bromocriptine (7.5 mg/night) was not effective.[92] In a recent case report, combined use of pergolide (0.3–0.5 mg/night) with domperidone reduced SB.[93] These medications are given at a low dosage in light of the side effects such as nausea, emesis, and dizziness.

In two open studies, the beta-adrenergic receptor antagonist propranolol has been administered to one severe SB patient (two doses of 60 mg/night)[94] and to two SB patients with antipsychotic drug exposure (less than 240 mg/day per os or 20 mg three times daily),[95] and a reduction of SB activity was noted. In a controlled, double-blind study, propranolol failed to reduce SB in patients with primary SB.[96] The same study reported that the alpha-adrenoreceptor agonist clonidine (0.3 mg/night) decreased SB by 60%. Since 20% of patients exhibited severe morning hypotension, clonidine cannot be recommended for the management of SB without close medical monitoring.

Botulinum toxin type A (BTX-A) is known to be symptomatically effective in patients with orofacial involuntary movements[97] and to reduce masseter muscle hypertrophy often associated with daytime clenching.[97a] It has been suggested that BTX-A is effective against secondary bruxism in patients with movement disorders (e.g., cranial dystonia).[98,99] In a recent small sample size study using ambulatory EMG recording, use of BTX-A as a treatment modality reduced jaw muscle EMG activity during sleep in SB patients.[100] Further studies, using quantitative sleep recordings, are needed to evaluate benefit/risk of botulinum toxin therapy when its duration of action is limited (3–6 months based on the results in the other types of movement disorders).

OTHER DISORDERS OR DISEASES WITH OROFACIAL MANIFESTATIONS DURING SLEEP

Several types of orofacial motor activity, including SB, have been reported to occur in patients with various medical conditions or movement disorders.[3,5]

OTHER SLEEP DISORDERS ASSOCIATED WITH SLEEP BRUXISM

Sleep Apnea

Sleep apnea (SA) is a sleep disorder that is characterized by repetitive cessation of respiration during sleep. SA is known to cause arousal or awakening from sleep, and it is correlated with multiple clinical symptoms, including excessive daytime sleepiness, fatigue, mood changes, snoring, and memory impairment.

In an epidemiologic study, patients with snoring and SA had SB more frequently than those without (odds ratio: 1.4 and 1.8, respectively).[7] Thus, SB occurrence may be correlated with SA in some patients. Approximately half of mild to severe obstructive SA patients were diagnosed as having SB.[101] More than 60% of slight tooth clenchings were associated with the termination of SA events,[102,103] but tooth clenching or tooth grinding with stronger masseter EMG activities, scored as SB events, were not related to SA events.[101] Another recent study has shown that SB is associated with the augmentation of respiration,[32] while an increase of respiration can be secondary to transient arousal activation. Thus, although SA may not be directly coupled with SB, the coexistence of SB and SA is possible.[104]

Another connection between SA and SB is the use of oral devices in the management of the two disorders. Mandibular advancement appliances or devices (MADs) that increase the upper airway space are known to be effective in the management of snoring and mild to moderate SA.[105–107] However, some reports have suggested that the use of these appliances may aggravate orofacial pain.[106,108,109] Oral devices (e.g., oral splints) used in SB management (see section on "Dental Strategies") exacerbate SA symptoms in some patients with mild SA.[75] It remains to be tested whether MADs can be useful for managing SB in OSA patients when appropriate titration is made.[76,77]

Sleep-Related Xerostomia and Gastroesophageal Reflux

The presence of sleep-related xerostomia can be suggested when patients' report dryness or discomfort in the mouth or throat that has wakened them to supplement water during the night.[110] This is an issue that may be relevant to sleep medicine because 23% of the North American population complains of a dry mouth during sleep.[110,111] Exacerbated oral parafunctional activities were reported in patients with burning mouth syndrome, a condition associated with xerostomia.[112] As a consequence of such parafunction in the absence of oral lubrication that normally helps to protect teeth from wear while they function (e.g., chewing), the harmful influence of SB could be worsened.[111] The relationship between daytime and sleep-related xerostomia as well as the impact of sleep-related xerostomia have yet to be elucidated.

During sleep, some patients may experience regurgitation of gastric contents that cause the sensation of heartburn and a sour taste. A similar condition is frequently seen in the patients with gastroesophageal reflux (GR) during daytime.[113] Tooth erosion in these patients is more likely to be related to the daytime influence of GR[114] and decreased daytime salivary function[115] because the oral pH of GR patients

is apparently not modified during sleep.[116] GR patients are disturbed by more sleep arousals than normal.[117] For GR patients, there is a higher risk that SB will produce tooth damage.[111] It has also been reported that GR events are often associated with swallowing-related pharyngeal activity during sleep.[117] A PSG analysis found that approximately 60% of RMMA episodes concomitantly occur with swallowing events in SB patients and normal subjects.[31] In SB subjects otherwise healthy, esophageal pH decreases can be associated with EMG bursts related to RMMA episodes.[118] A relationship between visceral functions and jaw motor activities needs further investigation in association with sleep arousal activities in healthy subjects and patients with GR.[119]

Repetitive water intake and the use of some oral devices, after a medical evaluation, may help protect the teeth of patients who suffer from both of the conditions. Pilocarpine drugs (e.g., Salagen) may increase salivary flow if not otherwise contraindicated (e.g., medical history of asthma or glaucoma).

Sleep Myoclonus in Masticatory Muscles to Epilepsy and Rhythmic Masticatory Muscle Activity Grinding

Sleep-related faciomandibular myoclonus, or oromandibular myoclonus, is characterized by tapping like vertical jaw movements during sleep.[51,120] Myoclonic movements of the jaw were characterized by muscle bursts (twitches) of short duration (0.25 second or less). We observed that 10% of subjects diagnosed with SB in our sleep laboratory had frequent twitches, and we named such activity idiopathic orofacial myoclonus during sleep since none of our patients showed epileptic spikes on our recordings (Fig. 41.2).[54] Moreover, we observed that 50% of the events occurred in clusters, in episodes of three or more twitches. Similar activities were also observed in patients with a history of tongue biting.[120] What is interesting to us is the report of a patient with RMMA and grinding with temporal lobe seizure.[121] Such an observation suggests that patients with tooth tapping or unusual RMMA grinding need to be examined in neurology to exclude epilepsy or other sleep disorders. Other concomitant or secondary medical conditions such as epilepsy, insomnia, or RBD should be ruled out.[121–124] As described later, we noted a high frequency of twitches in masseter muscles

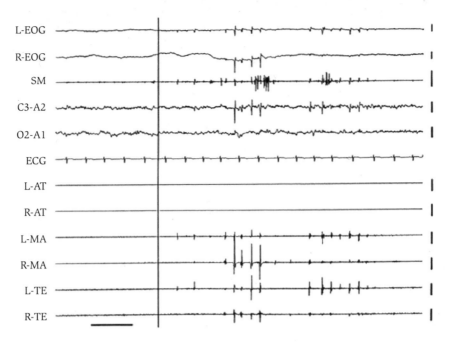

FIGURE 41.2 Records of an idiopathic myoclonic episode in masticatory muscles during sleep stage I. This subject was not diagnosed as a sleep bruxism (SB) patient. Tapping-like jaw movements occurred with short duration (<0.25 seconds) of muscle bursts in masseter and temporalis muscles. These contractions caused artifacts in electrooculographic (EOG) and electroencephalographic records. Full electroencephalographic montage revealed no epileptic spikes during the sleep of this subject. Vertical bars, 100 μV; horizontal bar, 2 seconds. Abbreviations are the same as those in Figure 41.1. The vertical line indicates the edges of the two scoring pages. (Reproduction from Figure 2 of the Kato et al., "Sleep bruxism and other disorders with orofacial activity during sleep" in *Sleep and Movement Disorders*, pp. 273–285, Copyright Elsevier, 2003.)

in a group of idiopathic RBD patients.[125] In a severe or high-frequency case, after excluding other neurological disorders, clonazepam could be used to reduce myoclonic events.[120] Again, controlled studies are needed to prove the efficacy of such management.

REM Sleep Behavior Disorder

RBD is characterized by excessive limb or body jerking and violent behavior in the REM sleep stage where muscle atonia is normally observed.[2] The loss of atonia in masticatory chin muscles during REM sleep is a common feature of RBD. RBD patients exhibit several orofacial movements such as chewing automatism (RMMA, see section on "Pathophysiology"), grimacing, and vocalization.[20] There is only one report describing SB in association with RBD.[126] In our laboratory, we found that older patients with idiopathic RBD showed a higher rate of brief masseter contractions (twice as many twitches

in REM sleep) than age-matched control subjects.[125] The relevance of such a finding is yet to be discerned. We must remind our readers that RBD is a condition at risk for neurodegenerative diseases. Clonazepam is reported to be effective since it suppresses phasic EMG activities in the RBD patient without restoring submental atonia during REM sleep.[127] RBD is a condition of importance in sleep medicine, and it is reviewed elsewhere in this volume (Chapters 29–31).

Restless Legs Syndrome and Periodic Limb Movement Syndrome

An epidemiologic study showed that the coexistence of SB and RLS was found only in 10% of the population.[6] With PSG recordings, PLMS was observed in a few patients with SB.[23] Through SB and these two conditions can coexist and there may be common risk factors, they seem pathophysiologically different. RLS and PLMS are reviewed elsewhere in this volume (Chapters 42–49).

Other Sleep Disorders

Sleep bruxism has been reported to occur concomitantly with other sleep disorders such as nocturnal groaning, sleep epilepsy, erunesis, insomnia, or parasomnias.[127–132]

OTHER DISORDERS OR DISEASES WITH OROFACIAL MANIFESTATIONS DURING SLEEP

Hyperkinetic Movement Disorders

Several hyperkinetic movement disorders affecting the orofacial region (e.g., Gilles de la Tourette syndrome [TS], cranial dystonia, hemifacial spasm [HFS], and Huntington's disease [HD]) have been reported to persist during sleep. Concomitant bruxism and involuntary movements are expected. In such a case, the concomitant bruxism might be referred to as tooth-grinding movements with audible sounds, and it should be called secondary bruxism if it was not present before. Sleep and hyperkinetic movement disorders are reviewed elsewhere in this volume.

Tics in TS occur frequently during sleep stage I, awakening, or a stage shift from deeper to lighter, but rarely in other sleep stages.[133,134] These patients have been suggested to suffer from arousal disorder.[133] In 62 TS patients with sleep disturbances, only 3 patients complained of SB.[135] Clonazepam, clonidine, pimozide, haloperidol, tetrabenazine, or fluphenazine have been suggested to be effective in TS management.[135] The clinician should be aware that xerostomia, probably an adverse effect of the drugs, and orofacial pain have been noted in TS patients who use these drugs.[136] TS and its relation to sleep are reviewed elsewhere in this volume.

Cranial dystonia is another condition that can persist during sleep, although its frequency decreases during sleep compared with wakefulness.[137] Most dystonic events have been reported to occur during non-REM sleep without EEG arousal; no events were recorded during REM sleep. SB has also been reported in patients with oromandibular dystonia (OMD)[138,139] and cranial-cervical dystonia.[99] The prevalence of bruxism was reported to be higher in patients with cranial-cervical dystonia than normal controls.[99] Some of these patients reported concomitant burning mouth sensations, TMJ symptoms, or muscle stiffness and pain.[99,138,139] Drugs commonly used for dystonia, such as clonazepam, were ineffective in management of OMD.[139] The injection of BTX-A has been reported to be effective for OMD.[97] The use of an appropriate dosage of BTX-A has resulted in a good treatment outcome. However, it can cause dysphagia or jaw muscle weakness in some patients.[99,138,139]

The prevalence of bruxism in HFS patients seems to be in the same range as the normal population (approximately 4%: 7 out of 158 HFS patients).[140] HFS persists during sleep, but its frequency shows a progressive decrease throughout sleep compared with that during wakefulness.[141] Bruxism, during sleep and wakefulness, was recently reported to occur in HD patients.[142] BTX-A was observed to be effective for reducing bruxism in these patients.

Neuroleptic-Induced Orofacial Movements

Neuroleptic-induced movement disorders, with self-reported SB or tooth grinding, have emerged as a significant clinical problem in psychiatry and neurology. Little objective data exist on the coexistence of neuroleptic-induced movement disorders and SB and on their valid management strategies. More data thereof and a better understanding of the disorders are becoming a matter of importance in light of the incidence of the disorders in the growing older population.

In patients with psychiatric problems, concomitant SB occurred shortly after the administration of the antidopaminergic drug haloperidol. SB developed with the appearance of neuroleptic-induced akathisia, and both responded to the beta-adrenergic receptor antagonist propranolol.[95] Tooth grinding has been reported to occur during wakefulness after administration of chronic antipsychotic drugs or calcium antagonist to patients with dementia as a dystonic manifestation.[95,143]

A study found that tardive dyskinesia induced by chronic neuroleptic exposure seemed to disappear during sleep, whereas neuroleptic-induced orolabial tremor, the so-called rabbit syndrome, may persist during sleep stage I but disappear during other stages.[144]

Parkinson's Disease

There are few reports available on the occurrence of orofacial activity during the sleep of Parkinson's disease (PD) patients. PD and its relation to sleep are reviewed elsewhere in this volume. SB[145] and facial dystonia during sleep[146] were reported in some PD patients undergoing the levodopa treatment. Many PD patients complain of joint or muscle pain in the body, although orofacial pain does not seem to be highly prevalent.[147] Orofacial pain remains to be fully characterized in PD patients because the patient's other complaints are more commonly drawn to the physician's attention. SB patients have no dopamine deficiency as typically seen in PD; the density of striatal D2 receptors in SB patients is similar to that of matched controls.[148] However, physicians should be aware that secondary or iatrogenic bruxism can occur in PD patients[145,149] or patients undergoing dopaminergic drug therapy (see Table 41.1).[95,143] To our knowledge, there is no evidence that SB patients aged 18 to 45 run a greater risk of developing PD when they get older than the normal population.

Other Medical Conditions and Drugs Relating to Bruxism

Bruxism, with or without tooth grinding, is known to occur in the presence of medical conditions other than the ones mentioned earlier. Bruxism occurring during wakefulness and sleep in one patient with Whipple's disease was associated with oculomasticatory myorhythmias, synchronous rhythmic contractions of the eyelids, mouth, and face.[150] Also, tooth grinding was observed in comatose patients afflicted with acute viral encephalitis, tuberculous meningitis, or cortical vein thrombosis.[151] SB is reported in patients with psychiatric problems such as attention-deficit/hyperactivity disorder, anxiety disorders, and depression.[7,131]

Alcohol, caffeine, and cigarettes have been suggested to exacerbate SB.[7,61,62] Cocaine, amphetamine, and amphetamine-related drugs (Ecstasy) have also been reported to induce bruxing or clenching during wakefulness.[152]

REFERENCES

1. Thorpy MJ. In: (ASDA) DCSC, ed. *The International Classification of Sleep Disorders. Diagnostic and Coding Manual.* Lawrence, KS: Allen Press; 1990:xx–xx.
2. American Academy of Sleep Medicine. *International Classification of Sleep Disorders: Diagnostic and Coding Manual.* 2nd ed. Westchester, IL: American Academy of Sleep Medicine; 2005.
3. Lavigne GJ, Manzini C, Huynh N. Sleep bruxism. In: Kryger MH, Roth T, and Dement C, eds. *Principles and Practice of Sleep Medicine.* 5th ed. Philadelphia, PA: Elsevier Saunders; 2011:1128–39.
4. Lavigne GJ, Khoury S, Abe S, et al. Bruxism physiology and pathology: an overview for clinicians. *J Oral Rehabil* 2008;35:476–94.
5. Kato T, Lavigne GJ. Sleep bruxism: a sleep related movement disorder. *Sleep Med Clin* 2010;5: 9–35.
6. Lavigne GJ, Montplaisir JY. Restless legs syndrome and sleep bruxism: prevalence and association among Canadians. *Sleep* 1994;17:739–43.
7. Ohayon MM, Li KK, Guilleminault C. Risk factors for sleep bruxism in the general population. *Chest* 2001;119:53–61.
8. Widmalm SE, Christiansen RL, Gunn SM. Oral parafunctions as temporomandibular disorder risk factors in children. *Cranio* 1995;13:242–6.
9. Laberge L, Tremblay RE, Vitaro F, et al. Development of parasomnias from childhood to early adolescence. *Pediatrics* 2000;106:67–74.
10. Carra MC, Huynh N, Morton P, et al. Prevalence and risk factors of sleep bruxism and wake-time tooth clenching in a 7- to 17-yr-old population. *Eur J Oral Sci* 2011;119:386–94.
11. Kato T, Velly AM, Nakane T, et al. Age is associated with self-reported sleep bruxism, independently of tooth loss. *Sleep Breath* 2012;16(4):1159–65.
12. Macaluso GM, Guerra P, Di Giovanni G, et al. Sleep bruxism is a disorder related to periodic arousals during sleep. *J Dent Res* 1998;77:565–73.
13. Kato T, Rompre P, Montplaisir JY, et al. Sleep bruxism: an oromotor activity secondary to micro-arousal. *J Dent Res* 2001;80:1940–4.
14. Huynh N, Kato T, Rompre PH, et al. Sleep bruxism is associated to micro-arousals and an increase in cardiac sympathetic activity. *J Sleep Res* 2006;15:339–46.
15. Rompré PH, Daigle-Landry D, Guitard F, et al. Identification of a sleep bruxism subgroup with a higher risk of pain. *J Dent Res* 2007;86: 837–42.
16. Reding GR, Zepelin H, Robinson JE, Jr., et al. Nocturnal teeth-grinding: all-night psychophysiologic studies. *J Dent Res* 1968;47:786–97.
17. Lavigne GJ, Rompre PH, Montplaisir JY. Sleep bruxism: validity of clinical research diagnostic criteria in a controlled polysomnographic study. *J Dent Res* 1996;75:546–52.

18. Lavigne GJ, Rompre PH, Poirier G, et al. Rhythmic masticatory muscle activity during sleep in humans. *J Dent Res* 2001;80:443–8.

19. Halász P, Ujszászi J, Gádoros J. Are microarousals preceded by electroencephalographic slow wave synchronization precursors of confusional awakenings? *Sleep* 1985;8:231–8.

20. Sforza E, Zucconi M, Petronelli R, et al. REM sleep behavioral disorders. *Eur Neurol* 1988;28:295–300.

21. Sato T, Harada Y. Electrophysiological study on tooth-grinding during sleep. *Electroencephalogr Clin Neurophysiol* 1973;35:267–75.

22. Sjöholm T, Lehtinen I, Helenius H. Masseter muscle activity in diagnosed sleep bruxists compared with non-symptomatic controls. *J Sleep Res* 1995;4:48–55.

23. Bader GG, Kampe T, Tagdae T, et al. Descriptive physiological data on a sleep bruxism population. *Sleep* 1997;20:982–90.

24. Lavigne GJ, Rompre PH, Guitard F, et al. Lower number of K-complexes and K-alphas in sleep bruxism: a controlled quantitative study. *Clin Neurophysiol* 2002;113:686–93.

25. Ikeda T, Nishigawa K, Kondo K, et al. Criteria for the detection of sleep-associated bruxism in humans. *J Orofac Pain* 1996;10:270–82.

26. Zucconi M, Oldani A, Ferini-Strambi L, et al. Arousal fluctuations in non-rapid eye movement parasomnias: the role of cyclic alternating pattern as a measure of sleep instability. *J Clin Neurophysiol* 1995;12:147–54.

27. Terzano MG, Parrino L, Boselli M, et al. CAP components and EEG synchronization in the first 3 sleep cycles. *Clin Neurophysiol* 2000;111:283–90.

28. Carra MC, Macaluso GM, Rompre PH, et al. Clonidine has a paradoxical effect on cyclic arousal and sleep bruxism during NREM sleep. *Sleep* 2010;33:1711–16.

29. Carra MC, Rompre PH, Kato T, et al. Sleep bruxism and sleep arousal: an experimental challenge to assess the role of cyclic alternating pattern. *J Oral Rehabil* 2011;38:635–42.

30. Kato T, Montplaisir JY, Guitard F, et al. Evidence that experimentally induced sleep bruxism is a consequence of transient arousal. *J Dent Res* 2003;82:284–8.

31. Miyawaki S, Lavigne GJ, Pierre M, et al. Association between sleep bruxism, swallowing-related laryngeal movement, and sleep positions. *Sleep* 2003;26:461–5.

32. Khoury S, Rouleau GA, Rompre PH, et al. A significant increase in breathing amplitude precedes sleep bruxism. *Chest* 2008;134:332–7.

33. Nashed A, Lanfranchi P, Rompré P, et al. Sleep bruxism is associated with a rise in arterial blood pressure. *Sleep* 2012;35:529–36.

34. Lobbezoo F, Naeije M. Bruxism is mainly regulated centrally, not peripherally. *J Oral Rehabil* 2001;28:1085–91.

35. Lobbezoo F, Rompré PH, Soucy J-P, et al. Lack of associations between occlusal and cephalometric measures, side imbalance in striatal D2 receptor binding, and sleep-related oromotor activities. *J Orofac Pain* 2001;15:64–71.

36. Kato T, Thie NM, Huynh N, et al. Topical review: sleep bruxism and the role of peripheral sensory influences. *J Orofac Pain* 2003;17:191–213.

37. Manfredini D, Lobbezoo F. Role of psychosocial factors in the etiology of bruxism. *J Orofac Pain* 2009;23:153–66.

38. Pierce CJ, Chrisman K, Bennett ME, et al. Stress, anticipatory stress, and psychologic measures related to sleep bruxism. *J Orofac Pain* 1995;9: 51–6.

39. Manfredini D, Fabbri A, Peretta R, et al. Influence of psychological symptoms on home-recorded sleep-time masticatory muscle activity in healthy subjects. *J Oral Rehabil* 2011;38:902–11.

40. Major M, Rompré PH, Guitard F, et al. A controlled daytime challenge of motor performance and vigilance in sleep bruxers. *J Dent Res* 1999;78:1754–62.

41. Schneider C, Schaefer R, Ommerborn MA, et al. Maladaptive coping strategies in patients with bruxism compared to non-bruxing controls. *Int J Behav Med* 2007;14:257–61.

42. Hublin C, Kaprio J, Partinen M, et al. Sleep bruxism based on self-report in a nationwide twin cohort. *J Sleep Res* 1998;7:61–7.

43. Abe Y, Suganuma T, Ishii M, et al. Association of genetic, psychological and behavioral factors with sleep bruxism in a Japanese population. *J Sleep Res.* 2012;21:289–96.

44. Velly Miguel AM, Montplaisir J, Rompre PH, et al. Bruxism and other orofacial movements during sleep. *J Craniomandib Disord: Fac Oral Pain* 1992;6:71–81.

45. Dutra KM, Pereira FJ, Jr., Rompre PH, et al. Oro-facial activities in sleep bruxism patients and in normal subjects: a controlled polygraphic and audio-video study. *J Oral Rehabil* 2009;36:86–92.

46. Abe S, Yamaguchi T, Rompre PH, et al. Tooth wear in young subjects: a discriminator between sleep bruxers and controls? *Int J Prosthodont* 2009;22:342–50.

47. Dao TTT, Lund JP, Lavigne GJ. Comparison of pain and quality of life in bruxers and patients with myofascial pain of the masticatory muscles. *J Orofac Pain* 1994;8:350–5.

48. Lobbezoo F, Lavigne GJ. Do bruxism and temporomandibular disorders have a cause-and-effect relationship? *J Orofac Pain* 1997;11:15–23.

49. Svensson P, Jadidi F, Arima T, et al. Relationships between craniofacial pain and bruxism. *J Oral Rehabil* 2008;35:524–47.

50. Ommerborn MA, Schneider C, Giraki M, et al. In vivo evaluation of noncarious cervical lesions in sleep bruxism subjects. *J Prosthet Dent* 2007;98:150–8.

51. Turp JC, Gobetti JP. The cracked tooth syndrome: an elusive diagnosis. *J Am Dent Assoc* 1996;127:1502–7.

52. Ekfeldt A, Johansson LA, Isaksson S. Implant-supported overdenture therapy: a retrospective study. *Int J Prosthodont* 1997;10:366–74.

53. Walters AS, Lavigne G, Hening W, et al. The scoring of movements in sleep. *J Clin Sleep Med* 2007;3:155–67.

54. Kato T, Montplaisir JY, Blanchet PJ, et al. Idiopathic myoclonus in the oromandibular region during sleep: a possible source of confusion in sleep bruxism diagnosis. *Mov Disord* 1999;14:865–71.

55. Kato T, Thie NM, Montplaisir JY, et al. Bruxism and orofacial movements during sleep. *Dent Clin North Am* 2001;45:657–84.

56. Gallo LM, Lavigne G, Rompre P, et al. Reliability of scoring EMG orofacial events: polosomnography compared with ambulatory recordings. *J Sleep Res* 1997;6:259–63.

57. American Academy of Sleep Medicine. *The AASM Manual for the Scoring of Sleep and Associated Events: Rules, Terminology and Technical Specifications*. Westchester, IL: American Academy of Sleep Medicine; 2007.

58. Smith MT, Wickwire EM, Grace EG, et al. Sleep disorders and their association with laboratory pain sensitivity in temporomandibular joint disorder. *Sleep* 2009;32:779–90.

59. Lobbezoo F, van der Zaag J, van Selms MK, et al. Principles for the management of bruxism. *J Oral Rehabil* 2008;35:509–23.

60. Morin CM. Psychological and behavioral treatments for primary insomnia. In: Kryger MH, Roth T, Dement C, eds. *Principles and Practice of Sleep Medicine*. 5th ed. Philadelphia, PA: Elsevier Saunders; 2005:726–48.

61. Lavigne GL, Lobbezoo F, Rompre PH, et al. Cigarette smoking as a risk factor or an exacerbating factor for restless legs syndrome and sleep bruxism. *Sleep* 1997;20:290–3.

62. Rintakoski K, Ahlberg J, Hublin C, et al. Tobacco use and reported bruxism in young adults: a nationwide Finnish Twin Cohort Study. *Nicotine Tob Res* 2010;12:679–83.

63. Clarke JH, Reynolds PJ. Suggestive hypnotherapy for nocturnal bruxism: a pilot study. *Am J Clin Hypn* 1991;33:248–53.

64. Cassisi JE, McGlynn FD, Belles DR. EMG-activated feedback alarms for the treatment of nocturnal bruxism: current status and future directions. *Biofeedback Self-Regulat* 1987;12:13–30.

65. Pierce CJ, Gale EN. A comparison of different treatments for nocturnal bruxism. *J Dent Res* 1988;67:597–601.

66. Nishigawa K, Kondo K, Takeuchi H, et al. Contingent electrical lip stimulation for sleep bruxism: a pilot study. *J Prosthet Dent* 2003;89:412–17.

67. Jadidi F, Castrillon E, Svensson P. Effect of conditioning electrical stimuli on temporalis electromyographic activity during sleep. *J Oral Rehabil* 2008;35:171–83.

67a. Jadidi F, Nørregaard O, Baad-Hansen L, et al. Assessment of sleep parameters during contingent electrical stimulation in subjects with jaw muscle activity during sleep: a polysomnographic study. *Eur J Oral Sci.* 2011;119:211–8.

68. Dao TTT, Lavigne GJ. Oral sprint: the crutches for temporomandibular disorders and bruxism? *Crit Rev Oral Biol Med* 1998;9:345–61.

69. Solberg WK, Clark GT, Rugh JD. Nocturnal electromyographic evaluation of bruxism patients undergoing short term splint therapy. *J Oral Rehabil* 1975;2:215–23.

70. Dube C, Rompre PH, Manzini C, et al. Quantitative polygraphic controlled study on efficacy and safety of oral splint devices in tooth-grinding subjects. *J Dent Res* 2004;83:398–403.

71. Harada T, Ichiki R, Tsukiyama Y, et al. The effect of oral splint devices on sleep bruxism: a 6-week observation with an ambulatory electromyographic recording device. *J Oral Rehabil* 2006;33:482–8.

72. Clark GT, Beemsterboer PL, Solverg WK, et al. Nocturnal electromyographic evaluation of myofascial pain dysfunction in patients undergoing occlusal splint therapy. *J Am Dent Ass* 1979;99:607–11.

73. Okesson JP. The effects of hard and soft occlusal splints on nocturnal bruxism. *J Am Dent Ass* 1987;114:788–91.

74. van der Zaag J, Lobbezoo F, Wicks DJ, et al. Controlled assessment of the efficacy of occlusal stabilization splints on sleep bruxism. *J Orofac Pain* 2005;19:151–8.

75. Gagnon Y, Mayer P, Morisson F, et al. Aggravation of respiratory disturbances by the use of an occlusal splint in apneic patients: a pilot study. *Int J Prosthodont* 2004;17:447–53.

76. Landry ML, Rompre PH, Manzini C, et al. Reduction of sleep bruxism using a mandibular advancement device: an experimental controlled study. *Int J Prosthodont* 2006;19:549–56.

77. Landry-Schonbeck A, de Grandmont P, Rompre PH, et al. Effect of an adjustable mandibular advancement appliance on sleep bruxism: a crossover sleep laboratory study. *Int J Prosthodont* 2009;22:251–9.

78. Baad-Hansen L, Jadidi F, Castrillon E, et al. Effect of a nociceptive trigeminal inhibitory splint on electromyographic activity in jaw closing muscles during sleep. *J Oral Rehabil* 2007;34:105–11.

79. Clark GT, Tsukiyama Y, Baba K, et al. Sixty-eight years of experimental occlusal interference studies: what have we learned? *J Prosthet Dent* 1999;82:704–13.

80. De Boever JA, Carlsson GE, Klineberg IJ. Need for occlusal theraepy and prosthodontic treatment in the management of temporomandibular disorders. Part I. Occlusal interferences and occlusal adjustment. *J Oral Rehabil* 2000;27:367–79.

81. Chasins AI. Methocarbamal (robaxin) as an adjunct in the treatment of bruxism. *J Dent Med* 1959;14:166–70.

82. Montgomery MT, Nishioka GJ, Rugh JD, et al. Effect of diszepam on nocturnal masticatory muscle activity. *J Dent Res* 1986;65:96.

83. Schenck CH, Mahowald MW. Long-term, nightly benzodiazepine treatment of injurious parasomnias and other disorders of disrupted nocturnal sleep in 170 adults. *Am J Med* 1996;100:333–7.

84. Saletu A, Parapatics S, Saletu B, et al. On the pharmacotherapy of sleep bruxism: placebo-controlled polysomnographic and psychometric studies with clonazepam. *Neuropsychobiol* 2005;51:214–25.

85. Mohamed SE, Christensen LV, Penchas J. A randomized double-blind clinical trial of the effect of amitriptyline on nocturnal masseteric motor activity (sleep Bruxism). *Cranio* 1997;15: 326–32.

86. Raigrodski AJ, Christensen LV, Mohamed SE, et al. The effect of four-week administration of amitriptyline on sleep bruxism. A double-blind crossover clinical study. *Cranio* 2001;19:21–5.

87. Ellison JM, Stanziani P. SSRI-associated nocturnal bruxism in four patients. *J Clin Psychiat* 1993;54:432–4.

88. Gerber PE, Lynd LD. Selective serotonin-reuptake inhibitor-induced movement disorders. *Ann Pharmacother* 1998;32: 692–8.

89. Lobbezoo F, van Denderen RJ, Verheij JG, et al. Reports of SSRI-associated bruxism in the family physician's office. *J Orofac Pain* 2001;15:340–6.

90. Leo RJ. Movement disorders associated with the serotonin selective reuptake inhibitors. *J Clin Psychiatr* 1996;57:449–54.

91. Lobbezoo F, Lavigne GJ, Tanguay R, et al. The effect of catecholamine precursor L-dopa on sleep bruxism: a controlled clinical trial. *Mov Disord* 1997;12:73–8.

92. Lavigne GJ, Soucy JP, Lobbezoo F, et al. Double-blind, crossover, placebo-controlled trial of bromocriptine in patients with sleep bruxism. *Clin Neuropharmacol* 2001;24:145–9.

93. Van der Zaag J, Lobbezoo F, Van der Avoort PG, et al. Effects of pergolide on severe sleep bruxism in a patient experiencing oral implant failure. *J Oral Rehabil* 2007;34: 317–22.

94. Sjöholm TT, Lehtinen I, Piha SJ. The effect of propranolol on sleep bruxism: hypothetical considerations based on a case study. *Clin Auton Res* 1996;6:37–40.

95. Amir I, Hermesh H, Gavish A. Bruxism secondary to antipsychotic drug exposure: a positive response to propranolol. *Clin Neuropharmacol* 1997;20:86–9.

96. Huynh N, Lavigne GJ, Lanfranchi PA, et al. The effect of 2 sympatholytic medications—propranolol and clonidine—on sleep bruxism: experimental randomized controlled studies. *Sleep* 2006;29:307–16.

97. Jankovic J. Botulinum toxin in movement disorders. *Curr Opin Neurol* 1994;7:358–66.

97a. Smyth AG. Botulinum toxin treatment of bilateral masseteric hypertrophy. *Br J Oral Maxillofac Surg* 1994;32:29–33.

98. Tan E-K, Jankovic J. Treating severe bruxism with botulinum toxin. *J Am Dent Ass* 2000;131:211–16.

99. Watts MW, Tan EK, Jankovic J. Bruxism and cranial-cervical dystonia: is there a relationship? *Cranio* 1999;17:196–201.

100. Lee SJ, McCall WD, Jr., Kim YK, et al. Effect of botulinum toxin injection on nocturnal bruxism: a randomized controlled trial. *Am J Phys Med Rehabil* 2010;89(1):16–23.

101. Sjöholm TT, Lowe AA, Miyamoto K, et al. Sleep bruxism in patients with sleep-disordered breathing. *Arch Oral Biol* 2000;45:889–96.

102. Okeson JP, Phillips BA, Berry DT, et al. Nocturnal bruxing events in subjects with sleep-disordered breathing and control subjects. *J Craniomandib Disord* 1991;5:258–64.

103. Phillips BA, Okeson J, Paesani D, et al. Effect of sleep position on sleep apnea and parafunctional activity. *Chest* 1986;90:424–9.

104. Kato T. Sleep bruxism and its relation to obstructive sleep apnea-hypopnea syndrome. *Sleep Biol Rhythm* 2004;2:1–15.

105. Hoekema A, Stegenga B, De Bont LG. Efficacy and co-morbidity of oral appliances in the treatment of obstructive sleep apnea-hypopnea: a systematic review. *Crit Rev Oral Biol Med* 2004;15:137–55.

106. de Almeida FR, Lowe AA, Tsuiki S, et al. Long-term compliance and side effects of oral appliances used for the treatment of snoring and obstructive sleep apnea syndrome. *J Clin Sleep Med* 2005;1:143–52.

107. Veasey SC, Guilleminault C, Strohl KP, et al. Medical therapy for obstructive sleep apnea: a review by the Medical Therapy for Obstructive Sleep Apnea Task Force of the Standards of Practice Committee of the American Academy of Sleep Medicine. *Sleep* 2006;29:1036–44.

108. Pantin CC, Hillman DR, Tennant M. Dental side effects of an oral device to treat snoring and obstructive sleep apnea. *Sleep* 1999;22:237–40.

109. Clark GT, Sohn J-W, Hong CN. Treating obstructive sleep apnea and snoring: assessment of an anterior mandibular positioning device. *J Am Dent Ass* 2000;131:765–71.

110. Fox PC, Busch KA, Baum BJ. Subjective reports of xerostomia and objective measures of salivary gland performance. *J Am Dent Assoc* 1987;115: 581–4.

111. Thie NM, Kato T, Bader G, et al. The significance of saliva during sleep and the relevance of oromotor movements. *Sleep Med Rev* 2002;6:213–27.

112. Paterson AJ, Lamb AB, Clifford TJ, et al. Burning mouth syndrome: the relationship between the HAD scale and parafunctional habits. *J Oral Pathol Med* 1995;24:289–92.

113. Orr WC. Gastrointestinal Physiology. In: Kryger MH, Roth T, Dement WC, eds. *Principles and Practices of Sleep Medicine*. 5th ed. Philadelphia, PA: Elsevier Saunders; 2005:283–91.

114. Järvinen V, Meurman JH, Hyvärinen H, et al. Dental erosion and upper gastrointestinal disorders. *Oral Surg Oral Med Oral Pathol* 1988;65:298–303.

115. Kao CH, Ho YJ, ChangLai SP, et al. Evidence for decreased salivary function in patients with reflux esophagitis. *Digestion* 1999;60:191–5.

116. Gudmundsson K, Kristlerfsson G, Theodors A, et al. Tooth erosion, gastroesophageal reflux, and salivary buffer capacity. *Oral Surg Oral Med Oral Pathol Oral Radiol Endodont* 1995;79:185–9.

117. Freidin N, Fisher MJ, Taylor W, et al. Sleep and nocturnal acid reflux in normal subjects and patients with reflux oesophagitis. *Gut* 1991;32:1275–9.

118. Miyawaki S, Tanimoto Y, Araki Y, et al. Association between nocturnal bruxism and gastroesophageal reflux. *Sleep* 2003;26: 888–92.

119. Ohmure H, Oikawa K, Kanematsu K, et al. Influence of experimental esophageal acidification on sleep bruxism: a randomized trial. *J Dent Res* 2011;90(5):665–71.

120. Vetrugno R, Provini F, Plazzi G, et al. Familial nocturnal facio-mandibular myoclonus mimicking sleep bruxism. *Neurology* 2002;58:644–7.

121. Meletti S, Cantalupo G, Volpi L, et al. Rhythmic teeth grinding induced by temporal lobe seizures. *Neurology* 2004;62:2306–9.

122. Bisulli F, Vignatelli L, Naldi I, Licchetta L, Provini F, Plazzi G, Di Vito L, Ferioli S, Montagna P, Tinuper P. Increased frequency of arousal parasomnias in families with nocturnal frontal lobe epilepsy: a common mechanism? Epilepsia. 2010 Sep;51(9):1852–60. doi: 10.1111/j.1528-1167.2010.02581.x.

123. Aguglia U, Gambardella A, Quattrone A. Sleep-induced masticatory myoclonus: a rare parasomnia associated with insomnia. *Sleep* 1991;14:80–2.

124. Frauscher B, Iranzo A, Hogl B, et al. Quantification of electromyographic activity during REM sleep in multiple muscles in REM sleep behavior disorder. *Sleep* 2008;31:724–31.

125. Abe S, Rompre PH, Gagnon JF, et al. Absence of tooth grinding in individuals with REM sleep behaior disorders. *87th Genral Session and Exhibitoin of the IADR* (abstract). 2009;210#74.

126. Tachibana N, Yamanaka K, Kaji R, et al. Sleep bruxism as a manifestation of subclinical rapid eye movement sleep behavior disorder. *Sleep* 1994;17:555–8.

127. Lapierre O, Montplaisir J. Polysomnographic features of REM sleep behavior disorder: development of a scoring method. *Neurology* 1992;42: 1371–4.

128. Ohayon MM, Caulet M, Priest RG. Violent behavior during sleep. *J Clin Psychiat* 1997;58:369–76.

129. Khatami R, Zutter D, Siegel A, et al. Sleep-wake habits and disorders in a series of 100 adult epilepsy patients—prospective study. *Seizure* 2006;15:299–306.

130. Ahlberg K, Jahkola A, Savolainen A, et al. Associations of reported bruxism with insomnia and insufficient sleep symptoms among media personnel with or without irregular shift work. *Head Face Med* 2008;4:4.

131. Ghanizadeh A. ADHD, bruxism and psychiatric disorders: does bruxism increase the chance of a comorbid psychiatric disorder in children with ADHD and their parents? *Sleep Breath* 2008;12:375–80.

132. Prihodova I, Sonka K, Kemlink D, et al. Arousals in nocturnal groaning. *Sleep Med* 2009;10:1051–5.

133. Glaze DG, Frost JD, Jankovic J. Sleep in Gilles de la Tourette's syndrome: disorders of arousal. *Neurology* 1983;33:586–92.

134. Fish DR, Sawyers D, Allen PJ, et al. The effect of sleep on the dyskinetic movements of Parkinson's disease, Gilles de la Tourette syndrome, Huntington's disease, and torsion dystonia. *Archives Neurology* 1991;48:210–14.

135. Jankovic J, Rohaidy H. Motor, behavioral and pharmacologic findings in Tourette's syndrome. *Can J Neurol Sci* 1987;14: 541–6.

136. Friedlander AH, Cummigs JL. Dental treatment of patients with Gilles de la Tourette's syndrome. *Oral Surg Oral Med Oral Pathol* 1992;73:299–303.

137. Sforza E, Montagna P, Defazio G. Sleep and cranial dystonia. *Electroencephal Clin Neurophysiol* 1991;79:166–9.

138. Ghika J, Regli F, Growdon JH. Sensory symptoms in cranial dystonia: a potential role in the etiology? *J Neurol Sci* 1993;116:142–7.

139. Sankhla C, Lai EC, Jankovic J. Peripherally induced oromandibular dystonia. *J Neurol Neurosurg Psyciatr* 1998;65:722–8.

140. Montagna P, Imbriaco A, Zucconi M, et al. Hemifacial spasm in sleep. *Neurology* 1986;36:270–3.

141. Wang A, Jankovic J. Hemifacial spasm: clinical findings and treatment. *Muscle Nerve* 1998;21:1740–7.

142. Tan EK, Jankovic J, Ondo W. Bruxism in Huntington's disease. *Mov Disord* 2000;15:171–3.

143. Micheli F, Fernandez Pardal M, Gatto M, et al. Bruxism secondary to chronic antidopaminergic drug exposure. *Clin Neuropharmacol* 1993;16:315–23.

144. Jus K, Jus A, Villeneuve A. Polygraphic profile of oral tardive dyskinesia and of rabbit syndrome: for quantitative and qualitative evaluation. *Dis Nerv Sys* 1973;34:27–32.

145. Magee KR. Bruxism related to levodopa therapy. *JAMA* 1970;214:147.

146. Lees AJ, Blackburn NA, Campbell VL. The nighttime problems of Parkinson's disease. *Clin Neuropharmacol* 1988;11:512–19.

147. Ford B, Louis ED, Greene P, et al. Oral and genital pain syndrome in Parkinson's disease. *Mov Disord* 1996;11:421–6.

148. Lobbezoo F, Soucy JP, Montplaisir JY, et al. Striatal D2 receptor binding in sleep bruxism: a controlled study with iodine-123-iodobenzamide and single-photon-emission computed tomography. *J Dent Res* 1996;75:1804–10.

149. Hauser RA, Olanow CW. Orobuccal dyskinesia associated with trihexyphenidyl therapy in a patient with Parkinson's disease. *Mov Disord* 1993;8:512–14.

150. Tison F, Louvet-Giendaj C, Henry P, et al. Permanent bruxism as a manifestation of the oculo-facial syndrome related to systemic Whipple's disease. *Mov Disord* 1992;7:82–5.

151. Pratap-Chand R, Gourie-Devi M. Bruxism: its significance in coma. *Clin Neurol Neurosurg* 1985;87:113–17.

152. Winocur E, Gavish A, Voikovitch M, et al. Drugs and bruxism: a critical review. *J Orofac Pain* 2003;17:99–111.

42

Restless Legs Syndrome
(Willis-Ekbom Disease)

An Introduction

RICHARD P. ALLEN, SUDHANSU CHOKROVERTY,
AND ARTHUR S. WALTERS

RESTLESS LEGS syndrome (RLS) after its first medical description by Willis in the 17th century[1,2] was largely ignored until the masterful synthesis of over 127 cases by Karl-Axel Ekbom.[3] He coined the name "restless legs" and provided the basic description of its symptoms. This condition gained increasing recognition with the development of the modern medical focus on not only prolonging life but also prolonging healthy living and maintaining quality of life. Thus, many chronic diseases have little impact on longevity but significantly curtail quality of life. RLS is one of these. At the same time, since the middle of the last century, there has been increasing awareness of the importance of sleep medicine. Disorders associated with sleep and arousal or waking have appropriately received attention as the long neglected silent third of life. Thus, the book you are currently reading: an entire book on movement disorders in sleep. It represents a compendium of information on this major subspecialty of the developing field of sleep medicine.

RLS, in particular, is the second or third most common sleep disorder, only less common than insomnia and perhaps slightly less common than sleep-disordered breathing. It also produces the most profound chronic sleep loss of any of the sleep disorders, reducing sleep times to an average of 5.5 hours a night for moderate to severe RLS.[4] Thus, about 1% to 3% of adults live with chronic profound sleep loss from RLS. This represents a major personal and public health problem that even today is only poorly recognized.[5,6]

RLS also intimately involves disruption of normal sensory-motor function in relation to the sleep state. The condition usually produces abnormal movements in sleep, and its primary symptom is an abnormal urge to move the legs related to inactivity and decreased alertness. Movement or arousal relieves the symptoms. It clearly deserves to be considered one of the major, if not *the* major movement-related disorder of sleep medicine.

The first edition of this book recognized the major developments in our understanding of RLS since the seminal work by Ekbom. Most of this occurred because of the pioneering studies of Wayne Hening and Arthur Walters, who essentially reintroduced RLS to the modern medical and sleep literature with their important descriptions of cases seen in their movement disorders clinic while working with Sudhansu Chokroverty. They published descriptions of the characteristics of these patients, including recognition of its presentation during resting while awake.[7] They went on to develop the currently used scale for evaluating the severity of RLS (the IRLS)[8] and set the basics for the diagnostic criteria for the disease.[9] The diagnostic criteria continued to evolve with a major clarification of the centrality of the urge to move at a consensus conference at the American National Institute of Health.[10] This standardization of diagnosis and severity evaluation permitted a virtual explosion of knowledge about the disorder that has continued since the first edition of this book and continues today. In fact, in the first 14 weeks of 2012, there were 107 articles related to RLS listed in Pub Med.

The first edition of this book noted important developments in epidemiology, pathophysiology, genetics, diagnosis, evaluation, and treatment of RLS. All of this has undergone major changes since the first edition was published. These advances have been well documented in this book mostly in the chapters in this section. Epidemiological studies have not only documented the variable prevalence of this disease but also factors contributing to its occurrence. Thus, as noted in the epidemiology (Chapter 43), RLS appears more common in women and in older individuals[10] and is less common in Japanese[11] but not Korean populations.[12] It occurs fairly commonly in children (about 0.25% to 1%), and there is no gender difference.[13] Chapter 46 on RLS in children notes several interesting characteristics of the presentation of this disease in children.

Curiously pregnancy appears to be a major factor contributing to occurrence of RLS even years after the pregnancy, so that nulliparous women have the same risk of RLS as men and significantly less risk than women who have been pregnant.[14,15] The major issue is that now epidemiology informs about significant risk factors for RLS that advance our understanding of the genetics and biology of the disease as well as areas for focusing treatment.

Perhaps the most remarkable advances in RLS have been in understanding the pathophysiology and genetics of RLS. As documented in the pathophysiology (Chapter 44), the RLS dopamine relation was not the expected decrease but rather an increase in dopaminergic production[16] with postsynaptic downregulation. In addition, data indicate likely increased glutamate[17] in RLS. Dopamine and glutamate would also both be increased with brain iron deficiency, linking these two abnormalities of RLS to one possible common cause. The noted anatomical changes in function with RLS appear to affect large parts of the brain and even peripheral muscles, and thus this is seen more as systemic or metabolic disease than the result of a specific loss of function in one area of the brain. The developing understanding of the RLS biology has now reached the point where it may guide treatment considerations, the opposite of the prior situation with treatment response guiding pathophysiological considerations.

The genetics of RLS have received considerable attention and are well documented in Chapter 8 on genetics of sleep included in an earlier section of this book. It remains a testimony to the coherence of the diagnostic criteria that RLS is well enough defined to permit identifying a small set of specific allelic variations associated with significant increased risk of developing RLS. These were discovered from modest size samples of patients with RLS compared to a large general population,[18,19] supporting the concept that RLS represents one coherent disease process.

Diagnosis has also advanced considerably with the recognition of both the importance of differential diagnosis and consideration of the course and clinical significance of the disorder. The differential diagnosis requires excluding disorders that produce symptoms closely mimicking those of RLS.[20] The RLS "mimics" can usually be easily identified in a clinical setting but are hard to exclude in population-based studies using questionnaires. These considerations led to the development of new diagnostic criteria for RLS that build on the prior criteria by adding a requirement that the RLS "mimics" are excluded. The new criteria also include clinical specifiers for clinical course and significance. Tools have also now been developed that are reasonably well-validated tools aides for making the diagnosis of RLS. These include a patient-completed questionnaire, a structured clinical inventory, and a structured diagnostic interview. These all permit more accurate diagnosis of RLS patients for clinical and epidemiological studies. They are included in Chapter 45 along with access to supplemental material to support expanding their use to enhance accuracy of diagnosis.

Chapter 47 on morbidity of RLS points out that the clinical consequences of RLS cannot be adequately explained as a response to primary symptoms. This rather profound appreciation of the scope of the impact of the disorder changes our focus from RLS symptoms to biology. The increased sleep loss, anxiety, depression.[21] and possible cardiovascular disease[22] seen with RLS appear to relate more to as yet unidentified underlying biological aspects of RLS than to the effects of the primary symptoms. The broad range of these morbidities of RLS serves to explain the profound effects RLS has on quality of life. Clearly, RLS is not only the thief of sleep but also of a healthy satisfactory life.

Finally, RLS treatments as described in Chapter 48 have advanced considerably with both a better understanding of the long-term consequences of the treatments, particularly the problems with RLS augmentation and an appreciation of the importance of nondopaminergic treatments. It is no longer the case that dopaminergic agonists should be considered the treatments of first choice for RLS; alternatives have now been demonstrated to work as well. Thus, we have a range of treatment options not previously available. Moreover, there are options for combined medications that may be needed to respond to morbidity as well as symptoms of the disease. Parenteral iron treatment documented as efficacious in one small controlled study,[23] despite holding great promise, remains poorly developed as a treatment option. Hopefully, understanding RLS biology will lead to better treatments.

The growing awareness of RLS biology and morbidity demonstrates that the current name for the condition is really inappropriate. The condition does not involve restlessness but rather a compelling specific urge to move; it is not a general restless feeling. This urge to move is not ubiquitous but rather develops under specific conditions. RLS has a very coherent pattern and now a better understood biology; thus, it is not a syndrome representing a collection of symptoms and problems but rather a neurological disease. It may, like many diseases, have multiple causes, but it has one central

symptomatic presentation and it appears to have a single unified biology. Given these issues, there has been a decision to add a new name for the disease that reduces the confusion introduced by the current name. The international restless legs syndrome study group (IRLSSG) and the patient groups in Europe and America have adopted *Willis-Ekbom disease* as a new alternate name for the disease. This new name recognizes the two neurologists who first characterized the disorder in the medical literature and avoids attempting to describe features of the disease. Willis-Ekbom disease may increasingly be used as the name for this disease in the future.

As noted previously, the continuing rapid development of scientific and clinical studies of Willis-Ekbom disease (RLS) bodes well for a better future for Willis-Ekbom patients. Much has been discovered, but there is much more to do.

REFERENCES

1. Willis T. *De Animae Brutorum*. London: Wells and Scott; 1672.
2. Willis T. *The London Practice of Physick*. London: Bassett and Crooke; 1685.
3. Ekbom KA. *Restless Legs*. Frey H, trans. Stockholm, Sweden: Ivar Haeggströms; 1945.
4. Allen RP, Stillman P, Myers AJ. Physician-diagnosed restless legs syndrome in a large sample of primary medical care patients in Western Europe: prevalence and characteristics. *Sleep Med* 2010;11(1):31–7.
5. Earley CJ, Silber MH. Restless legs syndrome: understanding its consequences and the need for better treatment. *Sleep Med* 2010;11(9):807–15.
6. Allen RP, Bharmal M, Calloway M. Prevalence and disease burden of primary restless legs syndrome: results of a general population survey in the United States. *Mov Disord* 2011;26(1):114–20.
7. Walters AS, Hening WA, Chokroverty S. Frequent occurrence of myoclonus while awake and at rest, body rocking and marching in place in a subpopulation of patients with restless legs syndrome. *Acta Neurol Scand* 1988;77(5):418–21.
8. Walters AS, Rosen R, Hening W, et al. A test of the reliability and validity of a brief, patient-completed severity questionnaire for the restless legs syndrome: The International

RLS Study Group Rating Scale. [abstract]. *Sleep* 2001;.

9. Walters A S, Aldrich MA, Allen RP, et al. Toward a better definition of the restless legs syndrome. *Mov Disord* 1995;10:634–42.

10. Allen RP, Picchietti D, Hening WA, et al. Restless legs syndrome: diagnostic criteria, special considerations, and epidemiology. A report from the restless legs syndrome diagnosis and epidemiology workshop at the National Institutes of Health. *Sleep Med* 2003;4(2):101–19.

11. Nomura T, Inoue Y, Kusumi M, et al. Prevalence of restless legs syndrome in a rural community in Japan. *Mov Disord* 2008;23(16):2363–9.

12. Cho YW, Shin WC, Yun CH, et al. Epidemiology of restless legs syndrome in Korean adults. *Sleep* 2008;31(2):219–23.

13. Picchietti D, Allen RP, Walters AS, et al. Restless legs syndrome: prevalence and impact in children and adolescents—the Peds REST study. *Pediatrics* 2007;120(2):253–66.

14. Pantaleo NP, Hening WA, Allen RP, et al. Pregnancy accounts for most of the gneder differences in prevalence of familial RLS. *Sleep Med* 2010;11(3):310–13.

15. Berger K, Luedemann J, Trenkwalder C, et al. Sex and the risk of restless legs syndrome in the general population. *Arch Intern Med* 2004;164(2):196–202.

16. Allen RP, Connor JR, Hyland K, et al. Abnormally increased CSF 3-Ortho-methyldopa (3-OMD) in untreated restless legs syndrome (RLS) patients indicates more severe disease and possibly abnormally increased dopamine synthesis. *Sleep Med* 2009;10(1):123–8.

17. Allen RP, Barker PB, Horska A. Restless legs syndrome: a hyperarousal disorder with a thalamic glutamate abnormality. *Neurology* 2011;76(Supp 4):A369.

18. Winkelmann J, Schormair B, Lichtner P, et al. Genome-wide association study of restless legs syndrome identifies common variants in three genomic regions. *Nat Genet* 2007;39(9):1000–6.

19. Stefansson H, Rye DB, Hicks A, et al. A genetic risk factor for periodic limb movements in sleep. *N Engl J Med* 2007;357(7):639–47.

20. Hening WA, Allen RP, Washburn M, et al. The four diagnostic criteria for the restless legs syndrome are unable to exclude confounding conditions ("mimics"). *Sleep Med* 2009;10(9):976–81.

21. Winkelmann J, Prager M, Lieb R, et al. "Anxietas tibiarum." Depression and anxiety disorders in patients with restless legs syndrome. *J Neurol* 2005;252(1):67–71.

22. Winkelman JW, Shahar E, Sharief I, et al. Association of restless legs syndrome and cardiovascular disease in the Sleep Heart Health Study. *Neurology* 2008;70(1):35–42.

23. Allen RP, Adler CH, Du W, et al. Clinical efficacy and safety of IV ferric carboxymaltose (FCM) treatment of RLS: a multi-centred, placebo-controlled preliminary clinical trial. *Sleep Med* 2011;12(9):906–13.

43

The Epidemiology of Restless Legs Syndrome

CLAUDIA DIEDERICHS AND KLAUS BERGER

THE FIRST description of specific clinical symptoms of the restless legs syndrome (RLS) dates back to the end of the 17th century.[1] Within the next two centuries RLS had an interesting history of attribution to different medical disciplines, until in 1945 the Swedish neurologist Ekbom established the name and provided a case description.[2] Fifty years later, the newly formed International Restless Legs Syndrome Study Group (IRLSSG) with 28 experts from seven countries developed a common set of minimal criteria for RLS,[3] which was revised in 2003.[4] The IRLSSG criteria, listed in Table 43.1, are essential for the diagnosis of RLS.

The IRLSSG also established criteria for the diagnosis of RLS in special populations, such as the cognitive impaired elderly and children. Today, most epidemiological studies published after 2003 use the minimal criteria to classify RLS case status.[5]

Although these criteria are well established and widely used in research, they have been criticized for their inability to exclude other conditions causing similar symptoms, for example, leg cramps, resulting in a specificity of 84%.[6] The specificity is defined as the ability of an instrument to correctly identify individuals without RLS. In combination with the sensitivity, it is a measure for the performance of a diagnostic instrument. Sensitivity describes the ability to correctly detect individuals suffering from RLS. However, other instruments, such as the Hopkins Telephone Diagnostic Interview (HDTI), with a higher sensitivity and specificity[7] have a limited practicability in epidemiological research because of the length of the questionnaire.

In other studies, the shortcomings of the IRLSSG definition are met by adding further symptoms, for example, the presence of sleep disruption[8,9] or the feeling of at least moderate distress,[10] which are not specific for but often observed in cases with RLS. An alternative approach is the determination of a minimum frequency of RLS symptoms, for example,

Table 43.1 International Restless Legs Syndrome Study Group Essential Diagnostic Criteria for Restless Legs Syndrome

1. The urge to move one's legs, usually accompanied or caused by an uncomfortable sensation in the legs

2. The urge to move or unpleasant sensations beginning or worsening during periods of rest or inactivity

3. The urge to move or unpleasant sensations that are either partially or totally relieved by movement

4. The urge to move or unpleasant sensations that worsen in the evening or at night compared to during the day or that occur only in the evening or night

more than once per week,[11] concentrating on those moderately to severely affected. Despite these various approaches to narrow the diagnostic definition for RLS, the four minimal criteria set up by the IRLSSG are still the most widely used tool to assess the prevalence of RLS symptoms.[5]

Thus, the establishment of a standardized instrument, in combination with the growing recognition of RLS as a neurological disorder, has prepared the ground for an increasing number of studies on the prevalence of RLS on the population level.[5] Population-based epidemiologic research is important because it complements knowledge gained in laboratory settings by providing precise estimates of disease prevalence and incidence, generating and testing etiologic hypotheses through the analysis of risk factors, clarifying the role of genetic markers in association studies of cases and controls sampled from the same source population and in evaluating disease outcomes from a population perspective. As with many other examples, in particular from cardiovascular disease, epidemiologic research contributes to better understand the etiology of RLS and thus will eventually lead to improved treatment options and, equally important, permit the development of preventive strategies.

PREVALENCE OF RESTLESS LEGS SYNDROME IN THE GENERAL POPULATION

The majority of population-based studies on the prevalence of RLS are conducted in the United States, Canada, Western Europe, and some Asian countries. Figure 43.1 summarizes the findings of studies, which used at least three criteria of the IRLSSG[7] to identify individuals with RLS. To further increase the comparability of prevalence, only studies that applied no age limits on the participants, except the exclusion of children and adolescents, were considered. Despite these uniform inclusion criteria, the population-based prevalence of RLS shows a high variability not only between countries but between different studies conducted in the same geographical location (Fig. 43.1).

On the European continent, the RLS prevalence ranges between 8.6%[16] and 4.6%[23] in the United Kingdom, 10.6%[19] and 2.4%[23] in Germany, and 10.8%[16] and 8.5%[22] in France. The highest RLS prevalence is found among patients in a primary care practice in Ireland (23.5%).[17] At the other end of the spectrum, especially Greece (3.9%)[25] and Turkey (3.2%)[26] have comparatively low prevalence. In one recent study directly comparing the prevalence of RLS between different European countries, the highest proportion was found in the Netherlands (6.3%), followed by Ireland, Spain, and the United Kingdom (each 4.6%).[23] Findings from the United States also show a high variability, which is partly caused by one study recruiting primary care practice patients with a very high RLS prevalence of 24.0%.[14] Population-based samples from Kentucky adults[15] and national US representatives[15,16] have a slightly narrower range with values between 19.4% and 7.6%.

Stratified by continents, the lowest prevalence is consistently found in East Asia. Only 1.8% of the Japanese population report symptoms of RLS,[27] followed by individuals in Taiwan (1.6%)[28] and Korea (1.1%).[29] One study conducted in a native South American population[13] also found very low prevalence (2.0%).

Possible explanations for the heterogeneous findings between studies especially from the same country include different assessment procedures, such as self-administered questionnaires sent by mail,[30] questionnaires completed in the clinic,[14] face-to-face interviews with a physician,[23] or by telephone.[31] The variability is further increased by different study populations, for example, patients

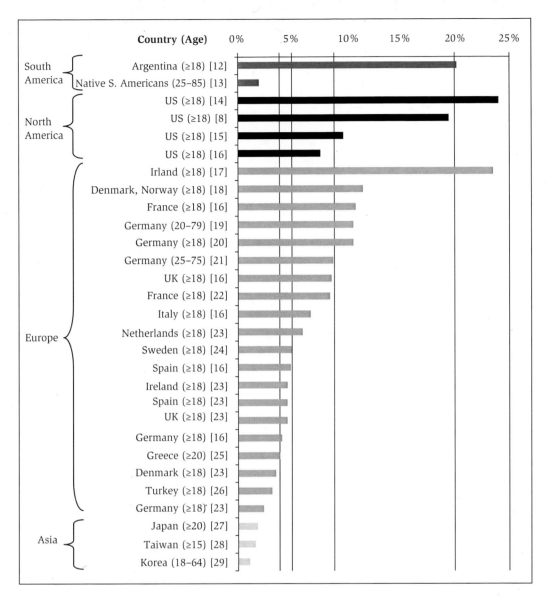

FIGURE 43.1   Population-based prevalence of restless legs syndrome by country with minimum International Restless Legs Syndrome Study Group criteria.

attending a rural practice[14,23,31] in contrast to random samples of the general population.[8,15,18] Furthermore, RLS prevalence is also determined by different age and sex compositions of the study populations, since RLS is associated with increasing age and female sex.

GENDER DIFFERENCES

Across all countries, the prevalence of RLS is considerably higher in women than in men (see Fig. 43.2). The average female-to-male ratio across 23 population-based studies which report sex-specific prevalence was 1.6, with six studies reporting prevalence at least twice as high in women.[5] The differences are observed both at high and low prevalence of RLS in the respective study population. Although the underlying reasons for these differences remain largely unexplored,[19] evidence exists that pregnancy and parity contribute to it.[32] During pregnancy, between 26% and 30% of women suffer from transient RLS symptoms with

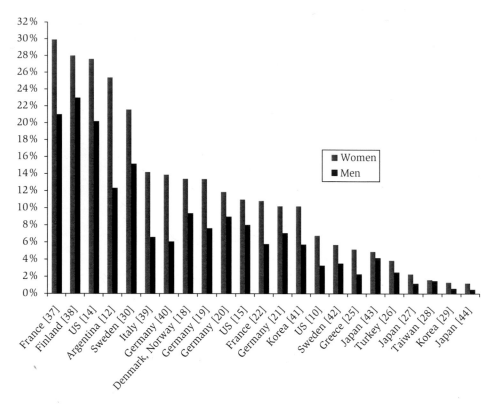

FIGURE 43.2   Population-based prevalence of restless legs syndrome by sex and country with minimum International Restless Legs Syndrome Study Group criteria.

the highest prevalence in the third trimester.[33,34] These women experience a four times higher risk to later develop the disease RLS in the long-term compared to pregnant women without transient RLS symptoms.[35] Furthermore, the risk of developing RLS is strongly associated with the number of children born. Compared to nulliparous women, the prevalence of RLS was twice as high in women with one child and gradually increased to a four times higher risk in women with three or more children.[19] Other studies also found a significant increase of RLS in parous women compared to nulliparous individuals, but there was no increase in the RLS prevalence beyond the first pregnancy. Furthermore, no differences were found between nulliparous women and men, suggesting a strong relationship between pregnancy and the occurrence of RLS.[36]

In addition to the role of pregnancy, a number of methodological aspects have to be considered in the analysis of gender differences. The assessment of RLS completely relies on self-report of symptoms. In general, women report a specific symptom already at a lower severity level, whereas men only consider something to be a "symptom" if it is really severe. These gender roles and symptom perceptions might also affect the observed frequencies of RLS.

AGE DIFFERENCES IN RESTLESS LEGS SYNDROME PREVALENCE

In general, age is one of the most important, independent risk factors for a majority of diseases and cannot be influenced, for example, by a healthy lifestyle or preventive measures. Regarding RLS, the majority of studies report a strong increase in RLS prevalence associated with age with a plateau in the sixth and seventh decades of life.[5] After this, the prevalence of RLS seems to slowly decrease.

While most studies focused on individuals aged 18 years and older, few studies have assessed the prevalence of RLS in children and adolescents.[45,46] By using the 2003 diagnostic criteria for definite RLS in a pediatric population,[16] 8- to 11-year old children in the United Kingdom and United States had a prevalence of 1.9%, whereas definite RLS was diagnosed in 2.0% of the 12- to 17-year old adolescent population.[46] In Turkish high school students aged 15 to 18 years, the diagnosis of RLS was confirmed in 3.6% with the IRLSSG criteria during a personal interview.[45]

INCIDENCE OF RESTLESS LEGS SYNDROME

To date, only two studies from Germany and one from Japan provide information about the incidence of RLS in the general population and its persistence over time.[47,48] In Germany, the incidence rates range from 9 RLS cases per 1000 person-years over a follow-up time of 5 years in a rural area close to the Baltic Sea to 22 per 1.000 person-years over a 2.2 years follow-up in the city of Dortmund. In both samples, the incidence rate was higher in women and increased with age.[47] In the Japanese cohort study, the incidence of RLS over a period of 2 years was 1.4% in a sample of adults. Regarding the persistence of RLS over time, 1.3% of the study participants in the follow-up had already reported to suffer from RLS in the baseline assessment.[48]

RISK FACTORS FOR RESTLESS LEGS SYNDROME

All existing information on risk factors for RLS to date comes from cross-sectional or case-control studies. A general limitation of cross-sectional studies is that no time sequence between occurrence of a risk factor and onset of RLS can be established. Case-control studies are prone to different types of bias that may strongly limit their interpretations. Thus, until results from prospective cohort studies become available that clearly allow for evaluating the time sequence between risk factors and incident RLS cases, definite conclusions on potential RLS risk factors are limited.

Apart from the positive relationships with female sex and increasing age, the prevalence of RLS differs by geographical regions as described earlier. Only very few studies have investigated the role of ethnicity in this context with controversial results.[5] Whereas two studies conducted in the United States found no differences between white and African American participants,[7,49] an assessment of health professionals reported a higher prevalence for white in comparison to non-white individuals.[50]

There is increasing evidence for a genetic disposition of RLS, which has long been recognized through observations of familial aggregation of RLS.[26,32,45] Between 50% and 92% of patients with primary RLS report a positive family history.[51] Siblings of patients with RLS have a 3.6 times higher relative risk to develop RLS compared to siblings of healthy individuals, whereas the offspring risk was found to be 1.8 times higher in children of RLS parents.[32]

The associations between different comorbidities and RLS on a population level have been researched in some detail. Good evidence exists for a strong relationship between RLS and depression.[9,27,29,41,52,53] Furthermore, many studies found an increased prevalence of hypertension and cardiovascular diseases in individuals with RLS.[9,15,19,42,54,55] The underlining mechanisms for this relationship are complex and currently follow three biological models. First, it is suggested that the sympathetic hyperactivity, which is often associated with RLS, causes daytime hypertension, which in turn leads to heart disease. Secondly, in case of the absence of daytime hypertension, the sympathetic hyperactivity contributes to atherosclerotic plaque formation and rupture as a direct risk factor for heart disease. And thirdly, other comorbidities that are associated with RLS, including renal failure, diabetes mellitus, iron deficiency, and insomnia, contribute to the development of cardiovascular diseases.[54] However, it has to be noted that other studies did not find associations between the comorbidities listed earlier and RLS. Furthermore, an increased risk for RLS has been linked to respiratory symptoms and airway obstruction,[28,56] diabetes mellitus,[20,57] and chronic kidney disease.[2]

The association between certain lifestyle factors and the prevalence of RLS is somehow clearer. The proportion of ex- and current smokers was consistently higher in individuals with RLS in comparison to subjects without RLS.[26,56,58] In the United States, Israel, and Taiwan, RLS was associated with obesity, measured either as body mass index[28,50] or hip[58] and waist circumference.[50]

In the last few years, research has focused on the role of iron deficiency in the onset of RLS. Some evidence exists that ferritin levels are significantly lower in individuals with RLS.[52,59] This theory is further supported by the fact that iron deficiency is often associated with the three most common secondary causes of RLS, namely end-stage renal disease, pregnancy, and anemia caused by a lack of iron.[59] In contrast to this, a population-based study from Ireland also reported lower ferritin levels in RLS participants, but these differences diminished after adjustment for study center, age, sex, and smoking history.[56] Two other studies from Korea and Germany found no difference in peripheral serum iron measurements[19,41] between individuals with and without RLS. Therefore, results concerning the relationship between RLS and other comorbidities remain controversial and prospective studies with longitudinal data are needed to assess the etiology of RLS. Furthermore, few reliable data exist to date on the influence of socioeconomic factors, including education, income, job and family status, on the incidence of RLS. This is another area of RLS research with a need for studies.

REFERENCES

1. Willis T. *The London Practice of Physick*. London: Bassett & Crooke; 1685.
2. Ekbom K. Restless legs: a clinical study. *Acta Med Scand Suppl* 1945;158:1–123.
3. Walters AS. Toward a better definition of the restless legs syndrome. The International Restless Legs Syndrome Study Group. *Mov Disord* 1995;10 634–42.
4. Allen RP, Picchietti D, Hening WA, et al. Restless legs syndrome: diagnostic criteria, special considerations, and epidemiology. A report from the restless legs syndrome diagnosis and epidemiology workshop at the National Institutes of Health. *Sleep Med* 2003;4:101–19.
5. Innes KE, Selfe TK, Agarwal P. Prevalence of restless legs syndrome in North America and Western European Populations: a systematic review. *Sleep Med* 2011;12(7):623–34.
6. Hening WA, Allen RP, Washburn M, et al. The four diagnostic criteria for restless legs syndrome are unable to exclude confounding conditions ("mimics"). *Sleep Med* 2009;10(9):976–81.
7. Hening WA, Allen RP, Washburn M, et al. Validation of the Hopkins telephone diagnostic interview for restless legs syndrome. *Sleep Medicine* 2008;9:283–9.
8. Phillips B, Young T, Finn L, et al. Epidemiology of restless legs symptoms in adults. *Arch Intern Med* 2000;160:2137–41.
9. Winkelman JW, Finn L, Yong T. Prevalence and correlates of restless legs syndrome symptoms in the Wisconsin Sleep Cohort. *Sleep Med* 2006;7:545–52.
10. Winkelman JW, Shahar E, Sharief I, et al. Association of restless legs syndrome and cardiovascular disease in the Sleep Heart Health Study. *Neurology* 2008;70:35–42.
11. Alattar M, Harrington JJ, Michell CM, et al. Sleep problems in primary care: a North Carolina family practice research network (NC-FP-RN) study. *J Am Board Fam Med* 2007;20(4):365–74.
12. Persi GG, Etcheverry JL, Vecchi C, et al. Prevalence of restless legs syndrome: a community-based study from Argentina. *Parkinsonism Relat Disord* 2009;15:461–5.
13. Castillo PR, Kaplan J, Lin SC, et al. Prevalence of restless legs syndrome among native South Americans residing in coastal and mountainous areas. *Mayo Clin Proc* 2006;81:1345–7.
14. Nichols DA, Allen RP, Grauke JH, et al. Restless legs syndrome symptoms in primary care: a prevalence study. *Arch Intern Med* 2003;163(19):2323–9.
15. Phillips B, Hening W, Britz P, et al. Prevalence and correlates of restless legs syndrome: results from the 2005 National Sleep Foundation Poll. *Chest* 2006;129(1):76–80.
16. Allen RP, Walters AS, Montplaisir J, et al. Restless legs syndrome prevalence and impact: REST general population study. *Arch Intern Med* 2005;165(11):1286–92.
17. O'Keeffe ST, Egan D, Myers A, et al. The frequency and impact of restless legs syndrome in primary care. *Ir Med J* 2007;100(7):539–42.
18. Bjorvatn B, Leissner L, Ulfberg J, et al. Prevalence, severity and risk factors of restless legs syndrome in the general adult population in two Scandinavian countries. *Sleep Med* 2005;6(4):307–12.
19. Berger K, Luedemann J, Trenkwalder C, et al. Sex and the risk of restless legs syndrome in the general population. *Arch Intern Med* 2004;164(2):196–202.
20. Moeller C, Wetter TC, Koester J, et al. Differential diagnosis of unpleasant sensations in the legs: prevalence of restless legs syndrome in a primary care population. *Sleep Med* 2010;11(2):161–6.
21. Happe S, Vennemann M, Evers S, et al. Treatment wish of individuals with known and unknown restless legs syndrome in the community. *J Neurol* 2008;255(9):1365–71.
22. Tison F, Crochard A, Leger D, et al. Epidemiology of restless legs syndrome in French adults. A nationwide

survey: the INSTANT Study. *Neurology* 2005;65:239–46.

23. Allen RP, Stillman P, Myers AJ. Physician-diagnosed restless legs syndrome in a large sample of primary medical care patients in western Europe: prevalence and characteristics. *Sleep Med* 2010;11(1):31–7.

24. Ulfberg J, Nystrom B, Carter N, et al. Prevalence of restless legs syndrome among men aged 18 to 64 years: an association with somatic disease and neuropsychiatric symptoms. *Mov Disord* 2001;16:1159–63.

25. Hadjigeorgiou GM, Stefanidis I, Dardiotis E, et al. Low RLS prevalence and awareness in central Greece. An epidemiological survey. *Eur J Neurol* 2007;14(11):1275–80.

26. Sevim O, Dogu O, Camdeviren H, et al. Unexpectedly low prevalence and unusual characteristics of RLS in Mersin, Turkey. *Neurology* 2003;61:1562–9.

27. Nomura T, Inoue Y, Kusumi M, et al. Prevalence of restless legs syndrome in a rural community in Japan. *Mov Disord* 2008;23(16):2363–9.

28. Chen NH, Chuang LP, Yang CT, et al. The prevalence of restless legs syndrome in Taiwanese adults. *Psychiatry Clin Neurosci* 2010;64:170–8.

29. Cho S-J, Hong JP, Hahm B-J, et al. Restless legs syndrome in a community sample of Korean adults: prevalence, impact on quality of life, and association with DSM-IV Psychiatric Disorders. *Sleep* 2009;32(8):1069–76.

30. Broman J-E, Mallon L, Hetta J. Restless legs syndrome and its relationship with insomnia symptoms and daytime distress: epidemiological survey in Sweden. *Psychiatry Clin Neurosci* 2008;62(4):472–5.

31. Hening W, Walters AS, Allen RP, et al. Impact, diagnosis and treatment of restless legs syndrome (RLS) in a primary care population: the REST (RLS epidemiology, symptoms, and treatment) primary care study [see comment]. *Sleep Med* 2004;5(3):237–46.

32. Xiong L, Montplaisir J, Desautels A, et al. Family study of restless legs syndrome in Quebec, Canada. *Arch Neurol* 2010;67(5):617–22.

33. Manconi M, Govoni V, De Vito A, et al. Restless legs syndrome and pregnancy. *Neurology* 2004;63:1065–9.

34. Tunc T, Karadag YS, Dogulu F, et al. Predisposing factors of restless legs syndrome in pregnancy. *Mov Disord* 2007;22:627–31.

35. Cesnik E, Casetta M, Turri M, et al. Transient RLS during pregnancy is a risk factor for the chronic idiopathic form. *Neurology* 2011;75:2117–20.

36. Pantaleo NP, Hening WA, Allen RP, et al. Pregnancy accounts for most of the gender difference in prevalence of RLS. *Sleep Med* 2010;11(3):310–13.

37. Celle S, Roche F, Kerleroux J, et al. Prevalence and clinical correlates of restless legs syndrome in an elderly French population: the synapse study. *J Gerontol A Biol Sci Med Sci* 2010;65(2):167–73.

38. Juuti AK, Läärä E, Rajala U, et al. Prevalence and associated factors of restless legs in a 57-year-old urban population in northern Finland. *Acta Neurol Scand* 2010;122(1):63–9.

39. Hoegl B, Kiechl S, Willeit J, et al. Restless legs syndrome: a community-based study of prevalence, severity, and risk factors. *Neurology* 2005;64(11):1920–4.

40. Rothdach AJ, Trenkwalder C, Haberstock J, et al. Prevalence and risk factors of RLS in an elderly population—The MEMO Study. *Neurology.* 2000;54:1064–8.

41. Kim KW, Yoon IY, Chung S, et al. Prevalence, comorbidities and risk factors of restless legs syndrome in the Korean elderly population—results from the Korean Longitudinal Study on Health and Aging. *J Sleep Res* 2010;19:87–92.

42. Ulfberg J, Bjorvatn B, Leissner L, et al. Comorbidity in restless legs syndrome among a sample of Swedish adults. *Sleep Med* 2007;8(7/8):768–72.

43. Mizuno S, Miyaoka T, Inagaki T, et al. Prevalence of restless legs syndrome in non-institutionalized Japanese elderly. *Psychiatry Clin Neurosci* 2005;59:461–5.

44. Tsuboi Y, Imamura A, Sugimura M, et al. Prevalence of restless legs syndrome in a Japanese elderly population. *Parkinsonism Relat Disord* 2009;15(8):598–601.

45. Yilmaz K, Kilincaslan A, Aydin N, et al. Prevalence and correlates of restless legs syndrome in adolescents. *Dev Med Child Neurol* 2011;53:40–7.

46. Piecchietti D, Allen RP, Walters AS, et al. Restless legs syndrome: prevalence and impact in children and adolescents—The Peds REST Study. *Pediatrics* 2007;120(2):253–66.

47. Szentkiralyi A, Fendrich K, Hoffmann W, et al. Incidence of restless legs syndrome in two population-based cohort studies in Germany. *Sleep Med* 2011;12(9):815–20.

48. Kagimura T, Nomura T, Kusumi M, et al. Prospective survey on the natural course of restless legs syndrome over two years in a closed cohort. *Sleep Med* 2011;12:821–6

49. Lee HB, Hening WA, Allen RP, et al. Race and restless legs syndrome symptoms in an adult community sample in east Baltimore. *Sleep Med* 2006;7(8):642–5.

50. Gao X, Schwarzschild MA, Wang H, et al. Obesity and restless legs syndrome in men and women. *Neurology* 2009;72(14):1255–61.

51. Montplaisir J, Boucher S, Poirier G, et al. Clinical, polysomnographic, and genetic characteristics of restless legs syndrome: a study of 133 patients diagnosed with new standard criteria. *Mov Disord* 1997;12:61–5.

52. Quinn C, Uzbeck M, Saleem I, et al. Iron status and chronic kidnex disease predict restless legs syndrome in an older hospital population. *Sleep Med* 2011;12:295–301.

53. Araujo SM, Sales des Bruin VM, Nepomuceno LA, et al. Restless legs syndrome in end-stage renal disease: clinical characteristics and associated comorbities. *Sleep Med* 2010;11:785–90.

54. Walters AS, Rye DB. Review of the relationship of restless legs syndrome and periodic limb movements in sleep to hypertension, heart disease and stroke. *Sleep* 2009;21(5):589–97.

55. Ohayon MM, Roth T. Prevalence of restless legs syndrome and periodic limb movement disorder in the general population. *J Psychosom Res* 2002;53:547–54.

56. Benediktsdottir B, Janson C, Lindberg E, et al. Prevalence of restless legs syndrome among adults in Iceland, Sweden: lung function, comorbidity, ferritin, biomarkers, quality of life. *Sleep Med* 2010;11(10):1043–8.

57. Cuellar NG, Ratcliffe SJ. Restless legs syndrome in type 2 diabetes: implications to diabetes educators. *Diabetes Educ* 2008;34(2):218–34.

58. Schlesinger I, Erikh I, Avizohar O, et al. Cardiovascular risk factors in restless legs syndrome. *Mov Disord* 2009;24(11):1587–92.

59. Allen RP. Controversies and challenges in defining the etiology and pathophysiology of restless legs syndrome. *Am J Med* 2007;120(1A):S13–21.

44

Pathophysiology

The Biology of Restless Legs Syndrome (Willis-Ekbom Disease)

RICHARD P. ALLEN

CHAPTERS ON pathophysiology or more generally biological factors of the restless legs syndrome (RLS; also Willis-Ekbom disease) usually start with the claim that the cause of RLS and its underlying biology remain unknown. This is far from the case. We know more about the neurobiology producing RLS than we do about many other common neurological and psychiatric disorders—certainly as much or more than we know about depression or essential tremor. The abundance of relevant human and animal studies providing insights into the neurobiology of RLS exceeds what can be presented fully in one chapter. They provide a somewhat unexpected but a reasonably integrated view of the neurobiology of RLS. Moreover, the results indicate metabolic factors producing RLS that alter biological functioning in various organs other than the brain. This chapter focuses on those studies with the most supportive data and does not attempt to list the many theoretical concepts or studies that have limited data support.

Seven major aspects of RLS studies have served to reveal significant aspects of RLS biology, namely pharmacological treatment responses and related clinical physiological and imaging studies, medically related conditions producing RLS, central nervous system (CNS) stimulation studies, genetics, autopsies, animal models, and finally peripheral nonneurological system studies. Although considered separately in the following, these diverse studies actually provide a converging description of the biological basis for RLS.

Biological considerations of a disease should provide guidance for treatment planning and developing new treatments. This has not been the case for RLS until now. As noted in the last section of this chapter, what we now understand about RLS biology indicates a need to reconsider our standard treatment approaches and suggests new directions for developing better treatments.

PHARMACOLOGICAL TREATMENT RESPONSE AND RELATED PHYSIOLOGICAL/IMAGING STUDIES

Four classes of medications each alone have been well documented to provide effective treatment for RLS, suggesting differing possible biological abnormalities, namely the following: drugs increasing dopamine stimulation (i.e., levodopa and dopamine agonists), glutamate inhibitors (i.e., gabapentin, gabapentin enacarbil, and pregabalin), opioids (e.g., hydrocodone, methadone), and intravenous iron (i.e., ferric carboxymaltose [FCM], iron dextran, iron sucrose).

Dopamine and Restless Legs Syndrome

Since levodopa and dopamine agonists provide immediate and dramatically effective treatment for RLS and dopamine antagonist can precipitate RLS symptoms it has long been assumed there is a primary dopamine abnormality in RLS leading to decreased extra-cellular dopamine.[1] Initial studies, however, failed to show reduction in dopamine metabolites in the cerebrospinal fluid (CSF).[2,3] Moreover, positron emission tomography (PET) brain imaging studies showed decreased striatal uptake of 11C-raclopride in the putamen and caudate[4] for both previously treated and untreated patients indicating decreased D2 receptors (D2R) unrelated to prior dopaminergic treatment and suggesting, if anything, a response to increased, not the expected decreased, extracellular dopamine. An autopsy study similarly reported decreased D2R in the putamen but also increased tyrosine hydroxylase (TH) in both the putamen and the substantia nigra,[5] most consistent with increased dopaminergic activation. Autopsy studies failed to show any indication for cell loss or any indication of neurodegeneration for nigrostriatal areas[6,7] or for the A11 dopamine neurons.[8] Two studies reported decreased uptake of fDOPA in the putamen and caudate.[4,9] Since there is neither cell loss nor indication for failure of amino acid transport of fDOPA, these results are also most consistent with increased dopamine turnover and increased extracellular dopamine. A report of two separate CSF studies found RLS patients compared to controls had increased CSF 3-OMD (3-ortho-methyldopa) that correlated with the amount of CSF HVA and the severity

of the RLS.[10] L-dopa is metabolized to either dopamine (DA) or 3-OMD, with both processes occurring essentially at the same metabolic step but involving different pathways. The increased L-dopa production suggested by increased TH in RLS would be expected to produce proportionally increased 3-OMD and DA. Thus, the significant correlation of the CSF 3-OMD to HVA reported in these studies further supports the putative increases for dopamine in RLS that is, as would be expected, greater with more severe RLS.[10]

Thus, we have a clear but somewhat surprising view that the dopaminergic abnormality in RLS involves increased DA production with increased turnover of dopamine in the dopamine-producing cells. There are two somewhat contrary findings that need to be considered. First, one study by Cervenka et al.[11] reported RLS patients not previously treated with dopaminergic agents showed increased not decreased 11C-raclopride binding in the striatum, indicating increased D2 receptors (D2R). This study, however, had very mild RLS patients, several with IRLS severity scores below the usual minimum level of 15–20 required for entry into a clinical treatment trial. The median IRLS was 18 with a range of 12 to 27; only one patient had a score over 25. The data from the autopsy study noted earlier indicated a strong inverse correlation between D2R and RLS severity with significant decreases occurring only for moderate to severe RLS with all IRLS scores at or over 25[5] (see Fig. 44.1). Thus, decreased D2R density would not be expected for the mild RLS patient sample used in the Cervenka et al. imaging study. Moreover, the changes in striatal D2R binding reported were small. Mild RLS may have only small intermittent increases in dopamine production that may cause a decrease in receptor affinity with a possible compensatory increase in overall number of receptors, including an increase in presynaptic D2R. Raclopride binding does not discriminate presynaptic versus postsynaptic location and thus does not inform about these likely changes with very mild RLS. Raclopride studies showing the decreased striatal binding described earlier[4] had patients who were not previously treated, and the patients had moderate to severe RLS similar to those in the autopsy study.

The second finding not totally consistent with increased dopamine is a decrease in membrane-bound striatal dopamine transporter (DAT). Three single-photon emission computed tomography (SPECT) studies and an

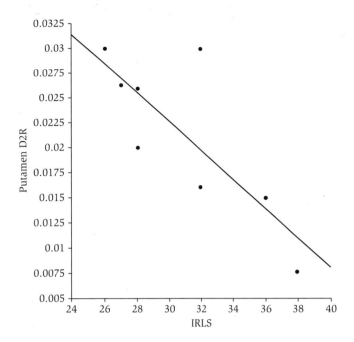

FIGURE 44.1 Correlation of autopsy staining for D2 receptors in putamen and IRLS score obtained within a few years of death. Note the strong inverse correlation ($r = -.80$, $p = .018$) between the amount of D2 expression measured in the autopsy samples of the putamen and the patient's score on the IRLS scale of restless legs syndrome (RLS) severity. The higher the score on the rating scale, the more severe the RLS symptoms; 40 is the maximum IRLS score. (From Connor et al.[5])

autopsy study failed to find any differences in DAT levels in the striatum, but these involved evaluation of all DAT, not just the functional DAT bound to the cellular membrane.[12–14] Another report of two separate studies, however, found that in both of these studies there was decreased[11] C-methylphenidate striatal binding, indicating decreased membrane-bound DAT,[15] a change consistent with animal models described later in this chapter. Decreased functional DAT would not be expected for increased extracellular DA, but this may reflect a pathological process in RLS, further supporting increased extracellular dopamine.

Overall, the data indicate RLS involves increased not decreased nigrostriatal dopamine production, leading to increased extracellular dopamine in the striatum but presumably also elsewhere in the CNS.

Glutamate and Restless Legs Syndrome

Medications that inhibit glutamate release (i.e., gabapentin, enacarbil, pregabalin) provide RLS treatment efficacy similar to dopamine agonists.[16–18]

Moreover, ketamine, an NMDA glutamate receptor antagonist, has been reported to provide effective treatment for two treatment-resistant cases of RLS.[19] The glutamate system involvement with RLS has not been studied largely because of the almost myopic focus in RLS research on the dopamine pathology but also because only recently have tools developed enabling imaging measurements of glutamate and glutamine. One recent study reported increased thalamic glutamate levels in RLS patients that correlated with the degree of waking during sleep but not the periodic limb movements in sleep (PLMS).[20] The glutamate-inhibiting drugs not only treat the primary RLS symptoms but also appear to improve sleep; in contrast, levodopa and the dopamine agonist treat the primary RLS symptoms, reduce the PLMS, but do not completely correct the sleep problems of RLS.

These data suggest two primary neurobiological abnormalities in RLS: (1) dopaminergic related to RLS sensory symptoms and PLMS, and (2) glutamatergic related to sensory symptoms and excessive arousal (hyperarousal) with sleep disturbance. These systems likely have complex interactions, but each appears to have a somewhat separate primary effect on RLS that may lead to a somewhat different RLS phenotype. The relative degree of PLM versus hyperarousal has not been carefully analyzed, but it deserves note that some fairly severe RLS patients have been found to have very few PLMS,[21,22] while in contrast some mostly milder RLS have been found to have reasonably normal nocturnal sleep but with excessive daytime sleepiness.[23] This may be a glimpse of important phenotype differences stemming from different degrees of these two biological abnormalities of RLS driving differing features of RLS symptoms.

Opioid System and Restless Legs Syndrome

One double-blinded and some open-label clinical trials have indicated that opioids provide effective treatment at least for some RLS patients,[24,25] but the opioid antagonism with naloxone fails to precipitate RLS symptoms.[26] A PET study with [11C] diprenorphine, a nonselective opioid receptor radioligand, also failed to show any significant difference between RLS and controls.[27] That study, however, revealed ligand uptake correlated with RLS severity and McGill pain scores indicating that greater degree of pain often occurring with more severe RLS produces a larger opioid release in the medial pain system. One very small pilot autopsy study of only five RLS and six controls reported 37.5% fewer thalamic cells staining for beta-endorphin and met-enkephalin but no difference for leu-enkephalin. They found no differences in the substantia nigra.[28] Aside from this one study, there have been no data indicating a primary opioid pathology in RLS, although it seems likely that the chronic sensory discomfort and pain associated with more severe RLS will alter in some way pain pathways and the opioid system as suggested by these studies. RLS and the RLS-related chronic sleep loss also alter nociception[29,30] and possibly the opioid system. The interaction of these effects complicates understanding the functioning of the opioid system in RLS. This remains a largely unexplored aspect of RLS despite the clinical and biological significance of the pain symptoms in RLS.

Overall, we currently have little understanding of the basis for the treatment benefits of the opioids except for one case study where the opioid benefit was largely reversed by a dopamine antagonist,[1] but specificity here is certainly not clear. Nonetheless, it may be that the opioid treatment benefits result from indirect effects on the dopamine system and thus are easily reversed by dopamine antagonists.

Iron and Restless Legs Syndrome

Oral iron treatment appears to benefit patients with low peripheral stores of iron as indicated by serum values of low ferritin, low transferrin saturation, or high total iron binding capacity. Usually the oral iron reduces the RLS symptoms but does not provide in itself complete relief from the symptoms.[31] Thus, low peripheral iron stores appear to exacerbate RLS symptoms but do not appear to be a primary cause of the symptoms except for some patients whose RLS appears only during the periods when they are iron deficient, usually associated with anemia. In contrast to oral, intravenous iron at total doses of about 1000 mg of iron has been shown to provide dramatic and long-lasting total remission from RLS in some but not all RLS. Unlike oral iron, the response to IV iron does not relate to peripheral iron stores but occurs also for those with high normal serum measures of iron status. Moreover, also unlike oral iron, IV iron alone appears to provide for some complete treatment benefit. The more tightly bound iron in dextran[32] or FCM[33] has significantly better treatment response than iron sucrose.[34] The latter releases iron readily and rather rapidly with possibly less taken up for distribution to tissues other than the liver, spleen, and bone marrow and in particular with less available for uptake into the brain. Thus, RLS may occur with brain iron deficiency despite normal peripheral iron, and the brain iron deficiency can for some be corrected by an IV iron formulation that promotes availability of the iron for uptake into the brain.

The presence of decreased brain iron is, in fact, the best-documented biological abnormality in RLS. It has been shown by both decreased CSF ferritin[35,36] (Fig. 44.2) and decreased iron in the substantia nigra on multiple magnetic resonance imaging (MRI) and ultrasound studies.[37,38,39] The CSF studies are particularly informative because they suggest that the brain iron is low in virtually all of the patients, even those with normal peripheral iron stores, but probably lower in those with lower peripheral brain iron (see Fig. 44.2). So why does IV iron only work for some and not most RLS patients? There may be significant difference between subjects in response of brain

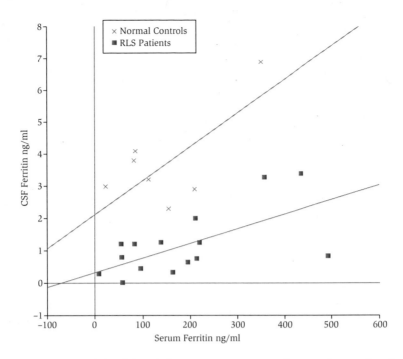

FIGURE 44.2 Cerebrospinal fluid (CSF) ferritin versus serum ferritin for restless legs syndrome (RLS) patients and matched (age and gender) normal controls. Note the much lower CSF ferritin for RLS despite serum ferritin values overlapping those for normal controls. Also note the extremely low CSF values for RLS patients with very low serum ferritin. (Reprinted with minor style modification from: Earley et al.[35])

iron status to changes in peripheral iron status. Some with RLS may also have too severe brain iron loss or iron pathology to benefit from IV iron, but others may have RLS for causes unrelated to brain iron status.

MAJOR SECONDARY CAUSES OF RESTLESS LEGS SYNDROME

While multiple medical factors have been associated with increased risk of RLS, there are only three conditions that are clearly associated with both development of new RLS with the condition and disappearance of RLS when the condition itself is resolved: iron deficiency, end-stage renal disease, and pregnancy. These three conditions have one common factor, that is, impaired iron status. Moreover, IV iron treatment has been shown to largely correct the RLS in end-stage renal disease.[40]

It deserves note that all medical conditions that compromise iron status, including very frequent blood donations,[41] inflammatory conditions,[42] lipoprotein apheresis,[43] gastric bypass surgery,[44] and Friedreich's ataxia,[45,46] are associated with an increased incidence of RLS in usually about 25% to 40% of the patients with the condition. Thus, it appears clear that compromised iron status, whenever it occurs, causes RLS in a large percentage but not all patients. It seems likely that those developing RLS are the ones who will have reduced brain iron with the condition, but to date this has not been adequately studied.

Some medical conditions that have been carefully documented to be associated with increased RLS do not, however, have a clear relation to iron status, particularly multiple sclerosis[47] and chronic obstructive pulmonary disease (COPD).[48] These suggest there are causes of RLS not related to iron status, presumably reflecting some other neurobiological pathway producing RLS symptoms that remains to be better determined.

CENTRAL NERVOUS SYSTEM STIMULATION STUDIES

Two studies have reported increased spinal cord excitability shown by lower threshold and greater spread of spinal flexor responses to stimulation of the medial plantar nerve for RLS/PLMS patients[49] and for RLS secondary to end-stage renal disease.[50] These findings were state dependent occurring in the first cycle of sleep but with little or no indication for spinal excitability in waking recordings during RLS symptom period of 21:00–00:00. It is important to note that RLS has a strong circadian component, but the spinal excitability depended on the sleep state and not the circadian time of RLS symptoms. This sleep-state dependency was seen as indicating the PLMS pathophysiology may involve loss of supraspinal inhibition during sleep, but spinal factors could not be excluded. The results overall support a relation between spinal cord excitability and the PLMS, which may be closely related to dopaminergic modulation. The relation of spinal excitability to RLS with its pronounced and defining daytime symptoms and circadian but not sleep modulation of symptoms is certainly not evident.

Several cortical stimulation studies evaluating motor cortex responses have demonstrated increased cortical excitability that unlike the spinal studies occur during the wakefulness in the day. Some (e.g.,[51]) but not all of these studies (e.g.,[52]), reported shortened cortical silent period in RLS. However, in contrast, all of the studies using transcranial paired-pulse magnetic stimulation report dramatic loss of intracortical inhibition (SICI) along with an increased intracortical facilitation (ICF).[53] ICF has been found to decrease with age to about 75% for older healthy adults (average age: 70.9).[54] This age-expected decrease in ICF has not been found for the RLS patients in any of these studies, further supporting the increased ICF for RLS. Nardone et al.[55] report standard RLS dopamine treatment increases the SICI (avr. ± sd) from 75% ± 15 to 52% ± 14 of baseline compared to controls at 44% ± 13 with a small nonsignificant reduction in ICF. The reduced SICI was still 0.6 SD above controls, and the sample sizes in that study of 14–15 had inadequate power to test for this effect size. Dopamine treatment partly reduces the loss of intracortical inhibition (SICI) but has little effect on the increased ICF. The former is considered to relate mostly to GABA neuronal activity, but increased dopamine stimulation would also be expected to add to cortical inhibitory activity, possibly through increased GABA activity. In contrast, ICF is considered to reflect glutamate as well as GABA activity,

and this measure may reflect a possible abnormally increased glutamatergic activity in RLS as suggested by treatment effects noted earlier. The critical factor here is that these changes reflect an abnormality that lies not with the spinal pathways but with subcortical and cortical pathophysiology producing motor-cortex excitability.[56]

Overall the CNS stimulation studies indicate that PLMS relate to a pathophysiology producing increased spinal cord excitability only during sleep, while the RLS symptoms relate to pathophysiology producing increased cortical excitability during waking. This is a critical distinction since it has now been well established that the PLM during waking (PLMW) on a SIT test or during the night polysomnography correlate very poorly if at all with the sleep PLMS.[57,58] PLMS and PLMW may appear somewhat similar in that both involve episodic leg movements, but the underlying pathophysiology, relative rates of occurrence across subjects, and the changes in rates with age[59] clearly differ. PLMS, while a very useful objective sign of RLS, may be a very secondary aspect of the primary biological features driving the RLS symptoms. In contrast, the cortical excitability may be more relevant.

GENETICS

A reasonably large number of linkage studies in families with RLS found significant linkages, but none found any specific gene or allelic variation related to RLS. In contrast, genome-wide association studies have identified 10 specific allelic variations on four genes associated with significant increased risk of RLS.[60] The relation of these genetic variations to biological factors related to RLS has only been shown for two of the genes. The RLS risk allele on BTBD9 was associated with lower serum ferritin,[61] and the degree of expression of MEIS1 has been reported to be associated with iron homeostasis for RLS lymphoblasts and brain tissue and for a common round worm (C. elegans).[62] The direction of the iron changes with MEIS1 expression appear to differ between studies, possibly related to methods or cells examined, but nonetheless suggest that MEIS1 has some relation to iron management. Further study of these genetic relations to iron homeostasis may provide some indication of the nature of the iron abnormalities that appear to be so common in RLS.

AUTOPSY STUDIES

As noted earlier, the RLS autopsy studies have largely confirmed the dopamine abnormalities expected from the ID animal model. These studies also demonstrated two other important findings. First, contrary to expectation, the mitochondrial ferritin in the substantia nigra (SN) is increased despite the profound decrease in H-ferritin.[63] This occurs with some indication for increased mitochondria in the RLS compared to control SN cells. The increased mitochondrial ferritin suggest increased iron requirement for mitochondria function in RLS, which will take up more of the cytosolic iron. If the conditions provide access to adequate iron stores, then the cytosolic iron balance can be maintained, but this requires increased input of iron to the cells. The decreased TfR found in these cells[6] indicates this is not happening for RLS and thus the increased mitochondrial demand for iron leads to cytosolic iron deficiency. It is interesting to note that this process will compromise the mitochondrial iron-sulfur complexes that have a critical role for producing the iron regulatory protein 1 (IRP-1). IRP-1 is also decreased in RLS SN.[6] Overall it appears that for RLS the iron deficiency at the cellular level is associated with increased priority for iron delivery to mitochondria to ensure cell life and maintain cell functioning with consequent decrease in cytosolic iron status. The increased tyrosine hydroxylase activity places further energy demands on the cell and may serve to exacerbate the cytosolic iron decreases. If the cell is provided access to adequate available iron, this may allow meeting the metabolic demands of the mitochondria without producing cytosolic iron deficiency, but compromised iron availability will produce cytosolic iron deficiency. Moreover, the increased energy demand for the dopamine-producing cells in RLS patients makes these particular cells vulnerable to the status of available brain iron stores (see Fig. 44.3).

The second major finding from RLS autopsy studies is the pervasive increase in hypoxic pathways in RLS shown by increased HIF-1 alpha in the substantia nigra[64] (see Fig. 44.4) and by increased HIF-2 alpha and vascular endothelial growth factor (VEGF) in the microvasculature of cortical brain tissue. Iron deficiency will activate hypoxic pathways, and in particular the messenger RNA encoding HIF-2 has an iron-responsive element.[65] Moreover, to some extent, activation of these pathways can also lead to decreased iron availability. Tyrosine hydroxylase will also be increased by HIF-1 alpha increase.

These results give us two pathways producing the neurobiological abnormalities of RLS: iron deficiency producing increased glutamate and dopamine abnormalities and hypoxic pathway activation with dopamine abnormalities.

Other conditions that produce significant activation of hypoxic pathways, including frank hypoxia, may also produce the dopamine

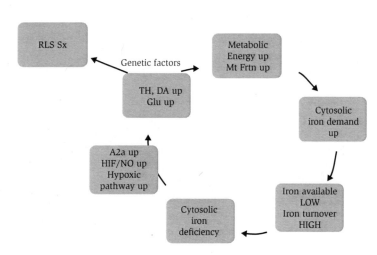

FIGURE 44.3 Iron-related metabolism changes produce a cycle that may increase degree of pathophysiology until it reaches a balance between the available iron and the increased energy and mitochondrial demands of the cell.

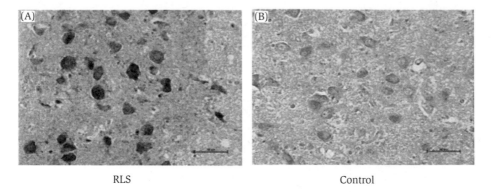

RLS   Control

FIGURE 44.4   HIF-1 alpha immunostaining in substantia nigra of control and restless legs syndrome (RLS) patients. This figure demonstrates inducible factor (HIF-1 alpha) staining is much increased in RLS compared to control tissue from the substantia nigra. (Reproduced from Patton et al.[64]) (*See* color insert.)

abnormalities even without significant iron deficiency, although the hypoxia will also serve to somewhat decrease iron. This may be the mechanism producing increased prevalence of RLS with COPD (see Fig. 44.5). It will be interesting to see whether the RLS with COPD has the same degree of hyperarousal as that seen with most RLS patients or whether this pathway produces more of the dopamine than glutamate changes. Overall the pathways from iron to RLS symptoms inform about other possible causes of RLS, and the pathways producing iron compromise also inform about significant biological factors of RLS, including increased TH (see Fig. 44.5).

ANIMAL MODELS

Since iron deficiency clearly causes RLS, it provides us with an experimental model for animal and cellular work that has produced very useful information about RLS neurobiology. Dietary iron deficiency either post weaning or starting at birth produces profound decreases in brain iron, particularly in the substantia nigra and striatum. These experimental brain-iron-deficient states produce decreased striatal D2 receptors proportional to the degree of iron loss and to a lesser extent decreased striatal D1 receptors.[66] DAT is also decreased but primarily membrane-bound DAT and not that in the cytosol.[67] Tyrosine hydroxylase (TH) is increased in both the nigra and the striatum.[5] Extracellular iron in the striatum is not only increased but the circadian variation in amplitude is as much as three to four times greater for the ID than control rat[68] (see Fig. 44.6).

The brain iron deficiency in RLS, while not as pronounced as that in these rat models, would be expected to produce similar changes in the nigrostriatal dopamine system. Indeed, the autopsy and imaging studies produce, as

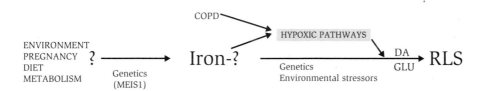

FIGURE 44.5   Significant pathways: genetic, environmental factors to iron abnormalities and iron abnormalities to changes (i.e., dopamine [DA], glutamate [Glu]) producing restless legs syndrome (RLS) symptoms. As the pathways from iron to RLS are better understood, other alternative causes may be found (e.g., chronic obstructive pulmonary disease [COPD] effect on hypoxic pathways producing RLS symptoms). As all of these pathways are better understood, treatments may be developed to alter them to reduce iron abnormalities or their effects, producing the RLS symptoms.

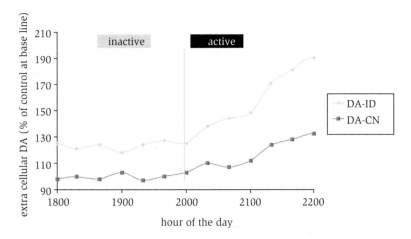

FIGURE 44.6   Extracellular dopamine (DA) in caudate is increased overall in iron-deficient rat at all times with the circadian change two to three times greater with iron deficiency. (Reproduced from Chen et al.[68])

noted earlier, the same changes observed in this animal model with the exception of the D1R, which is not reduced in RLS, but in the animal model this decrease is not related to the degree of iron loss and is less pronounced than the decrease in D2R. The D2R in the human autopsy was decreased but only for the more severe RLS, presumably related as in the animal model to the degree of iron deficiency. An important and striking finding from the dietary ID animal model is the increased striatal extracellular dopamine, consistent with the brain imaging and CSF results for RLS as noted earlier, and also the marked increased in the circadian variation of striatal dopamine (see Fig. 44.5). This corresponds to the RLS symptoms worse during the low part of the dopamine cycle (inactive period) with much improvement with dopamine increases in the beginning of the active period.

Iron-compromised animals also show increased striatal glutamate[69] and a particularly significant increased glutamate transporter (GLT-1) that provides astrocyte uptake of glutamate. These findings parallel the reported increased thalamic glutamate in RLS, indicating brain iron deficiency may also produce this aspect of RLS neurobiology.

PERIPHERAL, NONNEUROLOGICAL STUDIES

There have been two very important nonneurological studies of peripheral tissue in RLS patients. The first were the remarkable pair of studies by Wahlin-Larsson, who demonstrated that skeletal muscles of RLS patients show increased capillary proliferation with increased VEGF. She noted that the results were not consistent with increased exercise of the muscles. The RLS patients show instead decreased aerobic performance capacity. The results are most consistent with increased hypoxic pathway activation involving HIF-1 as also demonstrated in the brain autopsy study noted earlier. As noted, hypoxic pathway activation occurs with compromised iron status, and this appears to involve both the CNS and other systems.[70,71]

The second important nonneurological study evaluated iron-management proteins in lymphocytes of treated RLS patients compared to controls. The major iron proteins in the lymphocytes for 24 RLS females were compared to 35 controls matched with the RLS patients for age, hemoglobin, and serum iron profile. RLS had significantly higher transferrin receptor (TfR), divalent metal transporter-1 (DMT-1), and ferroportin. Both TfR and DMT-1 indicate increased iron influx, while ferroportin increased export from the cell, producing overall increased iron turnover. More fundamentally, these results, like the muscle biopsy results, indicate the pervasive nature of RLS pathophysiology at least for RLS related to iron. The iron pathophysiology appears as a pervasive disturbance of iron metabolism affecting not only the CNS but also major peripheral systems.

SUMMARY AND SIGNIFICANCE OF RESTLESS LEGS SYNDROME BIOLOGY FOR TREATMENT CONSIDERATIONS

Now we can ask the important question: how does the biology of RLS drive treatment developments? There are three features of RLS biology with significant implications for RLS treatment.

First, the iron metabolic changes in RLS are both pervasive involving peripheral as well as CNS changes and also persistent not showing the circadian patterns of RLS, although likely producing circadian dopamine changes that would account for the circadian cycles of RLS (see Fig. 44.5). The pathways from iron to RLS symptoms also identify mechanisms that could be produced by other conditions (see Fig. 44.4). Given the clear central role for iron in RLS, there should be much more animal and human research to determine better methods for iron treatments of RLS, including better studies of the options for increasing iron availability to the brain. This should be one major focus of RLS treatment research.

Second, the dopamine changes in RLS are contrary to those expected and challenge our current thinking about dopaminergic treatment. RLS clearly involves increased not decreased activation of presynaptic dopaminergic systems with an apparent increase in circadian amplitude and, as would be expected with increased stimulation, a downregulation of postsynaptic response. The occurrence of symptoms at the low point of dopamine activation can be corrected by adding more dopamine stimulation to the system during that time using levodopa or short-acting dopamine agonists (see Fig. 44.6). This, however, is adding fuel to the fire. The expected inevitable long-term consequence of adding dopamine stimulation is further downregulation of the postsynaptic response to dopamine and an overall increase in severity and daily duration of symptoms producing RLS augmentation, the well-described major problem of dopamine agonist treatment. An alternative approach of a constant, or better yet, continuous exogenous dopamine stimulation could with continued treatment serve to downregulate the presynaptic dopamine production and thereby at least partly reduce the underlying dopaminergic pathology of RLS. Thus, our understanding of the dopamine pathophysiology of RLS supports

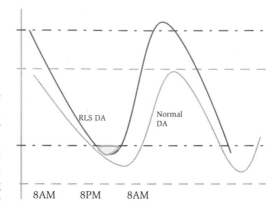

FIGURE 44.7 Concept of effects of restless legs syndrome (RLS) chronic increase in dopaminergic (DA) activity (solid red line) producing desensitized postsynaptic response (dashed red lines), which leaves a period at the low point of the dopamine cycle with inadequate dopamine activation corresponding to periods with RLS symptoms. Adding small amounts of dopamine stimulation during the symptomatic period will initially correct the problem but then lead to further postsynaptic desensitization and RLS augmentation with symptoms starting earlier in the day. Circadian dopamine cycle for normal (blue) and moderate RLS (red). Dashed lines indicate range for normal postsynaptic dopamine activity for normal (blue) and RLS (red). Filled pink indicates time with RLS symptoms. Dopamine falls below level needed to produce normal postsynaptic response. (*See* color insert.)

considering a shift in thinking about dopamine treatment away from short-duration palliative treatment during periods with symptoms to instead long-term continuous dopamine treatment addressing the underlying dopaminergic abnormalities in RLS.

Finally, the indications for glutamatergic activation noted earlier and the relation between iron deficiency and increased CNS glutamatergic activity support consideration of the medications reducing glutamate release as a possible primary treatment option for RLS. Gabapentin enacarbil, recently approved by the American Food and Drug Administration for treatment of RLS, and also gabapentin and pregabalin all reduce glutamate release and should be evaluated for first-line treatment of RLS. Given the dual effects of reduced iron on both glutamate and dopamine, the ideal treatment may involve some combination of dopaminergic and gluta-matergic treatment approaches at least for the more severe RLS cases.

REFERENCES

1. Montplaisir J, Lorrain D, Godbout R. Restless legs syndrome and periodic leg movements in sleep: the primary role of dopaminergic mechanism. *Eur Neurol* 1991;31(1):41–3.
2. Earley CJ, Hyland K, Allen RP. CSF dop-amine, serotonin, and biopterin metabolites in patients with restless legs syndrome. *Mov Disord* 2001;16(1):144–9.
3. Stiasny-Kolster K, Moller JC, Zschocke J, et al. Normal dopaminergic and serotonergic metabolites in cerebrospinal fluid and blood of restless legs syndrome patients. *Mov Disord* 2004;19(2):192–6.
4. Turjanski N, Lees AJ, Brooks DJ. Striatal dopaminergic function in restless legs syndrome: 18F-dopa and 11C-raclopride PET studies. *Neurology* 1999;52(5):932–7.
5. Connor JR, Wang X, Allen RP, et al. Altered dopaminergic profile in the putamen and substantia nigra in restless leg syndrome. *Brain* 2009;132(Pt 9):2403–12.
6. Connor JR, Boyer PJ, Menzies SL, et al. Neuropathological examination suggests impaired brain iron acquisition in restless legs syndrome. *Neurology* 2003;61:304–9.
7. Pittock SJ, Parrett T, Adler CH, et al. Neuropathology of primary restless leg syndrome: absence of specific tau- and alpha-synuclein pathology. *Mov Disord* 2004;19(6):695–9.
8. Earley CJ, Allen RP, Connor JR, et al. The dopaminergic neurons of the A11 system in RLS autopsy brains appear normal. *Sleep Med* 2009;10:1155–7.
9. Ruottinen HM, Partinen M, Hublin C, et al. An FDOPA PET study in patients with periodic limb movement disorder and restless legs syndrome. *Neurology* 2000;54(2):502–4.
10. Allen RP, Connor JR, Hyland K, et al. Abnormally increased CSF 3-Ortho-methyldopa (3-OMD) in untreated restless legs syndrome (RLS) patients indi-cates more severe disease and possibly abnor-mally increased dopamine synthesis. *Sleep Med* 2009;10(1):123–8.
11. Cervenka S, Palhagen SE, Comley RA, et al. Support for dopaminergic hypoactivity in restless legs syndrome: a PET study on D2-receptor binding. *Brain* 2006;129(Pt 8):2017–28.
12. Michaud M, Soucy JP, Chabli A, et al. SPECT imaging of striatal pre- and postsynaptic dopaminergic status in restless legs syndrome with periodic leg movements in sleep. *J Neurol* 2002;249(2):164–70.
13. Mrowka M, Jobges M, Berding G, et al. Computerized movement analysis and beta-CIT-SPECT in patients with rest-less legs syndrome. *J Neural Transm* 2005;112(5):693–701.
14. Eisensehr I, Wetter TC, Linke R, et al. Normal IPT and IBZM SPECT in drug-naive and levodopa-treated idiopathic restless legs syndrome. *Neurology* 2001;57(7):1307–9.
15. Earley CJ, Kuwabara H, Wong DF, et al. The dopamine transporter is decreased in the striatum of subjects with restless legs syndrome. *Sleep* 2011;34(3):341–7.
16. Walters AS, Ondo WG, Kushida CA, et al. Gabapentin enacarbil in restless legs syn-drome: a phase 2b, 2-week, randomized, double-blind, placebo-controlled trial. *Clin Neuropharmacol* 2009;32(6):311–20.
17. Lee DO, Ziman RB, Perkins AT, et al. A ran-domized, double-blind, placebo-controlled study to assess the efficacy and tolerability of gabapentin enacarbil in subjects with restless legs syndrome. *J Clin Sleep Med* 2011;7(3):282–92.
18. Bogan RK, Bornemann MA, Kushida CA, et al. Long-term maintenance treatment of restless legs syndrome with gabapentin enacarbil: a randomized controlled study. *Mayo Clin Proc* 2010;85(6):512–21.
19. Kapur N, Friedman R. Oral ketamine: a prom-ising treatment for restless legs syndrome. *Anesth Analg* 2002;94(6):1558–9, table of contents.
20. Allen RP, Barker PB, Horska A. Restless legs syndrome: a hyperarousal disorder with a thalamic glutamate abnormality *Neurology* 2011;76(Supp 4):A369.
21. Allen RP, Earley CJ. Validation of the Johns Hopkins restless legs severity scale. *Sleep Med* 2001;2:239–42.
22. Montplaisir J, Boucher S, Poirier G, et al. Clinical, polysomnographic, and genetic char-acteristics of restless legs syndrome: a study of 133 patients diagnosed with new standard criteria. *Mov Disord* 1997;12(1):61–5.
23. Kallweit U, Siccoli MM, Poryazova R, et al. Excessive daytime sleepiness in idiopathic

restless legs syndrome: characteristics and evolution under dopaminergic treatment. *Eur Neurol* 2009;62(3):176–9.

24. Walters AS, Wagner ML, Hening WA, et al. Successful treatment of the idiopathic restless legs syndrome in a randomized double-blind trial of oxycodone versus placebo. *Sleep* 1993;16(4):327–32.

25. Ondo WG. Methadone for refractory restless legs syndrome. *Mov Disord* 2005;20(3):345–8.

26. Winkelmann J, Schadrack J, Wetter TC, et al. Opioid and dopamine antagonist drug challenges in untreated restless legs syndrome patients. *Sleep Med* 2001;2(1):57–61.

27. von Spiczak S, Whone AL, Hammers A, et al. The role of opioids in restless legs syndrome: an [11C]diprenorphine PET study. *Brain* 2005;128(Pt 4):906–17.

28. Walters AS, Ondo WG, Zhu W, et al. Does the endogenous opiate system play a role in the restless legs syndrome? A pilot post-mortem study. *J Neurol Sci* 2009;279:62–5.

29. Edwards RR, Quartana PJ, Allen RP, et al. Alterations in pain responses in treated and untreated patients with restless legs syndrome: associations with sleep disruption. *Sleep Med* 2011;12(6):603–9.

30. Stiasny-Kolster K, Magerl W, Oertel WH, et al. Static mechanical hyperalgesia without dynamic tactile allodynia in patients with restless legs syndrome. *Brain* 2004;127(Pt 4):773–82.

31. Wang J, O'Reilly B, Venkataraman R, et al. Efficacy of oral iron in patients with restless legs syndrome and a low-normal ferritin: a randomized, double-blind, placebo-controlled study. *Sleep Med*. 2009;10(9):973–5.

32. Earley CJ, Heckler D, Horská A, et al. The treatment of restless legs syndrome with intravenous iron dextran. *Sleep Med* 2004;5(3):231–5.

33. Allen RP, Adler CH, Du W, et al. Clinical efficacy and safety of IV ferric carboxymaltose (FCM) treatment of RLS: a multi-centred, placebo-controlled preliminary clinical trial. *Sleep Med* 2011;12(9):906–13.

34. Grote L, Leissner L, Hedner J, et al. A randomized, double-blind, placebo controlled, multi-center study of intravenous iron sucrose and placebo in the treatment of restless legs syndrome. *Mov Disord* 2009;24(10):1445–52.

35. Earley CJ, Connor JR, Beard JL, et al. Abnormalities in CSF concentrations of ferritin and transferrin in restless legs syndrome. *Neurology* 2000;54(8):1698–700.

36. Mizuno S, Mihara T, Miyaoka T, et al. CSF iron, ferritin and transferrin levels in restless legs syndrome. *J Sleep Res* 2005;14(1):43–7.

37. Allen RP, Barker PB, Wehrl F, et al. MRI measurement of brain iron in patients with restless legs syndrome. *Neurology* 2001;56(2):263–5.

38. Godau J, Klose U, Di Santo A, et al. Multiregional brain iron deficiency in restless legs syndrome. *Mov Disord* 2008;23(8):1184–7.

39. Schmidauer C, Sojer M, Seppi K, et al. Transcranial ultrasound shows nigral hypoechogenicity in restless legs syndrome. *Ann Neurol* 2005;58(4):630–4.

40. Sloand JA, Shelly MA, Feigin A, et al. A double-blind, placebo-controlled trial of intravenous iron dextran therapy in patients with ESRD and restless legs syndrome. *Am J Kidney Dis* 2004;43(4):663–70.

41. Ulfberg J, Nystrom B. Restless legs syndrome in blood donors. *Sleep Med* 2004;5(2):115–18.

42. Weinstock LB, Walters AS. Restless legs syndrome is associated with irritable bowel syndrome and small intestinal bacterial overgrowth. *Sleep Med* 2011;12(6):610–13.

43. Happe S, Tings T, Schettler V, et al. Low-density lipoprotein apheresis and restless legs syndrome. *Sleep* 2003;26:A335–6.

44. Banerji N, Hurwitz L. Restless legs syndrome, with particular reference to its occurrence after gastric surgery. *Br Med J* 1970;4:774–5.

45. Synofzik M, Godau J, Lindig T, et al. Restless legs and substantia nigra hypoechogenicity are common features in Friedreich's ataxia. *Cerebellum* 2011;10(1):9–13.

46. Frauscher B, Hering S, Hogl B, et al. Restless legs syndrome in Friedreich ataxia: a polysomnographic study. *Mov Disord* 2011;26(2):302–6.

47. Manconi M, Ferini-Strambi L, Filippi M, et al. Multicenter case-control study on restless legs syndrome in multiple sclerosis: the REMS study. *Sleep* 2008;31(7):944–52.

48. Lo Coco D, Mattaliano A, Coco AL, et al. Increased frequency of restless legs syndrome in chronic obstructive pulmonary disease patients. *Sleep Med* 2009;10(5):572–6.

49. Bara-Jimenez W, Aksu M, Graham B, et al. Periodic limb movements in sleep: state-dependent excitability of the spinal flexor reflex. *Neurology* 2000;54(8):1609–16.

50. Aksu M, Bara-Jimenez W. State dependent excitability changes of spinal flexor reflex in patients with restless legs syndrome secondary to chronic renal failure. *Sleep Med* 2002;3(5):427–30.

51. Entezari-Taher M, Singleton JR, Jones CR, et al. Changes in excitability of motor cortical circuitry in primary restless legs syndrome. *Neurology* 1999;53(6):1201–5.

52. Kutukcu Y, Dogruer E, Yetkin S, et al. Evaluation of periodic leg movements and associated transcranial magnetic stimulation parameters in restless legs syndrome. *Muscle Nerve* 2006;33(1):133–7.

53. Tergau F, Wischer S, Paulus W. Motor system excitability in patients with restless legs syndrome. *Neurology* 1999;52(5):1060–3.

54. McGinley M, Hoffman RL, Russ DW, et al. Older adults exhibit more intracortical inhibition and less intracortical facilitation than young adults. *Exp Gerontol* 2010;45(9):671–8.

55. Nardone R, Ausserer H, Bratti A, et al. Cabergoline reverses cortical hyperexcitability in patients with restless legs syndrome. *Acta Neurol Scand* 2006;114(4):244–9.

56. Scalise A, Cadore IP, Gigli GL. Motor cortex excitability in restless legs syndrome. *Sleep Med* 2004;5(4):393–6.

57. Michaud M, Paquet J, Lavigne G, et al. Sleep laboratory diagnosis of restless legs syndrome. *Eur Neurol* 2002;48(2):108–13.

58. Garcia-Borreguero D, Larrosa O, de la Llave Y, et al. Correlation between rating scales and sleep laboratory measurements in restless legs syndrome. *Sleep Med* 2004;5(6):561–5.

59. Pennestri MH, Whittom S, Adam B, et al. PLMS and PLMW in healthy subjects as a function of age: prevalence and interval distribution. *Sleep* 2006;29(9):1183–7.

60. Winkelmann J, Czamara D, Schormair B, et al. Genome-wide association study identifies novel restless legs syndrome susceptibility loci on 2p14 and 16q12.1. *PLoS Genetics* 2011;7(7):e1002171.

61. Stefansson H, Rye DB, Hicks A, et al. A genetic risk factor for periodic limb movements in sleep. *N Engl J Med* 2007;357(7):639–47.

62. Catoire H, Dion PA, Xiong L, et al. Restless legs syndrome-associated MEIS1 risk variant influences iron homeostasis. *Ann Neurol* 2011;70(1):170–5.

63. Snyder AM, Wang X, Patton SM, et al. Mitochondrial ferritin in the substantia nigra in restless legs syndrome. *J Neuropathol Exp Neurol* 2009;68(11):1193–9.

64. Patton SM, Ponnuru P, Snyder AM, et al. Hypoxia-inducible factor pathway activation in restless legs syndrome patients. *Eur J Neurol* 2011;18(11):1329–35.

65. Sanchez M, Galy B, Muckenthaler MU, et al. Iron-regulatory proteins limit hypoxia-inducible factor-2alpha expression in iron deficiency. *Nat Struct Mol Biol* 2007;14(5):420–6.

66. Erikson KM, Jones BC, Hess EJ, et al. Iron deficiency decreases dopamine D1 and D2 receptors in rat brain. *Pharmacol Biochem Behav* 2001;69(3–4):409–18.

67. Erikson KM, Jones BC, Beard JL. Iron deficiency alters dopamine transporter functioning in rat striatum. *J Nutr* 2000;130(11):2831–7.

68. Chen Q, Beard JL, Jones BC. Abnormal rat brain monoamine metabolism in iron deficiency anemia. *J Nutritional Biochem* 1995;6:486–93.

69. Ill AM, Mitchell TR, Neely EB, et al. Metabolic analysis of mouse brains that have compromised iron storage. *Metab Brain Dis* 2006;21(2–3):77–87.

70. Larsson BW, Kadi F, Ulfberg J, et al. Skeletal muscle morphology in patients with restless legs syndrome. *Eur Neurol* 2007;58(3):133–7.

71. Wahlin-Larsson B, Ulfberg J, Aulin KP, et al. The expression of vascular endothelial growth factor in skeletal muscle of patients with sleep disorders. *Muscle Nerve* 2009;40(4):556–61.

45

Restless Legs Syndrome (Willis-Ekbom Disease)
Diagnosis, Differential Diagnosis (Mimics), and Evaluation

RICHARD P. ALLEN, ARTHUR S. WALTERS,
AND SUDHANSU CHOKROVERTY

THE FIRST basic clinical description of restless legs syndrome (RLS) was provided by Willis[1,2] in the 17th century, but it remained poorly defined until the seminal work by Karl-Axel Ekbom in the middle of the 19th century. The increasing recognition of RLS in the last 70 years since Ekbom's work occurred in the context of two important developments in medicine. First, there has been increasing emphasis not only on prolonging life but also on improving quality of life, particularly in the last half of life when medical problems tend to be more problematic. Thus, diseases that disrupt life quality and are significant problems in later adult life, such as RLS, have become seen as increasingly important, especially as life expectancy has increased. Second, sleep medicine has gained acceptance with recognition of the significant medical and social impacts of sleep. Disorders that disrupt sleep, such as RLS, have received increasing attention.

The emphasis in the diagnosis of RLS has evolved with increasing attention to the total pattern of the presenting symptoms. Willis in his description emphasized the excessive movements when resting and the associated sleep loss. Axel Ekbom in his large case series noted these but emphasized more the sensory phenomena of RLS, that is, the unusual, disturbing sensations in the legs and the associated movements of the legs. He also provided the name "restless legs" that is most commonly used today, although it is increasingly apparent it is somewhat of a misnomer. The American Academy of Sleep Medicine (then known as the Association of Sleep Disorder Centers) in its first nosology appropriately included RLS, emphasizing its disruption of sleep.[3] At about this time both the remarkable effectiveness of the newer dopaminergic treatments[4,5] and the unexpectedly high prevalence for RLS[6,7] were discovered. There developed a critical mass of clinicians treating these patients, and under the leadership of Arthur Walters they formed the International Restless Legs Syndrome Study Group (IRLSSG). The IRLSSG shared extensive clinical experience treating RLS that enabled the development by consensus of the first complete modern diagnostic criteria for RLS.[8] They were able to recognize the significance of both quiescegenic (rest-induced) and movement-responsive (relieved by activity) features of the disorder implicit but not so clearly stated before. They also emphasized the circadian nature of the symptoms, giving us the four basic essential criteria still used today for the diagnosis. This was further improved at a conference of the IRLSSG and American patient group (Restless Legs Foundation) at the American National Institutes of Health in 2003.[9] The akathisia (the urge to move or inability to sit still) focused on the legs was emphasized as the essential pathognomonic symptom, usually but not always accompanied by the dysesthesias (abnormal, unusual, uncomfortable leg sensations). The rest and activity effects were clearly separated. The primary diagnosis relies upon a subjective report of an abnormal sensory experience.

The National Institutes of Health (NIH) criteria provided the basis for a remarkable explosion of clinical science and effective diagnosis and treatment of thousands who suffered from RLS. Increasing clinical experience further identified two critical issues not covered in the 2003 NIH diagnostic criteria: differential diagnosis ("mimics") and degree of severity or frequency of the disease. These have now been addressed in the current IRLSSG diagnostic criteria posted on the IRLSSG Web site (http://www.irlssg.org/) and described here.

DIAGNOSIS: ESSENTIAL FEATURES

RLS diagnosis is based on the clinical history obtained by a well-trained clinician. It depends solely on subjective reports of the sensory symptoms defining the disorder, including subjective reports of the conditions affecting these symptoms. This requires attention to two major problems in making the diagnosis: differential diagnosis and identification of clinical course reflected in frequency-severity and clinical significance. These are both addressed in the 2012 IRLSSG diagnostic criteria for RLS.

Differential Diagnosis

The major problem faced by the patient and the clinician stems from the abnormal nature of the sensory symptoms of RLS. Since these are not normal sensory phenomena, there is no shared language to describe them. In this important way RLS differs from other movement disorders. Abnormal movements can be seen and measured; abnormal sensations are the private experience of the patient not seen, measured, or shared with those who do not have these. Patients have no trouble identifying their abnormal sensations and can provide reliable information about the factors affecting their expression. But describing the sensations is another matter. Patients generally report the sensations "feel like" and then describe some bizarre event involving their legs, for example, bugs crawling under the skin, Pepsi Cola in the veins, urge to move, or Elvis legs. These are clearly not normal sensory experience and the expressions carry some sense of the sensory reality experienced by the RLS patient, but without some common sensory experience language fails to adequately describe these sensory abnormalities. There are psychological tools for developing a language to describe these sensations, but work on this has been limited to some recent studies mostly from Bentley in South Africa.[10,11] The language problem leads to some confusing overlap with other conditions that produce sensory symptoms that "mimic" those of RLS.[12] The current IRLSSG diagnostic criteria have added a fifth essential criterion requiring differential diagnosis to exclude "mimics." These are discussed in more detail later, but the criterion itself serves to indicate the nature of these conditions.

Frequency, Severity, and Clinical Significance of Symptoms in Restless Legs Syndrome Diagnosis

The current diagnostic standard also addressed the thorny issue of the degree of frequency and severity of the symptoms needed to make a diagnosis. RLS symptoms occur episodically often with abrupt onset and limited duration of expression. Thus, they can be enumerated, but after considerable discussion among the members of the IRLSSG, both at a large diagnostic conference in Baltimore and in multiple subsequent reviews, *no consensus could be developed regarding minimum number of symptoms or severity needed to make a diagnosis of RLS.* It was felt first and foremost that this was a neurological condition. The sensory symptoms were not an extension of normal experience but rather an expression of an underlying neurological disease. Thus, any expression of the symptoms that suffices to meet the basic diagnostic criteria reflects the RLS disease process even if rare or of no clinical significance. Like many diseases, the process can be indolent, episodic, slowly progressive, or abruptly severe. The severity and time course of RLS varies considerably, but it is now identified as one neurological disease process based on basic neurological abnormalities (see Chapter 46). Moreover, any frequency-severity criteria would be arbitrary and likely exclude some who would benefit from treatment. It was also generally felt defining frequency and severity for the diagnosis really should come from the continuing scientific exploration of the biology of RLS supported by appropriate clinical population studies, rather than from some arbitrary criteria. None of the RLS diagnostic criteria are arbitrary and adding one now would serve to confuse rather than enhance RLS diagnosis. It was, in particular, noted that infrequent RLS symptoms can be clinically significant, requiring efforts to prevent their occurrence (e.g., oral iron treatments) or medications as needed to quickly relieve them (e.g., RLS limited to travel). Thus, treatment is appropriate even for patients with RLS symptoms occurring only a few times a year, or perhaps even on some years but not others. There was a clear consensus, however, that there was a large bulk of the patients treated for RLS who usually had symptoms occurring at least twice a week persisting for several months; some, however, had less persistent disease.

It was therefore decided not to make the severity or frequency some arbitrary absolute requirement for diagnosis but instead recognizing the somewhat arbitrary nature of this to add specifiers to the diagnosis to capture both the clinical course of the disease and the clinical significance. This leaves the diagnosis to the clinician's judgment whether the presentation suffices to make a diagnosis and separates, appropriately, the treatment decision from the diagnosis. RLS like many neurological conditions does not always need to be treated, and often the treatment can be behavioral or preventative. It is therefore appropriate to use specifiers to emphasize the importance of considering factors that impact treatment decision but do not have a role for diagnosis of the disease.

Essential Criteria for Restless Legs Syndrome Diagnosis

Table 45.1 gives the current IRLSSG diagnostic criteria that are accepted as the international standard for making the diagnosis. *No other criteria should be used for the clinical diagnosis of RLS.* These criteria can be summarized defining RLS as quiescegenic, nocturnal focal leg akathisia usually with dysesthesias that are not from RLS "mimics." These criteria have worked well for RLS diagnosis and evaluation, but they are somewhat deceptively simple. Each needs some careful elaboration.

Criteria 1: The pathognomonic sensory symptom of RLS: an urge to move or focal akathisia of the leg is a sensation often but not always associated with dysesthesia. The primary defining feature of RLS remains the strong, often irresistible, urge to move the leg occurring for no apparent reason other then possibly to respond to strange dysesthesias also occurring for no apparent reason. The urge to move appears to come from the leg and is focused on moving the leg not the whole body. In extreme cases other body parts become involved, and in extremis it may involve the whole body producing symptoms similar to drug-induced akathisia. The sensations generally, however, are limited to the leg. They rarely involve the feet and do not have the distill-proximal spread characteristic of peripheral neuropathy. They may occur in one or both legs and may have variable expression between the legs and even for location on the leg. If they occur exclusively for one leg, evaluation for possible radiculopathy contributing to the RLS is indicated. The urge to move should not be confused with unconscious movements such as anxious foot tapping. If the patient reports others tell him he is moving but he has no awareness of an urge to move, then this is not RLS. RLS patients are aware, usually painfully, of their need to move.

The dysesthesias that come with the urge to move follow the same pattern as the akathisia described earlier—coming from the leg, variable expression in the legs, and when extreme extended to other body parts. The sensations are rarely in the feet and are usually seen as inside the leg, not on the surface, nor in the joints. They usually have a dynamic quality to them. They are sometimes painful, and depending on severity and how pain is defined, are reported as painful by 30% to over 50% of clinical RLS patients.

The next three essential criteria for RLS diagnosis define conditions that must be shown to affect the expression of the RLS symptoms described in criterion 1.

Criteria 2: Quiescegenic symptoms start or get worse with rest. Rest here means not only physical

Table 45.1 Diagnostic Criteria for RLS (reprinted from the IRLSSG web site: www.IRLSSG.org)

Restless legs syndrome (RLS), a neurological sensorimotor disease often profoundly disturbing sleep and quality of life has variable expression influenced by genetic, environmental and medical factors. The symptoms vary considerably in frequency from less than once a month or year to daily and severity from mildly annoying to disabling. Symptoms may also remit for various periods of time. RLS is diagnosed by ascertaining symptom patterns that meet the following five essential criteria adding clinical specifiers where appropriate.

ESSENTIAL DIAGNOSTIC CRITERIA (ALL MUST BE MET)

1. An urge to move the legs usually but not always accompanied by or felt to be caused by uncomfortable and unpleasant sensations in the legs.[1,2]
2. The urge to move the legs and any accompanying unpleasant sensations begin or worsen during periods of rest or inactivity such as lying down or sitting.
3. The urge to move the legs and any accompanying unpleasant sensations are partially or totally relieved by movement, such as walking or stretching, at least as long as the activity continues.[3]
4. The urge to move the legs and any accompanying unpleasant sensations during rest or inactivity only occur or are worse in the evening or night than during the day.[4]
5. The occurrence of the above features are not solely accounted for as symptoms primary to another medical or a behavioral condition (e.g., myalgia, venous stasis, leg edema, arthritis, leg cramps, positional discomfort, habitual foot tapping).[5]

SPECIFIERS FOR CLINICAL COURSE OF RLS[6]

A. Chronic-persistent RLS: Symptoms when not treated would occur on average at least twice weekly for the past year.
B. Intermittent RLS: symptoms when not treated would occur on average <2/week for the past year, with at least 5 lifetime events.

SPECIFIER FOR CLINICAL SIGNIFICANCE FOR RLS

The symptoms of RLS cause significant distress or impairment in social, occupational, educational or other important areas of functioning by the impact on sleep, energy/vitality, daily activities, behavior, cognition or mood.

[1] Sometimes the urge to move the legs is present without the uncomfortable sensations and sometimes the arms or other parts of the body are involved in addition to the legs.

[2] For children, the description of these symptoms should be in the child's own words.

[3] When symptoms are very severe, relief by activity may not be noticeable but must have been previously present.

[4] When symptoms are very severe, the worsening in the evening or night may not be noticeable but must have been previously present.

[5] These conditions, often referred to as "RLS mimics," have been commonly confused with RLS particularly in surveys because they produce symptoms that meet or at least come very close to meeting all of the above criteria. The list here gives some examples of this that have been noted as particularly significant in epidemiological studies and clinical practice. RLS may also occur with any of these conditions, but the RLS symptoms will then be more in degree, conditions of expression or character than those usually occurring as part of the other condition.

[6] The clinical course criteria do not apply for pediatric cases nor for some special cases of provoked RLS such as pregnancy or drug induced RLS where the frequency may be high but limited to duration of the provocative condition.

inactivity but also decreased mental activity and decreased alertness. Sitting and lying still without cognitive stimulation defines the rest that engenders RLS symptoms. These not only occur with rest but also are more likely and more severe with the increasing duration of rest. The suggested immobilization test (SIT) relies upon this feature of the diagnosis. It requires the patient to sit upright in bed with the legs stretched, resting, relaxed, eyes open, without any cognitive stimulation for 1 hour. The subject indicates every 5 or 10 minutes the degree of leg discomfort, and leg movements are recorded continuously for the entire test. As shown in Figure 45.1 the leg movements of RLS reflecting inability to stay still increase dramatically with duration of the test,[13] validating this diagnostic criteria. Leg discomfort has also similarly been shown to increase with duration of test, further validating these diagnostic criteria.[14]

Criteria 3: Relief of symptoms occurs with movement of the legs. In contrast to the often gradual

development of symptoms with rest, the symptom relief with movement usually occurs rapidly. Patients often report some relief the minute they start walking, although some find that it takes a few minutes of walking before they sense any relief. Very severe cases may require more strenuous activity to relieve the symptoms, but there should always be some level of physical activity that rapidly provides relief. In most cases, reports that it takes more than 5 minutes of activity to produce any symptom relief raise serious doubts about the diagnosis. It is not exercise but rather increased alertness brought on by the activity that provides symptom relief. Other activities besides movement that serve to increase arousal such as computer games, sewing, exciting TV programs, or arguments also serve to reduce RLS symptoms. These, however, are much harder to assess or observe than actual movement; thus, the diagnosis here emphasizes the movement-related reduction of symptoms. It is important to note that

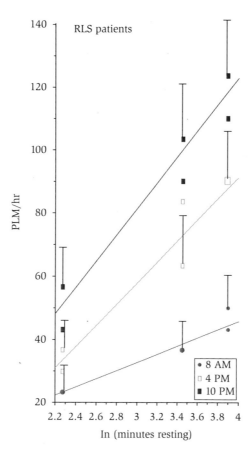

FIGURE 45.1   Average of PLMW/h on the SIT from each of two days for RLS patients by time-of-day vs. natural log of minutes resting. Larger points indicate two data points overlap. Bars = standard errors for repeated tests. (Reproduced from Allen et al. *Sleep Medicine* 6(2005) 429–34.)

although the immediate symptoms are reduced with movement of the legs, many patients may deny this. They may report movement had no effect since as soon as they stop moving the symptoms return. It is therefore important to determine whether there is any symptom relief at all while moving and that this relief continues while moving. Symptoms may return but only when movement stops or is reduced.

Criteria 4: Circadian pattern of RLS symptoms worse in the evening and night, generally with spontaneous remission of symptoms in the morning. RLS symptoms tend to occur more frequently and with greater severity later in the day. Thus, they may occur some in the late morning or afternoon but are less likely to occur then and if they occur will be less severe than in the evening. This is also shown in Figure 45.1, where the leg movements become more frequent as the time of day of the SIT becomes later, validating this diagnostic criteria. This has also been validated in two studies of RLS symptoms across the day with and without sleep deprivation. These studies showed worsening during the evening and night with improvement in the morning and day even if the patient was kept awake all night.[15,16] It deserves note that all of these 24-hour studies showed a "protected period" in the morning shortly after usual wake time when symptoms rarely if ever occur.

A major complication in evaluating this diagnostic criterion occurs because people are generally less active in the evening than the morning. The circadian worsening in the evening can become confused with the quiescegenic effects. It is therefore important to ask whether the symptoms when resting in the morning do not occur or are less than when resting in the evening or night. Those reporting symptoms that occur anytime when resting and are not more or less when resting in the morning than the night generally do not have RLS except for very severe cases when this circadian rhythm is overwhelmed by the overall severity of the symptoms.

Criteria 5: This last essential diagnostic criterion requires checking to ensure the RLS symptoms are not totally due to one of the conditions producing symptoms "mimicking" those of RLS. While this is usually a trivial matter in the clinic setting, it can sometimes be ignored. It is, in contrast, a difficult diagnostic problem when using only questionnaires in population studies. Possible mimics are presented in Table 45.2 modified from Hening et al.,[12] along with symptom features that help differentiate them from RLS.

Although patients with these conditions may report symptoms meeting the four prior diagnostic criteria, this usually occurs because of the linguistic problems describing the RLS symptoms. In the clinic setting asking added questions separates the mimics from RLS. Moreover, when the symptoms occur only with the other condition, they clearly are not RLS symptoms.

DIAGNOSIS: SPECIFIERS

Although the specifiers are not required as part of the diagnosis, it is strongly encouraged that they be applied in all cases where practical. The first specifier separates the more chronic and persistent cases from others. This serves to emphasize a category most likely to have daily medication treatment for RLS from those cases where other treatments, including no treatment, would more likely be considered. The clinical significance specifier is a particularly important guide for treatment decision. The guidance here is simply to specify whether this is a clinically significant issue in any or several of the identified areas. This provides useful information for considering change over time and treatment benefits.

DIAGNOSIS: OTHER CLINICAL FEATURES OF SIGNIFICANCE FOR DIAGNOSES

Three clinical features support the diagnosis of RLS as presented in Table 45.3. Periodic leg movements in sleep (PLMS) and wake (PLMW) are common in RLS, occurring frequently in about 85% of the clinical cases.[17] Thus, PLMS/PLMW provide objective motor signs of the disorder, and when not present the diagnosis should be reviewed to ensure accuracy. History of RLS in the family members of a patient serves to support the diagnosis if present, particularly for RLS patients whose symptoms started before age 45. RLS family history is about seven times more likely for an RLS patient whose symptoms started before age 45 than it is for non-RLS patients. While presence of others with RLS in the family supports the diagnosis, the lack of any RLS in family members has no significance. Finally, an initial positive response to levodopa or dopamine agonist is considered to be very supportive of the diagnosis. The clinical impression is that almost all RLS patients will improve in the initial

Table 45.2 RLS Mimics: Conditions Known to Produce Symptoms That Closely Mimic Those of RLS (modified from Hening et al. (2009)[12])

CONDITION	SIGNIFICANT DIFFERENCE FROM RLS
Leg cramps	Occur with muscle hardening not typical of RLS
Positional discomfort	Rapidly relieved with single simple body movement
Local leg injury	Not quickly relieved with walking
Arthritis	Not quickly relieved with walking
Positional ischemia	Numbness is not a symptom of RLS
Nerve damage	More localized, less variable than RLS (neuropathy/radiculopathy)
Sleep transition events	Limited to sleep transitions any time of day (hypnic jerks)
Leg shaking, jitters	Usually lack awareness
Habitual foot tapping	Lacks awareness
General nervousness	Pervades large areas of the body, not just legs Not quickly relieved with movement
Venuous stasis	Physical signs of stasis
Leg edema	leg swelling
Myalgia	Limited relief with movement
Drug induced akathisia	Less clearly focused on the legs Requires prior drug use
Pain syndromes	Not quickly relieved with movement
Painful legs and moving toes	Not circadian or quiescegenic

month of treatment with these medications, but this has only been demonstrated in a small 48-patient trial with levodopa.[18] The problem is that in large clinical trials the response rate for improved or much improved on dopamine agonists is about 60% to 80% and not 100%, so

Table 45.3 Clinical Features Supporting the Diagnosis of RLS

The following features, although not essential for diagnosis, are closely associated with RLS and should be noted when present.

1. Presence of periodic limb movements in sleep (PLMS) or resting wake (PLMW) at rates or intensity greater than expected for age.
2. Reduction in symptoms at least initially with dopaminergic treatment.
3. Family history of RLS among first-degree relatives.

this casts some doubt on the strength of this supportive feature for diagnosis. Nonetheless, this remains a reasonable clinical feature supporting the diagnosis.

There are six other clinical features of RLS that deserve note when present in relation to the diagnosis and treatment. (See Table 45.4.) First, some patients with more severe condition report a progressive development of their RLS severity. The course of this development should be noted when present. The sleep disturbance occurring with the condition is a marker of a primary morbidity and is expected to occur with most moderate-to-severe RLS. Failure to find this in more severe cases deserves note and special attention to the diagnosis. Age of onset of RLS less than 45 indicates increased risk of a familial pattern and when over 45 raises the possibility this is RLS associated with a medical condition. The degree of pain versus discomfort deserves note in relation to the overall severity of the symptoms. More severe symptoms tend to occur with pain, but mild symptoms are not

Table 45.4 Other Clinical Features of RLS Deserving Note

1. Progressive nature of symptom severity
2. Sleep disturbance
3. Age of onset
4. Degree of Pain vs. discomfort
5. Iron status
6. Lack of physical findings on medical or neurological exam

generally reported as painful. The iron status of the patient should always be checked, and either a low serum ferritin (below 75 mcg/l) or percent transferrin saturation (below 20) is consistent with RLS complicated by iron deficiency. Finally, RLS has no significant physical findings on the standard medical or neurological examination. Thus, finding physical abnormalities that might account for part of the symptoms requires carefully reviewing the full diagnosis.

DIAGNOSIS: DIAGNOSTIC TOOLS

There are three different tools available to assist in making an RLS diagnosis in different conditions.

The Hopkins telephone diagnostic interview (HTDI) and Hening clinical diagnostic interview (HCDI) are very similar structured interviews that provide the clinical information needed to make the diagnosis of RLS. This was initially developed to make the diagnosis by a telephone interview. It guides the questions to ensure obtaining the information needed to confirm the diagnosis and to exclude the most common possible "mimics." Thus, this interview covers all five of the essential diagnostic criteria for RLS. It has now been modified slightly, adding more instructions to support its use in the clinic setting. This was first validated in a clinical population of RLS patients and matched controls and there found to have 97% sensitivity and 92% specificity.[19] This has further been validated for a population of family members of clinical RLS patients or matched controls who unlike the first study had limited knowledge about RLS and no clinical diagnosis regarding the RLS prior to this study. Those with RLS represented a wide range of severity

of RLS. The HDTI compared to the independent diagnosis by two separate RLS experts had 90% sensitivity and 0.91% specificity. This compared to agreement between the two clinicians of 93%–96%,[20] giving for the HDTI 98% of achievable agreement. The clinical form of this diagnostic interview has been used successfully in major clinical trials in the United States, Spain, Germany, and Sweden. *This is the only validated clinical interview tool for making the RLS diagnosis and the only clinical diagnostic tool validated against a wide range of RLS severity.* It takes about 5–20 minutes to do the interview depending on the diagnostic complexity. Use of this interview schedule, however, requires training.

The RLS-DI is a diagnostic algorithm that provides an alternate approach for supporting the RLS diagnosis. Rather than guiding the clinician in making the diagnosis, this allows the clinician to check the accuracy of the diagnosis based on answering a series of 10 specific questions about the clinical status and laboratory test results for the patient. While this does not explicitly guide the diagnostic process, it requires ascertainment of critical information supporting the diagnosis and then provides a quantitative assessment of the probability an RLS diagnosis is correct along with a specific cutoff score for accepting the diagnosis. In a clinical sleep laboratory population (86 RLS patients and 93 patients with other sleep disorders) when compared to two independent clinical raters, this inventory had a 93% sensitivity and 99% specificity.[21] It should be noted though that this was not a general population of RLS patients and therefore was mostly patients with moderate to severe RLS, many of whom had been educated about RLS prior to this study. Specificity and sensitivity will likely be less in a more general population. The RLS-DI also does not specifically exclude RLS "mimics." This is, nonetheless, appropriate for use in a study of clinical patients. It is much easier to implement than the HTDI/HCDI and the quantitative score provides a more objective diagnostic basis than does the structured interview approach of the HTDI/HCDI.

The Cambridge-Hopkins RLS diagnostic questionnaire (CH-RLSq) is the only validated patient-completed diagnostic questionnaire for RLS. It has 11 critical items making the diagnosis and excluding two common "mimics" of leg cramps and positional discomfort. It also includes two extra items characterizing

RLS features that support the diagnosis and in its complete form also provides basic information about RLS features, including age of onset, frequency, and intensity of symptoms. It has been successfully used in several clinical trials, including an important study on social burden of RLS.[22] Since this was designed to maximize accuracy in a population where RLS prevalence would be expected to be 7% or less, the questionnaire was designed to maximize specificity over sensitivity. The CH-RLSq had an 87.2% sensitivity and 94.4% specificity when validated in a population of blood donors by comparison with diagnosis by expert clinical interviews using the HTDI.[23] This questionnaire is available from Richardjhu@me.com. It comes in the full form (CH-RLSq) and in the abbreviated 13-item form (CH-RLSq13) limited to mainly diagnostic questions and an abbreviated 11-item form (CH-RLSq11) that has the essential diagnostic information used in the validation study. The recommended forms that can be considered fully validated are the CH-RLSq and CH-RLSq13. One problem with this form is that it does consider RLS occurring during current or past pregnancies. If this is a concern, there is a version developed that adds the information about RLS in relation to pregnancy.

DIAGNOSIS: PHENOTYPES

The literature on RLS includes consideration of three different phenotypes based on familial occurrence, age of onset of symptoms, and primary versus secondary to another disorder.

Familial RLS is somewhat loosely defined by having RLS in a first-degree relative. This is often hard to reliably determine, and the probability of this increases with family size. Familial occurrence has been seen as an indication of a genetically determined RLS or one that is primary and not caused by another disorder. Thus, in one case series the RLS not associated with peripheral neuropathy occurred much more with familial RLS than nonfamilial RLS.[24]

Age of onset of RLS is also somewhat hard to determine since it relies upon patient recall of events that are sometimes several years earlier. The cutoff between early and late onset of RLS is also somewhat arbitrary, although data from brain and cerebrospinal fluid iron studies and from relative frequency of familial occurrence indicates that the critical cutoff should be somewhere between 30 and 45 years.[25-28]

In general, early-onset compared to late-onset RLS is more likely to be familial, has fewer comorbidities, and is less likely to be secondary. Early-onset RLS is more likely than late-onset RLS to be slowly progressive with frequent persisting symptoms, if they occur, usually developing after age 45.[25]

Secondary versus primary RLS is defined by clear indications that another condition caused the expression of the RLS. This can be documented by a patient's history of RLS developing and worsening in tandem with some other condition, or it can be documented by case studies showing that a specific condition not only commonly produces expression of RLS but when that condition resolves, the RLS also resolves. Secondary RLS can also be documented by indications that a condition produces the biological factors producing RLS. The primary biological factor know to cause RLS is brain iron deficiency as documented in Chapter 46. Thus, iron deficiency is not considered to be a secondary form of RLS, but rather a central part of the biology of primary RLS. In contrast, pregnancy and end-stage-renal disease cause RLS in a significant number of patients, but they probably do this primarily through their effects on brain iron status. Both of these are clearly secondary RLS since the RLS almost always resolves when the condition does, and they both have major effects impairing brain iron status. Other conditions that have been suggested as producing secondary RLS include rheumatoid arthritis, Friedreich's ataxia, chronic obstructive pulmonary disease, some peripheral neuropathies, some inflammatory conditions, and, for some patients, use of selective serotonin reuptake inhibitorsorserotonin–norepinephrinereuptake inhibitors.

There are also many conditions that appear to be comorbid with RLS. These occur more commonly than expected for patients with RLS but do not meet the pattern suggesting any causal relationship, for example. depression, anxiety disorders, attention-deficit disorder, multiple sclerosis, and some peripheral neuropathies. The distinction between secondary and comorbid can be at times uncertain, as shown here by consideration of peripheral neuropathy as either comorbid or a secondary cause. Studies support both considerations, and this may depend upon the type of peripheral neuropathy. In general, parsimony sides with seeing a condition as comorbid unless there is fairly strong evidence supporting a causal relation.

RESTLESS LEGS SYNDROME SEVERITY EVALUATION

Clinical severity is often roughly evaluated by determining the frequency of RLS symptoms and/or the degree of distress or intensity when the symptoms occur. Clinical significance can be assessed by the degree of RLS impact on significant aspects of functioning. The diagnostic specifiers noted earlier serve to support this clinical approach to RLS. Moreover, several epidemiological studies have defined as clinically significant those with RLS symptoms generally occurring twice a week or more with moderate to severe distress when present.[22,29,30] Three scales have also been developed to provide a quantitative assessment of RLS severity based on the patient's report of subjective experience.

The International RLS study group's RLS severity scale (IRLS) has become accepted as the gold standard for clinical evaluation of RLS severity. It has been used in almost all clinical trials, allowing some comparison between the trials. It has 10 items each with five responses for effectively no symptoms to severe symptoms occurring during the past week (scored 0–4). This questionnaire is to be administered by a clinician reading the items to the patient, including the possible answers, and writing down the patient's response on the questionnaire. The clinician is able to answer any patient questions about the test item and is encouraged to ensure that the patient understands the questionnaire item. The total score ranges from 0 to 40, and RLS severity is generally rated as mild for 0–10, moderate 11–20, severe 21–30, and very severe 31–40.[31] The minimal score required for entry to most clinical trials is 15, although some trials have required 20. This scale has excellent psychometric properties for inter- and intrarater reliability, internal consistency, and convergent validity with good responsiveness to changes in clinical status.[31–33]

Factor analysis has revealed two subscales of the IRLS, one for primary symptoms and the other for impact, as listed in Table 45.5. The scale also includes single items related to sleep, mood, and daytime fatigue, as well as both frequency and duration of symptoms. It has been modified slightly for the patient or research subject to complete, and in some forms the questions have been altered to remove reference to RLS. Usually the words "restless legs syndrome" are then replaced with "symptoms/feeling in your legs" or some other phrase related to the basis for identification of the subject for the study. Subject-completed forms have not been validated, but they obviously have considerable face validity. More needs to be done on development and validation of the patient-completed forms.

It is strongly recommended that all RLS research studies use the IRLS as a measure of RLS severity in order to permit comparison between studies. Versions of the IRLS are available in about 12 different languages. Each of these versions has been developed with careful linguistic validation by MAPI trust and has been used in prior clinical trials. The copyright for the scale is held by the IRLSSG, and there is a small fee for using the scale for commercial groups and studies funded by grants, but there is no fee for academic groups without outside funding. This scale and its validated translations can be obtained from MAPI by contacting PROinformation@mapi-trust.org or going to the MAPI Web site: http://www.mapi-trust.org/services/questionnairelicensing/catalog-questionnaires.

The RLS-6 severity questionnaire was developed to provide a scale that would separate daytime from evening and night symptoms. Despite the strong circadian feature of RLS with symptoms worse in the evening and night, most clinically significant RLS report some daytime symptoms. These become even more significant with RLS augmentation as discussed in Chapter 50. The RLS-6 is the only questionnaire that provides separate severity assessment by time of day and is recommended as a standard for clinical evaluation of the 24-hour pattern of RLS symptoms. The RLS-6 scale can be obtained from Ralf Khonen by e-mail at rkohnen@rpsweb.com.

The Johns Hopkins RLS Severity Scale (JHRLSS) was developed for a simple clinical evaluation of severity for patients who had symptoms most days and is based on the usual time of onset of symptoms when present. If symptoms occurred on average less than 5 days a week, it is scored as 0.5. Otherwise, it is scored for symptoms starting during sleep or at bedtime as 1, after 6 pm but before bedtime as 2, before 6 pm but after noon as 3, and before noon as 4. The JHRLSS has been validated against polysomnographic measures of PLMS/hr.[34] This scale has the advantage that patients can often recall the time of onset of symptoms several years ago, and thus it can provide

Table 45.5 Two Factors in the RLS Scale (modified from Allen et al. (2003)[35])

IRLS ITEMS	FACTOR LOADINGS	
	FACTOR 1	FACTOR 2
Factor 1 items		
Item 6: Overall, how severe is your RLS as a whole?	0.836	0.286
Item 1: Overall, how would you rate the RLS discomfort in your legs or arms?	0.820	0.147
Item 2: Overall, how would you rate the need to move around because of your RLS symptoms?	0.801	0.029
Item 4: Overall, how severe is your sleep disturbance from your RLS symptoms?	0.729	0.376
Item 8: When you have RLS symptoms how severe are they on an average day?	0.729	0.324
Item 7: How often do you get RLS symptoms?	0.687	0.110
Factor 2 items		
Item 9: Overall, how severe is the impact of your RLS symptoms on your ability to carry out your daily affairs?	0.398	0.757
Item 10: How severe is your mood disturbance from your RLS symptoms?	0.378	0.718
Item 3: Overall, how much relief of your RLS arm or leg discomfort do you get from moving around?	0.159	0.653
Item 5: How severe is your tiredness or sleepiness from your RLS symptoms?	0.562	0.614

a metric for change over time in symptoms. This is not, however, generally recommended for use in clinical research, particularly since it involves only one dimension of RLS severity and is not sensitive to differences in mild to moderate RLS with frequency less than 5 days a week.

Objective evaluations of RLS severity are unfortunately limited to evaluating either the degree of sleep disturbance or the frequency of PLMS or PLMW. As noted in Chapter 46, PLMS correlate poorly with the IRLS or other subjective evaluations of RLS severity, accounting at most for about 25% of the variance and in several studies the correlation was not statistically significant. There are patients with very severe daytime RLS who have few PLMS; nonetheless, PLMS remain the only objective sign of RLS and provide a reasonable objective measure of its severity. Its utility for evaluating treatment response has been noted to be very sensitive for dopaminergic drugs but appears to be less sensitive for the alpha-2-delta drugs. Sleep disturbance, particularly wake time during sleep, also shows a weak correlation with the PLMS and may be more sensitive to the treatment effects of the alpha-2-delta than dopaminergic medications. Thus, these two different objective markers of RLS severity tend to serve somewhat different benefits for treatment evaluations. The PLMS and PLMW have the advantage that leg activity monitors can measure these without the expense of all-night sleep studies.

The Multiple Suggested Immobilization Test (m-SIT) has recently been developed as an improved mixed subjective and objective severity test for RLS. Unlike other subjective assessments, this test involves response to the challenge of remaining still while sitting up in the bed. The test is conducted for 1 hour; a suggested immobilization test (SIT) is repeated four times with a 1-hour rest period in between each SIT. Thus, there are four specific SITs at 16:00, 18:00, 20:00, and 22:00. Each SIT includes measurement of the PLMW during the SIT and the subjective estimate of leg discomfort. This test has seen limited clinical use, but it has the major attraction of a standardized evaluation of RLS under specified conditions designed to elicit RLS symptoms. This is likely to become more accepted as a severity test in future research and clinical studies.

RESTLESS LEGS SYNDROME MEDICAL EVALUATION

The medical evaluation requires a careful medical history to make the diagnosis, meeting all five essential criteria mentioned earlier. In addition, possible secondary causes of RLS and common comorbid conditions should be evaluated and where present become part of the treatment considerations. Generally, however, the clinical neurological evaluation will fail to show any significant abnormality related to the disorder. The only medical test that must be obtained is that for iron status that ideally would be a morning fasting test for serum ferritin, percent transferrin saturation, total iron binding capacity, and iron levels. Low values of the iron measures are common in RLS and impact treatment decisions.

A full diagnostic evaluation requires evaluation to determine the specifiers noted earlier for clinical course and significance. In addition, defining phenotype of age of onset and familiality may help guide management.

SUMMARY

The remarkable successes of studies of the biology of RLS and its genetics have occurred to a large extent because of the clear definition of the disorder provided by the current IRLSSG diagnostic standard. Efforts to change the

diagnosis in any way should be avoided unless some biological factors dictate a need for a change. Similarly the current severity evaluations and the IRLS in particular have sufficed to provide a basis for comparing treatments that have proved clinically useful. Severity evaluation, however, clearly needs more careful consideration and development of better tools. The m-SIT may be a better laboratory test for RLS severity than the all-night polysomnogram, or it may be that these measure somewhat different aspects of RLS. At this point, the all-night sleep study remains a critical feature in evaluating clinical significance of RLS, and the m-SIT may add to this by evaluating the extent of sensory and motor symptoms during the afternoon and evening. Both serve different functions for severity evaluations. At some point it is hoped that a biological marker for the disease process will provide a better measure for diagnosis and severity. But clinical tools that have been developed certainly suffice, with future studies hopefully further refining these and expanding the context in which they can be used.

REFERENCES

1. Willis T. *De Animae Brutorum*. London: Wells and Scott; 1672.
2. Willis T. *The London Practice of Physick*. London: Bassett and Crooke; 1685.
3. Diagnostic Classification Steering Committee, Thorpy M. eds. *The International Classification of Sleep Disorders: Diagnostic and Coding Manual*. Lawrence, KS: Allen Press; 1990.
4. Akpinar S. Treatment of restless legs syndrome with levodopa plus benserazide [letter]. *Arch Neurol*, 1982;39(11):739.
5. Montplaisir J, Lorrain D, Godbout R. Restless legs syndrome and periodic leg movements in sleep: the primary role of dopaminergic mechanism. *Eur Neurol* 1991;31(1):41–3.
6. Allen R, Hening W, Montplaisir J, et al. Restless legs syndrome (RLS) a common disorder rarely diagnosed in Europe or USA: The REST (RLS Epidemiology, Symptoms and Treatment) study in primary care. *Mov Disord* 2002;17:S240.
7. Lavigne GJ, Montplaisir JY. Restless legs syndrome and sleep bruxism: prevalence and association among Canadians. *Sleep* 1994;17(8):739–43.

8. Walters AS, Aldrich MA, Allen RP, et al. Toward a better definition of the restless legs syndrome. *Mov Disord* 1995;10:634–42.

9. Allen RP, Picchietti D, Hening WA, et al. Restless legs syndrome: diagnostic criteria, special considerations, and epidemiology. A report from the restless legs syndrome diagnosis and epidemiology workshop at the National Institutes of Health. *Sleep Med* 2004;4(2):101–19.

10. Bentley AJ, Rosman KD, Mitchell D. Can the sensory symptoms of restless legs syndrome be assessed using a qualitative pain questionnaire? *Clin J Pain* 2007;23(1):62–6.

11. Kerr S, McKinon W, Bentley A. Descriptors of restless legs syndrome sensations. *Sleep Medicine* 2012;13(4):409–13.

12. Hening WA, Allen RP, Washburn M, et al. The four diagnostic criteria for the restless legs syndrome are unable to exclude confounding conditions ("mimics"). *Sleep Med* 2009;10(9):976–81.

13. Allen RP, Dean T, Earley CJ. Effects of rest-duration, time-of-day and their interaction on periodic leg movements while awake in restless legs syndrome. *Sleep Med* 2005;6(5):429–34.

14. Birinyi PV, Allen RP, Lesage S, et al. Investigation into the correlation between sensation and leg movement in restless legs syndrome. *Mov Disord* 2005;20(9):1097–103.

15. Hening WA, Walters AS, Wagner M, et al. Circadian rhythm of motor restlessness and sensory symptoms in the idiopathic restless legs syndrome. *Sleep* 1999;22(7):901–12.

16. Trenkwalder C, Hening WA, Walters AS, et al. Circadian rhythm of periodic limb movements and sensory symptoms of restless legs syndrome. *Mov Disord* 1999;14(1):102–10.

17. Montplaisir J, Boucher S, Poirier G, et al. Clinical, polysomnographic, and genetic characteristics of restless legs syndrome: a study of 133 patients diagnosed with new standard criteria. *Mov Disord* 1997;12(1):61–5.

18. Stiasny-Kolster K, Kohnen R, Moller JC, et al. Validation of the "L-DOPA test" for diagnosis of restless legs syndrome. *Mov Disord* 2006;21(9):1333–9.

19. Hening WA, Washburn T, Somel D, et al. Restless legs patients with a younger age of onset have an increased frequency of affected relatives (abstr). *Neurology* 2003;60:A11.

20. Hening WA, Allen RP, Washburn M, et al. Validation of the Hopkins telephone diagnostic interview for restless legs syndrome. *Sleep Med* 2008;9(3):283–9.

21. Benes H, Kohnen R. Validation of an algorithm for the diagnosis of restless legs syndrome: The Restless Legs Syndrome-Diagnostic Index (RLS-DI). *Sleep Med* 2009;10:515–23.

22. Allen RP, Bharmal M, Calloway M. Prevalence and disease burden of primary restless legs syndrome: results of a general population survey in the United States. *Mov Disord* 2011;26(1):114–20.

23. Allen RP, Burchell BJ, Macdonald B, et al. Validation of the self-completed Cambridge-Hopkins questionnaire (CH-RLSq) for ascertainment of restless legs syndrome (RLS) in a population survey. *Sleep Med* 2009;10(10):1097–100.

24. Ondo W, Jankovic J. Restless legs syndrome: clinicoetiologic correlates. *Neurology* 1996;47(6):1435–41.

25. Allen RP, Earley CJ. (2000). Defining the phenotype of the restless legs syndrome (RLS) using age-of-symptom-onset. *Sleep Med* 2000;1:11–19.

26. Allen RP, La Buda MC, Becker P, et al. Family history study of the restless legs syndrome. *Sleep Med* 2002;3(Suppl):S3–7.

27. Hening W, Allen RP, Thanner S, et al. The Johns Hopkins telephone diagnostic interview for the restless legs syndrome: preliminary investigation for validation in a multi-center patient and control population. *Sleep Med* 2003;4(2):137–41.

28. Mathias RA, Hening W, Washburn M, et al. Segregation analysis of restless legs syndrome: possible evidence for a major gene in a family study using blinded diagnoses. *Hum Hered* 2006;62(3):157–64.

29. Allen RP, Walters AS, Montplaisir J, et al. Restless legs syndrome prevalence and impact: REST general population study. *Arch Intern Med* 2005;165(11):1286–92.

30. Allen RP, Stillman P, Myers AJ. Physician-diagnosed restless legs syndrome in a large sample of primary medical care patients in western Europe: prevalence and characteristics. *Sleep Med* 2010;11(1):31–7.

31. Walters AS, LeBrocq C, Dhar A, et al. Validation of the International Restless Legs Syndrome Study Group rating scale for restless legs syndrome. *Sleep Med* 2003;4(2):121–32.

32. Abetz L, Vallow SM, Kirsch J, et al. Validation of the Restless Legs Syndrome Quality of Life questionnaire. *Value Health* 2005;8(2):157–67.

33. Abetz L, Arbuckle R, Allen RP, et al. The reliability, validity and responsiveness of the International Restless Legs Syndrome Study Group rating scale and subscales in a clinical-trial setting. *Sleep Med* 2006;7(4):340–9.

34. Allen RP, Earley CJ. Validation of the Johns Hopkins restless legs severity scale. *Sleep Med* 2001;2:239–42.

35. Allen RP, Kushida CA, Atkinson MJ. Factor analysis of the International Restless Legs Syndrome Study Group's scale for restless legs severity. *Sleep Med* 2003;4(2):133–135.

46

Restless Legs Syndrome and Periodic Limb Movement Disorder in Children and Adolescents

NARONG SIMAKAJORNBOON, LUNLIYA THAMPRATANKUL,
DENISE SHARON, AND ARTHUR S. WALTERS

RESTLESS LEGS syndrome (RLS) is a senso-rimotor disorder characterized by a strong irresistible urge to move, usually accompanied by a disagreeable sensation in the legs that commonly occurs prior to sleep onset. Periodic limb movements in sleep (PLMS) are characterized by periodic episodes of repetitive and highly stereotypic limb movements during sleep.[1] Periodic limb movement disorder (PLMD) is defined as the presence of periodic limb movement during sleep associated with symptoms of insomnia or excessive daytime sleepiness. Most patients with PLMD do not manifest RLS symptoms; however, approximately 80% of adults with RLS and 63%–74% of children with RLS have PLMS.[2-4] But there is no relation between their sleep status and the amount of PLMS.[2]

Although childhood RLS had been anecdotally mentioned in the literature, the first full case reports of RLS in children were published in pediatric literature in 1994.[5] While careful history revealed that 40% of adults suffering from RLS had the initial onset of symptoms before 20 years of age,[2,6] it was only until very recently that the initial epidemiological study of RLS was reported in children.[7] Based on this particular large-scale survey, it appears that RLS is common in children and adolescents, with moderate to severe RLS symptoms reported in 0.5% of school-aged children and 1% in adolescents in whom there were no significant gender differences.[7] Such figures, if confirmed by additional studies, would indicate that many children and adolescents are affected by RLS.

The etiology of pediatric RLS and PLMD is not well understood. It remains unclear which specific role(s) are played by genetic factors, dopamine dysfunction, and low iron stores in the pathophysiology of RLS and PLMD. There is also a significant proportion of shared comorbidity between attention-deficit/hyperactivity disorder (ADHD) and RLS and PLMD, implying the potential interactions between factors involved in the pathogenesis of ADHD and those underlying the onset and evolution of RLS and PLMD. The diagnosis of RLS in children can be quite challenging due to their inability to verbalize the presence of classic RLS symptoms. The International Restless Legs Study Group has published a set of proposed consensus criteria for reaching the diagnosis of RLS and PLMD in pediatric populations.[8] Although RLS is a clinical diagnosis, supportive evidence, such as presence of PLMS or family history of RLS, may be required in children. The management of RLS and PLMD may involve both nonpharmacologic and pharmacologic approaches. RLS children with evidence of low or even low-normal iron storage may benefit from iron therapy. There is overall limited experience regarding the use of dopaminergic agents in children with RLS and PLMD; other medications, including benzodiazepine, anticonvulsants, alpha-adrenergic, and opioid medications, have not been adequately studied in children. This chapter will emphasize clinical evaluation and management of RLS and PLMD in children.

EPIDEMIOLOGY

RLS is common in the adult population with estimated prevalence of 4%–10%.[8] Approximately 25%–40% of adult patients with RLS reported early onset of symptoms before the age of 20.[2,9] Several studies have evaluated the prevalence of RLS and PLMD in children in various settings. An initial cross-sectional study showed that RLS symptoms were noted in 17% of children aged 2–14 years in general pediatric clinics.[10] Childhood-onset RLS was diagnosed in 5.9% of children referred to pediatric sleep clinics.[3] Crabtree et al. evaluated prepubertal children and found that 8.4% of children who were referred to sleep clinics and 11.9% of children from community survey had PLMD.[11] Another study found PLMS (PLM index >5/hr) in 1.2% of children without comorbidity and 7.1% of children with ADHD who were referred for evaluation of sleep disorders.[12] A large-scale population study has shown that RLS is common in children and adolescents with an estimated prevalence of 1.9% in school-aged children and 2% in adolescents.[7] In addition, children with moderate to severe symptoms of RLS were found in 0.5%–1% of children and adolescents in the same cohort. Another recent study in high school students confirmed the prevalence of 2% in adolescents.[13] There is no significant difference in prevalence of RLS among boys and girls.[7] One study has suggested that PLMD is more common in Caucasian than African American children.[14]

PATHOPHYSIOLOGY

Several etiologies have been proposed to play a role in the pathophysiology of RLS and PLMD, including genetic factors, dopamine dysfunction, and low iron stores (see Chapter 44). This chapter will focus on genetic factors and low iron stores as they are related to RLS and PLMD in children. Many studies have shown the genetic influences in the pathogenesis of RLS and PLMD. Family history is common in patients with RLS and PLMD, especially the early onset.[15,16] In fact, parental history of RLS was found in 50%–80% of children with RLS and PLMD.[7,17,18] Recent studies in adult population have shown a significant association between PLMD and a common variant in an intron of BTBD9 on chromosome 6p21.1, emphasizing the potential for both genetic predisposition and genetic susceptibility to the occurrence of PLMD.[19,20] In addition, the serum ferritin was found to decrease in proportion to the number of mutant alleles of the at-risk variant in the same cohort.[19] Other genetic variants such as the homeobox gene MEIS1 on chromosome 2p and the genes encoding MAP2K5 and the transcription factor LBXCOR1 on chromosome 15q have been reported in adult RLS patients.[20] Interestingly, one study in childhood-onset RLS showed the association with MEIS1 and LBXCOR1, but not with BTBD9.[4] Another recent study demonstrated that carriers of both Parkin mutation and the RLS4 haplotype had an association with early age of onset of RLS, while Parkin mutation or RLS4 haplotype alone did not affect RLS age of onset, indicating the interaction between various gene mutations in modifying RLS age of onset.[21]

There is emerging evidence of the role of iron in the pathophysiology of RLS and PLMD. In children, low iron storage as evidenced by low ferritin, and iron deficiency were found in RLS children.[22,23] Low brain tissue iron concentration may lead to RLS and PLMD through alteration in the dopaminergic system.[24] In fact, iron is the cofactor for tyrosine hydroxylase, the rate-limiting enzyme, which converts tyrosine to dopamine. There is also a significant proportion of shared comorbidity between ADHD and RLS and PLMD, implying the potential interactions between factors involved in the pathogenesis of ADHD and those underlying the onset and evolution of RLS and PLMD. Iron deficiency may be a shared pathophysiologic finding in children with RLS, PLMD, and ADHD.[25] The relationship between RLS/PLMD and ADHD in children is discussed in a subsequent section.

CLINICAL MANIFESTATION

The clinical presentation of RLS and PLMD in children differs from that of the adult population. Children with RLS and PLMD may present with nonspecific symptoms such as growing pains, restless sleep, insomnia, and daytime sleepiness.[6,26] These symptoms may go unnoticed by their parents.[7,26,27] A history of growing pains is noted in 78%–85% of children and adolescents with RLS.[7] Sleep disturbances, including sleep onset and sleep maintenance insomnia, are common presentations in children with RLS and PLMD.[3,27] Young children may have difficulty describing symptoms of RLS and may describe these sensations with nonspecific but age-appropriate terms. Therefore, physicians and health care providers should be familiar with developmentally appropriate terms and descriptions. Some examples of description of sensory complaints in children are "oowies," "boo-boos," "tickle," "legs need to stretch," "ants crawling and aching feeling," "legs hurt and feel funny," "fidgety, restless, too much energy," and "spider in the legs" (see Table 46.1).[7,27] A family history of RLS is common in children with RLS. In fact, a positive family history of RLS is helpful as supportive evidence in making a diagnosis of RLS in children and in raising the possibility of developing RLS over time in children who do not meet criteria for RLS.[27]

Diagnosis

The diagnosis of RLS in children is challenging, particularly because young children may not be able to describe typical RLS symptoms or because these symptoms may not become manifest at very young ages. In fact, pediatrician and general practitioners often misdiagnose RLS in children as growing pain, hyperactivity, ADHD, and behavior problem.[4] The interval between the initial sleep consultation and the diagnosis of definite RLS revolves around 4.4 years.[27] In addition, the period of time elapsing between onset of clinical sleep disturbances and the diagnosis of definite RLS is 11.6 years.[27] RLS is underrecognized and therefore underdiagnosed, even among children whose family members seek medical advice.[7]

The International Restless Legs Syndrome Study Group has developed a set of diagnostic

Table 46.1 Description of Sensory Complaints in Children and Adolescents with Restless Legs Syndrome

"oowies"
"boo-boos"
"tingle"
"twitchy, jerky"
"legs need to stretch"
"ants crawling and aching feeling"
"legs hurt and feel funny"
"fidgety, restless, too much energy"
"spider in the legs"
"sand in toes"
"itchy feeling"
"legs hurt"
"legs feel funny"
"feel like moving"
"need to wiggle"
"legs want to kick"
"runaway legs, tweaky legs"
"crampy, uncomfortable legs"
"legs feeling giggly or jumpy"
"creepy or crawly legs"
"antsy, excited, exploding"

Source: From Picchietti et al. 2007.[7]

criteria for making diagnosis of RLS and PLMD in children.[8] The diagnosis was classified into three categories based on level of certainty, namely definite RLS, probable RLS, and possible RLS (Tables 46.2, 46.3, and 46.4). For clinical purposes, the pediatric RLS criteria should be used for children aged 2 through 12 years old, while for adolescents (>12 years old), the adult diagnostic criteria are considered more appropriate. The definite RLS criteria in children are more rigorous than those in adults with the aim to avoid overdiagnosing RLS in children (see Table 46.2). In addition to the four essential adult criteria, children should be able to describe RLS sensations in their own words. Therefore, adequate language development is essential to diagnose children with RLS. Children younger than 2 years old cannot be diagnosed with definite RLS because of the inability to describe their sensation. Other supportive evidence that can be used as part of the diagnostic criteria include the presence of sleep disturbances for age, a family history of RLS, and a polysomnographic finding of PLMS (PLM index >5/hr). Because the diagnostic criteria for RLS in children are still evolving, the probable and possible RLS categories are intended for research

Table 46.2 Diagnostic Criteria for Definite Restless Legs Syndrome (RLS) in Children

1. The child meets all four essential adult criteria for RLS (the urge to move the legs, is worse during rest, relived by movement and worse during the evening and at night); and
2. The child relates a description in his or her own words that is consistent with leg discomfort. The child may use terms such as "oowies," "tickle," "spiders," "boo-boos," "want to run," and "a lot of energy in my legs" to describe the symptoms. Age-appropriate descriptors are encouraged.

Or

1. The child meets all four essential adult criteria for RLS; and
2. Two of three following supportive criteria are present:
   (a) Sleep disturbance for age
   (b) A biologic parent or sibling has definite RLS
   (c) The child has a polysomnographically documented periodic limb movement index of 5 or more per hour of sleep.

Source: From Allen et al.[8] .

Table 46.3 Diagnostic Criteria for Probable Restless Legs Syndrome (RLS) in Children

1. The child meets all four essential adult criteria for RLS except criterion 4 (the urge to move or sensations are worse in the evening or at night than during the day); and
2. The child has a biologic parent or sibling with definite RLS.

Or

1. The child is observed to have behavior manifestations of lower-extremity discomfort when sitting or lying, accompanied by motor movement of the affected limbs, the discomfort has characteristic of adult criteria 2, 3, and 4 (i.e., is worse during rest and inactivity, relieved by movement, and worse during the evening and at night); and
2. The child has a biologic parent or sibling with definite RLS.

Source: From Allen et al.[8].

Table 46.4 Diagnostic Criteria for Possible Restless Legs Syndrome in Children

1. The child has periodic limb movement disorder; and
2. The child has a biologic parent or sibling with definite RLS, but the child does not meet definite or probable childhood RLS definitions.

Source: Allen et al.[8]

Table 46.5 Diagnostic Criteria for Periodic Limb Movement Disorder in Children

1. Polysomnographic study shows a periodic limb movement index of ≥5 per hour; and
2. Clinical sleep disturbance for age must be evident as manifested by sleep-onset problems, sleep-maintenance problems, or excessive daytime sleepiness; and
3. The leg movements cannot be accounted for by sleep-disordered breathing or medication effect (antidepressant medication).

Source: Allen et al.[8] .

purposes only in children aged 0 through 18 years, with the intent to capture the full spectrum of disease.[8,28] In fact, a recent retrospective study showed that some children with definite RLS had previously met the research criteria for diagnosis of probable or possible RLS.[27] Therefore, probable and possible RLS may be the early manifestation of RLS in children.

The diagnostic criteria for PLMD in children are shown in Table 46.5. Symptoms of sleep disturbance such as sleep onset and sleep maintenance insomnia and daytime sleepiness are required for the diagnosis of PLMD in children. In addition, it is important to exclude limb movements associated with medications or another disorders such as RLS, narcolepsy, or sleep-disordered breathing. Although RLS and PLMD in the adult population are separate entities, the relationship between RLS and PLMD in children is somewhat complex. The presence of PLMS is part of the supportive evidence for diagnosis of RLS in children. In addition, PLMD may be the early presentation of RLS, as many children with definite RLS have been previously diagnosed with PLMD.[27] The differences between adult and pediatric population could be due to normative data of PLMS across ages.[29] The high PLMS index is quite rare in children and adolescents, and therefore it is likely to indicate abnormality in children.[29]

Differential Diagnosis

The differential diagnosis for RLS includes other conditions that produce symptoms mimicking those of RLS. These mimic conditions include those associated with leg pain or leg discomfort such as positional discomfort, sore leg muscles, ligament sprain or tendon strain, arthritis, Osgood-Schlatter, chondromalacia patella, and various types of dermatitis.[8,27,30] Positional discomfort or transient nerve compression can superficially meet all the criteria for RLS. It is usually caused by pressure that compresses nerves and limits blood flow from lying down on one side, sitting on the leg, or crossing the leg. The discomfort is relieved by repositioning without requiring continued movement.[28,30,31] Other conditions such as sore leg muscles, arthritis, ligament or tendon injury, or Osgood-Schlatter are usually worse with movements.[30] Less common mimics in children include nocturnal leg cramp, peripheral neuropathy, radiculopathy, and myopathy.[30] In addition, several medical conditions can be associated with RLS (secondary RLS) such as pregnancy, renal failure, and children receiving dialysis.[32]

PLMS should be differentiated from other conditions such as sleep starts or hypnic jerks, phasic movements during REM sleep, fragmentary myoclonus, and myoclonic epilepsy.[31] Hypnic jerks typically occur at sleep onset or transition from awake to sleep. Phasic movements during REM sleep are normal electromyographic (EMG) activity, which is usually associated with bursts of rapid eye movements. Fragmentary myoclonus is an EMG diagnosis that is characterized by EMG activity that is briefer, variable in duration, and less periodic than PLMS.[31] The movements associated with myoclonic epilepsy are prominent during wakefulness.[28] PLMS can be seen in other sleep disorders such as narcolepsy, REM sleep behavior disorders, and sleep-disordered breathing.

Diagnostic Approach

The diagnostic approach should begin with a thorough and complete clinical history. The characteristic RLS symptoms include the urge to move the legs or unpleasant sensations, which are worse at night and at rest, and are partially or totally relieved by movement.[8] It is important to allow young children to give their own descriptions, not just rely on parental report. In some children, it is helpful to provide them with well-directed questions but to avoid introduction of bias. Examples of directed questions are "Do your legs bother you at night?" "Do your legs bother you at school?" "Do your legs ever hurt or feel funny?"[30] The history of growing pain is common and can be used as a "lead-in" question for a more specific description of RLS.[7] Physicians and pediatricians should be aware of the age-specific vocabulary and try to use the words that children understand.[30] Young children may not understand the word "urge," and they may describe their symptoms as "oowies," "boo-boos," "tickle," "leg pain," "leg hurt," or "funny feeling in the leg"[30] Some children may be able to better describe by drawing symptoms, which may encourage them to talk more about their RLS symptoms.[30]

It is important to ask for the typical topographic distribution of RLS symptoms in taking the history. Although true RLS can exist in almost any part of the body, the typical distribution is in the thighs and calves. The Pediatric RLS Severity Scale has recently been developed to grade severity of RLS in children.[33] On physical examination, certain conditions such as ligament/tendon injury, orthopedic condition, or dermatitis can be excluded. But most children will have normal findings. A complete neurological examination is essential to rule out other causes of leg discomfort, such as neuropathy.

Diagnosis of PLMD requires an overnight polysomnographic study to document PLMS and to exclude coexisting sleep-disordered breathing (Fig. 46.1). Previous study has shown that parental report of excessive leg movements or restless sleep is not a good predictor of PLMS in children.[34] A sleep study documenting PLMS is necessary in children suspected of RLS as supportive evidence when classic RLS symptoms are absent. The presence of periodic limb movements during wakefulness (PLMW) has been shown to be a sensitive and specific tool in evaluating and grading the severity of RLS in adult patients,[35,36] but the data on normal children indicate that PLMW rates are high in children and therefore not likely to have diagnostic value for RLS.[29] Physicians should be aware of

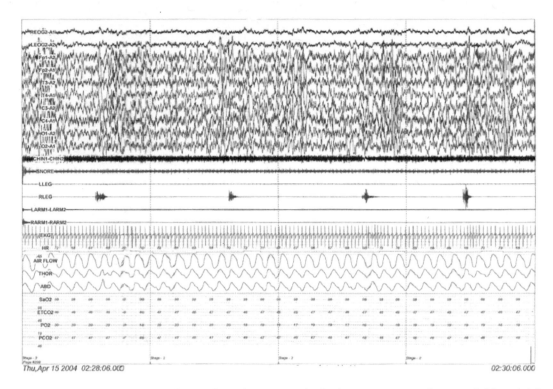

FIGURE 46.1 This 30-second recording shows periodic limb movement in sleep in children with restless legs syndrome and attention-deficit/hyperactivity disorder. There are four periodic bursts of electromyographic activity with 0.5- to 2-second duration and an interval of less than 90 seconds. (*See* color insert.)

random night-to-night variability of PLMS in children.[18] Therefore, children with negative sleep study who have clinical features highly suspicious of RLS and PLMD may warrant a repeated sleep study. The role of other diagnostic tools such as actigraphy remains uncertain. Although several studies have demonstrated that actigraphy is a sensitive and specific measure of PLMS in the adult population,[37–39] it is insufficient in making accurate assessment of PLMS in children.[40] This may be in part because of the high rates of PLMW noted in children,[29] but it also may reflect technical problems that could be corrected in the future. Because most children with RLS and PLMD have evidence of low-normal to low iron stores, it is important to obtain iron profiles, including complete blood count, preferably fasting morning serum measures of iron, ferritin, total iron binding capacity, and percent transferrin saturation. Any children with suspected neuropathy should have additional tests, including thyroid function, fasting blood sugar and insulin, and serum levels of vitamins B6, B9, and B12.[41]

CONSEQUENCES

The relationship between RLS/PLMD and hypertension in the adult population is discussed in other chapters. There are limited data on the cardiovascular consequences in children with RLS and PLMD. One study showed that the onset of leg movements of PLMS was associated with a rapidly occurring cardiac acceleration in children, suggesting evidence of vagal inhibition.[42] A recent study demonstrated the association between PLMS and nocturnal hypertension and higher blood pressure during the day.[43] The mechanism underlying blood pressure changes may be related to autonomic activation in the context of repeated arousals.[44] Dopamine dysfunction may also play a role in pathogenesis of hypertension in RLS and PLMD.[45,46]

Neurocognitive deficits have been reported in adults with RLS.[47,48] Several studies have shown the association between RLS in children and cognitive deficits. In a population study, children reported several adverse cognitive consequences of RLS such as difficulty sitting in the late afternoon or evening, a negative effect on mood, a lack of energy, and an inability to concentrate.[7] Adolescents with RLS have been shown to have poor school performance.[49] Children with RLS are also at risk for depression and anxiety disorder.[7,27] It has been speculated that sleep disruption in children with RLS may lead to neurocognitive deficits and affective disorders. The next section will discuss the association between RLS/PLMD and ADHD in children.

Other common comorbidities of RLS and PLMD in children are the parasomnias, such as confusional arousals, night terrors, sleepwalking, and nightmares. Several studies have shown that there is an increased frequency of parasomnias in children with RLS and PLMD.[26,50] The coexistence of RLS and PLMD and parasomnias and the resolution of parasomnias after treatment of RLS and PLMD suggest that sleep disruption associated with RLS and PLMD may trigger or facilitate the appearance of parasomnias.[51]

RESTLESS LEGS SYNDROME, PERIODIC LIMB MOVEMENT DISORDER, AND ATTENTION-DEFICIT/HYPERACTIVITY DISORDER

ADHD is common in children with a prevalence of 3%–5% in school-aged children.[52,53] Sleep disturbances ranging from insomnia, sleep-disordered breathing, and RLS are common in children with ADHD.[54] Several studies have shown the association between RLS, PLMD, and ADHD. The prevalence of RLS or RLS symptoms in children with ADHD is between 11.5% and 44% with some studies including children who had PLMD.[10,25,50,55,56] On the other hand, the prevalence of ADHD or ADHD symptoms in children with RLS is between 18% and 26%.[3,10,47,56]

The relationship between ADHD and RLS and PLMD is somewhat complex and can be explained by several possibilities.[56] First, sleep disruption associated with RLS and PLMD may lead to inattentiveness and hyperactivity. Second, RLS and PLMD may be a comorbidity of ADHD. Third, RLS and PLMD and a subset of ADHD may share common dopamine dysfunction.[57-60] In fact, improvement and even resolution of ADHD symptoms was noted after dopaminergic therapy in children with ADHD and RLS.[61,62] Fourth, diurnal manifestations of RLS and PLMD may mimic ADHD[56]

complicating the diagnosis and to some extent raising some doubt about the degree of comorbidity. Finally, iron deficiency may be a shared pathophysiologic finding in both children with RLS, PLMD, and ADHD.[25] Iron deficiency has been shown to contribute to the severity of ADHD symptoms in children with coexisting ADHD and RLS.[25]

MANAGEMENT

Nonpharmacologic

Many factors, including medications, sleep deprivation, nicotine, and alcohol, have been shown to precipitate or aggravate RLS and PLMD (Table 46.6).[28,41] Therefore, it is essential to identify and examine ways of avoiding these factors. Several medications, such as selective serotonin reuptake inhibitor (SSRI), metoclopramide, diphenhydramine, and dopamine antagonists, have been shown to aggravate RLS and PLMD.[28,41] Parents should be advised to avoid caffeine in their children. Adolescent patients should avoid smoking and drinking alcohol. Regular sleep routine and good sleep hygiene are essential for the management of RLS in children.[28,41] Sleep hygiene practices that should be encouraged include regular sleep and wake schedule, avoidance of heavy exercise and large meals close to bedtime, and eliminating stimulating activities at night. Regular exercise is beneficial and has been shown to improve RLS symptoms.[63]

Pharmacologic

Currently, there is no FDA-approved medication for RLS and PLMD in children. Although there are emerging literatures supporting medical therapy in children with RLS and PLMD,

Table 46.6 Aggravating Factors for Restless Legs Syndrome

Caffeine
Nicotine
Alcohol
Metoclopramide
SSRI medications
Diphenhydramine
Poor sleep hygiene
Irregular sleep routine

SSRI, selective serotonin reuptake inhibitor.

experience with the use of these medications in children is still limited. The guideline from the Standard of Practice Committee of the American Academy of Sleep Medicine states that no specific recommendations can be made regarding the use of dopaminergic medication in children with RLS or PLMD.[79] A recent population survey has shown that only 6.2% of children and 6.4% of adolescents with definite RLS received ongoing prescription medications. Furthermore, only 1.5% of patients received appropriate and specific medications for RLS treatment.[7]

Iron Treatment

As previously shown, iron deficiency and low iron stores play an important role in the pathophysiology of RLS and PLMD. Several studies have shown the benefit of iron therapy in reducing RLS symptoms in children.[22,23,64,65] Other studies have suggested the benefit of raising serum ferritin above 50 ng/ml.[22,23] The dose of iron therapy is 3 mg of elemental iron per kilogram per day corresponding to the dose used for iron deficiency anemia. Some children may benefit from vitamin C to improve iron absorption. The most common side effect is constipation. Other side effects are dark stool, nausea, and epigastric pain. Iron treatment should be avoided in children with hemolytic anemia and hemochromatosis. The duration of treatment used in our previous study was 3 months followed by slow tapering for a period of 1 year.[23] The preliminary long-term follow-up of these children treated with iron therapy showed sustained clinical improvements 1–2 years after iron therapy, with serum iron and ferritin remaining at adequate levels.[66] Iron therapy seems to produce long-lasting improvement in clinical symptoms and should be considered as the initial option when serum ferritin levels are <50 µg/L or percent transferrin saturation <20%. It is important to periodically check serum iron and ferritin after iron treatment, and adjust iron dose accordingly to reduce the risk of iron overload, particularly in cases of undiagnosed iron management problems, particularly hemochromatosis.

Medications

There is increasing literature on the use of dopaminergic mediations in children. Although ropinirole and pramipexole are FDA-approved medications in adults with RLS and PLMD, there is no approved medication in children. Published case reports show the effectiveness of levodopa,[61] ropinirole,[62] pramipexole,[51] and pergolide [61] in young children and adolescents. The use of dopaminergic medication was associated with clinical improvement of RLS symptoms and reduction of PLM index and associated arousals.[51,61] L-dopa and dopamine agonists resulted in long-term improvements in children with RLS and PLMD.[27,61,78] In children with RLS and ADHD, improvement and even resolution of ADHD symptoms was noted after dopaminergic therapy.[61,62] Although a recent double-blind, placebo-controlled study has demonstrated that L-dopa significantly improved RLS/PLMS, but not ADHD symptoms.[67] In addition, resolution of parasomnias was reported in children with RLS and parosomnias following treatment with dopaminergic medications.[51] One study has shown that clinical efficacy of ropinirole in patients with RLS is not affected by age of onset, suggesting that the early- and late-onset phenotypes of RLS share a common responsiveness to dopamine agonists.[68]

The potential side effects of dopaminergic medications include nasal congestion, nausea, vomiting, insomnia, daytime sleepiness, hallucinations, obsessive-compulsive behavior, and fluid retention.[41] Nausea is common with levodopa, but not with nonergot dopamine agonists. Compulsive behaviors such as impulsive gambling or shopping, although rare, have been reported in association with the use of dopaminergic medications.[69] Serious side effects, such as cardiac value fibrosis, have been reported to be associated with pergolide (an ergot dopamine agonist).[70] Worsening of RLS symptoms after initial improvement should raise the possibility of the phenomenon known as "augmentation." These patients usually manifest earlier symptoms during the day. Augmentation frequently occurs in patients using L-dopa but can occur with any of the dopamine agonists. Augmentation can occur in 70%–80% of patients using daily levodopa and in 15%–40% of those using dopamine agonists.[71-73] The management of augmentation involve reducing dose, withdrawing dopaminergic medication, and switching to another type of medication.[74] One study has suggested that augmentation is associated with low ferritin level.[75] The indications that childhood RLS is associated with low iron and commonly persists into adult life raise the potential for major problems with augmentation when the current standard dopaminergic medications are used as treatment over several years. This needs to be carefully followed in future studies.

Other medications, including benzodiazepines, anticonvulsants, alpha-adrenergic, and opioid medications, have not been adequately studied in children. Clonidine is commonly used for children with sleep-onset problems and can be effective in children with RLS and PLMD.[76] Another benefit of clonidine in RLS children is that it has been shown to improve ADHD symptoms. Clonazepam is commonly used for treatment of RLS and PLMD in children. However, it may aggravate hyperactivity in children with ADHD.[28]

It is important for children with RLS and PLMD to have regular follow-up visits to monitor clinical symptoms, side effects, and to adjust the dose of medication as needed. A wide range of optimal doses for dopaminergic medications has been reported.[28] Children receiving iron therapy should be periodically reassessed for their serum iron, percent transferrin saturation and ferritin, and the dose of iron supplement gradually adjusted to achieve the desired normalization of serum ferritin and iron levels. A repeated sleep study may be needed in children with PLMD who do not respond to iron before starting other medications. Since genetic factors play an important role in RLS and PLMD, parents may be affected and should be referred for further evaluation and treatment.

PROGNOSIS

Currently, there is limited information on the long-term consequences and outcomes associated with RLS and PLMD in children. In adults with early-onset RLS, there is a slow progression of the disease along with long periods of stability. A small percentage of patients can have a period of remission.[6,9,77] In children, the same pattern of slow progression has been reported.[27]

CONCLUSION

RLS and PLMD are common but underrecognized disorders in children and adolescents. Several factors, including genetics, brain dopaminergic dysfunction, and low iron stores, have been shown to play a role in the pathophysiology of RLS and PLMD. There is increasing evidence that RLS and PLMD, if left untreated, may lead to adverse cardiovascular and neurocognitive consequences. The diagnosis of RLS and PLMD in children is challenging, particularly because children may not be able to describe typical RLS symptoms. In addition to clinical description of RLS symptoms, supportive evidence, including the presence of clinical sleep disturbances, documented PLMS from overnight sleep study, and family history of RLS, may be required. The management of RLS and PLMD involves both nonpharmacologic and pharmacologic approaches. The importance of avoidance of aggravating factors and good sleep hygiene cannot be overemphasized. Children with evidence of low iron storage would benefit from iron therapy. While there is overall limited experience regarding the use of dopaminergic agents in children with RLS and PLMD, published reports have indicated the efficacy of compounds such as levodopa, ropinirole, and pramipexole. Other medications, including benzodiazepine, anticonvulsants, alpha-adrenergic and opioid medications, have not been adequately studied in children. Children with RLS and PLMD should have regular follow-up visits to evaluate clinical improvement and to monitor adverse effects of medical therapy. Further research is needed to further evaluate cardiovascular and neurocognitive consequences, to validate diagnostic and severity measures and the role of other diagnostic modalities, to examine iron metabolism, and to assess the long-term effect of iron and pharmacologic therapy in children with RLS and PLMD.

REFERENCES

1. Chesson AL, Jr., Anderson WM, Littner M, et al. Practice parameters for the nonpharmacologic treatment of chronic insomnia. An American academy of sleep medicine report. standards of practice committee of the American academy of sleep medicine. *Sleep* 1999;22(8):1128–33.
2. Montplaisir J, Boucher S, Poirier G, et al. Clinical, polysomnographic, and genetic characteristics of restless legs syndrome: a study of 133 patients diagnosed with new standard criteria. *Mov Disord* 1997;12(1):61–5.
3. Kotagal S, Silber MH. Childhood-onset restless legs syndrome. *Ann Neurol* 2004;56(6):803–7.
4. Muhle H, Neumann A, Lohmann-Hedrich K, et al. Childhood-onset restless legs syndrome: clinical and genetic features of 22 families. *Mov Disord* 2008;23(8): 1113–21; quiz 1203.

5. Walters AS, Picchietti DL, Ehrenberg BL, et al. Restless legs syndrome in childhood and adolescence. *Pediatric Neurol* 1994;11(3): 241–5.

6. Walters AS, Hickey K, Maltzman J, et al. A questionnaire study of 138 patients with restless legs syndrome: the "night-walkers" survey. *Neurology* 1996;46(1):92–5.

7. Picchietti D, Allen RP, Walters AS, et al. Restless legs syndrome: prevalence and impact in children and adolescents—the peds REST study. *Pediatrics* 2007;120(2):253–66.

8. Allen RP, Picchietti D, Hening WA, et al. Restless legs syndrome: diagnostic criteria, special considerations, and epidemiology. A report from the restless legs syndrome diagnosis and epidemiology workshop at the national institutes of health. *Sleep Med* 2003;4(2):101–19.

9. Bassetti CL, Mauerhofer D, Gugger M, et al. Restless legs syndrome: a clinical study of 55 patients. *Eur Neurol* 2001;45(2):67–74.

10. Chervin RD, Archbold KH, Dillon JE, et al. Associations between symptoms of inattention, hyperactivity, restless legs, and periodic leg movements. *Sleep* 2002;25(2):213–18.

11. Crabtree VM, Ivanenko A, O'Brien LM, et al. Periodic limb movement disorder of sleep in children. *J Sleep Res* 2003;12(1):73–81.

12. Kirk VG, Bohn S. Periodic limb movements in children: prevalence in a referred population. *Sleep* 2004;27(2):313–15.

13. Yilmaz K, Kilincaslan A, Aydin N, et al. Prevalence and correlates of restless legs syndrome in adolescents. *Dev Med Child Neurol* 2011;53(1):40–7.

14. O'Brien LM, Holbrook CR, Faye Jones V, et al. Ethnic difference in periodic limb movements in children. *Sleep Med* 2007;8(3):240–6.

15. Hanson M, Honour M, Singleton A, et al. Analysis of familial and sporadic restless legs syndrome in age of onset, gender, and severity features. *J Neurol* 2004;251(11):1398–401.

16. Whittom S, Dauvilliers Y, Pennestri MH, et al. Age-at-one in restless legs syndrome: a clinical and polysomnographic study. *Sleep Med* 2007;9(1):54–9.

17. Picchietti DL, Rajendran RR, Wilson MP, et al. Pediatric restless legs syndrome and periodic limb movement disorder: parent-child pairs. *Sleep Med* 2009;10(8):925–31.

18. Picchietti MA, Picchietti DL, England SJ, et al. Children show individual night-to-night variability of periodic limb movements in sleep. *Sleep* 2009;32(4):530–5.

19. Stefansson H, Rye DB, Hicks A, et al. A genetic risk factor for periodic limb movements in sleep. *N Engl J Med* 2007;357(7):639–47.

20. Winkelmann J, Schormair B, Lichtner P, et al. Genome-wide association study of restless legs syndrome identifies common variants in three genomic regions. *Nat Genet* 2007;39(8):1000–6.

21. Pichler I, Marroni F, Pattaro C, et al. Parkin gene modifies the effect of RLS4 on the age at onset of restless legs syndrome (RLS). *Am J Med Genet B, Neuropsychiatric Genet* 2010;153B(1):350–5.

22. Kryger MH, Otake K, Foerster J. Low body stores of iron and restless legs syndrome: a correctable cause of insomnia in adolescents and teenagers. *Sleep Med* 2002;3(2):127–32.

23. Simakajornboon N, Gozal D, Vlasic V, et al. Periodic limb movements in sleep and iron status in children. *Sleep* 2003;26(6):735–8.

24. Earley CJ, Connor JR, Beard JL, et al. Abnormalities in CSF concentrations of ferritin and transferrin in restless legs syndrome. *Neurology* 2000;54(8):1698–700.

25. Konofal E, Cortese S, Marchand M, et al. Impact of restless legs syndrome and iron deficiency on attention-deficit/hyperactivity disorder in children. *Sleep Med* 2007;8(7–8):711–15.

26. Picchietti DL, Walters AS. Moderate to severe periodic limb movement disorder in childhood and adolescence. *Sleep* 1999;22(3):297–300.

27. Picchietti DL, Stevens HE. Early manifestations of restless legs syndrome in childhood and adolescence. *Sleep Med* 2008;9(7):770–81.

28. Picchietti MA, Picchietti DL. Restless legs syndrome and periodic limb movement disorder in children and adolescents. *Sem Pediatric Neurol* 2008;15(2):91–9.

29. Pennestri MH, Whittom S, Adam B, et al. PLMS and PLMW in healthy subjects as a function of age: prevalence and interval distribution. *Sleep* 2006;29(9):1183–7.

30. Picchietti MA, Picchietti DL. Advances in pediatric restless legs syndrome: iron, genetics, diagnosis and treatment. *Sleep Med* 2010;11(7):643–51.

31. American Academy of Sleep Medicine. Restless leg syndrome and periodic limb movement disorder. In: *The International Classification of Sleep Disorders: Diagnostic and Coding Manual.* 2nd ed. Westchester, IL: American Academy of Sleep Medicine; 2005:178–186.

32. Davis ID, Baron J, O'Riordan MA, et al. Sleep disturbances in pediatric dialysis patients. *Pediatric Nephrol (Berlin)* 2005;20(1):69–75.

33. Arbuckle R, Abetz L, Durmer JS, et al. Development of the pediatric restless legs syndrome severity scale (P-RLS-SS): a patient-reported outcome measure of pediatric RLS symptoms and impact. *Sleep Med* 2010;11(9):897–906.

34. Martin BT, Williamson BD, Edwards N, et al. Parental symptom report and periodic limb movements of sleep in children. *J Clin Sleep Med* 2008;4(1):57–61.

35. Michaud M, Paquet J, Lavigne G, et al. Sleep laboratory diagnosis of restless legs syndrome. *Eur Neurol* 2002;48(2):108–13.

36. Allen RP, Dean T, Earley CJ. Effects of rest-duration, time-of-day and their interaction on periodic leg movements while awake in restless legs syndrome. *Sleep Med* 2005;6(5):429–34.

37. Kazenwadel J, Pollmacher T, Trenkwalder C, et al. New actigraphic assessment method for periodic leg movements (PLM). *Sleep* 1995;18(8):689–97.

38. Morrish E, King MA, Pilsworth SN, et al. Periodic limb movement in a community population detected by a new actigraphy technique. *Sleep Med* 2002;3(6):489–95.

39. King MA, Jaffre MO, Morrish E, et al. The validation of a new actigraphy system for the measurement of periodic leg movements in sleep. *Sleep Med* 2005;6(6):507–13.

40. Montgomery-Downs HE, Crabtree VM, Gozal D. Actigraphic recordings in quantification of periodic leg movements during sleep in children. *Sleep Med* 2005;6(4):325–32.

41. Gamaldo CE, Earley CJ. Restless legs syndrome: a clinical update. *Chest* 2006;130(5):1596–604.

42. Walter LM, Foster AM, Patterson RR, et al. Cardiovascular variability during periodic leg movements in sleep in children. *Sleep* 2009;32(8):1093–9.

43. Wing YK, Zhang J, Ho CK, et al. Periodic limb movement during sleep is associated with nocturnal hypertension in children. *Sleep* 2010;33(6):759–65.

44. Siddiqui F, Strus J, Ming X, et al. Rise of blood pressure with periodic limb movements in sleep and wakefulness. *Clin Neurophysiol* 2007;118(9):1923–30.

45. Hussain T, Lokhandwala MF. Renal dopamine receptors and hypertension. *Exp Biol Med* 2003;228(2):134–42.

46. Walters AS, Bye DB. Review of the relationship of restless legs syndrome an periodic limb movements in sleep to hypertension, heart disease, and stroke. *Sleep* 2009;32(5):589–87.

47. Wagner ML, Walters AS, Fisher BC. Symptoms of attention-deficit/hyperactivity disorder in adults with restless legs syndrome. *Sleep* 2004;27(8):1499–504.

48. Pearson VE, Allen RP, Dean T, et al. Cognitive deficits associated with restless legs syndrome (RLS). *Sleep Med* 2006;7(1):25–30.

49. Pagel JF, Forister N, Kwiatkowki C. Adolescent sleep disturbance and school performance: the confounding variable of socioeconomics. *J Clin Sleep Med* 2007;3(1):19–23.

50. Picchietti DL, England SJ, Walters AS, et al. Periodic limb movement disorder and restless legs syndrome in children with attention-deficit hyperactivity disorder. *J Child Neurol* 1998;13(12):588–94.

51. Guilleminault C, Palombini L, Pelayo R, et al. Sleepwalking and sleep terrors in prepubertal children: what triggers them? *Pediatrics* 2003;111(1):e17–25.

52. Dulcan M. Practice pameters for the assessment and treatment of children, adolescents, and adults with attention-deficit/hyperactivity disorder. *J Am Acad Child Adolesc Psychiatry* 1997;36(10 Suppl):85S–121S.

53. Polanczyk G, de Lima MS, Horta BL, et al. The worldwide prevalence of ADHD: A systematic review and metaregression analysis. *Am J Psychiatry* 2007;164(6):942–8.

54. Konofal E, Lecendreux M, Cortese S. Sleep and ADHD. *Sleep Med* 2010;11(7):652–8.

55. Chervin RD, Dillon JE, Bassetti C, et al. Symptoms of sleep disorders, inattention, and hyperactivity in children. *Sleep* 1997;20(12):1185–92.

56. Cortese S, Konofal E, Lecendreux M, et al. Restless legs syndrome and attention-deficit/hyperactivity disorder: A review of the literature. *Sleep* 2005;28(8):1007–13.

57. Sever Y, Ashkenazi A, Tyano S, et al. Iron treatment in children with attention deficit hyperactivity disorder. A preliminary report. *Neuropsychobiology* 1997;35(4):178–80.

58. Konofal E, Lecendreux M, Arnulf I, et al. Iron deficiency in children with attention-deficit/hyperactivity disorder. *Arch Pediatrics Adolesc Med* 2004;158(12):1113–15.

59. Oner P, Oner O. Relationship of ferritin to symptom ratings children with attention deficit hyperactivity disorder: effect

of comorbidity. *Child Psychiatry Human Dev* 2008;39(3):323–30.

60. Cortese S, Lecendreux M, Bernardina BD, et al. Attention-deficit/hyperactivity disorder, Tourette's syndrome, and restless legs syndrome: the iron hypothesis. *Med Hypotheses* 2008;70(6):1128–32.

61. Walters AS, Mandelbaum DE, Lewin DS, et al. Dopaminergic therapy in children with restless legs/periodic limb movements in sleep and ADHD. dopaminergic therapy study group. *Pediatric Neurol* 2000;22(3):182–6.

62. Konofal E, Arnulf I, Lecendreux M, et al. Ropinirole in a child with attention-deficit hyperactivity disorder and restless legs syndrome. *Pediatric Neurol* 2005;32(5):350–1.

63. Aukerman MM, Aukerman D, Bayard M, et al. Exercise and restless legs syndrome: A randomized controlled trial. *J Am Board Fam Med* 2006;19(5):487–93.

64. Mohri I, Kato-Nishimura K, Tachibana N, et al. Restless legs syndrome (RLS): an unrecognized cause for bedtime problems and insomnia in children. *Sleep Med* 2008;9(6):701–2.

65. Starn AL, Udall JN, Jr. Iron deficiency anemia, pica, and restless legs syndrome in a teenage girl. *Clin Pediatrics* 2008;47(1):83–5.

66. Simakajornboon N, Kheirandish-Gozal L, Gozal D, et al. A long term follow-up study of periodic limb movement disorders in children after iron therapy. Abstract. *Sleep* 2006;29(Suppl):A76.

67. England SJ, Picchietti DL, Couvadelli BV, et al. L-dopa improves restless legs syndrome and periodic limb movements in sleep but not attention-deficit-hyperactivity disorder in a double-blind trial in children. *Sleep Med* 2011;12(5):471–7.

68. Allen RP, Ritchie SY. Clinical efficacy of ropinirole for restless legs syndrome is not affected by age at symptom onset. *Sleep Med* 2008;9(8):899–902.

69. Tippmann-Peikert M, Park JG, Boeve BF, et al. Pathologic gambling in patients with restless legs syndrome treated with dopaminergic agonists. *Neurology* 2007;68(4):301–3.

70. Schade R, Andersohn F, Suissa S, et al. Dopamine agonists and the risk of cardiac-valve regurgitation. *N Engl J Med* 2007;356(1):29–38.

71. Allen RP, Earley CJ. Augmentation of the restless legs syndrome with carbidopa/levodopa. *Sleep* 1996;19(3):205–13.

72. Earley CJ, Allen RP. Pergolide and carbidopa/levodopa treatment of the restless legs syndrome and periodic leg movements in sleep in a consecutive series of patients. *Sleep* 1996;19(10):801–10.

73. Hening WA, Allen RP, Earley CJ, et al. An update on the dopaminergic treatment of restless legs syndrome and periodic limb movement disorder. *Sleep* 2004;27(3):560–83.

74. Silber MH, Ehrenberg BL, Allen RP, et al. An algorithm for the management of restless legs syndrome. *Mayo Clinic Proceedings* 2004;79(7):916–22.

75. Trenkwalder C, Hogl B, Benes H, et al. Augmentation in restless legs syndrome is associated with low ferritin. *Sleep Med* 2008;9(5):572–4.

76. Newcorn JH, Schulz K, Harrison M, et al. Alpha 2 adrenergic agonists. neurochemistry, efficacy, and clinical guidelines for use in children. *Pediatric Clin North Am* 1998;45(5):1099–22, viii.

77. Winkelmann J, Wetter TC, Collado-Seidel V, et al. Clinical characteristics and frequency of the hereditary restless legs syndrome in a population of 300 patients. *Sleep* 2000;23(5):597–602.

78. Martinez S, Guilleminault C. Periodic leg movements in prepubertal children with sleep disturbance. *Dev Med Child Neurol* 2004;46(11):765–70.

79. Littner MR, Kushida C, Anderson WM, et al. Practice parameters for the dopaminergic treatment of restless legs syndrome and periodic limb movement disorder. *Sleep* 2004;27(3):557–9.

47

The Morbidity of Restless Legs Syndrome
Sleep, Cognition, Mental and Physical Health, and Quality of Life

DIEGO GARCIA-BORREGUERO, DESISLAVA TZONOVA,
JANA VÂVROVÂ, LINDSAY BOOTHBY, AND RICHARD P. ALLEN

RESTLESS LEGS syndrome (RLS) is a disorder in which symptoms are observed mainly during wakefulness. However, the sensory symptoms may also occur during sleep and not be recognized except for their effects on sleep, that is, possible microarousals or even full awakenings. Similarly, the motor signs of RLS are expressed both while the patient is awake and resting (periodic limb movements during wakefulness [PLMW]) and during sleep (periodic limb movements during sleep [PLMS]). In both cases, a main consequence of RLS-related sensory and motor features is difficulty both in falling asleep and remaining asleep once sleep is started. The four RLS essential diagnostic criteria,[1] however, indicate symptoms depend not on the sleep state but rather on that of being awake while resting and inactive. Sleep disturbance is thus not part of the RLS diagnostic criteria; rather, it is a main consequence of the disorder. It has been assumed to relate mostly to the RLS symptoms disrupting starting or maintaining sleep, but it is now clear that some treatments can reduce these primary RLS symptoms but not adequately treat the RLS sleep disturbance. Thus, the situation is even more serious than expected from the symptoms. RLS disease itself directly impacts sleep independently of the primary symptoms. In this respect it reflects the severity of the overall disease, and the consequences of the chronic sleep loss is a primary factor contributing to the clinical impact of RLS.[2] Most patients with moderate to severe RLS complain of difficulties initiating and/or maintaining sleep, poor sleep quality, multiple awakenings, and unrefreshing sleep.[3] As a result of impaired sleep, those with RLS often experience daytime fatigue and may feel cognitively impaired, although curiously they are generally not excessively sleepy despite their sleep disruption.[4-6]

RLS morbidity, however, depends not only on the direct or indirect consequences of sleep disturbance but on multiple other factors.[7] Symptom onset during rest has many consequences on a patient's daily functioning, such as

624 •

difficulties concentrating, doing office work, sitting, driving, and so on.[3] More severe RLS is also associated with significant medical and mental health problems that do not have an obvious relation to the primary symptoms but like the profound sleep loss may relate more to aspects of the underlying RLS biology other than those producing the primary symptoms. This chapter describes the recognized major morbidities of RLS starting with the most obvious and possibly the most significant RLS morbidity of sleep disturbance.

SUBJECTIVE SLEEP DISTURBANCE

As already described, RLS effects peak in severity at night and often lead to chronic sleep loss. Depending on the time of night at which they occur, RLS effects interfere with the initiation and/or maintenance of sleep. RLS causes sleep fragmentation, prevents the patient from falling back to sleep, and leads to unrefreshing sleep. The degree of sleep disturbance experienced depends on disease severity, but chronic profound sleep loss occurs for even moderately severe RLS.[8]

Sleep disturbance in RLS has been evaluated in numerous large epidemiological studies. The REST study interviewed 16,202 adults (18 years of age and over) in five countries using accepted diagnostic questions to determine the presence, frequency, and severity of RLS symptoms; 61% reported disturbed sleep, 48% difficulties initiating sleep, and 39% difficulties maintaining sleep. A sleep-related symptom was reported in 38% of respondents as the most troublesome symptom.[9]

In another large survey performed in a primary care population ($n=23,052$), 88.4% of RLS patients reported at least one sleep-related symptom.[3] Other large multinational studies performed in Western countries[8,10,11] also found sleep disturbance to be among the most prevalent, if not the most severe, symptom of the disease. Moderately severe RLS patients report chronic persistent sleep durations of on average only 5.5 hours a night.[8] This degree of chronic sleep loss puts them at risk for medical problems and difficulties maintaining full alertness during the day.

Despite the significant chronic sleep loss, moderately severe RLS patients rarely report problems with excessive daytime sleepiness. Untreated RLS patients without other sleep problems report very short sleep durations but generally show Epworth Sleepiness Scale (ESS) scores of about five to eight, which are within the normal range.[12] A minority show Epworth scores above the customary normal value of ten,[12] but not the very high scores normally associated with their degree of profound sleep loss. Thus, healthy subjects in one study who did not have a sleep disorder but who had behaviorally or socially induced chronic sleep loss reported on average 5.5 hours of sleep,[13] matching that of moderately severe RLS and an average ESS of 13.6, considerably greater than for RLS. The lowest ESS for these healthy short sleepers was seven, which is about the average score for moderate to severe RLS patients who have equal or less sleep.[8] Moreover, 22% of these healthy chronic sleep-loss subjects reported sleepiness-related car accidents. In contrast, neither falling asleep while driving due to sleepiness nor increased risk of car accidents has been a finding in any of the clinical studies with untreated RLS subjects who have no other sleep disorders (e.g., sleep apnea).

Therefore, it seems likely that RLS patients suffer from some hyperarousal process maintaining wakefulness despite chronic sleep loss. This hyperarousal process could bring increased waking into the sleep period contributing to the short sleep times and sleep disturbance of RLS patients. It may also produce problems with maintained attention, fatigue, or disruption of cognitive brain functioning. These possible RLS morbidities have generally been ignored and not evaluated.

PHYSIOLOGICAL SLEEP DISTURBANCE

Sleep Architecture in Untreated Restless Legs Syndrome

In addition to evidence provided by epidemiological studies using subjective reports of RLS symptoms, a number of polysomnographic (PSG) studies have investigated the presence of objective abnormalities during sleep. Most studies included patients with moderate to severe RLS and found reduced total sleep time, sleep efficiency, increased wake after sleep onset time, number of awakenings, and a high arousal index.[14-18] Furthermore, most studies showed reduced non–rapid eye movement (non-REM) sleep, particularly Stage 2 time, while only a few studies with more severe patients reported increased Stage 1 time. REM sleep in particular appears not to be significantly altered in RLS, except when the disease is so severe that there is little total sleep time to allow normal expression of REM. In line with the common complaint of sleep-onset insomnia reported in epidemiological studies, a few studies generally with more severe RLS also found increased sleep latency.

A cyclic variation in central nervous system arousability, described as a cyclic alternating pattern (CAP),[19] has been found to be very disrupted in RLS, indicating disruption of the microstructure that appears to be important for sustaining sleep. This is not corrected by acute standard dopaminergic treatment with pramipexole.[20] CAP abnormality could account, at least in part, for the abnormal amount of electroencephalographic (EEG) and autonomic arousals and also the periodic limb movements in RLS.[21]

Periodic Limb Movements during Sleep

Sleep parameters reflecting motor dysfunction during sleep, such as the periodic limb movement (PLMS) per hour of sleep (PLMS/hr), PLMS arousal per hour of sleep (PLMA/hr), and sleep fragmentation indices are markedly elevated in RLS compared to controls (24–25).[14–18]

However, up to 12% of RLS patients show normal PLMS/hr after two consecutive PSG studies.[22] This might partially reflect the high day-to-day variability in PLM indices in RLS.[23,24] The use of leg actigraphy offers the advantage over a PSG of a simple measurement, which can easily be obtained over several nights.[25] One study using leg-activity meters found that it required averaging over five nights to reach a stable metric of PLMS/hr for a single RLS patient.[26]

PLMS are rhythmic leg and foot movements usually with at least extension of the big toe and dorsiflexion of the ankle. Flexion at the knee and hip may also occur, and many movements involve more complicated leg and foot movements. PLMS are only scored as such if they are part of four or more consecutive movements lasting 0.5 to 10 seconds with an inter-movement interval of 4 to 90 seconds.[27] PLMS can occur during sleep but also during relaxed wakefulness.[28] During sleep, PLMS are often associated with EEG signs of arousals and/or with autonomic arousals and as noted earlier are related to CAP and the microstructure of

sleep.[28,29] PLMS are described in more detail in Chapter 51.

PLMS arousals per hour of sleep (PLMSA/hr) in RLS typically decline progressively over the night (see Fig. 47.1). These variations over time occur for almost all RLS subjects regardless of the overall PLMS rate, microarousal occurrence, or slow-wave activity. This reflects the diagnostic circadian feature of RLS with disease expression more severe in the evening and night than in the early morning. Thus, the sleep disturbance itself is often more pronounced in the first than the last part of sleep period.

PLMS are not specific to RLS. They also occur in a wide range of disorders related to dopamine abnormalities, such as narcolepsy, rapid eye movement behavior disorder, and Parkinson's disease. PLMS are also often present in sleep apnea syndrome, in spinal cord lesions, and of course most healthy older individuals.[30]

The clinical significance of PLMS is uncertain. A high rate of PLMS/hr is associated with sleep fragmentation and is frequently associated with severe sensory symptoms and sleep disturbance,[31] but beside these extremes there is generally a weak, if any, significant correlation between the PLMS/hr and either the sleep disturbance or the severity of RLS.[31] PLMS have been associated with transient heart-rate and blood pressure increases with each movement. These transient changes in heart rate and blood pressure might relate to the increased risk for cardiovascular disease in RLS, but this putative association has not yet been confirmed.[23,32–34]

The PLMS themselves are also a clinical problem, particularly when disturbing bed partners even more than the RLS sufferer. The sleep disruption of bed partners, therefore, should be considered as one of the morbidities of RLS. Overall, PLMS provide a useful motor sign of RLS by objectively marking the severity of the disorder, but, except in extremis, do not clearly relate to other RLS morbidities, except possibly cardiovascular health.

COGNITIVE DYSFUNCTION

As already described, RLS symptoms often lead to chronic sleep loss. Sleep deprivation decreases cognitive function, particularly for tasks involving activation of the prefrontal lobes.[35] Studies found that RLS patients compared to controls[4] showed significant deficits in these same cognitive tests most affected by sleep loss. Thus, these RLS patients not reporting significant

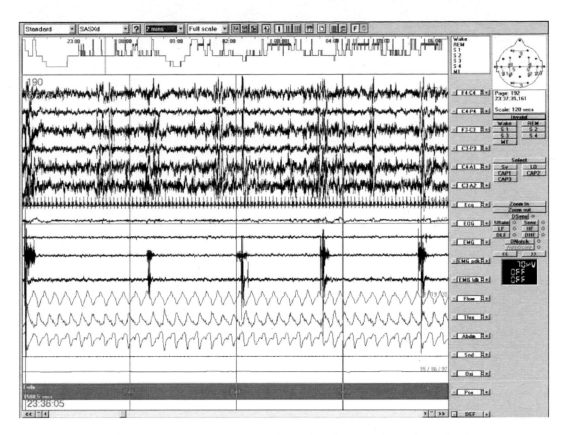

FIGURE 47.1 Polysomnogram of patients with restless legs syndrome/periodic leg movements during sleep. Duration of the hypnogram is 2 minutes. From the top to bottom: hypnogram (blue), EEG (six black leads), ECG (purple), EOG (two black leads), EMG (two black leads), with periodic leg movements. (*See* color insert.)

daytime sleepiness[36] despite significant chronic sleep loss still perform worse on cognitive tasks sensitive to sleep loss when compared to normal non-sleep-restricted subjects. However, in a study by Gamaldo et al.,[37] RLS patients performed statistically better on tasks sensitive to sleep loss than did controls, with experimental sleep restriction matching the sleep loss of the RLS patients. The authors suggested that the hyperarousal in RLS patients appears to reduce but not totally eliminate the expected cognitive impairment caused by chronic sleep loss.

MENTAL HEALTH

Depression

Several population-based studies[38–40] and those with patients presenting to medical clinics[41–43] provide information about the frequency of the symptoms of depression in adults with RLS. Each study suggests that the symptoms of depression are more common among adults with RLS than those without the disease. In their review, Picchietti et al.[44] suggested that the association between RLS and depression is likely complex: either RLS causes depression, depression causes RLS, or a third factor, possibly a shared biological abnormality, causes both RLS and depression.

Epidemiologic studies have demonstrated that insomnia and fatigue are risk factors for major depression.[45–47] In this way, sleep disruption, pain, and social isolation caused by RLS would be the mediating factors in producing depression.[48,49] Conversely, the sleep disruption caused by depression may exacerbate RLS sleep disturbance by intensifying the clinical impact of RLS. Finally, the treatment of depression with selective serotonin reuptake inhibitor or serotonin–norepinephrine reuptake inhibitor antidepressants can worsen RLS and PLMS.[50-52]

The association between RLS and depression could also be an artifact resulting from the many shared symptoms. Four of the DSM-IV criteria for major depression, "insomnia or hypersomnia," "fatigue/loss-of-energy," "diminished concentration," and "psychomotor retardation or agitation," are also experienced with RLS.[53] According to the DSM-IV, a diagnosis of major depression may be made if the patient meets only five out of nine possible criteria. Thus, patients with RLS may experience enough of the shared symptoms to easily exceed an abnormal score on a depression questionnaire, even in the absence of a major depressive episode. Although RLS patients could achieve high scores on depression scales, it seems as if somatic items (particularly those related to sleep disturbance) are the cause of their overall results.[15] In addition, a recent study found no evidence for cognitive dysfunction or depression in elderly patients with mild RLS.[54] Overall, however, regardless of cause, depression appears to be a common comorbidity of more severe RLS and certainly a major consideration for RLS treatment.

Anxiety Disorders

Less attention has been paid to the increased risk for anxiety disorders in RLS, but when evaluated they appear to be more closely associated with RLS than depression. One population-based study of untreated RLS patients used the research diagnostic interview schedule to diagnose major mental disorders according to the DSM-IV criteria. The trained lay interviewer also used seven basic questions to determine concurrent RLS symptoms. In this study, depression, general anxiety disorder, obsessive-compulsive disorder, and panic disorder were 2 to 5.6 times more frequent in RLS patients than in controls. In a prior study, patients in a German movement disorders clinic who had been clinically diagnosed with RLS were compared to controls from a community survey of the German general population. DSM-IV criteria for depression and anxiety disorders were both determined using a structured interview. The odds ratios (95% confidence interval) were as follows: depression, 2.6 (1.5–4.4); generalized anxiety disorder, 3.7 (1.8–7.4); and panic disorder, 5.2 (2.4–11.3).[43] In this last study RLS developed prior to the mental illness for most patients, and more RLS patients than controls

attributed these mental health problems to a medical disease mostly to RLS itself.

The striking features of these two well-done studies is not only the high rate of these mental illnesses in RLS patients but also that the increased risk for anxiety disorders was greater than for depression in both the general and clinical population of RLS. The much higher risk of panic disorder, and possibly obsessive-compulsive disorder, deserves special attention given the data indicating striatal dopamine abnormalities in RLS.[55,56]

Unlike depression, anxiety disorders and panic disorder in particular are not seen as resulting from sleep disturbance or any of the other clinical features of RLS. These may, therefore, reflect some shared common biological relationship. The increased risk for anxiety disorders in patients with RLS should be considered in treatment evaluations.

PHYSICAL HEALTH

A number of large studies have associated the presence of a strong and positive association between cardiovascular disease (CVD) and RLS.[57] Out of 15 large population-based studies that provided information on the association of RLS to CVD, the prevalence of RLS in adults reporting CVD was almost three-fold the prevalence observed in the general population without CVD.[49,58-61] Furthermore, a dose–response relationship between severity/frequency of RLS symptoms and CVD events was reported in two other studies.[57,60] However, due to the cross-sectional nature of these studies, any causal inferences are problematic. In addition, definitions of heart disease and RLS varied across studies, as did inclusion criteria. Yet despite study heterogeneity, these findings are remarkably consistent and robust. They show a positive association between RLS and CVD that persists after adjustment for multiple confounders (e.g., age, gender, body mass index [BMI], lifestyle factors, and other sleep disorders).[34] In contrast, in two large prospective studies of female and male health professionals, there was no evidence of an increased risk of any incident CVD in RLS patients.[62]

The relationship of hypertension and RLS seems less clear, although most (10 out of 17) studies have shown a positive association that persists after adjustment for BMI, smoking, and sleep disorders. Nevertheless, variations in population characteristics, definitions of both conditions, and the confounding effects of some antihypertensives (i.e., clonidine), which might help alleviate RLS, could have played a role in these results.[38,57,59,60,63,64] Particularly significant is the lack of any indication for the increased risk of stroke in RLS that would certainly be expected if there were a significant increase in blood pressure. Thus, at this point it seems doubtful there is any relation between high blood pressure and RLS.

Additionally, most but not all of the cross-sectional studies reviewed suggest a positive relationship between RLS and diabetes, which remained robust even after controlling for age, sex, BMI, smoking, or neuropathy. Furthermore, two out of three studies support an association between nondiabetic RLS and impaired glucose tolerance.[61,65,66] This may reflect the well-established relation between sleep loss and diabetes. Weaker evidence shows a modest association between RLS and BMI[67] and with dyslipidemia.[68,69]

QUALITY OF LIFE

Given the specific morbidities described earlier, it is hardly surprising to find that RLS has a significant negative impact on quality of life. All studies that have compared untreated RLS patients to matched or population controls have reported significantly worse quality of life for RLS. Moreover, this relates to the severity of the disease (see Fig. 47.2).[8,70] Given the severity of the RLS morbidities, it should also not have been surprising to find that RLS patients showed the same degree of impairment of quality of life as patients with other major chronic medical conditions, that is, type II diabetes, depression, arthritis, hypertension, angina, and history of myocardial infarction.[71] What is somewhat surprising is the discovery that despite the highly significant relation between RLS and depression and anxiety, the RLS quality of life is more impaired in physical than mental health domains. Role physical and vitality are the most impacted by RLS with role emotional and mental health showing impact only for the more severe cases (see Fig. 47.2).

This gives a picture of the continuum of RLS impact by its severity. When mild, it impacts mostly vitality and physical limitations on functioning with little impact on mental health, but as it becomes more severe mental health components also become a major feature of the disorder. It should be noted, however, that the SF36 mental health–related scales focus more on depressive than anxiety-related symptoms, so it is less clear whether the anxiety-related features of RLS will also, like depression, be evident mostly for the more severe cases.

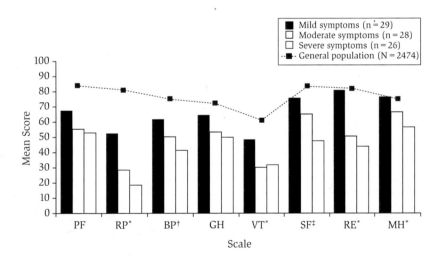

FIGURE 47.2 SF-36 scale scores for the restless legs syndrome group by patients' self-reported symptom severity (based on the overall score of the patient version of the International Restless Legs Scale). BP, bodily pain; GH, general health; MH, mental health; PF, physical functioning; RE, role limitations due to emotional problems; RP, role limitations due to physical problems; SF, social functioning; SF-36, Medical Outcomes Study 36-Item Short Form health survey; VT, vitality. Sample sizes varied by scale; however, sample sizes for each group always exceeded 25;* $p < .01$; $p < .05$; $p < .001$.

CONCLUSION: MORBIDITY SIGNIFICANCE AND RESTLESS LEGS SYNDROME TREATMENTS

The major morbidities of RLS are impressive both for the frequency with which they occur with RLS and the severe impact they have on the health and quality of life of the RLS patient. Viewing these, it is hard to dismiss RLS as a trivial disease of limited consequence. RLS, while not lethal, is indeed the thief of sleep, vitality, full physical functioning, mental health, and possibly physical health.

These morbidities also impact RLS treatment. The pharmacological treatments of RLS are discussed in Chapter 50, but it deserves note here that the treatments need to be adjusted to handle not only the primary RLS symptoms but also these RLS morbidities. *Reducing the RLS symptoms appears not to suffice for treating all of the morbidity of RLS.* Treatments that are equally effective in reducing the primary RLS symptoms have differing degrees of benefits for these morbidities of RLS. For example, dopaminergic treatments generally reduce PLMS more than any other, and to the extent these disturb the patient or the patient's bed partner or relate to development of cardiovascular disease, these treatments should be considered first. But dopaminergic treatment, despite dramatically reducing PLMS, fails to significantly reduce the RLS sleep disturbance. The dopamine agonists also provide some benefit for depression but may exacerbate any anxiety-related compulsive/impulsive behaviors. The alpha-2-delta anticonvulsants (gabapentin enacarbil, pregabalin, and gabapentin) provide particularly good relief for sleep disturbance more than any other treatment, but they also may exacerbate depression and have limited benefit for reducing PLMS. Thus, treatments should be tailored to deal with the differing morbidities of each RLS patient, and it may be important to consider combination treatments for many patients in order to reduce these very significant morbidities of RLS.

The major issue of the significance of the cardiovascular health risk for RLS patients remains uncertain. The possible impact of treatment for reducing this risk is even less clear given the lack of a clear mechanism accounting for the RLS relation. If the increased risk of cardiovascular disease is found to relate to effects of PLMS on blood pressure and heart rate, then the dopaminergic treatments may be more important. If, however, the sleep loss is the primary factor, then the alpha-2-delta drugs would be more important. It may be neither of these and instead some consequence of the hypoxic pathway activation or the iron metabolic disturbance that appears to be common in RLS. Hopefully, future studies will provide better guidance, but for now combination treatments addressing the recognized morbidities as well as symptoms of RLS may deserve more consideration than they currently receive.

REFERENCES

1. Allen RP, Picchietti D, Hening WA, et al. Restless legs syndrome: diagnostic criteria, special considerations, and epidemiology. A report from the restless legs syndrome diagnosis and epidemiology workshop at the National Institutes of Health. *Sleep Med* 2003;4(2):101–19.
2. Kushida CA, Allen RP, Atkinson MJ. Modeling the causal relationships between symptoms associated with restless legs syndrome and the patient-reported impact of RLS. *Sleep Med* 2004;5(5):485–8.
3. Hening W, Walters AS, Allen RP, et al. Impact, diagnosis and treatment of restless legs syndrome (RLS) in a primary care population: the REST (RLS epidemiology, symptoms, and treatment) primary care study. *Sleep Med* 2004;5(3): 237–46.
4. Pearson VE, Allen RP, Dean T, et al. Cognitive deficits associated with restless legs syndrome (RLS). *Sleep Med* 2006;7(1):25–30.
5. Gamaldo CE, Benbrook AR, Allen RP, et al. (2008). A further evaluation of the cognitive deficits associated with restless legs syndrome (RLS). *Sleep Med* 2008;9(5):500–5.
6. Calloway M, Bharmal M, Hill-Zabala C, et al. Development and validation of a subjective post sleep diary (SPSD) to assess sleep status in subjects with restless legs syndrome. *Sleep Med* 2011;12(7): 704–10.
7. Jung KY, Koo YS, Kim BJ, et al. Electrophysiologic disturbances during daytime in patients with restless legs syndrome: further evidence of cognitive dysfunction? *Sleep Med* 2011;12(4):416–21.
8. Allen RP, Stillman P, Myers AJ. Physician-diagnosed restless legs syndrome in a large sample of primary medical care patients in western

Europe: prevalence and characteristics. *Sleep Med* 2010;11(1):31–7.

9. Allen RP, Walters AS, Montplaisir J, et al. Restless legs syndrome prevalence and impact: REST general population study. *Arch Intern Med* 2010;165(11):1286–92.

10. McCrink L, Allen RP, Wolowacz S, et al. Predictors of health-related quality of life in sufferers with restless legs syndrome: a multi-national study. *Sleep Med* 2007;8(1):73–83.

11. Allen RP, Bharmal M, Calloway M. Prevalence and disease burden of primary restless legs syndrome: results of a general population survey in the United States. *Mov Disord* 2010;26(1):114–20.

12. Holmes R, Tluk S, Metta V, et al. Nature and variants of idiopathic restless legs syndrome: observations from 152 patients referred to secondary care in the UK. *J Neural Transm* 2007;114(7): 924–34.

13. Komada Y, Inoue Y, Hayashida K, et al. Clinical significance and correlates of behaviorally induced insufficient sleep syndrome. *Sleep Med* 2008;9(8):851–6.

14. Saletu M, Anderer P, Saletu B, et al. EEG mapping in patients with restless legs syndrome as compared with normal controls. *Psychiatry Res* 2002;115(1–2):49–61.

15. Hornyak M, Kopasz M, Berger M, et al. Impact of sleep-related complaints on depressive symptoms in patients with restless legs syndrome. *J Clin Psychiatry* 2005;66(9):1139–45.

16. Hornyak M, Feige B, Voderholzer U, et al. Polysomnography findings in patients with restless legs syndrome and in healthy controls: a comparative observational study. *Sleep* 2007;30(7):861–5.

17. Boehm G, Wetter TC, Trenkwalder C. Periodic leg movements in RLS patients as compared to controls: are there differences beyond the PLM index? *Sleep Med* 2009;10(5): 566–71.

18. Schilling C, Schredl M, Strobl P, et al. Restless legs syndrome: evidence for nocturnal hypothalamic-pituitary-adrenal system activation. *Mov Disord* 2010;25(8):1047–52.

19. Parrino L, Ferri R, Bruni O, et al. Cyclic alternating pattern (CAP): the marker of sleep instability. *Sleep Med Rev* 2012;16(1):27–45.

20. Ferri R, Manconi M, Aricò D, et al. Acute dopamine-agonist treatment in restless legs syndrome: effects on sleep architecture and NREM sleep instability. *Sleep* 2010;33(6):793–800.

21. Droste DW, Krauss JK, Hagedorn G, et al. Periodic leg movements are part of the B-wave rhythm and the cyclic alternating pattern. *Acta Neurol Scand* 1996;94(5):347–52.

22. Montplaisir J, Boucher S, Poirier G, et al. Clinical, polysomnographic, and genetic characteristics of restless legs syndrome: a study of 133 patients diagnosed with new standard criteria. *Mov Disord* 1997;12(1):61–5.

23. Sforza E, Pichot V, Barthelemy JC, et al. Cardiovascular variability during periodic leg movements: a spectral analysis approach. *Clin Neurophysiol* 2005;116(5):1096–104.

24. Haba-Rubio J, Sforza E. Test-to-test variability in motor activity during the suggested immobilization test in restless legs patients. *Sleep Med* 2006;7(7):561–6.

25. Allen RP. Improving RLS diagnosis and severity assessment: polysomnography, actigraphy and RLS-sleep log. *Sleep Med* 2007;8(Suppl 2):S13–18.

26. Trotti LM, Bliwise DL, Greer SA, et al. Correlates of PLMs variability over multiple nights and impact upon RLS diagnosis. *Sleep Med* 2009;10(6):668–71.

27. Zucconi M, Ferri R, Allen R, et al. The official World Association of Sleep Medicine (WASM) standards for recording and scoring periodic leg movements in sleep (PLMS) and wakefulness (PLMW) developed in collaboration with a task force from the International Restless Legs Syndrome Study Group (IRLSSG). *Sleep Med* 2006;7(2):175–83.

28. Ferri R, Manconi M, Plazzi G, et al. Leg movements during wakefulness in restless legs syndrome: time structure and relationships with periodic leg movements during sleep. *Sleep Med* 2012;13(5): 529–35.

29. Ferri R, Zucconi M. Heart rate and spectral EEG changes accompanying periodic and isolated leg movements during sleep. *Sleep* 2008;31(1):16–17; discussion 18–19.

30. Ferri R, Zucconi M, Manconi M, et al. Different periodicity and time structure of leg movements during sleep in narcolepsy/cataplexy and restless legs syndrome. *Sleep* 2006;29(12):1587–94.

31. Garcia-Borreguero D, Larrosa O, de la Llave Y, et al. Correlation between rating scales and sleep laboratory measurements in restless legs syndrome. *Sleep Med* 2004;5(6): 561–5.

32. Pennestri MH, Montplaisir J, Colombo R, et al. Nocturnal blood pressure changes in patients with restless legs syndrome. *Neurology* 2007;68(15):1213–18.

33. Walters AS, Rye DB. Evidence continues to mount on the relationship of restless legs syndrome/periodic limb movements in sleep to hypertension, cardiovascular disease, and stroke. *Sleep* 2010;33(3): 287.

34. Innes KE, Selfe TK, Agarwal P. Restless legs syndrome and conditions associated with metabolic dysregulation, sympathoadrenal dysfunction, and cardiovascular disease risk: a systematic review. *Sleep Med Rev* 2011;16(4):309–39.

35. Van Dongen HP, Baynard MD, Maislin G, et al. Systematic interindividual differences in neurobehavioral impairment from sleep loss: evidence of trait-like differential vulnerability. *Sleep* 2004;27(3):423–33.

36. Allen RP, Earley CJ. Restless legs syndrome: a review of clinical and pathophysiologic features. *J Clin Neurophysiol* 2001;18(2): 128–47.

37. Gamaldo C, Benbrook AR, Allen RP, et al. Evaluating daytime alertness in individuals with restless legs syndrome (RLS) compared to sleep restricted controls. *Sleep Med* 2009;10(1):134–8.

38. Ulfberg J, Nystrom B, Carter N, et al. Prevalence of restless legs syndrome among men aged 18 to 64 years: an association with somatic disease and neuropsychiatric symptoms. *Mov Disord* 2001;16(6):1159–63.

39. Sukegawa T, Itoga M, Seno H, et al. Sleep disturbances and depression in the elderly in Japan. *Psychiatry Clin Neurosci* 2003;57(3):265–70.

40. Sevim S, Dogu O, Kaleagasi H, et al. Correlation of anxiety and depression symptoms in patients with restless legs syndrome: a population based survey. *J Neurol Neurosurg Psychiatry* 2004;75(2): 226–30.

41. Bassetti CL, Mauerhofer D, Gugger M, et al. Restless legs syndrome: a clinical study of 55 patients. *Eur Neurol* 2001;45(2):67–74.

42. Vandeputte M, de Weerd A. Sleep disorders and depressive feelings: a global survey with the Beck depression scale. *Sleep Med* 2003;4(4):343–5.

43. Winkelmann J, Prager M, Lieb R, et al. (2005). Anxietas tibiarum. Depression and anxiety disorders in patients with restless legs syndrome. *J Neurol* 2005;252(1):67–71.

44. Picchietti D, Winkelman JW. Restless legs syndrome, periodic limb movements in sleep, and depression. *Sleep* 2005;28(7):891–8.

45. Breslau N, Roth T, Rosenthal L, et al. Sleep disturbance and psychiatric disorders: a longitudinal epidemiological study of young adults. *Biol Psychiatry* 1996;39(6):411–18.

46. Chang PP, Ford DE, Mead LA, et al. Insomnia in young men and subsequent depression. The Johns Hopkins Precursors Study. *Am J Epidemiol* 1997;146(2):105–14.

47. Addington AM, Gallo JJ, Ford DE, et al. Epidemiology of unexplained fatigue and major depression in the community: the Baltimore ECA follow-up, 1981–94. *Psychol Med* 2001;31(6):1037–44.

48. Bruce ML. Psychosocial risk factors for depressive disorders in late life. *Biol Psychiatry* 2002;52(3):175–84.

49. Ohayon MM, Schatzberg AF. Using chronic pain to predict depressive morbidity in the general population. *Arch Gen Psychiatry* 2003;60(1):39–47.

50. Damsa C, Bumb A, Bianchi-Demicheli F, et al. (2004). Dopamine-dependent side effects of selective serotonin reuptake inhibitors: a clinical review. *J Clin Psychiatry* 2004;65(8):1064–8.

51. Page RL, II, Ruscin JM, Bainbridge JL, et al. Restless legs syndrome induced by escitalopram: case report and review of the literature. *Pharmacotherapy* 2008;28(2):271–80.

52. Khalid I, Rana L, Khalid TJ, et al. Refractory restless legs syndrome likely caused by olanzapine. *J Clin Sleep Med* 2009;5(1):68–9.

53. American Psychiatric Association, American Psychiatric Association Task Force on DSM-IV. *Diagnostic and Statistical Manual of Mental Disorders*. Washington, DC, American Psychiatric Association; 2000.

54. Driver-Dunckley E, Connor D, Hentz J, et al. No evidence for cognitive dysfunction or depression in patients with mild restless legs syndrome. *Mov Disord* 2009;24(12):1840–2.

55. Connor JC, Boyer PJ, Menzies SL, et al. Neuropathological examination suggests impaired brain iron acquisition in restless legs syndrome. *Neurology* 2003;61(3):304–9.

56. Earley CJ, Kuwabara H, Wong DF, et al. The dopamine transporter is decreased in the striatum of subjects with restless legs syndrome. *Sleep* 2011;34(3):341–7.

57. Winkelman JW, Finn L, Young T. Prevalence and correlates of restless legs syndrome symptoms in the Wisconsin Sleep Cohort. *Sleep Med* 2006;7(7):545–52.

58. Berger K, Luedemann J, Trenkwalder C, et al. Sex and the risk of restless legs syndrome in the general population. *Arch Intern Med* 2004;164(2):196–202.

59. Wesstrom J, Nilsson S, Sundstrom-Poromaa I, et al. Restless legs syndrome among women: prevalence, co-morbidity and possible relationship to menopause. *Climacteric* 2008;11(5):422–8.

60. Winkelman JW, Shahar E, Sharief I, et al. Association of restless legs syndrome and cardiovascular disease in the Sleep Heart Health Study. *Neurology* 2008;70(1):35–42.

61. Juuti AK, Laara E, Rajala U, et al. Prevalence and associated factors of restless legs in a 57-year-old urban population in northern Finland. *Acta Neurol Scand* 2010;122(1):63–9.

62. Winter AC, Schurks M, Glynn RJ, et al. (2012). Restless legs syndrome and risk of incident cardiovascular disease in women and men: prospective cohort study. *BMJ* 2012;2:e000866.

63. Ohayon MM, Roth T. Prevalence of restless legs syndrome and periodic limb movement disorder in the general population. *J Psychosom Res* 2002;53(1):547–54.

64. Benediktsdottir B, Janson C, Lindberg E, et al. Prevalence of restless legs syndrome among adults in Iceland and Sweden: lung function, comorbidity, ferritin, biomarkers and quality of life. *Sleep Med* 2010;11(10):1043–8.

65. Bosco D, Plastino M, Fava A, et al. Role of the Oral Glucose Tolerance Test (OGTT) in the idiopathic restless legs syndrome. *J Neurol Sci* 2009;287:60–3.

66. Keckeis M, Lattova Z, Maurovich-Horvat E, et al. Impaired glucose tolerance in sleep disorders. *PLoS ONE* 2010;5(3):e9444.

67. Gao X, Schwarzschild MA, Wang H, et al. Obesity and restless legs syndrome in men and women. *Neurology* 2009;72(14):1255–61.

68. Banno K, Delaive K, Walld R, et al. Restless legs syndrome in 218 patients: associated disorders. *Sleep Med* 2000;1(3):221–9.

69. Schlesinger I, Erikh I, Avizohar O, et al. Cardiovascular risk factors in restless legs syndrome. *Mov Disord* 2009;24(11):1587–92.

70. Abetz L, Allen R, Follet A, et al. Evaluating the quality of life of patients with restless legs syndrome. *Clin Ther* 2004;26(6):925–35.

71. Abetz L, Arbuckle R, Allen RP, et al. (2006). The reliability, validity and responsiveness of the International Restless Legs Syndrome Study Group rating scale and subscales in a clinical-trial setting. *Sleep Med* 2006;7(4):340–9.

48

Treatment of Restless Legs Syndrome, Including Long-Term Management Issues

ANNE-MARIE WILLIAMS, DESISLAVA TZONOVA, AND DIEGO GARCIA-BORREGUERO

RESTLESS LEGS syndrome (RLS) has been shown to have a significant negative effect on general well-being, activities of daily living, and quality of life, and to be an important social and personal burden.[1-3] This effect is mainly considered to be due to the impact of RLS symptoms on sleep and the inability to remain still, even during the daytime.[2,4-9] Indeed, RLS is a sleep disorder that causes chronic loss of sleep, as shown in a recent survey, where over 50% of patients slept less than 5 hours a day on a chronic basis.[10] This is further illustrated in Figure 48.1, which shows that the RLS symptom patients find the most bothersome is the negative effect on sleep. Sleep loss by itself causes daytime drowsiness, difficulties concentrating, and loss of performance, and it negatively impacts mood.[7]

In addition to the loss of sleep, RLS symptoms occurring during the daytime, sometimes in the form of sudden attacks, are common in moderate to severe patients and might also play an important role in this deterioration of the quality of life.

Furthermore, studies have shown that there are health factors associated with RLS, such as diabetes, high blood pressure, and cardiovascular disease, as well as sleepiness, depression, and anxiety.[11-14]

TREATMENT

Although there is a 5%–15% prevalence of RLS, only about 25% of these require pharmacological treatment; that is, their symptoms are considered clinically significant because they impair the patient's quality of life, daytime functioning, social functioning, or they disrupt sleep. However, for patients with mild RLS, nonpharmacological treatment is recommended.

Nonpharmacological Treatment

A certain number of lifestyle behaviors are associated with RLS; these include caffeine intake,[15] alcohol consumption,[16] stress, shift

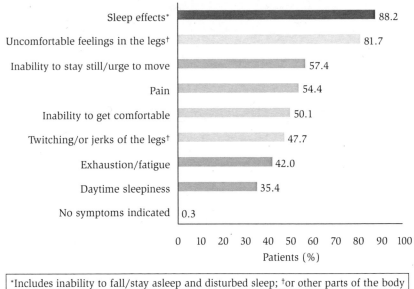

Sleep effects*	88.2
Uncomfortable feelings in the legs†	81.7
Inability to stay still/urge to move	57.4
Pain	54.4
Inability to get comfortable	50.1
Twitching/or jerks of the legs†	47.7
Exhaustion/fatigue	42.0
Daytime sleepiness	35.4
No symptoms indicated	0.3

Patients (%)

*Includes inability to fall/stay asleep and disturbed sleep; †or other parts of the body

FIGURE 48.1   Symptoms of restless legs syndrome (RLS) considered most troublesome by the RLS sufferer group (some sufferers ticked more than one option).[7]

work, and vigorous physical activity close to bedtime.[17] In general, before they consult a physician, patients will have already tried to relieve their symptoms nonpharmacologically. However, it is worthwhile to check whether patients with mild RLS have already changed their lifestyle in order to minimize symptoms; such changes include avoiding stimulants like caffeine, heavy meals, and vigorous exercise before bedtime, and keeping regular bedtime hours—sleep hygiene is important. Behavioral strategies that involve concentration, such as video games or crossword puzzles, may also reduce RLS symptoms at times of monotony, and tactile and temperature stimulation, including massage or hot baths, can also help to relieve mild symptoms.[18]

Certain medications are known to exacerbate RLS symptoms, and therefore the need for these medications should be reconsidered when possible. These medications include antihistamines, dopamine antagonists, antinausea medications, anxiolytics, antidepressants, serotonergic reuptake inhibitors,[19–24] neuroleptics,[25,26] beta-blockers, anticonvulsants, and lithium (see Table 48.1 for more details).[27–30]

In recent years there have been a number of studies examining the role of exercise,[22,31,32] pneumatic compression,[33,34] and near-infrared light[35] for the treatment of RLS. However, these treatments can only be considered investigational at the present time.[36]

Table 48.1 Drugs That May Exacerbate Restless Legs Syndrome

D2 antagonists (metoclopramide and prochlorperazine)
Diphenhydramine (and other over-the-counter cold remedies)
Certain benzodiazepines (chlordiazepoxide)
Traditional antipsychotics (phenothiazines)
Atypical neuroleptics (olanzapine and risperidone)
Antidepressants (especially selective serotonin or norephinephrine reuptake inhibitors)
Anticonvulsants (zonisamide, phenytoin, and methsuximide)
Antihistamines (diphenhydramine)

Source: Adapted from Garcia-Borreguero et al.[120]

Pharmacological Treatment

Pharmacological management of RLS depends upon whether the disorder is primary (idiopathic) or secondary (symptomatic). Those with primary RLS are likely to need treatment for the rest of their lives, particularly if the time course is continuous. In the case of secondary RLS, once the underlying causes (e.g., iron deficiency, chronic renal disease) are resolved, the symptoms usually remit (see later for more details).[37,38]

OVERVIEW OF PHARMACOLOGICAL MEDICATIONS

Dopaminergic Agents. Dopamine agents are one of the first-line treatment choices for RLS.[36] A response to dopaminergic therapy is considered a supportive diagnostic clinical feature, and in individual cases of lack of response to dopaminergic agents, the diagnosis of RLS can be eventually questioned.[39]

Levodopa has been investigated for the treatment of RLS in randomized, placebo-controlled trials.[40-42] However, the number of patients involved in the studies is not large and the duration of the trials is short, in most cases not exceeding 4 weeks. RLS augmentation, an increase in symptom severity as a result of long-term dopaminergic treatment,[43] can occur in up to 50% of the patients during treatment with levodopa.[44] Such is particularly likely when higher doses (200 mg or higher) of levodopa are used. In any case, long-term, prospective studies are needed in order to better assess and quantify the risk of augmentation.

Ropinirole is a nonergoline dopamine agonist with affinity for the D2 and D3 receptor subtypes. The mean elimination half-life of the drug is 6 hours with peak plasma concentration (Cmax) occurring at 1.5 hours. Ropinirole is generally used as a single dose 2 hours before bedtime, normally prior to the usual time of day RLS symptoms start, because once symptoms have started, the medication is less effective. The most common side effects are nausea, low blood pressure, dizziness, and headache. The role of ropinirole in RLS has been studied in several double-blind, placebo-controlled trials[45-51] that included patients with primary RLS. The duration of the studies was between 4 and 12 weeks, and the number of patients included reached 381 patients in the largest trial. At a mean dose of 2 mg/day, ropinirole was shown to be more effective than placebo in these short-term trials and was effective in reducing periodic limb movements during sleep (PLMS).[45,47,52] However, the efficacy of this drug has not been properly investigated over the long term. Reported side effects include nausea, somnolence, and dizziness. The incidence rate of augmentation has been investigated over periods of up to 1 year and has been reported to be 5.24%.[53] However, it is likely that, as with other dopaminergic drugs, such a rate accumulates over time.[54]

Pramipexole is a full agonist for the D2 receptor subfamily, with preferential affinity for the D3 receptor subtype. The elimination half-life of pramipexole is about 10 hours. The mean effective daily dose of pramipexole reported in clinical trials is between 0.25 and 0.75 mg as a single dose at night 2–3 hours before expected bedtime. The maximum approved dose is 0.50 mg/day in the United States and 0.75 mg/day in Europe. The efficacy of pramipexole for the treatment of RLS has been demonstrated in a large sample of patients and in controlled clinical trials lasting up to 6 months.[55-61] Apart from the improved RLS symptomatology measured by IRLS and CGI scores, pramipexole has also been shown to reduce the periodic limb movement index (PLMI).[60,61] The drug is well tolerated; however, side effects like nausea, headache, insomnia, somnolence, and dizziness have been described. Högl et al. studied the 6-month incidence of augmentation, confirming a rate of 9.2% for pramipexole and 6.0% for placebo. The rate increased with treatment duration for pramipexole but not placebo.[60] Previous retrospective studies have shown prevalence rates of 33%[62] and 32%.[63]

Rotigotine has D1, D2, and D3 receptor agonistic activity. It is administered once a day as an adhesive matrix-type transdermal patch because of a low oral bioavailability due to important first-pass effect. Using this form of administration, the drug release is continuous, providing stable plasma concentrations over 24 hours. The elimination half-life is approximately 7 hours. Independently of patch size, approximately 45% of the rotigotine from the patch is released within 24 hours. The change in the application site could lead to differences in the plasmatic concentration of rotigotine. Differences in bioavailability range from less than 2% (abdomen versus hip) to 46% (shoulder versus thigh) with shoulder application showing higher bioavailability. Nevertheless, there is no indication for a clinically relevant effect of this fluctuation on the patient's symptoms. RLS symptoms are generally improved by rotigotine in therapeutic doses between 1 mg and 3 mg. Rotigotine can be used in moderate to severe RLS patients who require daily treatment, but it is particularly indicated whenever daytime symptoms are present. All clinical trials with IRLS, CGI, RLS-6, and other approved-for-RLS assessments scales have demonstrated efficacy and safety of this drug in patients affected by moderate to severe RLS, both in the short and long term, the longest period of evaluation being 5 years.[64-70] The most frequent adverse events reported in the clinical trials were application site reactions, headache, and nausea. Clinically significant augmentation was observed in 13% of the participants in the 5-year follow-up trial.[64] Rotigotine patch has been approved recently by the FDA for treatment of moderate to severe RLS.

Pergolide has been studied in four randomized controlled trials,[71-74] and its short-term and long-term efficacy in primary RLS has been demonstrated. Pergolide has been shown to significantly improve sleep outcome measures such as PLMSI, sleep efficiency, total sleep time, and subjective sleep quality, compared with baseline or placebo. After 12 months of double-blind treatment, patients continued to show improvements in PLMI and PLMSA-I. The drug was withdrawn by the American Food and Drug Agency (FDA) following safety information[75] confirming the association of valvular heart disease in Parkinson's disease patients exposed to pergolide. So although pergolide is efficacious in RLS, it requires special monitoring due to increased incidence of valvular fibrosis and other fibrotic side effects.

The efficacy of cabergoline in patients with idiopathic RLS was assessed in three controlled trials.[76-78] The subject evaluation was performed using several validated RLS scales. These studies concluded that cabergoline is efficacious and generally well tolerated in a single-evening dose for sensorimotor symptoms of RLS. Common adverse effects were gastrointestinal symptoms, and augmentation was reported in 4% of patients over 6 months. Concerns about fibrosis have not been specifically addressed in RLS studies. Cardiopulmonary monitoring for fibrosis should also be performed in patients on cabergoline treatment.

Opioids. Opioids have not been investigated in large-scale trials for the treatment of RLS;

however, they are often used as an alternative following unsuccessful treatment with dopaminergic agents. In some countries opioids are administered with dopaminergic agents, but the efficacy or adverse effects of this combination has never been investigated.[79]

In the retrospective study by Walters et al.[26] based on the clinical records of 493 patients, 7.3% (n = 36) were on opioid monotherapy for an average of 5 years and 11 months. Of 16 patients who discontinued opioid monotherapy, in only one case was it due to addiction or tolerance problems. Furthermore, a polysomnogram (PSG) recording was performed on seven patients: development of sleep apnea was established in two cases and worsening of preexisting sleep apnea in one case. These facts supported the recommendation for periodical PSG recordings.

One double-blind randomized crossover trial performed with nighttime doses in 11 patients provided positive results regarding the use of oxycodone in refractory idiopathic RLS.[80] Statistically significant improvements in leg sensations, motor restlessness, PLMS, and PLMS arousals were achieved with a mean dose of 15.9 mg.

Methadone (5 to 40 mg/day) was administered to 29 RLS patients who failed to respond to dopaminergic agents. Seventeen of the initial 27 patients remained on methadone for 23 +/− 12 months (range, 4–44 months).[81] All patients who remained on methadone report at least a 75% reduction in symptoms, and none developed augmentation. Methadone shows neither augmentation nor major problems with continued efficacy, confirming that it is an efficient treatment for RLS that can be considered in RLS patients with an unsatisfactory response to dopaminergic agents. Due to its respiratory depressant effect, it should be used cautiously, especially in individuals with preexisting respiratory compromise.

A long-term open-label study (follow-up to 24 months) examined the efficacy of tramadol 50–150 mg in 12 RLS patients.[82] PSG measures improved and daytime sensory and motor symptoms disappeared after tramadol was stopped. Therefore, intermittent treatment with tramadol and careful monitoring are recommended. Both Vetrugno et al.[83] and also Earley and Allen[83a] each reported case of one patient developing RLS augmentation after long-term treatment with tramadol.

Morphine given intrathecally via infusion has been shown to be successful in a single case of RLS who had, severe leg pain resistant to any other analgesic medication.[84]

Opioid medications are usually well tolerated and demonstrate good long-term efficacy. The side effects described are nausea, sedation, dizziness, and constipation. There is a concern about the potential for abuse as well as addiction. This concern may be resolved through further studies, and it should be noted that a once nightly dose of an opioid has much less risk of addiction than the regular use of opioids for acute or chronic pain. Respiratory depression is another concern, especially at higher doses and in patients with preexisting respiratory compromise.

Alpha-2 Delta Ligands/Anticonvulsants. Studies have shown anticonvulsants to be effective for the treatment of RLS, possibly due to their action on the increased sensorimotor excitability, which accompanies this condition. When RLS symptoms are painful, and especially when the disease is associated with polyneuropathy, anticonvulsants approved for the treatment of pain, such as pregabalin, can be prescribed. Anticonvulsants are known to cause sedation; this may be an advantage of these agents in the treatment of RLS by improving sleep. Nevertheless, daytime sedation may be a problem with these agents, some of which have long half-lives.

Studies on the alpha-2-delta calcium channel blockers gabapentin enacarbil[85,86] and pregabalin[87-88a] have recently been reported. This class of drugs has been shown to improve both sensory symptoms and PLMS, and it appears to be as efficacious as dopaminergics. Their advantage lies in their greater therapeutic effects on sleep and sleep architecture. One double-blind long-term study (52 weeks) comparing pregabalin 300 mg with pramipexole 0.25 and 0.5 mg showed essentially no augmentation compared to significant augmentation occurring for treatment with pramipexole. This study also showed 300 mg pregabalin was more effective than 0.25 or 0.5 mg pramipexole for reducing RLS symptoms as assessed by the IRLS. The alpha-2-delta channel blocker drugs are now considered an alternative to dopamine agonists as a first-line treatment choice.

Pregabalin has been shown to be effective (mean effective dose was 322.50 mg/d) in the treatment of idiopathic RLS in two double-blind randomized studies.[87,88] In these studies, pregabalin significantly improved IRLS total score, CGI, RLS-6 sleep measures, and MOS scores for sleep disturbance, and sleep quantity. PLMI, PLM-AI, and PLM-W were also improved, and sleep stages 1 and 2 and slow-wave sleep also increased. In secondary RLS there is only one open-label case series in patients with polyneuropathy, where a mean dose of 305 mg/d was found to be effective in alleviation of RLS symptoms as measured by subjective self-rated patients' impression.[89]

Gabapentin enacarbil has been shown to improve IRLS and CGI-I investigator and patient scores, as well as sleep parameters.[90-92] Improvements in PLM parameters have also been reported.[93] The effective dose of gabapentin enacarbil for the treatment of RLS is 1200 mg/d. One study found gabapentin enacarbil to be effective at a dose of 600 mg/d as well as at 1200 mg/d, significantly improving RLS symptoms and sleep disturbance compared with placebo.[94] In all these studies the most common reported adverse events were somnolence and dizziness. Gabapentin enacarbil is approved by the FDA for the treatment of RLS.

Gabapentin has been found to be efficacious in patients with primary RLS and in secondary RLS in dialyzed patients or in iron-deficient subjects at doses ranging from 100 to 2400 mg.[45-51,95,96] Its clinical efficacy has been proven using the IRLS rating scale, CGI, PGI, PSQI, and PSG measures. In addition, gabapentin decreases stage-I sleep, increases slow-wave sleep, and is more beneficial for patients with painful symptoms.

Benzodiazepines. There is no consistent evidence of the clinical benefit of clonazepam for the treatment of RLS.[97-99] In the study by Saletu et al.[100] clonazepam significantly improved objective sleep efficiency and subjective sleep quality in patients with RLS and PLMD, but it failed to reduce the PLM per hour of sleep. The same drug, when compared to cognitive-behavioral therapy, showed a greater decrease in the periodic limb movement-arousals per hour of sleep. The two treatments were shown to be equal in improving subjective sleep quality as seen in sleep log measures of sleep-wake times and the Insomnia Symptom Questionnaire. In one study[101] of long-term benzodiazepine treatment of injurious parasomnias and other disorders of disrupted sleep, including PLMD, the authors described, low risk of dosage tolerance or abuse. Nonetheless, the withdrawal symptoms, habituation, and dependence potential of these medications (clonazepam) are well known.[102]

ASSESSMENT OF FREQUENCY

In the case of primary RLS, once the physician has established whether symptoms are clinically significant, it is necessary to assess the frequency of symptoms and to categorize them into intermittent, daily, and refractory RLS. A summary of treatment recommendations are provided next. These use the the categories of RLS from the treatment guidelines of the European Restless Legs Syndrome Study Group (EURLSSG) but the recommendations have been updated and more relevant to the world, not only Europe.

Intermittent RLS. (where the frequency of symptoms does not necessitate daily treatment): no FDA- or EMEA-approved treatment is available for the intermittent treatment of RLS; however, the EURLSSG states that the intermittent use of levodopa or pramipexole can be considered to be appropriate if an off-label treatment is warranted; other off-label treatment options include intermittent low-potency opioids.

Daily RLS. (moderate to severe RLS that negatively impacts daily living either every day or most days of the week): the dopamine agonists (pramipexole, ropinirole, and rotigotine) and the alpha-2-delta drugs (gabapentin, gabapentin enacarbil and pregabalin) are considered first-line treatment choice. Regulatory approval for treatment of RLS has been granted by the FDA for these dopamine agonists and gabapentin enacarbil. The EMEA has approved RLS treatment with these dopamine agonists.[36]

For nightime symptoms treatment can be initiated with a low nightly dose of any of these dopamine agonists or alpha-2-delta drugs Daytime symptoms should be treated preferentially with either gabapentin enacarbil or transdermal rotigotine as they have a longer duration of action.[68] Extended-release dopamine agonists are available for other indications but have not been approved for RLS. Second-line treatment consists of the alternate first-line treatment, combination of drugs or the opioid-like drugs (e.g., tramadol, tilidine, codeine, and methadone); however, their long-term use may lead to addiction issues as noted earlier.[36] In addition, painful forms of RLS or RLS associated with polyneuropathy (e.g., diabetic polyneuropathy) should be treated with alpha-2 delta agonists. Pramipexole has also been shown to improve painful symptoms in RLS patients.[103]

Refractory RLS. (defined as daily RLS that has been unsuccessfully treated with two classes of drugs, one dopaminergic and one nondopaminergic, at the correct dose and for an adequate length of time): a different dopamine agonist should be administered, as a suboptimal response to one agent does not rule out that another agent may be adequate.[104] Methadone has been used successfully in some very severe RLS refractory to other treatments[81]. It is also possible that iron deficiency is related to dopaminergic nonresponse in patients with RLS, so iron parameters need to be checked regularly.[105]

GENERAL TREATMENT CONSIDERATIONS

The drug dosages of dopaminergics given to RLS patients are far lower than those used to treat Parkinson's disease patients, and the maximum regulatory dose should not be exceeded. The dose for the alpha-2-delta drugs approximates that used to treat chronic pain. (see Table 48.2).

Table 48.2 Starting and Maximum Recommended Dosages

DRUG	STARTING DOSE AND MAXIMUM RECOMMENDED DOSAGE
Clonazepam	0.50 mg 2.0 mg
Gabapentin	300 mg 2700 mg
Gabapentin enacarbil	600 mg 1200 mg
Pramipexole	0.125 mg 0.75 mg
Pregabalin	25–300 mg
Levodopa	50 mg 200 mg
Ropinirole	0.25 mg 4 mg
Rotigotine	1–3 mg patches

It is also not recommended to divide dose if this increases the total daily dose; however, in some long-term RLS sufferers, it is necessary to divide the dose to ensure efficacy; such patients should be monitored to ensure that the total 24-hour dosage is kept low. Before switching drugs, it is recommended that the drug be given for a sufficient length of time to notice an effect on symptoms; this time varies from first dose (levodopa, clonazepam) to 10 days (ropinirole, gabapentin enacarbil). However, for all drugs, within 10 days it should be generally possible to see whether the drug has a sufficient effect on symptoms.

Treatment of Secondary Restless Legs Syndrome (Iron)

As mentioned earlier, secondary RLS occurs in the setting of iron deficiency, low serum ferritin values, pregnancy, end-stage renal disease (ESRD), rheumatoid arthritis, diabetes, neurological disorders such as polyneuropathy, and various forms of spinal disorders.

Iron deficiency is the most common cause of secondary RLS; not only is it implicated in the onset of secondary RLS but it is also implicated in the severity of RLS[106,107] and is common during pregnancy and ESRD.

All RLS patients should have their serum ferritin (SF) and transferrin saturation (TSAT) checked, and this is especially the case for patients with a history of gastrointestinal blood loss or those who give frequent blood donations. If SF or TSAT measurements are <50 μg/L or <20%, respectively, iron supplementation (325 mg ferrous sulphate three times daily with 100–200 mg of vitamin C) should be considered in order to replenish iron stores.[108] There is conflicting evidence concerning the efficacy of intravenous iron in improving RLS symptoms; however, intravenous iron is an alternative to oral iron in those patients with gastrointestinal problems that effect absorption.[109–112]

Treatment in Specific Populations

PREGNANCY

There is a high prevalence of RLS in pregnancy (26%) with a peak in prevalence and severity during the third trimester; however, symptoms often disappear shortly after delivery.[113] For RLS in pregnancy and breast-feeding, only iron and folic acid can be recommended. For FDA safety category and excretion in breast milk of some of the major RLS medications, see Table 48.3.

RESTLESS LEGS SYNDROME IN THE ELDERLY

There are no specific recommendations for the elderly (>75 years).

Table 48.3 Drug Safety in Pregnancy

MEDICATION NAME	FDA SAFETY CATEGORY	EXCRETED IN BREAST MILK
Levodopa/carbidopa	Class C	Yes
Pramipexole	Class C	No data
Clonazepam	Class D	Small amounts
Oxycodone	Class B; class D if chronic use	Yes
Methadone	Class B/C; class D if high dosage	Minimal
Gabapentin	Class C	Yes

FDA classification system: A, B, C, D, and X. A representing lowest risk and X representing highest risk of teratogenicity. Data are accurate as of April 2011. Please consult updated FDA data before proceeding.

PEDIATRIC RESTLESS LEGS SYNDROME

For children, as with adult sufferers of RLS, nonpharmacological treatment measures should be taken in the first instance, and iron parameters should be examined to rule out iron deficiency.

There are no FDA- or EMEA-approved drugs for the treatment of pediatric RLS. Furthermore, the Standards of Practice Committee of the American Academy of Sleep Medicine,[114,115] the Movement Disorder Society, the European Federation of Neurological Societies (EFNS), and the European Restless Legs Syndrome Study Group (EURLSSG) make no specific recommendations regarding treatment of children with RLS.

There are, however, data concerning the use of dopaminergic drugs in children, and they may be considered in children with severe RLS.[116] Nausea is a side effect for 20% of children. Long term effects, of these drugs given to children remain unknown.[117,118]

END-STAGE RENAL DISEASE

The prevalence of RLS in end-stage renal disease (ESRD) is between 6% and 83%. RLS often resolves following kidney transplantation.[38,119] As dopamine antagonists worsen RLS symptoms, it is important that patients are not treated with metoclopramide, which is often used to treat nausea in patients undergoing dialysis. As mentioned earlier, iron parameters need to be verified and iron deficiency corrected.

Urinary excretion is the major route of pramipexole elimination; thus, renal insufficiency can cause a large decrease in the ability to eliminate the drug, and dosage adjustment is needed in cases of renal failure. On the other hand, no difference was observed in the pharmacokinetics of ropinirole in patients with moderate renal impairment (creatinine clearance between 30 to 50 mL/min) compared to an age-matched population with creatinine clearance above 50 mL/min. Therefore, no dosage adjustment is necessary in moderately renally impaired patients.

FOLLOW-UP

RLS patients need to see their physician regularly, every 6–12 months, for follow-up. The physician needs to monitor treatment efficacy and be attentive to patients who are unresponsive to treatment, who suffer from rebound, or who develop augmentation (see Table 48.4). A treatment diary indicating when symptoms begin in the day can give the physician an indication of the severity of symptoms and the effect of treatment, and this will enable the identification of augmentation.[120]

Special Situations

REBOUND

Rebound is the development of RLS symptoms in the early morning when the half-life period of the drug has expired; it occurs in up to 35% of RLS patients.[121] The symptoms of rebound are worse than they were before treatment initiation, as is the case with augmentation; however, unlike augmentation where, symptoms appear earlier than their usual time of onset before treatment, with rebound symptoms usually reemerge in the early morning hours with no additional features typical of augmentation (such as spreading of symptoms to other body parts, shorter latency of symptoms at rest, or increased symptom intensity) present. Rebound is common in drugs with a short half-life such as rapid-release levodopa. If a patient suffers from rebound, then switching to another dopaminergic agent with a longer half-life, or to a different class of drugs (alpha-2-delta ligands, opioids), is recommended. Rebound can also be treated by adding a middle-of-the-night dose.[122]

TOLERANCE/LOSS OF EFFICACY

Tolerance is when the efficacy of a medication diminishes over time, and medication dose needs to be increased in order to maintain the original effect on symptoms. The symptoms are not worse than before treatment initiation. It needs to be differentiated from the natural progression of RLS, which occurs over several years. The relationship between tolerance and augmentation has yet to be clarified, as it is not clear whether patients develop tolerance of dopaminergic agents or whether tolerance precedes augmentation.[63] The International Restless Legs Syndrome Study Group (IRLSSG) recently approved a definition of clinically relevant response for the use in clinical trials (Table 48.5).[123]

Table 48.4 Differentiating Augmentation from Other Conditions

AUGMENTATION	TOLERANCE
Additional features (symptoms spread to other body parts, shorter latency to symptoms at rest, increased intensity of symptoms)	No additional features
Increase severity beyond baseline levels	Never worse than baseline
Symptom onset in afternoon or evening	Symptom onset in early morning
Anticipation of time of onset	Delayed onset of symptoms
Followed by usual course of symptoms	Followed by symptom-free interval in the morning/noon
Related to total daily dosage/severity of symptoms at baseline	Related to half-life. Occurs during the declining phase of plasma concentrations
Additional features (symptoms spread to other body parts, shorter latency to symptoms at rest, increased intensity of symptoms)	No additional features
Progresses within weeks/months	Natural progression of RLS is usually slow (years)
A reduction in the dose leads ultimately to a *decrease* in symptoms. An increase in the dose ultimately leads to an increase in symptoms.	A reduction in the dose leads to an *increase* in symptoms.
Increase beyond baseline severity	Increase beyond baseline severity

AUGMENTATION

A characteristic feature of augmentation is that symptoms are more severe than before initiation of treatment, and they improve when medication is discontinued. It was first described during treatment with levodopa, but it has since been reported during treatment with all dopaminergic agents.[124]

An operational definition of augmentation based on empirical data from clinical studies was generated in 2006, during a European Restless Legs Syndrome Study Group (EURLSSG)-sponsored Consensus Conference at the Max Planck Institute (MPI) in Munich (Germany). According to the MPI criteria, a reliable detection of augmentation could be obtained

Table 48.5 Definition of Loss of Clinically Relevant Response for Clinical Trials

A loss of response occurs when the patient meets both of the following two criteria:

Criterion A (defines initial clinically relevant response):
During the first 3 months of treatment, on any two consecutive evaluations at least 1 week apart:

1) There is a reduction in the IRLS total score by ≥40% from the baseline value, i.e., IRLS ≤ 60% of the baseline value. (*Example 1: a baseline IRLS score of 25 with decreases after treatment to ≤15*);

or

2) The IRLS score ≤10 (Example 2: regardless of the initial score, there is an improvement to ≤10)

Criterion B (defines clinically relevant loss of initial response):
Once clinically relevant response is established according to Criterion A, loss of response is defined as follows:

1) On any two consecutive evaluations at least 1 month apart, there is an increase of the IRLS score to >70% of the baseline score (*Example 1: baseline IRLS score of 25, treatment response of IRLS ≤15 followed by worsening with IRLS increased on two visits to ≥18*) and there is no re-establishment of response (defined as criterion A) afterward without a dose increase.

or

2) A dose increase occurring:
   • After the first 3 months of treatment

or

• Within the first 3 months of treatment and preceded by one evaluation with IRLS >70% of baseline

or

3) The patient drops out due to loss of response as determined by the investigator.

If the patient meets both criteria A and B indicating loss of response, the investigator should determine the presence of augmentation. The patient should be classified as one of the following:

• Loss of response with augmentation
• Loss of response without augmentation
• Loss of response—augmentation state not assessed

Source: From Garcia-Borreguero et al.[123]

based on a 4-hour time advance of symptoms, or a smaller (2–4 hour) advance of symptoms expressed in conjunction with other required clinical indications, such as a shorter latency of symptoms at rest, a spread of symptoms to other body parts in addition to the lower limbs, or a greater intensity of symptoms.[43] Furthermore, the paradoxical response to treatment—an increase in severity with increasing dose of medication, and an improvement following decrease in medication—was considered an alternative key feature for diagnosis (see Table 48.6).

Table 48.6 Max Planck Institute Criteria for Augmentation

Preamble

Augmentation is a worsening of RLS symptom severity experienced by patients undergoing treatment for RLS. The RLS symptoms in general are more severe than those experienced at baseline.

A. Basic features (all of which need to be met):

1. The increase in symptom severity was experienced on 5 out of 7 days during the previous week.
2. The increase in symptom severity is not accounted for by other factors such as a change in medical status, lifestyle, or the natural progression of the disorder.
3. It is assumed that there has been a prior positive response to treatment.

In addition, either B or C or both have to be met:

B. Persisting (although not immediate) paradoxical response to treatment: RLS symptom severity increases sometime after a dose increase and improves sometime after a dose decrease.

OR

C. Earlier onset of symptoms:

1. An earlier onset by at least 4 hours

OR

2. An earlier onset (between 2 and 4 hours) occurs with one of the following compared to symptom status before treatment:
   a. Shorter latency to symptoms when at rest
   b. Spreading of symptoms to other body parts
   c. Intensity of symptoms is greater (or increase in periodic limb movements [PLMs] if measured by polysomnography [PSG] or the suggested immobilization test [SIT])
   d. Duration of relief from treatment is shorter.

Augmentation requires criteria A + B, A + C, or A + B + C to be met.

Source: From Garcia-Borreguero et al.[43]
RLS, restless legs syndrome.

REFERENCES

1. Kushida C, Martin M, Nikam P, et al. Burden of restless legs syndrome on health-related quality of life. *Qual Life Res* 2007;16:617–24.
2. Allen RP, Bharmal M, Calloway M. Prevalence and disease burden of primary restless legs syndrome: results of a general population survey in the United States. *Mov Disord* 2011;26:114–20.
3. Phillips B, Hening W, Britz P, et al. Prevalence and correlates of restless legs syndrome: results from the 2005 National Sleep Foundation Poll. *Chest* 2006;129:76–80.
4. Kushida CA, Allen RP, Atkinson MJ. Modeling the causal relationships between symptoms associated with restless legs syndrome and the patient-reported impact of RLS. *Sleep Med* 2004;5:485–8.
5. Allen RP, Walters AS, Montplaisir J, et al. Restless legs syndrome prevalence and impact: REST general population study. *Arch Intern Med* 2005;165:1286–92.
6. Abetz L, Arbuckle R, Allen RP, et al. The reliability, validity and responsiveness of the Restless Legs Syndrome Quality of Life questionnaire (RLSQoL) in a trial population. *Health Qual Life Outcomes* 2005;3:79.
7. Hening W, Walters AS, Allen RP, et al. Impact, diagnosis and treatment of restless legs syndrome (RLS) in a primary care population: the REST (RLS epidemiology, symptoms, and treatment) primary care study. *Sleep Med* 2004;5:237–46.
8. Allen RP, Earley CJ. Validation of the Johns Hopkins restless legs severity scale. *Sleep Med* 2001;2:239–42.

9. Tison F, Crochard A, Leger D, et al. Epidemiology of restless legs syndrome in French adults: a nationwide survey: the INSTANT Study. *Neurology* 2005;65:239–46.

10. Kushida CA, Nichols DA, Simon RD, et al. Symptom-based prevalence of sleep disorders in an adult primary care population. *Sleep Breath* 2000;4:9–14.

11. Berger K, Luedemann J, Trenkwalder C, et al. Sex and the risk of restless legs syndrome in the general population. *Arch Intern Med* 2004;164:196–202.

12. Ulfberg J, Nystrom B, Carter N, et al. Prevalence of restless legs syndrome among men aged 18 to 64 years: an association with somatic disease and neuropsychiatric symptoms. *Mov Disord* 2001;16:1159–63.

13. Winkelman JW, Finn L, Young T. Prevalence and correlates of restless legs syndrome symptoms in the Wisconsin Sleep Cohort. *Sleep Med* 2006;7:545–52.

14. Winkelman JW, Shahar E, Sharief I, et al. Association of restless legs syndrome and cardiovascular disease in the Sleep Heart Health Study. *Neurology* 2008;70:35–42.

15. Lutz EG. Restless legs, anxiety and caffeinism. *J Clin Psychiatry* 1978;39:693–8.

16. Aldrich MS, Shipley JE. Alcohol use and periodic limb movements of sleep. *Alcohol Clin Exp Res* 1993;17:192–6.

17. Terao T, Terao M, Yoshimura R, et al. Restless legs syndrome induced by lithium. *Biol Psychiatry* 1991;30:1167–70.

18. Russell M. Massage therapy and restless legs syndrome. *J Bodywork Movement Ther* 2007;11:146–50.

19. Sanz-Fuentenebro FJ, Huidobro A, Tejadas-Rivas A. Restless legs syndrome and paroxetine. *Acta Psychiatr Scand* 1996;94:482–4.

20. Agargun MY, Kara H, Ozbek H, et al. Restless legs syndrome induced by mirtazapine. *J Clin Psychiatry* 2002;63:1179.

21. Paik IH, Lee C, Choi BM, et al. Mianserin-induced restless legs syndrome. *Br J Psychiatry* 1989;155:415–17.

22. Hargrave R, Beckley DJ. Restless leg syndrome exacerbated by sertraline. *Psychosomatics* 1998;39:177–8.

23. Markkula J, Lauerma H. Mianserin and restless legs. *Int Clin Psychopharmacol* 1997;12:53–8.

24. Dorsey CM, Lukas SE, Cunningham SL. Fluoxetine-induced sleep disturbance in depressed patients. *Neuropsychopharmacology* 1996;14:437–42.

25. Hening WA, Walters A, Kavey N, et al. Dyskinesias while awake and periodic movements in sleep in restless legs syndrome: treatment with opioids. *Neurology* 1986:1363–6.

26. Walters AS, Winkelmann J, Trenkwalder C, et al. Long-term follow-up on restless legs syndrome patients treated with opioids. *Mov Disord* 2001;16:1105–9.

27. Kraus T, Schuld A, PollmÑcher T. Periodic leg movements in sleep and restless legs syndrome probably caused by olanzapine. *Clin Psychopharmacol* 1999;19:478–9.

28. Wetter TC, Brunner J, Bronisch T. Restless legs syndrome probably induced by risperidone treatment. *Pharmacopsychiatry* 2002;35:109–11.

29. Morgan LK. Letter: Restless legs: precipitated by beta blockers, relieved by orphenadrine. *Med J Aust* 1975;2:753.

30. Drake ME. Restless legs with antiepileptic drug therapy. *Clin Neurol Neurosurg* 1988;90:151–4.

31. Ohayon MM, Roth T. Prevalence of restless legs syndrome and periodic limb movement disorder in the general population. *J Psychosom Res* 2002;53:547–54.

32. Phillips B, Young T, Finn L, et al. Epidemiology of restless legs symptoms in adults. *Arch Intern Med* 2000;160:2137–41.

33. Rajaram SS, Shanahan J, Ash C, et al. Enhanced external counter pulsation (EECP) as a novel treatment for restless legs syndrome (RLS): a preliminary test of the vascular neurologic hypothesis for RLS. *Sleep Med* 2005;6:101–6.

34. Eliasson AH, Lettieri CJ. Sequential compression devices for treatment of restless legs syndrome. *Medicine (Baltimore)* 2007;86:317–23.

35. Mitchell UH, Myrer JW, Johnson AW, et al. Restless legs syndrome and near-infrared light: an alternative treatment option. *Physiother Theory Pract* 2011;27:345–51.

36. Trenkwalder C, Hening WA, Montagna P, et al. Treatment of restless legs syndrome: an evidence-based review and implications for clinical practice. *Mov Disord* 2008;23:2267–302.

37. Lee KA, Zaffke ME, Baratte-Beebe K. Restless legs syndrome and sleep disturbance during pregnancy: the role of folate

and iron. *J Womens Health Gend Based Med* 2001;10:335–41.

38. Molnar MZ, Novak M, Ambrus C, et al. Restless legs syndrome in patients after renal transplantation. *Am J Kidney Dis* 2005;45:388–96.

39. Allen RP, Picchietti D, Hening WA, et al. Restless legs syndrome: diagnostic criteria, special considerations, and epidemiology. A report from the restless legs syndrome diagnosis and epidemiology workshop at the National Institutes of Health. *Sleep Med* 2003;4:101–19.

40. Benes H, Kurella B, Kummer J, et al. Rapid onset of action of levodopa in restless legs syndrome: a double-blind, randomized, multicenter, crossover trial. *Sleep* 1999;22:1073–81.

41. Trenkwalder C, Stiasny K, Pollmacher T, et al. L-dopa therapy of uremic and idiopathic restless legs syndrome: a double-blind, crossover trial. *Sleep* 1995;18:681–8.

42. Brodeur C, Montplaisir J, Godbout R, et al. Treatment of restless legs syndrome and periodic movements during sleep with L-dopa: a double-blind, controlled study. *Neurology* 1988;38:1845–8.

43. Garcia-Borreguero D, Allen RP, Kohnen R, et al. Diagnostic standards for dopaminergic augmentation of restless legs syndrome: report from a World Association of Sleep Medicine-International Restless Legs Syndrome Study Group consensus conference at the Max Planck Institute. *Sleep Med* 2007;8:520–30.

44. Hogl B, Garcia-Borreguero D, Kohnen R, et al. Progressive development of augmentation during long-term treatment with levodopa in restless legs syndrome: results of a prospective multi-center study. *J Neurol* 2010;257:230–7.

45. Happe S, Sauter C, Klosch G, et al. Gabapentin versus ropinirole in the treatment of idiopathic restless legs syndrome. *Neuropsychobiology* 2003;48:82–6.

46. Adler CH, Hauser RA, Sethi K, et al. Ropinirole for restless legs syndrome: a placebo-controlled crossover trial. *Neurology* 2004;62:1405–7.

47. Allen R, Becker PM, Bogan R, et al. Ropinirole decreases periodic leg movements and improves sleep parameters in patients with restless legs syndrome. *Sleep* 2004;27:907–14.

48. Trenkwalder C, Garcia-Borreguero D, Montagna P, et al. Ropinirole in the treatment of restless legs syndrome: results from a 12-week, randomised, placebo-controlled study in 10 European countries. *J Neurol Neurosurg Psychiatry* 2004;75:92–7.

49. Walters AS, Ondo WG, Dreykluft T, et al. Ropinirole is effective in the treatment of restless legs syndrome. TREAT RLS 2: a 12-week, double-blind, randomized, parallel-group, placebo-controlled study. *Mov Disord* 2004;19:1414–23.

50. Bliwise DL, Freeman A, Ingram CD, et al. Randomized, double-blind, placebo-controlled, short-term trial of ropinirole in restless legs syndrome. *Sleep Med* 2005;6:141–7.

51. Bogan RK, Fry JM, Schmidt MH, et al. Ropinirole in the treatment of patients with restless legs syndrome: a US-based randomized, double-blind, placebo-controlled clinical trial. *Mayo Clin Proc* 2006;81:17–27.

52. Walters AS, Ondo WG, Dreykluft T, et al. Ropinirole is effective in the treatment of restless legs syndrome. TREAT RLS 2: a 12-week, double-blind, randomized, parallel-group, placebo-controlled study. *Mov Disord* 2004;19:1414–23.

53. Garcia- Borreguero D, Högl B, Ferini Strambi L, et al. Systematic evaluation of augmentation during treatment with ropinirole in restless legs syndrome: results from a prospective, multicenter study over sixty-six weeks. *Mov Disord* 2012;27(2):277–83.

54. Allen RP, Ondo WG, Ball E, et al. Restless legs syndrome (RLS) augmentation associated with dopamine agonist and levodopa usage in a community sample. *Sleep Med* 2011;12:431–9.

55. Montplaisir J, Nicolas A, Denesle R, et al. Restless legs syndrome improved by pramipexole: a double-blind randomized trial. *Neurology* 1999;52:938–43.

56. Partinen M, Hirvonen K, Jama L, et al. Efficacy and safety of pramipexole in idiopathic restless legs syndrome: a polysomnographic dose-finding study—the PRELUDE study. *Sleep Med* 2006;7:407–17.

57. Winkelman JW, Sethi KD, Kushida CA, et al. Efficacy and safety of pramipexole in restless legs syndrome. *Neurology* 2006;67:1034–9.

58. Trenkwalder C, Stiasny-Kolster K, Kupsch A, et al. Controlled withdrawal of pramipexole after 6 months of open-label treatment in patients with restless legs syndrome. *Mov Disord* 2006;21:1404–10.

59. Oertel WH, Stiasny-Kolster K, Bergtholdt B, et al. Efficacy of pramipexole in restless legs syndrome: a six-week, multicenter, randomized, double-blind study (effect-RLS study). *Mov Disord* 2007;22:213–19.

60. Hogl B, Garcia-Borreguero D, Trenkwalder C, et al. Efficacy and augmentation during 6 months of double-blind pramipexole for restless legs syndrome. *Sleep Med* 2011;12:351–60.

61. Inoue Y, Hirata K, Kuroda K, et al. Efficacy and safety of pramipexole in Japanese patients with primary restless legs syndrome: a polysomnographic randomized, double-blind, placebo-controlled study. *Sleep Med* 2010;11:11–16.

62. Silber MH, Girish M, Izurieta R. Pramipexole in the management of restless legs syndrome: an extended study. *Sleep* 2003;26:819–21.

63. Winkelman JW, Johnston L. Augmentation and tolerance with long-term pramipexole treatment of restless legs syndrome (RLS). *Sleep Med* 2004;5:9–14.

64. Högl B, Trenkwalder C, Garcia-Borreguero D, et al. Long-term safety and efficacy of rotigotine in patients with idiopathic RLS: 5-year results from a prospective multinational open-label follow-up study. *Neurology* 2010;74:A106.

65. Oertel WH, Benes H, Garcia-Borreguero D, et al. Rotigotine transdermal patch in moderate to severe idiopathic restless legs syndrome: a randomized, placebo-controlled polysomnographic study. *Sleep Med* 2010;11:848–56.

66. Hening WA, Allen RP, Ondo WG, et al. Rotigotine improves restless legs syndrome: a 6-month randomized, double-blind, placebo-controlled trial in the United States. *Mov Disord* 2010;25:1675–83.

67. Benes H, Garcia-Borreguero D, Allen R, et al. Augmentation in long-term therapy of the restless legs syndrome with transdermal rotigotine—a retrospective systematic analysis of two large open-label 1-year trials. *Neurology* 2009;32.

68. Trenkwalder C, Benes H, Poewe W, et al. Efficacy of rotigotine for treatment of moderate-to-severe restless legs syndrome: a randomised, double-blind, placebo-controlled trial. *Lancet Neurol* 2008;7:595–604.

69. Oertel WH, Benes H, Garcia-Borreguero D, et al. Efficacy of rotigotine transdermal system in severe restless legs syndrome: a randomized, double-blind, placebo-controlled, six-week dose-finding trial in Europe. *Sleep Med* 2008;9:228–39.

70. Oertel WM, Benes H, Ferini-Strambi L, et al. Assessment of rotigotine in idiopathic RLS: results of a 7-week sleep lab trial. *Mov Disord* 2008;23:S370.

71. Staedt J, Wassmuth F, Ziemann U, et al. Pergolide: treatment of choice in restless legs syndrome (RLS) and nocturnal myoclonus syndrome (NMS). A double-blind randomized crosover trial of pergolide versus L-dopa. *J Neural Transm* 1997;104:461–8.

72. Earley CJ, Yaffee JB, Allen RP. Randomized, double-blind, placebo-controlled trial of pergolide in restless legs syndrome. *Neurology* 1998;51:1599–602.

73. Wetter TC, Stiasny K, Winkelmann J, et al. A randomized controlled study of pergolide in patients with restless legs syndrome. *Neurology* 1999;52:944–50.

74. Trenkwalder C, Hundemer HP, Lledo A, et al. Efficacy of pergolide in treatment of restless legs syndrome: the PEARLS Study. *Neurology* 2004;62:1391–7.

75. Zanettini R, Antonini A, Gatto G, et al. Valvular heart disease and the use of dopamine agonists for Parkinson's disease. *N Engl J Med* 2007;356:39–46.

76. Stiasny-Kolster K, Benes H, Peglau I, et al. Effective cabergoline treatment in idiopathic restless legs syndrome. *Neurology* 2004;63:2272–9.

77. Oertel WH, Benes H, Bodenschatz R, et al. Efficacy of cabergoline in restless legs syndrome: a placebo-controlled study with polysomnography (CATOR). *Neurology* 2006;67:1040–6.

78. Trenkwalder C, Benes H, Grote L, et al. Cabergoline compared to levodopa in the treatment of patients with severe restless legs syndrome: results from a multi-center, randomized, active controlled trial. *Mov Disord* 2007;22:696–703.

79. Trenkwalder C, Paulus W. Restless legs syndrome: pathophysiology, clinical presentation and management. *Nat Rev Neurol* 2010;6:337–46.

80. Walters AS, Wagner ML, Hening WA, et al. Successful treatment of the idiopathic restless legs syndrome in a randomized double-blind trial of oxycodone versus placebo. *Sleep* 1993;16:327–32.

81. Ondo WG. Methadone for refractory restless legs syndrome. *Mov Disord* 2005;20:345–8.

82. Lauerma H, Markkula J. Treatment of restless legs syndrome with tramadol: an open study. *J Clin Psychiatry* 1999;60:241–4.

83. Vetrugno R, La Morgia C, D'Angelo R, et al. Augmentation of restless legs syndrome with long-term tramadol treatment. *Mov Disord* 2007;22:424–7.

83a. Earley C, Allen R. Restless legs syndrome augmentation associated with tramadol. *Sleep Med* 2006;7:592–3.

84. Vahedi H, Kuchle M, Trenkwalder C, et al. [Peridural morphine administration in restless legs status]. *Anasthesiol Intensivmed Notfallmed Schmerzther* 1994;29:368–70.

85. Bogan RK, Bornemann MA, Kushida CA, et al. Long-term maintenance treatment of restless legs syndrome with gabapentin enacarbil: a randomized controlled study. *Mayo Clin Proc* 2010;85:512–21.

86. Agarwal P, Griffith A, Costantino HR, et al. Gabapentin enacarbil—clinical efficacy in restless legs syndrome. *Neuropsychiatr Dis Treat* 2010;6:151–8.

87. Garcia-Borreguero D, Larrosa O, Williams AM, et al. Treatment of restless legs syndrome with pregabalin. A double-blind, placebo-controlled study. *Neurology* 2010;74:1897–904.

88. Allen R, Chen C, Soaita A, et al. A randomized, double-blind, 6-week, dose-ranging study of pregabalin in patients with restless legs syndrome. *Sleep Med* 2010;11:512–19.

88a. Garcia-Borreguero D, Chen C, Allen R, et al. Long-term Efficacy and Augmentation Assessment of a Dopamine Agonist (Pramipexole) Compared with an Alpha-2-delta Ligand (Pregabalin) in Restless Legs Syndrome: Results of a Randomized, Double-Blinded, Placebo-Controlled Trial. American Academy of Neurology 2012, New Orleans, LA.

89. Sommer M, Bachmann CG, Liebetanz KM, et al. Pregabalin in restless legs syndrome with and without neuropathic pain. *Acta Neurol Scand* 2007;115:347–50.

90. Walters AS, Ondo WG, Kushida CA, et al. Gabapentin enacarbil in restless legs syndrome: a phase 2b, 2-week, randomized, double-blind, placebo-controlled trial. *Clin Neuropharmacol* 2009;32(6):311–20.

91. Kushida CA, Becker PM, Ellenbogen AL, et al. Randomized, double-blind, placebo-controlled study of XP13512/GSK1838262 in patients with RLS. *Neurology* 2009;72:439–46.

92. Ellenbogen AL, Thein SG, Winslow DH, et al. A 52-week study of gabapentin enacarbil in restless legs syndrome. *Clin Neuropharmacol* 2011;34:8–16.

93. Winkelman JW, Bogan RK, Schmidt MH, et al. Randomized polysomnography study of gabapentin enacarbil in subjects with restless legs syndrome. *Mov Disord* 2011;26:2065–72.

94. Lee DO, Ziman RB, Perkins AT, et al. A randomized, double-blind, placebo-controlled study to assess the efficacy and tolerability of gabapentin enacarbil in subjects with restless legs syndrome. *J Clin Sleep Med* 2011;7:282–92.

95. Micozkadioglu H, Ozdemir FN, Kut A, et al. Gabapentin versus levodopa for the treatment of restless legs syndrome in hemodialysis patients: an open-label study. *Ren Fail* 2004;26:393–7.

96. Saletu M, Anderer P, Saletu-Zyhlarz GM, et al. Comparative placebo-controlled polysomnographic and psychometric studies on the acute effects of gabapentin versus ropinirole in restless legs syndrome. *J Neural Transm* 2011;117:463–73.

97. Boghen D, Lamothe L, Elie R, et al. The treatment of the restless legs syndrome with clonazepam: a prospective controlled study. *Can J Neurol Sci* 1986;13:245–7.

98. Montagna P, de Bianchi LS, Zucconi M, et al. Clonazepam and vibration in restless leg syndrome. *Acta Neurol Scand* 1984;69:428–30.

99. Horiguchi J, Inami Y, Sasaki A, et al. Periodic leg movements in sleep with restless legs syndrome: effect of clonazepam treatment. *Jpn J Psychiatry Neurol* 1992;46:727–32.

100. Saletu M, Anderer P, Saletu-Zyhlarz G, et al. Restless legs syndrome (RLS) and periodic limb movement disorder (PLMD): acute placebo-controlled sleep laboratory studies with clonazepam. *Eur Neuropsychopharmacol* 2001;11:153–61.

101. Schenck CH, Mahowald MW. Long-term, nightly benzodiazepine treatment of injurious parasomnias and other disorders of disrupted nocturnal sleep in 170 adults. *Am J Med* 1996;100:333–7.

102. Roche. Klonopin tablets labeling information http://www.accessdata.fda.gov/drugsatfda_docs/label/2009/017533s045,020813s005lbl.pdf.

103. Partinen M, Hirvonen K, Jama L, et al. Open-label study of the long-term efficacy and safety of pramipexole in patients with restless legs syndrome

(extension of the PRELUDE study). *Sleep Med* 2008;9:537–41.

104. Silber MH, Ehrenberg BL, Allen RP, et al. An algorithm for the management of restless legs syndrome *Mayo Clin Proc* 2004;79 916–22.

105. Wang X, Wiesinger J, Beard J, et al. Thy1 expression in the brain is affected by iron and is decreased in restless legs syndrome. *J Neurol Sci* 2004;220:59–66.

106. Allen RP, Barker PB, Wehrl F, et al. MRI measurement of brain iron in patients with restless legs syndrome. *Neurology* 2001;56:263–5.

107. Connor JC, Boyer PJ, Menzies SL, et al. Neuropathological examination suggests impaired brain iron acquisition in restless legs syndrome. *Neurology* 2003;61:304–9.

108. Wang J, O'Reilly B, Venkataraman R, et al. Efficacy of oral iron in patients with restless legs syndrome and a low-normal ferritin: a randomized, double-blind, placebo-controlled study. *Sleep Med* 2009;10:973–5.

109. Earley CJ, Heckler D, Allen RP. The treatment of restless legs syndrome with intravenous iron dextran. *Sleep Med* 2004;5:231–5.

110. Earley CJ, Heckler D, Allen RP. Repeated IV doses of iron provides effective supplemental treatment of restless legs syndrome. *Sleep Med* 2005;6:301–5.

111. Earley CJ, Horska A, Mohamed MA, et al. A randomized, double-blind, placebo-controlled trial of intravenous iron sucrose in restless legs syndrome. *Sleep Med* 2009;10:206–11.

112. Grote L, Leissner L, Hedner J, et al. A randomized, double-blind, placebo controlled, multi-center study of intravenous iron sucrose and placebo in the treatment of restless legs syndrome. *Mov Disord* 2009;24:1445–52.

113. Manconi M, Govoni V, De Vito A, et al. Restless legs syndrome and pregnancy. *Neurology* 2004;63:1065–9.

114. Chesson AL, Jr., Wise M, Davila D, et al. Practice parameters for the treatment of restless legs syndrome and periodic limb movement disorder. An American Academy of Sleep Medicine Report.

Standards of Practice Committee of the American Academy of Sleep Medicine. *Sleep* 1999;22:961–8.

115. Littner MR, Kushida C, Anderson WM, et al. Practice parameters for the dopaminergic treatment of restless legs syndrome and periodic limb movement disorder. *Sleep* 2004;27:557–9.

116. England SJ, Picchietti DL, Couvadelli BV, et al. L-dopa improves restless legs syndrome and periodic limb movements in sleep but not attention-deficit-hyperactivity disorder in a double-blind trial in children. *Sleep Med* 2011;12:471–7.

117. Walters AS, Mandelbaum DE, Lewin DS, et al. Dopaminergic therapy in children with restless legs/periodic limb movements in sleep and ADHD. Dopaminergic Therapy Study Group. *Pediatr Neurol* 2000;22:182–6.

118. Konofal E, Arnulf I, Lecendreux M, et al. Ropinirole in a child with attention-deficit hyperactivity disorder and restless legs syndrome. *Pediatr Neurol* 2005;32:350–1.

119. Winkelmann J. The genetics of restless legs syndrome. *Sleep Med* 2002;(3 Suppl):S9–12.

120. Garcia-Borreguero D, Stillman P, Benes H, et al. Algorithms for the diagnosis and treatment of restless legs syndrome in primary care. *BMC Neurology* 2011;11:28.

121. Guilleminault C, Cetel M, Philip P. Dopaminergic treatment of restless legs and rebound phenomenon. *Neurology* 1993;43:445.

122. Garcia-Borreguero D, Odin P, Schwarz C. Restless legs syndrome: an overview of the current understanding and management. *Acta Neurol Scand* 2004;109:303–17.

123. Garcia-Borreguero D, Allen R, Kohnen R, et al. Loss of response during long-term treatment of restless legs syndrome: guidelines approved by the International Restless Legs Syndrome Study Group for use in clinical trials. *Sleep Med* 2010;11:956–7.

124. Garcia-Borreguero D, Williams AM. Dopaminergic augmentation of restless legs syndrome. *Sleep Med Rev* 2010;14:339–46.

49

Periodic Limb Movements in Sleep

ALEX DESAUTELS, MARTIN MICHAUD, PAOLA A. LANFRANCHI,
GILLES J. LAVIGNE, AND JACQUES Y. MONTPLAISIR

PERIODIC LIMB movements in sleep (PLMS) represent stereotyped repetitive movements of the lower and upper extremities that occur during sleep. These motor activities were originally documented in the lower limbs, especially in patients afflicted with the restless legs syndrome (RLS).[1] They were later reported in a wide variety of disorders and in normal subjects, especially among elderly individuals.

PERIODIC ARM MOVEMENTS

Several authors have mentioned the presence of arm paresthesia in patients with RLS.[2-5] In a study of 230 patients diagnosed with RLS, arm paresthesia was reported by 48.7% of the patients.[5] In rare cases, symptoms are reported in the arms before occurrence of any symptoms in the legs.[6] The presence of periodic arm movements (PAMs) has been evaluated in the sleep laboratory in 22 patients diagnosed with RLS, 15 of them showed PAMs during wakefulness but only three patients showed a PAM index

during sleep greater than 5.[7] However, PAMs have not been studied in diagnostic categories other than RLS, and in the latter they were not investigated systematically for patterns of motor activation or pathophysiology. Arm restlessness may appear during augmentation, which is a long-term adverse effect of dopaminergic treatments.[8] However, PAMs were not studied in this condition.

Therefore, the present chapter will focus on leg movements only, and the acronym "PLMS" will be used throughout the text to designate periodic leg movements in sleep.

PERIODIC LIMB MOVEMENTS IN SLEEP: DEFINITION AND CHARACTERISTICS

PLMS are best described as rhythmical extension of the big toe and dorsiflexion of the ankle, with occasional flexion of the knee and hip.[9] The quantification of PLMS is routinely performed in the sleep laboratory by the recording of bilateral surface electromyogram (EMG) of the anterior tibialis muscles.[9] The EMG picture of a single movement can vary from one sustained contraction to polyclonic bursts with a frequency of approximately 5 Hz.[10] PLMS cluster into episodes, each of which lasts several minutes and even hours. In general, these episodes are more numerous in the first half of the night, but they can also recur throughout the entire sleep period. Recently four normal subjects with a PLMS index >20 were studied in a forced desynchrony protocol with an imposed sleep-wake cycle of 20 hours for 12 "nights." A significant circadian rhythm of PLMS was found that peaked at the circadian phases when usual sleep onset occurs, preceding the evening rise in melatonin secretion.[11]

Sleep stages are known to modulate PLMS frequency and periodicity, at least in patients with RLS.[12–14] In a study of 100 patients diagnosed with RLS, PLMS were significantly shorter during rapid eye movement (REM) sleep. Indices (number of PLM per hour of sleep) calculated for stage 1, stage 2, stage 3, and stage 4 non-REM sleep were not statistically different from each other but were all significantly higher than the index of PLM in REM sleep.[14] The distribution of intermovement intervals (IMIs) was also clearly influenced by sleep stages. There was a progressive lengthening of IMI from stage 1 to stage 4 non-REM sleep, and the distribution during REM sleep was similar to that of stage 1 non-REM sleep.

PERIODIC LIMB MOVEMENTS IN SLEEP QUANTIFICATION

The standard method for recording PLMS was originally developed by Coleman[7] and was recently revised by a joined task force of the World Association of Sleep Medicine and the International RLS Study Group (IRLSSG).[15] According to these criteria, PLMS are scored only if they are part of a series of four or more consecutive movements lasting 0.5 to 10 seconds with an IMI of 5 to 90 seconds and amplitude greater than 8 microvolts above the baseline EMG signal. A PLMS index (number of PLMS per hour of sleep) greater than 5 for the entire night of sleep was previously considered pathological[7] and can still be used for children, but since elevated PLMS indices are found in a large percentage of healthy adults, an index greater than 15 is now used as a cutoff in older individuals.

The number of PLMS may vary considerably from one night to the other in the same individual in both children and adults, especially in individuals with less severe sleep complaints.[16–18] For this reason, it is recommended to record more than one night for optimal assessment of PLMS. An alternative strategy is to use actigraphic methods for recording PLMS during several consecutive nights.[19–21] Currently, there are still controversies over the diagnostic value of the actigraphic method, but actigraphy is currently used for follow-up evaluation and assessment of treatment outcome. In patients with hundreds of PLMS, visual scoring of each leg movement is a time-consuming task. Consequently, computer-assisted methods were developed and showed high concordance with visual scoring method.[22] Other methodological developments include procedures to better define the periodicity of PLMS.[23,24]

PERIODIC LIMB MOVEMENTS IN SLEEP AND MICROAROUSALS

PLMS are often associated with electroencephalographic (EEG) signs of arousal. In patients with RLS, the indices of PLMS associated with arousal were found to correlate with the international RLS severity score.[25] These arousals may be of short duration, insufficient for scoring an epoch as wakefulness, and are therefore named microarousals (MAs). The ASDA[26] provided rules to score for MA based on the visual analysis of the EEG. In non-REM sleep, MAs are defined as a return to alpha or theta activity lasting between 3 and 15 seconds. They are well differentiated from the background EEG activity. In REM sleep, criteria include, in addition to EEG changes, an increase in chin EMG amplitude. Using these criteria, almost 34% of PLMS seen in patients with RLS were associated with MA.[21] However, EEG spectral analysis revealed that PLMS with MA are associated with an increase in alpha, theta, and delta power, whereas PLMS without visually detected MA are associated with a significant increase in delta and theta activity.[27] Major differences can be found in the literature with regard to the percentage of PLMS associated with MA. This discrepancy may result from different definitions of MA but also from the low interrater reliability for scoring MA.[28]

Studies investigating sleep microstructure have identified the presence of a rhythmic sequence of EEG events during non-REM sleep (including delta bursts, EEG arousals or MAs, K-alpha complexes), which are distinct from the background EEG and occur with a periodicity of 2–60 seconds (mostly 20–40 seconds).[29] This pattern, so-called cyclic alternating pattern (CAP), is believed to represent an arousal rhythm and be a marker of unstable sleep. A CAP cycle consists of a phase A (the repetitive element) and a phase B (the intervening background). Typically, several cycles follow each other to form CAP sequences. Sequences are separated by non-CAP periods (i.e., absence of CAP for >60 seconds).[30] One study looking at EEG changes associated with PLMS in patients with insomnia found that compared to normal controls, insomniac subjects with PLMS had a significantly higher amounts of CAP time and CAP rate.[31] Ninety-two percent (92%) of the PLMS detected in non-REM sleep occurred during CAP with the great majority of limb movements (96%) associated with phase A (arousals and arousal-equivalent features). On the other hand, only 39% of CAP sequences were associated with PLMS, suggesting that CAP is not the generator of nighttime movements but, rather, operates as a gate-control rhythm that sets the pace of their periodic appearance.[31]

PERIODIC LIMB MOVEMENTS IN SLEEP AND CARDIOVASCULAR CHANGES

Recently, more attention has been paid to other signs of physiological activation associated with PLMS, both in patients with RLS and normal controls with PLMS. Regardless of the presence of MA, PLMS are associated with a tachycardia (decrease of R-R intervals) lasting approximately 5 to 10 beats after the onset of leg movements[27,32] followed by a bradycardia.[27] Both gender and age influence the magnitude of the cardiac activation associated with PLMS. The magnitude of electrocardiogram (ECG) changes (both tachycardia and bradycardia) appears to be higher in young males and to markedly decrease with age. In females, the amplitude of ECG activation shows no change across age groups. In addition to ECG changes, beat-to-beat monitoring of blood pressure (BP) during sleep conducted on RLS patients in our laboratory showed that PLMS are associated with a significant increase of systolic (mean increase of 22 mmHg) and diastolic (mean increase of 11 mmHg) BP (Fig. 49.1). Increments of SBP as high as 50 mmHg were seen in some individuals.[33] These BP changes were positively correlated with age and with the duration of RLS.

Interestingly, the investigation of cardiovascular changes in association with PLMS, and especially their temporal relationship with EEG changes, provides new insights into the physiological substrates of PLMS. Studies consistently reported that changes in heart rate and EEG activity precede the leg movement by several seconds. Specifically, the heart rate and EEG delta waves increase first, then motor activity appears, and eventually there is a progressive activation of the EEG.[27,34–37] The study of the time course of RR and EEG changes in association with leg movements confirmed that the low-frequency components of RR variability (an index of cardiac sympathetic influences) are the first physiological change to occur, followed by delta EEG, and finally the leg movement with or without faster EEG frequencies.[36] These data support the hypothesis of an integrative hierarchy of arousal responses primarily involving the autonomic system with sympathetic excitation, then EEG synchronization (phase A of CAP) progressing toward EEG arousal and eventually awakening.

Since RLS patients may have several hundred PLMS every night, PLMS-related BP fluctuations could contribute to the increased risk of cardiovascular diseases in RLS reported in two large epidemiological studies, that is the Wisconsin Sleep Cohort[38] and the Sleep Heart Health Study.[39] The contribution of PLMS to cardiovascular disease is supported by a series of recent findings.[40] For example, patients with a history of stroke have a greater prevalence and severity of PLMS,[41] and PLMS were associated with cerebral hemodynamic alterations measured by infrared spectroscopy.[42] PLMS are also frequent in patients with heart failure.[43–45] Recently it was shown that a PLMS index ≥ 5 was associated with a three-fold increase of mortality risk over a period of 39 months in patients with systolic heart failure.[45]

PREVALENCE OF PERIODIC LIMB MOVEMENTS IN SLEEP IN THE NORMAL POPULATION AND IN VARIOUS SLEEP AND OTHER MEDICAL DISORDERS

PLMS were first polygraphically documented in RLS patients.[46]

Most of what is known about PLMS comes from the study of RLS patients. In a study of

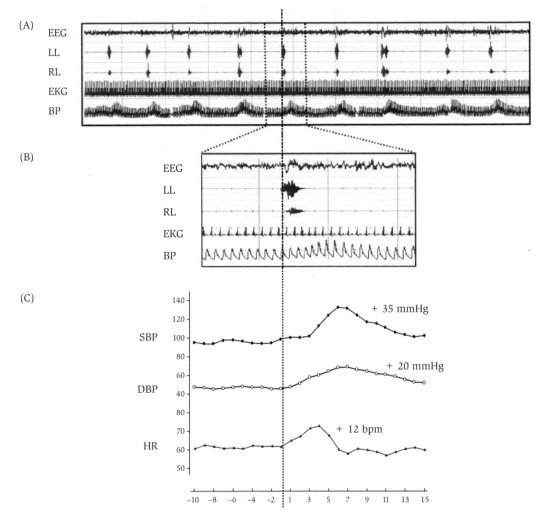

(A)

EEG
LL
RL
EKG
BP

(B)

EEG
LL
RL
EKG
BP

(C)

SBP

DBP

HR

+ 35 mmHg

+ 20 mmHg

+ 12 bpm

FIGURE 49.1 Periodic leg movements during sleep and related beat-to-beat blood pressure, electrocardiogram, and EEG signals, presented (A) in a compact window and (B) in a wider temporal window. The portion of signals shown in (B) represents the temporal window used for the analyses. (C) The corresponding measurements of systolic blood pressure, diastolic blood pressure, and heart rate. BP, blood pressure; DBP, diastolic blood pressure; EEG, electroencephalogram; EKG, electrocardiogram; HR, heart rate; LL, left leg; RL, right leg; SBP, systolic blood pressure. (Reproduced with permission from Pennestri et al.[33])

131 cases of RLS, a PLMS index greater than 5 was found in 82.2% of the patients during one night of polysomnographic recording. In 49 patients recorded for two consecutive nights, 87.8% were found to meet this criterion on either night.[4] In RLS, the mean PLMS index increases with age. In the study of 183 patients performed in our laboratory, the mean PLMS index was 15.1 for patients aged 20 to 39 years, 25.4 for those aged 40 to 59 years, and 44.4 for patients aged 60 years or older. The PLMS index

was also found to be correlated with RLS severity independently of age.[5]

PLMS also co-occur with a wide range of sleep-wake complaints, including sleep onset difficulty, nocturnal awakenings, and daytime sleepiness.[46] A multicenter collaborative study involving 18 sleep disorders clinics reported PLMS to be the primary polysomnographic finding in 18% of patients complaining of a trouble initiating and maintaining sleep and in 11% of hypersomniac patients complaining of excessive daytime sleepiness (EDS).[47] In the absence of any other cause, insomnia or hypersomnia with PLMS is referred to as periodic leg movements disorder (PLMD).

PLMS occurs in several sleep disorders, including narcolepsy, REM sleep behavior disorder (RBD), and obstructive sleep apnea syndrome (OSAS) (for review, see ref 48). Indeed, several studies have shown an increased prevalence of PLMS in adulthood and childhood narcolepsy.[49-53] For example, a PLMS index greater than 10 was found in 53% of 161 narcoleptic patients compared to 21% for 116 age-matched normal controls recorded in our laboratory.[50] Narcoleptic patients with an elevated PLMS index had a higher percentage of stage 1 sleep, a decrease of REM sleep percentage and REM sleep efficacy, and a shorter mean latency on the multiple sleep latency test performed the next day. Considering that PLMS are also found in narcoleptic dogs,[54] PLMS may be seen as an intrinsic component of narcolepsy.

PLMS are also highly prevalent in RBD,[49,55-58] a condition in which they were found to be more numerous in REM sleep compared to those seen in RLS patients or normal controls. Manconi and coworkers[53] reported PLMS in 17/20 patients with RBD. PLMS occurred more frequently during REM sleep, were shorter in duration, less often bilateral, and with a higher IMI in patients with RBD compared to those with RLS. Patients with RBD showed a lower LM periodicity compared with patients with RLS (Fig. 49.2). Fantini and coworkers[57] also reported a decreased autonomic response to PLMS in RBD patients.

PLMS were also repeatedly reported in patients with OSAS.[59-60] In this condition, leg movements may occur at the end of apneas in association with arousal responses. Patients with OSAS also have PLMS independent of apnea episodes. In one study, leg movements with long IMIs were found to be associated with respiratory events, while those with short intervals represented PLMS independent of respiration.[61] It should be noted that PLMS found in OSAS patients decrease but remain elevated when patients are treated with nasal continuous positive airway pressure.[61-63] The prevalence and characteristics of leg movements in OSAS and the relationship with respiratory events remain to be further elucidated.

PLMS are also found in a variety of other medical conditions and in patients treated with a variety of medications, especially tricyclic antidepressants, 5-HT reuptake blockers, and neuroleptics. Among medical conditions

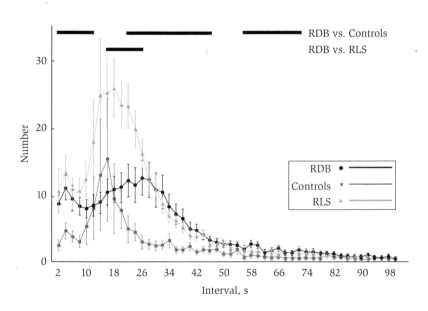

FIGURE 49.2   Distribution of intermovement intervals in controls, patients with REM sleep behavior disorder (RBD), and patients with restless legs syndrome (RLS); values are shown as mean and standard error. (Reproduced with permission from Manconi et al.[53])

associated with PLMS, renal failure, anemia, peripheral neuropathy, and rheumatoid arthritis are also associated with RLS.[64] PLMS seen in these conditions will not be discussed in detail here. The presence of PLMS was also recently reported in 6 out of 14 children (38%) with fibromyalgia.[65] In a study of 69 children who met the criteria for attention-deficit/hyperactivity disorder (ADHD), 27 were found to have clinical evidence of PLMS. When recorded in the sleep laboratory, 18 of these 27 children had a PLMS index greater than 5. The authors raised the possibility of comorbidity between ADHD and PLMS.[66] PLMS were also reported in five out of seven patients with Tourette's syndrome. Four of these patients also reported PAM.[67]

PLMS are also quite frequent in noncomplaining subjects. In a community-based sample of 593 subjects, Scofield and coworkers[68] found that 7.6% of the participants had a PLMS index >15. This prevalence was lower for African Americans compared to Caucasians (4.3 vs. 9.3%). This ethnic difference was also noted in other adults[69] and children populations.[70] PLMS also increases with advancing age. Whereas PLMS are rare in young individuals without RLS, they are relatively common in the elderly.[71-76] PLMS are rarely seen in subjects under the age of 40, but then the index increases dramatically.[76] The mean index is around 2 per hour of sleep in normal subjects between 30 and 40 years old, 11 in subjects age 40 to 50, 17 in subjects age 50 to 60, and 22 in subjects age 60 and older.[76] As in patients with RLS, PLMS seen in noncomplaining subjects exhibit a clear periodicity at intervals of 15 to 25 seconds.[76] One study found that PLMS seen in normal controls are of shorter duration than movements found in RLS.[77]

FUNCTIONAL SIGNIFICANCE OF PERIODIC LIMB MOVEMENTS IN SLEEP

The fact that PLMS are seen in patients who complain of primary sleep-onset, sleep-maintenance insomnia, or EDS suggests that PLMS may be responsible for the nonrestorative sleep and daytime somnolence reported by these patients. Although some studies have suggested that PLMS may be associated with sleep-wake complaints or with nocturnal sleep fragmentation,[78-79] a great majority of authors have concluded that PLMS have little impact on nocturnal sleep or daytime vigilance. As early as 1972, Lugaresi

and coworkers[80] concluded on the basis of their polysomnographic findings that PLMS were not responsible for sleep impairment. In 1980, Coleman[46] also suggested that there was no evidence that PLMS actually cause insomnia. More recently, several studies conducted on elderly individuals showed a lack of correlation between PLMS and subjective sleep complaints.[75,81,82] A study of younger insomniacs with and without PLMS also concluded that PLMS did not appear to be the primary cause of sleep disturbance in these patients.[83]

Similarly, in hypersomniac patients with PLMS there is no indication that these movements actually cause sleep disruption resulting in EDS. Two studies have shown a lack of correlation between the severity of PLMS and the mean sleep latency on the multiple sleep latency tests (MSLT) in patients with hypersomnia.[75,84-85] In one of these studies the mean sleep latency on the MSLT was negatively correlated with sleep efficiency at night; for example, the higher was sleep efficiency, the shorter was sleep latency during the day, suggesting that the propensity to fall asleep was present both at night and in the daytime and was independent of nocturnal sleep disruption. The same conclusion arises when one considers not only the PLMS index but also the PLMS with arousal index. In 1996, Mendelson[84] found no correlation between PLM arousal index and the subjective complaint of disturbed sleep, a sense of waking up refreshed in the morning, or an objective measure of daytime sleepiness. Clinical experience also reveals that hypersomniacs with PLMS respond positively to psychostimulants but not to treatment of PLMS with dopaminergic agents.

The question of the potential contribution of PLMS to nocturnal sleep disruption and impairment of daytime functioning remains unsettled and currently under investigation, especially those PLMS that are associated with EEG arousals.

PATHOPHYSIOLOGY

Neural Substrates

The decrease of PLMS index and duration noted during REM sleep is most likely the result of the motor inhibition characteristic of this stage. However, the presence of a significant number of PLMS during REM sleep suggests that REM sleep inhibition of spinal motor neurons is not complete throughout the REM sleep period, at least in patients with RLS-PLMS or PLMS only.

There is most likely a spinal cord contribution to PLMS. PLMS were found during epidural and spinal anesthesia.[86] They were also found in patients with spinal cord lesions or complete spinal cord transection.[87-91] These observations demonstrate that the spinal cord has all the neural substrates necessary for generating PLMS. Other motor rhythms originating from the spinal cord have been extensively studied, leading to the general idea of a central pattern generator.[92] The central pattern generator has been shown to be sensitive to both peripheral and central influences and to a variety of pharmacological agents, including levodopa.[93]

Videographic analyses revealed that PLMS have the same features as the abnormal plantar response (Babinsky response) noted during wakefulness in patients with pyramidal track lesion.[94] These features are a dorsiflexion of the ankle, of the small toes (with fanning), of the great toe, and, at times, a flexion of the knee and hip. On the other hand, a similar Babinsky response to plantar stimulation has been reported as a normal occurrence during non-REM sleep[95,96] and may represent a decrease of supraspinal descending inhibitory influences in non-REM sleep. Based on these findings, Smith[94] proposed in 1985 that PLMS are due to an exacerbation of the normal suppression of this sleep-related supraspinal inhibitory influence.

The contribution of the spinal cord to the pathophysiology of PLMS has been tested by Bara-Jimenez and coworkers.[97] They found a similarity between the pattern of muscle recruitment and spatial spread of late components of the flexor reflex elicited by stimulating medial plantar nerve and those of spontaneous PLMS. In addition, in comparison to control subjects, patients with both RLS and PLMS showed increased spinal cord excitability as indicated by a lower threshold and a greater spatial spread of the flexor reflex.[97] These results further support the hypothesis that PLMS result from a loss of supraspinal inhibitory influences. However, only patients with RLS-PLMS were tested, and further studies should include subjects with PLMS only. In a study of 26 syringomyelia patients, PLMS were found in 62% of patients even at a young age.[98] The authors concluded that the PLMS generator is located in the lumbar spinal cord and that propriospinal pathways are probably

involved. Wechsler and coworkers[99] studied the blink reflex in six patients with PLMS. Although only two components are normally found, three components were seen in five patients and four components in one patient. In addition, the second component of the blink reflex of these patients did not habituate as it normally does.[99,100] These electrophysiological abnormalities suggest a disorder of the central nervous system, producing increased excitability of segmental reflexes and operating at the pontine level or just rostral to it.[99,100]

Back-averaging techniques found no pre-movement potentials for PLMS.[10,101] Functional magnetic resonance imaging performed in patients with RLS and PLMS showed that PLMs in wakefulness were associated with pontine and red nucleus activation without cortical activation.[102] These results suggest that the motor cortex is not directly involved in triggering PLMS but that does not preclude to a role for the cerebral cortex in the hyperexcitability of the motor system found in patients with PLMS.

Finally, a significant genomewide association with a common variant of BTBD9 on chromosome 6p was found for PLMS in patients with or without RLS and no such association was found in RLS patients without PLMS.[103]

Neurotransmitter Dysfunction: Role of Dopamine

Several observations are consistent with the view that PLMS results from dopaminergic dysfunction. Placebo-controlled studies showed that levodopa[104,105] and dopaminergic agonists, especially pergolide[106-107] and pramipexole,[108] suppress PLMS in patients with RLS, whereas gamma-hydroxybutyrate,[109] a short-acting blocker of dopamine release, was found to increase PLMS, in both RLS and narcoleptic patients.

Brain imaging using single-photon emission computed tomography with D_2-receptor ligand, showed a decrease of D_2-receptor binding sites in the striatum of patients with RLS and PLMS or PLMS alone.[110-114] One of these studies also showed decreased binding to the presynaptic transporter of dopamine.[113] Two positron emission tomography (PET) studies measured nigrostriatal terminal dopamine storage with 18 F-DOPA and striatal D_2-receptor binding with 11 C-raclopride in RLS-PLMS patients.[115,116] Both pre- and postsynaptic bindings were found to be decreased in patients in comparison to controls. However, these PET studies were performed in patients with RLS and PLMS and not in patients with PLMS alone.

Another series of evidence supporting the dopaminergic hypothesis of PLMS comes from the study of conditions frequently associated with PLMS. As discussed previously, the prevalence of PLMS is higher in at least three sleep disorders, namely, RLS, narcolepsy, and RBD.[49] There are several indications that these three conditions are associated with impaired dopamine transmission. Evidence to support a dopamine hypothesis for RLS has been discussed earlier in this chapter and in other sections of this book. In narcolepsy, patients are best treated with psychostimulants that facilitate dopamine transmission in the central nervous system,[117] and there are several other evidence implicating dopamine in canine and human narcolepsy.[118] A brain imaging study emphasized a dopamine implication in RBD,[119] a condition associated with Parkinson's disease,[120,121] and with high prevalence of PLMS.

Other evidence in favor of the dopamine hypothesis of PLMS comes from the study of Parkinson's disease[122] and levodopa-responsive dystonia.[123] A study of unmedicated Parkinson's disease patients revealed an increase of PLM indices during both sleep and wakefulness in comparison to healthy controls of the same age.[122] Conversely, Ancoli-Israel and coworkers[124] have studied the prevalence of PLMS in schizophrenia, a condition characterized by an increase in dopamine in subcortical regions.[125] Only 14% of these patients (age 45–76) had elevated PLMS indices (PLMS index greater than 5). These authors concluded that elevated dopamine in subcortical areas in schizophrenia may be protective against PLMS.[124]

The dopamine hypothesis may also account for the increase in PLMS with advancing age. A decrease in D_2-receptor density and dopamine transporter binding occurs both in animals and in humans during the course of normal aging.[126,127] In this view, the increase in PLMS seen in elderly individuals may represent a biological marker of an age-related decrease in dopaminergic transmission.

In summary, neurophysiologic data suggest that PLMS may result from suprasegmental disinhibition at the brainstem and spinal cord levels. However, how a decreased dopamine transmission could lead to increased spinal cord excitability remains unclear. The presence of descending dopamine pathways in the central nervous system has been well identified, and these neuronal pathways may be involved. Most studies have looked at the dopaminergic diencephalospinal systems (A11).[128–130] In animals, experimental lesions of dopamine neurons in the diencephalon (A11)[131] and in the striatum[132] by 6-hydroxydopamine (6-OHDA) resulted in increased motor activity. Similarly, an injection of 6-OHDA into the striatum led to an increase in motor activity during sleep and especially during REM sleep.[132] These effects may mimic some of the symptoms of RLS, but no clear evidence of PLM was seen in these animals. These results are concordant with the hypothesis that dopamine, and possibly the dopaminergic diencephalospinal system, are involved in the pathophysiology of PLMS, although the periodicity of limb movements noted in these animals remains to be demonstrated, as stated by Bara-Jimenez and coworkers.[97] Understanding the role of dopamine in PLMS pathophysiology will depend on elucidating its mechanisms and the complex interaction between dopamine and other neurotransmitters at different levels of the neuraxis.[97]

TREATMENT

Most of what is known about PLMS treatment comes from the study of patients with RLS. The dopamine precursor levodopa,[104,105] and dopamine receptor agonists, especially pramipexole[108] and ropinirole,[133] are the most potent suppressing agents of PLMS seen in primary RLS or in RLS secondary to uremia. In patients with RLS, levodopa and dopaminergic agonists increase sleep efficiency and total sleep duration, but a recent study looking at the acute effect of pramipexole showed a decrease of PLMS but no effect on CAP rate or manifestation of sleep instability/continuity associated with RLS.[134] In the same study, acute treatment with pramipexole reduced the number of PLMS and the amplitude of the autonomic response associated with residual PLMS but did not influence heart rate variability during sleep. The authors concluded that pramipexole had no effect on abnormal sympathicovagal regulation associated with RLS and PLMS. Gabapentin and pregabaline were also found to decrease PLMS and improve sleep architecture in patients with RLS and may represent an alternative therapeutic approach.[135]

Dopaminergic medications were also found effective to treat PLMS in patients with narcolepsy.[136] However, no study has evaluated the effect of dopaminergic agents on PLMS seen in patients with a primary complaint of insomnia or hypersomnia (without narcolepsy). In the absence of controlled clinical trials, the indications of dopaminergic agents in the treatment of PLMS in non-RLS patients remain a question of clinical judgment. It should also be remembered that dopaminergic agents may exert a stimulant effect that might further disrupt nocturnal sleep in patients with insomnia and PLMS.

The most commonly used medications to treat PLMS in non-RLS patients are benzodiazepines, especially clonazepam.[137-141] These drugs have been shown to improve the quality of nocturnal sleep and to slightly decrease the number of PLMS and the number of arousals associated with leg jerks. Recently, clonazepam was found to lower the EEG instability during NREM sleep (CAP) without significantly reducing the number of PLMS indicating an indirect association between arousals and PLMS.[142]. Other treatments used for RLS, such as opiates, gabapentin, carbamazepine, and clonidine, have not been systematically studied in the treatment of PLMS in patients without RLS. In summary, the decision to treat PLMS in non-RLS patients is based on clinical expertise and not on any controlled study. The treatments of choice are most likely the dopaminergic agents, although these drugs may either exert an alerting effect, especially in insomniac patients, or worsen EDS.

REFERENCES

1. Lugaresi E, Coccagna G, Besti-Ceroni G, et al. Particularités cliniques et polygraphiques du syndrome d'impatiences des membres inférieurs. *Rev Neurol* 1965;113:545–55.
2. Ekbom KA. Restless legs syndrome. *Neurology* 1960;10:868–73.
3. Ondo W, Jankovic J. Restless legs syndrome: clinicoetiologic correlates. *Neurology* 1996;47:1435–41.
4. Montplaisir J, Boucher S, Poirier G, et al. Clinical, polysomnographic, and genetic characteristics of restless legs syndrome: a study of 133 patients diagnosed with new standard criteria. *Mov Disord* 1997;12:61–5.
5. Michaud M, Chabli A, Lavigne G, et al. Arm restlessness in patients with restless legs syndrome. *Mov Disord* 2000;15:289–93.
6. Freedom T, Merchut MP. Arm restlessness as the initial symptom in restless legs syndrome. *Arch Neurol* 2003;60(7):1013–15.
7. Chabli A, Michaud M, Montplaisir J. Periodic arm movements in patients with the restless legs syndrome. *Eur Neurol* 2000;44:133–8.
8. García-Borreguero D, Williams AM. Dopaminergic augmentation of restless legs syndrome. *Sleep Med Rev* 2010;14(5):339–46.
9. Coleman RM. Periodic movements in sleep (nocturnal myoclonus) and restless legs syndrome. In Guilleminault C, ed. *Sleeping and Waking Disorders: Indications and Techniques.* Menlo Park, CA: Addison-Wesley; 1982:265–95.
10. Lugaresi E, Cirignotta F, Coccagna G, et al. Nocturnal myoclonus and restless legs syndrome. *Adv Neurol* 1986;43:295–307.
11. Duffy JF, Lowe AS, Silva EJ, et al. Periodic limb movements in sleep exhibit a circadian rhythm that is maximal in the late evening/early night. *Sleep Med* 2011;12(1):83–8.
12. Montplaisir J, Godbout R, Boghen D, et al. Familial restless legs with periodic movements in sleep: electrophysiological, biochemical, and pharmacological study. *Neurology* 1985;35:130–4.
13. Pollmächer T, Schulz H. Periodic leg movements (PLM): their relationship to sleep stages. *Sleep* 1993;16(6):572–7.
14. Nicolas A, Michaud M, Lavigne G, et al. The influence of sex, age and sleep/wake state on characteristics of periodic leg movements in RLS patients. *Electroencephalogr Clin Neurophysiol* 1999;110(7):1168–74.
15. Zucconi M, Ferri R, Allen R, et al. The official World Association of *Sleep Medicine* (WASM) standards for recording and scoring periodic leg movements in sleep (PLMS) and wakefulness (PLMW) developed in collaboration with a task force from the International Restless Legs Syndrome Study Group (IRLSSG). *Sleep Med* 2006;7(2):175–83.
16. Sforza E, Haba-Rubio J. Night-to-night variability in periodic leg movements in patients with restless legs syndrome. *Sleep Med* 2005;6(3):259–67.
17. Picchietti MA, Picchietti DL, England SJ, et al. Children show individual night-to-night variability of periodic limb movements in sleep. *Sleep* 2009;32(4):530–5.
18. Trotti LM, Bliwise DL, Greer SA, et al. Correlates of PLMs variability over multiple

nights and impact upon RLS diagnosis. *Sleep Med* 2009;10(6):668–71.

19. Sforza E, Zamagni M, Petiav C, et al. Actigraphy and leg movements during sleep: a validation study. *J Clin Neurophysiol* 1999;16:154–60.

20. King MA, Jaffre MO, Morrish E, et al. The validation of a new actigraphy system for the measurement of periodic leg movements in sleep. *Sleep Med* 2005;6(6):507–13.

21. Allen RP. Improving RLS diagnosis and severity assessment: polysomnography, actigraphy and RLS-sleep log. *Sleep Med* 2007;8(Suppl 2):S13–18.

22. Ferri R, Zucconi M, Manconi M, et al. Computer-assisted detection of nocturnal leg motor activity in patients with restless legs syndrome and periodic leg movements during sleep. *Sleep* 2005;28(8):998–1004.

23. Ferri R, Zucconi M, Manconi M, et al. New approaches to the study of periodic leg movements during sleep in restless legs syndrome. *Sleep* 2006;29(6):759–69.

24. Rummel C, Gast H, Schindler K, et al. Assessing periodicity of periodic leg movements during sleep. *Front Neurosci* 2010;4. pii:58.

25. Hornyak M, Hundemer HP, Quail D, et al. Relationship of periodic leg movements and severity of restless legs syndrome: a study in unmedicated and medicated patients. *Clin Neurophysiol* 2007;118(7):1532–7.

26. American Sleep Disorders Association. EEG arousal: scoring rules and examples. *Sleep* 1992;15:174–84.

27. Sforza E, Nicolas A, Lavigne G, et al. EEG and cardiac activation during periodic leg movements in sleep: support for a hierarchy of arousal responses. *Neurology* 1999;52:786–91.

28. Bliwise DL, Keenan S, Burnburg D, et al. Inter-rater reliability for scoring periodic leg movements in sleep: scoring and clinical interpretation. *Sleep* 1991;14(3):249–51.

29. Terzano MG, Mancia D, Salati MR, et al. The cyclic alternating pattern as a physiologic component of normal NREM sleep. *Sleep* 1985;8:137–45.

30. Terzano MG, et al. Atlas, rules, and recording techniques for the scoring of cyclic alternating pattern (CAP) in human sleep. *Sleep Med* 2002;3:187–99.

31. Parrino L, Boselli M, Buccino GP, et al. The cyclic alternating pattern plays a gate-control on periodic limb movements during non-rapid

eye movement sleep. *J Clin Neurophysiol* 1996;13(4):314–23.

32. Winkelman JW. The evoked heart rate response to periodic leg movements of sleep. *Sleep* 1999;22:575–80.

33. Pennestri MH, Montplaisir J, Colombo R, et al. Nocturnal blood pressure changes in patients with restless legs syndrome. *Neurology* 2007;68(15):1213–18.

34. Ferrillo F, Beelke M, Canovaro P, et al. Changes in cerebral and autonomic activity heralding periodic limb movements in sleep. *Sleep Med* 2004;5:407–12.

35. Allena M, Campus C, Morrone E, et al. Periodic limb movements both in non-REM and REM sleep: relationships between cerebral and autonomic activities. *Clin Neurophysiol* 2009;120(7):1282–90.

36. Guggisberg AG, Hess CW, Mathis J. The significance of the sympathetic nervous system in the pathophysiology of periodic leg movements in sleep. *Sleep* 2007;30(6):755–66.

37. Sforza E, Jouny C, Ibanez V. Time course of arousal response during periodic leg movements in patients with periodic leg movements and restless legs syndrome. *Clin Neurophysiol* 2003;114(6):1116–24.

38. Winkelman WJ, Fynn L, Young T. Prevalence and correlates of restless legs syndrome symptoms in the Wisconsin Sleep Cohort. *Sleep Med* 2006;7(7):545–52.

39. Winkelman WJ, Shahar E, Sharief I, et al. Association of restless legs syndrome and cardiovascular disease in the Sleep Heart Health Study. *Neurology* 2008;70(1):35–42.

40. Walters AS, Rye DB. Review of the relationship of restless legs syndrome and periodic limb movements in sleep to hypertension, heart disease, and stroke. *Sleep* 2009;32(5):589–97.

41. Coelho FM, Georgsson H, Narayansingh M, et al. Higher prevalence of periodic limb movements of sleep in patients with history of stroke. *J Clin Sleep Med* 2010;6(5):428–30.

42. Pizza F, Biallas M, Wolf M, et al. Periodic leg movements during sleep and cerebral hemodynamic changes detected by NIRS. *Clin Neurophysiol* 2009;120(7):1329–34.

43. Javaheri S. Sleep disorders in systolic heart failure: a prospective study of 100 male patients. The final report. *Int J Cardiol* 2006;106(1):21–8.

44. Skomro R, Silva R, Alves R, et al. The prevalence and significance of periodic

leg movements during sleep in patients with congestive heart failure. *Sleep Breath* 2009;13(1):43–7.

45. Yumino D, Wang H, Floras JS, et al. Relation of periodic leg movements during sleep and mortality in patients with systolic heart failure. *Am J Cardiol* 2011;107(3):447–51.

46. Coleman RM, Pollak CP, Weitzman ED. Periodic movements in sleep (nocturnal myoclonus): relation to sleep disorders. *Ann Neurol* 1980;8:416–21.

47. Hornyak M, Feige B, Riemann D, et al. Periodic leg movements in sleep and periodic limb movement disorder: prevalence, clinical significance and treatment. *Sleep Med Rev* 2006;10(3):169–77.

48. Coleman RM, Bliwise DL, Sajben N, et al. Epidemiology of periodic movements during sleep. In: Guilleminault C, Lugaresi E, eds. *Sleep/Wake Disorders: Natural History, Epidemiology, and Long-Term Evolution.* New York: Raven Press; 1983:217–30.

49. Montplaisir J, Michaud M, Denesle R, et al. Periodic leg movements are not more prevalent in insomnia or hypersomnia but are specifically associated with sleep disorders involving a dopaminergic impairment. *Sleep Med* 2000;1:163–7.

50. Dauvilliers Y, Pennestri MH, Petit D, et al. Periodic leg movements during sleep and wakefulness in narcolepsy. *J Sleep Res* 2007;16(3):333–9.

51. Dauvilliers Y, Pennestri MH, Whittom S, et al. Autonomic response to periodic leg movements during sleep in narcolepsy-cataplexy. *Sleep* 2011;34(2):219–23.

52. Ferri R, Franceschini C, Zucconi M, et al. Sleep polygraphic study of children and adolescents with narcolepsy/cataplexy. *Dev Neuropsychol* 2009;34(5):523–38.

53. Manconi M, Ferri R, Zucconi M, et al. Time structure analysis of leg movements during sleep in REM sleep behavior disorder. *Sleep* 2007;30(12):1779–85.

54. Okura M, Fujiki N, Ripley B, et al. Narcoleptic canines display periodic leg movements during sleep. *Psychiatry Clin Neurosci* 2001;55(3):243–4.

55. Schenck CH, Hurwitz TD, Mahowald MW. REM sleep behaviour disorder: an update on a series of 96 patients and a review of the world literature. *Sleep Res* 1993;2:224–31.

56. Lapierre O, Montplaisir J. Polysomnographic features of REM sleep behavior disorder:

development of a scoring method. *Neurology* 1992;42:1371–4.

57. Fantini ML, Michaud M, Gosselin N, et al. Periodic leg movements in REM sleep behavior disorder and related autonomic and EEG activation. *Neurology* 2002;59(12):1889–94.

58. Dauvilliers Y, Rompré S, Gagnon JF, et al. REM sleep characteristics in narcolepsy and REM sleep behavior disorder. *Sleep* 2007;30(7):844–9.

59. Fry JM, DiPillipo MA, Pressman MR. Periodic leg movements in sleep following treatment of obstructive sleep apnea with nasal continuous positive airway pressure. *Chest* 1989;96:89–91.

60. Briellmann RS, Mathis J, Bassetti C, et al. Patterns of muscle activity in legs in sleep apnea patients before and during nCPAP therapy. *Eur Neurol* 1997;38:113–18.

61. Carelli G, Krieger J, Calvi-Gries F, et al. Periodic limb movements and obstructive sleep apneas before and after continuous positive airway pressure treatment. *J Sleep Res* 1999;8:211–16.

62. Yamashiro Y, Kryger MH. Acute effect of nasal CPAP on periodic limb movements associated with breathing disorders during sleep. *Sleep* 1994;17:172–5.

63. Morisson F, Decary A, Petit D, et al. Daytime sleepiness and EEG spectral analysis in apneic patients before and after treatment with continuous positive airway pressure. *Chest* 2001;119:45–52.

64. Montplaisir J, Nicolas A, Godbout R, et al. Restless legs syndrome and periodic limb movement disorder. In: Kryger MH, Roth T, Dement WC, eds. *Principles and Practice of Sleep Medicine.* Philadelphie, PA: WB Saunders; 2000:742–52.

65. Tayag-Kier CE, Keenan GF, Scalzi LV, et al. Sleep and periodic limb movement in sleep in juvenile fibromyalgia. *Pediatrics* 2000;106:E70.

66. Picchietti DL, England SJ, Walters AS, et al. Periodic limb movement disorder and restless legs syndrome in children with attention-deficit hyperactivity disorder. *J Child Neurol* 1999;13:588–94.

67. Voderholzer U, Muller N, Haag C, et al. Periodic limb movements during sleep are a frequent finding in patients with Gilles de la Tourette's syndrome. *J Neurol* 1997;244:521–6.

68. Scofield H, Roth T, Drake C. Periodic limb movements during sleep: population prevalence, clinical correlates, and racial differences. *Sleep* 2008;31(9):1221–7.

69. Lee JH, Parker KP, Ansari FP, et al. A secondary analysis of racial differences in periodic leg movements in sleep and ferritin in hemodialysis patients. *Sleep Med* 2006;7(8):646–8.

70. O'Brien LM, Holbrook CR, Faye Jones V, et al. Ethnic difference in periodic limb movements in children. *Sleep Med* 2007;8(3):240–6.

71. Bixler EO, Kales A, Vela-Bueno A, et al. Nocturnal myoclonus and nocturnal myoclonic activity in a normal population. *Res Commun Chem Pathol Pharmacol* 1982;36:129–40.

72. Ancoli-Israel S, Kripke D, Mason W, et al. Sleep apnea and periodic movements in an aging sample. *J Gerontol* 1985;40:419–25.

73. Bliwise D, Petta D, Seidel W, et al. Periodic leg movements during sleep in elderly. *Arch Gerontol Geriatr* 1985;4:273–81.

74. Bannerman C. Sleep disorders in the later years. *Postgrad Med J* 1988;84:265–74.

75. Youngstedt SD, Kripke DF, Klauber MR, et al. Periodic leg movements during sleep and sleep disturbances in elders. *J Gerontol* 1998;53A (5):M391–4.

76. Pennestri MH, Whittom S, Adam B, et al. PLMS and PLMW in healthy subjects as a function of age: prevalence and interval distribution. *Sleep* 2006;29(9):1183–7.

77. Boehm G, Wetter TC, Trenkwalder C. Periodic leg movements in RLS patients as compared to controls: are there differences beyond the PLM index? *Sleep Med* 2009:10(5):566–71.

78. Saskin P, Moldofsky H, Lue FA. Periodic movements in sleep and sleep-wake complaint. *Sleep* 1985;8:319–24.

79. Bastuji H, Garcia-Larrea L. Sleep/wake abnormalities in patients with periodic leg movements during sleep: factor analysis on data from 24-h ambulatory polygraphy. *J Sleep Res* 1999;8:217–23.

80. Lugaresi E, Coccagna G, Mantovani M, et al. Some periodic phenomena arising during drowsiness and sleep in man. *Electroencephalogr Clin Neurophysio* 1972;32:701–5.

81. Mosko SS, Dickel MJ, Paul T, et al. Sleep apnea and sleep-related periodic leg movements in community resident seniors. *J Am Geriatr Soc* 1988;36:502–8.

82. Dickel MJ, Mosko SS. Morbidity cut-offs for sleep apnea and periodic leg movements in predicting subjective complaints in seniors. *Sleep* 1990;13:155–66.

83. Karadeniz D, Ondze B, Besset A, et al. Are periodic leg movements during sleep (PLMS) responsible for sleep disruption in insomnia patients? *Eur J Neurol* 2000; 7:331–6.

84. Mendelson WB. Are periodic leg movements associated with clinical sleep disturbance? *Sleep* 1996;19:219–23.

85. Nicolas A, Lesperance P, Montplaisir J. Is excessive daytime sleepiness with periodic leg movements during sleep a specific diagnostic category? *Eur Neurol* 1998;40:22–6.

86. Watanabe S, Ono A, Naito H. Periodic leg movements during either epidural or spinal anesthesia in an elderly man without sleep-related (nocturnal) myoclonus. *Sleep* 1990;13(3):262–6.

87. Jackson J. Periodic movements of sleep in T10 paraplegic with failure to respond to parlodel. *Sleep Res* 1990;19:326.

88. Yokota T, Hirose K, Tanabe H, et al. Sleep-related periodic leg movements (nocturnal myoclonus) due to spinal cord lesion. *J Neurol Sci* 1991;104:13–18.

89. Dickel MJ, Renfrow SD, Moore T, et al. Rapid eye movement sleep periodic leg movements in patients with spinal cord injury. *Sleep* 1994;17(8):733–8.

90. De Mello MT, Lauro FAA, Silva AC, et al. Incidence of periodic leg movements and of the restless legs syndrome during sleep following acute physical activity in spinal cord injury subjects. *Spinal Cord* 1996;34:294–6.

91. Lee MS, Choi YC, Lee SH, et al. Sleep-related periodic leg movements associated with spinal cord lesions. *Mov Disord* 1996;11(6):719–22.

92. Grillner S, Ekeberg, El Manira A, et al. Intrinsic function of a neuronal network—a vertebrate central pattern generator. *Brain Res Brain Res Rev* 1998; 26:184–97.

93. Schomburg ED, Steffens H. Comparative analysis of L-dopa actions on nociceptive and non-nociceptive spinal reflex pathways in the cat. *Neurosci Res* 1998; 31:307–16.

94. Smith RC. Relationship of periodic movements in sleep (nocturnal myoclonus) and the Babinski sign. *Sleep* 1985;8:239–43.

95. Fujiki A, Shimizu A, Yamada Y, et al. The Babinski reflex during sleep and wakefulness. *Electroencephalogr Clin Neurophysiol* 1971;31:610–13.

96. Batini C, Fressy J, Gastaud H. A study of the plantar cutaneous reflex during different phases of sleep. *Electroencephalogr Clin Neurophysiol* 1964;16:412–13.

97. Bara-Jimenez W, Aksu M, Graham B, et al. Periodic limb movements in sleep: state-dependent excitability of the spinal flexor reflex. *Neurology* 2000;54:1609–16.

98. Nogues M, Cammarota A, Leiguarda R, et al. Periodic limb movements in syringomyelia and syringobulbia. *Mov Disord* 2000;15:113–19.

99. Wechsler LR, Stakes JW, Shahani BT, et al. Periodic leg movements of sleep (nocturnal myoclonus): an electrophysiological study. *Ann Neurol* 1986;19:168–73.

100. Briellmann RS, Rosler M, Hess CW. Blink reflex excitability is abnormal in patients with periodic leg movements in sleep. *Mov Disord* 1996;11:6:710–14.

101. Martinelli P, Coccagna G, Lugaresi E. Nocturnal myoclonus, restless legs syndrome, and abnormal electrophysiological findings. *Ann Neurol* 1987;21:515

102. Bucher SF, Seelos KC, Oertel WH, et al. Cerebral generators involved in the pathogenesis of the restless legs syndrome. *Ann Neurol* 1997;41:639–45.

103. Stefansson H, Rye DB, Hicks A, et al. A genetic risk factor for periodic limb movements in sleep. *N Engl J Med* 2007;357:639–47.

104. Brodeur C, Montplaisir J, Godbout R, et al. Treatment of restless legs syndrome and periodic movements during sleep with L-dopa: a double-blind, controlled study. *Neurology* 1988;38:1845–8.

105. Trenkwalder C, Stiasny K, Pollmacher T, et al. L-dopa therapy of uremic and idiopathic restless legs syndrome: a double-blind, crossover trial. *Sleep* 1995;18:681–8.

106. Earley CJ, Allen RP. Pergolide and carbidopa/levodopa treatment of the restless legs syndrome and periodic leg movements in sleep in a consecutive series of patients. *Sleep* 1997;19(10):801–10.

107. Wetter TC, Stiasny K, Winkelmann J, et al. A randomized controlled study of pergolide in patients with restless legs syndrome. *Neurology* 1999;52:944–50.

108. Montplaisir J, Nicolas A, Denesle R, et al. Restless legs syndrome improved by pramipexole: a double-blind randomized trial. *Neurology* 1999;52:938–43.

109. Bédard MA, Montplaisir J, Godbout R, et al. Nocturnal γ-hydroxybutyrate—effects on periodic leg movements and sleep organization of narcoleptic patients. *Clin Neuropharmacol* 1989;12:29–36.

110. Staedt J, Stoppe G, Kogler A, et al. Dopamine D2 receptor alteration in patients with periodic movements in sleep (nocturnal myoclonus). *J Neural Transm* 1993;93:71–4.

111. Staedt J, Stoppe G, Kogler A, et al. Nocturnal myoclonus syndrome (periodic movements in sleep) related to central dopamine D2-receptor alteration. *Eur Arch Psychiatry Clin Neurosci* 1995;245:8–10.

112. Staedt J, Stoppe G, Kogler A, et al. Single photon emission tomography (SPET) imaging of dopamine D2 receptors in the course of dopamine replacement therapy in patients with nocturnal myoclonus syndrome (NMS). *J Neural Transm* 1995;99:187–93.

113. Wetter TC, Linke R, Eisensehr I, et al. Iodine-123-IPT SPECT imaging in idiopathic restless les syndrome: preliminary findings. *Sleep* 2000;23(Supp 2):A130.

114. Michaud M, Soucy JP, Chabli A, et al. SPECT imaging of pre- and postsynaptic dopaminergic functions in patients with restless legs syndrome. *Sleep* 2000;23(Supp 2):A129–30.

115. Turjanski N, Lees AJ, Brooks DJ. Striatal dopaminergic function in restless legs syndrome. *Neurology* 1999;52:932–7.

116. Ruottinen HM, Partinen M, Hublin C, et al. An FDOPA PET study in patients with periodic limb movement disorder and restless legs syndrome. *Neurology* 2000;54:502–4.

117. Groves PM, Tepper JM. Neuronal mechanisms of action of amphetamine. In: Creese I, ed. *Stimulants: Neurochemical, Behavioral and Clinical Perspectives*. NewYork: Raven Press; 1983:81–129.

118. Guilleminault C, Heinzer R, Mignot E, et al. Investigations into the neurologic basis of narcolepsy. *Neurology* 1998;50(Supp1):S8–S15.

119. Eisensehr I, Linke R, Noachtar S, et al. Reduced striatal dopamine transporters in idiopathic rapid eye movement sleep behaviour disorder. Comparison with

Parkinson's disease and controls. *Brain* 2000;123(6):1155–60.

120. Comella CL, Nardine TM, Diederich NJ, et al. Sleep-related violence, injury, and REM sleep behavior disorder in Parkinson's disease. *Neurology* 1998;51:526–9.

121. Schenck CH, Bundlie SR, Mahowald MW. Delayed emergence of a Parkinsonian disorder in 38% of 29 older men initially diagnosed with idiopathic rapid eye movement sleep behavior disorder. *Neurology* 1996;46:388–93.

122. Wetter TC, Collado-Seidel V, Pollmacher T, et al. Sleep and periodic leg movement patterns in drug-free patients with Parkinson's disease and multiple system atrophy. *Sleep* 2000;23:361–7.

123. Gadoth N, Costeff H, Harel S, et al. Motor abnormalities during sleep in patients with childhood hereditary progressive dystonia, and their unaffected family members. *Sleep* 1989;12:233–8.

124. Ancoli-Israel S, Martin J, Jones DW, et al. Sleep-disordered breathing and periodic limb movements in sleep in older patients with schizophrenia. *Biol Psychiatry* 1999;45:1426–32.

125. Davis KL, Kahn RS, Ko G, et al. Dopamine in schizophrenia: a review and reconceptualization. *Am J Psychiatry* 1991;148:1474–86.

126. Wong DF, Wagner HN, Jr., Dannals RF, et al. Effects of age on dopamine and serotonin receptors measured by positron tomography in the living brain. *Science* 1984;226:1393–6.

127. van Dyck CH, Seibyl JP, Malison RT, et al. Age-related decline in striatal dopamine transporter binding with iodine-123-beta-CITSPECT. *J Nucl Med* 1995;36:1175–81.

128. Bjorklund A, Skagerberg G. Evidence for a major spinal cord projection from the diencephalic A11 dopamine cell group in the rat using transmitter-specific fluorescent retrograde tracing. *Brain Res* 1979;177:170–5.

129. Lundberg A. Multisensory control of spinal reflex pathways. *Prog Brain Res* 1979;50:11–28.

130. Weil-Fugazza J, Godefroy F. Dorsal and ventral dopaminergic innervation of the spinal cord: functional implications. *Brain Res Bull* 1993;30:319–24.

131. Ondo WG, He Y, Rajasekaran S, Le WD. Clinical correlates of 6-hydroxydopamine injections into A11 dopaminergic neurons in rats: a possible model for restless legs syndrome. *Mov Disord* 2000;15:154–8.

132. Decker M, Keating G, Freeman A, et al. Focal depletion of dopamine in the sensorimotor striatum of the rat recapitulates Parkinsonian-like sleep-wake disturbances. *Sleep* 2000;23(Supp 2):A136.

133. Allen R, Becker PM, Bogan R, et al. Ropinirole decreases periodic leg movements and improves sleep parameters in patients with restless legs syndrome. *Sleep* 2004;27(5):907–14.

134. Ferri R, Manconi M, Aricò D, et al. Acute dopamine-agonist treatment in restless legs syndrome: effects on sleep architecture and NREM sleep instability. *Sleep* 2010;33(6):793–800.

135. Garcia-Borreguero D, Larrosa O, Williams AM, et al. Treatment of restless legs syndrome with pregabalin: a double-blind, placebo-controlled study. *Neurology* 2010;74(23):1897–904.

136. Boivin DB, Montplaisir J, Poirier G. The effects of L-Dopa on periodic leg movements and sleep organization in narcolepsy. *Clin Neuropharmacol* 1989;12:339–45.

137. Moldofsky H, Tullis C, Quance G, et al. Nitrazepam for periodic movements in sleep (sleep-related myoclonus). *Can J Neurol Sci* 1986;13:52–4.

138. Oshtory MA, Vijayan N. Clonazepam treatment of insomnia due to sleep myoclonus. *Arch Neurol* 1980;37:119–20.

139. Ohanna N, Peled R, Rubin A-HE, et al. Periodic leg movements in sleep: effect of clonazepam treatment. *Neurology* 1985;35:408–11.

140. Mitler MM, Browman CP, Menn SJ, et al. Nocturnal myoclonus: treatment efficacy of clonazepam and temazepam. *Sleep* 1986;9:385–92.

141. Bonnet MH, Arand DL. The use of triazolam in older patients with periodic leg movements, fragmented sleep, and daytime sleepiness. *J Gerontol* 1990; 45:M139–M144.

142. Manconi M, Ferri R, Zucconi M, et al. Dissociation of periodic leg movements from arousals in restless legs syndrome. *Ann Neurol.* 2012 Jun;71(6):834–44.

50

Sleep and Tic Disorders

PHILIP A. HANNA, TASNEEM PEERAULLY,
AND JOSEPH JANKOVIC

THE CLASSIC form of tic disorder is Tourette syndrome (TS), a childhood-onset, genetic, neurobehavioral disorder characterized by multiple involuntary motor and phonic tics.[1-2] It is frequently associated with comorbidities, including obsessive-compulsive disorder (OCD) and attention-deficit (hyperactivity) disorder (ADHD).[1] In addition, TS patients often complain of sleep disturbances and sleep-related behavioral problems, which have been documented with polysomnographic (PSG) recordings.[3-7] These include alterations of arousal[3,4,7]; decreased percentage (up to 30%) of slow-wave sleep (SWS)[8,9]; increased or unaltered duration of SWS;[3,7,10,11] paroxysmal events in stage 4 sleep described as "sudden and intense arousal, apparent disorientation, confusion or combativeness or both, increase in tic activity, and occasional automatism-like activities"; decreased percentage of rapid eye movement (REM) sleep; increased awakenings; and persistence of tics during all stages of sleep.[3] Other reported disorders of sleep include sleep apnea, enuresis, sleepwalking (somnambulism), nightmares, myoclonus, bruxism,[4] sleep talking,[12] restless legs syndrome (RLS),[11-20] and periodic leg movements in sleep (PLMS).[10,19-22]

HISTORICAL BACKGROUND AND EPIDEMIOLOGY

In his classic monograph, George Gilles de la Tourette described disturbance of sleep in two of his nine patients, with three other patients manifesting disappearance of tics during sleep.[23] Despite this early reference to alterations of sleep in TS patients, there was little or no mention of any sleep disturbance in TS patients until Shapiro et al.,[24] in 1978, commented that tics lessen as patients enter drowsiness and "disappear with light sleep." Ten years later, additional work led the same authors to state that tics do persist during sleep, although they are diminished in frequency and severity.[25] In the same publication, however, these authors concluded that sleep disturbances "do not appear to us to

Table 50.1 Studies Evaluating Sleep Disturbance Complaint Data

REFERENCES	DIAGNOSIS	NUMBER	GENDER	AGE	CONTROLS	SLEEP DISORDER
Barabas[76]	TS	57	50M: 7F	5–21	58: epilepsy 53: LD	17.5%: sleepwalking (1.7% epilepsy controls and 3.8% LD controls) 15.8%: pavor nocturnus (1.7% epilepsy controls and 3.8% LD controls) 18.9%: enuresis (15.4% controls)
Barabas[33]	TS	65	54M:11F	10–12	TS with vs. TS without migraine	Sleepwalking and pavor nocturnus significantly higher in TS migraine group
Erenberg[12]	TS	58	N/A	15–25	None	22% (nightmares, rocking, talking, trouble falling/staying asleep), 14%: tics
Jankovic[4]	TS	112	3.8M:F	1–28	None	Tics ($n = 22$), enuresis (19), restless sleeper (12), insomnia (12), somnambulism (9), nightmares (8), myoclonus (6), bruxism (3)
Comings[28]	TS ± ADD	246:TS ± ADD 17:ADD 15:ADD secondary to TS gene	224M:54F	17 ± 12 9 ± 4 10 ± 9	47	50%: early awakening; 49.6%: trouble falling asleep; 46%: sleepwalking; 45.5%: pavor nocturns (of all patients with TS)
Allen[5]	TS ± ADHD	57: TS only 21: ADHD only 89: TS + ADHD	All M	7–14	146	Poor sleep: 48% in ADHD only 41% in TS + ADHD 26% in TS only 10% in controls
Freeman[29]	TS ± ADHD	967: TS only 3783: TS + ADHD 2055: TS: no ADHD	4:1 M:F	75% <18	None	17.8% of all patients with TS patients TS only: 9.4% children, 7.5% adults TS + ADHD: 22% of children. 18% of adults TS + no ADHD: 15% of children, 12% of adults

ADD, attention-deficit disorder: ADHD, attention-deficit/hyperactivity disorder; F, female; LD, learning disability; M, male; N/A, not assessed/reported; TS, Tourette syndrome.

be more frequent than expected in the population." The prevalence of sleep disturbances in the general population has been estimated at 1% to 6%.[26] A questionnaire study of parents of 146 healthy children (age 7 to 14 years) revealed that 10% of their children had sleep disturbances.[5] This observation was similar to the frequency in healthy students reported by Kahn, Van de Merckt, Rebuffat, et al.[27]

QUESTIONNAIRE STUDIES

Although not as accurate as PSG studies, questionnaire surveys provide some insight into the frequency and nature of sleep disturbances in patients with TS. Table 50.1 summarizes studies based primarily on questionnaire data, focusing on reported sleep complaints. Although the data must be interpreted cautiously, the most frequently reported sleep disturbances in TS patients include sleepwalking, sleep talking, night terrors (pavor nocturnus), nightmares, enuresis, and trouble falling or staying asleep. The studies, however, vary widely in number and age of subjects, inclusion of controls, comorbid features such as ADHD, and methodology. Considering the caveats noted before, these surveys suggest that the frequency of sleep-related disorders in TS patients is higher than in the general population.

The influence of comorbid features, such as ADHD, on sleep patterns of patients with TS has not been well studied. Comings and Comings[28] found that there was an increase in sleep difficulties, such as early awakening, difficulty falling asleep, pavor nocturnus, and sleepwalking (somnambulism) in patients with severe TS and in those with associated ADHD. Allen, Singer, Brown, et al.[5] analyzed four subgroups (TS only, ADHD only, TS and ADHD combination, or controls) and found that the incidence of sleep items t19 possible sleep items on the questionnaire, of which one was poor sleep; see Table 50.1) did not significantly differ for the majority of items between the TS-only group (5/19) and controls and between the ADHD-only group (6/19) and controls but was much higher (17/19) in the combined TS and ADHD subgroup. This suggests that the combination of TS and ADHD, and not TS alone, accounts for the sleep dysfunction observed in patients with TS.

Sleep problems were reported in 17.8% of 6805 cases contained in the Tourette Syndrome International Database Consortium, of which 65% had comorbid ADHD.[29] Moreover, sleep problems were more frequent in the combined inattentive-hyperactive subtype (37%) than in the inattentive subtype (24%). When divided into subsets comprised of TS + ADHD ($n = 3783$), TS without ADHD ($n = 2055$), and TS only (no comorbitities) ($n = 967$), current sleep problems were reported in 22%, 15%, and 9.4% of children, respectively, and 18%, 12%, and 7.5% of adults, respectively. However, while information from the dataset represents clinical reports by experienced clinicians, the ascertainment and referral biases are undetermined.

In a study comprising 84 children with tic disorder and 156 controls, Mlodzikowska-Albrecht et al. reported differing sleep habits between the two groups.[30] Naps were significantly more frequent in children with tics (29.8% vs. 12.8%), and controls were more likely to have a soft toy when falling asleep (44.9% vs. 6.0%), listen to bedtime stories read by a parent (31.4% vs. 3.6%), and sleep the whole night in the same position in bed (75% vs. 33.3%, $p < .005$).

Several authors have reported increased sleep disturbances, particularly parasomnias, in TS patients with a positive family history of TS or tic disorders.[3,31,32] In particular, of the 14 TS patients studied by Glaze, Frost, and Jankovic, 10 had a positive family history of TS. Six of these 10 patients reported sleep disturbances, whereas eight manifested disturbed sleep on PSG testing.[3] Conversely, none of the patients without a family history of TS either reported sleep disturbances or had PSG evidence of disordered sleep. In another study, 16 of 32 (50%) patients with TS and a family history of TS or tics reported a sleep disturbance compared with 5 of 18 (28%) patients without a family history.[32] Barabas and Matthews[33] found a higher frequency of sleep disturbances in patients with TS and migraine (or a family history of migraine) compared with patients with TS only.

The prevailing teaching is that tics, like other hyperkinetic disorders, decrease in severity and become less frequent[34] or disappear[35] with sleep. A number of researchers, however, have reported that tics do persist during sleep. Shapiro, Shapiro, Young, et al.[25] reported an incidence of 3% based on informant data. Burd and Kerbeshian[36] reported 8%, whereas 14% of TS patients reported tics during sleep in a study by Erenberg.[12] PSG studies, as discussed in the next section, have provided better quantification of the persistence of tics in sleep.

Table 50.2 Polysomnographic Data in Patients with Tourette Syndrome

REFERENCES	N	GENDER	AGE	CONTROLS	NIGHTS	D/EFF/L	SWS	REM	AR	TICS	RLS/PLMS	PARA
Mendelson[8]	6	5M:1F	10–20	9	4	0/0/0	↓	0	—	—	0	—
Glaze[3]	14	8M:4F	8–23	11	1	0/—/0	↑	↓	+	+	—	+
Jankovic[4]	34	—	—	Norms	—	—/—/—	—	—/↓	—/+	—/+	—/—	—/+
Drake[9]	7	—	10–36	Norms	—	—/↓/↑	↓	↓	+	—	—	—
Silvestri[10]	9	All M	11–32	42	3	↓/↓/—	↑	↓	+	+	—	—
Voderholzer[11]	7	6M:1F	31 ± 11	7	2	↓/↓/0	0	0	↑	—	PLMS↑	—
Rothenberger[7]	13	All M	8–16	13	2	0/↓/↓	0	(↑)	↑	+	—	—

ADHD, attention-deficit/hyperactivity disorder; Ar, arousals; D, duration of sleep; Eff, sleep efficiency; F, female; L, latency to sleep onset; M, male; para, parasomnias; PLMS, periodic leg movements in sleep; REM, rapid eye movement sleep; RLS, restless legs syndrome; SWS, slow-wave sleep; TS, Tourette syndrome.↑, Increased;↓, decreased,—not assessed/reported; 0, no change.

POLYSOMNOGRAPHIC EVALUATIONS

PSG has been a valuable tool in objectively evaluating patients (in conjunction with subjective self-reporting or family member questioning) with sleep disturbances, including arousal disorders such as parasomnias and alterations of sleep patterning. Yet differences in methodology, including age and number of patients, have led to varying results. Certain sleep parameters are highly dependent on methodology. For example, REM-sleep information may differ if the sleep laboratory evaluation is based on individualized time protocol (simulating the individual's usual time of going to bed and getting out of bed in the morning) compared with a fixed time pattern (same times for each subject). Furthermore, most early studies combined results of children and adults, whereas more recent reports[7,11] have separated the two groups, taking into account age-related differences in sleep profiles.

Table 50.2 summarizes some of the reported PSG data. Again, primarily because of methodologic differences, results vary widely. For example, SWS was decreased (up to 30%) in TS patients in three published studies[8,9,37] but was found to be either increased or unchanged in other studies.[3,7,10,11] REM sleep was either decreased[3,4,9,10] or unchanged.[11] Similarly, sleep efficiency was either decreased[3,7,10,11] or unaffected.[8]

Given the limitations of self-reporting and data based on informants regarding tics during sleep, PSG recordings are of particular help. In the study by Jankovic and Rohaidy,[4] motor tics were recorded by PSG in 23 of the 34 patients (68%) during all stages of sleep and vocal tics in 4 patients (12%). Similarly, Fish, Sawyers, Allen, et al.[38] and Silvestri, Raffaele, De Domenico, et al.[10] reported the occurrence of tics in all stages of sleep in their TS subjects. In the former study, tics most commonly appeared after an awakening or, less often, following a transition to a lighter stage of sleep. Although tics were rarely recorded during REM sleep in this study, Hashimoto et al. reported increased tics during REM sleep compared with non–rapid eye movement (non-REM) sleep in 4- to 12-year-old TS children.[31] In summary, the overall appearance of tics during sleep recordings is around 80% contrasted with the 3% to 14% frequency reported in the questionnaire studies.

RESTLESS LEGS SYNDROME AND PERIODIC LEG MOVEMENTS IN SLEEP

RLS is a neurologic disorder characterized by a desire to move the legs associated with discomfort of the legs (dysesthesias or paresthesias) and motor restlessness, worse at night and at rest, and at least partially and temporarily relieved by activity.[15–17,39] The prevalence is estimated to be 5% of the general population. RLS may be subdivided into two main subtypes, familial/idiopathic or sporadic/neuropathic.[17] Up to 80% of patients with RLS have PLMS. Muller, Voderholzer, Kurtz, et al.[14] reported a family in which the mother had RLS and the son had TS, but the coexistence of these relatively common disorders may be purely coincidental. In the study by Voderholzer, Muller, Haag, et al.,[11] five of seven TS patients had PLMS with high indices, whereas none had RLS. Although PLMS is reportedly rare in patients younger than 30 years, all except one of the patients in this series of TS patients was 35 years or younger. Picchietti, England, Walters, et al.[19] found that 18 of 69 (26%) ADHD children had PLMS versus 2 of 38 (5%) controls. There was no association between concomitant use of stimulants (for ADHD) and occurrence of PLMS. In a separate study,[20] the authors found that 117 of 129 (91%) children with PLMS had ADHD. However, Kirov et al. commented on the absence of PLMS in their study of 19 patients with comorbid TS and ADHD.[40]

With regard to treatment, one study found that five of seven children with both ADHD and RLS/PLMS had lessening of both nocturnal movements and daytime attentional difficulties with use of levodopa/carbidopa or pergolide.[41] Lipinski, Sallee, Jackson, et al.[18] reported a beneficial effect of pergolide in the reduction of tics, and this positive response was highly associated with the presence of RLS comorbidity.

Genetic studies can be of considerable import when searching for a common pathophysiology between associated conditions. Three genetic loci associated with risk alleles for RLS and PLMs were tested for an association with TS in a case control study involving 322 French Canadian TS cases conducted by the Montreal Tourette Study Group.[42] They found predisposing three alleles for RLS in the *BTBD9* gene to be strongly associated with TS, in particular TS without OCD. The authors felt that the findings were unlikely to be explained by RLS comorbidity as RLS was found in only 10% of those cases.[43] The study provides evidence of a molecular genetic link between RLS and TS, although these findings would need to be replicated in independent samples.

SLEEP APNEA

Two studies reported a high incidence of sleep apnea in adult TS patients, based on PSG. The study by Glaze, Frost, and Jankovic[3] found sleep apnea in 8 of 12 of their adult TS patients, and Jankovic and Rohaidy[4] reported sleep apnea in 8 of 34 in a larger study. By comparison, none of the unmedicated 19 patients or controls in Kirov's study exhibited any sleep-disordered breathing.[40]

A study by Sverd and Montero[44] raised the question of a possible causative or contributory role of TS in sudden infant death syndrome (SIDS) and childhood sleep apnea and concluded that there appears to be an increased prevalence (two to five times greater) of SIDS in TS families compared with the general population.

INFLUENCE OF MEDICATIONS ON SLEEP IN TOURETTE SYNDROME

In a number of the studies, particularly those based on questionnaire data, the influence of medications such as stimulants, anti-tic medications, and antidepressants on the sleep profile in TS patients was not evaluated adequately. Stimulants increase sleep latency but decrease total sleep time and sleep efficiency.[45–51] Mendelson, Caine, Goyer, et al.[8] reported that neuroleptics reduced overall nocturnal movements and normalized the decreased SWS in their TS patients. Specific effects on sleep parameters vary among the neuroleptic agents. Haloperidol has a hypnotic effect and increases REM latency and sleep efficiency[52,53]; pimozide may increase evening fatigue[51]; and risperidone improves sleep quantity and quality.[54,55] Fluphenazine appears to have a lower incidence of sedation compared with other neuroleptics, but this has not been formerly studied. In the study by Jankovic and Rohaidy,[4] tetrabenazine, a monoamine depleting and dopamine receptor blocking drug, reduced not only daytime tics but also tics during sleep, from 16.7 to 4.0 per recording session but had no distinct effect on REM sleep parameters. Another medication used often in TS, clonidine,

has a hypnotic effect and reduces REM sleep and sleep latency.[56–59] Selective serotonin reuptake inhibitors have caused nocturnal bruxism and increase REM latency and nocturnal awakenings while reducing REM sleep and overall sleep time and sleep efficiency.[60–63] Thus, many medications used to reduce tics or treat comorbid conditions such as ADHD and OCD may cause or increase daytime drowsiness in patients with TS.

PATHOPHYSIOLOGY

Lerner et al. performed PET neuroimaging in patients with TS to identify brain regions responsible for tic generation. They used stage 2 sleep as a baseline to eliminate normal wake state activity. They found that TS patients had increased blood flow in the premotor areas bilaterally, with decreased blood flow in the left inferior frontal gyrus, claustrum and superior temporal gyrus, and the putamina bilaterally.[64]

Decreased inhibition in the cortico-striatal pallidal-thalamic-cortical motor circuit, postulated to play a role in the production of tic in TS,[65] may promote not only the involuntary movements but also increased arousal, as well as movements during sleep such as PLMS, myoclonus, and sleepwalking. Arousal may be affected by alterations in dopaminergic and serotonergic metabolism.[5] Patients with TS often experience premonitory sensory symptoms, such as "pressure" or "tingling."[66–68] Tics may, to some degree, represent a voluntary motor response to an involuntary internal sensation.[1,66] In one study of 60 TS patients, 93% perceived their tics to be "irresistibly but purposefully executed."[69] It is possible that during daytime, compared with sleep, tic frequency and severity may be greater because patients' awareness of such premonitory sensations (which often are uncomfortable) is increased. The increased level of awareness, particularly of such premonitory sensations, in TS patients may contribute to difficulty falling asleep and increased sleep arousals.

In support of the dopaminergic hypothesis is the observation that treatment with dopamine-receptor blocking agents or dopamine-depleting agents ameliorates tics, whereas medications that augment central dopaminergic activity typically exacerbate tics.[1,4,70] While dopaminergic-receptor blocking medications haloperidol and pimozide are FDA-approved treatments for TS, blockade of dopaminergic systems may induce sleep disturbances. In analyzing the sleep characteristics on PSG of a 12-year-old

TS patient before and 6 months after treatment with risperidone was initiated, Arana-Lechuga et al. found the second study showed markedly decreased sleep latency, percent SWS, and total number of arousals and movements in both non-REM and REM. There was also an increase in sleep efficiency and light sleep. Noting that the patient's tics remitted in addition to the improvement in sleep parameter after treatment with the atypical antipsychotic drug, the authors suggested that the sleep disturbances resulted from the biochemical alterations of TS rather than an aggregated disease process.[71]

The association of TS with RLS and PLMS further points to alterations of dopamine metabolism as a common factor in these conditions. Furthermore, findings of low cerebrospinal fluid homovanillic acid provide additional support for the postulation that patients with TS and tic disorders have supersensitive dopamine receptors.[72-74] Postmortem studies, although limited, found evidence of increased presynaptic dopamine receptor binding.[72] A study using in vivo measurement of striatal vesicular monoamine transporter type-2 (VMAT2), however, found no evidence for increased binding to this transporter in the striatum of TS patients, leading the authors to conclude that dorsal striatal dopaminergic innervation density is normal in TS.[75] Postmortem studies of brains have revealed other biochemical abnormalities, including decreased serotonin, decreased glutamate in the globus pallidus internus, and decreased cortical cyclic AMP.[74]

Kirov et al. investigated the sleep patterns of 19 unmedicated children with TS and ADHD compared to 19 controls and found that the former displayed shortened REM sleep latency (105 minutes compared to 134 minutes) and increased REM sleep duration (25.7% compared to 21.8%).[40] The authors speculated that the increase in REM drive observed suggests common physiologic mechanisms underlying hypermotor symptoms and regulation of REM sleep.

DISCUSSION AND FUTURE ASPECTS

TS patients, in addition to their involuntary movements and vocalizations, are also beset by disturbances of sleep that often may be overlooked or not adequately assessed by medical practitioners. Sleep complaints are frequently based on questionnaire data, and PSG studies

have confirmed a number of sleep disturbances in TS patients, particularly decreased sleep efficiency, increased arousal phenomenon such as parasomnias, and alterations in duration and quality of REM and SWS. Furthermore, PSG studies confirm that tics do persist during all stages of sleep. Medications useful in diminishing daytime tics also appear to be useful in reducing nighttime tics and correcting the abnormal sleep profile of these patients. The observation that tics persist during sleep provides additional support to the involuntary nature and subcortical (basal ganglia) origin of tic phenomenon.

Are sleep disorders in TS intrinsic to this condition, representing part of the genetic spectrum, with variable expression including comorbidities such as obsessive-compulsive behavior and ADHD, or are the observed sleep disturbances secondary to a distinct yet associated disorder of arousal? Clearly, patients with combined TS and ADHD have increased sleep disorders, particularly parasomnias, suggesting that a combination of these conditions may be critical for the full manifestation of disorders of sleep, perhaps mostly explained by a general disturbance of arousal mechanisms. Studies by Allen, Singer, Brown, et al.[5] and Comings and Comings[28] indicate that sleep disturbances do not appear to be strictly intrinsic to TS. In Allen, Singer, Brown, et al.,[5] TS and ADHD combination and ADHD-only patients had a greater than normal occurrence of nearly all arousal-related sleep disturbances, whereas only sleep talking had an increased frequency in the TS-only group. Comings and Comings[28] reported that sleepwalking, sleep talking, and night terrors occur often in TS patients, with or without ADHD, but the TS-ADHD combination group had increased severity of these disturbances. Such evidence leads to the question of whether sleep disturbances of TS lead to ADHD symptomatology, whether ADHD symptomatology leads to sleep disturbances in TS patients, or both? Interestingly, the Montreal Tourette Study Group found that the genetic polymorphisms in the BTBD9 gene were predominantly associated with TS without psychiatric comorbidities.[42] However, only the TS without OCD and TS without OCD and ADHD groups reached statistical significance. Future genetic studies may clarify whether certain components of sleep disturbance in TS are independent of ADHD comorbidity.

Further refinements in methodology such as uniformity of age, gender, controls, and assessment of medication interactions and in PSG studies should help elucidate the relationship between TS and sleep. Studies assessing interactions between circadian rhythms, stages of sleep, and tics may give further insights into central nervous system motor control mechanisms. Genetic implications are intriguing given the association of TS with other genetic conditions such as RLS. Further revelations from genetic research will certainly lead to a greater understanding of the mechanisms of sleep disturbances in individuals with tic disorders.

REFERENCES

1. Jankovic J, Kurlan R. Tourette Syndrome: Evolving concepts. *Mov Disord* 2011;26:1149–56.
2. Tourette Syndrome Classification Study Group. Definitions and classifications of tic disorders. *Arch Neurol* 1993;50:1013.
3. Glaze DG, Frost JD, Jankovic J: Sleep in Gilles de la Tourette's syndrome: Disorder of arousal. Neurology 33:586, 1983.
4. Jankovic J, Rohaidy H. Motor, behavioral, and pharmacological findings in Tourette's patients. *Can J Neurol Sci* 1987;541.
5. Allen RP, Singer HS, Brown JE, et al. Sleep disorders in Tourette syndrome: A primary or unrelated problem? *Pediatr Neurol* 1992;8:275.
6. Comings DE. Tourette's syndrome: a behavioral spectrum disorder. In Weiner WJ, Lang AE, eds. Behavioral Neurology of Movement Disorders. Advances in Neurology. Vol 65. New York: Raven; 1995:293.
7. Rothenberger A, Kostanecka R, Kinkelbur J, et al. Sleep and Tourette syndrome. In Cohen D, Jankovic J, Goetz C, eds. Tourette Syndrome. *Adv Neurol* 2001;85:245.
8. Mendelson WB, Caine ED, Goyer P, et al. Sleep in Gilles de la Tourette syndrome. *Biol Psychiatry* 1980;15:339.
9. Drake ME, Hietter SA, Bogner JE, et al. Cassette EEG sleep recordings in Gilles de la Tourette syndrome. *Clin Electroencephalogr* 1992;23:142.
10. Silvestri R, Raffaele M, De Domenico P, et al. Sleep features in Tourette's syndrome, neuroacanthocytosis and Huntington's chorea. *Neurophysiol Clin* 1995;25:66.
11. Voderholzer U, Muller N, Haag C, et al. Periodic limb movements during sleep are a frequent finding in patients with Gilles de la Tourette's syndrome. *J Neurol* 1997;244:521.
12. Erenberg G. Sleep disorders in Gilles de la Tourette syndrome [Letter]. *Neurology* 1985;35:1397.
13. Ekbom KA. Restless legs syndrome. *Neurology* 1960;10:868.
14. Muller N, Voderholzer U, Kurtz F, et al. Tourette's syndrome associated with restless leg syndrome and akathisia in a family. *Acta Neurol Scand* 1994;89:429–32.
15. Walters A. Toward a better definition of the restless legs syndrome. *Mov Disord* 1995;10:634.
16. Ondo W, Jankovic J. Restless legs syndrome. In: Appel SH, ed. Current Neurology. Vol 17. Amsterdam, The Netherlands: IOS Press; 1998:207.
17. Ondo W, Jankovic J. Restless legs syndrome: clinicoetiologic correlates. *Neurology* 1996;47:1435.
18. Lipinski JF, Sallee FR, Jackson C, et al. Dopamine agonist treatment of Tourette disorder in children: results of an open-label trial of pergolide. *Mov Disord* 1997;12:402.
19. Picchietti DL, England SJ, Walters AS, et al. Periodic limb movement disorder and restless legs syndrome in children with attention-deficit hyperactivity disorder. *J Child Neurol* 1998;13:588.
20. Picchietti DL, Underwood DJ, Farris WA, et al. Further studies on periodic limb movement disorder and restless legs syndrome in children with attention-deficit hyperactivity disorder. *Mov Disord* 1999;14:1000.
21. Picchietti DL, Walters AS. Moderate to severe periodic limb movement disorder in childhood and adolescence. *Sleep* 1999;22:297.
22. Coleman RM, Pollak CP, Weitzman ED. Periodic movements in sleep (nocturnal myoclonus): relation to sleep disorder. *Ann Neurol* 1980;8:416.
23. Gilles de la Tourette G. Etude sur une affection nerveuse characterisee pa l'incoordination motrice accompagnee d'echolalie et de coprolalie (Jumping, Latah, Myriachit). *Arch Neurol* 1865 ;9:19–42, 158–200.
24. Shapiro AK, Shapiro ES, Bruun RD, et al. Gilles de la Tourette Syndrome. New York: Raven Press; 1978.
25. Shapiro AK, Shapiro ES, Young JG, et al. Gilles de la Tourette Syndrome. 2nd ed. New York: Raven Press; 1988.
26. Barabas G, Matthews WS, Ferrari M. Somnambulism in children with Tourette syndrome. *Dev Med Child Neurol* 1984;26:457.

27. Kahn A, Van de Merckt C, Rebuffat E, et al. Sleep problems in healthy preadolescents. *Pediatrics* 1989;84:542.

28. Comings DE, Comings BG. A controlled study of Tourette syndrome. VI. Early development, sleep problems, allergies and handedness. *Am J Hum Genet* 1987;41:822.

29. Freeman RD. Tic disorder and ADHD: answers from a world-wide clinical dataset on Tourette syndrome. *Eur Child Adolec Psychiatry* 2007;16:I/15–23.

30. Mlodzikowska-Albrecht J, Zarowski M, Steinborn B. The symptomatology of tic disorders and concomitant sleep habits in children. *Adv Med Sci* 2007;52;212–14.

31. Hashimoto T, Endo S, Fukuda K, et al. Increased body movements during sleep in Gilles de la Tourette syndrome. *Brain Dev* 1981;3:31.

32. Nee LE, Caine ED, Plinsky RJ, et al. Gilles de la Tourette Syndrome: clinical and family study of 50 cases. *Ann Neurol* 1998;7:41.

33. Barabas G, Matthews WS. Homogeneous clinical subgroups in children with Tourette syndrome. *Pediatrics* 1985;75:73.

34. American Psychiatric Association. Diagnostic and Statistical Manual of Mental Disorders. 4th ed. Washington, DC: American Psychiatric Association; 1994.

35. World Health Organization. Mental and behavioural disorders. Clinical descriptions and diagnostic guidelines. In: International Classification of Diseases. Geneva, Switzerland: World Health Organization; 1993.

36. Burd L, Kerbeshian J. Nocturnal coprolalia and phonic tics. *Am J Psychiatry* 1988;145:132.

37. Moeller AA, Krieg JC. Sleep EEG in Gilles de la Tourette's syndrome. *J Neurol* 1993;239:113.

38. Fish DR, Sawyers D, Allen PJ, et al. The effect of sleep on the dyskinetic movements of Parkinson's disease, Gilles de la Tourette syndrome, Huntington's disease, and torsion dystonia. *Arch Neurol* 1991;48:210.

39. Chokroverty S, Jankovic J. Restless legs syndrome. A disease in search of identity. *Neurology* 1999;52:907.

40. Kirov R, Banaschewski T, Uebel H, et al. REM-sleep alterations in children with co-existence of tic disorders and attention-deficit/hyperactivity disorder: impact of hypermotor symptoms. *Eur Child Adolec Psychiatry* 2007;16:I/45–50.

41. Walters AS, Mandelbaum DE, Lewin DS, et al. Dopaminergic therapy in children with restless legs/periodic limb movements in sleep and ADHD. *Pediatr Neurol* 2000;22:182.

42. Rivere JB, Xiong L, Levchenko A, et al. Association of intronic variants of the BTBD9 gene with Tourette Syndrome. *Arch Neurol* 2009;66(10):1267–72.

43. Lesperance P, Djerroud N, Diaz Anzaldua A, et al. Restless legs in Tourette's syndrome. *Mov Disord* 2004;19(9):1084–7.

44. Sverd J, Montero G. Is Tourette syndrome a cause of sudden infant death syndrome and childhood obstructive sleep apnea? *Am J Med Genetics* 1993;46:494.

45. Roehrs R, Papineau K, Rosenthal L, et al. Sleepiness and the reinforcing and subjective effects of methylphenidate. *Exp Clin Psychopharm* 1999;7:145.

46. Stein M. Unravelling sleep problems in treated and untreated children with ADHD. *J Child Adolesc Psychopharm* 1999;9:157.

47. Stein MA, Blondis RA, Schnitzler ER, et al. Methylphenidate dosing: twice daily versus three times daily. *Pediatrics* 1996;98:748.

48. Kent JD, Blader JC, Koplewicz HS, et al. Effects of late-afternoon methylphenidate administration on behavior and sleep in attention-deficit hyperactivity disorder. *Pediatrics* 1995;96:320.

49. Oken BS, Kishiyama SS, Salinsky MC. Pharmacologically induced changes in arousal: effects on behavioral and electrophysiologic measures of alertness and attention. *Electroencephalogr Clin Neurophysiol* 1995;95:359.

50. Tirosh E, Sadeh A, Munvez R, et al. Effects of methylphenidate on sleep in children with attention-deficit hyperactivity disorder. An activity monitor study. *Am J Dis Child* 1993;147:1313–5.

51. Nicholson AN, Pascoe PA. Dopaminergic transmission and the sleep-wakefulness continuum in man. *Neuropharm* 1990;4:411.

52. Maixner S, Tandon R, Eiser A, et al. Effects of antipsychotic treatment on polysomnographic measures in schizophrenia: a replication and extension. *Am J Psychiatry* 1998;55:1600.

53. Frieboes RM, Murck H, Antonijevic I, et al. Characterization of the sigma ligand panamesine, a potential antipsychotic, by immune response in patients with schizophrenia and by sleep-EEG changes in normal controls. *Psychopharmacology* 1999;141:107.

54. Dursun SM, Patel JK, Burke JG, et al. Effects of typical antipsychotic drugs and risperidone

on the quality of sleep in patients with schizo-phrenia: a pilot study. *J Psychiatry Neurosci* 1999;24:333.

55. Ostroff RB, Nelson JC. Risperidone augmentation of selective serotonin reuptake inhibitors in major depression. *J Clin Psychiatry* 1999;60:256.

56. Wagner ML, Walters AS, Coleman RG, et al. Randomized, double blind, placebo-controlled study of clonidine in restless legs syndrome. *Sleep* 1996;19:52.

57. Danchin N, Genton P, Atlas P, et al. Comparative effects of atenolol and clonidine on polygraphically recorded sleep in hypertensive men: a randomized, double-blind, cross-over study. *Int J Clin Pharmacol Ther* 1995;33:52.

58. Prince JB, Wilens TE, Biederman J, et al. Clonidine for sleep disturbances associated with attention-deficit hyperactivity disorder: a systematic chart review of 62 cases. *J Am Acad Child Adolesc Psychiatry* 1996;35:599.

59. Gentili A, Godschalk MF, Gheorghiu D, et al. Effect of clonidine and yohimbine on sleep in healthy men: a double-blind, randomized, controlled trial. *Eur J Clin Pharmacol* 1996;50:463.

60. Schlosser R, Roschke J, Rossbach W, et al. Conventional and spectral power analysis of all-night sleep EEG after subchronic treatment with paroxetine in healthy male volunteers. *Eur Neuropsychopharmacol* 1998;8:273.

61. Ellison JM, Stanziani P. SSRI-associated nocturnal bruxism in four patients. *J Clin Psychiatry* 1993;54:432.

62. Sharpley AL, Williamson DJ, Attenburrow ME, et al. The effects of paroxetine and nefazodone on sleep: a placebo controlled trial. *Psychopharmacology* 1996;126:50.

63. Vasar V, Appelberg B, Rimon R, et al. The effect of fluoxetine on sleep: a longitudinal, double-blind polysomnographic study of healthy volunteers. *Int Clin Psychopharmacol* 1994;9:203.

64. Lerner A, Bagic A, Boudreau EA, et al. Neuroimaging of neuronal circuits involved in tic generation in patients with Tourette syndrome. *Neurology* 2007;68:1979–87.

65. Ziemann U, Paulus W, Rothenberger A. Decreased motor inhibition in Tourette's disorder: evidence from transcranial magnetic stimulation. *Am J Psychiatry* 1997;154:1277.

66. Cohen AJ, Leckman JF. Sensory phenomena associated with Gilles de la Tourette's syndrome. *J Clin Psychiatry* 1992;53:319.

67. Scahill LD, Leckman JF, Marek KL. Sensory Phenomena in Tourette's Syndrome. Advances in Neurology. Vol 65. New York: Raven Press; 1995:273.

68. Chee KY, Sachdev P. A controlled study of sensory tics in Gilles de la Tourette syndrome and obsessive-compulsive disorder using a structured interview. *J Neurol Neurosurg Psychiatry* 1997;62:188.

69. Lang A. Patient perception of tics and other movement disorders. *Neurology* 1991;41:223.

70. Jankovic J, Beach J. Long-term effects of tetrabenazine in hyperkinetic movement disorders. *Neurology* 1997;48:358.

71. Arana-Lechuga Y, Sanchez-Escandon O, de Santigo-Trevino N, et al. Risperidone treatment of sleep disturbances in Tourette's syndrome. *J Neuropsychiatry Clin Neurosci* 2008;20:3:375–6.

72. Singer HS, Wendlandt JT. Neurochemistry and synaptic neurotransmission in Tourette syndrome. In: Cohen DJ, Jankovic J, Goetz CG, eds. *Tourette Syndrome. Advances in Neurology.* Vol. 85. 2001;163.

73. Singer HS. Neurobiology of Tourette syndrome. In: Jankovic J, ed. Tourette Syndrome. *Neurological Clinics of North America.* Vol. 15. 1997;1618.

74. Singer HS, Hahn IH, Krowiak E, et al. Tourette's syndrome: a neurochemical analysis of postmortem cortical brain tissue. *Ann Neurol* 1990;27:443.

75. Meyer P, Bohnen NI, Minoshima S, et al. Striatal presynaptic monoaminergic vesicles are not increased in Tourette's syndrome. *Neurology* 1999;53:371.

76. Barabas G, Matthews WS, Ferrari M. Disorders of arousal in Gilles de la Tourette's syndrome. *Neurology* 1984;34:815.

51

Sleep Disturbances in Parkinson's Disease

NICO J. DIEDERICH AND CYNTHIA L. COMELLA

Sleep becomes much disturbed; the tremulous motion of the limbs occurs during the sleep
and augments until they awaken the patient.... [In the final stages of the disease there is]
constant sleepiness, with slight delirium and other marks of extreme exhaustion.

—James Parkinson *(1817)*

Although James Parkinson[86] defined the hallmarks of the disease that bears his name as *daytime* disturbances, he also recognized that PD patients frequently suffer from sleep disturbances. Other early authors like Charcot[16] and Gowers[39] emphasized the fluctuating expression of tremor at nighttime. Pronounced daytime sleepiness was a striking feature in postencephalitic parkinsonism, with impressive awakening by levodopa treatment. However, until today the full impact of sleep on Parkinson's disease (PD) and vice versa is not yet known. In fact, the causes of sleep disturbances are multifactorial, multilayered, and often confusing. Their impact on disease expression and progression remains controversial. It is difficult to distinguish the consequences of *primary* involvement of sleep-regulating centers from *secondary* sleep signs due to motor and autonomic involvement and *tertiary* signs due to medical treatment.[6] In this chapter we shall try to distinguish among the different causes in a theoretical way, understanding that in the individual patient, there is likely a combination of causes. In each section, we shall indicate where the theory is being presented rather than clinical evidence.

PREVALENCE

There is considerable debate on the prevalence of sleep disturbances and their impact on a patient's quality of life. In an early community-based study,[55,107] with comparison of 245 PD patients with 100 patients with diabetes mellitus and 100 healthy elderly controls, two thirds of the PD patients were complaining of sleep problems compared to 46% of the patients with diabetes mellitus and 33% of the healthy controls. Sleep fragmentation and early awakening were the most frequent complaints. The percentage of sleep complaints was over 90% in a national survey study, which may have selected the most affected PD patients.[35] Two recent multicenter observational studies of nonmotor symptoms in PD recruited a much larger number of patients. A nationwide German study on 1449

PD outpatients, which was representative of the disease spectrum, reported sleep disturbances in 49% of the patients.[94] An Italian study on 1072 patients (PRIAMO study) showed fatigue to be the most common symptom (58%), followed by insomnia (37%), urgency and nocturia (35%), REM sleep behavior disorder (RBD) (30%), excessive daytime sleepiness (EDS) (21%), and restless legs syndrome (RLS) (15%).[11] However, there have also been studies showing no difference between PD patients and age-matched controls for sleep initiation and sleep maintenance.[114].

ASSESSMENT SCALES

Validity and usefulness of different sleep scales used in PD have been controversially discussed. The Task Force on Sleep Disorders, organized by the Movement Disorder Society, examined the clinimetric properties and the clinical adequacy of 36 questionnaires.[47] Only six could be recommended, among them the Epworth sleepiness scale (ESS) to evaluate daytime sleepiness and the Pittsburgh sleep quality index (PSQI) to evaluate nocturnal sleep problems. Two scales specially designed for PD were recommended. The Parkinson's Disease Sleep Scale (PDSS) can provide an indication of the causes of sleep abnormalities in PD and has modest information about daytime sleepiness. The Scales for Outcomes in PD-Sleep Scale (SCOPA-S) assesses both, nocturnal

dysfunction and daytime sleepiness, without investigating possible causes.[61]

IMPACT ON QUALITY OF LIFE

It is possible to explain almost any sleep event in the parkinsonian patient in more than one way with little to indicate which, if any, explanation is correct.
—Nausieda PA (1993)

Sleep disturbance is one of the most important nonmotor signs in terms of impact on health-related quality of life (Hr-QL). In a large study Hr-QL scores correlated similarly with mood and fatigue ($r = .74$), followed by daytime somnolence ($r = .65$) and nocturnal sleep dysfunction ($r = .55$). In contrast, the UPDRS motor score or the dyskinesias scored much lower, each with $p < .5$.[36] Depression and anxiety are contributing factors to reduced QL in PD patients and, at the same time, powerful predictors of poor sleep quality in PD.[40] For causes of sleep disturbances, see Figure 51.1.

PRIMARY INVOLVEMENT OF SLEEP-REGULATING STRUCTURES

PD is a disorder that typically affects the elderly. Thus, just by their age, PD patients are already at risk for regulatory sleep dysfunction. Several neuroanatomical studies in PD have shown that,

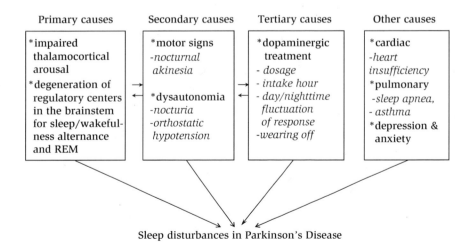

FIGURE 51.1 Causes of sleep impairment in Parkinson's disease: interactive model. (Reprinted from Diederich and McIntyre.[28])

in addition to these age-related changes, there is primary degeneration of structures responsible for maintenance of sleep and physiological REM sleep. The structure mainly involved is the cholinergic *pedunculopontine nucleus (PPN)*; the number of the neurons in the pars compacta of this nucleus is reduced by 40%–53% in PD patients in comparison to age-matched control patients.[49,50,124] The essential role of the PPN in control of sleep has been shown in animal studies. In some PD patients, deep brain stimulation of the PPN has increased REM sleep, as well as cortical arousal during the day. This effect, however, is variable in these small observational studies and may depend on the frequency of stimulation. Additional studies are needed before the role of the PPN in disturbed sleep of PD is elucidated.[1,2,7] Other areas involved in the degenerative process include the noradrenergic *locus coeruleus*, the serotonergic *raphe nuclei*, and the dopaminergic *tegmental area of the mesencephalus*.[15,49,50,87,98] There may be only transient deficiency of the respective transmitters, and pharmacotherapy may overcome the problem. The nuclei may also have partially or totally lost their physiological function, thus becoming unresponsive to endogenous (neurotransmitters) or exogenous stimulation (pharmacotherapy). There are little data to indicate that in PD, the degeneration of these nuclei follows a distinguishable temporal or spatial course, or whether this occurs as a primary or secondary event (Wallerian degeneration).

PD patients have been shown in pathological studies to have a reduction of hypocretin neurons in the hypothalamus.[33,108] Although cerebrospinal fluid shows variable results in hypocretin levels, it may be that the degeneration of these neurons may have effects on sleep and wakefulness, as has been demonstrated in narcolepsy in which there is much more marked degeneration.[22,29,42,121]

Rye and coworkers have postulated that the mesocorticolimbic dopamine system, originating in the ventral tegmental area (VTA), "modulates wakefulness and sleep."[96,97,112] Although there are only scarce neuropathological data evidencing changes of the major nuclei of this system (nuclei paranigralis and interfasciculatis),[31] it is thought that dysfunctional *thalamocortical arousal induces* a lack of normal thalamocortical rhythms during nighttime, with loss of slow-wave sleep and loss of sleep spindles, and at the same time, excessive sleepiness during daytime.[96] Studies have shown that PD patients

do show progressive sleep "destructuring" during nighttime,[25] echoed by impaired wakefulness state during daytime. Furthermore, abrupt intrusions of REM sleep into wakefulness have been reported.[26] Intriguingly, these phenomena may occur simultaneously, with thus shorter mean sleep latencies during daytime *and* longer total nocturnal sleep time.[97] Finally, there may be circadian variations of the dopamine receptor sensitivity with increased sensitivity at nighttime.[38]

In summary, unexplained microsleeps during the day, the tendency toward taking frequent naps, daytime hypersomnia, reversal of the day-night sleep pattern, and REM sleep behavior disorders may all arise from underlying degenerative changes[18] (Table 51.1).

SECONDARY SLEEP DISTURBANCES DUE TO CLINICAL SIGNS

The motor symptoms, including bradykinesia, rigidity, and tremor, are the cardinal features of PD. These symptoms may recur at night during the lighter stages of sleep, resulting in *nocturnal akinesia*. Of the PD patients included in one survey, 65% considered nocturnal akinesia as the most troublesome symptom, giving rise to discomfort and fragmented sleep.[35] During REM sleep, *tremor* practically disappears, and during non-REM sleep, the tremor tends to have a reduced amplitude.[8] *Rigidity* and *cogwheeling* are reduced but present during sleep.[8] *Nocturia* is the most frequent autonomic nocturnal disturbance in PD. Other autonomic features influencing sleep quality at a late stage of the disease are nocturnal blood pressure variability (paradoxical hypertension) and orthostatic hypotension.

RLS is often reported by PD patients. Some have hypothesized that there is an increased frequency of RLS due to dopamine deficiency, and they have proposed that RLS may be inherent to PD. Others have observed that RLS and akathisia may be confused and account for the increased frequency. Indeed, RLS can be easily mimicked by motor restlessness.[67] Thus, in a cohort of 269 PD patients, the prevalence of RLS was only 11%, similar to that in the general population,[116] while a survey study of 303 patients demonstrated an RLS frequency of 21% in PD. When further evaluating the PD patients with RLS, it was seen that they also had a lower ferritin level, which is a known risk factor for RLS.[80]

Table 51.1 Sleep-Regulating Nuclei Possibly Underlying Primary Sleep Disturbances in Parkinson's Disease

NUCLEUS/AREA	MAIN TRANSMITTER	FUNCTION	CONSEQUENCE OF DYSFUNCTION IN PD
Nucleus pedunculopontinus	Ach	Regulation of REM-S	RBD
Locus coeruleus	NA	Regulation of REM-S	Reduction/absence of REM sleep
Area peri-locus coeruleus	?	Inhibition of spinal motoneurons via nucleus magnocellularis	Loss of muscle atonia during REM => RBD
Raphe nuclei in midbrain and pons	5HT	Regulation of SWS	Reduction of SWS
Midbrain tegmental area	DA	Thalamocortical arousal	Reduction of SWS Excessive sleepiness during daytime
Hypothalamus	Orexin/ hypocretin	Maintenance of daytime vigilance	Abrupt napping and microsleeps during daytime

PD, Parkinson's disease; REM-S, REM sleep; RBD, REM sleep behavior disorder; SWS, slow-wave sleep.

Sleep-related *respiratory muscle dysfunction* can reflect the fluctuations in motor function arising from intermittent use of antiparkinsonian medication (peak-dose or end-dose dysrhythmia). Patients and physicians often misinterpret these phenomena as related to cardiac or pulmonary problems. The immediate sensation upon awakening is a sensation of suffocation interpreted as *sleep apnea syndrome* (SAS). However, when comparing PD patients with non-PD subjects, matched for apnea/hypopnea indices (AHI), PD patients demonstrate significantly less oxygen desaturation.[26] Whether there is an increased frequency of SAS in PD is not yet clear. It does appear that PD patients with SAS also do not have increased body mass and therefore may not be suspected of having SAS. Hence, there may be many factors that contribute to a history suggestive of sleep apnea, and polysomnography may be indicated to make the distinction.[20,59,113]

Depression and *anxiety* are strongly correlated with nocturnal sleep abnormalities in general, and both can cause nightly awakenings and the feeling of unrefreshing sleep.[63,72,84,104]

TERTIARY SLEEP DISTURBANCES DUE TO PHARMACOLOGIC TREATMENTS

Pharmacological treatment influences sleep in different ways, depending on the specific drug and its administration schedule. Antiparkinsonian medications can both *relieve and aggravate* nocturnal symptoms. The effect of *levodopa* has been studied most extensively, and it shows a dual effect: low dosages of levodopa have a sedating, sleep-enhancing effect, while large doses have a stimulating, sleep-inhibiting effect. It is speculated that at low dosage, levodopa primarily stimulates self-inhibitory dopamine autoreceptors, while at high dosage it induces a postsynaptic stimulation.[23] However, the applicability of these laboratory-based findings to treatment in PD patients remains controversial. Thus, a case-control study, investigating the impact of 200 mg controlled-release levodopa, given at bedtime, on sleep microstructure in PD patients, found no impact on various sleep parameters.[117]

Similarly, a polysomnogram-based retrospective study did not evidence a correlation between total dosage of diurnal dopaminergic medication and the amount of slow-wave sleep,[27] whereas another study did show an increase of sleep stages 1 and 2 with the administration of dopaminergic drugs.[54] As the levodopa wears off in the early morning hours, akinetic episodes may recur, causing early morning awakening. Levodopa also causes nighttime hallucinations. It has been shown that the dose-dependent sleep disruption caused by levodopa predominates in the early stages of the disease and that the beneficial effects on nocturnal akinesia and stiffness predominate in the late stages.[115]

THE SYMPTOMS

Insomnia

Self-reported insomnia is one of the factors that most strongly predict poor quality of life in PD patients.[53] *Sleep initiation insomnia* is uncommon and may reflect an amphetamine-like effect of selegiline or an alerting effect of levodopa. This effect wanes after a short time. *Sleep maintenance insomnia* is more common, and PD patients rate this symptom among the five most troublesome symptoms at a late stage of the disease.[89] They awake after 2–3 hours, feeling relatively refreshed and unable to fall back to sleep. The sleep remains *fragmented* throughout the night. Secondary factors may contribute to maintenance insomnia as well, including decreased body movement and reduced positional shifts, nocturia, altered dream content, pain, anxiety, and depression. During daytime, sleepiness recurs and the patient takes multiple short naps. Although sleep is not consolidated, the total quantity of sleep over a 24-hour period is normal.[74] As is seen in other elderly people, PD patients may *advance* their sleeping hours, with earlier bedtimes and morning awakenings. Depressed PD patients may also have an altered sleep perception or *pseudoinsomnia*. In advanced cases there may be transitory *overlapping of sleep and wakefulness*, and in this setting, one is hard pressed to define whether the patient is awake or asleep the majority of the time.[77]

Hypersomnia

Drowsiness and tiredness in PD can have different clinical expressions that have to be distinguished because different therapeutic approaches are applied.

Fatigue or lassitude is defined as an overwhelming sense of tiredness, lack of energy, or feeling of exhaustion. As a purely subjective parameter, it is difficult to quantify fatigue. A community-based study found fatigue in 44% of the PD patients, in contrast to only 18% of healthy elderly controls.[53] *Excessive daytime sleepiness (EDS)* is defined as symptomatic daytime somnolence with frequent sleep periods. EDS is severe in 15% of PD patients in a community-based setting, and mild *daytime sleepiness* is found in another 10%.[107] In an university outpatient setting, 44% of the PD patients complained of EDS.[114] EDS in PD patients has been associated with more severe PD, with higher frequency of cognitive decline.

It has been known for many years that somnolence can develop as a side effect of levodopa.[52] Likewise, the nonergot dopamine agonists can cause sleepiness and have been associated with *abrupt and irresistible onset of sleep* or "*sleep attacks.*"[34,35,85] In an early report,[34] eight patients were reported with sudden irresistible naps that resulted in car accidents; all were taking pramipexole and one has similar episodes when switched to ropinirole. These attacks stopped after discontinuation of the drug. In a second retrospective study, 21 of 37 patients taking pramipexole reported some level of somnolence and 7 of them felt asleep while driving. The dose of pramipexole was relatively high.[77] The authors suggested a specific soporific effect of D2/D3 agonists based on observations that the direct application of D2/D3 agonists into the ventral tegmental dopaminergic nucleus induces narcolepsy in an animal model.[92] In addition, these DA agents are thought to downregulate dopaminergic input to the reticular activating system by preferentially acting on presynaptic receptors. Thus, it was thought that this class of dopaminergic agents imparts a particular risk for EDS. Two multicenter studies, however, suggested that any dopaminergic agent could be at fault. A study with over 600 PD patients reported a correlation between the Epworth sleepiness score and levodopa-equivalent daily doses, independently of the drug chosen.[43] Another study conducted phone interviews in almost 3000 PD patients and showed that sleep attacks could occur with both direct dopamine agonists and levodopa. The odds ratio for dopamine agonist therapy was 2.9 compared to 1.9 with levodopa therapy. It was also 1.05 for a 1-year-longer disease duration.[88] Other clinicians also found that EDS was associated with the onset of autonomic failure, presence of advanced disease, and male gender, but not with use of any specific DA agonist.[68,79,85] Thus, the specificity and the pathophysiological background of sleep attacks due to dopamine agonists are far from being resolved.[3,44,76,88,118] It is therefore prudent to caution patients about excessive daytime sleepiness and falling asleep at the wheel, whenever any dopaminergic agent is initiated.[76,122]

Parasomnias

In 1986 Schenck et al.[99] described a new parasomnia, called *REM-sleep behavior disorder (RBD)* and defined as loss of muscle atonia during REM sleep, in association with complex, vigorous, or violent movements (acting out of dreams). Idiopathic PD and other forms of Parkinsonism were identified among the associated causes. Ten years later the same authors[101] showed that RBD can *precede the onset* of PD; 11 out of 29 male PD patients (38%) developed symptoms of RBD a mean of 3.7 years prior to the onset of PD. The maximal interval between RBD onset and PD diagnosis was 12.7 years. These findings have since been confirmed by other investigators and suggest that from 50% to 70% of the subjects with primary RBD are at risk of having a parkinsonian syndrome within two decades. This interval may be as long as 50 years. However, these observations are limited by the lack of objective polysomnographic data to diagnose RBD.[19,37,48]

Prevalence, incidence, and additional clinical characteristics of RBD are described extensively in Chapter 29. Briefly, the patients show aggressive behavior, involving complex movements like gesturing, arm flailing, kicking, sitting, crawling, and punching that occur during REM sleep. When awakened, they recall vivid, action-packed, violent dreams. Self-injuries include ecchymoses, lacerations, and fractures. Bed partners are also at risk for injuries at the hands of the sleeping patient. However, not all behaviors are violent. Nonviolent elaborate behaviors have been observed as well.[83] An association between RBD and visual hallucinations (has been proposed, as visual hallucinations may represent REM fragments exported in wakefulness and thus correspond to dream imagery.[5] Finally, *formes frustes*, just documented by loss of muscle atonia during REM, may be the most common form of REM sleep dysfunction in PD patients.[70]

More recently, another parasomnia, *sleepwalking*, has been shown to be associated with PD. It has first been reported that in a PD cohort of 165 patients, 6 patients (4%) experienced new-onset sleepwalking, emerging with or after PD onset.[90] Later the same authors reported that in a survey of 417 PD patients, 9% indicated sleepwalking, with 5% having first experienced this symptom as an adult. The first study confirmed the syndrome by polysomnography in five out of six patients, while the second study was only questionnaire based.[75]

Caregiver Concerns

Self-reported sleep disturbances have been reported by 27% of male and 48% of female spouses in one large questionnaire-based survey of 153 PD patient/spouse pairs. The spouses not only complained about poor sleep quality related to their own rating of depression but also about frequent awakenings in order to assist the patient. These surprising findings suggest that a major contributing factor to the caregiver distress is the patient's sleep disturbances.[103]

POLYSOMNOGRAPHIC FINDINGS

Our knowledge of polysomnographic findings in *untreated* PD is limited, as there are only a few studies from the 1970s and one recent study, all with limited description of the clinical stage.[12,119,120] Other abnormalities of sleep architecture are disease inherent, even when lacking direct clinical consequences. PD patients have a reduction of total sleep time and frequent awakenings.[12,119] Concerning *non-REM sleep*, they show a reduction of sleep spindles and K complexes in stage 2.[32] Interestingly enough, it has been advocated that a reduction in K-complexes is equivalent to a reduction of synchronizing, oscillatory rhythms, which could produce poor gating and filtering of sensory input and thus be a risk factor for hallucinations.[58] Actually a reduction of K complexes has been found in late-stage hallucinating PD patients, but we lack data on nonhallucinating PD patients.[21] PD patients produce less deep sleep, especially of stage 4. Concerning *REM sleep*, increased alpha activity has been shown in de novo patients during the first one third of the night. This finding possibly indicates a deficient "REM sleep pressure" as an early sign of a functional disconnection between generators of REM and non-REM sleep in PD.[120] EMG atonia can be periodically abolished in REM sleep, as a precursor sign of RBD. Nevertheless, trained scorers show high

Table 51.2 Typical Polysomnographic Findings in Parkinson's Disease

POLYSOMNOGRAPHY

Repeated blinking (blepharospasm) at sleep onset
Reduction of sleep spindles in stage II
Reduction of K complexes in stage II
Reduction of sleep III/IV
Blepharospasm and rapid eye movements during slow-wave sleep
Intermittent loss of muscle atonia during REM sleep
Phasic muscle bursts in non-REM sleep
Intermixture of sleep stages (rhythm in REM; REM in non-REM)
No normal cycling of REM/non-REM
Pronounced sleep fragmentation

Multiple sleep latency test

REM sleep onsets
Reduced sleep onset latency

interrater reliability for identification of REM sleep in PD.[13] Bursts of phasic muscle activity can be seen in non-REM sleep stages as well.[14] REM sleep can intrude in other sleep stages, α rhythm reappear during REM periods, and the normal REM/non-REM cycling can be abolished. Finally, hemiparkinsonism does not cause nocturnal EEG asymmetry.[71]

EDS has also been assessed during *multiple sleep latency tests* (MSLTs) in PD patients. Patients with RBD may have REM-sleep onsets,[4,95] although this has not been confirmed in a more recent study realizing MSLT in 30 patients. In this latter study EDS could well have been documented with 11 patients (37%), having a mean sleep latency under 5 minutes. However, none showed sleep-onset REM episodes.[91] Typical polysomnographic findings are summarized in Table 51.2.

THERAPEUTIC STRATEGIES

There is still a substantial lack of evidence-based guidelines concerning the treatment of sleep disorders in PD. In its report on treatment of nonmotor symptoms in PD, the Quality Standards Subcommittee of the American Academy of Neurology did not find any treatment with a level A recommendation.[123] The paucity of evidence-supported guidelines is noted by others, although their conclusions are less restrictive.[10,17,64,69] Objective evaluation of treatment strategies is also hampered by the lack of objective polysomnogram-driven data. For instance, continuous dopaminergic stimulation has been proposed as a best treatment option in general (see later). However, in two studies, providing also objective polysomnogram criteria, no change was found in terms of the number of hours slept, sleep latency, total sleep quantity, or number of awakenings.[30,105]

IMPACT OF SLEEP ON PARKINSONIAN SYMPTOMS

Not all PD daytime symptoms persist in the same amount at nighttime. For example, the alternating PD *resting tremor* becomes *subclinical* at nighttime; its amplitude and duration decrease gradually from stage 1 to stage 4 and tremor completely vanishes during REM.[8] On the other hand, sleep can improve the parkinsonian signs of the next morning. The so-called *sleep benefit* phenomenon is defined as motor improvement after sleep and before drug intake. The term has been coined by Marsden et al. in 1981.[60] who observed a transient amelioration, especially of the tremor in up to 20% of the subjects (treated or untreated). Recent surveys found evidence of sleep benefit in even 33% to 55% of the patients.[24,66] These patients tend to have good cognitive and functional levels, but they do not show a different polysomnographic pattern than those without sleep benefit.[45] Sleep benefit lasts from 30 minutes to 3 hours, and some patients can delay or even skip the first morning dose of their antiparkinsonian medication. Pathogenesis remains unclear. There is no pharmacological evidence for nocturnal *presynaptic accumulation* of levodopa or *postsynaptic sensibilization* for levodopa.

CONVENTIONAL TREATMENT

General principles of sleep hygiene are especially applicable to PD patients. Because of the fluctuating motor impairment, PD patients may acquire poor sleep habits over time, like frequent and extended naps during the day, irregular bedtimes, and irregular meals. A sleep diary can be a first step for assessment. In addition to sleep hygiene concerns, causes of sleep disturbances that affect the elderly populations should be considered. Obstructive sleep apnea, although not more common in PD patients than in age-matched controls, may cause significant sleep disruption with consequent excessive daytime sleepiness. It is highly treatable if correctly diagnosed. Pain from arthritis, nocturia due to urinary tract disorders, as well as the effect of medications used to treat concurrent medical conditions may all cause sleep disruption. One randomized controlled study has compared the nonbenzodiazepine hypnotic eszoplicone versus placebo in insomniac PD patients and found improved quality and maintenance of sleep, reduced number of awakenings, but no difference in total sleep time in the treated group.[65] In a small, open-trial study, quetiapine, an atypical second-generation neuroleptic, has improved subjective sleep quality.[51] Thus, the frequent use of benzodiazepines or atypical neuroleptics in the PD population requires further confirmation by additional studies.

SPECIFIC PHARMACOTHERAPY

Global Subjective Sleep Quality

Two recent studies have focused on global subjective sleep quality. The first study was a double-blind, randomized, placebo-controlled study and applied rotigotine by transdermal patch. There was a significant treatment effect on the PDSS-2 score, in particular for the items "difficulty falling asleep," "urge to move arms and legs," and "uncomfortable and immobile."[111] The second study compared prolonged-release versus immediate-release ropinirole in 33 patients.[30] Prolonged-release formula showed better scores on different sleep-related questionnaires than immediate-release formula; sleep attacks completely disappeared in 8 patients. However, as already mentioned earlier, objective data, obtained in a small subgroup of patients, did not show any difference.

Nocturnal Akinesia

At low dosages, levodopa can improve sleep continuity, while higher dosages have an awakening effect. With high dopaminergic dosages, nighttime hallucinations and nightmares can develop. Optimization of daytime antiparkinsonian treatment may also improve sleep efficiency.[9] For *nocturnal akinesia*, levodopa is equally

efficient, when given a standard or slow-release formula. Nocturnal disability improves in 57% and 61%, respectively, and a similar percentage of patients continue the treatment.[110] In refractory cases, overnight apomorphine infusion has been effective.[93]

Excessive Daytime Sleepiness and Fatigue

In selected patients *very pronounced EDS* be treated by modafinil or sodium oxybate,[41,46,81,82] while methylphenidate or modafinil has been suggested to treat *fatigue*.[57,62] However, the experience for both treatment options is still limited.

Other Specific Treatment Options

Periodic leg movements are very sensitive to late-day intake of pergolide or another dopamine agonist. The dosage is usually very low, so that the orthostatic side effects of these drugs do not occur. *REM sleep behavior disorder* usually responds well to clonazepam given at bedtime.[78,101] It is unknown whether this benzodiazepine has a specific effect in RBD or whether other benzodiazepines are equally effective. The cessation of mirtazepine, venlafaxine, or fluoxetine has been reported to be efficient in improving RBD.[73,100,102] Tan et al.[106] reported improvement of RBD by dopaminergic treatment. *Nocturnal hallucinations* have to be distinguished from RBD, as they respond to other treatment strategies. Despite its application restrictions, the atypical neuroleptic clozapine has become the treatment of choice, if reduction of the dopaminergic treatment is not possible or inefficient. The direct impact of clozapine on the sleep architecture of PD patients has not been studied specifically, but individual patients and their caregiver normally report a better sleep. There is no increase of fatigue or daytime somnolence, if the nocturnal dosage remains lower or equal to 25 mg.[109]

DEEP BRAIN STIMULATION

The impact of deep brain stimulation (DBS) at different localizations has been studied in relation to its effect on sleep. In general, DBS improves nocturnal akathisia as well as axial and early morning dystonia; consequently total sleep time is increased. Bilateral STN-DBS has been studied most thoroughly; it increases total sleep time and reduces sleep problems, as subjectively reported by the patient. This effect is maintained for at least 2 years. However, despite dosage reduction of the dopaminergic treatment, EDS is not reduced.[56] Thalamic-generated sleep spindles are also not modified by this treatment, and there is no reduction of PLM and RBD, confirming the current concept that these symptoms are not mediated by nigro-striato-pallido-cortical pathways.[4]

Despite these therapeutic strategies, it is not uncommon for sleep in the advanced PD patient to remain very disrupted, with numerous arousals, turnings, nightmares, or vocalizations due to RBD. To prevent undue caregiver stress, it is wise to suggest that the caregiver move to another room to obtain a good night sleep, if possible.[84,103]

FUTURE RESEARCH AVENUES

Prospective and longitudinal sleep-related data over the course of the disease are needed to clarify the role of the multiple causes of sleep disturbances in PD and its consequences on daily life. These issues are highlighted in the recent modification of the Unified Parkinson's Disease Rating Scale (the MDS-UPDRS). In MDS-UPDRS, part II, specific questions address daytime sleepiness and nighttime sleep problems. Potentially there is differential effect of different dopamine receptors on sleep modulation, as recently suggested by the debate on sleep attacks provoked by D2/D3 agonists. Daytime sleepiness needs to be more systematically investigated by MSLT, mean wakefulness tests, and standardized questionnaires. The effect of EDS on driving safety also requires further investigation. Additional studies of sleep and daytime sleepiness in PD will provide not only improved ways to diagnose and treat patients but also insights into the underlying pathophysiology of this degenerative disorder.

REFERENCES

1. Alessandro S, Ceravolo R, Brusa L. Non-motor functions in parkinsonian patients implanted in the pedunculopontine nucleus: focus on sleep and cognitive domains. *J Neurol Sci* 2010;289:44–8.
2. Amara AW, Watts RL, Walker HC. The effects of deep brain stimulation on sleep in Parkinson's disease. *Ther Adv Neurol Disord* 2011;4:15–24.
3. Arellano FM, Corrigan M. Falling asleep at the wheel: motor vehicle mishaps in persons taking pramipexole and ropinirole. *Neurology* 2000;54:275.
4. Arnulf I, Bejjani B, Garma L, et al. Improvement of sleep architecture in PD with subthalamic nucleus stimulation. *Neurology* 2000;55:1732–4.
5. Arnulf I, Bonnet AM, Damier P, et al. Hallucinations, REM sleep, and Parkinson's disease. *Neurology* 2000;55:281–8.
6. Arnulf I, Konofal E, Merino-Andreu M, et al. Parkinson's disease and sleepiness: an integral part of PD. *Neurology* 2002;58:1019–24.
7. Arnulf I, Ferraye M, Fraix V, et al. Sleep induced by stimulation in the human pedunculopontine nucleus area. *Ann Neurol* 2010;67:546–9.
8. Askenasy JJ, Yahr MD. Parkinsonian tremor loses its alternating aspect during non-REM sleep and is inhibited by REM sleep. *J Neurol Neurosurg Psychiatry* 1990;53:749–53.
9. Askenasy JM. Approaching disturbed sleep in late Parkinson's disease: first step toward a proposal for a revised UPDRS. *Parkinsonism Relat Disord* 2001;8:123–31.
10. Aurora RN, Zak RS, Maganti RK, et al. Best practice guide for the treatment of REM sleep behavior disorder (RBD). *J Clin Sleep Med* 2010; 6: 85–95.
11. Barone P, Antonini A, Colosimo C, et al. The PRIAMO study: a multicenter assessment of nonmotor symptoms and their impact on quality of life in Parkinson's disease. *Mov Disord* 2009;24:1641–9.
12. Bergonzi P, Chiurulla C, Gambi D, et al. L-dopa plus dopa-decarboxylase inhibitor. Sleep organization in Parkinson's syndrome before and after treatment. *Acta Neurol Belg* 1975;75:5–10.
13. Bliwise DL, Williams ML, Irbe D, et al. Inter-rater reliability for identification of REM sleep in Parkinson's disease. *Sleep* 2000;23:671–7.
14. Bliwise DL, Trotti LM, Greer SA, et al. Phasic muscle activity in sleep and clinical features of Parkinson disease. *Ann Neurol* 2010;68:353–9.
15. Braak H, Del Tredici K, Rüb U, et al. Staging of brain pathology related to sporadic Parkinson's disease. *Neurobiol Aging* 2003;24:197–211.
16. Charcot JM. *Lectures on the Diseases of the Nervous System. Lecture V.* Sigerson G, trans. London: The New Sydenham Society; 1877.
17. Chaudhuri KR, Schapira AHV. Non-motor symptoms of Parkinson's disease:

dopaminergic pathophysiology and treatment. *Lancet Neurol* 2009;8:464–74.

18. Chokroverty S. Sleep and degenerative neurologic disorders. *Neurologic Clinics* 1996;14:807–26.

19. Claassen DO, Josephs KA, Ahlskog JE, et al. REM sleep behavior disorder preceding other aspects of synucleinopathies by up to half a century. *Neurology* 2010;75:494–9.

20. Cochen De Cock V, Abouda M, Leu S, et al. Is obstructive sleep apnea a problem in Parkinson's disease? *Sleep Med* 2010;11:247–52.

21. Comella CL, Tanner CM, Ristanovic RK. Polysomnographic sleep measures in Parkinson's disease patients with treatment-induced hallucinations. *Ann Neurol* 1993;34:710–14.

22. Compta Y, Santamaria J, Ratti L, et al. Cerebrospinal hypocretin, daytime sleepiness and sleep architecture in Parkinson's disease dementia. *Brain* 2009;132:3308–17.

23. Corsini GU, Del Zompo M, Manconi S, et al. Evidence for dopamine receptors in the human brain mediating sedation and sleep. *Life Sci* 1977;20:1613–18.

24. Currie LJ, Bennett JP, Jr., Harrison MB, et al. Clinical correlates of sleep benefit in Parkinson's disease. *Neurology* 1997;48:1115–17.

25. Diederich NJ, Vaillant M, Mancuso G, et al. Progressive sleep "destructuring" in Parkinson's disease. A polysomnographic study in 46 patients. *Sleep Med* 2005;6:313–18.

26. Diederich NJ, Vaillant M, Leischen M, et al. Sleep apnea syndrome in Parkinson's disease. A case-control study in 49 patients. *Mov Disord* 2005;20:1413–18.

27. Diederich NJ, Paolini V, Vaillant M. Slow wave sleep and dopaminergic treatment in Parkinson's disease. A polysomnographic study. *Acta Neurol Scand* 2009;120:308–13.

28. Diederich NJ, McIntyre DJ. Sleep disorders in Parkinson's Disease. Many causes, few therapeutic options. *J Neurol Sci* 2012;314:12–9.

29. Drouot X, Moutereau S, Nguyen JP, et al. Low levels of ventricular CSF orexin/hypocretin in advanced PD. *Neurology* 2003;61:540–3.

30. Dusek P, Buskova J, Ruzicka E, et al. Effects of ropinirole prolonged-release on sleep disturbances and daytime sleepiness in Parkinson's disease. *Clin Neuropharmacol* 2010;33:186–90.

31. Dymecki J, Lechowicz W, Bertrand E, et al. Changes in dopaminergic neurons of the mesocorticolimbic system in Parkinson's disease. *Folia Neuropathol* 1996;34:102–6.

32. Emser W, Brenner M, Stober T, et al Changes in nocturnal sleep in Huntington's and Parkinson's disease. *J Neurol* 1988;235:177–9.

33. Fronczek R, Overeem S, Lee SY, et al. Hypocretin (orexin) loss in Parkinson's disease. *Brain* 2007;130:1577–85.

34. Frucht SJ, Rogers JD, Greene PE, et al. Falling asleep at the wheel: motor vehicle mishaps in persons taking pramipexole and ropinirole. *Neurology* 1999;52:1908–10.

35. Frucht SJ, Greene PE, Fahn S. Sleep episodes in Parkinson's disease: a wake-up call. *Mov Disord* 2000;15:601–3.

36. Gallagher DA, Lees AJ, Schrag A. What are the most important nonmotor symptoms in patients with Parkinson's disease and are we missing them? *Mov Disord* 2010;25:2493–500.

37. Gagnon JF, Postuma RB, Mazza S, et al. Rapid-eye-movement sleep behaviour disorder and neurodegenerative diseases. *Lancet Neurol* 2006;5:424–32.

38. Garcias-Borregueroa D, Larrosa O, Granizo JJ, et al. Circadian variation in neuroendocrine response to L-dopa in patients with restless legs syndrome. *Sleep* 2004;27:669–73.

39. Gowers WR. *A Manual of Diseases of the Nervous System.* 2nd ed. Philadelphia, PA: P. Blakiston; 1893:643–4.

40. Happe S, Schrodl B, Faltl M, et al. Sleep disorders and depression in patients with Parkinson's disease. *Acta Neurol Scand* 2001;104:275–80.

41. Happe S, Pirker W, Sauter C, et al. Successful treatment of excessive daytime sleepiness in Parkinson's disease with modafinil. *J Neurol* 2001;248:632–4.

42. Haq IZ, Naidu Y, Reddy P, et al. Narcolepsy in Parkinson's disease. *Expert Rev Neurother* 2010;10:879–84.

43. Hobson DE, Lang AE, Martin WR, et al. Excessive daytime sleepiness and sudden-onset sleep in Parkinson disease: a survey by the Canadian Movement Disorders Group. *JAMA* 2002;287:455–63.

44. Hoehn MM. Falling asleep at the wheel: motor vehicle mishaps in persons taking pramipexole and ropinirole. *Neurology* 2000;54:275.

45. Högl BE, Gómez-Arévalo G, García S, et al. A clinical, pharmacologic, and polysomnographic study of sleep benefit in Parkinson's disease. *Neurology* 1998;50:1332–9.

46. Högl B, Saletu M, Brandauer E, et al. Modafinil for the treatment of daytime sleepiness in

Parkinson's disease: a double-blind, randomized, crossover, placebo-controlled polygraphic trial. *Sleep* 2002;25:905–9.

47. Högl B, Arnulf I, Comella C, et al. Scales to assess sleep impairment in Parkinson's disease: critique and recommendations. *Mov Disord* 2010;25:2704–16.

48. Iranzo A, Molinuevo JL, Santamaria J, et al. Rapid eye-movement sleep behavior disorder as an early marker for a neurodegenerative disorder: a descriptive study. *Lancet Neurol* 2006;5:572–7.

49. Jellinger K. The pedunculopontine nucleus in Parkinson' disease, progressive supranuclear palsy and Alzheimer's disease. *J Neurol Neurosurg Psychiatr* 1988;51:540–3.

50. Jellinger KA. Neuropathological correlates of mental dysfunction in Parkinson's disease: an update. In: Wolters EC, Scheltens P, Berendse HW, eds. *Mental Dysfunction in Parkinson's Disease II*. Utrecht, The Netherlans: Academic Pharmaceutical Productions BV; 1999:82–105.

51. Juri C, Chaná P, Tapia J, et al. Quetiapine for insomnia in Parkinson disease: results from an open-label trial. *Clin Neuropharmacol* 2005;28:185–7.

52. Kales A, Ansel RD, Markham CH, et al. Sleep in patients with Parkinson's disease and normal subjects prior to and following levodopa administration. *Clin Pharmacol Ther* 1971;12:397–406.

53. Karlsen K, Larsen JP, Tandberg E, et al. Fatigue in patients with Parkinson's disease. *Mov Disord* 1999;14:237–41.

54. Kaynak D, Kiziltan G, Kaynak H, et al. Sleep and sleepiness in patients with Parkinson's disease before and after dopaminergic treatment. *Eur J Neurol* 2005;12:199–207.

55. Lees AJ, Blackburn NA, Campbell VL. The nighttime problems of Parkinson's disease. *Clin Neuropharm* 1988;11:512–19.

56. Lyons KE, Pahwa R. Effects of bilateral subthalamic nucleus stimulation on sleep, daytime sleepiness, and early morning dystonia in patients with Parkinson disease. *J Neurosurg* 2006;104:502–5.

57. Lou JS, Dimitrova DM, Park BS, et al. Using modafinil to treat fatigue in Parkinson disease: a double-blind, placebo-controlled pilot study. *Clin Neuropharmacol* 2009;32:305–10.

58. Mahowald MW. Synchrony, sleep, dreams, and consciousness: clues from K-complexes. *Neurology* 1997;49:909–11.

59. Maria B, Sophia S, Michalis M, et al. Sleep breathing disorders in patients with idiopathic Parkinson's disease. *Respir Med* 2003;97:1151–7.

60. Marsden CD, Parkes J, Quinn N. Fluctuations of disability in Parkinson's disease: clinical aspects. In: Marsden CD, Fahn S, eds. *Movement Disorders*. London: Butterworth Scientific; 1981:96–122.

61. Martinez-Martin P, Visser M, Rodriguez-Blazquez C, et al. SCOPA-sleep and PDSS: two scales for assessment of sleep disorder in Parkinson's disease. *Mov Disord* 2008;23:1681–8.

62. Mendonça DA, Menezes K, Jog MS. Methylphenidate improves fatigue scores in Parkinson disease: a randomized controlled trial. *Mov Disord* 2007;22:2070–6.

63. Menza MA, Rosen RC. Sleep in Parkinson's disease. The role of depression and anxiety. *Psychosomatics* 1995;36:262–6.

64. Menza M, Dobkin RD, Marin H, et al. Sleep disturbances in Parkinson's disease. *Mov Disord* 2010;25(Suppl 1):S117–22.

65. Menza M, Dobkin RD, Marin H. Treatment of insomnia in Parkinson's disease: a controlled trial of eszopiclone and placebo. *Mov Disord* 2010;25:1708–14.

66. Merello M, Hughes A, Colosimo C, et al. Sleep benefit in Parkinson's disease. *Mov Disord* 1997;12:506–8.

67. Möller JC, Unger M, Stiasny-Kolster K, et al. Restless legs syndrome (RLS) and Parkinson's disease (PD)-related disorders or different entities? *J Neurol Sci* 2010;289:135–7.

68. Montastruc JL, Brefel-Courbon C, Senard JM, et al. Sleep attacks and antiparkinsonian drugs: a pilot prospective pharmacoepidemiologic study. *Clin Neuropharmacol* 2001;24:181–3.

69. Morgenthaler TI, Kapur VK, Brown T, et al. Practice parameters for the treatment of narcolepsy and other hypersomnias of central origin. *Sleep* 2007;30:1705–11.

70. Mouret J. Differences in sleep in patients with Parkinson's disease. *Electroencephalogr Clin Neurophysiol* 1975;38:653–7.

71. Myslobodsky M, Mintz M, Ben-Mayor V, et al. Unilateral dopamine deficit and lateral EEG asymmetry: sleep abnormalities in hemi-Parkinson's patients. *Electroencephalogr Clin Neurophysiol* 1982;54:227–31.

72. Naismith SL, Hickie IB, Lewis SJ. The role of mild depression in sleep disturbance and quality of life in Parkinson's disease. *J Neuropsychiatry Clin Neurosci* 2010;22:384–9.

73. Nash JR, Wilson SJ, Potokar JP, et al. Mirtazapine induces REM sleep behavior disorder (RBD) in Parkinsonism. *Neurology* 2003;61:1161.

74. Nausieda PA. Sleep in Parkinson's disease. In: Koller WC, ed. *Handbook of Parkinson's Disease*. 2nd ed. New York: Marcel Dekker; 1993:451–67.

75. Oberholzer M, Poryazova R, Bassetti CL. Sleepwalking in Parkinson's disease: a questionnaire-based survey. *J Neurol* 2011;258(7):1261–7.

76. Olanow CW, Schapira HV, Roth T. Waking up to sleep episodes in Parkinson's disease. *Mov Disord* 2000;2:212–15.

77. Olanow CW, Schapira HV, Roth T. Falling asleep at the wheel: motor vehicle mishaps in persons taking pramipexole and ropinirole. *Neurology* 2000;54:274.

78. Olson EJ, Boeve BF, Silber MH. Rapid eye movement sleep behaviour disorder: demographic, clinical and laboratory findings in 93 cases. *Brain* 2000;123:331–9.

79. Ondo WG, Dat-Vuong K, Khan H, et al. Daytime sleepiness and other sleep disorders in Parkinson's disease. *Neurology* 2001;57:1392–6.

80. Ondo WG, Dat-Vuong K, Jankovic J. Exploring the relationship between Parkinson disease and restless legs syndrome. *Arch Neurol* 2002;59:421–4.

81. Ondo WG, Fayle R, Atassi F, Jankovic J. Modafinil for daytime somnolence in Parkinson's disease: double blind, placebo controlled parallel trial. *J Neurol Neurosurg Psychiatry* 2005;76:1636–9.

82. Ondo WG, Perkins T, Swick T, et al. Sodium oxybate for excessive daytime sleepiness in Parkinson disease: an open-label polysomnographic study. *Arch Neurol* 2008;65:1337–40.

83. Oudiette D, De Cock VC, Lavault S, et al. Nonviolent elaborate behaviors may also occur in REM sleep behavior disorder. *Neurology* 2009;72:551–7.

84. Pal PK, Thennarasu K, Fleming J, et al. Nocturnal sleep disturbances and daytime dysfunction in patients with Parkinson's disease and in their caregivers. *Parkinsonism Relat Disord* 2004;10:157–68.

85. Pal S, Bhattacharya KF, Agapito C et al. A study of excessive daytime sleepiness and its clinical significance in three groups of Parkinson's disease patients taking pramipexole, cabergoline and levodopa mono

86. Parkinson J. *An Essay on the Shaking Palsy*. London: Whittingham and Rowland for Sherwood, Neely, and Jones; 1817.

87. Paulus W, Jellinger K. The neuropathologic basis of different clinical subgroups of Parkinson's disease. *J Neuropathol Exp Neurol* 1991; 50: 743–55.

88. Paus S, Brecht HM, Köster J et al. Sleep attacks, daytime sleepiness, and dopamine agonists in Parkinson's disease. *Mov Disord* 2003; 18: 659–67.

89. Politis M, Wu K, Molloy S. Parkinson's disease symptoms: the patient's perspective. *Mov Disord* 2010;25:1646–51.

90. Poryazova R, Waldvogel D, Bassetti CL. Sleepwalking in patients with Parkinson disease. *Arch Neurol* 2007;64:1524–7.

91. Poryazova R, Benninger D, Waldvogel D, et al. Excessive daytime sleepiness in Parkinson's disease: characteristics and determinants. *Eur Neurol* 2010; 63:129–35.

92. Reid MS, Tafti M, Nishino S, et al. Local administration of dopaminergic drugs into the ventral tegmental area modulates cataplexy in the narcoleptic canine *Brain Res* 1996;733:83–100.

93. Reuter I, Ellis CM, Chaudhuri K. Nocturnal subcutaneous apomorphine infusion in Parkinson's disease and restless legs syndrome. *Acta Neurol Scand* 1999;100:163–7.

94. Riedel O, Klotsche J, Spottke A, et al. Frequency of dementia, depression, and other neuropsychiatric symptoms in 1449 outpatients with Parkinson's disease. *J Neurol* 2010;257:1073–82.

95. Rye DB, Johnston LH, Watts RL, et al. Juvenile Parkinson's disease with REM sleepbehavior disorder, sleepiness, and daytime REM onset. *Neurology* 1999;53:1868–70.

96. Rye DB, Bliwise DL, Dihenia B, et al. Daytime sleepiness in Parkinson's disease. *J Sleep Res* 2000;9:63–9.

97. Rye DB. The two faces of Eve: dopamine's modulation of wakefulness and sleep. *Neurology* 2004;63(Suppl 3):S2–S7.

98. Scarnati E, Florio T. The pedunculopontine nucleus and related structures. *Adv Neurol* 1997;74:97–110.

99. Schenck CH, Bundlie SR, Ettinger MG, et al. Chronic behavioral disorders of human REM sleep: a new category of parasomnia. *Sleep* 1986;9:293–308.

and combination therapy. *J Neural Transm* 2001;108:71–7.

100. Schenck CH, Mahowald MW, Kim SW, et al. Prominent eye movements during NREM sleep and REM sleep behavior disorder associated with fluoxetine treatment of depression and obsessive-compulsive disorder. *Sleep* 1992;15:226–35.

101. Schenck CH, Bundlie SR, Mahowald MW. Delayed emergence of a Parkinsonian disorder in 38% of 29 older men initially diagnosed with idiopathic rapid eye movement sleep behavior disorder. *Neurology* 1996;46:388–93.

102. Schutte S, Doghramji K. REM behavior disorder seen with venlafaxine (Effexor). *Sleep Res* 1996;25:364.

103. Smith MC, Ellgring H, Oertel WH. Sleep disturbances in Parkinson's disease patients and spouses. *J Am Geriatr Soc* 1997;45:194–9.

104. Starkstein SE, Preziosi TJ, Robinson RG. Sleep disorders, pain and depression in Parkinson's disease. *Eur Neurol* 1991;31:352–5.

105. Stocchi F, Barbato L, Nordera G, et al. Sleep disorders in Parkinson's disease. *J Neurol* 1998;245(Suppl 1):S15–8.

106. Tan A, Salgado M, Fahn S. Rapid eye movement sleep behavior disorder preceding Parkinson's disease with therapeutic response to levodopa. *Mov Disord* 1996;11:214–16.

107. Tandberg E, Larsen JP, Karlsen K. Excessive daytime sleepiness and sleep benefit in Parkinson's disease: a community-based study. *Mov Disord* 1999;14:992–7.

108. Thannickal TC, Lai YY, Siegel JM. Hypocretin (orexin) cell loss in Parkinson's disease. *Brain* 2007;130:1586–95.

109. The Parkinson Study Group. Low-dose clozapine for the treatment of drug-induced psychosis in Parkinson's disease. *N Eng J Med* 1999;340:757–63.

110. The U.K. Madopar CR Study Group. A comparison of madopar CR and standard madopar in the treatment of nocturnal and early-morning disability in Parkinson's disease. *Clin Neuropharma* 1989;12:498–503.

111. Trenkwalder C, Kies B, Rudzinska M. Rotigotine effects on early morning motor function and sleep in Parkinson's disease: a double-blind, randomized, placebo-controlled study (RECOVER). *Mov Disord* 2011;26:90–9.

112. Trotti LM, Rye DB. Neurobiology of sleep: the role of dopamine in Parkinson's disease. In: Chaudruri, KR, Tolosa E, Schapira A, Poewe W, eds. *Non-Motor Symptoms in Parkinson's Disease*. New York: Oxford University Press; 2009:165–76.

113. Trotti LM, Bliwise DL. No increased risk of obstructive sleep apnea in Parkinson's disease. *Mov Disord* 2010;25:2246–9.

114. Van Hilten JJ, Weggeman M, van der Velde EA, et al. Sleep, excessive daytime sleepiness and fatigue in Parkinson's disease. *J Neural Transm* 1993;5:235–44.

115. Van Hilten B, Hoff JI, Middelkoop HAM, et al. Sleep disruption in Parkinson's disease. Assessment by continuous activity monitoring. *Arch Neurol* 1994;51:922–8.

116. Verbaan D, van Rooden SM, van Hilten JJ, et al. Prevalence and clinical profile of restless legs syndrome in Parkinson's disease. *Mov Disord* 2010;25:2142–7.

117. Wailke S, Herzog J, Witt K, et al. Effect of controlled-release levodopa on the microstructure of sleep in Parkinson's disease. *Eur J Neurol* 2011;18:590–6.

118. Weiner WJ. Falling asleep at the wheel: motor vehicle mishaps in persons taking pramipexole and ropinirole. *Neurology* 2000;54:274–5.

119. Wetter TC, Collado-Seidel V, Pollmaecher T, et al. Sleep and periodic leg movement patterns in drug-free patients with Parkinson's disease and multiple system atrophy. *Sleep* 2000;23:361–7.

120. Wetter TC, Brunner H, Högl B, et al. Increased alpha activity in REM sleep in de novo patients with Parkinson's disease. *Mov Disord* 2001;16:928–33.

121. Yasui K, Inoue Y, Kanbayashi T, et al. CSF orexin levels of Parkinson's disease, dementia with Lewy bodies, progressive supranuclear palsy and corticobasal degeneration. *J Neurol Sci* 2006;250:120–3.

122. Zesiewicz TA, Cimino CR, Gardner NM, et al. Driving safety in Parkinson's disease. *Neurology* 2000;54(Suppl 3):A472.

123. Zesiewicz TA, Sullivan KL, Arnulf I, et al. Practice parameter: treatment of nonmotor symptoms of Parkinson's disease. Report of the Quality Standards Subcommittee of the American Academy of Neurology. *Neurology* 2010;74:924–31.

124. Zweig RM, Jankel WR, Hedreen JC, et al. The pedunculopontine nucleus in Parkinson's disease. *Ann Neurol* 1989;26:41–6.

52

Sleep Dysfunction in Parkinson's Plus Syndrome

MICHAEL H. SILBER

PARKINSON'S PLUS syndrome refers to a group of neurodegenerative disorders with the common feature of parkinsonism not due to Lewy body pathology. Some of the conditions, such as multiple-system atrophy, are synucleinopathies, whereas others, such as progressive supranuclear palsy, are tauopathies. Generally, other neurologic manifestations are present in addition to parkinsonism, such as dysautonomia, cerebellar dysfunction, oculomotor abnormalities, and dementia. Sleep disorders are common in many of these conditions.

MULTIPLE-SYSTEM ATROPHY

Multiple-system atrophy (MSA) is a sporadic, adult-onset neurodegenerative disorder characterized by autonomic failure and combinations of parkinsonism (poorly responsive to levodopa) and dysfunction of the cerebellar and corticospinal systems.[1-3] When autonomic failure predominates, the condition is often referred to as Shy-Drager syndrome. When parkinsonism predominates, the subtype is named MSA-P (sometimes called striatonigral degeneration), whereas the subtype characterized by predominant cerebellar dysfunction is named MSA-C (sometimes called sporadic olivopontocerebellar atrophy).[2] The incidence in a community-based study was found to be 0.6 per 100,000 (3.0 for ages 50–99 years).[1] MSA, like Parkinson's disease, is a synucleinopathy with characteristic oligodendroglial cytoplasmic inclusions due to accumulation of the protein alpha-synuclein.[3] Degenerative cell loss and gliosis occur in the basal ganglia, brainstem, cerebellum, and spinal cord.[4] Respiratory and motor disturbances during sleep are common and important manifestations of MSA.

Sleep-Related Respiratory Problems

VOCAL CORD DYSFUNCTION

Nocturnal stridor is the most characteristic sleep-related breathing problem in MSA.[5]

Observers will often describe a harsh or strained, high-pitched, inspiratory sound, usually distinguishable from snoring, but occasionally stridor is only detected after listening to a recording.[6] It may develop at any stage of the disease and may even be the initial manifestation.[7-9] Stridor may also be present during wakefulness.[10] In small series, the frequency of stridor in MSA varies between 20% and 42%.[11-13] In a larger series of 100 consecutive patients with clinically probable MSA, 34% had stridor (95% confidence intervals: 25–44).[14] A report of 203 pathologically proven cases of MSA gleaned from 108 publications indicated stridor present in 13%.[15]

Laryngoscopy during wakefulness may reveal normal vocal cords, weakness of abduction on inspiration, paradoxical adduction on inspiration, or complete abduction paralysis with cords fixed in the paramedian position.[5,10,16,17] Cord involvement may initially be unilateral[17] but later progress to bilateral dysfunction.[18] During sleep, video-laryngoscopy reveals adduction of the cords in inspiration with downward displacement of the larynx.[19]

A number of studies have addressed the pathogenesis of vocal cord dysfunction in MSA. Pathologic studies of the laryngeal muscles have shown fiber atrophy, usually neurogenic in type, in the posterior cricoarytenoid (PCA) muscles, the sole abductors of the cords.[5,20-22] Studies of the recurrent laryngeal nerve (which innervates the PCA muscles) have shown reduced numbers of myelinated fibers compared to controls.[5,22] The branchiomotor neurons of the medullary vagal nucleus, nucleus ambiguus, innervate the laryngeal muscles. Pathologic studies of the nucleus in small numbers of patients have yielded contradictory results: in a few studies neuronal loss has been reported,[23,24] whereas in others the branchiomotor neurons remained normal in number and morphology.[5,25]

Electromyographic studies of individual laryngeal muscles, using esophageal,[26] concentric needle,[27] or wire electrodes,[28] have provided another approach to the understanding of laryngeal dysfunction in MSA. No evidence of denervation was noted in 10 patients studied.[27,28] In a total of 20 patients,[26-29] some studied during wakefulness and some during sleep, strong activity of the thyroaretenoid (TA) muscles, sometimes with co-contraction of the PCA muscles, was detected during inspiration, although the TA muscle are normally abductors of the cords and

active only during expiration. These data suggest that in most MSA patients, vocal cord dysfunction is caused by a defect in central control mechanisms, resulting in dystonic overactivity of the adductor muscles during inspiration. It is possible that selective neuronal degeneration in nucleus ambiguus may contribute to stridor by inducing weakness of the PCA muscles in some cases, especially as the disease advances and complete vocal cord paralysis ensues.

What are the possible consequences of untreated vocal cord dysfunction in MSA? There are reports of at least eight MSA patients dying suddenly, usually during sleep, within days to weeks of a diagnosis of stridor.[6,7,10,16,30,31] One of these patients had a normal laryngoscopic examination during wakefulness 2 weeks earlier,[16] and another had only unilateral vocal cord paralysis.[32] In one study,[33] five out of eight untreated patients died suddenly, a mean of 1.1 years after diagnosis.

OTHER RESPIRATORY PROBLEMS IN SLEEP

In addition to nocturnal stridor, sleep apnea is common in MSA. Case reports have documented snoring and obstructive sleep apneas (OSAs),[30,32,34] as well as central sleep apneas (CSAs).[35,36] Case series suggest that OSA is more common than CSA. In a study of 39 patients with MSA,[11] 6 specifically referred for sleep complaints, 15% had five or more obstructive events per hour (range: 7–16). Another study[37] found OSAs or hypopneas in 6 of 21 (28.6%) consecutive MSA patients. More than five apneas or hypopneas per hour (mean: 22.4 per hour) were noted in 20 of 29 patients with MSA specifically referred for sleep disturbances.[10] In all but one patient, the events were predominantly obstructive.

Abnormal breathing patterns have been described both during wakefulness and sleep. Irregularity of respiratory rate and tidal and minute volumes has been reported.[36,38,39] A case of cluster breathing during wake and sleep has been described,[40] as well as cases of apneustic breathing.[5] Periodic breathing associated with central apneas during sleep can occur,[10,39] as well as in the erect position during tilt-table testing.[41]

In some MSA patients, alveolar hypoventilation occurs, presumably on a central neurogenic basis. Three of seven patients with vocal cord abductor paralysis were hypercapnic in one study,[42] and death from hypercapnic respiratory failure has been reported despite tracheostomy, often at night.[5,10,43,44] Reduction of ventilatory responsiveness to CO_2 and O_2 has been reported.[39,43,45] Respiratory failure from central neurogenic hypoventilation may be an initial presentation of MSA.[9,46]

Autopsy studies of the brainstem of patients dying with respiratory disturbances have shown extensive abnormalities. Extensive gliosis and neuronal loss in the medulla and pons have been noted.[32,36,40,41] Severe loss of chemosensitive glutaminergic and serotonergic neurons in the ventral medullary arcuate nucleus has been demonstrated in MSA.[47] These pathologic findings provide further evidence for centrally mediated respiratory disturbances in MSA.

MANAGEMENT OF SLEEP-RELATED RESPIRATORY PROBLEMS IN MULTIPLE-SYSTEM ATROPHY

MSA patients have a median survival from onset of symptoms of 8.5[1] to 9.5[14] years, and respiratory dysfunction is probably a major cause of death.[44] The management of the nocturnal respiratory problems associated with MSA is challenging, but optimal treatment may well increase survival.

It is clear that some patients with vocal cord dysfunction die in their sleep, sometimes very soon after diagnosis.[7,10,16,30,32] The standard recommended treatment has traditionally been tracheostomy. However, not being aware of the presence of stridor themselves, many patients have trouble accepting that this is necessary. In addition, care of a tracheostomy may be challenging for patients who are often elderly and disabled. Central sleep apnea has been reported following tracheostomy,[16,48] but the clinical significance is uncertain. Death despite tracheostomy has been reported, sometimes during sleep.[5,43,44] An alternative approach, more acceptable to most patients, has been to use nasal continuous positive airway pressure (CPAP). The available data on which to base optimal treatment decisions are summarized next.

In one study,[33] five of eight patients with vocal cord paralysis who did not undergo tracheostomy died suddenly a mean of 1.1 years after diagnosis, while 9 of 11 patients who underwent tracheostomy were alive, a maximum of 5 years later. In another study,[10] 9 of 11 patients with stridor died, a median of 1.8 years after the sleep evaluation. Tracheostomy had been performed in both survivors. Four of five patients with daytime stridor died, a mean of only 0.8 years after the sleep evaluation, with the survivor having undergone tracheostomy. Of three patients with immobile cords on laryngoscopy, two died and the survivor had undergone tracheostomy. Two patients with stridor refused all treatment; both died, one as early as 1 month after evaluation. However, tracheostomy did not entirely prevent death in this series. Two of four patients with tracheostomy died, both 1 year after presentation. One was noted to be hypoxemic and the other hypercapnic on presentation. Six of 19 patients without stridor died, two from pneumonia and three from respiratory failure, a mean of 2.4 years after presentation. Kaplan-Meier statistics showed a significantly shorter survival from the sleep evaluation for patients with stridor compared to those without.

Three of four patients with MSA and stridor tolerated CPAP well and were alive with elimination of stridor 6 months after commencement of therapy.[49] In contrast, all five patients in another series treated with CPAP for stridor died, a mean of 2.4 years after presentation. However, one had immobile vocal cords and daytime stridor, one had poor CPAP compliance, one had audible stridor despite CPAP use, and one died of pneumonia. In a series of 14 patients with stridor,[50] three refused or discontinued treatment and died. The remaining 11 were treated with CPAP; two subsequently developed daytime stridor and received tracheostomies. After 3–28 months follow-up, three of the nine still on CPAP were alive and six died, five from pneumonia. In another study,[51] 5 of 10 patients treated with CPAP discontinued therapy; three died. Of the remaining five, one died of pneumonia and the other four were alive a mean of 24.8 months after initiating treatment.

Another possible surgical approach is vocal cord lateralization, which has been reported to successfully alleviate stridor in one patient.[52] A single study of unilateral injection of botulinum toxin into the thyroarytenoid muscle reported improvement of the stridor and reduction in tonic electromyographic activity in the muscle 1 month later in three of four patients.[27] Nocturnal ventilation has been used in hypercapnic respiratory failure.[38]

The available data suggest that there are at least two major causes of death in MSA. One is laryngeal obstruction as a result of vocal cord abductor dysfunction, often resulting in death during sleep. However, death also occurs in patients successfully treated with tracheostomy and in those without stridor, often from respiratory failure, respiratory arrest, or pneumonia, again often during the night. These patients may die as a result of progressive central alveolar hypoventilation from neuronal loss and gliosis of pontomedullary respiratory centers. Based on the available data, the following management is recommended,[53] with the reservation that prospective studies are needed to confirm that this approach improves outcome.

All patients with MSA and their bed partners should be questioned about stridor, snoring, apneas, daytime dyspnea, and daytime sleepiness. If stridor or sleep apnea is suspected, a polysomnogram should be performed with application of CPAP if either is detected. Arterial blood gasses should be checked if daytime or nighttime dyspnea is present. Overnight oximetry should be performed if a polysomnogram is not planned. If stridor is heard on polysomnogram, laryngoscopy should be performed. CPAP should be considered the first-line treatment for stridor occurring only during sleep as long as it is shown to eliminate stridor during the sleep study and laryngoscopy does not show bilaterally immobile vocal cords. Tracheostomy should be strongly recommended if daytime stridor is present, the vocal cords are immobile, CPAP does not eliminate stridor, or CPAP compliance is incomplete. If arterial blood gas analysis or overnight oximetry reveals hypercapnic respiratory failure with nocturnal hypoxemia unrelated to obstructive sleep apnea syndrome, nocturnal ventilation, either via a nasal mask or tracheostomy, should be considered. This approach has been successfully used in patients with amyotrophic lateral sclerosis, with improvement in quality of life and survival.[54]

For patients without evidence of respiratory problems, the patient's bed partner should be urged to report if stridor is subsequently heard. Arterial blood gas analysis and overnight oximetry should be performed should dyspnea subsequently develop.

Motor and Other Disturbances of Sleep

REM SLEEP BEHAVIOR DISORDER

Rapid eye movement (REM) sleep behavior disorder (RBD) is characterized by loss of normal voluntary muscle atonia during REM sleep with excessive motor activity while dreaming. Motor activity ranges from excessive twitching of the limbs to violent activity resulting in injuries to the patient and bed partner.[55] Polysomnography reveals either pathologically increased transient (phasic) muscle activity in the chin or limbs or complete elimination of atonia with tonic elevation of the chin electromyogram. RBD occurs when descending pontomedullary pathways resulting in presynaptic inhibition of anterior horn cells are interrupted.[56] As autopsy studies of MSA have shown extensive degeneration of pontine nuclei with gliosis,[4] it is not surprising that RBD is common in MSA. In large series of RBD patients (96–151 subjects), MSA has been noted in 5%–30%.[55,57,58] In a consecutive series of MSA patients, REM sleep without atonia has been noted in 90%–95% and RBD with dream enactment behavior in 69%–90% of subjects.[11,61] Thus, motor disturbances in REM sleep may be the commonest sleep disturbance seen in MSA patients.

The frequency of episodes of RBD in MSA patients has been reported to vary from three per month to more than once a night.[11] RBD is a predominantly male disorder (87% of each of two large series), but this gender specificity is less marked in MSA, with 36%–39% of MSA patients with RBD reported to be women.[55,57] RBD often precedes other symptoms of neurodegenerative disease, including MSA. Symptoms of RBD were reported before other symptoms in 36%–54% of MSA patients[11,56,58] by 1–19 years.[11,56] In some patients with pure autonomic failure, the development of RBD may predict subsequent evolution of MSA.[59]

The standard medication for the treatment of RBD is clonazepam, completely or partially successful in 87%–90% of patients.[55,58] Caution should be exercised in the use of benzodiazepines in patients with MSA because of the occurrence of laryngeal and oropharyngeal obstruction during sleep, central respiratory failure, and gait instability. As an alternative, melatonin can be used in doses of 3–12 mg.[60] It is also important to improve the safety of the sleep environment with such techniques as moving furniture away from the bed and placing mattresses on the floor alongside the bed.

SLEEP DISTURBANCE AND PERIODIC LIMB MOVEMENTS IN SLEEP

In addition to episodes of dream enactment behavior, MSA patients report disturbed nocturnal sleep because of stiffness, back pain, and nocturia.[11] Sleep efficiency and total sleep time are reduced.[11,34] Motor dyscontrol in non-REM sleep is also common. In a series of 39 consecutive cases of MSA, 26% had periodic limb movements in sleep (PLMS) with electroencephalographic (EEG) arousals.[11] In 28 MSA patients referred to a sleep center, but not specifically for PLMS or restless legs syndrome, 79% had PLM indices greater than 20 per hour, and 71% had indices greater than 90 per hour.[10] The frequency of PLMS was significantly higher in a series of 26 MSA patients with RBD compared to controls with either Parkinson's disease and RBD or idiopathic RBD.[57] However, in a series of 10 MSA patients compared to 10 age-matched controls, the frequency of PLMS was not significantly different.[61] Impaired cortical and autonomic arousals following PLMS have been reported compared to PLMS in subjects with restless legs syndrome.[62]

Excessive Daytime Sleepiness

Excessive daytime sleepiness, measured by the Epworth Sleepiness Scale, was more frequent in 86 MSA patients compared to age- and sex-matched controls.[63] Multivariate analysis showed that only sleep efficiency and sleep-disordered breathing predicted sleepiness. An autopsy study of seven MSA patients showed marked reduction in the number of hypocretin neurons with glial inclusions in the hypothalamus compared to controls,[64] suggesting the possibility that hypocretin deficiency might contribute to daytime somnolence. However, in another study cerebrospinal fluid hypocretin-1 levels were found to be normal in 12 MSA patients.[65]

PROGRESSIVE SUPRANUCLEAR PALSY

Progressive supranuclear palsy (PSP) (Richardson-Steele-Olszewski syndrome) is a neurodegenerative disorder characterized by a rigid akinetic parkinsonian syndrome with prominent axial rigidity and lack of responsiveness to levodopa, early gait instability with falls, supranuclear (especially downward) vertical gaze palsies, pseudobulbar palsy, and a frontal lobe type dementia.[1,66,67] The disorder commences after 40 years of age[1,67] with a median survival from onset of 5.3–5.6 years. The community-based incidence has been calculated as 1.1 per 100,000 (5.3 for ages 50–99 years).[1] In contrast to MSA, PSP is a tauopathy with deposition of tau protein in neurons before degeneration and their subsequent presence in neurofibrillary tangles and neuropil threads.[3,67] Neuronal loss and gliosis occur in the basal ganglia and brainstem with relative preservation of the cortex and hippocampus.

Sleep disturbances appear to be an integral part of PSP, but the frequency of sleep complaints is uncertain. In a questionnaire study of 437 patients with a clinical diagnosis of PSP, 50% of patients more than 3 years after diagnosis reported changed sleeping patterns or difficulty sleeping.[68] At least 9 of 11 patients with PSP reported frequent nocturnal awakenings and immobility in bed, and these symptoms occurred more frequently than in age- and sex-matched controls.[66]

Sleep architecture in PSP has been investigated in four studies[69–72] (6–20 subjects), with reasonably consistent findings. Marked insomnia was noted, with low sleep efficiency, increased wake time after sleep onset, and, in most studies, reduced total sleep time. Light non-REM sleep was increased with reduction in REM sleep. Reduction in abundance and amplitude of sleep spindles has been noted.[69,70] Patients with advanced disease have been reported with EEG rhythms during behavioral sleep indistinguishable from those of wakefulness (status dissociatus).[73] The pathophysiology of the sleep disturbances is presumably linked to the extensive brainstem pathology.

It has been suggested that RBD and REM sleep without atonia are relatively specific to synucleinopathies.[74] Thus, the question whether RBD occurs in PSP, a tauopathy, is of particular interest. The electromyographic tone in REM sleep appeared to be normal in an EEG study of four patients.[73] Five case series, all with patients diagnosed clinically with PSP, have examined the topic with varying results. Quantitative assessment of muscle tone in six patients revealed REM sleep atonia in 99.2% of REM sleep time, findings not significantly different from those of age- and sex-matched controls.[70] A clinical assessment of 10 patients found none with RBD.[75] A questionnaire study of 30 patients suggested that 20% had RBD.[76] A study of 15 patients found 27% with quantitative increased muscle tone in REM sleep compared to controls, with 13% diagnosed with RBD.[71] A similar study of 20 patients found 85% with loss of REM sleep atonia and 35% with a diagnosis of RBD.[72] There has been a single case report of polysomnographically confirmed RBD in an autopsy-proven case of PSP.[77] The reason for the discrepancy between different studies is uncertain. It would appear that RBD and REM sleep without atonia do occur in some patients with PSP, but the frequency seems lower than in patients with synucleinopathies. Confirmation that RBD can occur in some tauopathies is found in a study of nine patients with guadeloupian parkinsonism, seven of whom had RBD.[78] Presumably the pathologic anatomy of the different disorders dictates whether the REM sleep atonia system is compromised.

Nocturnal respiratory disturbances do not appear to be prominent in PSP. The frequency of apneas and hypopneas was not significantly different from controls[69] or Parkinson's disease patients[69,72] in two studies. In an oximetry study of 11 patients, infrequent decreases of 4% or more in oxyhemoglobin saturation were noted in three patients, but all were at a frequency of less than 4 per hour.[66] In another series, 2 of 10 patients had sleep apneas, one predominantly central and one predominantly obstructive.[69] A patient with what appears to be apneustic breathing has been described.[79] Failure of 11 patients to adequately perform spirometry was ascribed to a supranuclear impairment of voluntary respiratory control.[66] Periodic limb movements of sleep were not more frequent than in normal controls or Parkinson's disease patients in one study of 15 patients,[71] but periodic limb movements of sleep and wakefulness were both more frequent than in Parkinson's disease in another study of 20 patients.[72] Cerebrospinal fluid hypocretin-1 levels were lower in 16 patients with PSP compared to 62 with Parkinson's disease.[80]

CORTICOBASAL DEGENERATION

Corticobasal degeneration (CBD) is another neurodegenerative disorder with tau protein inclusions.[3] It is characterized by an asymmetric akinetic-rigid syndrome, motor apraxia, cortical sensory loss, alien limb phenomenon, and dementia.[81] Neuronal loss, gliosis, and intracytoplasmic inclusion bodies are found, especially in the cortex and substantia nigra. In a series of five clinically diagnosed cases, total sleep time and sleep efficiency were reduced.[82] Only one patient had an apnea hypopnea index of >10/hour and multiple sleep latency tests were normal. Cerebrospinal fluid hypocretin-1 levels were lower in seven CBD patients compared to 62 with Parkinson's disease.[80] Unilateral or

asymmetric periodic limb movements have been described in a few patients, worse on the more affected side.[82,83]

RBD and REM sleep without atonia have been described in case reports of clinically diagnosed CBD without pathologic confirmation.[61,84,85] However, in a series of 10 clinically diagnosed cases, none had RBD by history.[75] In a similar series of 14 patients, RBD was diagnosed by questionnaire in only one patient.[76] In a series of five patients, quantitative assessment of muscle tone revealed normal REM sleep atonia in all.[82] Thus, it appears that disturbances of REM muscle tone are rare in CBD.

REFERENCES

1. Bower JH, Maraganore DM, McDonnell SK, et al. Incidence of progressive supranuclear palsy and multiple system atrophy in Olmsted County, Minnesota, 1976 to 1990. *Neurology* 1997;49:1284–8.
2. Gilman S, Wenning GK, Low PA, et al. Second consensus statement on the diagnosis of multiple system atrophy. *Neurology* 2008;71:670–6.
3. Goedert M. Filamentous nerve cell inclusions in neurodegenerative diseases: tauopathies and alpha-synucleinopathies. *Phil Trans R Soc Lond* 199;354:1101–18.
4. Papp MI, Lantos PL. The distribution of oligodendroglial inclusions in multiple system atrophy and its relevance to clinical symptomatology. *Brain* 1994;117:235–43.
5. Bannister R, Gibson W, Michaels L, et al. Laryngeal abductor paralysis in multiple system atrophy. A report on three necropsied cases, with observations on the laryngeal muscles and the nuclei ambigui. *Brain* 1981;104:351–68.
6. Katsikuba N, Sadaoka T, Fujiwara Y, et al. Peculiar snoring in patients with multiple system atrophy: its sound source, acoustic characteristics, and diagnostic significance. *Ann Otol Rhinol Laryngol* 1987;106:380–4.
7. Hughes RGM, Gibbon KP, Lowe J. Vocal cord abductor paralysis as a solitary and fatal manifestation of multiple system atrophy. *J Laryngol Otol* 1998;112:177–8.
8. Martinovits G, Leventon G, Goldhammer Y, et al. Vocal cord paralysis as a presenting sign in the Shy-Drager syndrome. *J Laryngol Otol* 1988;102:280–1.
9. Glass GA, Josephs KA, Alhskog JE. Respiratory insufficiency as the primary

presenting symptom of multiple-system atrophy. *Arch Neurol* 2006;63:978–81.

10. Silber MH, Levine S. Stridor and death in multiple system atrophy. *Mov Disord* 2000;15:699–704.

11. Plazzi G, Corsini R, Provini F. REM sleep behavior disorders in multiple system atrophy. *Neurology* 1997;48:1094–7.

12. Vertrugno R, Provini F, Cortelli P, et al. Sleep disorders in multiple system atrophy: a correlative video-polysomnographic study. *Sleep Med* 2004;5:21–30.

13. Shimohata T, Shinoda H, Nakayama H, et al. Daytime hypoxemia, sleep-disordered breathing, and laryngopharyngeal findings in multiple system atrophy. *Arch Neurol* 2007;64:856–61.

14. Wenning GK, Ben Shlomo Y, Magalhaes M, et al. Clinical features and natural history of multiple system atrophy. An analysis of 100 cases. *Brain* 1994;117:835–45.

15. Wenning GK, Tison F, Shlomo B, et al. Multiple system atrophy: a review of 203 pathologically proven cases. *Mov Disord* 1997;12:133–47.

16. Kavey NB, Whyte J, Blitzer A, et al. Sleep-related laryngeal obstruction presenting as snoring or sleep apnea. *Laryngoscope* 1989;99:851–4.

17. Williams A, Hanson D, Calne DB. Vocal cord paralysis in the Shy-Drager syndrome. *J Neurol Neurosurg Psychiatr* 1979;42:151–3.

18. Hanson DG, Ludlow CL, Bassich CJ. Vocal fold paresis in Shy-Drager syndrome. *Ann Otol Rhinol Laryngol* 1983;92:85–90.

19. Kuzniar TJ, Morgenthaler TI, Prakash UB, et al. Effects of continuous positive airway pressure on stridor in multiple system atrophy-sleep laryngoscopy. *J Clin Sleep Med* 2009;5:65–7.

20. DeReuck J, Van Landegem W. The posterior crico-arytenoid muscle in two cases of Shy-Drager syndrome with laryngeal stridor. Comparison of the histological, histochemical and biometric findings. *J Neurol* 1987;234:187–90.

21. Hayashi M, Isozaki E, Oda M, et al. Loss of large myelinated nerve fibres of the recurrent laryngeal nerve in patients with multiple system atrophy and vocal cord palsy. *J Neurol Neurosurg Psychiatr* 1997;62:234–8.

22. Isozaki E, Hayashi M, Hayashida T, et al. Myopathology of the intrinsic laryngeal muscles in neurodegenerative disorders, with reference to the mechanism of vocal

cord paralysis. *Rinsho Shinkeigaku—Clinical Neurology* 1998;38:711–18.

23. Lapresle J, Annabi A. Olivopontocerebellar atrophy with velopharyngeal paralysis: a contribution to the somatopy of the nucleus ambiguus. *J Neuropathol Exp Neurol* 1979;38:401–6.

24. Isozaki E, Matsubara S, Hayashida T, et al. Morphometric study of nucleus ambiguus in multiple system atrophy presenting with vocal cord abductor paralysis. *Clin Neuropath* 2000;19:213–20.

25. Benarroch EE, Schmeichel AM, Parisi JE. Preservation of branchiomotor neurons of the nucleus ambiguus in multiple system atrophy. *Neurology* 2003;61:722–3.

26. Isozaki E, Osanai R, Horiguchi S, et al. Laryngeal electromyography with separated surface electrodes in patients with multiple system atrophy presenting with vocal cord paralysis. *J Neurol* 1994;241:551–6.

27. Merlo IM, Occhini A, Pacchetti C, et al. Not paralysis, but dystonia causes stridor in multiple system atrophy. *Neurology* 2002;58:649–52.

28. Vertrugno R, Liguori R, Cortelli P, et al. Sleep-related stridor due to dystonic vocal cord motion and neurogenic tachypnea/tachcardia in multiple system atrophy. *Mov Disord* 2007;22:673–8.

29. Simpson DM, Kaufmann H, Sanders I, et al. Laryngeal dystonia in multiple system atrophy. *Muscle Nerve* 1992;15:1212–15.

30. Briskin JG, Lehrman K, Guilleminault C. Shy-Drager syndrome and sleep apnea. In: Guilleminault C, Dement WC, eds. *Sleep Apnea Syndromes*. New York: Allan R. Liss; 1978:317–22.

31. Guilleminault C. Obstructive Sleep apnea syndrome: the clinical syndrome and historical perspectives. *Med Clin North Am* 1985;69:1187–203.

32. Guilleminault C, Tilkian A, Lehrman K, et al. Sleep apnoea syndrome: states of sleep and autionomic dysfunction. *J Neurol Neurosurg Psychiatr* 1977;40:718–25.

33. Isozaki E, Miyamoto K, Osanai R, et al. [Clinical studies of 23 patients with multiple system atrophy presenting with vocal cord paralysis]. *Rinsho Shinkeigaku—Clinical Neurology* 1991;31:249–54.

34. Manni R, Morini R, Matignoni E, et al. Nocturnal sleep in multiple system atrophy with autonomic failure: polygraphic findings in ten patients. *J Neurol* 1993;240:247–50.

35. Chokroverty S, Sachdeo R, Masdeu J. Autonomic dysfunction and sleep apnea in olivopontocerebellar degeneration. *Arch Neurol* 1984;41:926–31.

36. Munschauer FE, Loh L, Bannister R, et al. Abnormal respiration and sudden death during sleep in multiple system atrophy with autonomic failure. *Neurology* 1990;40:677–9.

37. Tachibani N, Kimura K, Kitajima K, et al. REM sleep motor dysfunction in multiple system atrophy: with special emphasis on sleep talk as its early clinical manifestation. *J Neurol Neurosurg Psychiatr* 1997;63:678–81.

38. Apps MC, Sheaff PC, Ingram DA, et al. Respiration and sleep in Parkinson's disease. *J Neurol Neurosurg Psychiatr* 1985;48:1240–5.

39. McNicholas WT, Rutherford R, Grossman R, et al. Abnormal respiratory pattern generation during sleep in patients with autonomic dysfunction. *Am Rev Respir Dis* 1983;128:429–33.

40. Lockwood AH. Shy-Drager syndrome with abnormal respirations and antidiuretic hormone release. *Arch Neurol* 1976;33:292–5.

41. Chokroverty S, Sharp JT, Barron KD. Periodic respiration in erect posture in Shy-Drager syndrome. *J Neurol Neurosurg Psychiatr* 1978;41:980–6.

42. Isozaki E, Naito A, Horiguchi S, et al. Early diagnosis and stage classification of vocal cord abductor paralysis in patients with multiple system atrophy. *J Neurol Neurosurg Psychiatr* 1996;60:399–402.

43. Chester GS, Gottfried SB, Cameron DI, et al. Pathophysiologic findings in a patient with Shy-Drager and alveolar hypoventilation syndromes. *Chest* 1988;94:212–14.

44. Shimohata T, Ozawa T, Nakayama H, et al. Frequency of nocturnal sudden death in patients with multiple system atrophy. *J Neurol* 2008;255:1483–5.

45. Tsuda T, Onodera H, Okabe S, et al. Impaired chemosensitivity to hypoxia is a marker of multiple system atrophy. *Ann Neurol* 2002;52:367–71.

46. Cormican LJ, Higgins S, Davidson AC, et al. Multiple system atrophy presenting as central sleep apnoea. *Eur Respir J* 2004;24:323–5.

47. Benarroch EE, Schmeichel AM, Low PA, et al. Depletion of putative chemosensitive respiratory neurons in the ventral medullary surface in multiple system atrophy. *Brain* 2007;130:469–75.

48. Jin K, Okabe S, Chida K, et al. Tracheostomy can fatally exacerbate sleep-disordered breathing in multiple system atrophy. *Neurology* 2007;68:1618–21.

49. Iranzo A, Santamaria J, Tolosa E. Continuous positive airway pressure eliminates nocturnal stridor in multiple system atrophy. *Lancet* 2000;356:1329–30.

50. Iranzo A, Santamaria J, Tolosa E, et al. Long-term efect of CPAP in the treatment of nocturnal stridor in multiple system atrophy. *Neurology* 2004;63:930–2.

51. Ghorayeb I, Yekhlef F, Bioulac B, et al. Continuous positive airway pressure for sleep-related breathing disorders in multiple system atrophy: long-term acceptance. *Sleep Med* 2005;6:359–62.

52. Kenyon GS, Apps MC, Traub M. Stridor and obstructive sleep apneain Shy-Drager syndrome trated with laryngofissure and cord lateralization. *Larygoscope* 1984;94(8):1106–8.

53. Iranzo A. Management of sleep-disordered breathing in multiple system atrophy. *Sleep Med* 2005;6:297–300.

54. Piepers S, van den Berg JP, Kalmijn S. Effect of non-invasive evntilation on survival, quality of life, repsirtaory function and cognition: a review of the literature. *Amyotroph Lateral Scler* 2006;7:195–200.

55. Olson EJ, Boeve BF, Silber MH. Rapid eye movement sleep behavior disorder: demographic, clinical and laboratory findings in 93 cases. *Brain* 2000;123:331–9.

56. Boeve B, Silber MH, Saper CB, et al. Pathophysiology of REM sleep behaviour disorder and relevance to neurodegenerative disease. *Brain* 2007;130:2770–88.

57. Iranzo A, Santamaria J, Rye DB, et al. Characteristics of idiopathic REM sleep behavior disorder and that associated with MSA and PD. *Neurology* 2005;65:247–52.

58. Schenck CH, Mahowald MW. REM sleep parasomnias. *Neurologic Clinics* 1996;14:697–720.

59. Plazzi G, Cortelli P, Montagna P. REM sleep behaviour disorder differentiates pure autonomic failure from multiple system atrophy with autonomic failure. *J Neurol Neurosurg Psychiatr* 1998;64:683–5.

60. Aurora RN, Zak RS, Maganti RK, et al. Best practice guide for the treatment of REM sleep behavior disorder (RBD). *J Clin Sleep Med* 2010;6:85–95.

61. Wetter TC, Collado-Seidel V, Pollmacher T, et al. Sleep and periodic leg movement patterns in drug-free patients with Parkinson's

disease and multiple system atrophy. *Sleep* 2000;23:361–7.

62. Vertrugno R, D'Angelo R, Cortelli P, et al. Impaired cortical and autonomic arousal during sleep in multiple system atrophy. *Clin Neurophysiol* 2007;118:2512–18.

63. Moreno-Lopez C, Santamaria J, Salamero M, et al. Excessive daytime sleepiness in multiple system atrophy (SLEEMSA study). *Arch Neurol* 2011;68:223–30.

64. Benarroch EE, Schmeichel AM, Sandroni P, et al. Involvement of hypocretin neurons in multiple system atrophy. *Acta Neuropathol* 2007;113:75–80.

65. Abdo WF, Bloem BR, Kremer HPH, et al. CSF hypocretin-1 levels are normal in multiple system atrophy. *Parkinsonism Relat Disord* 2008;14:342–4.

66. De Bruin VS, Machado C, Howard RS, et al. Nocturnal and respiratory disturbances in Steele-Richardson-Olszewski syndrome (progressive supranuclear palsy). *Postgrad Med J* 1996;72:293–6.

67. Verny M, Jellinger KA, Hauw J-J, et al. Progressive supranuclear palsy: a clinicopathological study of 21 cases. *Acta Neuropathol* 1996;91:427–31.

68. Santacruz P, Uttl B, Litvan I, et al. Progressive supranuclear palsy. A survey of the disease course. *Neurology* 1998;50:1637–47.

69. Aldrich MS, Foster NL, White RF, et al. Sleep abnormalities in progressive supranuclear palsy. *Ann Neurol* 1989;25:577–81.

70. Montplaisir J, Petit D, Decary A, et al. Sleep and quantitative EEG in patients with progressive supranuclear palsy. *Neurology* 1997;49:999–1003.

71. Arnulf I, Merino-Andreu M, Bloch F, et al. REM sleep behavior disorder and REM sleep without atonia in patients with progressive supranuclear palsy. *Sleep* 2005;28:349–54.

72. Sixel-Doring F, Schweitzer M, Mollenhauer B, et al. Polysomnographic findings, video-based sleep analysis and sleep perception in progressive supranuclear palsy. *Sleep Med* 2009;10:407–15.

73. Gross RA, Spehlman R, Daniels JC. Sleep disturbances in progressive supranuclear palsy. *Electroenceph Clin Neurophysiol* 1978;45:16–25.

74. Boeve BF, Silber MH, Ferman TJ, et al. Association of REM sleep behavior disorder and neurodegenerative disease may reflect an underlying synucleinopathy. *Mov Disord* 2001;16:622–30.

75. Cooper AD, Josephs KA. Photophobia, visual hallucinations, and REM sleep behavior disorder in progressive supranuclear palsy and progressive supranuclear palsy. *Parkinsonism Rel Disord* 2009;15:59–61.

76. Diederich NJ, Leurgans S, Fan W, et al. Visual hallucinations and symptoms of REM sleep behavior disorder in Parkinsonian tauopathies. *Int J Geriatr Psychiatr* 2008;23:598–603.

77. Compta Y, Marti MJ, Rey MJ, et al. Parkinsonism, dysautonomia, REM behaviour disorder and visual hallucinations mimicking synucleinopathy in a patient with progressive supranuclear palsy. *J Neurol Neurosurg Psychiatr* 2009;80:578–9.

78. De Cock VC, Lannuzel A, Verhaeghe S, et al. REM sleep behavior disorder in patients with guadeloupean pakinsonism, a tauopathy. *Sleep* 2007;30:1026–32.

79. Collins SJ, Ahlskog JE, Parisi JE, et al. Progressive supranuclear palsy: neuropathologically based diagnostic criteria. *J Neurol Neurosurg Psychiatr* 1995;58:167–73.

80. Yasui K, Inoue Y, Kanbayashi T, et al. CSF orexin levels of Parkinson's disease, dementia with Lewy bodies, progressive supranuclear palsy and corticobasal degeneration,. *J Neurol Sci* 2006;250:120–3.

81. Kompoliti K, Goetz CG, Boeve BF, et al. Clinical presentation and pharmacological therapy in corticobasal degeneration. *Arch Neurol* 1998;55:957–61.

82. Roche S, Jacquesson J-M, Destee A, et al. Sleep and vigilance in corticobasal degeneration: a descriptive study. *Clin Neurophysiol* 2007;37:261–4.

83. Iriarte J, Alegre M, Arbizu J, et al. Unilateral periodic limb movements during sleep in corticobasal degeneration. *Mov Disord* 2001;16:1180–3.

84. Kimura K, Tachibana N, Aso T, et al. Subclinical REM sleep behavior disorder in a patient with corticobasal degeneration. *Sleep* 1997;20:891–4.

85. Gatto EM, Uribe Roca MC, Martinez O, et al. Rapid eye movement (REM) sleep without atonia in two patients with corticobasal degeneration (CBD). *Parkinsonism Relat Disord* 2007;13:130–2.

53

Sleep Disorders in Other Hyperkinetic Syndromes

MARK ERIC DYKEN AND ROBERT L. RODNITZKY

THIS CHAPTER will address the relationship between sleep and a few disorders associated with chorea/ballismus, dystonia, tremor, and myoclonus. The specific topics to be addressed include Huntington's disease (HD), focal and generalized dystonia, Tourette syndrome (TS), palatal tremor, and hemifacial spasm.

The phenomena to be discussed are primarily waking (diurnal) movement disorders, whose characteristic movements generally decrease or resolve in sleep. These entities can lead to secondary sleep problems when movements result in difficulties initiating and/or maintaining sleep, and excessive sleepiness. In addition, associated medical, psychological, and otherwise common intrinsic sleep problems may also result in sleep-related complaints. As such, a complete assessment requires a waking and sleep history, review of an accurate sleep diary, a careful physical and neurologic examination, laboratory investigations dictated by the specific illness, and possibly polysomnography (PSG) and multiple sleep latency testing (MSLT)

with extended electromyogram (EMG)-video monitoring.

CHOREA

Chorea is an abnormal movement disorder or dyskinesia, which is caused by an overactivity of dopamine in areas of the brain that control movement. It is characterized by brief, irregular contractions that are not repetitive or rhythmic but seem to flow from one muscle to another. It often occurs with athetosis (writhing/twisting movements). Chorea is a primary feature of HD, an autosomal dominant hereditary disorder that is associated with atrophy of the caudate nucleus, dementia, and behavioral changes. It is caused by a cytosine/adenine/guanine (CAG) trinucleotide repeat in the "interesting transcript 15" (IT15 gene) located on the short arm of chromosome 4.[1]

Although PSG studies have shown that chorea, in a variety of disorders, decreases in severity during sleep, it generally persists to some

696 •

extent, all the while retaining the clinical and electrophysiologic characteristics appreciated during wakefulness.[2-4] Nevertheless, the information gleaned from these studies has often been compromised due to limitations in monitoring techniques.

In 1982, Mano et al. analyzed four patients with choreoathetosis: two with HD and two with drug-induced movements.[5] They did not monitor airflow, respiratory effort, or oximetry, nor did they use video analysis of movements. EMG activity of affected musculature was graded on a scale of 0 to 4 and plotted every minute during sleep. The mean number of movements per minute of each specific sleep stage was reported as a mean percent value of waking movements. There was an average reduction in movements to 44.0% of wake-level movements in stage 1, to 16.9% of wake-level movements in stage 2, and to 5.7% of wake-level movements early in stage 3 non–rapid eye movement (non-REM or N) sleep. Early stage N3 sleep can be considered to occur when only 20% to 50% of every 30-second scoring period, or epoch, is comprised of slow-wave activity (SWA; waves of frequency 0.5 to 2.0 Hz, with a peak-to-peak amplitude >75 μv). No movements were noted in the later stages of N3 sleep. Later stage N3 sleep can be considered when >50% of every 30-second scoring epoch is comprised of SWA.

Hoffmann (H) reflex studies performed during sleep were reported as a percent amplitude change compared to waking. In two patients with HD the recovery cycles indicated prolonged silent periods and reduced excitability in sleep. These findings were most impressive in rapid eye movement (stage REM or R) sleep. As such, it was of particular interest that in REM sleep, EMG activity believed to represent "choreo-athetotic discharges" was relatively high, averaging 33.7% of that seen in wakefulness. With the exception of stage N1 sleep, this was higher than all non-REM stages. It is possible that normal phasic REM movements were overinterpreted as there was no concomitant video analysis, EMG monitoring was limited to "the submental muscles and muscles affected by the involuntary movements," and no controls were used.

In a controlled study, Wiegand et al. investigated the relationship between sleep and severity of HD as determined by caudate nucleus atrophy demonstrated on cranial computed tomography (CT).[6] Of 16 patients studied, there was an overall long sleep latency, reduced sleep efficiency with frequent prolonged arousals, and a reduction in SWA. In addition, there was an increase in sleep spindle density. Sleep spindles characteristically appear in stage N2 sleep, as a centrally dominant train of distinct waveforms that are spindle-like in appearance, with a frequency of 11 to 16 Hz, and a duration ≥0.5 seconds. Sleep spindle density is determined by the ratio of the number of spindles occurring in stage N2 to the duration of N2 sleep. These findings were most significant in individuals with chronic and severe disease associated with extensive atrophy of the caudate nuclei. However, there were significant limitations to the Wiegand study. Only a single submental EMG, electrode was used without video monitoring, and as such, the effects of intrinsic sleep disorders such as periodic limb movements could not be appreciated. In addition, as respiration was not monitored, movements resulting from arousals associated with underlying sleep-related breathing disorders could not be differentiated.

In a controlled study, Fish and colleagues studied the movements in sleep of five patients with HD.[7] After allowing one night of adaptation to the sleep study environment, a PSG, using split-screen video analysis with a low-light-intensity camera, was performed for each patient. Six channels were used to record sleep, of which up to three were used for EMG monitoring. Accelerometry was used for monitoring movements in some individuals.

Some movements occurred after sleep stage transitions. Movements also tended to occur after phenomena such as K-complexes (in stage N2 sleep, a K-complex is the combination of a frontally dominant negative sharp wave and an immediately following positive component that has a total duration ≥0.5 seconds) and hypersynchronous bursts, and less frequently after sleep spindles or SWA. The infrequent dyskinetic movements in REM sleep generally followed periods of fragmentary myoclonus or elevated EMG activity.

In the patients with HD, diurnal "characteristic movements" decreased progressively during the transition from wake to stage N1 and N2 sleep to REM sleep. No characteristic movements were reported for stage N3 sleep. The dyskinesias in sleep were of shorter duration, lower amplitude, and more fragmented compared to those appreciated while awake. Movements common in stage N1 sleep often followed brief arousals after sleep spindles or SWA.

The authors hypothesized that although different dyskinesias probably originate from unique central nervous system (CNS) generators, sleep exerts an inhibitory effect on all sites either by a general effect or through inactivation of a common pathway. As a support for their hypothesis, they cited the example of the REM sleep behavior disorder (RBD) that can follow lesions in descending inhibitory pathways of the brainstem.

In a study attempting to address the potential effects of medical concomitants, seven drug-free patients with moderately severe HD were studied during sleep.[8] These individuals were found to have reduced sleep efficiencies, SWA and REM sleep, and prolonged REM latencies. Nevertheless, anecdotal reports have documented relatively short REM sleep latencies, or increased REM sleep, and increased sleep associated with SWA. On the other hand, some studies have found no differences in many sleep parameters when compared to normal individuals.[5,9]

In a relatively recent controlled study from 2008, 25 subjects with HD underwent nighttime video and sleep monitoring and daytime MSLTs.[10a] The HD patients had early sleep onset, increased stage N1 sleep, delayed and shortened REM sleep, and increased periodic limb movements, with three individuals showing evidence for RBD. No sleep abnormality was found to correlate with CAG repeat length, and reduced REM duration worsened with severity of disease. Four subjects had MSLTs with sleep latencies <8 minutes and none had sleep-onset REM periods.

Whether a result of degenerative CNS processes, or by chance occurrence, patients with HD may be subject to a variety of intrinsic sleep disorders. Patients with juvenile-onset HD can experience sleep disturbance from difficulties initiating and maintaining sleep due to a variety of motor-related sleep phenomena, including rigidity, choreoathetoid movements, and generalized seizures (reported in up to 35% of this patient population).[11,12] We performed a PSG on a patient with juvenile-onset HD, who complained of insomnia and daytime sleepiness. The overnight study was remarkable for relatively short sleep onset and REM latencies (of only 2 minutes and 28.0 minutes, respectively) and brief periods of rhythmic body rocking arising from stage N1 sleep (minimally suggestive of a rhythmic movement disorder). The following MSLT revealed borderline pathological daytime sleepiness with a mean sleep latency of 6.5 minutes during four daytime naps, with no sleep-onset REM periods.

Finally, in another relatively recent study the authors proposed that circadian disturbance is an important feature of HD that results from pathology in the suprachiasmatic nucleus (SCN), the biological clock.[12] They indicated that patients with HD have a reversal of normal daytime/nighttime activity patterns, a situation that predisposes to "sundowning." It was observed that similar behaviors are appreciated in a transgenic model of HD (R6/2 mice) in association with a disrupted expression of the circadian clock genes mPer2 and mBmal1 in the SCN. The authors concluded that treating this sleep-wake disturbance should bring appreciable benefits to patients with HD.

HEMIBALLISM

Ballistic movements are involuntary flinging motions involving the extremities that are often violent in nature with wide swings in amplitude that can be exacerbated by activity and decrease with relaxation. Ballistic movements are associated with injury to the basal ganglia with the most severe hemiballistic movements noted with subthalamic nucleus injury but also reported with damage/degeneration in the globus pallidus, putamen, and caudate nucleus.

Although stroke of the subthalamic nucleus is the most common cause of hemiballism, this movement disorder has been reported with basal ganglia lesions associated with trauma, amyotrophic lateral sclerosis, nonketotic hyperglycemia, tumors, vascular malformations, demyelinating lesions, and infections.[13] In severe hemiballism, early surgical treatments included paralyzing the limb with alcohol injection and even amputation of affected limbs, as potential death associated with fatigue (especially in patients with multiple medical problems) was often reported as justification for such drastic therapeutic measures.[14] Functional stereotactic surgery on thalamic and pallidal targets is now used in a limited number of patients. In cases other than stroke (where the hemiballismus might be particularly severe), the movements are often relatively minimal and tend to resolve over time without specific treatment, other than aggressively addressing the primary precipitating disorder. Antidopaminergic medications such as perphenazine, pimozide, haloperidol, and chlorpromazine have been reported to be effective in approximately 90% of the cases associated with hemiballismus.[13] Other potential therapies include anticonvulsants (such as topiramate),[15] intrathecal baclofen,[16] botulinum injections,[13,16] and tetrabenazine.[17]

Mano et al. studied the movements in sleep of an individual with ballism secondary to basal ganglia stroke.[5] The "discharge groupings" approximating diurnal ballism were found to decrease in sleep. Compared to waking ballism, the mean amount of activity was 56.0% in stage N1, 7.1% in stage N2, and 4.4% in early stage N3 sleep, whereas no movement was appreciated in the deeper stages of N3 sleep and REM sleep. We have reported similar findings in a patient with a right thalamic infarction and left hemiballism[18] (see Fig. 53.1 and video).

The authors inferred that the paucity of movements in REM may have been an artifact of stroke-induced oculomotor paresis.[5] They imply that the subsequent absence of rapid eye movements (as a result of stroke) may have resulted in an underscoring of REM sleep when using classic sleep scoring criteria, which require the presence of rapid eye movements to define REM sleep. As such, REM-associated ballism would have also been underreported. Nevertheless, in our report, oculomotor paresis was not a complicating factor in the analysis of sleep-stage-associated movements.

DYSTONIA

Generalized Dystonia

Dystonia is disordered tonicity of muscles in which sustained contractions may cause twisting and repetitive movements or abnormal postures. Generalized dystonia occurs in a variety of disorders. In idiopathic (primary) torsion dystonia, the common genetic form typically begins in childhood and often presents with gastrocnemius hypertonia and progression to plantar flexion and internal rotation of the foot, thigh adduction, hip flexion, and knee extension, ultimately involving the upper extremities

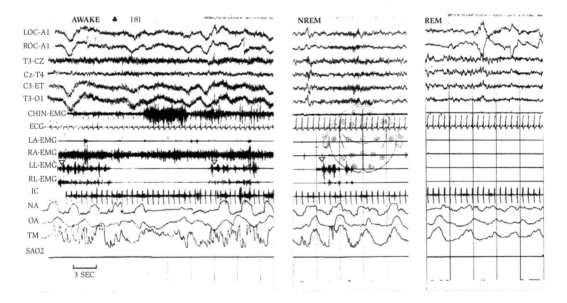

FIGURE 53.1 Polysomnography of a patient with a right thalamic infarction demonstrated the changes associated with clinically impressive left hemiballismus that improved in non–rapid eye movement (non-REM) sleep and disappeared in REM sleep. Hemiballismic movements are indicated by the open arrowheads. Less impressive increases in muscle tone and movement artifactual changes are noted in the electromyographic channels on the supporting right extremities when the patient was lying on the right side. A_1 (left ear) + A_2 (right ear); C, central; ET, ear tied; IC, intercostal electromyogram; LA, left arm; LL, left leg; LOC, left outer canthus; NA, nasal airflow; O, occipital; RA, right arm; RL, right leg; ROC, right outer canthus; SAO_2, oxygen saturation; T, temporal; TM, thoracic movement. (From Figure 1, Dyken ME, Rodnitzky RL. Periodic, aperiodic, and rhythmic motor disorders of sleep. *Neurology* 1992;42(suppl 6):68–74; with permission.)

as well. The more severely afflicted patients exhibit prolonged sleep latencies.[3]

Fish and colleagues studied 14 patients with primary generalized torsion and 10 individuals with secondary torsion dystonia.[7] Dystonic events were most frequent while awake, decreased markedly from stage N1 to stage N2 sleep, and were absent in stage N3 and REM sleep. The authors expressed concern over interpreting these results as patients were taking a variety of medications, including benzodiazepines, anticholinergics, dopaminergics, and antidopaminergics. In addition, two individuals with primary torsion dystonia had previously received bilateral thalamotomies.

After a thorough screen for a possible postencephalitic state, cerebral palsy, Wilson's disease, and Hallervorden-Spatz disease, Jankel and colleagues studied four individuals with severe torsion dystonia, three of whom had family histories of the disorder.[19] These patients were compared with gender- and age-matched controls. EMG activity in controls and patients showed similar "stage-appropriate" reductions in chin EMG, while biceps and triceps occasionally showed greater EMG reductions in stage N2 sleep when compared to REM sleep. The patients had increased sleep latencies, frequent awakenings, a decreased number of REM periods, and reduced total sleep times and sleep efficiencies. Video analysis and respiratory monitoring was not performed. All patients had extremely large sleep spindles in stage N2 sleep. Although the quantity of spindle activity was similar between controls and patients, controls had significantly more sleep spindles with amplitudes less than or equal to 50 μv, while patients had a greater number of spindles from 50 to over 100 μv. All patients received medications, including trihexyphenidyl hydrochloride, diazepam, dantrolene sodium, and chloral hydrate. Three individuals had prior "neurosurgical procedures." Nevertheless, two patients observed off diazepam had prolonged sleep latencies with reduced sleep efficiencies and large-amplitude sleep spindles. In addition, benzodiazepines and anticholinergics might be expected to improve these sleep parameters without affecting spindle amplitude. In the one patient without surgery the spindle activity was symmetrical, and asymmetries noted in the others were believed to be the result of their stereotactic brain surgery.

The authors hypothesized that reduced norepinephrine from the locus coeruleus could result in relative overactivity of the serotonergic raphe system. This could accentuate non-REM sleep phenomena and lead to large sleep spindles.[20] Excellent figures in this publication allay concerns that K-complexes might have been mistaken for high-amplitude sleep spindles.

Mano and colleagues analyzed five individuals with secondary dystonia due to Wilson's disease, encephalitis, or basal ganglia stroke.[5] Prolonged EMG discharges from nonreciprocal agonist/antagonist musculature characteristic for diurnal dystonia progressively decreased in the deeper stages of non-REM sleep and REM sleep. The mean dystonic EMG activity during sleep compared to waking was 41.8% in stage N1, 8.4% in stage N2, 5.9% in early stage N3, 1.6% in late stage N3, and 9.8% in REM sleep. It was suggested that normal phasic REM elevations in EMG might have accounted for the relatively high, apparently dystonic activity in REM sleep.

Hoffmann (H) reflexes were reduced in non-REM sleep, averaging only 15.2% of waking amplitudes. Prolonged H-reflex recovery and silent periods were most significant in REM sleep. The tendon (T) reflex studies during sleep were reported as percent amplitude change compared to waking. In Wilson's disease this was 33.0% in non-REM and 30.5% in REM. The tonic stretch and vibration reflexes (induced by 100 Hz activity) were also markedly reduced in non-REM and REM sleep.

Focal Dystonia

The etiology of idiopathic cervical dystonia (spasmodic torticollis), the most common focal dystonia, is unknown. Nevertheless, it is generally considered a disease of the basal ganglia.[21] Pain associated with involuntary contractions and sustained movements has been reported to be significantly reduced during sleep, but some reports indicate that EMG activity persists throughout sleep, suggesting that it is muscular activity, not pain, that is primarily responsible for interfering with sleep continuity in this disorder.[22–24]

In a review by Lobbezoo et al., there has been a documentation of prolonged REM latencies, reduced total REM sleep times, and decreased sleep efficiencies in patients with idiopathic cervical dystonia.[25] With regard to dystonia, they indicate that some investigators have found no decrease in cervical muscular activity in sleep in studies that were primarily descriptive, and without detailed statistical analysis or full controls. Nevertheless, Forgasch and colleagues reported short bursts of asynchronous EMG activity over the sternocleidomastoid during REM sleep in 8 of 16 individuals with spasmodic torticollis.[20]

In 1996, Lobbezoo et al. studied nine patients and gender- and age-matched controls with PSG after a first night habituation study.[25] The examinations were performed without respiratory or lower-extremity EMG monitoring. Activity of the upper trapezius and sternocleidomastoid muscles was analyzed with bipolar surface disc electrodes and videotape monitoring using infrared cameras. Scoring of sleep stages and muscular activity was performed in a blinded fashion by experienced technologists. Waking EMG activity was recorded with the patient sitting upright without head support and when lying down, with the intention of remaining awake. No significant differences between patients and controls were found in regard to total sleep time spent in stages N1 through N3 and REM sleep, wake time after sleep onset, sleep efficiency, sleep and REM latency, number of awakenings, and sleep stage shifts.

It was noted, however, that the variance in sleep latency was significantly larger in this patient population, probably due to variability in pain reduction expected during the transition from wake to sleep. Cervical discomfort was rated by sensory/intensity and affective scales, before and after the second sleep recording, as 0 = none, 1 = little, 2 = moderate, and 3 = a lot. In the patients, ratings of cervical spinal pain intensity and cervical spinal pain unpleasantness improved by 53.5% and 54.2%, respectively, when comparisons were made between the evening prior to sleep and the morning after the sleep periods.

Grading of EMG activity, using a four-point rating scale as normal, low, medium, or high abnormal, had very high intraobserver reliability. In six patients, cervical EMG activity normalized during the first sleep cycle prior to stage N2. One individual exhibited a low level of abnormal muscular contraction in the left sternocleidomastoid muscle only to the first epoch of stage N2 sleep.

In a controlled study from 2009, Trotti et al. examined sleepiness, using the Epworth Sleepiness Scale (ESS), in 43 consecutive patients with cervical dystonia.[26] They found a higher percentage of cervical dystonia patients had abnormal ESS scores of >11 than did either of two control groups (21%, versus 0% [in 19 patients with other focal movement disorders], versus 4% [in 49 healthy, age- and gender-matched controls], $p < .05$ for each pairwise comparison with the cervical dystonia group). Using the Toronto Western Spasmodic Torticollis Rating Scale and subscores, age, gender, race, severity, disability, and pain, and other common medication use (benzodiazepines and antidepressants) were not associated with increased ESS scores. This suggested that excessive sleepiness was due to a disturbance of intrinsic sleep mechanisms, rather than a direct effect of dystonic muscle activity.

Nevertheless, a subsequent controlled study from 2011, by Paus et al., showed that only 6% of 221 subjects with cervical dystonia and blepharospasm had excessive daytime sleepiness using the ESS.[27] Be that as it may, impaired quality of sleep, as defined by the Pittsburgh Sleep Quality Index, was found in 44% of the subjects with cervical dystonia and was appreciated in 46% of individuals with blepharospasm (as compared to only 20% of the 93 neurologically healthy controls). Impaired quality of sleep in the dystonia population was not associated with severity of dystonic symptoms, but it did associate with symptoms of depression (as defined by the Beck's Depression Inventory, 26%; $p < .001$) and restless legs syndrome (RLS; defined using the minimal criteria of the International RLS Study Group; 19%; $p < .01$). In addition, bruxism (teeth grinding) was noted in 28% of the subjects with cervical dystonia and 18% of those with blepharospasm. The authors concluded that the impaired quality of sleep in this study was probably due to an intrinsic mechanism of sleep disturbance rather than a direct effect of dystonic muscle activity.

TOURETTE SYNDROME

Glaze and colleagues noted that patients with Tourette syndrome (TS) frequently complained of insomnia.[28] They inferred that the report of frequent nocturnal arousals might have been related to tics that persisted in sleep. This group subsequently performed a controlled study of 14 subjects with TS, using overnight PSG to characterize nocturnal tics using technician visual reports, videotape analysis, and a triaxial accelerometer placed on areas of tics.

The younger patients (ages 8 to 23 years) had an increase in the percentage of stage N3 sleep, a reduction in the percentage of REM sleep, and an increase in the number of nocturnal arousals compared to controls. Sixty-seven percent of the subjects also had either central or obstructive sleep apneic events. In addition, 58% had sleep terrors associated with hypersynchrony. Hypnagogic hypersynchrony is not unusual in young children, and electroencephalographically it is formally defined as paroxysmal bursts of diffuse, high-amplitude (75 to 350 µv), sinusoidal, 3 to 4.5 Hz waves, which begin abruptly in a widely distributed manner, with a maximum over the central, frontal, or frontocentral regions.[29]

Ninety-two percent of these patients had persistent tics that were characteristic of their diurnal events, with rare vocalizations noted in all sleep stages. There was an average of 12 events for every 8 hours of sleep recorded. Two older patients (both 48 years of age) showed a reduction in stage N2 and the deeper portions of stage N3 sleep compared to controls. Neither of these adults exhibited persistent tics in sleep or sleep terror–like episodes.

Jankovic et al. indicated that quantifying tics in TS simply by observation in the waking state was inaccurate as voluntary suppression is possible.[30] As such, they suggested the utility of quantifying tics in the sleeping state to avoid this potential pitfall. They further proposed that such quantification pre and post the institution of therapy might allow a very sensitive way of monitoring medication efficacy.

In the preliminary work of this group, they compared the sleep of young patients pre and post therapy with tetrabenazine. Significant changes noted with medication included a general reduction in the percentage of total sleep, a decrease in the number of nocturnal arousals, and a reduction in the number of sleep-related tics. A cumulative total of 50 tics were captured in sleep prior to therapy, whereas only 12 were recorded while the three individuals were receiving tetrabenazine.

Fish and colleagues found that among the dyskinesias, TS could involve unique "predormitory" movements during the transition from waking to sleeping.[7] In a population of 10 patients, which included young adults and children, a total of 143 tics were documented, with a median number of 11.5, a mean of 12, and a range of 0 to 57 per patient. There was a median number of 43 epochs containing tics per 100 waking epochs reviewed, 32 epochs of tics for every 100 epochs of the transition from sleep to wake reviewed, 14 epochs of tics for every 100 epochs of the transition from deeper to lighter sleep reviewed, 1.9 epochs of tics for every 100 epochs of tics of stage N1 sleep reviewed, and 0.5 epochs of tics for every 100 epochs of stage N2 sleep reviewed. No tics were reported in stage N3 and REM sleep. In addition, no tics occurred during sleep in patients who were 37 years of age or older.

A controlled study by Cohrs et al. showed an increase in sleep-related movements in patients with TS.[31] Twenty-five patients with TS were studied with PSG and simultaneous split-screen video monitoring. Sleep was significantly more disturbed in TS compared to controls with decreased sleep efficiency and slow-wave sleep percentage, increased sleep latency, percentage of stage N1, percentage of awakeness, number of awakenings, and sleep stage changes and more overall movements during sleep. The severity of TS during the day, as assessed using the TS severity scale, correlated positively with the number of awakenings and sleep stage changes and negatively with sleep efficiency. In contrast to the Fish study, tic frequency, as well as the frequency of regular movements, was significantly higher in REM than in non-REM sleep, with no associated disturbance of either the REM sleep percentage or REM latency.

TREMOR

Tremor is an involuntary, slightly rhythmical pattern of muscle contraction/relaxation that leads to oscillating body movements. Tremor in a variety of extrapyramidal disorders tends to persist in sleep. Although tremor with cerebellar disease and Parkinson's disease may decrease by 50% in sleep, it generally retains its diurnal electrophysiologic and clinical characteristics, although in some instances this can be a variable and controversial issue.[32,33] Parkinsonian tremor routinely decreases in amplitude and duration in early non-REM sleep, is rarely seen in stage N3 sleep, and often disappears in REM sleep.[34] However, isolated movements may resolve in stage N1 sleep, and then reappear in stage N2 sleep and during sleep stage transitions and burst of rapid eye movements in REM sleep.[35,36] It is implied that these reported movements may actually represent otherwise normal periodic limb movements in sleep, frequently found in stage N2 sleep, and muscle twitches normally appreciated in phasic REM sleep.

Palatal tremor, also known as palatal myoclonus, is one of the rarest of the rhythmic hyperkinesias.[37] The tremor is often associated with simultaneous contractions of the tongue, lips, cheek, eyelids, diaphragm, and extremities.

Palatal tremor can present in essential and symptomatic forms (often related to ischemic, traumatic, or demyelinating interruption of the dentato-rubral-olivary pathways [Mollaret's triangle]). The essential type is usually associated with ear clicks and has no identifiable etiology, while symptomatic palatal tremor is related to brainstem pathology and may present with significant brainstem and cerebellar signs and in association with oscillopsia.

Prior to PSG studies, visual observation of apparently sleeping individuals with known palatal tremor suggested that this form of tremor persisted in sleep.[38,39] Jacobs and Bender reported the effects of sleep on one patient with palato-ocular synchrony.[40] Movement in the first and last 3-hour periods of sleep was similar to waking and occurred with a frequency of 2.5 Hz. Between 3 and 4½ hours into the study tremor frequency reduced to half of the waking rate. Vertical ocular tremor persisted in stage N1 and N2 sleep, was absent during stage N3 sleep, and recurred in REM sleep. This pattern of eye tremor was reported by Tahmoush et al., but in their study it did not show the same synchronous association with palatal tremor that was appreciated during the waking hours.[41]

Kayed et al. examined three subjects with palatal tremor.[42] Two of these patients had essential palatal tremor (with normal electroencephalograms [EEGs], brainstem auditory evoked responses [BAERs], visual evoked potentials [VEPs], and brain computed tomography scans [CTs]) ranging from 180 to 240 beats per minute, and the other subject was thought to have the symptomatic form at 90 beats per minute. Despite a normal VEP, BAER, and head CT, this individual had a positive family history of tremor and exhibited involvement of the masseter and periorbital muscles with dysphagia, vertigo, ataxia, and diplopia.

These patients received full PSG examinations with respiratory monitoring. During these studies a piezoceramic transducer was placed over the cricothyroid to record the palatal tremor. The rate of tremor was reported at the beginning, at 5-minute intervals, and at the end of each specific sleep stage. The frequency and amplitude of tremor gradually diminished, without complete resolution, from stage N1 to N3 to REM sleep. In REM sleep the tremor developed a characteristic clustering of two to four high-amplitude movements at variable intervals with no relationship to rapid eye movements or respiratory phenomena.

In one patient, a specific movement type limited to stage N2 sleep was associated with repetitive bursts of submental EMG activity lasting 2–3 seconds and recurring at 30-second intervals. This activity had no relationship to periodic limb movements in sleep. A figure provided in the original report suggested that K-complexes preceded these movements, and as such they may have been K-alpha microarousals.

MYOCLONUS

Myoclonic movements are sudden, brief involuntary movements of a muscle or muscle group. Myoclonic movements in sleep should not be mistaken for periodic limb movements in sleep (previously referred to as "sleep myoclonus" as part of the "nocturnal myoclonus syndrome").[43] Periodic limb movements in sleep are longer in duration than myoclonic jerks, 0.5 to 10 seconds, respectively, as compared to 50 to 150 milliseconds.

Mano and colleagues performed PSG studies on 11 patients with myoclonus associated with a variety of neurologic problems.[5] These included seizures, focal cortical atrophy, anoxic encephalopathy, mercury poisoning, olivopontocerebellar atrophy, brainstem encephalitis, Behcet's disease, cervical spondylosis, and spinal arterial-venous malformation. The analysis grouped patients according to their proposed, primary neurological injury into potentially epileptogenic cortex and upper brainstem lesions and lower brainstem or spinal cord lesions.

In five patients with potential epileptic discharges, myoclonus occurred with and without EEG spikes. Simultaneous spikes and myoclonus were found to occur most frequently in the waking state. In these individuals myoclonus tended to decrease in sleep while spike activity persisted relatively unabated or increased in sleep, frequently without the previously appreciated simultaneously occurring myoclonic activity. The mean frequency of characteristic EMG discharges characteristic for the movements of interest compared to the frequency during wakefulness averaged 63.4% for stage N1, 26.8% for stage N2, 7.3% for stage N3, and 17.5% for REM sleep.

An interesting observation was reported in one patient with myoclonus related to a spinal cord lesion, where H and T reflex and EMG recordings of clonus were performed. The number of EMG discharges indicating ankle clonus compared to waking was 33% in stage N1, 28%

in stage N2, 17% in stage N3, and 12% in REM sleep. The soleus H-reflex amplitude compared to waking was 88% in non-REM and 28% in REM sleep. The T-reflex amplitude compared to awake was 48% in stages N1 and N2 sleep, 20% in stage N3 sleep, and 21% in REM sleep.

It was a unique finding that myoclonus associated with lesions in the lower brainstem and spinal cord tended to increase in sleep, specifically in stage N1 and N2 sleep. In lesions of the pons and medulla, the mean frequency of myoclonus in sleeping compared to waking averaged 185.3% in stage N1 sleep, 201.3% in stage N2, 109.0% in early stage N3, 80.0% in deeper stage N3 sleep, and 49.7% in REM sleep.

Shiozawa hypothesized that sleep-related myoclonus with spinal cord lesions might be due to dissociation of spinal alpha and gamma motor neuron activity or to hypnic disinhibition of spinal interneurons, which mediate the polysynaptic flexor reflex.[44] He suggested that lesions in descending inhibitory pathways (probably the inhibitory reticulo-spinal tract) which innervate spinal interneurons accentuated this mechanism.

HEMIFACIAL SPASM

There is controversy concerning peripheral and central elements responsible for hemifacial spasm. Although resolution of hemifacial spasm after vascular decompression suggests a peripheral origin, studying sleep, which is a state of modified "central" excitability, presented an avenue where "nuclear" theories can be directly assessed.

Montagna et al. performed PSG studies on 13 individuals with idiopathic and 3 patients with postparalytic hemifacial spasm; one suffered the disorder as a result of trauma.[45] Ten women and six men, from 44 to 74 years of age, had PSG studies during EMG monitoring of the submental, frontalis, orbicularis oculi, and orbicularis oris musculature of the affected side. In six cases, simultaneous assessment of the unaffected side was also performed. To avoid inadvertently recording activity from the opposite side of the face, special care was made to place the recording electrodes far from midline. Scoring epochs of 20 seconds were used to grade facial EMG activity on an "arbitrary" six-point scale. The absence of muscular activity was graded as 0, while continuous activity noted throughout an epoch received a score of 5.

Patients showed prolonged sleep latencies and frequent awakenings with 29.9% of the total study time being scored as awake. The total sleep time percentages revealed 14.1% stage N1, 51.7% stage N2, 18.0% stage N3, and 17.6% as REM sleep. As there were no differences noted in EMG activity between idiopathic and postparalytic hemifacial spasm, the data were pooled. In an apparent attempt to avoid scoring normal phasic REM movements as spasm, the authors analyzed movements independently in phasic REM (77% of REM) and tonic REM (23% of total REM) sleep.

During wakefulness the degree of typical clonic activity was found to synchronously affect all affected facial muscles monitored in each individual patient, but the magnitude of activity was found to vary markedly from patient to patient. In general, hemifacial spasm was associated with intermittent prolonged periods silent for muscular activity, although in two individuals clonus was continuous when awake. Abnormal muscular activity in sleep progressively decreased in amplitude and duration. Compared to waking, the EMG activity of hemifacial spasm was 74.0% in stage N1, 53.0% in stage N2, 51.0% in the early stages of N3, 56% in the deeper stages of N3, and 42.0% in REM sleep. The amount of spasm was not different between phasic and tonic REM sleep. Variability in the amount of spasm was greatest in wakefulness, and progressively decreased through stages N1 to N3 sleep, with the least variability in REM sleep.

The authors concluded that a combination of peripheral and central mechanisms explained hemifacial spasm. They surmised that hemifacial spasm originated from ectopic activity in the peripheral nerve with synkinetic spread to other facial musculature. The progressive, partial reduction in hemifacial spasm with sleep may be due to central inhibitory effects on the facial nerve similar to the motoneuron hyperpolarization documented in animal experiments and H-reflex studies.

GENERAL THERAPEUTICS

It is paramount to distinguish between sleep disturbance resulting from hyperkinetic movements and the variety of other commonly occurring sleep disorders that may be associated with specific movement disorders. As such, a thorough sleep-wake history and neurologic examination is mandatory. Insomnia is ubiquitous in depression, and a common problem in HD and a variety of the dementing and physically disabling disorders. Expert evaluation and treatment by a psychiatrist/psychologist familiar with sleep disorders and the use of medications with minimal side effects are often useful in such circumstances.

Nocturnal tremor, dystonia, chorea, ballism, and muscle spasm should be addressed using the same pharmacological approaches as used with the corresponding diurnal problems. However, adverse effects on sleep, of otherwise essential medications are common. Levodopa for parkinsonian tremor can, for example, increase sleep latency and produce nightmares and nocturnal hallucinations, making drug dose and timing an important part of therapy.

In general, the standard treatments are used when common intrinsic sleep disorders are encountered in this population. For example, if obstructive sleep apnea is present, continuous positive airway pressure therapy should be considered. However, if there is difficulty with compliance due to associated behavioral problems, dementia, or significant medical concomitants, uvulopalatopharyngoplasty or tracheostomy may be viable therapeutic alternatives.

DISCUSSION

The 1997, revised edition of the *International Classification of Sleep Disorders* defines some of the hyperkinetic syndromes described in this chapter as "slowly progressive conditions characterized by abnormal behaviors or involuntary movements, often with evidence of other motor system degeneration."[46] In patients with sleep complaints it is important to carefully assess for intrinsic sleep disorders that are commonly associated with degenerative diseases, such as restless legs syndrome, periodic limb movements in sleep, RBD, and central and obstructive sleep apnea. In many cases, a PSG with extended EMG monitoring and an MSLT can be invaluable.[18]

Volitional movements and diurnal hyperkinesias (primarily associated with the waking state) generally decrease in sleep. Animal and human H and T reflex studies have shown a progressive hyperpolarization of anterior horn cell alpha motor neurons during sleep in otherwise normal subjects.[47-49] It has been hypothesized that in some patients with neurodegenerative processes there can be a reduction in the normal inhibitory effect of sleep due to lesions

that might exist at many levels of the CNS. This may explain why diurnal dyskinesias tend to improve only incompletely in sleep in some individuals.[2,5]

Disinhibition has been hypothesized to explain palatal tremor. It has been demonstrated that stimulation of the central tegmental fasciculus in the inferior olive can produce palatal tremor. Clinically, palatal tremor may occur when lesions in the cerebellar dentate nucleus result in a disinhibition of the central tegmental tract of the brainstem.[42,50,51]

Myoclonus with lower brain stem and spinal cord lesions, and periodic limb movements in sleep are unique among the dyskinesias as they tend to be exacerbated by, or occur only in, sleep. We and others have reported individuals with unilateral hemispheric stroke with frequent, periodic limb movements in the otherwise paretic limbs.[18,52] This reinforces the hypothesis that sleep-activated limb movements may result after lesions at many CNS levels due to the loss of excitatory influence upon inhibitory subcortical systems (see Fig. 53.2).

Description inconsistencies due to relatively incomplete monitoring methods and variable scoring techniques can lead to a misinterpretation of movements associated with the arousals and microarousals routinely seen in the associated sleep-related breathing disorders and variety of medical and psychiatric concomitants that patients with cerebral degenerative processes may manifest.[53-55] As such, the use of infrared video analysis with full PSG testing utilizing adequate monitoring of airflow, respiratory effort, and oximetry has allowed for a more confident physiological characterization of a variety of diurnal hyperkinetic syndromes.

In some cases, CNS centers, which generate non-REM and REM sleep and normal circadian rhythms, may be affected. HD has been associated with a low-amplitude EEG with a reduction in alpha activity that parallels cortical atrophy and disease progression, prolonged awakenings, with reductions in sleep efficiency, SWA and REM sleep and REM density, and abnormally slow rapid eye movements.[6,56,57]

Degenerative effects in many CNS areas could also produce respiratory problems. Lesions rostral to the upper cervical spinal cord and caudal to the fifth cranial nerve in the pons can lead to failure of automatic respiration.[58,59] Damage to the nucleus ambiguus and nucleus tractus solitarius in the medulla has been associated with obstructive and central apneas,

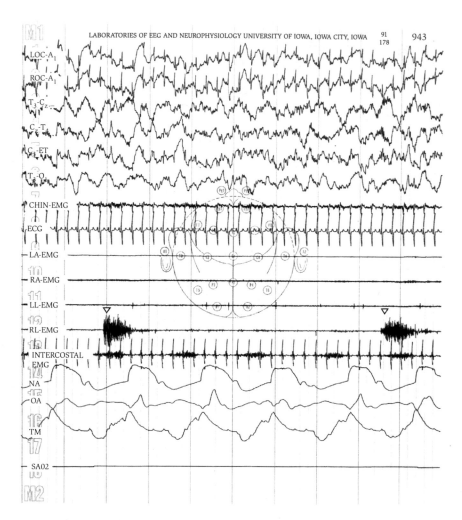

FIGURE 53.2   Polysomnogram of a patient with a left occipital infarction associated with a small left cerebellar hemorrhage; the two, small open arrowheads in this 3-second sample of the patient's sleep study give a small demonstration of what are periodic limb movements during stage 2–3 sleep, almost exclusively occurring in the right lower extremity. A_1 (left ear) + A_2 (right ear); C, central; ET, ear tied; IC, intercostal electromyogram; LA, left arm; LL, left leg; LOC, left outer canthus; NA, nasal airflow; O, occipital; RA, right arm; RL, right leg; ROC, right outer canthus; SAO_2, oxygen saturation; T, temporal; TM, thoracic movement. (From Figure 2, Dyken ME, Rodnitzky RL. Periodic, aperiodic, and rhythmic motor disorders of sleep. *Neurology* 1992;42(suppl 6):68–74; with permission.)

respectively.[54,55,58,60–63] Other centers for respiratory control have been reported in mesencephalic and diencephalic nuclei, and fronto-orbital, anterior-temporal, cingulate, insular, and sensorimotor cortices.[64,65]

Although not proposed as a generalized scoring technique, Fish's group and others have introduced modifications to Rechtschaffen and Kales's classic *A Manual of Standardized Terminology, Techniques and Scoring Systems for Sleep Stages of Human Subjects*[7,66] and the updated 2012 American Academy of Sleep Medicine's Manual for the Scoring of Sleep and Associated Events; Rules, Terminology and Technical Specifications, Version 2.0,[29] which have allowed finer analysis of a variety of nocturnal dyskinesias. Although the Rechtschaffen manual was intended to provide a uniform method for describing sleep, the definition of discrete physiological events such as "body movements" was left to the individual investigator using a 30-second epoch scoring system, whereas the 2012 updated manual does include rules governing the scoring of periodic limb movements in sleep, alternating leg muscle activation, hypnagogic foot tremor, fragmentary myoclonus, bruxism, the RBD, and the rhythmic movement disorder.

As movements are often associated with a sleep stage change, Fish proposed scoring "amendments" to include transition epochs. A "predormitory" epoch contains a transition from wake to sleep; "lightening" contains a transition from a deeper to lighter stage of sleep; "deepening" contains a transition from a lighter to deeper sleep; and an epoch scored as "awakening" includes a transition from sleep to wake.

Some investigators have used "miniepoch" scoring systems to more accurately associate specific sleep stages with movements of interest. Fish et al. have scored movements as occurring during the stage of sleep that was seen 2 seconds prior to the movement of interest. A 2-second epoch was chosen as they found movements during episodes of unequivocal sleep usually followed a 2-second epoch of arousal. In the classically used epoch scoring system for adults, movements would be considered to occur in the sleep stage that comprises 50% or more of the 30-second period temporally associated with the movement. This would lead to scoring most movements in the drowsy or waking state.

SUMMARY

There is a tremendous paucity of knowledge in regard to the effect of hyperkinetic syndromes on sleep. Nevertheless, dramatic advances in technology with PSG have provided insight into the basic physiology underlying a variety of these disorders. This has improved the diagnosis of a variety of associated sleep abnormalities, allowing implementation of specific therapies that have improved sleep and subsequently patient quality of life. It should be remembered that with the exception of periodic limb movements and myoclonus associated with lower brainstem and spinal cord lesions, most diurnal hyperkinesias generally improve in sleep. As such, although it makes sense that successful treatment of the primary movement abnormality should improve sleep, improving sleep by also directly addressing a variety of intrinsic sleep problems may reduce the clinical effects of diurnal movements.

REFERENCES

1. The Huntington's Disease Collaborative Research Group. A novel gene containing a trinucleotide repeat that is expanded and unstable on Huntington's disease chromosomes. *Cell* 1993;72:971–83.
2. Tassinari CA, Broughton R, Roger J, et al. A polygraphic study of the evolution of abnormal movements during sleep. *Electroenceph Clin Neurophysiol* 1964;17:721.
3. Tassinari CA, Broughton R, Poire R, et al. An electro-clinical study of nocturnal sleep in patients presenting abnormal movements. *Electroenceph Clin Neurophysiol* 1965;19: 95.
4. Marsden CD, Quinn NP. The dystonias. *Br Med J* 1990;300:139–44.
5. Mano T, Schiozawa Z, Sobue I. Extrapyramidal involuntary movements during sleep. In: Broughton RJ, ed. *Henri Gastaut and the Marseilles School's Contribution to the Neurosciences* (EEG Suppl 35). Amsterdam, The Netherlands: Elsevier;1982:431–42.
6. Wiegand M, Moller AA, Lauer CJ, et al. Nocturnal sleep in Huntington's disease. *J Neurol* 1991;238:203–8.
7. Fish DR, Sawyers D, Allen PJ, et al. The effect of sleep on the dyskinetic movements of Parkinson's disease, Gilles de la Tourette syndrome, Huntington's disease, and torsion dystonia. *Arch Neurol* 1991;48:210–14.
8. Hansotia P, Wall R, Berendes J. Sleep disturbances and severity of Huntington's disease. *Neurology* 1985;35:1672–4.
9. Emser W, Brenner M, Stober T, et al. Changes in nocturnal sleep in Huntington's and Parkinson's disease. *J Neurol* 1988;235:177–9.
10. Arnulf I, Nielsen J, Lohmann E, et al. Rapid eye movement sleep disturbances in Huntington disease. *Arch Neurol* 2008;65:482–288.
11. Weiner WJ, Lang AE. Huntington's disease. In: Weiner WJ, Lang AE, eds. *Movement Disorders;A Comprehensive Survey*. New York: Futura;1989:300–1.
12. Morton AJ, Wood NI, Hastings MH, et al. Disintegration of the sleep-wake cycle and circadian timing in Huntington's disease. *J Neurosci* 2005;25:157–63.
13. Postuma RB, Lang AE. Hemiballism: revisitng a classic disorder. *Lancet Neurol* 2003;2:661–8.
14. Krauss JK, Grossman RG. Surgery for hyperkinetic movement disorders. In: Jankovic J Tolosa E, eds. *Parkinson's Disease and Movement*

Disorders. 5th ed. Philadelphia, PA: Lippincott Williams & Wilkins;2006:1017–48.

15. Driver-Dunckley E, Evidente VG. Hemichorea-hemiballismus may respond to topiratmate. *Clin Neuropharmacol* 2005;3:142–4.

16. Francisco GE. Successful treatment of posttraumatic hemiballismus with intrathecal baclofen. *Am J Phys Med Rehabil* 2006;85:779–82.

17. Sitburana O, Ondo WG. Tetrabenazine in hyperglycemic induced hemichorea hemiballismus. *Mov Disord* 2006;21:2023–5.

18. Dyken MD, Rodnitzky RL. Periodic, aperiodic, and rhythmic motor disorders of sleep. *Neurology* 1992;42(Suppl 6):68–74.

19. Jankel WR, Niedermeyer E, Graf M, et al. Polysomnography of torsion dystonia. *Arch Neurol* 1984;41:1081–3.

20. Forgach L, Eisen A, Fleetham J, et al. Studies on dystonic torticollis during sleep. *Neurology* 1986;36(Suppl 1):120.

21. Truong DD, Dubinsky R, Hermanowicz N, et al. Posttraumatic torticollis. *Arch Neurol* 1991;48:221–3.

22. Chan J, Brin MF, Fahn S. Idiopathic cervical dystonia: clinical characteristics. *Mov Disord* 1991;6:119–26.

23. Claypool DW, Duane DD, Ilstrup DM, et al. Epidemiology and outcome of cervical dystonia (spasmotic torticollis) in Rochester, Minnesota. *Mov Disord* 1995;10:608–14.

24. Marsden CD, Harrison MJ. Idiopathic torsion dystonia (dystonia musculorum deformans). A review of forty-two patients. *Brain* 1974;97:793–810.

25. Lobbezoo F, Thon TM, Remillard G, et al. Relationship between sleep, neck muscle activity, and pain in cervical dystonia. *Can J Neurol Sci* 1996;23:285–90.

26. Trotti LM, Esper CD, Feustel PJ, et al. Excessive daytime sleepiness in cervical dystonia. *Parkinsonism Relat Disord* 2009;15:784–6.

27. Paus S, Gross J, Moll-Müller M, et al. Impaired sleep quality and restless legs syndrome in idiopathic focal dystonia: a controlled study. *J Neurol* 2011;258:1835–40.

28. Glaze DG, Frost JD, Jr., Jankovic J. Sleep in Gilles de la Tourette's syndrome: disorder of arousal. *Neurology* 1983;33:586–92.

29. Berry RB, Brooks R, Gamaldo CE, et al. for the American Academy of Sleep Medicine. The AASM Manual for the Scoring of Sleep and Associated Events: Rules, Terminology and Technical Specifications, Version 2.0.

www.aasmnet.org, Darien, Illinois: American Academy of Sleep Medicine, 2012.

30. Jankovic J, Glaze DG, Frost JD, Jr. Effect of tetrabenazine on tics and sleep of Gilles de la Tourette's syndrome. *Neurology* 1984;34:688–92.

31. Cohrs S, Rasch T, Altmeyer S, et al. Decreased sleep quality and increased sleep related movements in patients with Tourette's syndrome. *J Neurol Neurosurg Psychiatry* 2001;70:192–7.

32. April R. Observations on Parkinsonian tremor in all night sleep. *Neurology* 1966;16:72–4.

33. Mano T, Schiozawa Z, Sobue Y. Polygraphic study of extrapyramidal involuntary movements in man during sleep. *Proc Third Internat Cong Sleep Research* Tokyo;1979:220.

34. Askenasy JJ, Yahr MD. Parkinsonian tremor loses its alternating aspect during non-REM sleep and is inhibited by REM sleep. *J Neurol Neurosurg Psychiatr* 1990;53:749–53.

35. Stern M, Roffwarg H, Duvoisin R. The Parkinsonian tremor in sleep. *J Nerv Ment Dis* 1968;147:202–10.

36. Aldrich MS. Parkinsonism. In: Kryger MH, Roth T, Dement WC. Principles and Practice of Sleep Medicine. Philadelphia: WB Saunders, 2000;1051–7.

37. Deuschl G, Toro C, Valls-Sole J, et al. Symptomatic and essential palatal tremor. *Brain* 1994;117:775–88.

38. Bonduelle M. The myoclonias. In: Vinken PJ, Bruyn GW, eds. *Handbook of Clinical Neurology*. Vol 6. Amsterdam, The Netherlands: North Holland;1970:761–81.

39. Nathanson M. Palatal myoclonus. Further clinical and pathophysiological observations. *Arch Neurol Psychiatry* 1956;75:285–95.

40. Jacobs L, Bender B. Palato-ocular synchrony during eyelid closure. *Arch Neurol* 1976;33:289–91.

41. Tahmoush AJ, Brooks JE, Keltner JL. Palatal myoclonus associated with abnormal ocular and extremity movements: a polygraphic study. *Arch Neurol* 1972;27:431–40.

42. Kayed K, Sjaastad O, Magnussen I, et al. Palatal myoclonus during sleep. *Sleep* 1983;6:130–6.

43. American Academy of Sleep Medicine. International Classification of Sleep Disorders. Diagnostic and Coding Manual. 2nd ed. Westchester, IL: American Academy of Sleep Medicine;2005:182–6.

44. Shiozawa Z. Sleep and Internal Medicine. *Int Med* 1996;35:45–7.

45. Montagna P, Imbriaco A, Zucconi M, et al. Hemifacial spasm in sleep. *Neurology* 1986;36:270–3.

46. American Sleep Disorders Association. *International Classification of Sleep Disorders. Diagnostic and Coding Manual.* Rev. Rochester, MN: American Sleep Disorders Association;1997:235.

47. Dagnino N, Loeb C, Massazza G, et al. Hypnic physiological myoclonias in man: an EEG-EMG study in normals and neurological patients. *Eur Neurol* 1969;2:47–58.

48. Gassell MM, Marchiafava PL, Pompeiano O. Tonic and phasic inhibition of spinal reflexes during deep, desynchronized sleep in unrestrained cats. *Arch Ital Biol* 1964;102:471–99.

49. Hodes R, Dement WC. Depression of electrically induced reflexes ("H-reflexes") in man during low voltage EEG "sleep." *Electroencephalogr Clin Neurophysiol* 1964;17:617–29.

50. Lapresle J. Rhythmic palatal myoclonus and the dentato-olivary pathway. *J Neurol* 1979;220:223–30.

51. Lapresle J, Hamida MB. The dentato-olivary pathway. Somatotropic relationship between the dentate nucleus and the contralateral inferior olive. *Arch Neurol* 1970;22:135–43.

52. Kang SY, Sohn, YH, Lee IK, et al. Unilateral periodic limb movement in sleep after supratentorial cerebral infarction. *Parkinsonism Relat Disord* 2004;10:429–31.

53. Dyken ME. The relationship between stroke and obstructive sleep apnea. *Arteres Veines* 1997;16:226–39.

54. Merrill EG. The lateral respiratory neurones of the medulla: their associations with nucleus ambiguus, nucleus retroambigualis, the spinal accessory nucleus and the spinal cord. *Brain Res* 1970;24:11–18.

55. Berger AJ, Mitchell RA, Severinghaus JW. Regulation of respiration. *N Engl J Med* 1977;297:92–7,138–43,194–201.

56. Margerison JH, Scott DF. Huntington's chorea;clinical, EEG and neuropathological findings. *Electroencephalogr Clin Neurophysiol* 1965;19:314.

57. Scott DF, Heathfield KWG, Toone B, et al. The EEG in Huntington's chorea: a clinical and neuropathological study. *J Neurol Neurosurg Psychiatry* 1972;35:97–102.

58. Levin BE, Margolis G. Acute failure of automatic respirations secondary to a unilateral brainstem infarct. *Ann Neurol* 1977;1:583–6.

59. Severinghaus JW, Mitchell RA. Ondine's curse-failure of respiratory center automaticity while awake. *Clin Res* 1962;10:122.

60. Chaudhary BA, Elguindi AS, King DW. Obstructive sleep apnea after lateral medullary syndrome. *South Med J* 1982;75:65–7.

61. Askenasy JJ, Goldhammer I. Sleep apnea as a feature of bulbar stroke. *Stroke* 1988;19:637–9.

62. Guilleminault C, Dement W. eds. *Sleep Apnea Syndromes.* New York: Alan R. Liss; 1978:11.

63. Beal MF, Richardson EP, Brandstetter R, et al. Localized brainstem ischemic damage and Ondine's curse after near-drowning. *Neurology* 1983;33:717–21.

64. Hugelin A. Forebrain and midbrain influence on respiration. In: Fishman AP, Cheniak NS, Widdicombe JG, Geige SR, eds. *Handbook of Physiology, Section 3. The respiratory system, Vol. II. Control of Breathing.* Bethesda, MD: American Physiological Society; 1986:69–91.

65. Lee MC, Klassen AC, Heaney LM, et al. Respiratory rate and pattern disturbance in acute brain stem infarction. *Stroke* 1976;7:382–5.

66. Rechtschaffen A, Kales A. *A Manual of Standardized Terminology, Techniques and Scoring Systems for Sleep Stages of Human Subjects.* Bethesda, MD: *National Institutes of Health*; 1968:204.

54

Unusual Movement Disorders

SUDHANSU CHOKROVERTY

INTENSIVE ATTENTION is now given to the sleep problems and phenomena of the well-described movement disorders; however, a few miscellaneous abnormal movement disorders, including some newly described entities, also have an interaction with sleep/wake states. Often, these disorders are known only from a few reports. However, in a number of cases, it is already established that these predominantly diurnal dyskinetic disorders persist during sleep or are associated with disordered sleep.

In this section I briefly describe fasciculations, palatal myoclonus, respiratory myoclonus, "belly dancer's" dyskinesia, spinal and propriospinal myoclonus, and "bobble-head doll" syndrome and indicate their relation to sleep. In addition, I also briefly mention paroxysmal hypnogenic dyskinesias, rhythmic limb movements resembling rhythmic movement disorder (RMD) on termination of apnea-hypopnea, rhythmic leg movements in wakefulness, non–rapid eye movement (non-REM) and REM sleep, and hyperekplexia.

Fasciculations can be defined as brief, involuntary, twitch-like movements that result from contractions of a few fascicles or bundles of muscle fibers. The most common condition in which fasciculations are seen consists of slowly progressive anterior horn cell disease (e.g., amyotrophic lateral sclerosis [ALS]). Fasciculations can be positively diagnosed by electromyography. Fasciculations persist during sleep and these malignant manifestations may be confused with a benign condition such as excessive fragmentary myoclonus (EFM).[1] EFM generally does not cause gross body or limb movements and is seen in the electromyographic recordings of the polysomnographs. Currently, EFM is thought to be a nonspecific condition and is seen in a variety of sleep disorders. There is another condition, so-called benign fasciculation syndrome, which could be mistaken with these malignant fasciculations associated with anterior horn cell disease or, sometimes, with polyradiculoneuropathies. Benign fasciculations are seen in many normal individuals, creating intense anxiety, particularly in those with a medical background or relatives of patients with ALS. These are not associated with muscle wasting, weakness, or reflex abnormalities. The subjects need reassurance that these are benign and do not progress to the development of ALS.[2] Sometimes it is difficult to distinguish benign from malignant fasciculations clinically, and electromyographic examination may be helpful. Malignant fasciculations fire randomly and irregularly at a rate of less than 1–2 Hz (voluntary potential begin firing at around 6 Hz), whereas benign fasciculations fire faster and may be seen repetitively in the same place (e.g., eyelids, calves). A rare condition called muscular pain-fasciculation syndrome[3] sometimes may be misdiagnosed as ALS because of the presence of widespread fasciculation that is often made worse by exercise, consumption of coffee, or anxiety accompanied by occasional cramps at night and dull aching pain in the limbs.

Palatal myoclonus, currently renamed palatal tremor, is characterized by rhythmic movements of the palate at a rate of 1 to 3 Hz that persists during sleep and wakefulness, although they may become somewhat arrhythmic and show a slight change in frequency and amplitude during sleep (see also Chapter 16).[4,5] This condition results from a lesion affecting any part of the Guillain-Mollaret triangle, which comprises projections from the inferior olivary nucleus to the contralateral dentate nucleus, pathways from the dentate nucleus to the contralateral mesencephalic tegmentum in the region of the interstitial nucleus of Cajal, the nucleus of Darkschewitsch, and the posterior commissural nucleus from which originates the central tegmental tract that then projects to the ipsilateral inferior olivary nucleus to complete the triangle. Palatal myoclonus or tremor may be primary (no cause found) resulting from rhythmic contractions of tensor veli palatini muscle or secondary (resulting from a variety of brainstem lesions) caused by rhythmic contractions of the levator veli palatini muscle, associated with lesions anywhere in the Guillain-Mollaret triangle.

Respiratory or diaphragmatic myoclonus (Leeuwenhoek's disease) is characterized by rhythmic diaphragmatic contractions at a rate of 4 to 5 Hz.[6,7] The generator source most likely resides in the respiratory centers in the rostral medulla, and conceivably the movements may persist during sleep at night.

Spinal and propriospinal myoclonus may consist of oligosegmental myoclonus in which myoclonus is limited to the muscles innervated by a few adjacent spinal segments and plurisegmental (propriospinal) myoclonus.[8,9] Propriospinal myoclonus is a special form of spinal myoclonus originating from a generator, usually within the midthoracic region of the spinal cord with propagation up and down the spinal cord via slowly conducting propriospinal pathways. The movements can be rhythmic or arrhythmic, causing flexor or extensor jerks that involve several contiguous segments of the spinal cord. The rhythmic variety of spinal and propriospinal myoclonus may persist during sleep, causing diagnostic confusion with other sleep-related movement disorders. The condition may be symptomatic or idiopathic. This is different from propriospinal myoclonus at sleep onset, which is described in Chapter 27.

Iliceto, Thompson, Day, et al.[10] described five patients with focal abnormal involuntary movements of the abdominal wall under the heading of "belly dancer's" dyskinesia, diaphragmatic flutter, and the moving umbilicus syndrome. They did not find cause in any of the patients. The authors stated that the movements associated with belly dancer's dyskinesia were unlike the movements of spinal myoclonus or axial torsion dystonia.

"Bobble-head doll" syndrome[11] is a condition described in infants with mental retardation resulting from obstructive hydrocephalus caused by lesions in or around the aqueduct or third ventricle. The characteristic 2 to 4 Hz oscillations of the head may be confused with other infantile rhythmic movement disorders during sleep (e.g., head banging). The condition may also be mistaken for spasmus nutans,[12] which is characterized by pendular hystagmus, up and down or lateral head nodding, and occasionally twisted neck position. This is a benign condition occurring during the first 2 years of life lasting for weeks or up to 6 months—its etiology is unknown.

Paroxysmal hypnogenic dyskinesias include nocturnal paroxysmal dystonia (now known as nocturnal frontal lobe epilepsy), described in Chapters 26 and 35, familial paroxysmal choreothetosis, and posttraumatic paroxysmal nocturnal dystonia. In 1969, Horner and Jackson[13] described two families with several members having paroxysmal hypnogenic choreoathetosis. In one family member the hypnogenic episodes eventually disappeared, but several members had paroxysmal kinesigenic dyskinesias in the daytime. It is uncertain whether these nocturnal dyskinesias were similar to what Lugaresi et al. and Scheffer and coworkers later described as nocturnal paroxysmal dystonia or nocturnal frontal lobe epilepsy (see Chapters 26 and 35). There is one case described by Biary et al.[14] of posttraumatic paroxysmal nocturnal hemidystonia showing base ganglia lesion in the magnetic resonance imaging of the brain and improvement on acetazolamide treatment.

Stereotyped repetitive and rhythmic movements of the body and head occurring predominantly during drowsiness or sleep and accompanied by significant clinical consequences are currently categorized as rhythmic movement disorder (see Chapters 12, 26, 27, and 40). Recently, however, there have been brief reports of rhythmic limb and body movements on termination of apneas-hypopneas, which are eliminated by positive pressure therapy.[15,16,17]

Rhythmic leg movements in wakefulness, non-REM sleep, and REM sleep are frequently noted during polysomnographic recording in the sleep laboratory[15] resembling hypnagogic foot tremor but are different. In a retrospective study Yang and Winkelman[18] recently used the term "high-frequency leg movements" to describe similar phenomena noted both in wakefulness (two thirds) and sleep (one third). Their significance remains undetermined. We need further clinical-physiological correlation establishing scoring criteria in a prospective manner to understand their pathophysiology and clinical significance.

Hyperekplexia or exaggerated startle syndrome was originally described as an autosomal dominant hereditary disorder in a number of Dutch family members by Suhren et al. in 1966.[19] The infants showed exaggerated startle response with unexpected stimuli followed by muscle stiffness and hypertonia. Sudden infant death and recurrent apneas during sleep had been described in infants with hyperekplexia.[20] Another sleep-related characteristic consists of spontaneous myoclonic jerks. Five causative genes have been identified, but primarily the condition is caused by mutations in the genes encoding the inhibitory neurotransmitter glycine receptor alpha subunit (GLRA1) and the presynaptic glycine transporter GlyT2 (SLC6A5).[21] Sporadic cases may occur from recessive mutations of the same glycine receptor gene. A spectrum of clinical severity from minor brief jerks to major tonic startle spasms exists.[21] The essential sporadic startle syndrome could be a variant of hereditary hyperekplexia. Symptomatic hyperekplexia may result from structural brainstem lesions. The characteristic physiological finding is hyperactive startle reflex with impaired habituation.[22,23] This condition resembles startle epilepsy, Jumping Frenchmen of Maine, Myriachit, and Latah.[20] Clonazepam is the treatment of choice. Alternatively valproic acid may be useful.

The movement disorder specialists caring for patients presenting with diurnal movements during wakefulness and sleep specialists treating patients with nocturnal abnormal movements and behavior during sleep must be knowledgeable about all of the conditions described in this and other sections for a correct diagnosis and treatment of such patients.

REFERENCES

1. Broughton R, Tolentino MA, Krelina M. Excessive fragmentary myoclonus in NREM sleep: a report of 38 cases. *Electroencephalogr Clin Neurophysiol* 1985;61:123.
2. Blexrud MD, Windebank AJ, Baube JR. Long-term follow-up of 121 patients with benign fasciculations. *Ann Neurol* 1993;34:622–5.
3. Hudson AJ, Brown WF, Gilbert JJ. The muscular pain fasciculation syndrome. *Neurology* 1978;28:1105–9.
4. Deuschl G, Mischke G, Schenck E, et al. Symptomatic and essential rhythmic palatal myoclonus. *Brain* 1990;113:1645.
5. Chokroverty S, Barron KD. Palatal myoclonus and rhythmic ocular movements: a polygraphic study. *Neurology* 1969;19:975.
6. Phillips JR, Eldridge FL. Respiratory myoclonus (Leeuwenhoek's disease). *N Engl J Med* 1973;289:1390.
7. Chen R, Remtulla H, Bolton CF. Electrophysiological study of diaphragmatic myoclonus. *J Neurol Neurosurg Psychiatry* 1995;58:480.
8. Brown P, Thompson PD, Rothwell JC, et al. Axial myoclonus of propriospinal origin. *Brain* 1991;114:197.
9. Chokroverty S, Walters A, Zimmerman T, et al. Propriospinal myoclonus: a neurophysiological analysis. *Neurology* 1992;42:1591.
10. Iliceto G, Thompson PD, Day BL, et al. Diaphragmatic flutter, the moving umbilicus syndrome, and "belly dancer's" dyskinesia. *Mov Disord* 1990;5:15.
11. Mussel' GH, Dure LS, Percy AK, et al. Bobble-head doll syndrome: report of a case

and review of the literature. *Mov Disord* 1997;12:810.

12. Anthony JH, Ouvrier RA, Wise G. Spasmus nutans, a mistaken identity. *Arch Neurol* 1980;37:373–5.

13. Horner FH, Jackson LC. Familial paroxysmal choreoathetosis. In: Barbeau A, Brunette J-R, eds. *Progress in Neurogenetics*. Amsterdam, The Netherlands: Experta Medica Foundation; 1969:745–51.

14. Biary N, Singh B, Bahou Y, et al. A case of post-traumatic paroxysmal nocturnal hemidystonia. *Mov Disord* 1994;9(1):98–9.

15. Chokroverty S, Thomas R, Bhatt M. *Atlas of Sleep Medicine*. Philadelphia, PA: Butterworth-Heinemann; 2005.

16. Gharagozlou P, Seyffert M, Santos R, et al. Rhythmic movement disorder associated with respiratory arousals and improved by CPAP titration in a patient with restless legs syndrome and sleep apnea. *Sleep Med* 2009;10:501–3.

17. Chirakalwasan N, Hassan F, Kaplish N, et al. Near resolution of sleep related rhythmic movement disorder after CPAP for OSA. *Sleep Med* 2009;10:497–500.

18. Yang C, Winkelman JW. Clinical and polysomnographic characteristics of high frequency leg movements. *J Clin Sleep Med* 2010;6:431–8.

19. Suhren O, Bruyn GW, Tuynman JA. Hyperekplexia: a hereditary startle syndrome. *J Neurol Sci* 1966;3:577–605.

20. Amdermann F, Anderman E. Startle disorders of man: hyperekplexia, jumping and startle epilepsy. *Brain Dev* 1988;10:214–22.

21. Mineyko A, Whiting S, Graham GE. Hyperekplexia: treatment of a severe phenotype and review of the literature. *Can J Neurol Sci* 2011;38:411–16.

22. Matsumoto J, Fuhr P, Nigro M, et al. Physiological abnormalities in hereditary hyperekplexia. *Ann Neurol* 1992;32:41–50.

23. Chokroverty S, Walczak T, Hening W. Human startle reflex: technique and criteria for abnormal response. *Electroencephalogr Clin Neurophysiol* 1992;85:236–42.

55

Drug-Related Movement Disorders during Sleep

JACOB I. SAGE

THE DRUG-RELATED movement disorders discussed in this chapter are chorea, dystonia, myoclonus, akathisia, tics, tremor, and abnormal oral and facial movements. Much attention is directed at the drug-related abnormalities of movement that occur during the treatment of Parkinson's disease (PD). Until recently, it has been accepted dogma that (with a few notable exceptions) abnormal involuntary movements were not present during sleep. It has now become clear that abnormal movements do persist during the hours of sleep, although usually not with the same force, duration, or frequency as in the day. When they occur during the night, movement disorders, including those related to drugs, generally occur during the transitions from sleep to wakefulness and during the lighter stages of non–rapid eye movement (non-REM) sleep.[1] Underlying cerebral pathologic conditions, most commonly PD and Alzheimer's disease, predispose to drug-related movement disorders. This is also true of movements occurring during sleep.

LEVODOPA, DOPAMINE AGONIST, AND OTHER DOPAMINETIC SLEEP-ASSOCIATED MOVEMENTS IN PARKINSON'S DISEASE

The most common drug-related movement disorders occurring during sleep are those associated with the treatment of PD. To have a better understanding of how these movements arise and of their treatment, I briefly review several features of the pathophysiology and pharmacology of PD.

Clinical symptoms and signs of PD begin when patients have lost 50% to 80% of their dopamine-producing neurons in the substantia nigra. Orally ingested levodopa (LD) crosses from the gut to the blood and then crosses the blood–brain barrier by neutral amino acid carrier systems. Once in the brain, LD is converted to dopamine, which, at least in the earlier stages of disease, is stored in the presynaptic terminals of the nigral cell processes for release onto the postsynaptic dopamine receptors in the striatum. Normal functioning of the basal ganglia output system is generally thought to require tonic stimulation of the postsynaptic dopamine receptors.[2]

On average, peripheral pharmacokinetic parameters for LD absorption do not change throughout the course of PD. Immediate-release preparations of LD produce peak plasma concentrations within 30 to 60 minutes after oral ingestion, which then return to baseline within 2 to 3 hours after ingestion. Controlled-release products such as carbidopa-levodopa (Sinemet CR) produce much lower peak plasma concentration at between 1 and 2 hours after oral dosing, which then return to baseline by 4 to 6 hours after ingestion. It is important to keep in mind that as nigral cell loss continues with disease progression, central storage capacity and central buffering capacity for dopamine diminish accordingly. The clinical response then begins to rely on synaptic dopamine concentrations, which are critically dependent on plasma LD levels. It is at this point that factors affecting peripheral pharmacokinetics become important in the timing and type of motor fluctuation that may be observed in any individual patient. Of particular note for this discussion are nighttime abnormalities of movement that are related to the timing and preparation type (immediate or controlled release) of the last LD dose before bed.

Variability in the absorption patterns of all available LD preparations is an important additional factor in the origin and frequency of day and nighttime motor fluctuations. Differences in the peak plasma LD concentrations, the lag time to peak concentration, and the duration of therapeutic levels with evening and nighttime doses may vary considerably between patients and for any given patient on different nights. Under similar conditions, patients may show a lag time to peak plasma concentrations of LD that varies from 10 minutes to several hours. Plasma concentrations from a given dose of immediate-release LD may remain within the therapeutic range for as little as less than an hour to more than 4 hours. Some patients may even display a biphasic absorption pattern from a single dose of LD. With the addition of various generic forms of immediate and now controlled-release LD, the potential consequences of this variability begin to increase rapidly.

Disease progression and prolonged use of LD in patients with PD often result in motor fluctuations characterized by a variable response to medications for Parkinson's symptoms and the appearance of difficult-to-control dyskinesias. Within a year of the introduction of LD use in clinical practice, peak dose choreiform and dystonic movements were noted in some patients. Typically, LD-induced chorea occurs as a peak dose phenomenon. This pattern has been referred to as "I-D-I" (improvement-dyskinesia improvement) because a patient's Parkinson's symptoms initially improve after a dose of LD is ingested and the plasma LD concentration rise into the therapeutic range.[3] Then chorea occurs as the peak plasma concentration rises above the therapeutic range. Third, as concentrations fall back into a therapeutic range, patients remain improved without supervening chorea until the effect of that dose wears off and Parkinson's symptoms reemerge.[3] We prefer high dopa dyskinesia (HDD) as the term for this pattern.[4] HDD can be defined as dyskinesias that occur above a specific plasma LD threshold, continue to worsen as plasma LD concentrations increase, and disappear when plasma LD declines below a second (usually lower) threshold.

More important for nighttime occurrence of drug-related motor disturbances in PD are low dopa dyskinesias (LDDs).[4] These were initially referred to as demonstrating the "D-I-D" (dyskinesia-improvement-dyskinesia) pattern of motor response.[3] Because the dyskinesias occurred at the beginning and end of each dosing cycle, they were also called biphasic dyskinesias. LDDs are dyskinesias that begin at a certain low-threshold plasma LD concentration and then disappear above another higher threshold concentration. This second threshold is where the "on" effect for a particular dose kicks in. LDD is in fact usually monophasic as an end-of-dose phenomenon, sometimes lasting for hours after the last LD dose of the day and not disappearing until plasma LD concentrations approach zero. These newer terms (LDD and HDD) clarify the relationship of the patterns to LD concentration and do not necessarily imply an association of the phenomenon to the timing of the dose or the presence of biphasic or monophasic patterns of dyskinesias. The current understanding of the anatomic and biochemical connections in the basal ganglia does not permit a simple or even complex explanation for the genesis of dyskinesias by both high and subtherapeutic concentrations of LD. Speculation, however, may focus on the agonist or antagonist activity at high and low dopamine concentrations at different receptor subtypes in different anatomic pathways.

HDD is the most common dyskinesia type seen during the day but can also be present in some patients during the hours of sleep. When occurring during the night, HDD is often associated with relatively high and frequent doses of LD taken in the evening hours or in patients who take LD doses periodically during the night, both of which may result in increased plasma LD concentrations during the night. Some patients who have trouble sleeping because of extreme bradykinesia take controlled-release LD preparations during the night or just before bed to help with sleep. These preparations are prone to causing nighttime chorea, particularly if they are taken close together during the evening and night and thereby cause plasma LD concentrations to rise above the threshold for causing HDD. The movements are often noted by spouses as patients go through the lighter stages of sleep and may not interfere with the patients' sleep pattern. On the other hand, some patients are awakened by the involuntary movements and cannot go back to sleep until the movements have diminished.

Another more dramatic and more common movement associated with high intake of LD is kicking and flailing of the arms during sleep. These motions can be so violent that they often awaken the sleep partner; the victim may involuntarily injure the sleep partner. These motions are usually associated with nightmares, yelling, screaming, or even moaning but may not awaken the patient, who often has no recollection of the event on awakening the next morning.[5] Attempts should be made to reduce the nighttime and evening doses of LD in such patients because this sort of behavior may be a prelude to hallucinations and other psychotic phenomena. In some cases, these episodes continue for long periods, with the sleep partner moving to another room for sleep and safety.

Although I have concentrated on LD, it is clear that all dopaminergic drugs used in the treatment of PD can produce effects that mimic high-dopa phenomena. The new catechol-O-methyltransferase (COMT) inhibitors (tolcapone and entacapone) are particularly prone to exacerbate dyskinesias. The direct-acting dopamine receptor agonists (pergolide, bromocriptine, pramipexole, and ropinirole) are less likely to worsen dyskinesia at night than are the COMT inhibitors, but they can certainly increase other high-dopa nighttime movements.

LDDs can be the most severe and long lasting of all LD-associated involuntary movements.[6] Typically choreiform and/or dystonic movements develop as an end-of-dose phenomenon appearing after the last LD dose of the day when plasma concentrations have dropped below the therapeutic range but have not yet approached zero. When patients take their last dose of LD several hours before bedtime, dyskinesias begin just as the patient is going to sleep. Some patients who have difficulty sleeping because of severe bradykinesia or rigidity may take LD just before bedtime.

In patients on controlled-release preparations in which the decline in plasma LD concentrations is slow and may take several hours to reach zero, taking the dose at bedtime or in the late evening may produce LDD during the night. These evening or nighttime dyskinesias may be prolonged, lasting up to 4 or 5 hours without stop. Occasionally, adding a direct-acting dopamine receptor agonist to the last LD dose of the evening minimizes the duration and severity of these movements.

Other debilitating movements that can occur during sleep as a low-dopa phenomenon are dyskinetic breathing patterns with dyspnea (gasping for breath), hyperpnea, and shortness of breath. Painful dystonia, usually with cramping of the legs or feet, can be severe enough to awaken a patient from sleep, although the more usual dystonic cramps occur early in the morning on rising. Akathisia in which the patient feels the need to get up and walk during the night is also not infrequently seen as a low-dopa phenomenon. Restless legs syndrome (RLS), unlike akathisia, is generally accompanied by a variety of sensory phenomena in the legs. These include paresthesia, formication, aching, itching, stabbing, heaviness, burning, or coldness. Symptoms may be worse in the evening, while awake, and while lying down. They are often associated with insomnia. Laryngeal stridor associated with cranial or cervical dystonia has been reported and can occur during the night as the effectiveness of the last LD dose from the previous evening wanes.[7]

LD administration to PD patients seems to exacerbate nighttime myoclonus. LD-induced myoclonus is usually associated with chronic use and often does not awake the patient but is disturbing to the spouse. It may predict mental changes in patients with PD. The mechanism is unclear, although an effect on the serotonergic system has been postulated. Some animal studies have shown that administration of LD depletes central serotonin. Methysergide, however, a serotonin antagonist, reportedly decreases LD-induced myoclonus. This suggests that DA-related myoclonus may only be partially related to serotonergic mechanisms, and an effect on other neurotransmitter systems is necessary to fully explain the clinical observation.[8,9]

PERSPECTIVE ON OTHER DRUGS CAUSING MOVEMENT DISORDERS DURING SLEEP

The frequency of abnormal movements during sleep associated with drugs other than LD is not high.[10] With the exception of tremor and myoclonus, the long lists of drugs included in the tables are mostly taken from anecdotal evidence published as case reports. Many of these reports have been written by psychiatrists and internists not trained in movement disorders, making the description and reliability of the information somewhat suspect. Most of the drugs included in these tables must therefore be considered as possibly causing the movement in question but are certainly open to challenge and revision. Some of the tables list neuroleptics and also include various neuroleptic agents specifically reported to cause the movement in question. In most reports, it is probable that neuroleptic-associated movements refer to tardive dyskinesias that persist in sleep. The following text consists of comments on the drugs listed in the accompanying tables (Tables 55.1 to 55.7).

Table 55.1 Myoclonus

Opiates
Meperidine
Morphine
Methadone
Oxycodone
Norphidine
Trazodone
Buspirone
Verapamil
Nifedipine
Cocaine
Lithium
Monoamine oxidase (MAO) inhibitors
l-Tryptophan
Tricyclic antidepressants
Monoamine reuptake (MARU) inhibitors
Neuroleptics
Penicillin
Cephalosporins

MYOCLONUS

In PD patients, amitriptyline may increase nighttime myoclonus.[8] L-Tryptophan or 5-hydroxytryptophan may be of some benefit, although clinical efficacy for these two agents has not been demonstrated in rigorous studies. Myoclonus is the most common movement disorder related to the use of opiate drugs. In patients with renal failure, meperidine causes stimulus-sensitive myoclonus that must be distinguished from that caused by uremic encephalopathy.[11,12] Lithium often causes myoclonus at toxic serum concentrations but can do so even at therapeutic levels.[13]

SOMNAMBULISM

Sleepwalking (somnambulism), particularly in older adults, can be related to medications.[14,15]

Table 55.2 Chorea

Methsuximide
Phenobarbital
Primidone
Pemoline
Cocaine
Methylphenidate
Amphetamine
Lithium
Imipramine
Amitriptyline
Amoxapine
Monoamine reuptake (MARU) inhibitors
Neuroleptics (also tardive)
Digoxin
Oxymetholone
Flecainide
Disulfiram
Trazodone
Anticholinergics
Cimetidine
Oral contraceptives
Ethosuximide
Phenytoin
Carbamazepine

Table 55.3 Tremor

Lithium
Monoamine reuptake (MARU) inhibitors
Monoamine oxidase (MAO) inhibitors

Table 55.4 Dystonia

Doxepin
Amitriptyline
Neuroleptics
Prochlorperazine
Promethazine
Metoclopramide
Molindone
Phenytoin
Chloroquine
Amodiaquine
Disulfiram
Diazepam
Cimetidine
H2 receptor blockers
Verapamil
Cinnarizine
Flunarizine
Cocaine
Amphetamine
Tranylcypromine
Amoxapine
Alpha-methyl para-tyrosine

Table 55.5 Akathisia

Midazolam
Cyproheptadine
Methysergide
Buspirone
Diltiazem
Cinnarizine
Flunarizine
Alcohol
Amoxapine
Neuroleptics
Promethazine
Droperidol
Metoclopramide
Prochlorperazine

Table 55.6 Tics

Carbamazepine
Cocaine
Pemoline
Methylphenidate
Amphetamine
Tricyclic antidepressants
Neuroleptics

Table 55.7 Oral/Facial Dyskinesias

Antihistamines
Chlorpheniramine
Brompheniramine
Phenindamine
Mebhydroline
Verapamil
Ethanol (withdrawal)
Neuroleptics
Anticholinergics
Metoclopramide
Prochlorperazine

Medications reportedly associated with somnambulism include thioridazine, lithium, diphenhydramine, chlorpromazine, thioxanthene, methylphenidate, chlorprothixene, methaqualone, propanolol, and zolpidem.

RESTLESS LEGS SYNDROME, PERIODIC MOVEMENTS IN SLEEP, AND AKATHISIA

Tricyclics may induce or worsen periodic leg movements in sleep (PLMS).[16,17] Exacerbation of PLMS may occur with LD, probably related to the short duration of action of LD and the subsequent rebound effect when the effect of the drug wears off.[18] Drugs that are more likely to cause or exacerbate RLS or PLMS are lithium, caffeine, terbutaline, and nifedipine. Other drugs that cause RLS include ethanol, methsuximide, phenytoin, amitriptylene, serotonin reuptake blockers such as paroxetene, beta-blockers, H_2 blockers, antihistamines, droperidol, and neuroleptics such as compazine and metoclopramide.[19-37] Neuroleptics are the most likely agents to cause akathisia. Withdrawal from vasodilators, sedative, tricyclics, and opiates are reported to exacerbate RLS. The incidence of PLMS is probably higher in patients with neuroleptic-induced akathisia.[1]

TICS

Tics can persist during all stages of sleep. Drugs that can produce tics persisting in sleep include stimulants, LD, neuroleptics (tardive Tourette's), and anticonvulsants.[25]

BRUXISM

Bruxism is increased in patients with PD receiving LD therapy. Tricyclic antidepressants may increase bruxism. In a placebo-controlled trial, four alcoholic drinks at bedtime significantly increased bruxism during the night. Cocaine and amphetamines may also worsen bruxism.[26-30]

Sleep-Related Eating Disorder

Sleep-related eating disorder (SRED), also known as nocturnal sleep-related eating disorder (NSRED), is a combination of a parasomnia and an eating disorder (see Chapter 48). Binge eating occurs during the night during periods of altered consciousness. SRED is thought to be different from night eating disorder (NES) because in the latter, the patient is fully awake during the eating binge. Zolpidem seems to be the most common drug that increases the occurrence of SRED. Oddly enough, both dopaminergic drugs used to treat RLS and olanzapine have been reported to increase SRED.[44-58] Topiramate may be of benefit in treating this problem.[58]

REM Sleep Behavior Disorder

Many antidepressants,[59] particularly selective serotonin reuptake inhibitors (SSRIs), are known to cause REM sleep behavior disorder (RBD), and in fact are a very common cause of acute RBD.

REFERENCES

1. Hening WA, Walters AS, Chokroverty S. Motor functions and dysfunctions of sleep. In: Chokroverty S, ed. *Sleep Disorders Medicine*. 3rd ed. Philadelphia, PA: Saunders/Elsevier; 2009:295–335.
2. Sage JI, Mark MH. Basic mechanisms of motor fluctuations. *Neurology* 1994;44(Suppl 6):S10–4.
3. Muenter MD, Sharpless NS, Tyce GM, et al. Patterns of dystonia ("I-D-I" and "D-I-D") in response to L-dopa therapy for Parkinson's disease. *Mayo Clin Proc* 1977;52:163.
4. Sage JI, Mark MH, McHale DM, et al. Benefits of monitoring plasma levodopa in Parkinson's disease patients with drug-induced chorea. *Ann Neurol* 1991;89:623.
5. Riley DE, Lang AE. The spectrum of levodopa-related fluctuations in Parkinson's disease. *Neurology* 1993;43:1459.
6. Zimmerman TR, Sage JI, Lang AE, et al. Severe evening dyskinesias in advanced Parkinson's disease: clinical description, relations to plasma levodopa and treatment. *Mov Disord* 1994;9:173.
7. Corbin DO, Williams AC. Stridor during dystonic phases of Parkinson's disease [Letter]. *J Neurol Neurosurg Psychiatry* 1987;50:821.
8. Klawans HL, Goetz CG, Bergen D. Levodopa-induced myoclonus. *Arch Neurol* 1975;32:331.
9. Comella CL, Tanner CM. The side effects of chronic treatment in Parkinson's disease. In: Joseph AB, Young RL, eds. *Movement Disorders in Neurology and Neuropsychiatry*. Boston, MA: Blackwell Scientific; 1992:336.
10. Riley DE. Antidepressant therapy and movement disorders. In: Lang AE, Weiner WJ, eds. *Drug-Induced Movement Disorders*. Mount Kisco, NY: Futura; 1992:231.
11. Reutens DC, Stewart-Wynn, EG. Norpethidine-induced myoclonus in a patient with renal failure. *J Neurol Neurosurg Psychiatry* 1989;52:1450.
12. Hochman MS. Meperidine-associated myoclonus and seizures in long-term hemodialysis patients. *Ann Neurol* 1983;14:593.
13. Rosen PB, Stevens R. Action myoclonus in lithium toxicity. *Ann Neurol* 1983;13:221.
14. Masand P, Weilburg JB. Sleepwalking (somnambulism). In: Joseph AB, Young RL, eds. *Movement Disorders in Neurology and Neuropsychiatry*. Boston, MA: Blackwell Scientific; 1992:631.
15. Hupaya LVM. Seven cases of somnambulism induced by drugs. *Am J Psychiatry* 1979;136:985.
16. Ware JC, Brown FW, Moorad PJ, et al. Nocturnal myoclonus and tricyclic antidepressants. *Sleep Res* 1984;13:72.
17. Ehrenberg BL. Sleep pathologies associated with nocturnal movements. In: Joseph AB, Young RL, eds. *Movement Disorders in Neurology and Neuropsychiatry*. Boston, MA: Blackwell Scientific; 1992:634.
18. Montplaisir J, Godbout R, Poirier G, et al. Restless legs syndrome and periodic movements in sleep: physiopathology and treatment with L-dopa. *Clin Neuropharmacol* 1986;9:456.
19. Ehrenberg BL. Sleep pathologies associated with nocturnal movements. In: Joseph AB, Young RL, eds. *Movement Disorders in Neurology and Neuropsychiatry*. Boston, MA: Blackwell Scientific; 1992:634.
20. Barnes TRE, Braude WM. Akathisia variants and tardive dyskinesia. *Arch Gen Psychiatry* 1985;42:874.

21. Heiman EM, Christie M. Lithium-aggravated nocturnal myoclonus and restless legs syndrome. *Am J Psychiatry* 1986;143:1191.

22. Lutz EG. Restless legs, anxiety and caffeinism. *J Clin Psychiatry* 1978;39:693.

23. Zelman S. Terbutaline and muscular symptoms. *JAMA* 1978;239:930.

24. Keidar S, Binenboim C, Palant A. Muscular cramps during treatment with nifedipine. *Br Med J* 1982;285:1241.

25. Hargrave R, Beckley DJ. RLS exacerbated by sertraline. *Psychosomatics* 1998;39:177.

26. Duggal HS, et al. Clozapine and RLS. *J Clin Psychopharmacol* 2007;27:89.

27. Wetter TC, Brunner J, Bronisch T. Restless leg syndrome probably induced by risperidone treatment. *Pharmacopsychiatry* 2002;35:109–11.

28. Terao T, Terao M, Yoshimura R, et al. Restless leg syndrom induced by lithium. *Biol Psychiatry* 1991;30:1167–70.

29. Kraus T, Schuld A, Pollmacher T. Periodic leg movements in sleep and restless legs syndrome probably caused by olanzapine. *J Clin Psychopharmacol* 1999;19:478.

30. Pinninti NR, Mago R, Townsend J, et al. Periodic restless legs syndrome associated with quetiapine use: a case report. *J Clin Psychopharmacol* 2005;25:617.

31. Perroud N, Lazignac C, Baleydier B, et al. Restless legs syndrome induced by citalopram: a psychiatric emergency?. *Gen Hosp Psychiatry* 2007;29:72–4.

32. Bakshi R. Fluoxetine and restless leg syndrome. *J Neurol Sci* 1996;142:151–2.

33. Bahk WM, Pae CU, Chae JH, et al. Mirtazapine may have the propensity for developing a restless legs syndrome? A case report. *Psychiatry Clin Neurosci* 2002;56:209–10.

34. Bonin B, Vandel P, Kantelip JP. Mirtazapine and restless leg syndrome: a case report. *Therapie* 2000;55:655.

35. Agargun MY, Kara H, Ozbek H, et al. Restless leg syndrome induced by mirtazapine. *J Clin Psychiatry* 2002;63:1179.

36. Allen RP, et al. Antihistamines excacerbating RLS. *Sleep* 2005;28:A279.

37. Abril B, Carlander B, Touchon J, et al. Restless legs syndrome in narcolepsy: a side effect of sodium oxybate? *Sleep Med* 2007;8:181.

38. Lang AE. Movement disorder symptomatology. In: Bradley WG, Daroff RB, Fenichel GM, Marsden CD, eds. *Neurology in Clinical Practice.* Boston, MA: Butterworth-Heinemann; 1991:315.

39. Hartmann E, Mehta N, Forgione A, et al. Bruxism: effects of alcohol. *Sleep Res* 1987;16:351.

40. Hartmann E. Bruxism. In: Kryger MH, Roth T, Dement WC, eds. *Principles and Practice of Sleep Medicine.* Philadelphia, PA: WB Saunders; 1989:385.

41. Coleman R, Pollak CP, Weitzman ED. Periodic movements of sleep (nocturnal myoclonus): relation to sleep disorders. *Ann Neurol* 1980;8:416.

42. Magee KR. Bruxism related to levodopa therapy. *JAMA* 1970;214:147.

43. Ehrenberg BL. Bruxism. In: Joseph AB, Young RL, eds. *Movement Disorders in Neurology and Neuropsychiatry.* Boston, MA: Blackwell Scientific; 1992:649.

44. Stunkard AJ, Grace WJ, Wolff HG. The night-eating syndrome: a pattern of food intake among certain obese patients. *Am J Med* 1955;19:78.

45. Schenck CH, Hurwitz Td, Bundlie SR, et al. Sleep-related eating disorders: polysomnographic correlated of a heterogeneous syndrome distinct from daytime eating disorders. *Sleep* 1991;14:419.

46. American Academy of Sleep Medicine. *The International Classification of Sleep Disorders. Diagnostic and Coding Manual.* 2nd ed. Westchester, IL: American Academy of Sleep Medicine; 2005.

47. Allison KC, Lundgren JD, O'Reardon JP, et al. Proposed diagnostic criteria for night eating syndrome. *Int J Eat Disord* 2010;43:241.

48. O'Reardon JP, Peshek A, Allison KC. Night eating syndrome: diagnosis, epidemiology and management. *CNS Drugs* 2005;19:997.

49. Stunkard AJ, Allison KC. Two forms of disordered eating in obesity: binge eating and night eating. *Int J Obes Relat Metab Disord* 2003;27:1.

50. Striegel-Moore RH, Franko DL, Garcia J. The validity and clinical utility of night eating syndrome. *Int J Eat Disord* 2009;42:720.

51. Vetrugno R, Manconi M, Ferini-Strambi L, et al. Nocturnal eating: sleep-related eating disorder or night eating syndrome? A video-polysomnographic study. *Sleep* 2006;29:949.

52. Provini F, Antelmi E, Vignatelli L, et al. Association of restless legs syndrome with nocturnal eating: a case-control study. *Mov Disord* 2009;24:871.

53. Pourcher E, Rémillard S, Cohen H. Compulsive habits in restless legs syndrome patients

under dopaminergic treatment. *J Neurol Sci* 2010;290:52.

54. Morgenthaler TI, Silber MH. Amnestic sleep-related eating disorder associated with zolpidem. *Sleep Med* 2002;3:323.

55. Hoque R, Chesson AL, Jr. Zolpidem-induced sleepwalking, sleep related eating disorder, and sleep-driving: fluorine-18-flourodeoxyglucose positron emission tomography analysis, and a literature review of other unexpected clinical effects of zolpidem. *J Clin Sleep Med* 2009;5:471.

56. Paquet V, Strul J, Servais L, et al. Sleep-related eating disorder induced by olanzapine. *J Clin Psychiatry* 2002;63:597.

57. Winkelman JW. Clinical and polysomnographic features of sleep-related eating disorder. *J Clin Psychiatry* 1999;59:14–19.

58. Winkelman JW. Treatment of nocturnal eating syndrome and sleep-related eating disorder with topiramate. *Sleep Med* 2003;4:243–6.

59. Mahowald MW, Schenck CH, Bornemann MA. Pathophysiologic mechanisms in REM sleep behavior disorder. *Cur Neurol Neurosci Rep* 2007;7:167–72.

56

Psychiatric Aspects of Movement during Sleep

CHARLES R. CANTOR AND RICHARD J. ROSS

IN THIS chapter we examine abnormalities of motor control during sleep that may be manifested in a range of psychiatric disorders, as well as psychiatric symptoms that may be encountered in the major sleep-related movement disorders. We review psychiatric aspects of idiopathic restless legs syndrome (RLS) and periodic limb movements (PLMs), as well as sleep paralysis and cataplexy. We discuss parasomnias emerging from both non-rapid eye movement (non-REM) sleep and rapid eye movement (REM) sleep, including disorders of arousal, sleep-related eating, bruxism, and REM sleep behavior disorder. We next review the evidence for alterations in motor control during sleep in the dementias, the mood disorders, the anxiety disorders, schizophrenia, attention-deficit/hyperactivity disorder (ADHD), and the substance-related disorders. Finally, we discuss the various ways in which psychoactive drugs can influence motor activity during sleep. Throughout, we offer speculations on the mechanisms of hypnoid motor dysfunction in mental illness.

MOTOR FUNCTION DURING NORMAL SLEEP

Although the details of motor function during normal REM and non-REM sleep are described in detail elsewhere in this volume, we summarize those points that bear directly on this chapter. REM sleep is notable as a behavioral state characterized by atonia of the body musculature. In the normal adult, spinal motoneurons are inhibited postsynaptically during REM sleep by pathways originating in the caudal brainstem.[1] Excitatory barrages from supraspinal regions intermittently override this potent motoneuronal inhibition, producing phasic twitches of the extraocular muscles and the distal muscles of the extremities.[1] Thus, isolated motor unit action potentials can be a prominent feature of normal REM sleep, whereas sustained bursts of potentials (>600 milliseconds in duration) rarely occur.[2]

Conjugate, saccadic eye movements, resulting from phasic activation of the extraocular muscles, are a defining property of REM sleep. This REM activity, typically recorded during clinical polysomnography, can be quantified as REM density (number of rapid eye movements/ REM sleep time). Burst neurons in the pontine reticular formation generate saccades, whereas omnipause neurons in the caudal pons and rostral bulbar region inhibit saccades and permit ocular fixation. Forebrain modulation of saccade generation depends on the superior colliculus and the frontal cortical eye fields.[3] Saccades during REM sleep have a lower velocity and shorter duration than those during wake.[4] Although the notion that REM activity during REM sleep indicates a true scanning of dream imagery now appears unlikely, the view that REM activity correlates positively with the vividness of dream mentation continues to find wide support.[5]

A body movement is defined as "a massive movement of the body generally associated with the presence of artifacts on the polygraphic tracing." Body movements are intrinsic to sleep, and they recur regularly throughout the sleep period, with a periodicity approximating 90 minutes; they also can be elicited by external stimuli.[6] Body movements occur most commonly at non-REM sleep to REM sleep transitions, and they have been viewed as a manifestation of a change in arousal level.[6]

RESTLESS LEGS SYNDROME AND PERIODIC LIMB MOVEMENTS

Restless legs syndrome (RLS) and periodic limb movements (PLMs) are sensorimotor sleep-related phenomena that are commonly encountered in clinical practice. RLS is estimated to affect 5%–10% of adults, with a female predominance.[7] It can be characterized as a sensory disturbance with a volitional motor response. Individuals with RLS experience a compelling urge to move their legs. This urge is usually associated with dysesthesias that are variously described; the urge is temporarily relieved by movement. It is symptomatic when the individual is at rest or in a confined space, and it has a pronounced circadian pattern, typically reaching a peak in the evening and at bedtime, when it can interfere with sleep onset.

PLMs consist of periodic lower-extremity movements that resemble triple flexion. These are repetitive movements, each between 0.5 and 10 seconds in duration, that are part of a train of at least four movements occurring at intervals of

5 to 90 seconds.[8] Periodic upper-extremity flexions are also occasionally observed. Although asymptomatic PLMs are frequently noted during routine polysomnography in patients who do not have RLS, 80% to 90% of patients with RLS exhibit PLMs.[7] Detailed discussion of the clinical manifestations, pathophysiology, and treatment of these disorders is presented elsewhere in this volume.

Psychiatric Aspects of Restless Legs Syndrome

Both RLS and PLMs have been associated with psychiatric symptoms. Although Driver-Dunckley et al.[9] did not find evidence of a mood disorder in individuals with mild RLS, several studies indicate an increased prevalence of anxiety and depression among RLS patients.[10–12] In the Wisconsin Sleep Cohort, the presence of anxiety or depression appears to correlate with frequency of RLS symptoms.[11] Whether RLS predisposes to depression, or whether depression predisposes to RLS, has not been established. Cognitive deficits potentially consistent with insufficient sleep also have been identified in RLS patients.[13] Several studies have found a higher rate of depression in individuals who have PLMs without RLS.[14]

In children, both RLS and PLMs have been associated with Attention-deficit/hyperactivity disorder (ADHD). In a 2005 review of the literature, Cortese et al.[15] noted RLS in 44% of ADHD patients, and ADHD in 26% of RLS patients. As discussed later in this chapter (see section on "Attention-Deficit/Hyperactivity Disorder"), there is a high prevalence of PLMs in children with ADHD.[16] Although the mechanism of the relationship is not clear, dopaminergic dysfunction is thought to have a role in the pathophysiology of both disorders. Iron supplementation can be effective in treating both RLS and ADHD, suggesting another possible etiologic connection.[17]

Restless Legs Syndrome in Patients with Psychiatric Disorders

There is an increased susceptibility to RLS in patients who are treated with antipsychotic agents, as might be expected on the basis of the dopamine antagonist properties of these drugs. However, there are few data to determine the prevalence of RLS and PLMs in untreated individuals with schizophrenia.[18,19]

A higher prevalence of RLS has been noted among patients with depression compared to healthy controls,[14] but the use of antidepressants in this population may be confounding. Although data on the effect of antidepressants on RLS are conflicting, both selective serotonin reuptake inhibitors (SSRIs) and serotonin/norepinephrine reuptake inhibitors (SNRIs) appear to induce or worsen PLMs, and there is anecdotal evidence that tricyclic antidepressants and lithium have a similar effect.[14,20,21] Bupropion, trazodone, and nefazodone do not.[14] Bupropion is regarded as the drug of choice in treating depressed patients with RLS.[14] There are also case reports of amelioration of depression with successful treatment of RLS using dopamine agonists.[22,23]

Psychiatric Complications of Treatment for Restless Legs Syndrome

The dopamine agonists ropinirole and pramipexole are widely used in the treatment of RLS. Prescribers should be aware, however, of the possibility that, as is the case with Parkinson's disease patients,[24] a subset of patients receiving dopamine agonists may develop impulse control disorders. Two recent studies have demonstrated a range of behaviors, including compulsive eating, shopping, gambling, spending, and hypersexuality, among RLS patients. Pourcher et al.[25] identified compulsive behaviors in 10% of respondents to a questionnaire. Using both a questionnaire and a phone interview, Cornelius et al.[26] found such behaviors in 17% of their sample, with a statistically significant dose effect.

SLEEP PARALYSIS AND CATAPLEXY

Sleep paralysis and cataplexy are among the cardinal manifestations of narcolepsy, which is discussed in detail elsewhere in this volume. Although sleep paralysis and cataplexy are most commonly encountered in patients with narcolepsy, both can exist as idiopathic familial disorders.[27,28] Sleep paralysis also occurs sporadically in the general population, with a prevalence that has not been well established.

Individuals frequently experience anxiety during episodes of sleep paralysis, sometimes associated with visual hallucinations or a sense of suffocation.[29,30] High rates of sleep paralysis have been noted in patients with anxiety disorders, including panic attacks and posttraumatic stress disorder (PTSD).[31,32] The association between anxiety and cataplexy has not been well studied. The risk of cataplexy may prompt individuals with narcolepsy to avoid social situations that could provoke a cataplectic attack.[33,34] A preliminary investigation found an increased rate of cataplexy among patients with anxiety, raising the question of whether narcolepsy may be underdiagnosed in this population.[35]

Episodes associated with anxiety and resembling sleep paralysis have been reported in patients with schizophrenia.[36] Psychogenic episodes resembling cataplexy and termed "pseudocataplexy" have been observed in narcoleptic patients who also had genuine attacks of cataplexy.[37,38]

PARASOMNIAS

The term "parasomnia" refers to a variety of motor, sensory, and behavioral phenomena that arise from sleep or occur during the sleep period. Included in this category are disorders of arousal, nocturnal seizures, REM sleep behavior disorder, dissociative states, and bruxism. Although these phenomena (with the exception of dissociation) are currently understood as neurologic disorders, they may present clinically with symptoms or behaviors, including anxiety, hallucinations, confusion, and aggression, that suggest psychopathology.

Disorders of Arousal

The disorders of arousal are characterized by partial awakenings from non-REM sleep. They are typically described as existing on a continuum of severity. In the mildest disorder of this type, the confusional arousal, the individual appears to awaken briefly, exhibits disorientation (sometimes associated with agitation), and then returns to sleep. If he or she arises from bed, the activity is broadly referred to as sleepwalking, although more elaborate behaviors such as eating and sexual advances can occur.[39] The most dramatic disorder of arousal is the night terror, often heralded with a scream and associated with fearful behaviors and autonomic activation. Affected individuals typically have a family history of disorders of arousal, and there is usually limited recall of specific episodes, with bed partners or other observers providing much of the history. Sleep deprivation, noise, touch, stress, alcohol ingestion, and sedative hypnotics—notably zolpidem—have been identified as provocative factors in the disorders of arousal.[40,41]

Violence during sleep, including acts of homicide, has been reported in individuals with a disorder of arousal.[42–45] Early investigations suggested a high frequency of psychopathology in sleepwalkers[46] and those with sleep terrors,[47] but the current consensus is that violent behavior in sleep is not associated with any psychiatric disorder.[44,48] Conversely, we are not aware of reports of a higher incidence of sleepwalking or night terrors in patients with psychopathology.

REM SLEEP BEHAVIOR DISORDER

Patients with REM sleep behavior disorder (RBD) have a dysfunction of the normal atonia-generating mechanisms of REM sleep and can display vigorous and sometimes violent motor activity during REM sleep consistent with dream enactment.[49] RBD appears to be an early manifestation of a synucleinopathy in more than half of patients who present with a seemingly idiopathic disorder. Patients are predominantly male. Although the dreams described by patients with RBD have a greater percentage of aggressive content than do the dreams of controls, Fantini et al.[50] have noted that these patients have normal daytime levels of aggressiveness as assessed by questionnaire. Idiopathic RBD has not been associated with psychopathology[51]; however, neuropsychological deficits, including impaired attention and visual perception, and an increased frequency of visual hallucinations, have been observed in RBD patients with Parkinson's disease.[52,53] Of note, a number of psychoactive medications can produce secondary RBD, as discussed later (see section on "Effects of Psychoactive Drugs on Sleep-Related Movement").

PARASOMNIA OVERLAP SYNDROME

Schenck et al.[54] have described a parasomnia overlap syndrome, with combined features of sleepwalking, sleep terrors, and RBD. They did not find an increased prevalence of psychiatric disorders in their series but noted that 45% of these patients had previously been treated unsuccessfully for a presumed psychiatric disorder.

DISSOCIATIVE DISORDERS

Dissociative disorders, including dissociative amnesia, dissociative fugue, and dissociative identity disorder (formerly called multiple personality disorder), can manifest during the sleep period.[48] Making the diagnosis of nocturnal dissociation often depends on polysomnographic evidence of the emergence of elaborate behaviors during wake, typically at the wake-sleep transition or shortly after awakening from stages N1, N2, or REM sleep. Dissociation may sometimes occur exclusively during the sleep period, so that the clinician cannot always expect to obtain an additional history of daytime dissociative episodes. For example, Schenck et al.[48] described exclusively nocturnal "animalistic" episodes arising from well-defined electroencephalographic wake epochs after variable intervals of sleep in a 19-year-old man with dissociative identity disorder. The patient would suddenly leave the bed, "growling, hissing, crawling, leaping about, and biting objects," while assuming the alter ego of a large jungle cat. Of note, the *DSM-IV-TR*[55] does not include any mention of dissociation occurring during the sleep period; this lowers the likelihood that such events will be recognized. However, care must be taken to avoid prematurely coming to the diagnosis of a dissociative disorder when sleepwalking, sleep terrors, and/or RBD may be implicated.[56]

BRUXISM

Bruxism, stereotypical grinding of the teeth during non-REM sleep, occurs in many normal adults, but it can be associated with mental retardation and acute psychoses.[57] Manfredini and Lobezzo[58] distinguish between bruxism during wake, which consists primarily of clenching, and bruxism during sleep, consisting of tooth grinding. They observed an association between daytime clenching and both anxiety and depression but found no relationship between "psychosocial disorders" and bruxism during sleep.

NOCTURNAL EATING DISORDERS

The spectrum of nocturnal eating disorders includes night-eating syndrome (NES) and sleep-related eating disorder (SRED), which combines features of both a sleep disorder and an eating disorder.[59] In NES the individual eats while fully awake and has good recall for the event, whereas in SRED the level of alertness is altered and varying degrees of amnesia for eating are present. Both NES and SRED must be distinguished from nocturnal manifestations of bulimia nervosa and anorexia nervosa.

Stunkard et al.[60] first identified NES, which they considered a new eating disorder characterized by nocturnal hyperphagia, insomnia, and morning anorexia.[60] Most patients suffered from refractory obesity and 92% were female. Individuals with this disorder were noted to eat large quantities of high-calorie foods, particularly sweets, between dinner and bedtime. Diagnostic criteria have varied since the disorder was first described, but the essential features include the following: (1) at least 25% of the individual's caloric intake occurs during the evening before bedtime and (2) awakenings from sleep followed by the consumption of food occur at least twice weekly.[61] Estimates of the prevalence of NES range from 1.1% to 1.6% in the general population, with a higher rate in obese people.[61]

Exacerbations of NES may coincide with stressful life events.[60] Low self-esteem has been noted in night-eaters.[62] Their mood has been characterized as mildly depressed and, unlike the mood in melancholic depression, has been found to worsen during the evening and night. These individuals compared to controls may have higher rates of substance abuse.[63] Eating episodes, which involve only edible substances, are described as snacks, with a carbohydrate to protein ratio of 7:1.[64] This composition is thought to increase the transport of tryptophan across the blood–brain barrier and to facilitate the production of serotonin, with its sleep-promoting and mood-enhancing properties. Twenty-four-hour studies of night-eaters indicate that melatonin and leptin fail to show their usual nighttime rise, suggesting a neuroendocrine mechanism leading to delayed food intake.[65] Consistent with a postulated serotonergic mechanism in NES, the selective serotonin reuptake inhibitor sertraline has been used effectively in treating the syndrome. Topirimate has also shown promising results.[66]

Chronic, compulsive nocturnal eating in a state that can be described as partially or fully asleep characterizes SRED. Consistent or occasional morning amnesia for the events is usually reported. Unlike patients with NES, those with SRED do not experience either problematic eating in the evening between dinner and bedtime or initial insomnia. They have partial arousals from sleep, usually 2–3 hours after sleep onset, and then proceed directly to the kitchen possessed by an uncontrollable urge to eat. Consumption of inappropriate foods or nonnutritive substances is frequent; Schenck and Mahowald[67] mention "raw, frozen, or spoiled foods; salt or sugar sandwiches; buttered cigarettes; cat food; and odd mixtures prepared in a blender." Most patients are careless with nocturnal food handling, and some eat large meals with their bare hands. Many patients, finding that they are unable to alter their night eating, restrict daytime eating and overexercise, but rarely do they engage in purging. SRED is reported to have a prevalence of 4.6% in a college population and a higher prevalence among those with identified eating disorders.[68]

Polysomnographic studies of patients with SRED have demonstrated that other primary sleep disorders are common in this population.[59,67] Among 38 patients, Schenck and associates[67,69] diagnosed 70% with sleepwalking, 13% with RLS and PLMs, and 10% with a sleep-related breathing disorder. In addition, one case was attributed to triazolam abuse and two cases were viewed as anorexia nervosa with nocturnal bulimia. Most patients were obese. About half had comorbid psychiatric illnesses, primarily mood or anxiety disorders. Psychoactive drug regimens used to treat such conditions (see section on "Effects of Psychoactive Medications on Sleep-Related Movement") may have provoked sleepwalking and led to sleep-related eating. Medications that have been implicated include tricyclic antidepressants, lithium, triazolam, and atypical antipsychotic drugs. Recent reports have focused on zolpidem as a precipitant of both sleepwalking and SRED.[70,71]

Winkelman[59] has also documented an association between SRED and other primary sleep disorders. Among 23 consecutive SRED cases, approximately 50% were diagnosed with sleepwalking, about 25% exhibited PLMs, and 13% had a sleep-related breathing disorder. Fully 35% had a current or past history of a daytime eating disorder. This contrasts with Schenck and colleagues'[67,69] finding of a daytime eating disorder in only 5% of their SRED patients. Notably, 70% of Winkelman's patients were taking psychotropic agents, primarily benzodiazepines, antidepressants, and antipsychotic drugs, possibly confounding the polysomnographic data.[59]

Schenck and associates[67,69] have found that SRED can often be controlled with treatment of any associated sleep disorder that may predispose to arousal. SRED associated with sleep apnea was controlled with the addition of continuous positive airway pressure (CPAP) in two reported cases.[67] For SRED associated with RLS/PLMs, treatment at bedtime with a dopaminergic agent combined with an opiate appeared most effective. The addition of clonazepam was sometimes required to achieve full control. In cases of SRED associated with sleepwalking, clonazepam monotherapy may be sufficient. Patients with SRED alone have been effectively treated with dopaminergic agents or topiramate.[66]

MOOD DISORDERS

An elevated REM density (number of rapid eye movements/REM sleep time) in individuals with major depression is among the earliest seminal findings in biological psychiatry.[72] Subsequently, REM density was reported to correlate positively with severity of depression in some, but not all, studies (reviewed in ref. 73). It is now recognized that an increase in REM density during the first REM sleep episode of the sleep period may be most specific to major depression.[74] A potential neuropharmacological mechanism for the increase in first REM sleep period REM activity (number of rapid eye movements) in major depression is suggested by the finding that, compared to placebo, the muscarinic agonist RS 86 increased REM density in depressed patients, but not other groups, including healthy controls.[75]

The observation that REM activity can remain high as long as 6 months into the remission from a depressive episode raised the question of whether an elevated REM density might be a trait marker for major depression or alternatively a slow-to-normalize sequela of the disorder.[76] Reports that REM density tended to normalize as depression remitted favored the latter explanation.[77,78] However, a reduction of REM activity following nonpharmacologic treatment of depression has not consistently been observed.[79] Furthermore, evidence that REM density in the first cycle of the sleep period as well as during the entire night is higher in healthy individuals at risk for major depression (by dint of family history) than in controls suggests that an elevated REM density is a trait biomarker.[80] Reports that patients experiencing a manic episode and patients in remission from an episode of bipolar depression also have heightened REM activity suggest that an increased REM density may also be a biologic marker of the full bipolar mood disorder diathesis.[81,82]

Thase et al.[83] found that depressed patients with greater sleep dysregulation, including heightened REM activity, showed a poorer response to cognitive-behavioral therapy. On this basis they argued that disturbed sleep indicated a form of depression that warranted pharmacotherapy. An increased REM density also has been associated with a poor response

to treatment with one night of late-night partial sleep deprivation.[84] The potential significance of an increased REM density in major depression was mitigated by a meta-analysis of polysomnographic data in mental disorders in which no increase in REM density across studies of subjects with mood disorders was found.[85] Consistent with this synthesis are reports that the REM densities of two groups of military veterans, with major depression and schizophrenia, respectively, substantially overlapped the normal range.[86]

ANXIETY DISORDERS: PANIC DISORDER, OBSESSIVE-COMPULSIVE DISORDER, AND POSTTRAUMATIC STRESS DISORDER

Panic Disorder

A panic attack is a discrete psychophysiological event including extreme fear or anxiety. The experiencing of recurrent, unexpected panic attacks is the defining feature of panic disorder. Up to two thirds of patients with panic disorder report symptoms during sleep as well as wake. There is evidence that this subgroup, compared to panic disorder patients overall, has a more severe disease diathesis, with more comorbid mood and anxiety disorders.[87]

Nocturnal panic attacks are associated with intense physiologic arousal and, when the individual awakens, a feeling of impending doom. Unlike sleep terrors, episodes of nocturnal panic often are well recalled. Nocturnal panic attacks emerge at the transition from stage N2 to stage N3 sleep, and they may be initiated by a brief muscle twitch that develops into a large body movement precipitating awakening.[88]

Different from major depression (see earlier) and posttraumatic stress disorder (PTSD) (see later), panic disorder is associated with an unchanged, or even reduced, REM density.[89,90] Increased movement time during sleep and increased "intermediate length body movements (2.5 to 15 seconds)" during stage N2 sleep have been observed in individuals with panic disorder, but there have been contradictory reports, one showing that panic disorder patients without nighttime panic compared to both those with this symptom and to normal control subjects had the highest level of movement time.[91] Uhde[92] subsequently suggested that increased movement time during sleep might in fact prevent nocturnal panic. Noting that "highly anxious sleep" could, as a manifestation of "agitation or restlessness," be expected to contain increased movements, Sheikh et al.[93] proposed instead that a suppression of movement during sleep in panic disorder is consistent with the well-known association between freezing and fear. They proceeded to speculate that sleep with little movement and frequent brief awakenings could be adaptive "where heightened vigilance is required in a dangerous environment."

Obsessive-Compulsive Disorder

Individuals with obsessive-compulsive disorder (OCD) have recurrent thoughts, images, or impulses that produce anxiety relieved by mental or behavioral rituals. Sleep in OCD is thought to have neurobiological mechanisms different from those identified in major depression.[94] However, in a large group of individuals with OCD, most free of psychotropic medication for at least 14 days, REM density during the first REM sleep episode of the sleep period was higher than in a group of healthy control subjects.[94] Although "many" of these patients also "suffered from mild or moderate depressive symptoms," the investigators noted that "depression occurred in the course of the underlying OCD and did not precede the OC symptoms according to the clinical judgment."

Posttraumatic Stress Disorder

Recurring nightmares, that is, long, frightening dreams that awaken one from REM sleep, are one of the definining symptoms of PTSD, and there has been great interest in determining the polysomnographic correlates of this parasomnia. The results of two studies suggested that nightmares in PTSD are associated with non-REM sleep. In one of these, subjects who reported a nightmare upon awakening in the morning were noted to have demonstrated body movement during stage 2 sleep.[95] Subsequent observations in the literature are more consistent with a relation between nightmares in PTSD and REM sleep. The one spontaneous awakening from a nightmare observed by Ross et al.[96] in combat veterans with PTSD and all three of those recorded by Mellman et al.[97] were preceded by REM sleep.

Similarly, the polysomnographic abnormalities most often described in PTSD relate to REM sleep. An increased REM density was the strongest finding in a meta-analysis of polysomnographic studies of PTSD.[98] Compared to a healthy control group, a group of combat veterans with chronic PTSD, five of whom had comorbid major depression, had an elevated REM density throughout the sleep period.[96] This increase was viewed as distinct from the high REM density that is confined to the first REM sleep episode of the night in major depression. Therefore, an increased REM density may be an inherent feature of PTSD but related to circadian factors in major depression. An emphasis on heightened REM density in PTSD is consistent with the early observation of a direct relation between REM activity and the intensity of dream mentation in healthy subjects.[5]

In the same group of veterans mentioned earlier, Ross et al.[99] also noted a greater frequency of phasic leg muscle twitches (calculated as the percentage of REM sleep epochs with at least one prolonged tibialis anterior twitch and defined as the REM sleep phasic leg activity [RPLA] index). The only nightmare observed in this study emerged from a REM sleep episode with an exceedingly high RPLA index (Fig. 56.1). Although no clear association between RPLA and REM activity was seen overall, this single recorded nightmare occurred out of a REM sleep episode with a particularly high REM density as well (Fig. 56.2). Thus, as a nightmare unfolds, diverse REM sleep phasic processes, which can otherwise be uncoupled, may possibly be recruited en masse.

In contradistinction to the evidence for increased phasic muscle activity during REM sleep in PTSD stands the report that combat veterans with chronic PTSD showed a significant reduction of sleep movement time, defined as 30-second sleep epochs occupied more than half the time by "dense, large-amplitude artifacts in electroencephalogram (EEG), electrooculogram (EOG), and electromyogram EMG channels."[100] Interestingly, sleep movement time in this population was inversely correlated with the severity of trauma-related nightmares. Because of the uncertain relation between movement time and brief limb and other body movements, Woodward et al.[100] suggested that there was no incompatibility between their finding and previous reports of elevated REM sleep phasic activity.

An early report of polysomnographic findings in "trauma survivors" anecdotally noted extreme motor activity, including excessive and at times "violent" movements during REM sleep.[101] This suggests a possible link between PTSD and

RBD, discussed earlier in this chapter. RBD is generally thought not to be associated with psychopathology[49]; however, a recent report on veterans by Husain et al.[102] suggested a high rate of comorbidity between RBD and PTSD.

Individuals with RBD may also show motor dysregulation during non-REM sleep, in the form of PLMs.[49] Ross et al.[99] reported an increased occurrence of PLMs in combat veterans with chronic PTSD compared to a healthy control

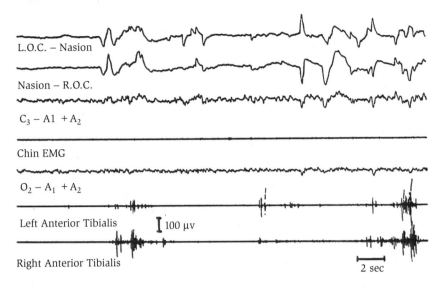

FIGURE 56.1   Polygraphic recording in a posttraumatic stress disorder (PTSD) subject of a rapid eye movement (REM) sleep epoch from a REM sleep episode that culminated in an arousal out of a nightmare. A_1, left auricular electrode; A_2, right auricular electrode; C_3, left central electrode; L.O.C., left outer canthus electrode; O_z, midline occipital electrode; R.O.C., right outer canthus electrode. (Reprinted with permission from Ross RJ, Ball WA, Dinges DF, et al: Motor dysfunction during sleep in posttraumatic stress disorder. Sleep 17:723, 1994.)

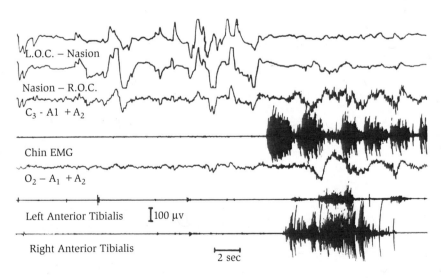

FIGURE 56.2   Polygraphic recording of the arousal of a posttraumatic stress disorder (PTSD) subject from a nightmare. Abbreviations as in Fig. 56.1. (Reprinted with permission from Ross RJ, Ball WA, Dinges DF, et al: Rapid eye movement sleep disturbance in posttraumatic stress disorder. Biol Psychiatry 35:195, 1994.)

group. A potential link between the mechanisms of PLMs and PTSD can be seen in the observation that PLMs patients have an abnormal blink reflex[103]; the latter comprises one component of the startle reflex, which is often exaggerated during wake in PTSD.[104] Krakow et al.[105] detected a high prevalence of symptoms of RLS/PLMs among sexual assault survivors with PTSD and emphasized the importance of considering these conditions in the differential diagnosis of insomnia in PTSD patients. Comparing the sleep of subjects with PTSD and frequent nightmares, that of nontraumatized subjects with "idiopathic" nightmares, and that of healthy controls, Germain and Nielsen[106] adduced that PLMs may be a general correlate of aversive dreaming rather than a marker of hyperarousal during sleep in PTSD.

SCHIZOPHRENIA

There is a strong association between disturbed sleep and reduced quality of life in individuals with schizophrenia, a group reported to demonstrate diverse polysomnographic abnormalities.[107] These include an increased sleep onset latency, reduced total sleep time, sleep fragmentation, decreased REM sleep time and REM sleep latency, and decreased slow-wave sleep. REM density findings have been inconsistent, perhaps owing to a number of potentially confounding factors.

Emphasizing that most previous polysomnographic investigations of schizophrenia had been carried out in patients withdrawn from antipsychotic medications, which may themselves have long-term effects on sleep, Poulin[108] reported on a comparison of 11 drug-naïve patients and 11 healthy control subjects. Although there was no difference in REM density, the Brief Psychiatric Rating Scale (BPRS) score correlated negatively with REM density. Similarly, Riemann et al.[109] found that, independent of depression, REM density correlated inversely with negative symptoms (alogia, flattened affect, avolition) of schizophrenia. On the other hand, REM density has also been found to correlate positively with negative symptom severity[110] and with a specific hallucinatory symptom item from the Brief Psychiatric Rating Scale.[86] There are two reports that total REM activity during REM sleep is higher in patients with schizophrenia who are displaying suicidal behavior.[111,112] Given these discrepant findings, it may be possible only to conclude that "REM density is closely associated with symptom severity in schizophrenia."[113] Some investigators have taken such an association as evidence that schizophrenia and REM sleep share a common neurobiological substrate.[19]

The involvement of dopaminergic mechanisms in the pathophysiology of both schizophrenia and RLS/PLMs suggests that individuals with schizophrenia compared to healthy controls might show a different prevalence of sleep-related movement disorders. However, this has not been demonstrated.[19]

ATTENTION-DEFICIT/HYPERACTIVITY DISORDER

There have been reports of increased movement time in children with ADHD (reviewed in ref. 114). Picchietti et al.[115] reported a five-fold higher occurrence of PLMs in children with ADHD compared with age- and gender-matched controls. These investigators speculated that the sleep disruption produced by PLMs, along with the motor restlessness of RLS, could explain the symptoms during wake in certain children with ADHD. However, Mick et al.[116] inferred from family history data that ADHD does not simply represent the consequences during the day of disturbed sleep at night. Yet Picchietti et al.[117] provided evidence for a genetic linkage between ADHD and PLMs/RLS, and many children with moderate to severe PLMs may have ADHD.[115] Because pharmacotherapy with L-dopa or a dopamine agonist improved both PLMs/RLS and ADHD in a small group of children, Walters et al.[118] hypothesized that these disorders may share a dopamine deficiency.

There is evidence for eye movement dyscontrol during wake in ADHD (reviewed in ref. 119). It has been suggested that a reduction in the fine control of eye movements may relate to the attentional difficulties in ADHD.[119] Noting that saccadic eye movements during wake and REM sleep have similar control mechanisms, involving dopaminergic pathways, Grissom et al.[119] reported lower frequency, higher amplitude rapid eye movements in the REM sleep of children (ages 6–10) with ADHD compared to control subjects.

DEMENTIA

Common manifestations of disturbed sleep in patients with dementia include fragmented sleep, agitation with the approach of night, disruption of the normal circadian rhythm, and excessive daytime sleepiness. As discussed later, patients with specific subtypes of dementia may develop specific sleep-associated behaviors; conversely—as demonstrated by the association between RBD and extrapyramidal disorders—certain nocturnal behaviors may be the harbinger of specific neurodegenerative syndromes.

Alzheimer's Disease

Alzheimer's disease (AD) patients often exhibit disrupted sleep at night and involuntary dozing during the daytime. These two phenomena are mutually reinforcing. Motor disturbances may include nocturnal wandering, vocalizations, and combativeness. These behaviors, often referred to as sundowning, tend to emerge in the late afternoon and early evening. Sleep fragmentation is manifested with an increase in stage N1 sleep and a decrease in slow-wave sleep greater than expected for age.[120] A decreased REM sleep percentage and a decreased REM density have also been reported in AD.[121]

The circadian rhythm disturbances observed in AD have been speculatively attributed to decreased melatonin secretion as well as to degenerative changes in the suprachiasmatic nucleus; lack of bright light exposure may exacerbate these disturbances.[122,123] Degenerative changes in the cholinergic nuclei of the basal forebrain and brainstem may underlie the observed changes in sleep architecture.[121]

In contrast to patients with synucleinopathies, AD patients typically do not develop RBD, although they may manifest it when treated with cholinesterase inhibitors.[124] The diagnosis of RBD in the setting of AD should therefore prompt reconsideration of the diagnosis or consideration of a coexisting synucleinopathy. A variety of approaches have been utilized to treat the sleep disturbances of AD. Bright light therapy and melatonin have shown benefit in some reports.[123,125,126]

Frontotemporal Dementia

Frontotemporal dementia (FTD) is a term that encompasses syndromes characterized by focal degeneration of the frontal and temporal lobes. In these disorders, psychiatric symptoms are more prominent than memory loss. Patients may exhibit executive dysfunction, apathy, socially inappropriate behavior, and language dysfunction.

Harper et al.,[127] in a study of institutionalized AD and FTD patients, found evidence for an advanced sleep phase uncoupled from core body temperature in FTD. In contrast, a more recent study in noninstitutionalized patients suggested a delayed sleep phase with a decreased sleep efficiency and decreased total sleep time.[128] Although assessment of sleep in FTD is limited by small sample sizes and the diverse manifestations of the disorder, there are no reports of specific motor disturbances or unusual behaviors during sleep.

Huntington's Disease

Huntington's disease (HD) is a hereditary neurodegenerative disorder characterized by progressive dementia and involuntary movements. It also has prominent psychiatric features, including depression, compulsivity, and aggressiveness. To date, only a few studies have examined sleep in HD. Increased sleep spindles have been noted,[129,130] Reduced sleep efficiency is consistently reported; however, the chorea that is a hallmark of the disease decreases during sleep and is not thought to be a significant factor in sleep disruption.[131,132] Arnulf[133] found evidence of early sleep onset in a sample of 25 patients, but this has not been consistently described in other studies. RBD has been reported in a small number of HD patients.[133,134] There appears to be an association between disturbed sleep and depression in HD.[135]

Corticobasal Ganglionic Degeneration

Corticobasal ganglionic degeneration (CBD) is a rare progressive neurodegenerative disorder characterized by an asymmetric akinetic-rigid syndrome with gait impairment and dysarthria, accompanied in most patients by cognitive dysfunction. Data on sleep disturbances in this illness are limited. An early report noted subclinical RBD in a CBD patient.[136] This has not subsequently been observed. Several small series evaluating sleep in CBD have demonstrated the presence of PLMs.[137-139] Although there was a low sleep efficiency in the patients described by Roche et al.,[137] these patients did not appear excessively sleepy when objectively assessed by the Multiple Sleep Latency Test.

Creutzfeld-Jakob Disease

Creutzfeld-Jakob disease (CJD) is a subacute spongiform encephalopathy associated with an abnormal configuration of the prion protein. Clinical manifestations include progressive dementia, ataxia, behavioral disturbances, myoclonus, and rapid deterioration leading to death within months.

Sleep has not been extensively studied in this disorder. Wall et al.[140] have noted that insomnia, as well as depression and psychosis, are common symptoms. In their small series, Landolt et al.[141] found a reduced sleep efficiency and a loss of both sleep spindles and REM sleep, prompting the authors to compare sleep in CJD to sleep in fatal familial insomnia, another prion disease with more specific thalamic involvement. Periodic sharp wave complexes, which are present on EEG in two thirds of patients in the advanced stages of CJD, are decreased in sleep.[142]

Lewy Body Dementia/Parkinson's Disease

Hallucinations, depression, and cognitive dysfunction are encountered in individuals with Parkinson's disease, Lewy body dementia (LBD), and other parkinsonian syndromes. The sleep-related aspects of these disorders are discussed in detail elsewhere in this volume.

SUBSTANCE-RELATED DISORDERS

Alcohol

Alcoholism is associated with prominent sleep changes that can have motor manifestations. Compared with a control group, middle-aged men with primary alcoholism, withdrawn from alcohol for approximately 17 days, had a heightened REM density during the first REM sleep episode of the sleep period.[143] Although this finding resembled observations in major depression, REM density correlated with the amount of prior alcohol use and not with the depression rating. The potential clinical significance of an elevated REM density in individuals recently abstinent from alcohol derives from observations that it can predict relapse within 3 months of discharge from a 1-month inpatient treatment program.[144] REM density also served to predict relapse in a group with primary alcoholism and comorbid lifetime secondary

depression; the elevation of REM activity was thought to exceed that seen in major depression and possibly to reflect alcohol withdrawal specifically.[145] In a subsequent study, comparing individuals with primary alcoholism (with and without lifetime secondary depression) to individuals with current primary major depression, Clark et al.[146] found REM density to be more elevated by alcoholism than by depression. "REM pressure," a variable that includes REM density as well as REM percent and REM latency,[144] was observed to be higher in alcohol-dependent compared to depressed patients.[147]

Frequent body movements, often punctuating REM sleep, have been described in young adults newly abstinent from alcohol,[148] and the discontinuation of alcohol use can precipitate RBD.[49] There is evidence that, after at least 1 year of sobriety, the amount of movement time during sleep may return to normal.[149] A higher frequency of PLMs has been associated with current alcohol use,[150] but not with alcoholism in recent remission.[151]

Marijuana

The psychological effects of marijuana are thought be due to Δ-9-tetrahydrocannabinol (THC; reviewed in Schierenbeck et al.[152]). In one study, the administration of THC reduced REM density, with the development of some tolerance; the abrupt withdrawal of THC led to an extremely high REM density compared to baseline.[153] In a study of experienced marijuana users, THC smoked in marijuana cigarettes over 10 days was at first associated with a decrease in body movements, which then increased and decreased again during recovery sessions.

Psychostimulants

Psychostimulants used recreationally (cocaine, nicotine, and methamphetamine) as well as therapeutically (amphetamine and methylphenidate) cause sleep-onset insomnia during usage and rebound hypersomnia during withdrawal. These drugs reduce both total sleep time and REM sleep percent. Their effect on REM density has not been established.[154] However, in a polysomnographic study of individuals addicted to cocaine and hospitalized for detoxification, a very high REM density was observed during the first week of withdrawal.[155] Body movements during sleep are increased by amphetamine.[51,154]

Caffeine has minimal abuse potential but can produce motor and cardiovascular side effects. It increases sleep latency and decreases sleep efficiency and stage N2 sleep, with relative sparing of REM sleep.[156] High doses have been associated with secondary RBD.[51]

Unlike the conventional psychostimulants, the newer wake-promoting agents modafinil and armodafinil have a low abuse potential, although they occasionally cause anxiety and restlessness.[157,158] They have minimal impact on normal sleep architecture.[158]

Opiate Agents

Opiates induce relaxation, drowsiness, and psychomotor retardation.[159] They are used in the treatment of RLS and PLMs.[159] However, other data suggest that single opiate doses may produce an initial activation, which persists, although attenuated, during chronic administration. A single dose of heroin increased "muscle tension" in abstinent individuals with a history of opiate dependence; at the same time, REM density was decreased.[160] A single dose of morphine or methadone had comparable effects in similar populations.[160,161] On the other hand, chronic morphine, but not chronic methadone, administration increased REM density.[162] Thirty percent of a group of opiate-dependent patients stabilized on methadone vocalized during REM sleep (reviewed in ref. 163).

Sodium Oxybate

Sodium oxybate, the sodium salt of gamma hydroxybate (GHB), is approved for the treatment of cataplexy and excessive sleepiness in narcolepsy. GHB has a history as a drug of abuse. It has been used by weightlifters for effects on muscle growth and by recreational drug users to produce euphoria and to enable sexual assault ("date rape").

The mechanism by which sodium oxybate is effective in narcolepsy is incompletely understood. A pilot study conducted by Mamelak et al.[164] demonstrated an increase in slow-wave sleep and improved daytime alertness. After increasing initially, REM sleep and REM density subsequently decreased in a dose-dependent fashion over the course of the study.

Adverse effects of sodium oxybate have included agitation, excessive sedation, nausea, vomiting, enuresis, and respiratory depression leading in some cases to death.[165] Confusion and sleepwalking have been reported anecdotally.[166] Despite the potential for abuse of sodium oxybate, a review by Wang et al.[167] of postmarketing clinical experience concluded that there is low risk for abuse or misuse of the drug.

EFFECTS OF PSYCHOACTIVE MEDICATIONS ON SLEEP-RELATED MOVEMENT

Antidepressant Drugs

Acutely, nearly all the tricyclic antidepressant drugs (TCAs) suppress REM sleep, and the impression exists that REM sleep is persistently, if not completely, reduced with chronic drug administration.[74] In contrast, there is evidence that any suppression of rapid eye movement activity (REM activity; number of rapid eye movements) shows marked tolerance over time in antidepressant-treated depressed patients.[168] For example, the effective treatment of elderly depressed individuals with the TCA nortriptyline markedly increased REM activity throughout the night, even into the maintenance phase of treatment.[169] Treatment with second-generation antidepressant drugs that selectively block serotonin reuptake (SSRIs) also appears to increase REM activity.[170] The SSRI fluoxetine, administered together with interpersonal psychotherapy or fluoxetine alone, increased the frequency of rapid eye movements during REM sleep (REM density).[171,172] Armitage et al.[170] found that depressed men and women treated with fluoxetine showed increases in the number and amplitude of rapid eye movements during non-REM as well as REM sleep. Increases in REM activity and rapid eye movement amplitude have been shown to persist for weeks after drug discontinuation.[172] Treatment of depressed unipolar and bipolar patients with another SSRI, paroxetine, also increased REM density.[173] It is not known how second-generation antidepressant drugs that block both serotonin and norepinephrine reuptake (SNRIs) influence REM density. Bupropion, which has effects on norepinephrine and dopamine reuptake, increased REM density in patients with major depressive disorder, but unlike most other antidepressants, did not suppress REM sleep.[174]

Not all antidepressant drugs produce an increase in REM activity. The antidepressant tranylcypromine, a nonhydrazine monoamine oxidase inhibitor (MAOI), did not affect REM density in patients with bipolar depression.[175]

Phenelzine, a hydrazine MAOI, increased "tonic EMG activity" (measured in all sleep stages) in a small group of patients with major depressive disorder and abolished the ultradian variation in eye movement activity during the non-REM sleep/REM sleep cycle.[176]

Although the SSRIs are effective in the treatment of a range of mood and anxiety disorders, they can affect sleep adversely by inducing RBD.[177] The TCAs, SNRIs, and the antidepressant mirtazapine may act similarly (reviewed in refs. 178 and 179). Antidepressant drugs also can increase PLMs during sleep.[20]

Antipsychotic Drugs

Although they have other indications, including the treatment of certain mood, anxiety, and personality disorders, first- and second-generation antipsychotic drugs are used primarily in the treatment of schizophrenia. The therapeutic mechanism of the first-generation drugs is thought to involve the antagonism of dopamine's action at type 2 dopamine receptors. Second-generation (atypical antipsychotic) drugs (including clozapine, olanzapine, quetiapine, risperidone, and ziprasidone) act as well as antagonists at type 2a and 2c serotonin receptors. Both classes can have additional blocking actions at alpha-1 adrenergic, histaminergic, and cholinergic receptors. There is no firm evidence that atypical antipsychotic drugs have greater therapeutic efficacy. Some have a potential to cause serious metabolic disturbances. There is an emerging consensus, however, that these newer medications are less likely to produce parkinsonian side effects and to cause tardive dyskinesia.

No double-blind, placebo-controlled studies of the effects of antipsychotic medications on sleep have been carried out in individuals with schizophrenia.[180] Furthermore, existing investigations are compromised by small sample sizes, inadequate drug washout periods, and additional medications. Most studies of low-potency, first-generation antipsychotic drugs, which generally have anticholinergic, antihistaminergic, and alpha-1 adrenergic antagonist activity, showed no effect on REM density. The same is true of high-potency, first-generation drugs, which are less anticholinergic and less sedating. The atypical antipsychotic drug clozapine, which can show efficacy in patients unresponsive to other medications, has been demonstrated to increase REM density in healthy individuals as well as patients with schizophrenia (reviewed in ref. 19), and olanzapine had a similar effect.[181,182] The investigators viewed these findings as unexpected because clozapine and olanzapine are highly anticholinergic, and muscarinic activation has been associated with increased REM activity.[183] Quetiapine and risperidone have not been shown to alter REM density (reviewed in ref. 19). Ziprasidone decreased REM density in a small group of healthy young adult males.[184]

Probably because of their dopaminergic antagonist properties, first-generation antipsychotic drugs have been associated with RLS after chronic administration.[19] Krystal et al.[180] have suggested that RLS in schizophrenic patients could lead to difficulty initiating sleep at night and a consequent circadian rhythm disturbance. Largely on the basis of case reports, first-generation antipsychotic drugs, alone or in combination with other psychotropic agents, including lithium, anticholinergic medications, antidepressants, benzodiazepines, and antihistamines, also have been implicated in the development of sleepwalking. Chlorprothixene in one patient, thioridazine in another, thioridazine combined with methaqualone in another, and thioridazine in combination with chloral hydrate in a fourth were associated with sleepwalking.[185-187] Sleepwalking resulting from chlorpromazine and fluphenazine was reduced by clonazepam in one patient.[188] A case in which sleepwalking occurred only when an anticholinergic medication was added to a regimen of chlorpromazine, lithium, and triazolam suggested to the authors that REM sleep suppression could be essential to the promotion of slow-wave-sleep-related behaviors.[189] Comorbid sleepwalking, as well as night eating, should be considered in the differential diagnosis of disturbed sleep in individuals with schizophrenia receiving pharmacotherapy.[19]

Benzodiazepine Receptor Agonists

The effects of benzodiazepines on sleep architecture include a reduction in slow-wave sleep, a mild reduction in REM sleep, and a lengthening of REM sleep latency (time from sleep onset to the first REM sleep episode of the sleep period[190,191]).

In addition to their use as hypnotics, benzodiazepines provide a therapeutic approach to several of the sleep-related movement disorders. They are employed in the treatment of disorders of arousal. They also have been used in the treatment of RLS and PLMs, primarily to suppress arousals.[51] Clonazepam has gained wide acceptance for controlling RBD, conceivably through a serotonergic mechanism.[49] Schenck and Mahowald[192] have made the important observation that, for a period equal to or greater than 6 months, benzodiazepines can maintain their efficacy in managing injurious parasomnias, including sleepwalking, night terrors, and RBD. These investigators also reported a low incidence of adverse effects, tolerance, and abuse.

In the treatment of insomnia, adverse effects of benzodiazepines can include daytime sedation, impaired psychomotor performance and vigilance, and short-term memory loss.[193] Rebound insomnia upon discontinuation of these drugs is common, but dependence and abuse among patients without a substance abuse history are rare.[194,195]

Impairment of memory and psychomotor performance has also been reported with the newer nonbenzodiazepine receptor agonists, including zolpidem, zaleplon, and eszoplicone. Residual sedation is uncommon, and these drugs have a low potential for abuse and tolerance. Sleepwalking, sleep-driving, sleep-related eating, and other complex sleep-related behaviors have been reported with zolpidem, but the incidence of such behaviors has not been well studied.[196] Factors that may predispose to complex sleep-related behaviors include coadministration with alcohol[196] and a dose greater than 10 mg.[197]

Mood Stabilizers

The mood stabilizers lithium, carbamazepine, and valproic acid are commonly used in the management of bipolar disorder. As noted earlier (see section on "Antipsychotic Drugs"), lithium in combination with an antipsychotic drug has been associated with sleepwalking, which occurred within days of the initiation of combination treatment and could be self-limited. Drug-induced electroencephalographic irregularities during wake, involving nonspecific, diffuse, excessive slow-and sharp-wave activity that sometimes was more prominent than expected with a lithium-antipsychotic drug combination, were associated with the persistence of sleepwalking.[198] Lithium alone also may increase the prevalence of sleepwalking-like behavior. The effect, which occurred independently of psychiatric diagnosis, could be self-limited or could persist over years; of clinical significance, there was a potential for self-injury.[199] Forty-four percent of the patients described by Landry et al.[199] had a history of

sleepwalking during childhood, which might therefore be an identifiable risk factor. Lithium can exacerbate RLS.[179] In one open-label study, valproate was demonstrated to promote sleep consolidation in a small group of patients with PLMs.[200]

Mood stabilizers generally do not have prominent effects on REM sleep (reviewed in ref. 73). Unlike the antidepressant drugs, lithium has been reported to decrease REM activity in healthy individuals, depressed patients, and manic patients (reviewed in ref. 201). To our knowledge, there is practically no information about the effects of carbamazepine and valproic acid on REM activity. In one small group of healthy subjects, 400 mg carbamazepine administered daily for 5 days led to a reduction in REM density.[202] There are as yet insufficient data to suggest that, in contradistinction to antidepressant-induced rapid eye movement activation, mood stabilization involves a reduction in REM density.

Cognitive Enhancers

Medications approved for the treatment of cognitive dysfunction in AD include the acetylcholinesterase inhibitors donepezil, galantamine, and rivastigmine and the N-methyl-d-aspartate (NMDA) receptor antagonist memantine. As might be expected on the basis of increased cholinergic tone, studies in healthy individuals have shown that donepezil can increase REM density and decrease REM sleep latency.[203] A similar effect has been noted in patients with AD.[204] Donepezil has reportedly induced nightmares in the setting of both mild cognitive impairment and AD.[205,206] No significant differences in REM sleep percentage were noted by Cooke et al.[207] in a comparison among the acetylcholinesterase inhibitors in 76 patients with AD.

Although RBD is rare in AD, the induction of RBD with both donepezil and rivastigmine in AD patients has been described.[208] In a single case report, rivastigmine reduced nocturnal agitation and wandering in a patient with LBD.[209] In RBD patients without dementia, the acetylcholinesterase inhibitors may actually have a therapeutic benefit in treating the parasomnia.[210, 211]

The effects of memantine on sleep architecture have not been well studied. In patients with LBD or dementia associated with PD, Larsson et al.[212] have found memantine to be helpful in reducing physical activity in patients with suspected RBD.

SUMMARY

Among sleep-related movements, REM activity has been the best studied across a range of mental disorders. There is substantial evidence for an elevated REM density in PTSD, bereavement, and major depression. Although the functional significance of these findings remains uncertain, the relative specificity of increased REM activity for these few disorders suggests other than an epiphenomenal mechanism. Particular significance may be attached to the heightened REM activity seen in PTSD, perhaps as a physiologic correlate of the repetitive, stereotypical anxiety dreams characteristic of this disorder, and to the increased REM activity predictive of relapse among recovering alcoholics.

Dopaminergic mechanisms have been invoked to explain a possible relationship between RLS/PLMs and schizophrenia, as well as ADHD. The disorders of arousal and RBD have generally not been found to show an association with psychopathology of any type; they must be distinguished from a dissociative disorder, which may on occasion manifest only at night. Nocturnal eating has a differential diagnosis that includes SRED and NES, an eating disorder. Certain medications used in treating psychiatric disorders can precipitate motor abnormalities during sleep, sometimes with overt clinical consequences, and medications used to treat sleep disorders can occasionally have adverse consequences manifested as psychiatric symptoms.

REFERENCES

1. Chase MH, Morales FR. The atonia and myoclonia of active (REM) sleep. *Annu Rev Psychol* 1990;41:557–84.
2. Askenasy JJ, Yahr MD. Different laws govern motor activity in sleep than in wakefulness. *J Neural Transm Gen Sect* 1990;79(1–2):103–11.
3. Fuchs AF, Kaneko CR, Scudder CA. Brainstem control of saccadic eye movements. *Annu Rev Neurosci* 1985;8:307–37.
4. Steriade M, McCarley RW. *Brainstem Control of Wakefulness and Sleep.* New York: Plenum Press; 1990:307.
5. Rechtschaffen A. The psychophysiology of mental activity during sleep. In: McGuigan FJ, Schoonover RA, eds. *The Psychophysiology of Thinking.* New York: Academic; 1973:153.
6. Terzano MG, Parrino L, Mennuni GF, eds. *Eventi Fasici e Microstruttura del Sonno.* Lecce, Italy: Martano Editore Lecce; 1997:123.
7. American Academy of *Sleep Medicine,* ed. *International Classification of Sleep Disorders. Diagnostic and Coding Manual.* 2nd ed. Westchester, IL: American Academy of Sleep Medicine; 2005.
8. Coleman RM. Periodic movements in sleep. In: Guilleminault C, ed. *Sleeping and Waking Disorders: Indications and Techniques.* Boston, MA: Butterworths; 1982:265.
9. Driver-Dunckley E, Connor D, Hentz J, et al. No evidence for cognitive dysfunction or depression in patients with mild restless legs syndrome. *Mov Disord* 2009;24(12):1840–2.
10. Hornyak M, Kopasz M, Berger M, et al. Impact of sleep-related complaints on depressive symptoms in patients with restless legs syndrome. *J Clin Psychiatry* 2005;66(9):1139–45.
11. Winkelman JW, Finn L, Young T. Prevalence and correlates of restless legs syndrome symptoms in the Wisconsin sleep cohort. *Sleep Med* 2006;7(7):545–52.
12. Winkelmann J, Prager M, Lieb R, et al. "Anxietas tibiarum." Depression and anxiety disorders in patients with restless legs syndrome. *J Neurol* 2005;252(1):67–71.
13. Pearson VE, Allen RP, Dean T, et al. Cognitive deficits associated with restless legs syndrome (RLS). *Sleep Med* 2006;7(1):25–30.
14. Picchietti D, Winkelman JW. Restless legs syndrome, periodic limb movements in sleep, and depression. *Sleep* 2005;28(7):891–8.
15. Cortese S, Konofal E, Lecendreux M, et al. Restless legs syndrome and attention-deficit/hyperactivity disorder: a review of the literature. *Sleep* 2005;28(8):1007–13.
16. Sadeh A, Pergamin L, Bar-Haim Y. Sleep in children with attention-deficit hyperactivity disorder: a meta-analysis of polysomnographic studies. *Sleep Med Rev* 2006;10(6):381–98.
17. Konofal E, Lecendreux M, Deron J, et al. Effects of iron supplementation on attention deficit hyperactivity disorder in children. *Pediatr Neurol* 2008;38(1):20–6.
18. Kang SG, Lee HJ, Jung SW, et al. Characteristics and clinical correlates of restless legs syndrome in schizophrenia. *Prog Neuropsychopharmacol Biol Psychiatry* 2007;31(5):1078–83.
19. Cohrs S, Rodenbeck A, Hornyak M, et al. Restless legs syndrome, periodic limb movements, and psychopharmacology. *Nervenarzt* 2008;79(11):1263–4, 1266–72.

20. Yang C, White DP, Winkelman JW. Antidepressants and periodic leg movements of sleep. *Biol Psychiatry* 2005;58(6):510–14.

21. Terao T, Terao M, Yoshimura R, et al. Restless legs syndrome induced by lithium. *Biol Psychiatry* 1991;30(11):1167–70.

22. Montagna P, Hornyak M, Ulfberg J, et al. Randomized trial of pramipexole for patients with restless legs syndrome (RLS) and RLS-related impairment of mood. *Sleep Med* 2011;12(1):34–40.

23. Benes H, Mattern W, Peglau I, et al. Ropinirole improves depressive symptoms and restless legs syndrome severity in RLS patients: a multicentre, randomized, placebo-controlled study. *J Neurol* 2011;258(6):1046–54.

24. Weintraub D, Siderowf AD, Potenza MN, et al. Association of dopamine agonist use with impulse control disorders in Parkinson disease. *Arch Neurol* 2006;63(7):969–73.

25. Pourcher E, Remillard S, Cohen H. Compulsive habits in restless legs syndrome patients under dopaminergic treatment. *J Neurol Sci* 2010;290(1–2):52–6.

26. Cornelius JR, Tippmann-Peikert M, Slocumb NL, et al. Impulse control disorders with the use of dopaminergic agents in restless legs syndrome: a case-control study. *Sleep* 2010;33(1):81–7.

27. Hartse KM, Zorick FJ, Sicklesteel JM, et al. Isolated cataplexy: a familial study. *Henry Ford Hosp Med J* 1988;36(1):24–7.

28. Mignot E. Genetics of narcolepsy and other sleep disorders. *Am J Hum Genet* 1997;60(6):1289–302.

29. Ohayon MM, Zulley J, Guilleminault C, et al. Prevalence and pathologic associations of sleep paralysis in the general population. *Neurology* 1999;52(6):1194–200.

30. Cheyne JA, Newby-Clark IR, Rueffer SD. Relations among hypnagogic and hypnopompic experiences associated with sleep paralysis. *J Sleep Res* 1999;8(4):313–17.

31. Otto MW, Simon NM, Powers M, et al. Rates of isolated sleep paralysis in outpatients with anxiety disorders. *J Anxiety Disord* 2006;20(5):687–93.

32. Sharpless BA, McCarthy KS, Chambless DL, et al. Isolated sleep paralysis and fearful isolated sleep paralysis in outpatients with panic attacks. *J Clin Psychol* 2010;66(12):1292–306.

33. Daniels E, King MA, Smith IE, et al. Health-related quality of life in narcolepsy. *J Sleep Res* 2001;10(1):75–81.

34. Ervik S, Abdelnoor M, Heier MS, et al. Health-related quality of life in narcolepsy. *Acta Neurol Scand* 2006;114(3):198–204.

35. Flosnik DL, Cortese BM, Uhde TW. Cataplexy in anxious patients: is subclinical narcolepsy underrecognized in anxiety disorders? *J Clin Psychiatry* 2009;70(6):810–16.

36. Krahn LE. Reevaluating spells initially identified as cataplexy. *Sleep Med* 2005;6(6):537–42.

37. Plazzi G, Khatami R, Serra L, et al. Pseudocataplexy in narcolepsy with cataplexy. *Sleep Med* 2010;11(6):591–4.

38. Krahn LE, Black JL, Silber MH. Narcolepsy: new understanding of irresistible sleep. *Mayo Clin Proc* 2001;76(2):185–94.

39. Schenck CH, Arnulf I, Mahowald MW. Sleep and sex: what can go wrong? A review of the literature on sleep related disorders and abnormal sexual behaviors and experiences. *Sleep* 2007;30(6):683–702.

40. Pressman MR. Factors that predispose, prime and precipitate NREM parasomnias in adults: clinical and forensic implications. *Sleep Med Rev* 2007;11(1):5,30, discussion 31–3.

41. Mendelson WB. Sleepwalking associated with zolpidem. *J Clin Psychopharmacol* 1994;14(2):150.

42. Siclari F, Khatami R, Urbaniok F, et al. Violence in sleep. *Brain* 2010;133(Pt 12):3494–509.

43. Bornemann MA, Mahowald MW, Schenck CH. Parasomnias: clinical features and forensic implications. *Chest* 2006;130(2):605–10.

44. Moldofsky H, Gilbert R, Lue FA, et al. Sleep-related violence. *Sleep* 1995;18(9):731–9.

45. Cartwright R. Sleepwalking violence: a sleep disorder, a legal dilemma, and a psychological challenge. *Am J Psychiatry* 2004;161(7):1149–58.

46. Kales A, Soldatos CR, Caldwell AB, et al. Somnambulism: clinical characteristics and personality patterns. *Arch Gen Psychiatry* 1980;37(12):1406–10.

47. Kales JD, Kales A, Soldatos CR, et al. Night terrors: clinical characteristics and personality patterns. *Arch Gen Psychiatry* 1980;37(12):1413–17.

48. Schenck CH, Milner DM, Hurwitz TD, et al. A polysomnographic and clinical report on sleep-related injury in 100 adult patients. *Am J Psychiatry* 1989;146(9):1166–73.

49. Schenck CH, Bundlie SR, Ettinger MG, et al. Chronic behavioral disorders of human REM sleep: a new category of parasomnia. *Sleep* 1986;9(2):293–308.

50. Fantini ML, Corona A, Clerici S, et al. Aggressive dream content without daytime aggressiveness in REM sleep behavior disorder. *Neurology* 2005;65(7):1010–15.

51. Mahowald MW, Schenck CH. REM sleep parasomnias. In: Kryger M, Roth T, Dement WC, eds. *Principles and Practice of Sleep Medicine.* 5th ed. St Louis, MO: Elsevier Saunders; 2011:1083.

52. Pacchetti C, Manni R, Zangaglia R, et al. Relationship between hallucinations, delusions, and rapid eye movement sleep behavior disorder in Parkinson's disease. *Mov Disord* 2005;20(11):1439–48.

53. Onofrj M, Thomas A, D'Andreamatteo G, et al. Incidence of RBD and hallucination in patients affected by Parkinson's disease: 8-year follow-up. *Neurol Sci* 2002; 23 Suppl 2:S91–4.

54. Schenck CH, Boyd JL, Mahowald MW. A parasomnia overlap disorder involving sleepwalking, sleep terrors, and REM sleep behavior disorder in 33 polysomnographically confirmed cases. *Sleep* 1997;20(11):972–81.

55. American Psychiatric Association. *Diagnostic and Statistical Manual of Mental Disorders. 4th ed., tex rev.* Arlington, VA: American Psychiatric Association; 2000.

56. Bokey K. Conversion disorder revisited: severe parasomnia discovered. *Aust NZ J Psychiatry* 1993;27(4):694–8.

57. Dyken ME, Rodnitzky RL. Periodic, aperiodic, and rhythmic motor disorders of sleep. *Neurology* 1992;42(7 Suppl 6):68–74.

58. Manfredini D, Lobbezoo F. Role of psychosocial factors in the etiology of bruxism. *J Orofac Pain* 2009;23(2):153–66.

59. Winkelman JW. Clinical and polysomnographic features of sleep-related eating disorder. *J Clin Psychiatry* 1998;59(1):14–19.

60. Stunkard AJ, Grace WJ, Wolff HG. The night-eating syndrome; a pattern of food intake among certain obese patients. *Am J Med* 1955;19(1):78–86.

61. Stunkard AJ, Allison KC, Geliebter A, et al. Development of criteria for a diagnosis: lessons from the night eating syndrome. *Compr Psychiatry* 2009;50(5):391–9.

62. Gluck ME, Geliebter A, Satov T. Night eating syndrome is associated with depression, low self-esteem, reduced daytime hunger, and less weight loss in obese outpatients. *Obes Res* 2001;9(4):264–7.

63. Lundgren JD, Allison KC, Crow S, et al. Prevalence of the night eating syndrome in a psychiatric population. *Am J Psychiatry* 2006;163(1):156–8.

64. Birketvedt GS, Florholmen J, Sundsfjord J, et al. Behavioral and neuroendocrine characteristics of the night-eating syndrome. *JAMA* 1999;282(7):657–63.

65. Stunkard AJ, Allison KC, Lundgren JD, et al. A biobehavioural model of the night eating syndrome. *Obes Rev* 2009;10(Suppl 2): 69–77.

66. Howell MJ, Schenck CH, Crow SJ. A review of nighttime eating disorders. *Sleep Med Rev* 2009;13(1):23–34.

67. Schenck CH, Mahowald MW. Review of nocturnal sleep-related eating disorders. *Int J Eat Disord* 1994;15(4):343–56.

68. Winkelman JW, Herzog DB, Fava M. The prevalence of sleep-related eating disorder in psychiatric and non-psychiatric populations. *Psychol Med* 1999;29(6):1461–6.

69. Schenck CH, Hurwitz TD, O'Connor KA, et al. Additional categories of sleep-related eating disorders and the current status of treatment. *Sleep* 1993;16(5):457–66.

70. Yun CH, Ji KH. Zolpidem-induced sleep-related eating disorder. *J Neurol Sci* 2010;288(1–2):200–1.

71. Najjar M. Zolpidem and amnestic sleep related eating disorder. *J Clin Sleep Med* 2007;3(6):637–8.

72. Kupfer DJ. REM latency: a psychobiologic marker for primary depressive disease. *Biol Psychiatry* 1976;11(2):159–74.

73. Riemann D, Berger M, Voderholzer U. Sleep and depression—results from psychobiological studies: an overview. *Biol Psychol* 2001;57(1–3):67–103.

74. Reynolds CF, Gillin JC, Kupfer DJ. Sleep and affective disorders. In: Meltzer HY, ed. *Psychopharmacology: The Third Generation of Progress.* New York: Raven Press; 1987:647.

75. Sitaram N, Nurnberger JI, Jr., Gershon ES, et al. Cholinergic regulation of mood and REM sleep: potential model and marker of vulnerability to affective disorder. *Am J Psychiatry* 1982;139(5):571–6.

76. Rush AJ, Erman MK, Giles DE, et al. Polysomnographic findings in recently drug-free and clinically remitted depressed patients. *Arch Gen Psychiatry* 1986;43(9):878–84.

77. Giles DE, Jarrett RB, Rush AJ, et al. Prospective assessment of electroencephalographic sleep in remitted major depression. *Psychiatry Res* 1993;46(3):269–84.

78. Thase ME, Reynolds CF,3rd, Frank E, et al. Polysomnographic studies of unmedicated depressed men before and after cognitive behavioral therapy. *Am J Psychiatry* 1994;151(11):1615–22.

79. Jindal RD, Thase ME, Fasiczka AL, et al. Electroencephalographic sleep profiles in single-episode and recurrent unipolar forms of major depression: II. comparison during remission. *Biol Psychiatry* 2002;51(3):230–6.

80. Modell S, Ising M, Holsboer F, et al. The Munich vulnerability study on affective disorders: premorbid polysomnographic profile of affected high-risk probands. *Biol Psychiatry* 2005;58(9):694–9.

81. Hudson JI, Lipinski JF, Frankenburg FR, et al. Electroencephalographic sleep in mania. *Arch Gen Psychiatry* 1988;45(3):267–73.

82. Riemann D, Voderholzer U, Berger M. Sleep and sleep-wake manipulations in bipolar depression. *Neuropsychobiology* 2002;45(Suppl 1):7–12.

83. Thase ME, Simons AD, Reynolds CF,3rd. Abnormal electroencephalographic sleep profiles in major depression: association with response to cognitive behavior therapy. *Arch Gen Psychiatry* 1996;53(2):99–108.

84. Clark C, Dupont R, Golshan S, et al. Preliminary evidence of an association between increased REM density and poor antidepressant response to partial sleep deprivation. *J Affect Disord* 2000;59(1):77–83.

85. Benca RM, Obermeyer WH, Thisted RA, et al. Sleep and psychiatric disorders. A meta-analysis. *Arch Gen Psychiatry* 1992;49(8):651,68; discussion 669–70.

86. Benson KL, Zarcone VP,Jr. Rapid eye movement sleep eye movements in schizophrenia and depression. *Arch Gen Psychiatry* 1993;50(6):474–82.

87. Labbate LA, Pollack MH, Otto MW, et al. Sleep panic attacks: an association with childhood anxiety and adult psychopathology. *Biol Psychiatry* 1994;36(1):57–60.

88. Hauri PJ, Friedman M, Ravaris CL. Sleep in patients with spontaneous panic attacks. *Sleep* 1989;12(4):323–37.

89. Uhde TW, Roy-Byrne P, Gillin JC, et al. The sleep of patients with panic disorder: a preliminary report. *Psychiatry Res* 1984;12(3):251–9.

90. Dube S, Jones DA, Bell J, et al. Interface of panic and depression: clinical and sleep EEG correlates. *Psychiatry Res* 1986;19(2):119–33.

91. Mellman TA, Uhde TW. Sleep panic attacks: new clinical findings and theoretical implications. *Am J Psychiatry* 1989;146(9):1204–7.

92. Uhde TW. Anxiety disorders. In: Kryger MH, Roth T, Dement WC, eds. *Principles and Practice of Sleep Medicine*. 3rd ed. Philadelphia, PA: Saunders; 2000:1123.

93. Sheikh JI, Woodward SH, Leskin GA. Sleep in post-traumatic stress disorder and panic: convergence and divergence. *Depress Anxiety* 2003;18(4):187–97.

94. Voderholzer U, Riemann D, Huwig-Poppe C, et al. Sleep in obsessive compulsive disorder: polysomnographic studies under baseline conditions and after experimentally induced serotonin deficiency. *Eur Arch Psychiatry Clin Neurosci* 2007;257(3):173–82.

95. van der Kolk B, Blitz R, Burr W, et al. Nightmares and trauma: a comparison of nightmares after combat with lifelong nightmares in veterans. *Am J Psychiatry* 1984;141(2):187–90.

96. Ross RJ, Ball WA, Dinges DF, et al. Rapid eye movement sleep disturbance in posttraumatic stress disorder. *Biol Psychiatry* 1994;35(3):195–202.

97. Mellman TA, Kulick-Bell R, Ashlock LE, et al. Sleep events among veterans with combat-related posttraumatic stress disorder. *Am J Psychiatry* 1995;152(1):110–15.

98. Kobayashi I, Boarts JM, Delahanty DL. Polysomnographically measured sleep abnormalities in PTSD: a meta-analytic review. *Psychophysiology* 2007;44(4):660–9.

99. Ross RJ, Ball WA, Dinges DF, et al. Motor dysfunction during sleep in posttraumatic stress disorder. *Sleep* 1994;17(8):723–32.

100. Woodward SH, Leskin GA, Sheikh JI. Movement during sleep: associations with posttraumatic stress disorder, nightmares, and comorbid panic disorder. *Sleep* 2002;25(6):681–8.

101. Lavie P, Hertz G. Increased sleep motility and respiration rates in combat neurotic patients. *Biol Psychiatry* 1979;14(6):983–7.

102. Husain AM, Miller PP, Carwile ST. REM sleep behavior disorder: potential relationship to post-traumatic stress disorder. *J Clin Neurophysiol* 2001;18(2):148–57.

103. Wechsler LR, Stakes JW, Shahani BT, et al. Periodic leg movements of sleep (nocturnal myoclonus): an electrophysiological study. *Ann Neurol* 1986;19(2):168–73.

104. Grillon C, Morgan CA,3rd, Davis M, et al. Effects of experimental context and explicit threat cues on acoustic startle in Vietnam veterans with posttraumatic stress disorder. *Biol Psychiatry* 1998;44(10):1027–36.

105. Krakow B, Germain A, Warner TD, et al. The relationship of sleep quality and posttraumatic stress to potential sleep disorders in sexual assault survivors with nightmares, insomnia, and PTSD. *J Trauma Stress* 2001;14(4):647–65.

106. Germain A, Nielsen TA. Sleep pathophysiology in posttraumatic stress disorder and idiopathic nightmare sufferers. *Biol Psychiatry* 2003;54(10):1092–8.

107. Tandon R, Shipley JE, Taylor S, et al. Electroencephalographic sleep abnormalities in schizophrenia. relationship to positive/negative symptoms and prior neuroleptic treatment. *Arch Gen Psychiatry* 1992;49(3):185–94.

108. Poulin J, Daoust AM, Forest G, et al. Sleep architecture and its clinical correlates in first episode and neuroleptic-naive patients with schizophrenia. *Schizophr Res* 2003;62(1–2):147–53.

109. Riemann D, Hohagen F, Krieger S, et al. Cholinergic REM induction test: Muscarinic supersensitivity underlies polysomnographic findings in both depression and schizophrenia. *J Psychiatr Res* 1994;28(3):195–210.

110. Tandon R, Shipley JE, Eiser AS, et al. Association between abnormal REM sleep and negative symptoms in schizophrenia. *Psychiatry Res* 1989;27(3):359–61.

111. Keshavan MS, Reynolds CF, Montrose D, et al. Sleep and suicidality in psychotic patients. *Acta Psychiatr Scand* 1994;89(2):122–5.

112. Lewis CF, Tandon R, Shipley JE, et al. Biological predictors of suicidality in schizophrenia. *Acta Psychiatr Scand* 1996;94(6):416–20.

113. Yang C, Winkelman JW. Clinical significance of sleep EEG abnormalities in chronic schizophrenia. *Schizophr Res* 2006;82(2–3):251–60.

114. Galland BC, Tripp EG, Taylor BJ. The sleep of children with attention deficit hyperactivity disorder on and off methylphenidate: a matched case-control study. *J Sleep Res* 2010;19(2):366–73.

115. Picchietti DL, England SJ, Walters AS, et al. Periodic limb movement disorder and restless legs syndrome in children with attention-deficit hyperactivity disorder. *J Child Neurol* 1998;13(12):588–94.

116. Mick E, Biederman J, Jetton J, et al. Sleep disturbances associated with attention deficit hyperactivity disorder: the impact of psychiatric comorbidity and pharmacotherapy. *J Child Adolesc Psychopharmacol* 2000;10(3):223–31.

117. Picchietti DL, Walters AS. Moderate to severe periodic limb movement disorder in childhood and adolescence. *Sleep* 1999;22(3):297–300.

118. Walters AS, Mandelbaum DE, Lewin DS, et al. Dopaminergic therapy in children with restless legs/periodic limb movements in sleep and ADHD. Dopaminergic therapy study group. *Pediatr Neurol* 2000;22(3):182–6.

119. Grissom EM, Brubaker B, Capdevila OS, et al. Eye movement during REM sleep in children with attention deficit hyperactivity disorder. *Dev Neuropsychol* 2009;34(5):552–9.

120. Prinz PN, Vitaliano PP, Vitiello MV, et al. Sleep, EEG and mental function changes in senile dementia of the Alzheimer's type. *Neurobiol Aging* 1982;3(4):361–70.

121. Montplaisir J, Petit D, Lorrain D, et al. Sleep in Alzheimer's disease: further considerations on the role of brainstem and forebrain cholinergic populations in sleep-wake mechanisms. *Sleep* 1995;18(3):145–8.

122. Bliwise DL. Sleep disorders in Alzheimer's disease and other dementias. *Clin Cornerstone* 2004;6(Suppl 1A):S16–28.

123. Weldemichael DA, Grossberg GT. Circadian rhythm disturbances in patients with Alzheimer's disease: a review. *Int J Alzheimers Dis* 2010;2010:716453.

124. Yeh SB, Yeh PY, Schenck CH. Rivastigmine-induced REM sleep behavior disorder (RBD) in a 88-year-old man with Alzheimer's disease. *J Clin Sleep Med* 2010;6(2):192–5.

125. Salami O, Lyketsos C, Rao V. Treatment of sleep disturbance in Alzheimer's dementia. *Int J Geriatr Psychiatry* 2010;26(8):771–82.

126. de Jonghe A, Korevaar JC, van Munster BC, et al. Effectiveness of melatonin treatment on circadian rhythm disturbances in dementia. are there implications for delirium? A systematic review. *Int J Geriatr Psychiatry* 2010;25(12):1201–8.

127. Harper DG, Stopa EG, McKee AC, et al. Differential circadian rhythm disturbances in men with Alzheimer disease and frontotemporal degeneration. *Arch Gen Psychiatry* 2001;58(4):353–60.

128. Anderson KN, Hatfield C, Kipps C, et al. Disrupted sleep and circadian patterns in frontotemporal dementia. *Eur J Neurol* 2009;16(3):317–23.

129. Emser W, Brenner M, Stober T, et al. Changes in nocturnal sleep in Huntington's and Parkinson's disease. *J Neurol* 1988;235(3):177–9.

130. Wiegand M, Moller AA, Lauer CJ, et al. Nocturnal sleep in Huntington's disease. *J Neurol* 1991;238(4):203–8.

131. Silvestri R, Raffaele M, De Domenico P, et al. Sleep features in Tourette's syndrome, neuroacanthocytosis and Huntington's chorea. *Neurophysiol Clin* 1995;25(2):66–77.

132. Fish DR, Sawyers D, Allen PJ, et al. The effect of sleep on the dyskinetic movements of Parkinson's disease, Gilles de la Tourette syndrome, Huntington's disease, and torsion dystonia. *Arch Neurol* 1991;48(2):210–14.

133. Arnulf I, Nielsen J, Lohmann E, et al. Rapid eye movement sleep disturbances in Huntington disease. *Arch Neurol* 2008;65(4):482–8.

134. Videnovic A, Leurgans S, Fan W, et al. Daytime somnolence and nocturnal sleep disturbances in Huntington disease. *Parkinsonism Relat Disord* 2009;15(6):471–4.

135. Aziz NA, Anguelova GV, Marinus J, et al. Sleep and circadian rhythm alterations correlate with depression and cognitive impairment in Huntington's disease. *Parkinsonism Relat Disord* 2010;16(5):345–50.

136. Kimura K, Tachibana N, Aso T, et al. Subclinical REM sleep behavior disorder in a patient with corticobasal degeneration. *Sleep* 1997;20(10):891–4.

137. Roche S, Jacquesson JM, Destee A, et al. Sleep and vigilance in corticobasal degeneration: a descriptive study. *Neurophysiol Clin* 2007;37(4):261–4.

138. Wetter TC, Brunner H, Collado-Seidel V, et al. Sleep and periodic limb movements in corticobasal degeneration. *Sleep Med* 2002;3(1):33–6.

139. Iriarte J, Alegre M, Arbizu J, et al. Unilateral periodic limb movements during sleep in corticobasal degeneration. *Mov Disord* 2001;16(6):1180–3.

140. Wall CA, Rummans TA, Aksamit AJ, et al. Psychiatric manifestations of Creutzfeldt-Jakob disease: a 25-year analysis. *J Neuropsychiatry Clin Neurosci* 2005;17(4):489–95.

141. Landolt HP, Glatzel M, Blattler T, et al. Sleep-wake disturbances in sporadic Creutzfeldt-Jakob disease. *Neurology* 2006;66(9):1418–24.

142. Wieser HG, Schindler K, Zumsteg D. EEG in Creutzfeldt-Jakob disease. *Clin Neurophysiol* 2006;117(5):935–51.

143. Gillin JC, Smith TL, Irwin M, et al. EEG sleep studies in "pure" primary alcoholism during subacute withdrawal: relationships to normal controls, age, and other clinical variables. *Biol Psychiatry* 1990;27(5):477–88.

144. Gillin JC, Smith TL, Irwin M, et al. Increased pressure for rapid eye movement sleep at time of hospital admission predicts relapse in nondepressed patients with primary alcoholism at 3-month follow-up. *Arch Gen Psychiatry* 1994;51(3):189–97.

145. Clark CP, Gillin JC, Golshan S, et al. Increased REM sleep density at admission predicts relapse by three months in primary alcoholics with a lifetime diagnosis of secondary depression. *Biol Psychiatry* 1998;43(8):601–7.

146. Clark CP, Gillin JC, Golshan S, et al. Polysomnography and depressive symptoms in primary alcoholics with and without a lifetime diagnosis of secondary depression and in patients with primary major depression. *J Affect Disord* 1999;52(1–3):177–85.

147. Gann H, van Calker D, Feige B, et al. Polysomnographic comparison between patients with primary alcohol dependency during subacute withdrawal and patients with a major depression. *Eur Arch Psychiatry Clin Neurosci* 2004;254(4):263–71.

148. Johnson LC, Burdick JA, Smith J. Sleep during alcohol intake and withdrawal in the chronic alcoholic. *Arch Gen Psychiatry* 1970;22(5):406–18.

149. Adamson J, Burdick JA. Sleep of dry alcoholics. *Arch Gen Psychiatry* 1973;28(1):146–9.

150. Aldrich MS, Shipley JE. Alcohol use and periodic limb movements of sleep. *Alcohol Clin Exp Res* 1993;17(1):192–6.

151. Le Bon O, Verbanck P, Hoffmann G, et al. Sleep in detoxified alcoholics: impairment of most standard sleep parameters and increased risk for sleep apnea, but not for myoclonias—a controlled study. *J Stud Alcohol* 1997;58(1):30–6.

152. Schierenbeck T, Riemann D, Berger M, et al. Effect of illicit recreational drugs

upon sleep: cocaine, ecstasy and marijuana. *Sleep Med Rev* 2008;12(5):381–9.

153. Feinberg I, Jones R, Walker J, et al. Effects of marijuana extract and tetrahydrocannabinol on electroencephalographic sleep patterns. *Clin Pharmacol Ther* 1976;19(6):782–94.

154. Kay DC, Samiuddin Z. Sleep disorders associated with drug abuse and drugs of abuse. In: Williams RL, Karacan I, Moore CA, eds. *Sleep Disorders: Diagnosis and Treatment*. New York: Wiley; 1988:315.

155. Kowatch RA, Schnoll SS, Knisely JS, et al. Electroencephalographic sleep and mood during cocaine withdrawal. *J Addict Dis* 1992;11(4):21–45.

156. Drapeau C, Hamel-Hebert I, Robillard R, et al. Challenging sleep in aging: the effects of 200 mg of caffeine during the evening in young and middle-aged moderate caffeine consumers. *J Sleep Res* 2006;15(2):133–41.

157. Bogan RK. Armodafinil in the treatment of excessive sleepiness. *Expert Opin Pharmacother* 2010;11(6):993–1002.

158. Valentino RM, Foldvary-Schaefer N. Modafinil in the treatment of excessive daytime sleepiness. *Cleve Clin J Med* 2007;74(8):561,6, 568–71.

159. Obermeyer WH, Benca RM. Effects of drugs on sleep. *Neurol Clin* 1996;14(4):827–40.

160. Kay DC, Pickworth WB, Neider GL. Morphine-like insomnia from heroin in nondependent human addicts. *Br J Clin Pharmacol* 1981;11(2):159–69.

161. Kay DC, Pickworth WB, Neidert GL, et al. Opioid effects on computer-derived sleep and EEG parameters in nondependent human addicts. *Sleep* 1979;2(2):175–91.

162. Kay DC. Human sleep during chronic morphine intoxication. *Psychopharmacologia* 1975;44(2):117–24.

163. Wang D, Teichtahl H. Opioids, sleep architecture and sleep-disordered breathing. *Sleep Med Rev* 2007;11(1):35–46.

164. Mamelak M, Black J, Montplaisir J, et al. A pilot study on the effects of sodium oxybate on sleep architecture and daytime alertness in narcolepsy. *Sleep* 2004;27(7):1327–34.

165. Zvosec DL, Smith SW, Porrata T, et al. Case series of 226 gamma-hydroxybutyrate-associated deaths: lethal toxicity and trauma. *Am J Emerg Med* 2011;29(3):319–32.

166. Mamelak M. Narcolepsy and depression and the neurobiology of gammahydroxybutyrate. *Prog Neurobiol* 2009;89(2):193–219.

167. Wang YG, Swick TJ, Carter LP, et al. Safety overview of postmarketing and clinical experience of sodium oxybate (Xyrem): abuse, misuse, dependence, and diversion. *J Clin Sleep Med* 2009;5(4):365–71.

168. Kupfer DJ, Spiker DG, Rossi A, et al. Nortriptyline and EEG sleep in depressed patients. *Biol Psychiatry* 1982;17(5):535–46.

169. Reynolds CF,3rd, Buysse DJ, Brunner DP, et al. Maintenance nortriptyline effects on electroencephalographic sleep in elderly patients with recurrent major depression: double-blind, placebo- and plasma-level-controlled evaluation. *Biol Psychiatry* 1997;42(7):560–7.

170. Armitage R, Trivedi M, Rush AJ. Fluoxetine and oculomotor activity during sleep in depressed patients. *Neuropsychopharmacology* 1995;12(2):159–65.

171. Hendrickse WA, Roffwarg HP, Grannemann BD, et al. The effects of fluoxetine on the polysomnogram of depressed outpatients: a pilot study. *Neuropsychopharmacology* 1994;10(2):85–91.

172. Buysse DJ, Kupfer DJ, Cherry C, et al. Effects of prior fluoxetine treatment on EEG sleep in women with recurrent depression. *Neuropsychopharmacology* 1999;21(2):258–67.

173. Murck H, Nickel T, Kunzel H, et al. State markers of depression in sleep EEG: dependency on drug and gender in patients treated with tianeptine or paroxetine. *Neuropsychopharmacology* 2003;28(2):348–58.

174. Ott GE, Rao U, Lin KM, et al. Effect of treatment with bupropion on EEG sleep: relationship to antidepressant response. *Int J Neuropsychopharmacol* 2004;7(3):275–81.

175. Jindal RD, Fasiczka AL, Himmelhoch JM, et al. Effects of tranylcypromine on the sleep of patients with anergic bipolar depression. *Psychopharmacol Bull* 2003;37(3):118–26.

176. Landolt HP, Raimo EB, Schnierow BJ, et al. Sleep and sleep electroencephalogram in depressed patients treated with phenelzine. *Arch Gen Psychiatry* 2001;58(3):268–76.

177. Schenck CH, Mahowald MW, Kim SW, et al. Prominent eye movements during NREM sleep and REM sleep behavior disorder associated with fluoxetine treatment of

depression and obsessive-compulsive disorder. *Sleep* 1992;15(3):226–35.

178. Lam SP, Zhang J, Tsoh J, et al. REM sleep behavior disorder in psychiatric populations. *J Clin Psychiatry* 2010;71(8):1101–3.

179. Roux FJ, Kryger MH. Medication effects on sleep. *Clin Chest Med* 2010;31(2):397–405.

180. Krystal AD, Goforth HW, Roth T. Effects of antipsychotic medications on sleep in schizophrenia. *Int Clin Psychopharmacol* 2008;23(3):150–60.

181. Salin-Pascual RJ, Herrera-Estrella M, Galicia-Polo L, et al. Olanzapine acute administration in schizophrenic patients increases delta sleep and sleep efficiency. *Biol Psychiatry* 1999;46(1):141–3.

182. Muller MJ, Rossbach W, Mann K, et al. Subchronic effects of olanzapine on sleep EEG in schizophrenic patients with predominantly negative symptoms. *Pharmacopsychiatry* 2004;37(4):157–62.

183. Riemann D, Hohagen F, Fleckenstein P, et al. The cholinergic REM induction test with RS 86 after scopolamine pretreatment in healthy subjects. *Psychiatry Res* 1991;38(3):247–60.

184. Cohrs S, Meier A, Neumann AC, et al. Improved sleep continuity and increased slow wave sleep and REM latency during ziprasidone treatment: a randomized, controlled, crossover trial of 12 healthy male subjects. *J Clin Psychiatry* 2005;66(8):989–96.

185. Huapaya L. Somnambulism and bedtime medication. *Am J Psychiatry* 1976;133(10):1207.

186. Luchins DJ, Sherwood PM, Gillin JC, et al. Filicide during psychotropic-induced somnambulism: a case report. *Am J Psychiatry* 1978;135(11):1404–5.

187. Scott AI. Attempted strangulation during phenothiazine-induced sleep-walking and night terrors. *Br J Psychiatry* 1988;153:692–4.

188. Goldbloom D, Chouinard G. Clonazepam in the treatment of neuroleptic-induced somnambulism. *Am J Psychiatry* 1984;141(11):1486.

189. Glassman JN, Darko D, Gillin JC. Medication-induced somnambulism in a patient with schizoaffective disorder. *J Clin Psychiatry* 1986;47(10):523–4.

190. Parrino L, Terzano MG. Polysomnographic effects of hypnotic drugs. A review. *Psychopharmacology (Berl)* 1996; 126(1):1–16.

191. Borbely AA, Akerstedt T, Benoit O, et al. Hypnotics and sleep physiology: a consensus report. European Sleep Research Society, Committee on Hypnotics and Sleep Physiology. *Eur Arch Psychiatry Clin Neurosci* 1991;241(1):13–21.

192. Schenck CH, Mahowald MW. Long-term, nightly benzodiazepine treatment of injurious parasomnias and other disorders of disrupted nocturnal sleep in 170 adults. *Am J Med* 1996;100(3):333–7.

193. Roth T, Roehrs TA. Issues in the use of benzodiazepine therapy. *J Clin Psychiatry* 1992;(53 Suppl):14–18.

194. Mendelson WB, Roth T, Cassella J, et al. The treatment of chronic insomnia: drug indications, chronic use and abuse liability. Summary of a 2001 new clinical drug evaluation unit meeting symposium. *Sleep Med Rev* 2004;8(1):7–17.

195. Griffiths RR, Johnson MW. Relative abuse liability of hypnotic drugs: a conceptual framework and algorithm for differentiating among compounds. *J Clin Psychiatry* 2005;66(Suppl 9):31–41.

196. Zammit G. Comparative tolerability of newer agents for insomnia. *Drug Saf* 2009;32(9):735–48.

197. Hwang TJ, Ni HC, Chen HC, et al. Risk predictors for hypnosedative-related complex sleep behaviors: a retrospective, cross-sectional pilot study. *J Clin Psychiatry* 2010;71(10):1331–5.

198. Charney DS, Kales A, Soldatos CR, et al. Somnambulistic-like episodes secondary to combined lithium-neuroleptic treatment. *Br J Psychiatry* 1979;135:418–24.

199. Landry P, Warnes H, Nielsen T, et al. Somnambulistic-like behaviour in patients attending a lithium clinic. *Int Clin Psychopharmacol* 1999;14(3):173–5.

200. Ehrenberg BL, Eisensehr I, Corbett KE, et al. Valproate for sleep consolidation in periodic limb movement disorder. *J Clin Psychopharmacol* 2000;20(5):574–8.

201. Hudson JI, Lipinski JF, Frankenburg FR, et al. Effects of lithium on sleep in mania. *Biol Psychiatry* 1989;25(5):665–8.

202. Riemann D, Gann H, Hohagen F, et al. The effect of carbamazepine on endocrine and sleep EEG variables in a patient with 48-hour rapid cycling, and healthy controls. *Neuropsychobiology* 1993;27(3):163–70.

203. Schredl M, Hornung O, Regen F, et al. The effect of donepezil on sleep in elderly, healthy

persons: a double-blind placebo-controlled study. *Pharmacopsychiatry* 2006;39(6):205–8.

204. Moraes Wdos S, Poyares DR, Guilleminault C, et al. The effect of donepezil on sleep and REM sleep EEG in patients with Alzheimer disease: a double-blind placebo-controlled study. *Sleep* 2006;29(2):199–205.

205. Kitabayashi Y, Ueda H, Tsuchida H, et al. Donepezil-induced nightmares in mild cognitive impairment. *Psychiatry Clin Neurosci* 2006;60(1):123–4.

206. Ross JS, Shua-Haim JR. Aricept-induced nightmares in Alzheimer's disease: 2 case reports. *J Am Geriatr Soc* 1998;46(1):119–20.

207. Cooke JR, Loredo JS, Liu L, et al. Acetylcholinesterase inhibitors and sleep architecture in patients with Alzheimer's disease. *Drugs Aging* 2006;23(6):503–11.

208. Carlander B, Touchon J, Ondze B, et al. REM sleep behavior disorder induced by cholinergic treatment in Alzheimer's disease. *J Sleep Res* 1996;5(Suppl 1):28.

209. Terzaghi M, Rustioni V, Manni R, et al. Agrypnia with nocturnal confusional behaviors in dementia with Lewy bodies: immediate efficacy of rivastigmine. *Mov Disord* 2010;25(5):647–9.

210. Ringman JM, Simmons JH. Treatment of REM sleep behavior disorder with donepezil: a report of three cases. *Neurology* 2000;55(6):870–1.

211. Simmons J. Treatment of REM sleep behavior disorder with acetylcholinesterase inhibitors. *Sleep* 2009;32:A292.

212. Larsson V, Aarsland D, Ballard C, et al. The effect of memantine on sleep behaviour in dementia with Lewy bodies and Parkinson's disease dementia. *Int J Geriatr Psychiatry* 2010;25(10): 1030–8.

57

Pediatric Sleep-Related Movement Disorders

TIMOTHY F. HOBAN

Although clinical descriptions of sleep-related movement disorders in children date from the late nineteenth century,[1] this category of sleep disorders has received only limited scientific study in the pediatric age group, primarily during the last fifteen years. This chapter provides a concise overview of sleep-related movement disorders in children intended to supplement the disorder-specific reviews provided in earlier chapters, with particular focus upon how clinical presentation and treatment differ for children compared to adults.

CHILDHOOD RESTLESS LEGS SYNDROME (RLS) AND PERIODIC LIMB MOVEMENTS IN SLEEP (PLMS)

As is the case for adults, childhood restless legs syndrome (RLS) and periodic limb movement disorder (PLMD) represent distinct but frequently coinciding conditions that may impact the duration, quality, and continuity of nighttime sleep. Symptoms of RLS in children include urges to move the legs, transient relief of these urges with movement, and paresthesias that range from ill defined to distinctly painful. Because younger or developmentally disabled children may have limited ability to describe the essential symptoms of RLS, specific pediatric criteria for diagnosis were established at a National Institutes of Health consensus conference on RLS diagnosis and epidemiology,[2] which were subsequently incorporated in the International Classification of Sleep Disorders, second edition.[3] (See Table 57.1 for diagnostic criteria.) Description of RLS symptoms by children and their parents may include unusual or age-dependent terms such as oowies, crazy legs, bugs, shark bites, and need to run.[2] Many children with "growing pains" actually meet diagnostic criteria for RLS based on nighttime predominance of symptoms and the concurrent presence of urges to move the legs, which are ameliorated by movement.[4]

Table 57.1 Diagnostic Criteria for the Diagnosis of Pediatric Restless Legs Syndrome (RLS)

Diagnosis in pediatric patients aged 2–12 years (A alone or B plus C satisfy the criteria)

A. The child meets all four essential adult criteria for RLS (urge to move or dysesthesias involving the legs, worsening of symptoms with rest or inactivity, temporary relief of symptoms with movement, and symptoms are present or worse in the evening or night) and describes symptoms consistent with leg discomfort in his or her own words.

OR

B. The child meets all four essential adult criteria for RLS but does not relate symptoms consistent with leg discomfort in his or her own words.

AND

C. The child demonstrates at least two of the following three findings:
  a. A sleep disturbance for age
  b. A biological parent or sibling with definite RLS
  c. A periodic limb movement index of at least five movements per hour during nocturnal polysomnography

Diagnosis of RLS requires that symptoms are not better explained by another sleep, medical, psychiatric, or neurological disorder; or by medication or substance use.

Source: From Allen, Picchietti et al. and AASM.[2,3]

In contrast to RLS, the *ICSD-2* diagnostic criteria for PLMD are applied uniformly to both children and adults, since they rely on polysomnography (PSG) and easily identifiable symptoms rather than subjectively reported complaints.[5] Although it is not unusual for affected children to have comorbid RLS and PLMD, either condition may present independently.

A clinically significant sleep disturbance that is thought to be caused by the PLMS and not some other disorder such as RLS or Narcolepsy is required for the diagnosis of PLMD.[3] Common sleep disturbances in affected children include insomnia, excessive night waking, restlessness before or during sleep, and increased limb movements.[6] Symptoms often evolve over time, and many children exhibit disturbed sleep for years prior to meeting criteria for the diagnosis of RLS.[7]

Although restlessness during sleep affected 17% of children and growing pains affected 8% in one community-based survey, the prevalence of clinically definite RLS in a large population-based study was 1.9% for children and 2.0% for adolescents.[8,9] Growing pains was a misdiagnosis given to children with RLS in one series.[4] A majority of children with RLS have at least one affected parent, suggesting dominant inheritance, but genetic linkage studies of families with early-onset RLS have yielded inconsistent results.[9–12]

Several studies have reported pediatric RLS to be frequently associated with low blood levels of ferritin, consistent with the hypothesis that deficiency or disturbed metabolism of iron in the basal ganglia may play a role in the pathogenesis of the condition.[6,7,13] High rates of RLS have also been identified in children with chronic kidney disease[14] and PLMD in Williams syndrome.[15]

The consequences of pediatric RLS and PLMD remain poorly understood and seemingly variable in nature and severity. Some affected children exhibit clearly referable daytime tiredness, inattention, hyperactivity, or emotional lability, which is proportionate to the severity of sleep disruption and improves with treatment of the underlying sleep disorder. In contrast, other children are sometimes found to have significantly elevated periodic limb movements of sleep during PSG in the absence of any clinical sleep disturbance or referable sequelae during wakefulness.

Available data suggest some association between childhood RLS/PLMD and attention-deficit/hyperactivity disorder (ADHD). Several studies have reported high rates of daytime inattention or hyperactivity among children and adolescents with RLS symptoms.[6,16] Conversely, studies of children with ADHD have reported high rates of both RLS symptoms and periodic limb movements during sleep for affected children.[17–19] It has not been established whether the association between RLS/PLMD and ADHD is necessarily causative in nature, and some authors have postulated that underlying disturbances of brain iron or dopaminergic metabolism could represent a root cause for these and other disorders.[20,21]

Clinical treatment practices for pediatric RLS and PLMD vary widely, and no outcome-based treatment guidelines exist at present. Nonpharmacologic treatment options may be appropriate for children with mild or intermittent symptoms. These include gentle massage of the legs or judicious use of warm or cool compresses. In light of adult reports associating use of selective serotonin reuptake inhibitors (SSRIs) and other medications with increased risk for PLMD, careful review of the medication history is indicated in affected pediatric patients.[22]

For children with more significant or frequent symptoms, it is appropriate to screen for underlying iron deficiency states, which represent common and treatable conditions in the pediatric population.[23] Although the serum ferritin level represents the most commonly administered screening measure for patients with RLS/PLMD, and low ferritin levels are thought to be indicative of low body iron stores, ferritin is also an acute phase reactant for which serum levels may transiently increase during or following acute illness. Since this effect can complicate interpretation of serum ferritin levels, this author's practice is to perform a complete blood count (CBC), iron level, and total iron binding capacity (TIBC) in conjunction with serum ferritin level to provide a more complete view of the child's hematologic iron status.

Limited data suggest that children with RLS/PLMD and ferritin levels of less than 50 μg/L or other evidence of iron deficiency may benefit from treatment with ferrous sulfate, even in the absence of anemia.[24,25] Although some authors have assessed and recommended ferrous sulfate doses at 3 mg/kg per day (based on elemental iron), optimal dosing for the pediatric population is not well established, so treatment should be carefully monitored.[25,26] Potential side effects of treatment include constipation, staining of the teeth, and iron overload. Enteral absorption of iron is inefficient but may be enhanced by concurrent administration of vitamin C.[23] The response of RLS/PLMD symptoms and lab parameters to iron therapy tends to be gradual. This author's practice is to recheck CBC, iron, TIBC, and ferritin levels after the first 3 months of treatment and correlate these results with any clinical changes reported by the family.

Some children with significant sleep disruption due to RLS/PLMD are treated with prescription medications, particularly if they do not have evidence of iron deficiency, or have symptoms that have persisted despite correction of underlying iron deficiency. Although dopaminergic agents pramipexole and ropinirole have been labeled by the United States Food and Drug Administration (FDA) for the treatment of moderate to severe RLS in adults, no FDA-approved agents for the treatment of pediatric RLS exist, so all drug treatment in this age group is off label.

Published case reports and case series have documented successful treatment of pediatric RLS using dopaminergic agents pramipexole,[27] ropinirole,[28,29] levodopa,[4,30] and pergolide.[30] A recent double-blind study assessing children with RLS/PLMD and ADHD reported that treatment with levodopa was associated with improvement of RLS/PLMD symptoms but no effect on ADHD symptoms.[31] Treatment of pediatric RLS/PLMD should be carefully titrated and supervised due to the potential for significant gastrointestinal and behavioral side effects and because of the lack of long-term data regarding use of these agents in the pediatric age group.[32]

Case reports also exist regarding treatment of childhood RLS using nondopaminergic agents such as clonidine[4] and—in children with Williams syndrome and PLMD—clonazepam.[15]

SLEEP-RELATED RHYTHMIC MOVEMENT DISORDER

Childhood sleep-related rhythmic movement disorder (RMD) is characterized by recurrent episodes of stereotypical movements that may occur during wakefulness, the wake-sleep transition, sustained sleep, or following arousal from sleep. Movements involve the head, body, or limbs either independently or in combination, often accompanied by synchronous humming or moaning vocalizations. The movements of RMD occur at a frequency to 0.5–2 Hz.[33] The duration of movement episodes may be as short as a few seconds or as long as 20 minutes. Cumulative duration of rhythmic movements during a single night can sometimes be measured in hours.

Published accounts of RMD date to the late 19th and early 20th centuries.[33–36] The term "jactatio capitis nocturna," first used by Zappert to describe sleep-associated head banging, remains in use today.

RMD is often categorized according to the predominant pattern of body movement observed. *Head banging* (*jactatio capitis nocturna*) is characterized by forward-and-backward head movement, which is sometimes vigorous in nature. Depending on body position, the head may strike the pillow, bed, or less commonly solid surfaces such as the wall or side of a crib. *Head rolling* and *body rolling* involve rhythmic side-to-side turning form the lateral position. *Body rocking* consists of forceful rocking movements while elevated upon the hands and knees.

ICSD-2 diagnostic criteria for RMD are uniform for children and adults.[37] Diagnosis of the condition requires that the stereotypical movements involve large muscle groups, be predominantly sleep-related, and be clearly associated with sleep disruption, impaired daytime function, or risk for injury.

Sleep-related rhythmic movements have been reported to affect nearly two thirds of infants, but most of these children experience only mild or intermittent sleep disruption, and the great majority outgrow the condition by 5 years of age.[38] Clinically significant RMD may be more common in children with developmental disabilities or those with a family history of the condition.[39-41]

The consequences of childhood RMD are variable in nature and severity. Milder forms of the condition may be associated with self-limited sleep disruption in the form of delayed sleep onset or increased wake after sleep onset. Children with more vigorous RMD behaviors sometimes sustain minor injuries such as abrasions or bruising. Although diurnal head banging in developmentally disabled children may be associated with substantial risk for traumatic injury, serious injury is only rarely observed in sleep-related RMD affecting otherwise healthy children.[42,43] Several small case series assessing pediatric RMD subjects have reported relatively high rates of ADHD, but the consistency of this finding has not been verified in larger, controlled trials.[32,41]

Although the diagnosis of RMD is established primarily on the basis of the medical history, polysomnography (PSG) may be helpful when the diagnosis is uncertain, when concurrent sleep disorders are suspected, or where objective data are needed to assess sleep quality or duration in affected patients. The addition of sixteen-lead electroencephalography (EEG) to standard PSG may be appropriate in situations where sleep-related seizures represent a diagnostic consideration.

RMD episodes recorded during PSG are associated with monomorphic, high-amplitude, rhythmic movement artifact on EEG or limb leads (Fig. 57.1). Many subjects exhibit synchronous humming or moaning vocalizations that may be evident on the snore channel or audio recording. Episodes most commonly occur during wakefulness and light non-REM sleep and less frequently arise during REM sleep.[33,44]

The pathophysiology of childhood RMD remains poorly understood at present. Earlier theories that the condition might represent self-directed aggression, autoerotic gratification, or a manifestation of underlying anxiety have not been validated.[45-49] Contemporary hypotheses postulate that sleep-related RMD may represent self-soothing behavior which is positively reinforced via repetition over time or that the condition may result from activation of central motor pattern generators by arousal fluctuations.[50,51]

Most children with RMD do not require specific treatment, since the clinical manifestations are mild or intermittent in most cases and because the condition spontaneously remits for most affected children. For children whose movements are sufficiently severe to pose risk for injury, use of a protective helmet or judicious use of padding over hard surfaces adjacent to the bed may be appropriate.

Drug therapy for children with RMD has not been systematically studied, although case reports have documented clinical improvements with use of clonazepam,[52-54] oxazepam,[49] imipramine,[55,56] and citalopram.[57] Proposed behavioral therapies for childhood RMD include use of a water bed[58] and sleep restriction,[59] which were both reported to be effective in small case series. Hypnosis and forced awakening have also been investigated for the treatment of sleep-related RMD in children.[60,61]

SLEEP-RELATED BRUXISM

Sleep-related bruxism in children has received scant scientific study. The condition appears to be common in children, with population-based surveys reporting prevalence rates of 35.3% in Brazilian schoolchildren and 22.9% in school-aged Chinese children.[62,63]

The prevalence of clinically significant bruxism in children remains unknown. One small pilot study reported higher arousal indices for children with sleep bruxism compared to controls, with otherwise comparable sleep architecture.[64] Bruxism episodes recorded during

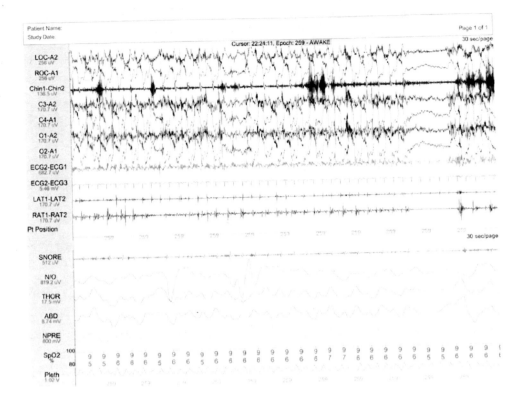

FIGURE 57.1 Rhythmic head banging (jactation capitis nocturna) during wake-sleep transition in a 9-year-old girl. Rhythmic movement artifact is present in the electroencephalographic leads (C3, C4, O1, and O2) and eye movement leads (LOC, ROC) on this 30-second polysomnogram epoch.

PSG arose most frequently during stage 2 and REM sleep. Attention and behavior concerns were reported for 4 of the 10 affected children in this cohort.

Case reports have identified sleep bruxism in association with methylphenidate and fluoxetine use in children.[65,66] A cross-sectional study of Mexican children with Down syndrome reported a high 42% prevalence of bruxism.[67]

Treatment of childhood bruxism has not been systematically studied. Although mouth guards represent the most commonly administered treatment for affected adults, this treatment is used cautiously in children due to concern that long-term use might adversely affect growth of the dental arches.

REM SLEEP BEHAVIOR DISORDER

Although REM sleep behavior disorder (RBD) most commonly affects older adults, the condition may rarely affect children. Most pediatric and adolescent reports of the condition have occurred in the context of associated sleep or neurological disorders such as narcolepsy,[68] autism,[69] juvenile Parkinson's disease,[70] Tourette syndrome,[71] or brainstem tumor.[72] A detailed review of pediatric and adolescent RBD was recently published by Stores.[73]

Treatment data in the pediatric population are extremely limited, although a few reports document successful treatment using clonazepam.[69,74]

HYPNAGOGIC BEHAVIOR DISORDER

Pareja and colleagues reported a distinctive pattern of complex motor behaviors affecting two young boys at wake-sleep transition.[75] Behaviors included prolonged periods of nonrhythmic movements variably associated with vocalizations or laughter. Video-EEG studies were unremarkable and symptoms eventually remitted as both children grew older. Identical sleep-related behaviors have been rarely observed in young children meeting diagnostic criteria for the diagnosis of PLMD (Hoban, unpublished data).

OTHER CHILDHOOD PARASOMNIAS ASSOCIATED WITH PROMINENT SLEEP-RELATED MOVEMENTS

Benign sleep myoclonus of infancy is characterized by repetitive and often vigorous myoclonic jerks of the trunk affecting young infants exclusively during sleep.[76] The condition spontaneously remits by 6 months of age for most affected infants. Because benign sleep myoclonus cannot be reliably distinguished from myoclonic seizure by history or observation alone, video EEG or video PSG studies are usually required for confirmation of the diagnosis.

Excessive limb or body movements sometimes represent a prominent feature of other parasomnias, particularly in sleep terrors, where running or physically violent behaviors are sometimes observed. *Parasomnia overlap disorder*—characterized by features of both RBD and non-REM arousal parasomnias—is occasionally encountered in children.[77] Tremulous movements may also occur as a transient and nonspecific feature of arousal or forced awakening in children.

OTHER CONDITIONS THAT CAN MIMIC SLEEP-RELATED MOVEMENT DISORDERS IN CHILDREN

Several varieties of nonconvulsive seizures are associated with events and movements that may resemble parasomnias.[78] *Nocturnal frontal lobe epilepsy (NFLE)* may present with episodes of agitation or ambulation arising from sleep, dystonic episodes during sleep, or paroxysmal arousals. The fact that nocturnal frontal lobe seizures are often stereotyped and may occur multiple times per night helps distinguishes them from parasomnias, but PSG with full EEG is usually required for definitive diagnosis.[79]

Benign epilepsy of childhood with centrotemporal spikes (BECT) may be associated with facial twitches during drowsiness or sleep that are sometimes not immediately recognized as a variety of focal seizure. Similarly, children with *juvenile myoclonic epilepsy* may exhibit prominent myoclonic jerks of the extremities upon awakening before other clinical manifestations

of their underlying seizure disorder become clearly evident.

REFERENCES

1. Putnam-Jacobi, M. Case of nocturnal rotary spasm . *J Nerv Ment Dis* 1880;7:390–402.
2. Allen RP, Picchietti D, Hening WA, et al. Restless legs syndrome: diagnostic criteria, special considerations, and epidemiology. A report from the restless legs syndrome diagnosis and epidemiology workshop at the National Institutes of Health. *Sleep Med* 2003;4(2):101–19.
3. American Academy of Sleep Medicine. Restless legs syndrome. In: *The International Classification of Sleep Disorders*. 2nd ed. Westchester, IL: American Academy of Sleep Medicine; 2005:178–81.
4. Rajaram SS, Walters AS, England SJ, et al. Some children with growing pains may actually have restless legs syndrome. *Sleep* 2004;27(4):767–73.
5. American Academy of Sleep Medicine. Periodic limb movement disorder. *The International Classification of Sleep Disorders*. 2nd ed. Westchester, IL: American Academy of Sleep Medicine; 2005:182–6.
6. Kotagal S, Silber MH. Childhood-onset restless legs syndrome. *Ann Neurol* 2004;56(6):803–7.
7. Picchietti DL, Stevens HE. Early manifestations of restless legs syndrome in childhood and adolescence. *Sleep Med* 2008;9(7):770–81.
8. Chervin RD, Archbold KH, Dillon JE, et al. (2002). Associations between symptoms of inattention, hyperactivity, restless legs, and periodic leg movements. *Sleep* 2002;25(2):213–18.
9. Picchietti D, Allen RP, Walters AS, et al. Restless legs syndrome: prevalence and impact in children and adolescents—the Peds REST study. *Pediatrics* 2007;120(2):253–66.
10. Lohmann-Hedrich K, Neumann A, Kleensang A, et al. Evidence for linkage of restless legs syndrome to chromosome 9p: are there two distinct loci? *Neurology* 2008;70(9):686–94.
11. Muhle H, Neumann A, Lohmann-Hedrich K, et al. Childhood-onset restless legs syndrome: clinical and genetic features of 22 families. *Mov Disord* 2008;23(8):1113–21; quiz 1203.

12. Sas AM, Di Fonzo A, Bakker SL, et al. Autosomal dominant restless legs syndrome maps to chromosome 20p13 (RLS-5) in a Dutch kindred. *Mov Disord* 2010;25(11):1715–22.

13. Picchietti MA, Picchietti DL. Advances in pediatric restless legs syndrome: iron, genetics, diagnosis and treatment. *Sleep Med* 2010;11(7):643–51.

14. Applebee GA, Guillot AP, Schuman CC, et al. Restless legs syndrome in pediatric patients with chronic kidney disease. *Pediatric Nephrol* 2009;24(3):545–8.

15. Arens R, Wright B, Elliott J, et al. Periodic limb movement in sleep in children with Williams syndrome. *J Pediatrics* 1998;133(5):670–4.

16. Yilmaz K, Kilincaslan A, Aydin N, et al. Prevalence and correlates of restless legs syndrome in adolescents. *Dev Med Child Neurol* 2011;53(1):40–7.

17. Picchietti DL, Underwood DJ, Farris WA, et al. Further studies on periodic limb movement disorder and restless legs syndrome in children with attention-deficit hyperactivity disorder. *Mov Disord* 1999;14(6):1000–7.

18. Cortese S, Konofal E, Lecendreux M, et al. Restless legs syndrome and attention-deficit/hyperactivity disorder: a review of the literature. *Sleep* 2005;28(8):1007–13.

19. Silvestri R, Gagliano A, Arico I, et al. Sleep disorders in children with attention-deficit/hyperactivity disorder (ADHD) recorded overnight by video-polysomnography. *Sleep Med* 2009;10(10):1132–8.

20. Cortese S, Lecendreux M, Bernardina BD, et al. Attention-deficit/hyperactivity disorder, Tourette's syndrome, and restless legs syndrome: the iron hypothesis. *Med Hypotheses* 2008;70(6):1128–32.

21. Konofal E, Lecendreux M, Deron J, et al. Effects of iron supplementation on attention deficit hyperactivity disorder in children. *Pediatric Neurol* 2008;38(1):20–6.

22. Yang C, White DP, Winkelman JW. Antidepressants and periodic leg movements of sleep. *Biological Psychiatry* 2005;58(6):510–14.

23. Borgna-Pignatti C, Marsella M, et al. Iron deficiency in infancy and childhood. *Pediatric Ann* 2008;37(5):329–37.

24. Kryger MH, Otake K, Foerster J. Low body stores of iron and restless legs syndrome: a correctable cause of insomnia in adolescents and teenagers. *Sleep Med* 2002;3(2):127–32.

25. Simakajornboon N, Kheirandish-Gozal L, Gozal D, et al. Periodic limb movements in sleep and iron status in children. *Sleep* 2003;26(6):735–8.

26. Simakajornboon N, Kheirandish-Gozal L, Vlasic V, et al. Diagnosis and management of restless legs syndrome in children. *Sleep Med Rev* 2009;13(2):149–56.

27. Mohri I, Kato-Nishimura K, Kagitani-Shimono K, et al. [Restless-leg syndrome—possible unrecognized cause for insomnia and irritability in children]. *No to Hattatsu [Brain Dev]* 2008;40(6):473–7.

28. Konofal E, Arnulf I, Lecendreux M, et al. Ropinirole in a child with attention-deficit hyperactivity disorder and restless legs syndrome. *Pediatric Neurol* 2005;32(5):350–1.

29. Cortese S, Konofal E, Lecendreux M, et al. Effectiveness of ropinirole for RLS and depressive symptoms in an 11-year-old girl. *Sleep Med* 2009;10(2):259–61.

30. Walters AS, Mandelbaum DE, Lewin DS, et al. Dopaminergic therapy in children with restless legs/periodic limb movements in sleep and ADHD. Dopaminergic Therapy Study Group. *Pediatric Neurol* 2000;22(3):182–6.

31. England SJ, Picchietti DL, Couvadelli BV, et al. L-dopa improves restless legs syndrome and periodic limb movements in sleep but not attention-deficit-hyperactivity disorder in a double-blind trial in children. *Sleep Med* 2011;12(5):471–7.

32. Harris MA, Harris MA. Too soon for dopaminergics in the management of restless legs syndrome in children. *Sleep Med Rev* 2009;13(4):299–300; author reply 301–292.

33. Dyken ME, Lin-Dyken DC, Yamada T. Diagnosing rhythmic movement disorder with video-polysomnography. *Pediatric Neurol* 1997;16(1):37–41.

34. Cruchet R. Tics et sommeil. *Presse Medicale* 1905;13:33–6.

35. Cruchet R. Six nouveaux cas de rhythmies du sommeil (les rhythmies a la caserne). *Gaz Hebd Sci Med* 1912;33:303–8.

36. Zappert J. Uber nactliche Kopfbewegungen bei kindern (jactatio capitis nocturna). *Jahrbuch fuer Kinderheilkunde* 1905;62:70–83.

37. Anonymous. Sleep related rhythmic movement disorder. In: *The International Classification of Sleep Disorders*. 2nd ed. Westchester, IL: American Academy of Sleep Medicine; 2005:193–5.

38. Klackenberg G. Rhythmic movements in infancy and early childhood: head banging, head turning, and rocking. *Acta Paediatrica* 1971;60(s224):74–83.

39. Mitchell R, Etches P. Rhythmic habit patterns (stereotypies). *Dev Med Child Neurol* 1977;19(4):545–50.

40. Matin MA, Rundle AT. Physiological and psychiatric investigations into a group of mentally handicapped subjects with self-injurious behaviour. *J Ment Defic Res* 1980;24(2):77–85.

41. Stepanova I, Nevsimalova S, Hanusova J. Rhythmic movement disorder in sleep persisting into childhood and adulthood. *Sleep* 2005;28(7):851–7.

42. Sormann GW. The headbangers tumour. *Br J Plast Surg* 1982;35(1):72–4.

43. Whyte J, Kavey NB, Gidro-Frank S. (1991). A self-destructive variant of jactatio capitis nocturna. *J Nerv Ment Dis* 1991;179(1):49–50.

44. Mayer G, Wilde-Frenz J, Kurella B. Sleep related rhythmic movement disorder revisited. *J Sleep Res* 2007;16(1):110–16.

45. Levy DM. On the problem of movement restraint (tics, stereotyped movements, hyperactivity). *Am J Orthopsychiatry* 1944;14:651–69.

46. Evans J. Rocking at night. *J Child Psychol Psychiatry* 1961;2:71–85.

47. Silberstein RM, Blackman S, Mandell W. Autoerotic head banging; a reflection on the opportunism of infants. *J Am Acad Child Psychiatry* 1966;5(2):235–42.

48. Freud A, Burlingham DT. *Infants without Families*. New York: International Universities Press; 1973.

49. Walsh JK, Kramer M, Skinner JE. (1981). A case report of jactatio capitis nocturna. *Am J Psychiatry* 1981;138(4):524–6.

50. Manni R, Tartara A. Clonazepam treatment of rhythmic movement disorder. *Sleep* 1997;20(9):812.

51. Hoban TF. Sleep-related rhythmic movement disorder. In: Thorpy MJ, Plazzi G, eds. *The Parasomnias and Other Sleep-Related Movement Disorders*. New York: Cambridge University Press; 2010:270–7.

52. Manni R, Terzaghi M. Rhythmic movements during sleep: a physiological and pathological profile. *Neurological Sci* 2005;26(Suppl 3):S181–5.

53. Hashizume Y, Yoshijima H, Uchimura N, et al. Case of head banging that continued to adolescence. *Psychiatry Clin Neurosci* 2002;56(3):255–6.

54. Su C, Miao J, Liu Y, et al. Multiple forms of rhythmic movements in an adolescent boy with rhythmic movement disorder. *Clin Neurol Neurosurg* 2009;111(10):896–9.

55. Freidin MR, Jankowski JJ, Singer WD. Nocturnal head banging as a sleep disorder: a case report. *Am J Psychiatry* 1979;136:1469–70.

56. Drake ME, Jr. Jactatio nocturna after head injury. *Neurology* 1986;36(6):867–8.

57. Vogel W, Stein DJ. Citalopram for head-banging. *J Am Acad Child Adolesc Psychiatry* 2000;39(5):544–5.

58. Garcia J. Waterbeds in treatment of rhythmic movement disorders: experience with two cases. *Sleep Res* 1996;25:243.

59. Etzioni T, Katz N, Hering E, et al. Controlled sleep restriction for rhythmic movement disorder. *J Pediatrics* 2005;147(3):393–5.

60. Rosenberg C. Elimination of a rhythmic movement disorder with hypnosis—a case report. *Sleep* 1995;18(7):608–9.

61. Jeannet PY, Kuntzer T, Deonna T, et al. Hirayama disease associated with a severe rhythmic movement disorder involving neck flexions. *Neurology* 2005;64(8):1478–9.

62. Serra-Negra JM, Ramos-Jorge ML, Flores-Mendoza CE, et al. Influence of psychosocial factors on the development of sleep bruxism among children. *Intl J Paediatric Dentistry* 2009;19(5):309–17.

63. Serra-Negra JM, Paiva SM, Seabra AP, et al. Prevalence of sleep bruxism in a group of Brazilian schoolchildren. *Euro Arch Paediatric Dentistry* 2010;11(4):192–5.

64. Herrera M, Valencia I, Grant M, et al. Bruxism in children: effect on sleep architecture and daytime cognitive performance and behavior.[Erratum appears in *Sleep*. November 1, 2006;29(11):1380]. *Sleep* 2006;29(9):1143–8.

65. Mendhekar DN, Andrade C. Bruxism arising during monotherapy with methylphenidate. *J Child Adol Psychopharmacol* 2008;18(5):537–8.

66. Sabuncuoglu O, Ekinci O, Berkem M. Fluoxetine-induced sleep bruxism in an adolescent treated with buspirone: a case report. *Spec Care Dentistry* 2009;29(5):215–17.

67. Lopez-Perez R, Lopez-Morales P, Borges-Yanez SA, et al. Prevalence of bruxism among Mexican children with Down syndrome. *Down Syndrome Res Prac* 2007;12(1):45–9.

68. Nevsimalova S, Prihodova I, Kemlink D, et al. REM behavior disorder (RBD) can be one of the first symptoms of childhood narcolepsy. *Sleep Med* 2007;8(7–8):784–6.

69. Thirumalai SS, Shubin RA, Robinson R. Rapid eye movement sleep behavior disorder in children with autism. *J Child Neurol* 2002;17(3):173–8.

70. Rye DB, Johnston LH, Watts RL, et al. Juvenile Parkinson's disease with REM sleep behavior disorder, sleepiness, and daytime REM onset. *Neurology* 1999;53(8):1868–70.

71. Trajanovic NN, Voloh I, Shapiro CM, et al. REM sleep behaviour disorder in a child with Tourette's syndrome. *Can J Neurol Sci* 2004;31(4):572–5.

72. De Barros-Ferreira M, Chodkiewicz JP, et al. Disorganized relations of tonic and phasic events of REM sleep in a case of brain-stem tumour. *Electroencephal Clin Neurophysiol* 1975;38(2):203–7.

73. Stores G. Rapid eye movement sleep behaviour disorder in children and adolescents. *Dev Med Child Neurol* 2008;50(10):728–32.

74. Blaw ME, Leroy RF, Steinberg JB, et al. Hereditary quivering chin and REM behavioral disorder. *Ann Neurol* 1989;26(3):471.

75. Pareja JA, Cuadrado ML, Garcia-Morales I, et al. Hypnagogic behavior disorder: complex motor behaviors during wake-sleep transitions in 2 young children. *J Child Neurol* 2008;23(8):959–63.

76. American Academy of Sleep Medicine. Benign sleep myoclonus of infancy. In: *The International Classification of Sleep Disorders*. 2nd ed. Westchester, IL: American Academy of Sleep Medicine; 2005: 211–2.

77. Schenck CH, Boyd JL, Mahowald MW. A parasomnia overlap disorder involving sleepwalking, sleep terrors, and REM sleep behavior disorder in 33 polysomnographically confirmed cases. *Sleep* 1997;20(11):972–81.

78. American Academy of Sleep Medicine. Sleep related epilepsy. In: *The International Classification of Sleep Disorders*. 2nd ed. Westchester, IL: American Academy of Sleep Medicine; 2005:232–5.

79. Provini F, Plazzi G, Tinuper P, et al. Nocturnal frontal lobe epilepsy. A clinical and polygraphic overview of 100 consecutive cases. *Brain* 1999;122(Pt 6):1017–31.

Index

children
  respiratory events in
    scoring of, 157–8
  SRMDs in, 745–53
    BSMI, 750
    conditions mimicking, 750
    hypnagogic behavior disorder, 749–50
    leg cramps, 547
    PLMD, 612–23. *see also* periodic limb movement disorder
      (PLMD), in children and adolescents
    PLMS, 745–7, 746*t*
    RBD, 749
    RLS, 745–7, 612–23, 746*t*. *see also* restless legs syndrome
      (RLS), in children and adolescents
    RMD, 550, 747–8, 749*f*
    SB, 748–9
    sleep talking, 551–2
chin EMG amplitude
  in muscle activity of RBD
    automatic analysis of, 172–3
cholinergic-monoaminergic mechanisms
  in REM sleep, 49
cholinesterase inhibitors
  in RBD management, 417
chorea
  clinical neurophysiology of, 222
  sleep disturbances in, 696–8
    drugs causing, 717*t*
choreoacanthocytosis
  amyotrophic
    movement disorders during sleep in, 538
Chokroverty, S., v
circadian activity cycles, 108
circadian dysrhythmia
  in patients with movement disorders, 356
circadian entrainment, 83–4, 85*f*, 84*f*
circadian neurobiology, 80–100. *see also* circadian timing
    system
  melatonin in, 84–6
  ontogeny in, 86
  SCN in, 80–100. *see also* suprachiasmatic nucleus (SCN)
circadian pacemaker
  SCN as, 80
circadian rhythm(s), 30–1
  ambulatory activity monitoring in determination of, 210
  movement disorders related to, 89
  regulation of
    genes in, 116–17
circadian rhythm sleep disorders (CRSDs), 87–9, 88*f*
  types of, 41, 39*t*
circadian timing system, 80–1
  components of, 81–2, 81*f*
  genetic regulation of, 82–4, 85*f*, 84*f*
  in sleep regulation, 86–7
  sleep–wake cycle disorders related to, 87–9, 88*f*
  in wakefulness regulation, 86–7
CJD. *see* Creutzfeld-Jakob disease (CJD)
clinical neurophysiology
  of movement disorders, 216–29. *see also* specific disorders
    and movement disorder(s), clinical neurophysiology of
clinical science, 313–753
clonazepam
  in PLMS management, 658
  in RBD management, 433, 690, 416
  in RLS management, 638, 639*t*
CNS. *see* central nervous system (CNS)
cognitive-behavioral therapy

in NES management, 468
cognitive dysfunction
  RLS and, 626–7
cognitive enhancers
  effects on sleep-related movements, 735
complex (including violent) sleep behavior, 386–7, 512–23
  non–REM parasomnias, 512–20
  in non–REM sleep
    general limitation on, 513
    organic changes in brain function underlying, 513
  release of primitive drives in, 516–18
  REM sleep parasomnias, 519–20
    functional changes in brain function underlying, 520
    general limitation on, 520
    organic changes in brain function underlying, 519–20
computed tomography (CT)
  in SRMDs, 339
computer-assisted scoring
  PSG in, 158–9
computerized polysomnography (PSG)
  scoring by, 158–9
confusional arousals, 325, 397–8, 513–14, 326*t*, 324*t*
  clinical presentation of, 397
  defined, 397
  diagnosis of, 397–8
  epidemiology of, 397
  genetics of, 397
  pathophysiology of, 397
  treatment of, 398
continuous spike-and-wave discharges during slow-wave sleep
    (CSWS)
  neuroimaging of, 289, 287
continuous spike-wave(s)
  during non–REM sleep
    and Landau-Kleffner syndrome, 506–7
cortical arousal, 183–4
corticobasal degeneration (CBD), 692
corticobasal ganglionic degeneration
  sleep-related movements in
    psychiatric aspects of, 731
corticospinal projections
  startle reaction effects of, 237–8
Creutzfeld-Jakob disease (CJD)
  sleep-related movements in
    psychiatric aspects of, 732
CRSDs. *see* circadian rhythm sleep disorders (CRSDs)
CSAs. *see* central sleep apneas (CSAs)
CSWS. *see* continuous spike-and-wave discharges during
    slow-wave sleep (CSWS)
CT. *see* computed tomography (CT)
cyclic alternating pattern (CAP)
  absence of, 179
  described, 179
  generators of
    arousals and, 188–90, 189*f*
  in sleep, 28–9, 179–93, 25*f*
    amplitude limits, 181
    arousals and, 188–90, 183–4, 189*f*
    body movements and, 184–6, 185*f*
    parasomnias, 187–8
    phase A subtypes, 188, 184, 181, 182*f*
    phase B, 188, 184
    PLMs and, 186–7
    recording techniques and montages, 181
    REM sleep, 180–1
    response of complex networks to stimuli, 182–3
    time limits, 181

neuroleptic-induced orofacial movements, 566

neurologic disorders
  negative motor phenomena and, 316–17
  positive motor phenomena and, 317–19

neurologic history
  in SRMDs, 336, 334t

neuromodulator(s)
  in maintaining wakefulness, 35

neuron(s)
  MnPN
    in non–REM sleep regulation, 48–9
  nucleus reticularis pontis caudalis
    physiological mechanisms of, 231–2, 231f
  VLPO
    in non–REM sleep regulation, 48–9

neuropathic tremor
  clinical neurophysiology of, 226

neuroprotective agents
  in RBD management, 418

neuropsychiatric disorders
  motor system effects of
    during sleep, 109

neurotransmitter(s)
  dysfunction of
    in PLMS pathophysiology, 656–7
  in inhibitory synaptic control of motoneurons during REM
    sleep, 67, 64–5, 66f
  in maintaining wakefulness, 35
  in sleep
    in animal model of narcolepsy, 116

newborn(s)
  sleep patterns in, 29

NFLE. see nocturnal frontal lobe epilepsy (NFLE)

Night Eating Questionnaire (NEQ), 467

night eating syndrome (NES), 462–6, 464f
  assessment of, 467–8, 467f
  differential diagnosis of, 467–8
  epidemiology of, 466–7
  obesity and, 466
  prevalence of, 467
  psychiatric aspects of, 725–7
  treatment for, 468

night terrors, 514

nightmare(s), 327, 324t
  in patients with movement disorders, 358
  prevalence of, 322

nigrostriatal dopaminergic deficiency
  RBD related to, 442–3

nitric oxide (NO)
  in sleep regulation, 53

NO. see nitric oxide (NO)

nocturnal akinesia, 676
  in PD
    treatment of, 681

nocturnal dyskinesias
  drug-induced, 332, 325t

nocturnal eating disorders. see night eating syndrome (NES)

nocturnal epilepsy(ies)
  neuroimaging of, 286–9, 288f
    BECTS, 287
    Landau-Kleffner syndrome, 289, 287
    NFLE, 286–7, 288f

nocturnal frontal lobe epilepsy (NFLE), 329, 190, 501–5, 330t,
    329t, 324t, 501f–3f
  causes of, 504–5
  clinical and video-PSG features of, 366t–7t
  diagnosis of, 504–5

differential diagnosis of, 505, 364–8, 506t, 366t–7t
  disorders of arousal vs., 402
  evaluation of, 363–4
  features of, 505, 502–3, 329t, 501f–3f
  gender predilection for, 504
  neuroimaging of, 286–7, 288f
  nocturnal paroxysmal, 379
  non–REM arousal disorders vs., 506t
  risk factors for, 504
  SRMDs in children vs., 750
  treatment of, 504–5

nocturnal jerks, 332, 325t

nocturnal leg cramps. see sleep-related leg cramps

nocturnal myoclonus. see periodic limb movements in sleep
    (PLMS)

nocturnal paroxysmal dystonia (NPD), 329, 136, 325t
  in NFLE, 501
  recent clinical advances in, 379

nocturnal polysomnography (PSG)
  in EDS assessment, 197

nocturnal seizures, 328–30, 496–511, 330t, 329t, 324t–5t.
    see also epilepsy(ies); epilepsy syndromes,
    sleep-associated
  abnormal movements during sleep vs., 5
  benign focal epilepsy of childhood, 329, 324t
  case examples, 507–8, 508f
  described, 496–7
  frontal lobe seizures, 329, 325t
  generalized epilepsies: symptomatic and cryptogenic, 499
  generalized tonic-clonic seizures on awakening, 498–9
  historical background of, 496
  JME, 498
  juvenile myoclonic seizures, 328, 324t
  NFLE, 329, 329t, 330t, 324t
  nocturnal paroxysmal dystonia, 329, 325t
  partial complex seizures, 329, 324t
  partial epilepsies: idiopathic, 499–500, 500f
  partial epilepsies: symptomatic and cryptogenic, 501–6,
    506t, 501f–3f
  primary generalized tonic-clonic seizures, 328, 324t
  prognosis of, 509
  pseudoseizures, 330, 330t
  psychogenic nonepileptic seizures, 330, 330t
  tonic seizures, 328–9, 324t

nocturnal temporal lobe epilepsy (NTLE), 506

non-CAP. see non–cyclic alternating pattern (CAP)

non–cyclic alternating pattern (non-CAP)
  during sleep, 28–9, 25f

nonepileptic myoclonus
  clinical neurophysiology of, 219–22, 221f, 219f

noninvasive EEG, 257–8
  limitations of, 258

non–rapid eye movement (REM) sleep. see non–REM sleep

non–REM arousal disorders
  NFLE vs., 506t

non–REM parasomnias, 512–20. see also disorders of arousal,
    during non–REM sleep
  causes of, 5
  clinical and video-PSG features of, 366t–7t
  neuroimaging of, 278

non–REM sleep
  ATP concentration and, 11–17, 13f–17f
    ATP level regulation by AMPK, 16–17, 18f, 17f
    discussion, 17
    future directions in, 19
    introduction to, 11–12
    response to data/hypothesis, 18–19, 19t